FIRST AID FOR THE®

EMERGENCY MEDICINE BOARDS

BARBARA K. BLOK, MD
Assistant Professor, Division of Emergency Medicine
Department of Surgery
University of Colorado Denver School of Medicine
Aurora, Colorado

Assistant Program Director
Denver Health Residency in Emergency Medicine
Denver, Colorado

DICKSON S. CHEUNG, MD, MBA, MPH
Department of Emergency Medicine
Sky Ridge Medical Center
Carepoint, P.C.
Denver, Colorado

TIMOTHY F. PLATTS-MILLS, MD
Department of Emergency Medicine
University of North Carolina at Chapel Hill
Chapel Hill, North Carolina

SERIES EDITOR:

TAO LE, MD, MHS
Assistant Professor of Pediatrics
Division of Allergy and Clinical Immunology
Department of Pediatrics
University of Louisville
Louisville, Kentucky

Assistant Professor of Medicine
Division of Allergy and Clinical Immunology
Department of Medicine
Johns Hopkins University
Baltimore, Maryland

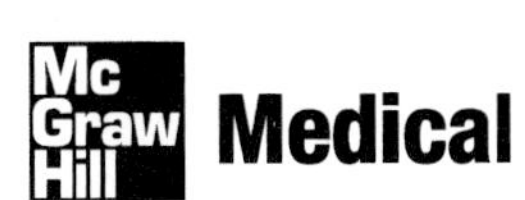

New York / Chicago / San Francisco / Lisbon / London / Madrid / Mexico City

Milan / New Delhi / San Juan / Seoul / Singapore / Sydney / Toronto

The McGraw·Hill Companies

First Aid for the® Emergency Medicine Boards

1 2 3 4 5 6 7 8 9 0 QPD/QPD 12 11 10 9

ISBN 978-0-07-147771-0
MHID 0-07-147771-3

NOTICE

Medicine is an ever-changing science. As new research and clinical experience broaden our knowledge, changes in treatment and drug therapy are required. The authors and the publisher of this work have checked with sources believed to be reliable in their efforts to provide information that is complete and generally in accord with the standards accepted at the time of publication. However, in view of the possibility of human error or changes in medical sciences, neither the authors nor the publisher nor any other party who has been involved in the preparation or publication of this work warrants that the information contained herein is in every respect accurate or complete, and they disclaim all responsibility for any errors or omissions or for the results obtained from use of the information contained in this work. Readers are encouraged to confirm the information contained herein with other sources. For example and in particular, readers are advised to check the product information sheet included in the package of each drug they plan to administer to be certain that the information contained in this work is accurate and that changes have not been made in the recommended dose or in the contraindications for administration. This recommendation is of particular importance in connection with new or infrequently used drugs.

This book was set in Electra LH by International Typesetting and Composition.
The editors were Catherine A. Johnson and Christie Naglieri.
The production supervisor was Sherri Souffrance.
Project management was provided by Aparna Shukla, International Typesetting and Composition.
Quebecor World Dubuque was printer and binder.

This book is printed on acid-free paper.

Library of Congress Cataloging-in-Publication Data

First aid for the emergency medicine boards / [edited by] Barbara K.
Blok, Dickson S. Cheung, Timothy Fortescue Platts-Mills.
p. ; cm.
Includes index.
ISBN-13: 978-0-07-149617-9 (pbk.)
ISBN-10: 0-07-149617-3 (pbk.)
1. Emergency medicine—Examinations, questions, etc. I. Blok, Barbara K. II. Cheung, Dickson S. III. Platts-Mills, Timothy Fortescue.
[DNLM: 1. Emergency Treatment—methods—Examination Questions. 2. Emergency Treatment—methods—Handbooks. 3. Emergency Medicine—methods—Examination Questions. 4. Emergency Medicine—methods—Handbooks. WB 18.2 F5263 2008]
RC86.9.F57 2008
616.02'5076—dc22

2008008603

DEDICATION

To our families, friends, and loved ones, who endured and assisted in the task of assembling this guide,

and

To the contributors to this and future editions, who took time to share their knowledge, insight, and humor for the benefit of residents and clinicians

CONTENTS

CONTRIBUTING AUTHORS

Hagop M. Afarian, MD, MS
Chief Resident
Department of Emergency Medicine
University of California, San Francisco-Fresno
Fresno, California

Mashal Ahmadi, MD
Department of Emergency Medicine
Kaiser Permanente
San Jose, California

Formerly, Senior Resident
Denver Health Residency in Emergency Medicine
Denver, Colorado

Kenny V. Bahn, MD
Clinical Instructor
Department of Emergency Medicine
University of California, San Francisco-Fresno
Fresno, California

Kelly Bookman, MD
Assistant Professor
Division of Emergency Medicine
University of Colorado Denver School of Medicine
Aurora, Colorado

Charles H. Brown IV, MD
Resident
Department of Anesthesiology and Critical Care Medicine
Johns Hopkins Hospital
Baltimore, Maryland

Jennie A. Buchanan, MD
Fellow, Medical Toxicology
Rocky Mountain Poison & Drug Center
Denver, Colorado

Formerly, Chief Resident
Denver Health Residency in Emergency Medicine
Denver, Colorado

Gregory W. Burcham, MD, FACEP
Attending Physician
Department of Emergency Medicine
Swedish Medical Center
Englewood, Colorado

Liza J. Cadnapaphornchai, MD
Department of Emergency Medicine
Kaiser Permanente Medical Centers
Fremont/Hayward, California

Formerly, Senior Resident
Denver Health Residency in Emergency Medicine
Denver, Colorado

Emilie J. B. Calvello, MD, MPH
Senior Resident
Department of Emergency Medicine
Johns Hopkins Hospital
Baltimore, Maryland

Danielle D. Campagne, MD
Chief Resident
Department of Emergency Medicine
University of California, San Francisco-Fresno
Fresno, California

Aaron E. Chen, MD
Assistant Professor
Department of Pediatric Emergency Medicine
Johns Hopkins University
Baltimore, Maryland

Lisa Cheng, MD
Staff Physician
Berkeley Emergency Medicine Group
Berkelely, California

Formerly, Senior Resident
Denver Health Residency in Emergency Medicine
Denver, Colorado

Jonathan Claud, MD
Department of Emergency Medicine
Legacy Salmon Creek Hospital
Vancouver, Washington

Ann C. Czarnik, MD
Private Practice
Union Memorial Hospital
Baltimore, Maryland

Formerly, Chief Resident
Department of Emergency Medicine
Johns Hopkins Hospital
Baltimore, Maryland

Mitzi A. Dillon, MD
Clinical Assistant Professor
Emergency Department
University of Nevada, School of Medicine
University Medical Center
Las Vegas, Nevada

Ross I. Donaldson, MD, MPH
Assistant Clinical Professor Medicine
David Geffen School of Medicine at UCLA
Assistant Director of Process and Quality Improvement
Department of Emergency Medicine
Harbor-UCLA Medical Center
Los Angeles, California

Kim Fredericksen, MD
Resident Physician
Department of Emergency Medicine
Johns Hopkins University
Baltimore, Maryland

Lauren Grossman, MD, MS
Clinical Instructor of Surgery
University of Colorado Health Sciences Center
Denver, Colorado

Staff Physician
Emergency Department
Swedish Medical Center
Englewood, Colorado

Attending Staff Physician
Department of Emergency Medicine
Denver Health Medical Center
Denver, Colorado

Hugh F. Hill III, MD, JD, FACEP, FCLM
Assistant Professor
Johns Hopkins University
Baltimore, Maryland

Alex Ho, MD
Bixler Emergency Center
Tallahassee Memorial Hospital

Formerly, Resident,
Department of Emergency Medicine
University of North Carolina
Chapel Hill, North Carolina

Allison L. Hobelmann, MD
Chief Resident
Department of Emergency Medicine
Johns Hopkins University
Baltimore, Maryland

Jason Hoppe, DO
Clinical Instructor
Division of Emergency Medicine
University of Colorado Denver School of Medicine
Aurora, Colorado

Formerly, Fellow Medical Toxicology
Rocky Mountain Poison & Drug Center
Denver, Colorado

Manon Kwon, MD
Assistant Clinical Professor of Emergency Medicine
University of California, San Francisco-Fresno

Medical Student Clerkship Director
Director of Clinical Skills Lab
Fresno, California

Carrie D. Mendoza, MD
Clinical Instructor
Division of Emergency Medicine
University of Colorado Denver School of Medicine
Aurora, Colorado

Fellow, Medical Toxicology
Rocky Mountain Poison & Drug Center
Denver, Colorado

Christian Merlo, MD, MPH
Assistant Professor of Medicine
Division of Pulmonary and Critical Care Medicine
Johns Hopkins University, School of Medicine
Baltimore, Maryland

Hardin A. Pantle, MD
Department of Emergency Medicine
Johns Hopkins University
Baltimore, Maryland

Sean H. Rhyee, MD, MPH
Assistant Professor of Emergency Medicine
Division of Medical Toxicology
University of Massachusetts Medical School
Worchester, Massachusetts

Formerly, Fellow, Medical Toxicology
Rocky Mountain Poison & Drug Center
Denver, Colorado

Jeffrey Sankoff, MD
Assistant Professor
Division of Emergency Medicine
University of Colorado Denver School of Medicine
Aurora, Colorado

Attending Physician
Denver Health Medical Center Emergency Department
Denver, Colorado

Maryam B. Shapland, MD
Resident
Department of Emergency Medicine
Johns Hopkins Hospital
Baltimore Maryland

Ana Paola Uranga, MD, MBA
Department of Emergency Medicine
University of California, San Francisco-Fresno
Fresno, California

Jacqueline Ward-Gaines, MD, FACEP
Assistant Professor
Division of Emergency Medicine
University of Colorado Denver School of Medicine
Aurora, Colorado

SENIOR REVIEWERS

Amin N. Azzam, MD
Assistant Clinical Professor
University of California, San Francisco

Department of Psychiatry
University of California
Berkeley School of Public Health
Berkeley, California
Chapter 16: Psychobehavioral Disorders

Scott Biggins, MD, MAS
Assistant Professor
Department of Medicine
University of California, San Francisco
San Francisco, California
Chapter 11: Abdominal and Gastrointestinal Emergencies

Michael D. Burg, MD, FACEP
Assistant Clinical Professor
Department of Emergency Medicine
Medical Education Program
University of California, San Francisco-Fresno
Fresno, California
Chapter19: Procedures and Skills

Christopher Chen, MD
Orthopaedic Surgeon
Pacific Bone and Joint Clinic
Berkley, California
Chapter 4: Orthopedics

Bryan Cho, MD, PhD
Clinical Instructor
University of California, San Francisco
San Francisco, California

Staff Dermatologist
Camino Medical Group
Sunnyvale, California
Chapter 17: Dermatology

James Comes, MD
Program Director
Health Sciences Associate Clinical Professor
University of California, San Francisco

School of Medicine
Emergency Medicine Residency Program
Fresno, California
Chapter 7: Endocrine, Metabolic, Fluid, and Electrolyte Disorders

Jeffrey Druck, MD
Assistant Professor
Division of Emergency Medicine
University of Colorado Denver School of Medicine
Aurora, Colorado

Associate Program Director
Denver Health Residency in Emergency Medicine
Denver, Colorado
Chapter 15: Neurology

Madonna Fernandez-Frackelton, MD, FACEP
David Geffen School of Medicine at UCLA
Assistant Director of Process and Quality Improvement
Department of Emergency Medicine
Harbor-UCLA Medical Center
Los Angeles, California
Chapter 8: Infectious Disease

Kennon Heard, MD
Associate Professor
Division of Emergency Medicine
University of Colorado Denver School of Medicine
Aurora, Colorado

Director
Medical Toxicology Fellowship Program
Rocky Mountain Poison and Drug Center
Denver, Colorado
Chapter 6: Toxicology

Gregory W. Hendey, MD
Medical Education Program
University of California, San Francisco-Fresno
Fresno, California
Chapter 12: Obstetrics and Gynecology

Mark Kozlowski, MD
Medical Director
Emergency Department
Swedish Medical Center
Englewood, Colorado
Chapter 21: Ethics, Legal Issues, and Emergency Department Administration

Todd Larabee, MD
Assistant Professor
Division of Emergency Medicine
University of Colorado Denver School of Medicine
Aurora, Colorado
Chapter 1: Resuscitation

Charles M. Little, DO, FACEP
Program Coordinator, Pandemic Taskforce
University of Colorado Hospital

Associate Professor
Division of Emergency Medicine
University of Colorado Denver School of Medicine
Aurora, Colorado
Chapter 20: EMS and Disaster Medicine

Kristen Nordenholz, MD
Associate Professor
Division of Emergency Medicine
University of Colorado Denver School of Medicine
Aurora, Colorado
Chapter 2: Cardiovascular Emergencies

Jennifer A. Schaffner, Esq.
Attorney at Law
Denver, Colorado
Chapter 21: Ethics, Legal Issues, and Emergency Department Administration

Fred Severyn, MD
Associate Professor
Division of Emergency Medicine
University of Colorado Denver School of Medicine
Aurora, Colorado
Chapter 13: Environmental Emergencies

Hugo St-Hilaire, DDS, MD
Assistant Professor of Surgery
Division of Plastic & Reconstructive Surgery
Louisiana State University Health Science Center
New Orleans, Louisiana
Chapter 14: Head, Eye, Ear, Nose and Throat Emergencies

Dave M. Stocker, MD
Division of Pediatric Emergency Medicine
Carepoint, PC
Denver, Colorado
Chapter 5: Pediatrics

Meg Wolfe, MD
Associate Professor of Surgery
Department of Surgery
University of California, San Francisco-Fresno
Fresno, California
Chapter 3: Trauma

Lynne M. Yancey, MD, FACEP
Assistant Professor
Division of Emergency Medicine
University of Colorado Denver School of Medicine
Aurora, Colorado
Chapter 18: Renal and Genitourinary Emergencies

Mark Yoder, MD
Assistant Professor
Pulmonary and Critical Care Medicine
Rush University Medical Center
Chicago, Illinois
Chapter 10: Thoracic and Respiratory Disorders

INTRODUCTION

Passing the emergency medicine written certification examination is an important milestone in the process of becoming a board certified emergency physician. The written exam, formerly called the Written Certification Examination and now referred to by the American Board of Emergency Medicine (ABEM) as the "Qualifying Examination," is used to identify candidates who are ready to take the oral exam, the final step in becoming board certified. The Qualifying Examination measures core knowledge, and, to many who must take it, it is an intimidating hurdle. Every year approximately ten percent of examinees fail the test and must retake it the following year. Given that many test takers are completing their residency and may be moving to start a new job in the months leading up to the test, it is clear that there is a need for a focused, easy-to-use review book to help them prepare.

First Aid for the Emergency Medicine Boards is such a book. The First Aid series is based on the idea that people who have recently prepared for and taken the test know best how to teach others to study for it. We have drawn on the experience of 31 individual chapter authors and nearly as many senior reviewers, integrating clinical experience, information from existing review books, and the ABEM practice questions to create a book designed to improve your score on the Qualifying Examination. *First Aid for the Emergency Medicine Boards* contains dozens of challenging cases ("minicases") and reinforces important information in highlighted "key facts" and "mnemonics." Filled with tables and figures, it presents key findings and must-know information in a clear, concise, and highly accessible format that makes it easy to recall both on test day and in the emergency department.

ABOUT THE QUALIFYING EXAMINATION

The Qualifying Examination consists of approximately 305 questions. Candidates are given six-and-a-half hours of time in which to complete the test. All questions are the multiple choice, **single-best-answer** type. You will be presented with a case scenario and a question, followed by five answer options. Approximately 10% of the questions include a figure (radiograph, photograph, ECG, rhythm strip, or ultrasound image). There are no penalties for wrong answers, so if you find a question unanswerable, make your best guess and move on. Candidates who achieve a score of 75% or higher pass.

The exam is given in the fall of each year at one of 200 PearsonVUE professional computer-based testing centers. Test locations can be found by selecting "Locate a Test Center" on www.pearsonvue.com. Information on registration, fees, and test composition can be obtained from the ABEM website, www.abem.org.

Exam content is defined by ABEM's Model of the Clinical Practice of Emergency Medicine (EM Model). The table lists the relative weight given to different elements of the exam.

Relative Weight of EM Model Elements

Condition/Component	Relative Weight
Signs, Symptoms, and Presentations	9%
Abdominal and Gastrointestinal Disorders	9%
Cardiovascular Disorders	10%
Cutaneous Disorders	2%
Endocrine, Metabolic, and Nutritional Disorders	3%
Environmental Disorders	3%
Head, Ear, Eye, Nose, and Throat Disorders	5%
Hematologic Disorders	2%
Immune System Disorders	2%
Systemic Infectious Disorders	5%
Musculoskeletal Disorders (Nontraumatic)	3%
Nervous System Disorders	5%
Obstetrics and Gynecology	4%
Psychobehavioral Disorders	3%
Renal and Urogenital Disorders	3%
Thoracic-Respiratory Disorders	8%
Toxicologic Disorders	4%
Traumatic Disorders	11%
Procedures and Skills	6%
Other Components (EMS, Administration, Legal)	3%

HOW TO USE THIS BOOK

As we have done with other books in the First Aid series, we encourage you to read this book early on and throughout your residency, and to supplement it with margin notes. As with general medicine, mastering emergency medicine does not result from a single reading of a textbook but from many readings and multiple experiences treating patients. For common conditions, such as blunt trauma, CHF, and pneumonia, we focus on the kinds of complicated scenarios that you will find on the test. At this point in your career, you will not be tested on your knowledge of basic information. You will not be asked *What is the most common cause of community acquired pneumonia?* for example. Instead, you are tested on your ability to apply that basic knowledge in the far more challenging situations you are likely to encounter in the ED, where the question is more likely to be *What is the cause of pneumonia in this patient who has just returned from a rat-infested cabin in New Mexico?* For rare conditions, such as an organophosphate overdose, ciguatera toxicity, or high-altitude pulmonary edema, our goal has been to provide simple, clear, memorable explanations. By the time you have read this book two or three times, you should be well prepared to make the right decisions on the exam and in real life.

Some young physicians say that practicing medicine is intuitive and experience based, that once you have done a residency, studying and memorizing are things of the past. For most of us, this is not true. When a patient comes into the emergency department 15 minutes after eating dark-meat fish with flushing and palpitations, you might know that you need to initiate treatment with diphenhydramine for scombroid poisoning. But this knowledge is hardly intuitive. And, unless you had trained in Florida, you would probably never have seen this disease. For most examinees, study and memorization are a necessary part of test preparation.

In preparing for the exam, take an expansive and a reductionist approach. Be expansive by studying with your reference books and internet resources readily at hand. Supplementing your clinical knowledge with pictures and detailed descriptions of illnesses will help you remember how to identify and manage complex and rare diseases. Be reductionist by preparing notes on the subjects you have difficulty remembering. Linking key words together on paper, "dendritic ulcer → herpes keratitis," for example, and reviewing them regularly is often enough to help you "capture" an important piece of knowledge—and ensure the right answer—on test day.

Most cases you see in an emergency department will require more complex thinking than can be presented in a multiple choice question. We encourage you to accept that the test simplifies complexities in order to provide an objective measure of your knowledge. For evolving and complex situations, such as evaluating the source of chest pain, we describe the current, generally accepted approaches. Please be aware that medicine continually changes, and there are many situations for which we still do not know the best approach.

TEST-PREPARATION STRATEGIES

When you work in the emergency department, knowledge and experience are your friends. The greater your experience with and understanding of a given complaint, the faster you will be able to help your patient. And while it may seem that the amount of information that could be included on an emergency medicine certification exam is unlimited, it is not. Like most of the exams you have taken in the past, this one tests a finite body of knowledge. The material on the exam is readily identifiable and studying can greatly improve your competency with it. In short, you *can* master the content of this exam. What's more, preparing for the exam should make you a more confident and capable emergency physician. You are no longer simply studying for an organic chemistry test; you are preparing for a career as an emergency physician.

How much time you allow for test preparation will depend on your interest in the formal study of the material and how likely you are to pass the exam with minimal preparation. If you consistently score above 85% on in-service or practice examinations and are currently practicing emergency medicine and reading regularly, you probably won't need to study too much. Most people, however, need 2 to 3 months to study for the exam. Giving yourself adequate time makes the experience richer and more enjoyable, and enables you to integrate your clinical experience with what you are studying. We recommend that you read this book in its entirety at least two months before the exam date. Use this initial read to identify the gaps in your knowledge and facts that you want to memorize. Use practice test questions, such as those found in PEER VII, to improve your test-taking skills, to further identify knowledge gaps, and to add to your list of facts to memorize. Two weeks before the test, review the book again, focusing on areas of weakness. Avoid trying to cover new ground, and instead spend your time reviewing core knowledge and memorizing your list of facts.

TEST-TAKING STRATEGIES

Knowing the right answers is the most obvious way to pass the test, but studying is not the only way to prepare. Knowing how to take a multiple choice test can also help. There are five key components.

First, anticipate the answer as you read the question. With most questions, you should already have an answer in mind before you look at the choices. For example, a question might describe a young lady who presents with odd neurologic complaints. She is not obviously sick, and she reports that she had a different neurologic problem two months ago. Just as when you listen to real patients describe their symptoms, a differential should form in your mind. At the top of the list for the test patient should be multiple sclerosis. If you are confident in your answer, you can avoid wasting the time it takes to carefully consider the merits of each answer choice. Instead, you can scan for the one you know is right, check the alternatives to make sure they don't compete with your anticipated answer, and move on.

Second, when you cannot anticipate the answer, use the following guidelines to help you make your choice:

1. **Opposites attract**. If two of the answers are the opposites of each other, one of them is usually the right answer.
2. **Similars attract.** If two answers are similar, one of them is usually the right answer. Test writers don't usually create two similar wrong answers.
3. **Grammar is a guide.** Sometimes wrong answers can be identified through minor grammatical inconsistencies between the question and the answer choice. The right answer should link to the question without grammatical errors, as if it is part of a sentence that was cut neatly in half.
4. **Avoid "always" and "never."** Answers that include *always* and *never* are almost never correct. This fact has become so well known that you will probably not see these words on the test. If you do, be wary.
5. **Worst-case answers are often right.** One of the goals of emergency medicine training is to teach you to consider life-threatening illnesses first. Be always on the look out for the pulmonary embolus or the ectopic pregnancy, and anticipate the need for immediate surgical consultation and early intubation. The diagnoses of GERD, gastroenteritis, or musculoskeletal low-back pain should be made only after you have ruled out more serious diseases with similar presentations.

Third, don't be flustered if you have difficulty interpreting a figure on the test. Like diagnostic tests in the emergency department, images on the written exam should be used to confirm or refute a clinical suspicion. The question will often guide you to the answer without the image. Use the picture to strengthen your confidence in your answer choice. For example, a 72-year-old male presents with hip pain and difficulty walking after a ground-level fall at home. What is his diagnosis? If you were seeing this patient in the emergency department, you would put hip fracture at the top of the differential. The purpose of the radiograph would be to exclude a hip dislocation (although your exam will usually do this) and to identify the location of the fracture. If the radiograph is negative and the patient really cannot walk without a lot of pain, you will probably proceed to a CT or an MRI to find the fracture that you cannot see on radiograph. Take the same approach to this patient on the test as you would in the emergency department. Determine the answer from the story, and look to the image to confirm your diagnosis. If you can't interpret the image, answer the question without it.

Fourth, read the question carefully. As in the emergency department, there is a danger in being overly confident in a diagnosis. It is good to anticipate an answer as you read, but be sure to read the entire question. Don't be so certain about your diagnosis of glaucoma that you miss the sulfa allergy, the history of sickle cell disease, or COPD. Paying attention to such details can mean the difference between choosing the right answer and a wrong one.

Fifth, be aware that test writers like to mislead test takers. It has been said that writing good test questions is easy—it is writing good test answers that is difficult. A good test answer choice captures the imagination of unprepared test takers, and lures them down the wrong path. Here, again, knowledge is your friend. In this book, we include information about unusual problems to help you hone in on the correct diagnosis and alert you when you are being led astray. For example, strychnine causes muscle convulsions leading to asphyxia two hours after ingestion and is therefore unlikely to be the right answer to any question, but if you don't know that, you might end up choosing it. Of course, good foils sometimes are right answers; knowing the key information covered by each question should help you tell the difference.

Finally, good luck and enjoy your time studying. There are few careers that offer as much opportunity to positively impact the lives of others as that of the emergency physician. The investment you make in yourself by studying will make you a stronger test taker and a more competent emergency physician.

OTHER RESOURCES

There are a number of excellent books that will help you prepare for the written exam. They are listed below, along with sources of practice questions and review courses you can take.

Books for Review

Harwood-Nuss A, Wolfson AB, Linden CH, et al, (Eds). *Harwood-Nuss' Clinical Practice of Emergency Medicine*, 4th ed. New York: Lippincott Williams & Wilkins; 2005.

Marx JA, Hockberger RS, Walls RM (Eds). *Rosen's Emergency Medicine Concepts and Clinical Practice*, 6th ed. St Louis, MO: Mosby; 2006.

Rivers C (Ed). *Preparing for the Written Board Exam in Emergency Medicine*, 5th ed. Milford, OH: EMEE, Inc.; 2006.

Tintinalli JE, Galen DK, Stapcyzinski JS. *Emergency Medicine: A Comprehensive Study Guide*, 6th ed. New York: McGraw-Hill; 2004.

Practice Questions

PEER VII: Physician's Evaluation and Educational Review in Emergency Medicine, 7th ed. Dallas, TX: American College of Emergency Physicians; 2006.

Pennsylvania Chapter, American College of Emergency Physicians Written Board Practice Examination. www.paacep.org.

Promes S. *Emergency Medicine Examination and Board Review*, 3rd ed. New York: McGraw-Hill; 2005.

Written Exam Review Courses

Emergency Medicine Review: The Comprehensive CORE CONTENT Board Review Course. Education Medical Services, Inc.
P.O. Box 510222
St. Louis, MO 63151
1-800-MED-TEST

Illinois College of Emergency Physicians, Written Board Review Course
1 S 280 Summit Avenue, Court B-2
Oakbrook Terrace, IL 60181
1-630-495-6400
www.icep.org

LSU Emergency Medicine Written Board Review Course and Clinical Update
Department of Medicine, Section of Emergency Medicine
Louisiana State University School of Medicine
LSUHSC Institute of Professional Education
1600 Canal Street, Suite 1034
New Orleans, LA 70112
1-504-568-5272

Medical University of South Carolina Intensive Review in Emergency Medicine
Office of Continuing Medical Education
261 Calhoun St., Ste. 301
P.O. Box 250189
Charleston, SC 29425
(843) 876-1925

National Emergency Medicine Board Review
4535 Dressler Road NW
Canton, OH 44718
1-800-651-CEME
www.emboards.com

Ohio Chapter American College of Emergency Physicians, Emergency Medicine Review Course
3510 Snouffer Road, Suite 100
Columbus, OH 43235
1-888-OHA-CEP4
www.ohacep.org

Pennsylvania Chapter American College of Emergency Physicians, PaACEPs
Emergency Medicine Written Board Review Course
777 East Park Drive, P.O. Box 8820
Harrisburg, PA 17105-8820
1-888-633-5784
www.paacep.org

Preparing for the Written Board Exam in Emergency Medicine
Emergency Medicine Educational Enterprises
200 TechneCenter Drive, #103
Milford, OH 45150
1-800-878-5667
www.emeeinc.com

CHAPTER 1

Resuscitation

Jeffrey Sankoff, MD and Lisa Cheng, MD

AIRWAY MANAGEMENT

Indications for Definitive Airway

- **Failure to maintain a patent airway and protect against aspiration**
  - Inadequate gag reflex and inability to handle secretions
  - Decreased mental status (GCS < 8) not due to a rapidly reversible cause (eg, hypoglycemia, opioid overdose)
  - Severe maxillofacial trauma
- **Failure to adequately oxygenate or ventilate**
  - Hypoxemia unresponsive to supplemental oxygen, as measured by pulse oximetry with good waveform
  - Hypercapnea, as measured by ABG or end tidal CO_2 ($ETCO_2$) with decreased mental status or other adverse effect
- **Anticipated clinical deterioration**
  - Status epilepticus, multiple trauma +/– head injury, certain overdoses (TCA), penetrating neck trauma, tiring asthmatic, etc.

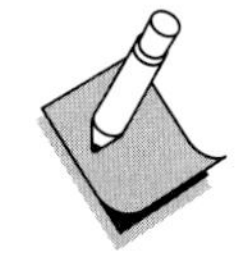

Be sure to correlate ABG findings with the patient's clinical status.

EMS presents with an obese 34-year-old male with cerebral palsy who is unconscious after a fall. On examination, he is unresponsive, GCS 6, with shallow sonorous respirations. He has obvious facial trauma, a receding mandible and a short neck, but his beard is well lubricated to facilitate bagging. How do you prepare for his intubation?

This patient has several markers of a difficult airway, including obesity, facial trauma, facial hair, receding mandible, and a short neck. This is a patient for whom you want to have back-up plans in case endotracheal intubation attempts fail. Preparation for advanced airway procedures is key.

Recognizing the Difficult Airway

Routinely evaluating patients for markers of difficult intubation, bag mask ventilation, and cricothyrotomy allows the emergency physician to thoughtfully plan alternative approaches.

- **Difficult bag-valve mask (BVM)**
  - Difficult mask placement
    - Edentulous, bearded, abnormal facies, facial trauma
  - Difficult mask ventilation
    - Obese, airway obstruction, stiff lungs, advanced pregnancy
- **Difficult laryngoscopy and intubation**
  - Abnormal neck mobility
    - Immobilization, surgery, ankylosing spondylitis
  - Limited mouth opening
    - Less than three patient fingerbreadths between the upper and lower teeth.
  - Poor oral access
    - Mallampati score (see Table 1.1 and Figure 1.1)
    - Prominent incisors
    - Receding mandible: Less than three patient fingerbreadths from the mentum to the hyoid bone

TABLE 1.1. Mallampati Score for Oral Access

Class	Visible on Mouth Opening	Difficulty With Oral Access
I	Soft palate, uvula, fauces, tonsillar pillars	None
II	Soft palate, uvula, fauces	None
III	Soft palate, base of uvula	Moderate
IV	Hard palate only	Severe

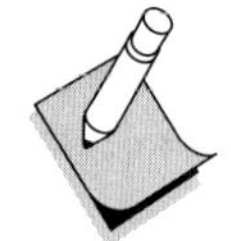

Predictors of difficult laryngoscopy and intubation include:

Abnormal neck mobility

Limited mouth opening

Poor oral access

High larynx

Upper airway obstruction

- High larynx
    - Distance from the undersurface of the mandible to the laryngeal prominence < 2 patient fingerbreadths
- Upper airway obstruction
    - Epiglottitis, angioedema, neck hematoma/masses

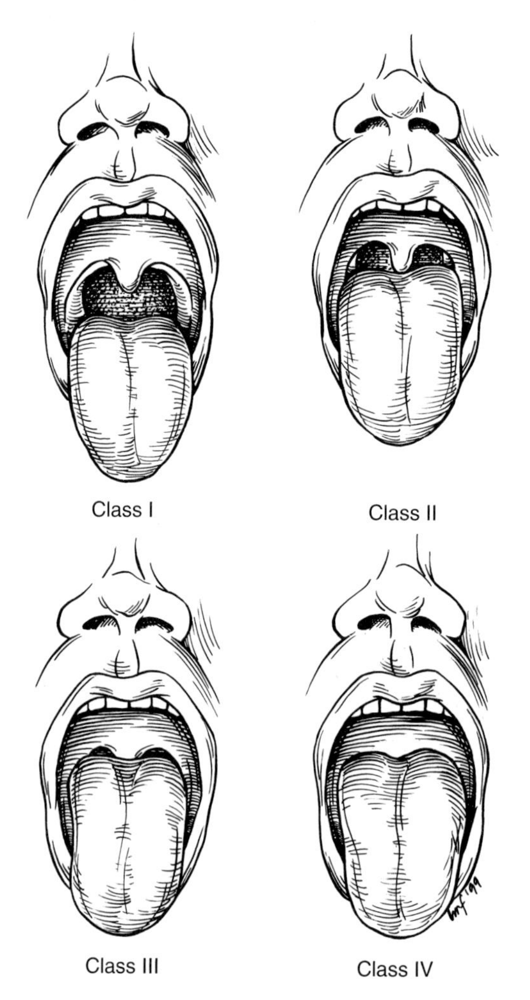

FIGURE 1.1. Mallampati score for oral access.

(Reproduced, with permission, from Tintinalli JE, Kelen GD, Stapczynski JS. *Emergency Medicine: A Comprehensive Study Guide*, 6th ed. New York: McGraw-Hill, 2004:117.)

- **Difficult cricothyrotomy**
  - Predictors include: Short/obese neck, prior surgery or radiation, presence of mass or hematoma.

Pediatric Versus Adult Anatomy

Besides the obvious smaller size of the pediatric airway, there are other important anatomic differences compared to the adult airway (see Table 1.2). These differences gradually decrease with age. Adult proportions are seen at 8–10 years.

Airway Equipment

ENDOTRACHEAL (ET) TUBE

- Adult male: 7.5–9.0 mm tube
- Adult female: 7.0–8.0 mm tube
- **Pediatrics: (4 + age in years)/4**
- Traditional practice is to use uncuffed tube if <8 years old.
- Nasal intubation: Use slightly smaller tube (by 0.5–1.0 mm).

The narrowest part of the adult airway = vocal cords. The narrowest part of the pediatric airway = cricoid ring.

LARYNGOSCOPE BLADES

- **MacIntosh**
  - Curved, fits into the vallecula
  - Indirectly lifts the epiglottis via the *hypoepiglottic ligament*
- **Miller**
  - Straight, goes under the epiglottis to lift it directly
  - Preferred in pediatric patients (especially <3 years old) or if larynx is fixed by scar tissue

The MacIntosh blade indirectly lifts the epiglottis via the hypoepiglottic ligament.

TABLE 1.2. Differences Found in Pediatric Versus Adult Anatomy

VARIABLE	PEDIATRIC ANATOMY	EFFECT
Size of occiput	Larger	Flexed neck when supine, obstructing airway
Smallest airway diameter	At cricoid ring (vs vocal cords in adult)	ET tube may pass through cords but go no further
Larynx	More superior and anterior	Better visualized with straight blade
Epiglottis	Larger and floppy	Best displaced with straight blade
Tongue	Larger	↑ Risk of obstruction
Length of trachea	Infant = 5 cm 18 month = 7 cm (vs adult = 12 cm)	Depth at teeth = 3 × the ET tube size *or* (0.5 × age [yrs]) + 12

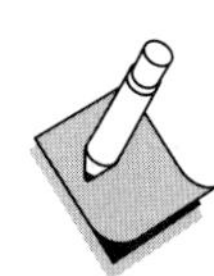

Elevating the child's torso with blankets will correct for the larger occiput and the more anterior anatomy, making visualization easier.

- **Sizing**
  - Premature infants: Size 0
  - Normal infants: Size 1
  - Older children: Size 2
  - Adults: Size 3–4

BAG-VALVE MASK

A BVM with reservoir bag (to increase delivered O_2) is essential for airway management.

For pediatrics:

- Should have a minimum volume of 450 mL
- Pop-off valves should be avoided (pressures required to ventilate are often higher than the pop-off threshold).

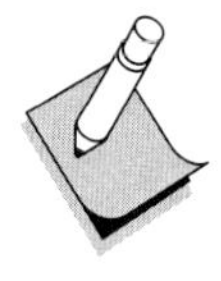

*$ETCO_2$ should be confirmed after **six** manual breaths.*

END TIDAL CO_2 ($ETCO_2$) DETECTOR

Detecting $ETCO_2$ (yellow color change or 5% CO_2) after **six manual breaths** is the 1° means of confirming ET tube placement.

- False-positive $ETCO_2$
  - May occur if tube is in the supraglottic region, with gastric distention or immediately following sodium bicarbonate administration
- Indeterminate or false-negative result
  - May occur in patient with poor pulmonary perfusion (cardiac arrest, massive pulmonary embolism [PE])
    - Level > 2% (tan or yellow) = correct placement in cardiac arrest
    - No $ETCO_2$ → tube could be anywhere!

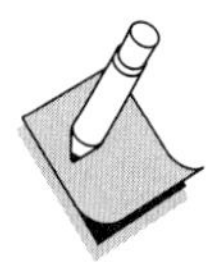

False-negative $ETCO_2$ may occur with low pulmonary perfusion states (massive PE, cardiac arrest).

GUM ELASTIC BOUGIE

- Helpful when only arytenoids are seen or cord opening is narrow
- Secures a path into the trachea, over which an ET tube can be guided in

A 23-year-old male arrives to the ED via EMS after having a witnessed seizure at home. On examination, he is lying supine on the stretcher and has sonorous respirations with loud upper airway noises during inspiration. What is the first step in managing this patient's airway?

This patient likely has an upper airway obstruction from his tongue falling back against his posterior pharynx. The first step is to perform a chin-lift and jaw-thrust maneuver, which will relieve the obstruction. This can be followed by nasopharyngeal (not oropharyngeal) airway placement.

Basic Airway Procedures

OROPHARYNGEAL AND NASOPHARYNGEAL AIRWAY PLACEMENT

The **tongue** is the most common cause of upper airway obstruction in the supine unconscious or semiconscious patient.

Indication

- Relieve upper airway obstruction from tongue in the unconscious or semi-conscious patient.
- Adjunct to BVM ventilation

A patient who easily tolerates an oral airway needs intubation.

Contraindication

- The oropharyngeal airway should **not** be used on the patient with an **intact gag reflex** (risk of vomiting).

Procedure

- Oropharyngeal airway
  - Insert the device while inverted → rotate 180° once well into the mouth → advance distal end into the hypopharynx.
    - This technique is **not recommended for pediatric patients.**
  - **Or** compress the tongue with a tongue depressor and advance the device without inversion.
- Nasopharyngeal airway
  - Gently advance into a nostril until the flared end is resting against the nasal orifice.

Complications

- Epistaxis (nasopharyngeal airway)
- Vomiting and aspiration
- Worsened obstruction from improper placement (oropharyngeal airway)

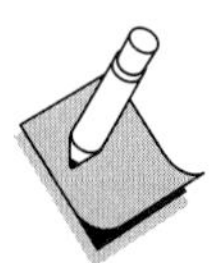

What is the appropriate volume to administer with BVM? One that achieves chest rise.

Bag-Valve Mask Ventilation

Indication

- Inadequate oxygenation or ventilation, as bridge to intubation

Procedure

- Open airway via jaw thrust and naso- or oropharyngeal airway.
- Position mask to cover mouth and nose.
  - **Single-handed mask hold**: Thumb and index fingers on mask with remaining fingers wrapped around mandible. This is a difficult technique but may be necessary for a single rescuer.
  - **Two-handed technique**: Thumb and index fingers on either side of mask with remaining fingers wrapped around mandible.
- **Lift mandible** into mask to form seal.
  - Two-handed mask hold obtains better seal!
- Squeeze bag and administer **volume necessary to achieve chest rise.**
  - Verify oxygen flow rate of 15 L/min.
  - Avoid pop-off valves (if present).

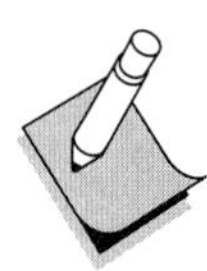

Avoid pop-off valves as airway pressure in emergency conditions often exceeds the valve pressure.

Complications

- Inadequate mask seal
- Inadequate ventilation
- Gastric distention → emesis and aspiration.
- Insufflation of vomitus/blood/debris into trachea

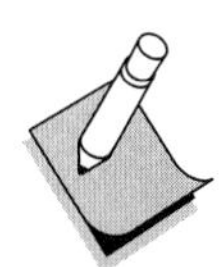

If you can't bag a patient, add naso- and oropharyngeal airways, reposition head, and try again.

- Air trapping or pneumothorax
  - From overaggressive ventilation or too large a bag (pediatrics)
  - If you suspect air trapping (eg, history of asthma or COPD), stop bagging and squeeze the chest to help the patient exhale, then bag at a slower rate.

OROTRACHEAL INTUBATION

INDICATIONS

- Failure to maintain or protect the airway
- Failure of oxygenation or ventilation
- Anticipated deterioration

CONTRAINDICATIONS

- There are no absolute contraindications.

PROCEDURE

> ***Tracheal manipulation of the thyroid and cricoid cartilages—***
>
> ***BURP***
>
> **B**ackward
> **U**pward
> **R**ightward
> **P**ressure

- Position the patient.
  - Sniffing position of head
- Open patient's mouth.
- Insert blade (using left hand) and **sweep patient's tongue** to left.
  - Final position—in vallecula if curved blade
  - Underneath epiglottis if straight blade
- Elevate epiglottis.
  - Lift the blade upward and forward at a 45° angle in the direction of the handle.
- **Tracheal manipulation**
  - **BURP: B**ackward, **U**pward, **R**ightward **P**ressure on thyroid and cricoid cartilages
  - **Bimanual laryngoscopy: Intubator moves trachea into view with right hand.** Assistant should then hold trachea in preferred position.
  - Brings the larynx further posterior and superior for better visualization of cords
  - Improves visualization by one full grade, on average

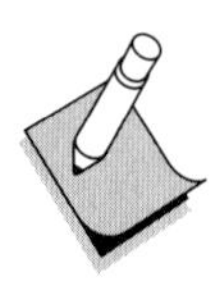

BURP can improve laryngoscopic visualization by one full grade, on average.

- Insert ET tube through cords. Inflate ET tube balloon.
  - Depth at teeth:
    - 23 cm for adult males
    - 21 cm for adult females
    - Children = (0.5 × age in years) + 12 cm or 3 × the ET tube size.
- Confirm tube placement.
  - **$ETCO_2$ = best method.**
  - Gold standard = fiberoptic visualization of tracheal rings through ET tube.
  - Esophageal detector device
    - Syringelike aspiration device that is inserted into the end of ET tube
      - No resistance to pulling plunger = tracheal intubation.
      - Resistance = esophageal intubation.
  - Other methods: Direct visualization, physical examination, pulse oximetry, CXR

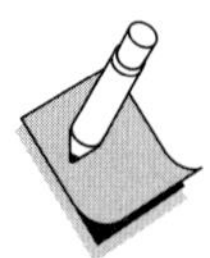

Confirmation of $ETCO_2$ is the best method of confirming ET tube placement.

COMPLICATIONS

- Broken teeth
- Laryngospasm
- Mainstem intubation

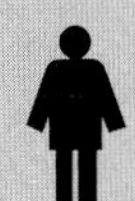

A patient who was unable to escape a burning building that collapsed on him 3 days ago is decompensating and developing respiratory failure. What paralytic would you use for intubation?

A nondepolorizing agent (eg, vecuronium, rocuronium) should be used. Upregulation of acetylcholine receptors in the setting of recent (3 days to 6 months) burns or crush injury may lead to exaggerated K^+ release and hyperkalemia with the use of succinylcholine.

RAPID SEQUENCE INTUBATION

PREPARATION

- Monitors, IV, equipment
- Positioning of patient

6 P's of RSI:

Preparation
Preoxygenation
Pretreatment
Paralysis with induction
Placement of tube
Postintubation management

PREOXYGENATION

- **Three minutes** of 100% O_2 **or six vital capacity breaths.**

PRETREATMENT

- Pretreatment medications include lidocaine, opioid, atropine and defasciculating agent (LOAD).
- Indications for pretreatment medications include (see Table 1.3):
  - ↑ Intracranial or intraocular pressure (lidocaine, opioid, defasciculating agent)
  - Mitigate tachycardic response to intubation in dissection, CAD (opioid).
  - Mitigate bronchospasm with laryngoscopy (lidocaine).
  - Prevent reflex bradycardia in the pediatric age group (atropine).
- Administer approximately 3 minutes before induction medications.

Pretreatment medications—

LOAD

Lidocaine
Opioid
Atropine
Defasciculator

Paralysis with induction:

- Administer induction medication (see Table 1.4), then paralytic (see Table 1.5).
- Avoid succinylcholine in patients who may have preexisting hyperkalemia (eg, patient with ESRD).
- **Also avoid succinylcholine in patients at risk for succinylcholine-induced hyperkalemia.**
  - Neuromuscular diseases (eg, ALS, muscular dystrophy)
  - Skeletal muscle denervation (stroke, spinal cord injury): Of <6 months
  - Multiple trauma: From day 3 to 6 months
  - Major burns: From day 2 to 6 months
  - Prolonged abdominal sepsis >3 days

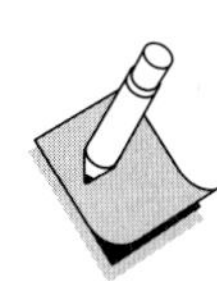

Risk of hyperkalemia with succinylcholine if:
Neuromuscular disease
Denervation disease
Crush injury
Major burn
Prolonged abdominal sepsis

TABLE 1.3. Pretreatment Medications for Rapid Sequence Intubation

DRUG	MECHANISM	INDICATION
Lidocaine	↓ Intracranial pressure (ICP) ↓ Bronchospastic response to intubation	↑ ICP ↑ Intraocular pressure (IOP) Reactive airway disease
Fentanyl	↓ Sympathetic response to intubation	↑ ICP Intracranial bleed or aneurysm Heart disease Aortic dissection
Atropine	↓ Bradycardia due to succinylcholine ↓ Bronchorrhea due to ketamine	< 10 years old
Defasciculating dose of: Vecuronium, pancuronium, *or* rocuronium	↓ ICP response to succinylcholine	↑ ICP/IOP

PLACEMENT OF TUBE (INTUBATION)

Postintubation Management

- Sedation with benzodiazepines or propofol to minimize agitation
- Pain control with narcotics to blunt sympathetic response to being intubated
- Paralysis if needed for patient control during imaging or invasive procedures

TABLE 1.4. Induction Medications for Rapid Sequence Intubation

DRUG	CLASS	BENEFIT	SIDE EFFECT
Etomidate	Imidazole derivative	↓ ICP Hemodynamically stable	Brief myoclonus
Ketamine	PCP derivative	Bronchodilator Dissociative amnesia Short acting	↑ Secretions ↑ ICP Emergence phenomenon
Midazolam	Benzodiazepine	↓ ICP	Negative inotropy → hypotension.
Thiopental	Barbiturate	↓ ICP	Negative inotropy and vasodilation → hypotension.

TABLE 1.5. Paralytic Agents for Rapid Sequence Intubation

DRUG	ONSET	DURATION	COMPLICATION
Depolorizing Agent			
Succinylcholine	45–60 sec	5–9 min	Hyperkalemia Fasciculations Increased ICP/IOP Malignant hyperthermia Prolonged action if ↓ pseudo-cholinesterase activity
Nondepolorizing Agents			
Vecuronium	2–4 min	40–60 min	Prolonged action in obese/elderly/hepatorenal dysfunction
Rocuronium	1–3 min	30–45 min	Tachycardia
Pancuronium	2–5 min	40–60 min	Tachycardia Hypertension

Advanced Airway Procedures

Used in the management of the difficult or failed airway

Difficult Airway

- Difficult mask ventilation or endotracheal intubation
- If anticipated by preintubation assessment → perform awake (**no paralysis**) intubation

Failed Airway

- Failed intubation ("can't intubate") and failed BVM ventilation ("can't ventilate")

Advanced airway procedures include:

- Awake intubation
- Supraglottic airway (eg, laryngeal mask airway)
- Fiberoptic intubation
- Translaryngeal jet ventilation
- Retrograde tracheal intubation
- Lighted stylet
- Cricothyrotomy
- Tracheostomy

Awake Intubation

Indications

- Spontaneously breathing patients with an anticipated difficult airway

Procedure

- Administer local airway anesthetic.
  - Options include nebulized or atomized 4% lidocaine and topical benzocaine gel to base of tongue.
- Sedate to blunt airway reflexes.
  - Ketamine (10–20 mg/dose): Muscle tone is maintained.
- Perform direct laryngoscopy and intubation once sedated.
- Confirm placement.

Fiberoptic Awake Intubation

Indication

- Spontaneously breathing patient with an anticipated difficult airway
  - Suspected laryngeal abnormalities
  - Poor mouth opening

Contraindications

- Copious blood or secretions
- Inadequate oxygenation or ventilation (because of time required for procedure)

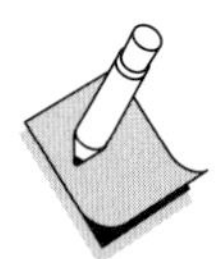

The nasal approach is better tolerated than the oral approach in fiberoptic awake intubation.

Procedure

- Anesthetize nasal and/or oral mucosa as with awake intubation.
  - Nasopharyngeal approach is preferred.
    - Easier angle of insertion
    - More defined path of insertion
    - Better tolerated by patient
- Insert scope "loaded" with ET tube and advance through cords under direct visualization.
- Advance ET tube.
- Confirm placement.

Blind Nasotracheal Intubation

Indications

- Spontaneously breathing patient with an anticipated difficult airway

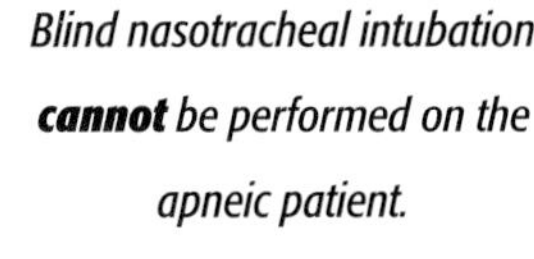

Blind nasotracheal intubation ***cannot*** *be performed on the apneic patient.*

Contraindications

- Pediatric patient <10 years old
- Midface trauma or basilar skull fracture
- ↑ intracranial pressure
- Anticoagulation or anticipated need for thrombolysis
- Combative patient
- Apnea

Procedure

- Preoxygenate.
- Administer nasal anesthetic and vasoconstrictor.
- Administer nasal lubricant.
- Insert ET tube with **bevel away from septum** and gently advance until breath sounds are heard best through tube.

- Advance the tube during **inspiration**.
- If successful, there is usually associated coughing and/or stridor and cessation of vocalization.
- Inflate cuff and confirm placement.

COMPLICATIONS

- Epistaxis
- Esophageal intubation
- Sinusitis, turbinate damage

LARYNGEAL MASK AIRWAY (LMA)

The LMA is available in the following sizes:

- 1–3: Newborn to 30–50 kg child, in .5 increments
- 4: 50–70 kg adult
- 5: Larger adults

INDICATIONS

- Rescue device for "can't intubate" situations

CONTRAINDICATIONS

- Significant oropharyngeal pathology, trauma, or bleeding.

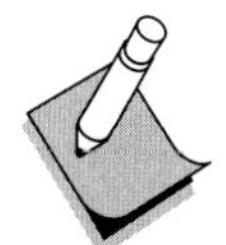

Ease of use and potential to transition to a definitive airway make the LMA useful in the difficult airway but doesn't protect against aspiration.

PROCEDURE

- Open airway via head tilt.
- Insert LMA with opening facing the tongue and advance along the hard palate until tip is well into hypopharynx.
- Inflate cuff with 20–40 mL air (amount listed on device).
  - Forms seal around glottic opening
- With the intubating LMA, an ET tube can be advanced through the lumen of the LMA for blind tracheal intubation.

COMPLICATIONS

- Aspiration
- Limited utility in patients who require high pressures to ventilate (eg, obese, severe asthma)

RETROGRADE TRACHEAL INTUBATION

INDICATION

- Rescue device for "can't intubate" situations

PROCEDURE

- Via Seldinger technique place needle in cricothyroid membrane or a high tracheal space.
- Pass a wire through the needle until it emerges from the mouth. Remove the needle and secure the percutaneous part of the wire with a hemostat.
- Advance the ET tube over wire into trachea.

COMPLICATIONS

- Hemorrhage if the cricothyroid artery is lacerated
- Soft-tissue infection

A 50-year-old male is brought to ED by EMS after being found with agonal respirations in a closed garage with the car running. On arrival, the patient is being ventilated via a Combitube, but waking up and regaining spontaneous respiratory effort. How do you want to manage his airway now?

If you want to keep the patient intubated, an ET tube should be inserted (with Combitube in place) after deflation of the pharyngeal balloon. If you want to let the patient wake up, he should be rolled to the side, both cuffs deflated, and the Combitube removed.

ESOPHAGEAL TRACHEAL COMBITUBE

An esophageal tracheal combitube consists of a twin-lumen tube with a proximal low-pressure cuff that seals the pharyngeal area, a distal cuff that seals the esophagus (or the trachea), and ports for ventilation in-between (see Figure 1.2).

The pharyngeal lumen and KING LT supraglottic airways have similar function.

It is available in two sizes only.

- 37F: Small adult/large child
- 41F: Larger adults

INDICATIONS

- Apneic and unconscious adult with
  - Failed intubation
  - Limited mouth opening

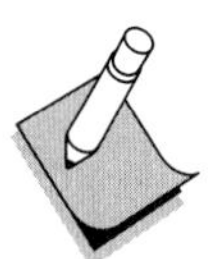

The Combitube can be used in the setting of upper GI bleed, but not if there is expected esophageal pathology.

CONTRAINDICATIONS

- Patient with intact airway reflexes
- Esophageal disease
- Caustic ingestion
- Upper airway obstruction
- Children ≤4 feet tall

PROCEDURE

- Grab and elevate the tongue and jaw with nondominant hand.
- Pass the tube blindly into the pharynx until the marker on the tube is between the patient's teeth.
  - Placement is facilitated by neck flexion.

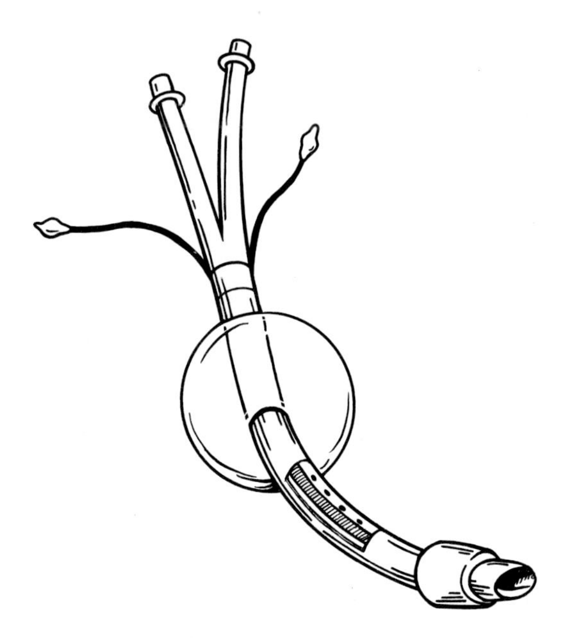

FIGURE 1.2. Esophageal tracheal Combitube.

(Reproduced, with permission, from Tintinalli JE, Kelen GD, Stapczynski JS. *Emergency Medicine: A Comprehensive Study Guide*, 6th ed. New York: McGraw-Hill, 2004:105.)

- Inflate the pharyngeal balloon with 100 mL of air.
- Inflate the distal white balloon with 5–15 mL of air.
- Begin ventilation through the longer (blue) connector.
  - Air entry to lungs → confirms esophageal placement.
  - Air entry into stomach → tracheal placement (rare), in which case confirm with ventilation through shorter (clear) tube.

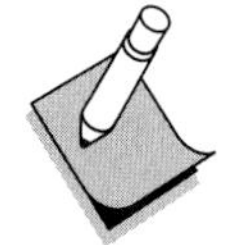

"A blue patient is bad": Begin ventilation through the Combitube's blue connector. Air entry into lungs confirms correct (esophageal) placement of device.

LIGHTED STYLET

INDICATIONS

- Difficult airway
- Limited mouth opening
- Limited cervical spine mobility

CONTRAINDICATION

- Failed airway: Because of time required
- Laryngeal pathology

PROCEDURE

- Grab and elevate the tongue and jaw with nondominant hand.
- Insert lighted stylet "loaded" with ET tube into oropharynx, with curved tip midline and pointing inferiorly, until it sits in the posterior pharynx.
- Rock tip forward while lifting jaw and tongue.

A lateral or poorly defined glow indicates improper lighted stylet placement.

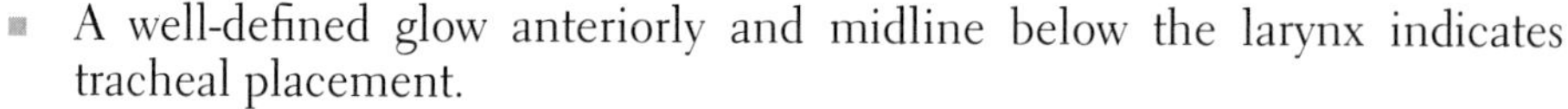

- A well-defined glow anteriorly and midline below the larynx indicates tracheal placement.
- Advance ET tube.
- Confirm placement.

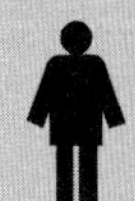

An 8-year-old boy is in respiratory arrest after being ejected from a car during a rollover accident. He has obvious head and face trauma. You are unable to intubate or BVM ventilate. What should you do next?

This child has a failed airway ("can't intubate, can't ventilate"). You should immediately perform a needle cricothyrotomy to provide oxygenation. While you prep and initiate the procedure, another provider can attempt to place an LMA as a rescue maneuver.

NEEDLE CRICOTHYROTOMY

Surgical airway of choice in children <10 years old. Allows for oxygenation, but ventilation is often inadequate.

Needle cricothyrotomy will provide oxygenation, but ventilation may be inadequate.

INDICATIONS

- Rescue device for **oxygenation** in failed airway

CONTRAINDICATION

- Tracheal transection with retraction of the distal end
- Cricoid or laryngeal damage

PROCEDURE

- Attach a 12- or 14-gauge needle catheter to a 3-mL syringe.
- Locate and stabilize the cricoid membrane.
- Direct the needle catheter inferiorly and insert it (aspirating continuously) through the cricoid membrane into the trachea.
- Once in trachea, advance the catheter over the needle.
- Attach catheter to jet-ventilation system and oxygenate.
  - Deliver 100% O_2 for 1 second, then release for 4 seconds and repeat.

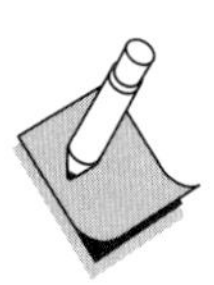

Advantages of needle cricothyrotomy over surgical cricothyrotomy: Simpler, faster, less bleeding, fewer long-term complications, can be done in patients of all ages!

COMPLICATIONS

- Common
  - Subcutaneous emphysema, catheter kinking/obstruction, coughing if patient is conscious, CO_2 retention
- Uncommon but serious
  - Barotrauma, pneumothorax, pneumomediastinum

CRICHOTHYROTOMY

Equipment needed at a minimum: Scalpel, tracheal hook, 5.5 or 6.0 cuffed endotracheal tube

INDICATIONS

- Failed airway

Contraindications

- Difficult to perform in patients < 10 years old

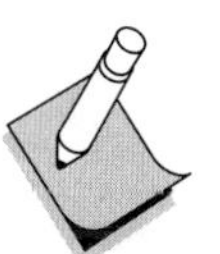

Surgical cricothyrotomy is difficult to perform in children <10 years old. Needle cricithyrotomy is a better choice in this age group.

Procedure

- Locate the cricothyroid membrane with nondominant hand.
- Make a midline longitudinal skin incision at the level of the cricothyroid membrane.
- Stabilizing the larynx with thumb and middle finger of nondominant hand, make an horizontal incision in the cricothyroid membrane.
- Use the tracheal hook to maintain control of trachea.
- Bluntly widen the cricothyroid membrane orifice with finger or blunt end of scalpel/hemostat.
- Insert the tracheostomy or endotracheal tube.
- Confirm placement with $ETCO_2$.

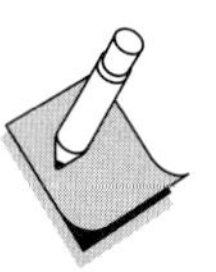

Surgical cricothyrotomy: Longitudinal (vertical) skin incision. Horizontal incision through cricoid membrane.

Complications

- More likely in pediatric population due to lack of laryngeal prominence, superior larynx, and small cricothyroid membrane
- Bleeding
- Airway injury

Management of Airway Obstruction

Heimlich Maneuver

Indication

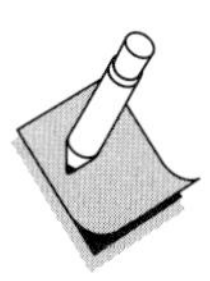

Do not perform the Heimlich maneuver on a patient who is breathing or coughing and appears to have adequate oxygenation.

- Complete airway obstruction due to tracheal foreign body

Contraindication

- Breathing/coughing patient with adequate oxygenation

Procedure

- Child/adult
  - Subdiaphragmatic thrusts
    - Arms wrapped around victim if conscious
- Infant/small toddler: 5 back blows followed by 5 chest thrusts
- Direct laryngoscopy with foreign body removal, when available

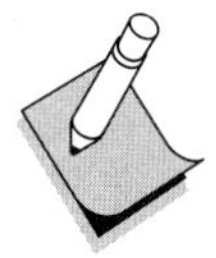

Abdominal thrusts are relatively contraindicated in pregnant patients. Use chest compressions instead.

VENTILATION TECHNIQUES

Noninvasive Ventilation

Requirements: Patent airway, patient cooperation, and intact respiratory drive

Allows time to treat the cause of respiratory distress, avoid ET intubation and its associated complications, and ↓ length of stay

Continuous Positive Airway Pressure (CPAP)

- Provides constant airway pressure to **prevent upper airway collapse**
- Need properly fitted mask
- Reduces work of breathing, increases oxygenation and CO_2 clearance

BiPAP is a combination of CPAP and inspiratory assist.

Bi-Level Positive Airway Pressure (BiPAP)

- It is a combination of CPAP and inspiratory assist.
- Inspiratory positive pressure (8–10cm H_2O) exceeds that of expiratory positive pressure (3–5cm H_2O) provided.
- **It provides extrinsic PEEP.**
- Each cycle is triggered by patient initiation of inhalation.

Complications

- Volutrauma, pressure necrosis of the skin from an ill-fitting mask, gastric distention, delayed definitive airway management.

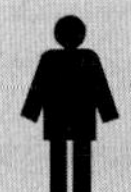

A 60-year-old smoker in COPD exacerbation is failing aggressive noninvasive therapy. He is now orotracheally intubated. What should his initial ventilator settings be?

In a patient with COPD, the initial selected tidal volume and rate should be slightly reduced to avoid hyperinflation and hyperventilation. Begin with 10 mL/kg of patient's ideal body weight at 10 breaths per minute and 100% FiO_2 and wean as tolerated.

Mechanical Ventilation

Initial ventilator setting should be based on review of the underlying pulmonary process (see Table 1.6).

Complications

- Volutrauma
  - Overdistention of alveoli
  - Prevented by using smaller tidal volumes

TABLE 1.6. Initial Ventilator Settings

Pulmonary Process	Ventilator Settings
Pulmonary contusion	Low tidal volume (5–10 mL/kg) to prevent barotrauma PEEP of 5–15 cm H_2O to prevent alveoli collapse
Asthma/COPD	Slow respiratory rate and prolonged exhalation phase PEEP
ARDS	Low respiratory rate (maximize recruitment) Low tidal volume (6 mL/kg) to prevent volutrauma PEEP
Neonates	Best setting = pressure controlled ventilation
Acidosis	Continue respiratory compensation with a high respiratory rate
Head injury	Avoid hypercapnea, which causes cerebral vasodilation and ↑ ICP.

- **Barotrauma**
  - Caused by excessive pressure
  - Prevented by lowering inspiratory pressures
- **Ventilator associated pneumonia**
  - Risk increases exponentially in relationship to duration of intubation.
  - Decrease risk by sitting patients up in bed by at least 30 degrees if not contraindicated.
  - **Early pneumonias** (< 72 hours postintubation): Community acquired pathogens
  - **Late pneumonias** (> 72 hours postintubation): Nosocomial pathogens, more resistant strains
- **Hemodynamic instability**
  - High respiratory rate, PEEP, or inverse ratio ventilation may increase intrathoracic pressure, decreasing venous return → decreased cardiac output → hypotension.
  - May also increase cerebral venous pressure → cerebral ischemia

BLOOD GASES

Blood gases are a useful tool in the evaluation of the patient with respiratory failure. The use of blood gases to evaluate acid-base status is covered separately (see Chapter 7).

Basic Principles of Pulmonary Physiology

VENTILATION

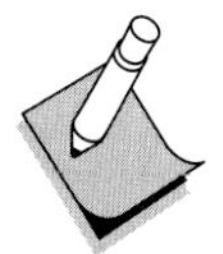

Decreased ventilation OR an increase in dead space → increased CO_2 on blood gas.

- The **clearance of CO_2** from the body is primarily determined by **ventilation.**
- Ventilation is primarily a function of the rate and depth (tidal volume) of breathing.
- The air that does not participate in gas exchange (approximately 30% in normal conditions) = **dead space.**
  - An increase in dead space (picture breathing through a snorkel) requires increased ventilation to maintain CO_2 clearance.
  - Diseases with ↑ dead space include: COPD, PE.

An increase in dead space (COPD, PE) requires increased ventilation to maintain CO_2 clearance.

DIFFUSION

- Diffusion = **movement of O_2** (or other gases) across the **alveolar-capillary membrane.**
  - ↑ Solubility of gases → better diffusion.
  - O_2 is much less soluble than CO_2, therefore more easily affected by diseases of the alveolar-capillary membrane.
  - Diseases affecting the alveolar-capillary membrane include: Pulmonary edema, interstitial fibrosis.
- ↓ Diffusion → low P_aO_2 and an increased Alveolar-arterial (A-a) gradient on blood gas, which **improve with supplemental oxygen.**

Oxygenation is adversely affected by diseases of the alveolar-capillary membrane that decrease diffusion (eg. interstitial fibrosis).

SHUNT

- **Physiologic right-to-left shunt** = blood flow (perfusion) to alveoli that cannot participate in gas exchange (therefore no oxygenation).
  - Occurs in setting of nonfunctioning alveoli, such as ARDS, pneumonia

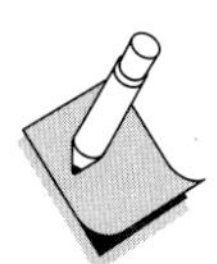

Hypoxemia due to an anatomic shunt does not correct with 100% O_2.

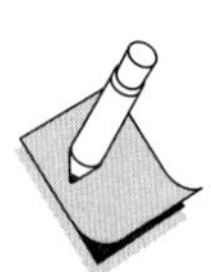

Carbon monoxide replaces O_2 by binding to hemoglobin AND shifts the oxyhemoglobin dissociation curve to the left, decreasing the availability of O_2 to tissues.

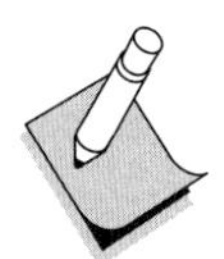

Four rhythms produce cardiac arrest: Ventricular fibrillation, pulseless ventricular tachycardia, pulseless electrical activity, and asystole.

- **Anatomic right-to-left shunt** = blood flow that bypasses the lungs altogether as in a VSD with pulmonary hypertension.
- Right-to-left shunt → low P_aO_2 and an increased A-a gradient on blood gas. If anatomic, it will not improve **with supplemental oxygen**.

O_2 Delivery to Tissues

- Three principal components determine O_2 delivery to tissues:
  - **O_2 content:** Amount of O_2 dissolved in blood and carried on hemoglobin
  - **Cardiac output**
  - **Oxyhemoglobin saturation** at a given P_aO_2
    - Demonstrated in the oxyhemoglobin dissociation curve
    - **Right shift of curve = O_2 more readily given up to tissue.**
    - **Causes of right shift:** Acidosis, hyperthermia, increased 2,3-DPG
    - **Causes of left shift:** Alkalosis, hypothermia, abnormal hemoglobin, decreased 2,3-DPG

CARDIAC CONDUCTION AND RHYTHM ASSESSMENT

General Approach

Arrhythmias are a problem encountered frequently by the emergency physician. A general approach to assessing rhythms is essential in determining management.

Is the patient in cardiac arrest?

- Four rhythms produce cardiac arrest: **Ventricular fibrillation, pulseless ventricular tachycardia, pulseless electrical activity, and asystole**
- See "Management of Cardiac Arrest."

Is the rhythm stable or unstable?

The definition of stability relates to the ability of the heart to produce sufficient cardiac output.

Signs of instability:

- Cardiac ischemia manifested by chest pain or acute CHF
- Circulatory compromise (hypotension, diaphoresis, weak pulses)
- Neurologic dysfunction caused by decreased cerebral blood flow
  - Generally global with altered mental status; rarely (if ever) focal

Is the rhythm too fast (> 100 bpm) or too slow (< 60 bpm)?

Is the rhythm wide or narrow complex?

Rhythm complex width is defined as the width of the QRS. QRS ≥ 0.12 seconds is considered wide complex.

- Wide complex rhythms result from conduction outside the normal pathways (bundle branch block, pacemaker, initiation below the AV node) or the presence of a metabolic abnormality or toxin (hyperkalemia, TCA overdose).
- Narrow complex rhythms are conducted through normal pathways and almost always begin above or within the AV node.

Is the rhythm regular or irregular?

Regular rhythms include:

- Sinus
- Some AV-node blocks (first-degree AV block, second-degree AV block with fixed conduction.)
- Paroxysmal supraventricular tachycardia (PSVT)
- Atrial flutter with fixed block
- Atrial tachycardia
- Ventricular tachycardia

Irregular rhythms include:

- Atrial fibrillation
- Atrial flutter with variable block
- Multifocal atrial tachycardia with or without conduction blocks
- Some AV-node blocks (Wenckebach, second-degree AV block with variable conduction)

Are P waves present? If so, are they associated with QRS complexes?

The presence or absence of P waves as well as whether or not they conduct is important to understanding the origin of the rhythm.

Once a rhythm is diagnosed, specific therapy may be instituted.

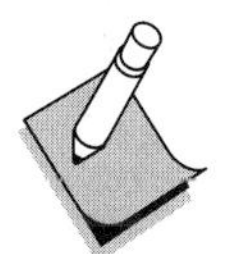

Unstable rhythm = rhythm with associated signs or symptoms of inadequate cardiac output.

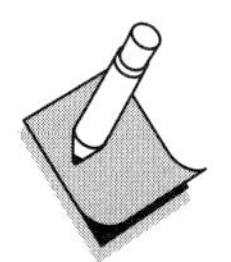

Unstable cardiac rhythms require immediate intervention. Stable rhythms may be further delineated via more investigation.

Rhythm with QRS ≥ 0.12 sec = wide complex.

A 55-year-old male presents to the ED with acute onset of chest pain, shortness of breath, and diaphoresis. His initial ECG shows acute ST elevation in the anterior leads. You initiate ACS protocols and activate the cath lab. Shortly thereafter he complains of lightheadedness. The monitor now shows third-degree AV block with a ventricular escape rhythm at 35 bpm. What should you do first?

Anterior MI is associated with infranodal conduction damage that is often permanent. Transcutaneous pacing should be initiated and the patient prepped for transvenous pacer placement. Atropine may actually WORSEN the conduction ratio, and therefore should **not** be used in this setting. Isoproterenol may also be used to increase the ventricular rate.

Conduction Abnormalities

Conduction abnormalities can occur above the atrioventricular node (supranodal blocks), at the level of atrioventricular conduction, or within the ventricles (intraventricular blocks). Intraventricular blocks are described in detail in the section "ECG Essentials" in Chapter 2.

Supranodal Blocks

- Sinoatrial block
- Intra-atrial block

Atrioventricular (AV) Blocks

- Involve the AV node and/or proximal His bundle ("infranodal" AV block)
- Are measured as degrees with increasing conduction abnormality

- First-degree AV block
- Second-degree AV block type I (Wenckebach, Mobitz I)
- Second-degree AV block type II (Mobitz II)
- Third-degree AV block (complete heart block)

INTRAVENTRICULAR BLOCKS

- Unilateral fascicular blocks
  - Right bundle branch block (RBBB)
  - Left anterior fascicular block (LAFB)
  - Left posterior fascicular block (LPFB)
- Bifascicular blocks
  - RBBB + LAFP *or* LPFB
  - Left bundle branch block (LBBB)
- Trifascicular blocks
  - Any bifascicular block + first-degree AV block
  - Alternating RBBB and LBBB

FIRST-DEGREE AV BLOCK

First-degree AV block is common and is often a normal variant in a healthy heart. It results from prolonged conduction of the atrial impulse, typically at the AV node.

CAUSES

Causes include:

- Increased vagal tone in healthy heart
- ACS (usually **inferior MI**)
- Infectious disease (eg, Lyme disease, rheumatic fever)
- Infiltrative myocardial disease (eg, sarcoidosis)
- Structural heart disease (congenital or surgical)
- Medications

ECG FINDINGS (SEE FIGURE 1.3)

- All P waves conducted (QRS for every P wave)
- PR interval > 0.2 seconds
- PR interval constant

TREATMENT

- Does **not** cause serious signs or symptoms
- Treat underlying condition.

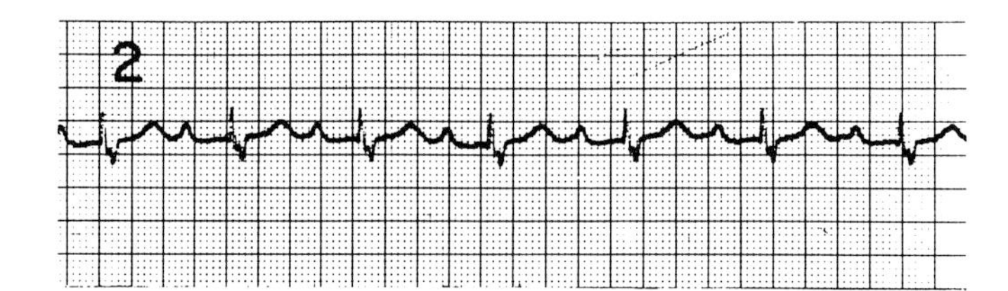

FIGURE 1.3. First-degree AV block.

(Reproduced, with permission, from Tintinalli JE, Kelen GD, Stapczynski JS. *Emergency Medicine: A Comprehensive Study Guide*, 6th ed. New York: McGraw-Hill, 2004:193.)

SECOND-DEGREE AV BLOCK TYPE I (WENCKEBACH, MOBITZ I)

Characterized by gradually increasing block **at the AV node** due to prolongation of the AV-nodal refractory period; can occur in normal hearts

CAUSES

Similar to first-degree AV block. In ACS, it is commonly associated with **inferior MI**.

ECG FINDINGS (SEE FIGURE 1.4)

- PR progressively elongates until one QRS complex is dropped.
- P waves regular
- Not all P waves conducted past AV node
- PR interval generally > 0.2 seconds.
- QRS complexes appear "grouped."

First-degree heart block, Wenckebach, and RBBB can all occur in a healthy heart.

TREATMENT

- Unlikely to cause serious signs or symptoms
- Treat underlying condition.

SECOND-DEGREE AV BLOCK TYPE II (MOBITZ II)

A significant rhythm since it is associated with damage to the conducting system below the AV node (**infranodal**) and can progress without warning to complete heart block.

CAUSES

Mobitz II does **not** occur in healthy hearts. Causes include:

- ACS (commonly **anteroseptal MI**)
- Infectious disease (eg, Lyme disease, rheumatic fever)
- Infiltrative myocardial disease (eg, sarcoidosis)
- Structural heart disease (congenital or surgical)
- Medications

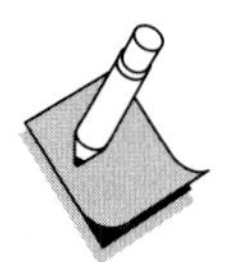

Second-degree AV block type II (Mobitz II) = damage to the infranodal conducting system.

ECG FINDINGS (SEE FIGURE 1.5)

- PR interval constant
- P waves regular
- QRS complex regularly or randomly dropped

TREATMENT

- Symptomatic bradycardia → transcutanous pacing.
- Transvenous pacemaker placement (required, unless chronic)
- Atropine is **not** helpful (may actually worsen conduction ratio).
- Admission (unless chronic)

Inferior MI → reversible AV block.
Anteroseptal MI → permanent infranodal conduction system damage.

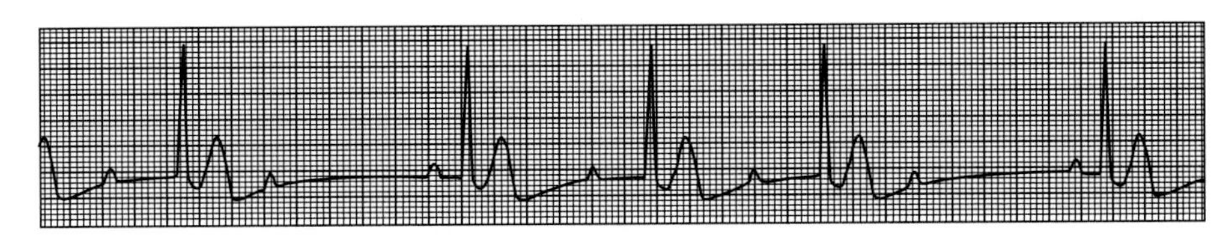

FIGURE 1.4. Second-degree AV block type I.

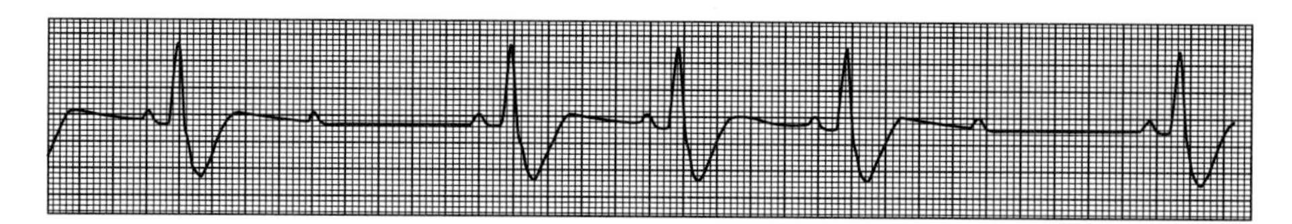

FIGURE 1.5. **Second-degree AV block type II.**

THIRD-DEGREE AV BLOCK

Generally unstable rhythm resulting in syncope and often hypotension. Third-degree AV block (third-degree heart block) can be due to damage at the AV node or at the infranodal conducting system.

CAUSES

Causes are similar to second-degree AV block. Be sure to consider medications such as β-blockers and Ca channel blockers as a cause.

In the setting of ACS, third-degree AV block may be either nodal or infranodal.

- **Nodal** third-degree AV block is seen primarily with inferior MI and is typically transient.
- **Infranodal** third-degree AV block is seen in large anteroseptal MI from damage to the infranodal conducting system and is often permanent.

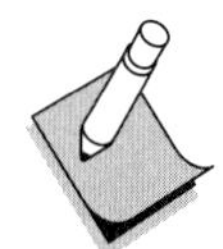

Inferior MI → third-degree AV block with junctional escape (40–60 bpm) and narrow complexes.

Anterior MI → third-degree AV block with ventricular escape (<40 bpm) and wide complexes.

ECG FINDINGS (SEE FIGURE 1.6)

- No P waves conducted
- Nodal block → junctional escape rhythm, narrow complexes.
- Infranodal block → ventricular escape rhythm, wide complexes.

TREATMENT

- Nodal
  - Atropine and transcutaneous pacing if symptomatic
  - Temporary transvenous pacemaker often required
- Infranodal
  - **Avoid: Atropine** (may worsen the conduction rate).
  - Isoproterenol (to increase ventricular rate) and transcutaneous pacing if symptomatic, until
  - Transvenous pacemaker placement
- If congenital and asymptomatic, may not require immediate therapy

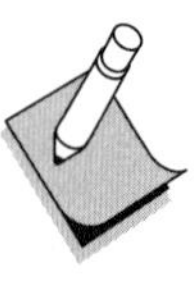

Atropine may actually worsen the conduction ratio with infranodal AV block (Mobitz II or infranodal third degree).

EXTRASYSTOLES

Extrasystoles are ectopic impulses occurring in addition to regular sinus beats.

- Premature atrial contraction
- Premature ventricular contraction

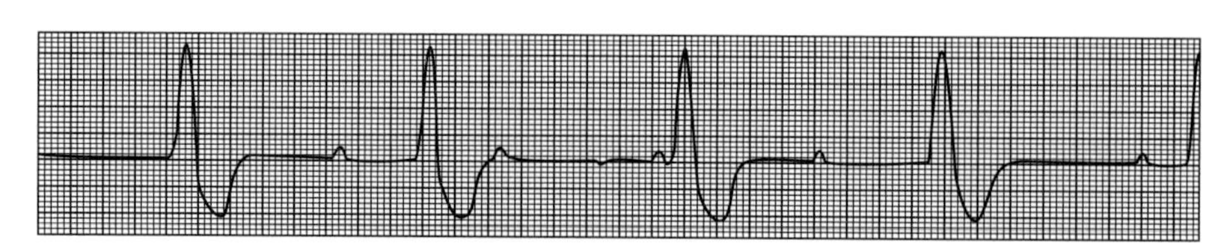

FIGURE 1.6. **Third-degree AV block.**

PREMATURE ATRIAL CONTRACTION (PAC)

ECG FINDINGS

- Premature beat with preceding P wave
  - Narrow or wide QRS complex depending on timing
- P wave different from normal sinus P wave
- Noncompensatory pause (sinus node is depolarized → next normal beat is earlier than expected)

PREMATURE VENTRICULAR CONTRACTION (PVC)

ECG FINDINGS (SEE FIGURE 1.7)

- Premature wide QRS without preceding P wave
- Appropriate discordance present
- Interpolated between normal beats **or**
- Fully compensatory pause (one missed sinus beat, but sinus node **not** reset)

> A 52-year-old male is brought to the ED by EMS complaining of palpitations with shortness of breath and chest pain. At presentation he is diaphoretic and pale. He speaks three words at a time and is clutching his chest. After being transferred to a gurney he is placed on a cardiac monitor that demonstrates a wide complex rhythm at 175 bpm. His BP is 110/80 and his RR is 30. How should you proceed?
>
> This patient has a wide complex tachycardia and is symptomatic with chest pain and shortness of breath. Because you are not given any further information to differentiate this rhythm from SVT with aberrancy you should treat it as VT. Start with immediate synchronized cardioversion at 100J.

Dysrhythmias

Dysrhythmias can be grouped based on whether the resulting rate is too slow or too fast.

Rates that are too slow (bradydysrhythmias) can result from the following:

- Depression of sinus node activity
- Conduction blocks (see above)

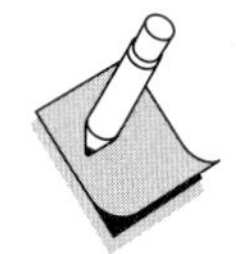

Three mechanisms of tachydysrhythmias:
Increased automaticity
Reentry
Triggered rhythm

Rates that are too fast (tachydysrhythmias) may result from three mechanisms:

- Increased automaticity of a sinus or ectopic focus
- Reentry via AV node or accessory pathway
- Triggered rhythm (eg, R on T)

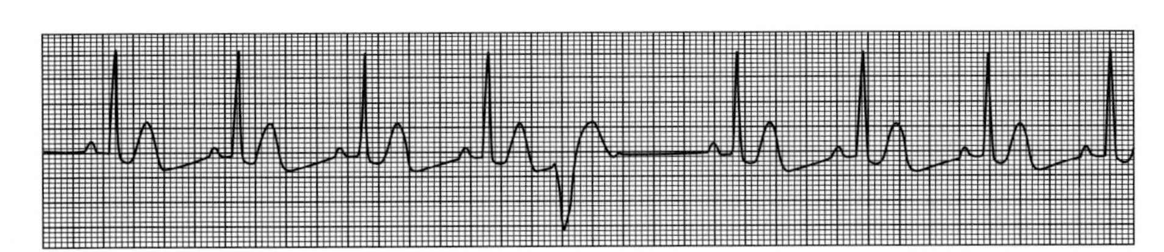

FIGURE 1.7. Premature ventricular contraction.

Bradydysrhythmias

- Sick sinus syndrome
- Sinus arrest

Tachydysrhythmias

- Atrial tachycardia
- Multifocal atrial tachycardia
- Atrial flutter
- Atrial fibrillation
- Paroxysmal supraventricular tachycardia
  - Wolfe-Parkinson-White syndrome
  - Brugada syndrome
  - AV-nodal reentrant tachycardia
- Ventricular tachycardia
- Torsades de pointes
- Ventricular fibrillation
- Sinus tachycardia

Sick Sinus Syndrome (SSS)

Causes

- Occurs as a result of disease in the sinoatrial node
- May cause tachycardia-bradycardia syndrome in which sinus rate varies from fast to slow and back again
- Often manifests as syncope

ECG Findings

- Irregular rhythm with pauses in sinus activity

Treatment

- Depends on presentation
- Too slow: Rate stimulation with atropine or pacing
- Too fast: Rate control with calcium channel or β-blockers
- Definitive therapy: Typically a combination of permanent pacemaker placement plus rate control medications

Sinus Arrest (Sinus Block)

Left untreated, SSS leads to complete cessation of SA activity.

ECG Findings (See Figure 1.8)

- No P waves
- Escape pacemaker activity
  - Usually from the AV node or bundle of His (40–60 bpm) but may be ventricular escape (< 40 bpm).

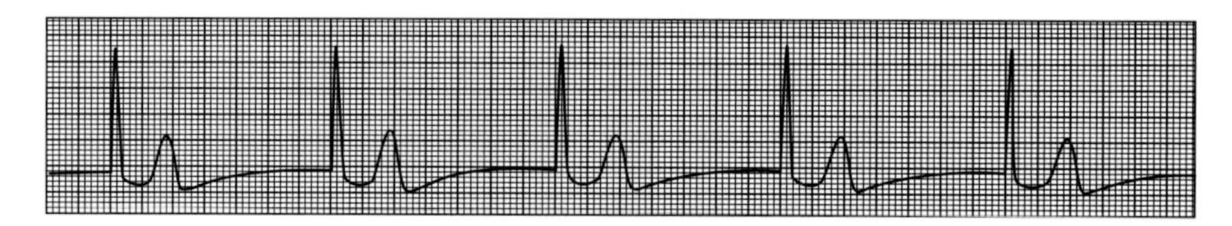

FIGURE 1.8. Sinus arrest with junctional escape rhythm.

Treatment

- Atropine
- Often requires emergent temporary transcutaneous or transvenous pacing
- Permanent pacemaker insertion is definitive therapy.

Sinus arrest or sinus block is often the result of untreated sick sinus syndrome.

Sinus Tachycardia

Diagnosis and Causes

A diagnosis of exclusion

There are many causes of sinus tachycardia, including:

- **HR increase to maintain cardiac output**
  - Decreased effective circulating volume (bleeding, volume loss, anemia, or abnormal hemoglobin function)
  - Impaired cardiac function (MI, ACS, valvular disease, tamponade)
  - PE
  - Hypoxia
- **Metabolic/endocrine derangements**
  - DKA
  - Hyperthyroidism
  - Adrenal insufficiency
  - Fever/sepsis
  - SIRS
  - Drug ingestions (sympathomimetics)
  - Drug/alcohol withdrawal
- Anxiety or pain

ECG Findings

- P waves precede all QRS complexes.
- Regular rhythm

Treatment

- Treat underlying condition.

Atrial Tachycardia

Atrial tachycardia results when an ectopic atrial focus takes over either due to increased autonomic activity or intra-atrial reentry. These atrial impulses are conducted to the ventricles.

Causes

Causes include:

- Triggered by a PAC
- Electrolyte imbalance
- Drugs (think **Digoxin**!)
- Fever
- Hypoxia

ECG Findings

- Regular narrow complex tachycardia
- P wave before each QRS

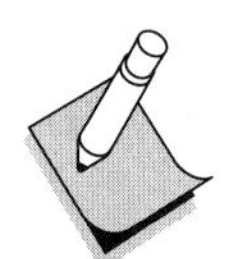

Atrial tachycardia is typically due to an underlying medical (not a cardiac) condition.

- P different from normal sinus P waves
- **Atrial tachycardia with AV block** is classic for digoxin toxicity!

TREATMENT

- Usually a stable rhythm, not requiring therapy
- Treat underlying condition.
- When treatment is needed because of signs of instability
  - Rate control with diltiazem, β-blockers

MUTIFOCAL ATRIAL TACHYCARDIA (MAT)

A subset of atrial tachycardia, MAT occurs when multiple ectopic foci stimulate the atria.

CAUSES

Often associated with **chronic lung disease and hypoxemia**

ECG FINDINGS (SEE FIGURE 1.9)

- Irregular narrow complex tachycardia
- P wave before each QRS
- Multiple unique P waves present

TREATMENT

- Usually a stable rhythm not requiring therapy (treat the pulmonary condition)
- When treatment is needed because of signs of instability
  - Rate control with diltiazem, β-blockers

ATRIAL FLUTTER

Atrial flutter is organized atrial electrical activity, usually without contractile action.

CAUSES

- Idiopathic
- Hyperthyroidism or metabolic abnormalities
- Stimulant use
- Pericarditis
- CHF
- Valvular dysfunction
- Acute or chronic lung disease

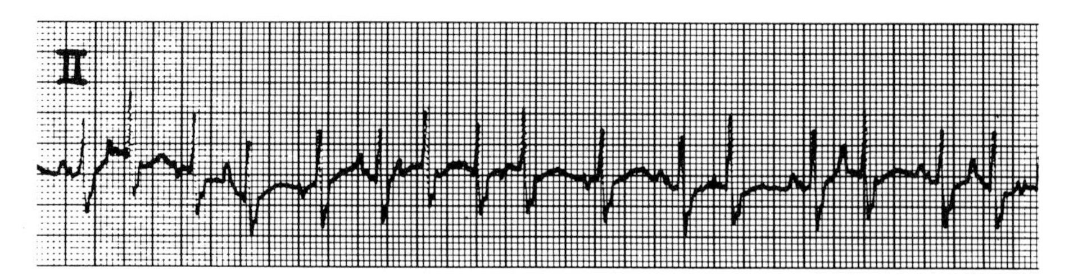

FIGURE 1.9. Multifocal atrial tachycardia.

(Reproduced, with permission, from Tintinalli JE, Kelen GD, Stapczynski JS. *Emergency Medicine: A Comprehensive Study Guide*, 6th ed. New York: McGraw-Hill, 2004:184.)

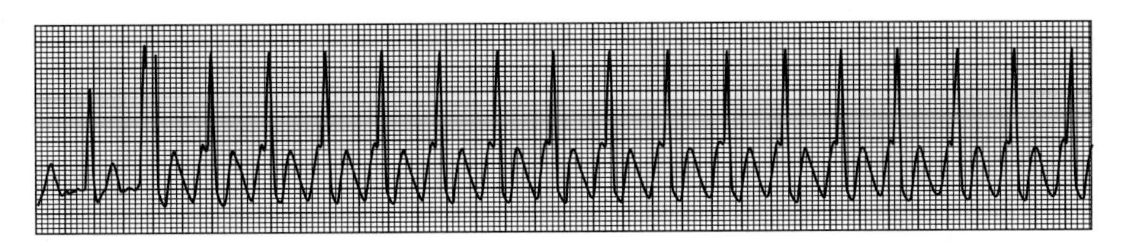

FIGURE 1.10. Atrial flutter.

ECG Findings (See Figure 1.10)

- Atrial rate ranges from 250 to 300 bpm.
- AV-node conduction of every 2 or 3 atrial impulses
  - Ventricular rate is classically 150 (2:1 conduction).
- P waves have characteristic "saw tooth pattern."

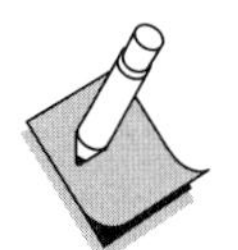

The ventricular rate in untreated atrial flutter is typically 150 bpm due to 2:1 conduction of atrial impulses.

Diagnosis

- If in question may use **adenosine** to block the AV node and "uncover" the underlying atrial rhythm

Treatment

- If patient unstable → electrical cardioversion.
  - Synchronized
  - May be successful with 25–50J
  - Sedation, if possible
- Otherwise → rate control with AV-node blocking agents.
  - Diltiazem
  - β-Blockers
- Chemical cardioversion may then be tried.
  - Choices include:
    - Amiodarone
    - Ibutilide
    - Procainamide
    - Quinidine
- **Avoid**: AV-nodal blocking drugs if accessory pathway suspected.

Atrial Fibrillation (AFib)

Atrial fibrillation is disorganized atrial electrical activity (rate >400 bpm) with **no** organized atrial contraction. Ventricular rate is limited by the AV node (or accessory pathway refractory period).

Alcohol use is commonly associated with AFib.

Causes

Causes are similar to atrial flutter. Alcohol use is commonly associated with AFib ("holiday heart").

ECG Findings (See Figure 1.11)

- Irregularly irregular QRS complexes
- No P waves
- Variable rates of ventricular response (as high as 175 bpm)
- QRS complex narrow unless
  - Preexisting conduction blocks
  - Accessory pathway (eg, Wolfe-Parkinson-White)

QRS complexes are narrow in AFib unless there is a preexisting conduction block or an accessory pathway.

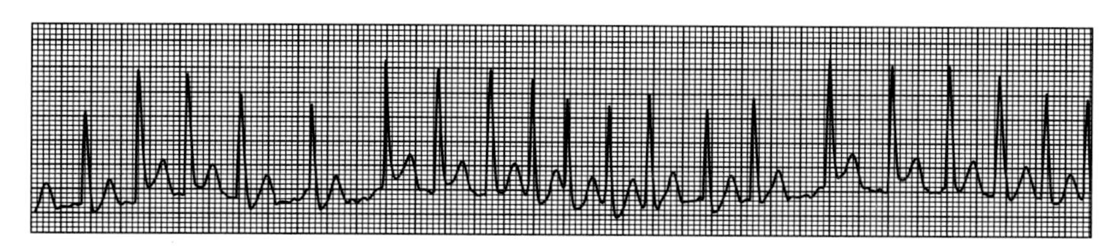

FIGURE 1.11. Atrial fibrillation.

Treatment

- If rapid ventricular response and patient is unstable → electrical cardioversion.
  - Synchronized
  - Start with 50–100J
  - Sedation, if possible
- Otherwise, rate control with AV-node blocking agents
  - Diltiazem
  - β-Blockers
- Chemical cardioversion
  - Indicated for **acute (<24 hours of symptoms) AFib only** or after transeophageal echocardiogram excludes atrial thrombus.
  - If clot present, patient needs 3–4 weeks of anticoagulation prior to cardioversion.
  - Choices include:
    - Amiodarone
    - Ibutilide
    - Procainamide
    - Quinidine
- **Avoid:**
  - AV-nodal blocking drugs **if accessory pathway suspected**
  - Chemical or elective electrical cardioversion in chronic atrial fibrillation until **after** 3–4 weeks of systemic anticoagulation

AV-nodal blocking drugs should be avoided in AFib or a-flutter if an accessory pathway is suspected.

Complications

- Cardiovascular collapse: If accessory pathway and AV-nodal blocking agents given
- Embolic stroke
  - >24 hours of symptoms associated with higher risk of intra-atrial clot and possible resultant stroke
  - The risk of embolus and risk-based treatment for patients with chronic/recurrent atrial fibrillation is summarized in Table 1.7.

AV-Nodal Reentrant Tachycardia (AVNRT)

AVNRT is the most common cause of paroxysmal SVT and results from the formation of a "circus reentrant" pathway within the AV node. It is usually clinically stable.

Pathophysiology

- Requires presence of **two limbs** within the AV node with different refractory times
- PAC arrives when only one limb is fully recovered → impulse travels down this limb to distal AV node → refractory second limb is now recovered → impulse travel retrograde up this limb → reentry circuit now established.

TABLE 1.7. CHADS2 Score to Predict Risk of Stroke in Patients With Chronic Atrial Fibrillation

	VARIABLE	POINTS
C	CHF	1
H	Hypertension	1
A	Age > 75 years	1
D	Diabetes	1
S	Prior TIA or Stroke	2
Low risk (0–1 points): Aspirin Moderate risk (2 points): Aspirin or warfarin High risk (≥ 3 points): Warfarin (aspirin, if warfarin contraindicated)		

ECG FINDINGS (SEE FIGURE 1.12)

- Narrow QRS complexes at rate of 120–200 bpm
- Absence of visible P waves
  - Retrograde P waves are buried in QRS.
- Regular rhythm

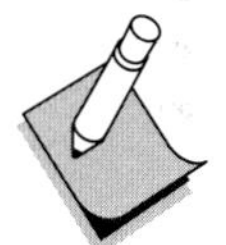

Adenosine will be effective in the vast majority of patients with AVNRT.

TREATMENT

- If patient unstable → electrical cardioversion:
  - Synchronized
  - Begin with 50–100J
- Other therapy focused on interrupting circuit within AV node
- Vagal maneuvers
  - Valsalva
  - Carotid sinus massage
    - Be wary in elderly.
    - Ensure no carotid bruits first.
  - Immerse face in cold water → dive reflex (more effective in infants).
- AV-node blockers
  - Adenosine
  - Diltiazem
  - β-Blockers

WOLFE-PARKINSON-WHITE SYNDROME (WPW)

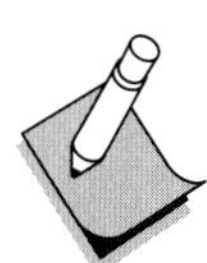

WPW accessory pathway = bundle of Kent, connecting the atrium directly to the ventricle.

A very small percentage of the population has an accessory pathway that allows sinus impulses to bypass the AV node and be conducted directly to the ventricles. WPW is the most common accessory pathway syndrome.

In WPW, the accessory tract = bundle of Kent

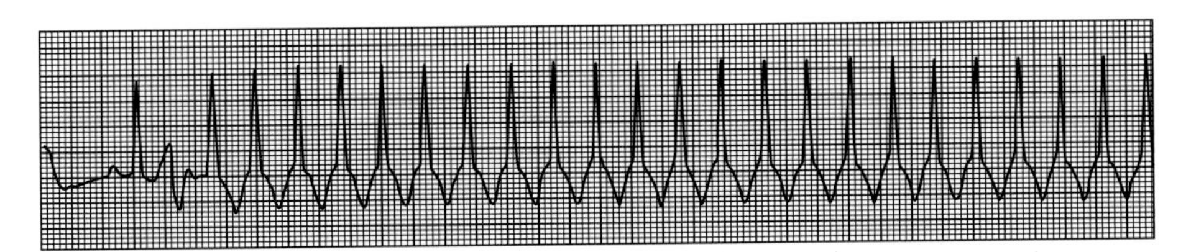

FIGURE 1.12. AV-nodal reentrant tachycardia.

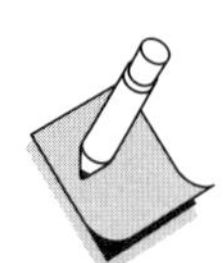

A bypass tract may be completely hidden on the resting ECG.

The orthodromic circuit travels down the AV node (good). The antidromic circuit travels down the accessory pathway (bad).

Pathophysiology

- Bundle of Kent connects atrium directly to ventricle.
- **"Normal" conduction**
  - Impulses travel down both the accessory pathway AND the AV node to the ventricle → slurred QRS complex on the resting ECG.
  - In some, bypass tract is *completely hidden* during normal conduction.
- **AFib or a-flutter**
  - If short refractory period in accessory pathway → **many** impulses reach ventricle → very high ventricular rates (wide complexes).
- **Orthodromic reentry tachycardia**
  - Reentry circuit with impulse traveling down the AV node and up the accessory pathway → narrow complexes.
  - Rate controlled by AV node **(good)**
- **Antidromic reentry tachycardia**
  - Reentry circuit with impulse traveling down the accessory pathway and up the AV node → wide complexes.
  - Rate controlled by accessory pathway **(bad)**

ECG Findings

- Resting ECG = preexcitation (see Figure 1.13)
  - Short PR interval
  - Slurred R wave (the delta wave) → wide QRS.
- Orthodromic reentry tachycardia
  - Narrow QRS complexes
  - No P waves
  - Rates > 200 bpm
- Antidromic reentry tachycardia
  - Wide QRS complexes
  - No P waves
  - Rates often > 200 bpm

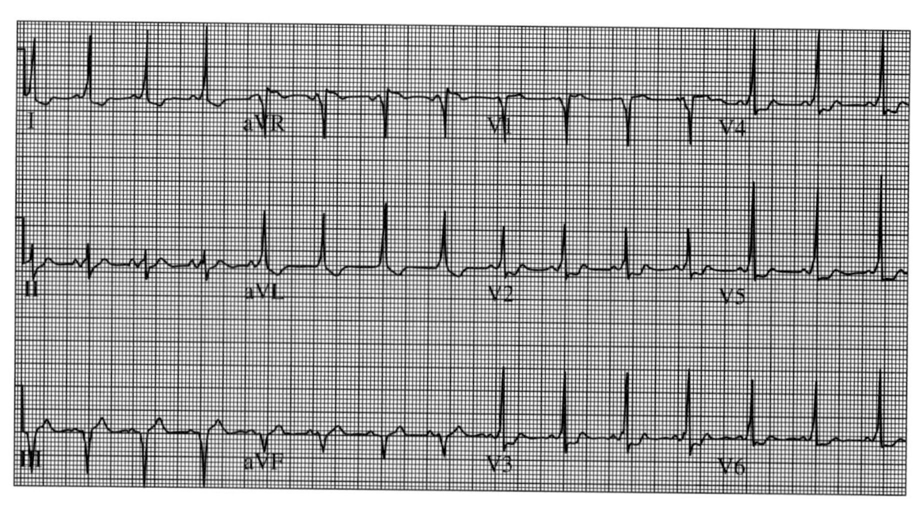

FIGURE 1.13. Delta wave on resting ECG.

- WPW with atrial flutter and accessory pathway conduction
  - Regular wide QRS complexes
  - 1:1 conduction possible
  - Rates may reach 300 bpm.
- WPW with atrial fibrillation and accessory pathway conduction (see Figure 1.14)
  - Irregular wide QRS complexes
  - No P waves
  - Rates often > 250 bpm

DIFFERENTIAL

Other accessory pathway syndromes include:

- **Lown-Ganong-Levine (LGL) syndrome**
- Accessory pathway = James fibers.
- Pathway connects the atria to the His bundle.
  - → Short PR and normal QRS on resting ECG
- **Mahaim bundles**
  - Connect AV node, His bundle, *or* bundle branches to the ventricle
    - → Normal PR with initial slurred QRS (delta wave) on resting ECG

TREATMENT

- Narrow complex tachycardia
  - Implies conduction through the AV node → can treat similar to AVNRT (above)
- Wide complex rhythm
  - Treatment of choice = synchronized electrical cardioversion (50–100J).
  - Implies AV conduction through the accessory pathway
  - **Avoid all AV blocking agents** (may precipitate ventricular fibrillation [VFib]).

*WPW with **narrow** complex tachycardia → treatment is similar to AVNRT (AV blocking drugs are OK).*

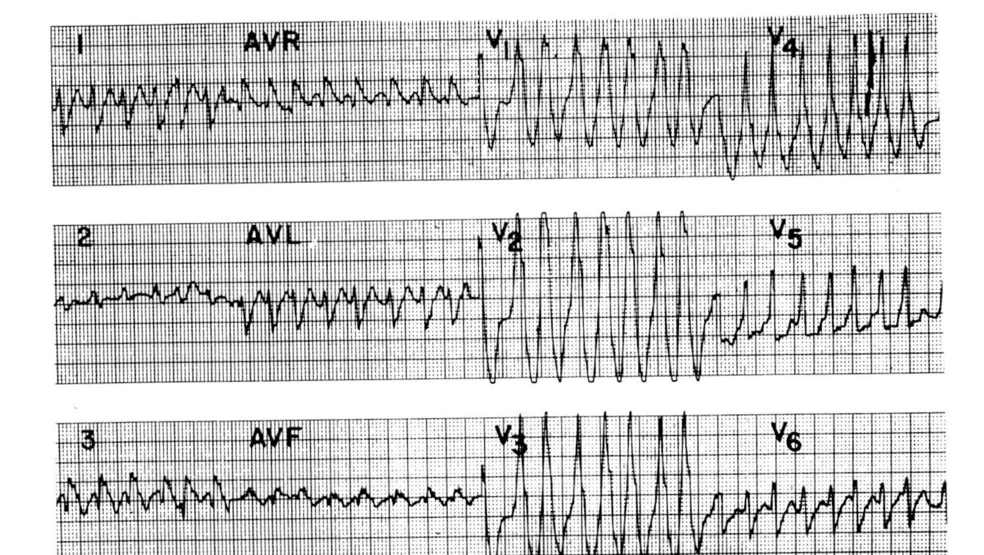

FIGURE 1.14. WPW with atrial fibrillation and accessory pathway conduction.

(Reproduced, with permission, from Tintinalli JE, Kelen GD, Stapczynski JS. *Emergency Medicine: A Comprehensive Study Guide*, 6th ed. New York: McGraw-Hill, 2004:200.)

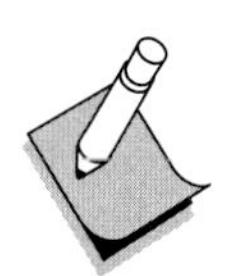

Therapeutic options for patients with WPW who present with rapid AFib are procainamide, amiodarone, or electrical cardioversion.

- Stable patient: Medical therapy with procainamide or amiodarone may be tried.
  - Blocks the accessory pathway
  - Increases transmission through the AV node
  - Hold for hypotension, 50% QRS widening

A 45-year-old male presents to the ED complaining of palpitations. He has a history of alcohol abuse and chronic pain, for which he takes a tricyclic antidepressant. He is awake and alert with a BP of 120/60 and an initial pulse of 80. The monitor shows intermittent runs of torsades de pointes. What is your initial treatment for this patient?

Torsades is a type of polymorphic VT that occurs in the setting of prolonged repolarization, which in this patient is likely due to hypokalemia, hypomagnesemia, and/or tricyclic antidepressant use. Since he is stable, begin treatment with a magnesium sulfate infusion. If this is unsuccessful, try shortening repolarization by increasing the ventricular rate via isoproterenol infusion or overdrive pacing.

VENTRICULAR TACHYCARDIA (VT)

Ventricular tachycardia is defined as >3 consecutive ectopic ventricular beats. It is grouped according to ECG pattern.

- **Monomorphic VT**
  - Ectopic beats are morphologically the same.
- **Polymorphic VT**
  - QRS complexes have many different shapes.
  - Sicker heart

Common variants of VT include:

- **Torsades de pointes (atypical VT)**
  - Type of polymorphic VT occurring in a patient with a long QT (> 600 msec)
  - QRS axis shifts from positive to negative in a single lead.
- **Bidirectional VT**
  - Unique form of VT where QRS axis changes periodically
  - Associated with digitalis toxicity
- **Brugada syndrome**
  - Hereditary syndrome characterized by structurally normal heart, abnormal resting ECG, and sudden cardiac death from polymorphic VT or VFib
  - Resting ECG is characterized by RBBB pattern and ST elevation in V_1-V_3 (see Figure 1.15).

CAUSES

Causes include

- Virtually any form of structural heart disease
- Trauma
- Hypothermia
- Severe electrolyte abnormalities
- Familial disorders (eg, Brugada syndrome, congenital long QT syndrome)
- Medications that prolong the QT interval

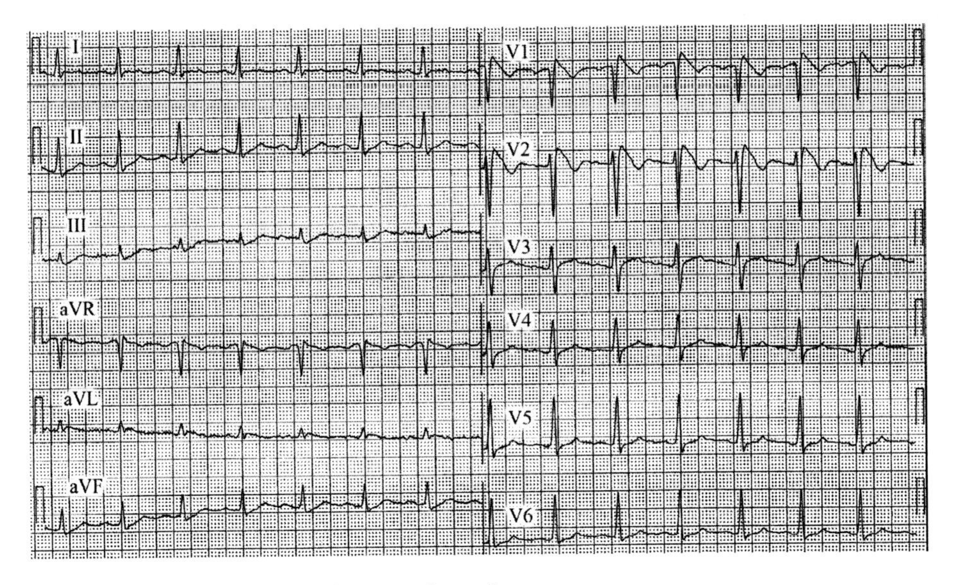

FIGURE 1.15 Typical ECG for Brugada syndrome.

(Reproduced, with permission, from Fuster V, Walsh RA, O'Rourke RA, Poole-Wilson P. *Hurst's The Heart*, Vol.2, 12th ed. New York: McGraw-Hill, 2008:1661.)

ECG Findings (See Figure 1.16)

- Regular wide complex tachycardia
- Inappropriately concordant QRS complexes across the precordial leads
- AV dissociation
- Fusion complexes

Differential

- VT must be differentiated from SVT with aberrant conduction.
- An approach using a combination of historical clues, general ECG characteristics, and the Brugada ECG criteria (see Table 1.8) will diagnose VT with reasonable accuracy.

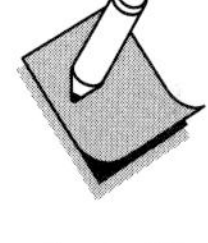

In the patient with prior MI, wide complex tachycardia is nearly always VT.

Treatment

- Pulseless → immediate cardioversion. See "Management of Cardiac Arrest."
- Unstable → cardioversion.
  - Synchronized
  - Start with 100J
  - Sedation, if possible

When in doubt, treat any wide complex tachycardia as ventricular tachycardia!

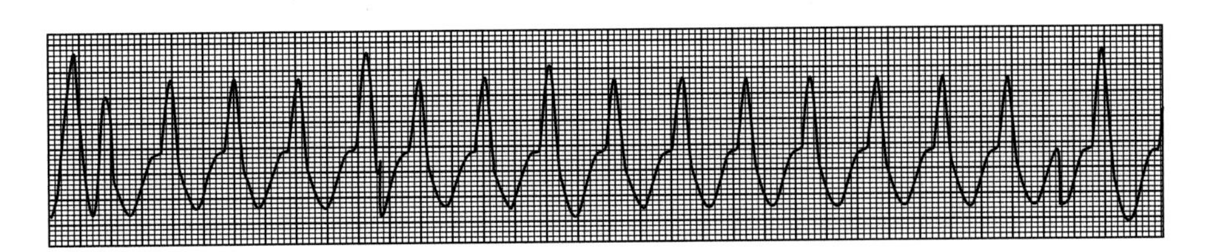

FIGURE 1.16. Ventricular tachycardia.

TABLE 1.8. Differentiating Ventricular Tachycardia (VT) From SVT With Aberrancy

Historical Clues That Suggest VT
Age > 35 years
History of heart disease
Prior history or family history of VT
General ECG Characteristics That Suggest VT
AV dissociation
Fusion beats
Concordance
Extreme left axis
QRS duration > 0.14 seconds
No response to vagal maneuvers
Brugada ECG Criteria That Suggest VT
Absence of RS complexes in all V leads
If RS complex present → RS duration > 0.1 sec
Presence of AV dissociation
Presence of VT QRS morphology

- Stable
  - Trial of amiodarone or lidocaine **OR** synchronized cardioversion
  - Refractory stable VT → synchronized cardioversion as above.

TORSADES DE POINTES

Torsades is a form of polymorphous VT in which the axis of the heart rotates, creating a sinusoidal appearance of the ventricular rhythm. Definition requires long QT (>600 msecs) seen on resting ECG or rhythm strip.

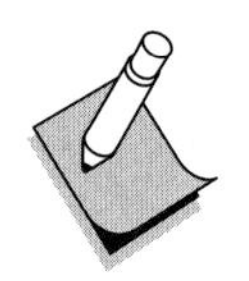

Torsades is due to prolongation of repolarization (QT interval).

CAUSES

- **Prolongation of the QT interval**
  - Medications (eg, class IC agents, TCAs)
  - Hypomagesemia
  - Hypokalemia

ECG FINDINGS (SEE FIGURE 1.17)

- Sinusoidal variation in amplitude and duration of wide QRS complexes
- AV dissociation

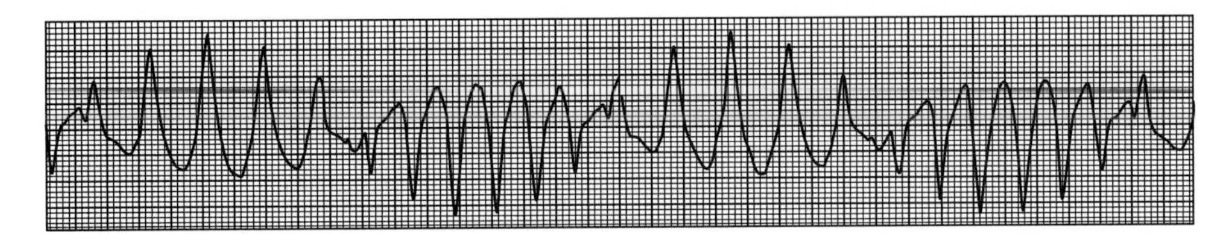

FIGURE 1.17. Torsades de pointes (atypical ventricular tachycardia).

Treatment

- Unstable → immediate cardioversion
  - Synchronized
  - Begin with 50–100J
- Magnesium infusion
- Increase the ventricular rate (to shorten repolarization).
  - Isoproterenol infusion **or**
  - Overdrive pacing (external or transvenous)
  - To ventricular rate of 100–120 bpm
- Amiodarone may be tried, if patient is stable.
- **Avoid**: Any drugs that can prolong repolarization (eg, procainamide).

Ventricular Fibrillation (VFib)

Ventricular fibrillation is totally disorganized ventricular depolarization. Causes are similar to VT (above).

ECG Findings (See Figure 1.18)

- Zig-zag pattern without P waves or QRS complexes

Treatment

- See "Management of Cardiac Arrest."

MANAGEMENT OF CARDIAC ARREST

The four causes of pulseless cardiac arrest include VFib, pulseless VT, pulseless electrical activity, and asystole.

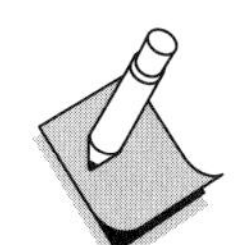

Pediatric cardiac arrest is most commonly due to progressive hypoxia or shock.

In comparison to the adult population, a primary cardiac cause (sudden cardiac death) of cardiac arrest is uncommon in the pediatric population. Pediatric arrest is most commonly **secondary** to progressive hypoxia or shock.

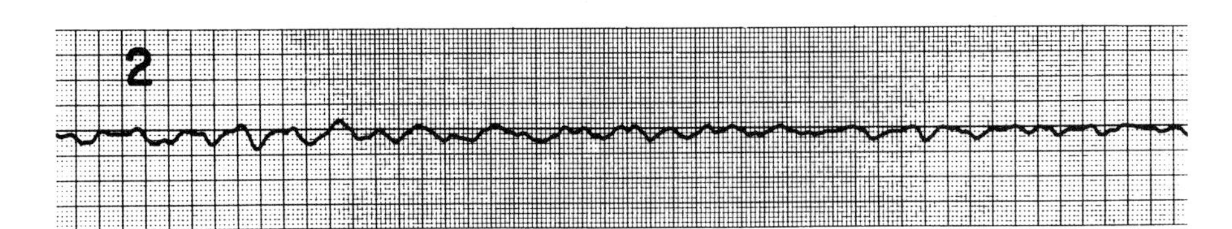

FIGURE 1.18. Ventricular fibrillation.

(Reproduced, with permission, from Tintinalli JE, Kelen GD, Stapczynski JS. *Emergency Medicine: A Comprehensive Study Guide*, 6th ed. New York: McGraw-Hill, 2004:191.)

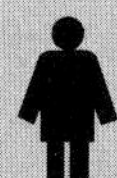

During resuscitation of a witnessed arrest, you ensured that CPR was minimally interrupted and proper technique was employed. However, the patient still suffered hypoxic cerebral and cardiac injury. Why?

Even properly performed closed chest CPR only provides 25% of pre-arrest cardiac output. Coronary and cerebral blood flow also fall, to 5% and 10%, respectively.

Basic Cardiopulmonary Resuscitation (CPR)

The basic tenet of CPR is to generate enough **coronary perfusion pressure (CPP)** to produce the myocardial blood flow necessary for return of spontaneous circulation.

$$\text{CPP} = \text{aortic diastolic pressure} - \text{R atrial diastolic pressure}$$

Initial step for health care providers:

- For sudden, collapse (all ages) → phone or call for defibrillator prior to initiating CPR.
- For arrest likely due to asphyxia → immediate CPR prior to calling for help.

The technique for adult and pediatric CPR in the ED assumes that multiple providers are present (see Table 1.9).

TABLE 1.9. Basic CPR in the Emergency Department

	PEDIATRIC	ADULT
Ventilation		
Rate (breaths/min)	Bag-valve mask (BVM): 20 ET tube: 12–20	BVM: 10–12 ET tube: 8–10
Compression		
Position	Lower half of sternum Infant: 2 thumb-encircling hands Child: Heel of hand or as for adults	Lower half of sternum Heel of one hand, other hand on top
Depth	1/3–1/2 depth of chest	$1^1/_2$–2 inches
Rate	100/min	100/min
Ratio to ventilation	BVM: 15:2 (pause for 2 breaths every 15 compressions) ET tube: No pauses for ventilation	BVM: 30:2 ET tube: No pauses for ventilation
Defibrillation	Use pediatric pads when possible. No recommendations for infants	Use adult pads.

Airway and breathing:

All basic CPR begins with opening the airway with a head tilt and chin lift (jaw thrust alone if suspected trauma) and administration of two rescue breaths.

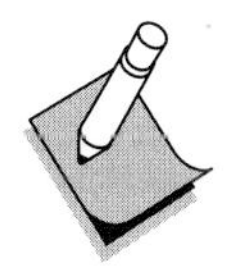

Factors that worsen CPP:

Interrupting chest compressions

Overventilation

Improper CPR technique

Chest compressions:

Chest compressions may either push the blood out by direct compression of the heart (*cardiac pump theory*) or produce blood flow via a pressure gradient between the thorax and body (*thoracic pump theory*).

Factors that can worsen CPP:

- Not allowing full recoil of chest ("push hard, push fast")
  - Limits the "thoracic pump"
- Interruptions in chest compression
  - Even brief interruption cause significant declines in CPP.
- Overventilation
  - Decreases venous return and perfusion pressures

You are called to assess a newborn who just delivered on your ambulance bay. He has been placed under a warmer and is being dried. On rapid examination he has spontaneous respirations, poor tone, and an HR of 90 bpm. There was no meconium present on delivery. What is your first step in the management of this neonate?

This neonate needs further resuscitation as his HR is < 100. The focus should initially be on airway and breathing, beginning with (if no meconium is present) positive pressure ventilation with 100% O_2 via BVM at a rate of 40–60 breaths/min. If the HR is not improved after 15–30 seconds, intubate, and provide further positive pressure ventilation. A persistent low HR after this is indication for chest compressions followed by cardiac drugs, glucose, and narcan if indicated.

Neonatal Resuscitation

Newborn resuscitation is unique compared to adult and pediatric resuscitation in that the initial approach focuses almost entirely on management of the airway and breathing. A primary cardiac etiology is uncommon.

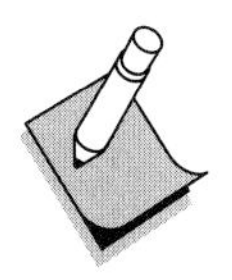

Indications for neonatal resuscitation:

Apnea

HR < 100

Immediately after delivery the infant airway should be suctioned with a bulb syringe (mouth, then nares); placed under warmer, dried, and positioned to open airway (head tilt); stimulated; and assessed for respiratory effort and HR.

Indications for further neonatal resuscitation:

- Apnea
- HR < 100 bpm

TREATMENT

- Airway
  - **If meconium present** → immediate **intubation and endotracheal** suctioning.
  - Otherwise, provide **positive pressure ventilation** via BVM (100% O_2) at 40–60 breaths/min.

- **Reassess breathing and heart rate (HR)** after 15–30 seconds.
- If apnea or HR < 100 bpm (by umbilical pulse or auscultation of precordium) → **intubate** and ventilate.
- **Reassess HR** after 15–30 seconds.
- If HR < 60 bpm → begin **chest compressions**.
  - Thumbs just below nipple line with hands encircling the chest
  - Depth = 1/3–1/2 depth of chest
    - Rate = 120/min
  - Compression: ventilation ratio 3:1 (with pauses for ventilation)
- **Reassess HR** after 15–30 seconds.
- If HR < 60 bpm → begin **drug therapy**.
  - Epinephrine
  - Narcan (as indicated)
  - Glucose
  - Normal saline (NS) bolus

Drug therapy in neonatal resuscitation:
Epinephrine
Narcan (as indicated)
Glucose
NS fluid bolus

Pulseless Ventricular Tachycardia and Ventricular Fibrillation

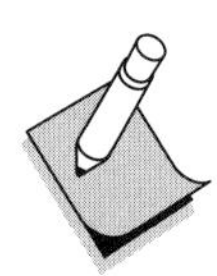

A shorter time from onset of VFib to defibrillation = single best determinant of successful outcome in cardiac arrest.

TREATMENT

- The goal of treatment is to rapidly provide defibrillation while minimizing interruptions in CPR.
- Provide O_2 via BVM when available, but do not delay CPR.
- **Immediate CPR AND rapid defibrillation.**
  - Critical interventions in first minute.
  - 360J monophasic (120–200J biphasic) asynchronous.
  - Administer *one shock only* at this time.
- **Immediately resume CPR** after defibrillation (don't pause to check rhythm).
- After **2 minutes of CPR → check rhythm.**
- Defibrillate again, if needed.
- Administer epinephrine. Repeat every 3–5 minutes for three doses **or** a single dose of vasopressin may be substituted for the first or second epinephrine.
- After **2 minutes of CPR → check rhythm.**
- Defibrillate again, if needed.
- Administer lidocaine or amiodarone as antidysrhythmic therapy.
  - Evaluate for shockable rhythm. If present, administer shock.
- If any of the above is successful, check pulse and → postresuscitation therapy.
- Change of rhythm to pulseless electrical activity or asystole should initiate those algorithms (see below).

Pulseless Electrical Activity (PEA)

PEA patients may be differentiated into two groups:

- Those with electrical activity and echocardiographic evidence of cardiac motion
- Those with electrical activity in the absence of any cardiac motion
  - Patients in this group have a worse outcome than those with cardiac motion.

PEA often results from reversible causes. These must be aggressively pursued and managed if present:

- Hypovolemia
- Hypothermia
- Hypoxia
- Hypoglycemia
- Acidosis
- Electrolyte disturbances
- Cardiac tamponade
- Overdoses
- Tension pneumothorax
- Massive PE
- MI

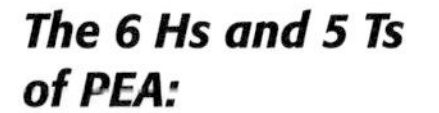

The 6 Hs and 5 Ts of PEA:

Hypoxia
Hydrogen ion overload (acidosis)
Hyperkalemia/hypokalemia
Hypoglycemia
Hypothermia
Hypovolemia
Toxins
Tamponade (cardiac)
Tension pneumothorax
Thromboembolism (PE)
Thrombosis (coronary)

ECG Findings

- Will vary with underlying cause and duration of systemic abnormality
  - Hyperkalemia → sinusoidal rhythm.
  - Hypovolemia or tamponade → marked sinus tachycardia.
  - Severe acidosis or hypoxia → bradyasystolic rhythm.
  - ACS → idioventricular rhythm.

Treatment

- Administer immediate CPR and **limit interruptions in CPR.**
- Provide O_2 via BVM, when available, but do not delay CPR.
- Treat reversible causes, as for PEA (see page 40).
- Epinephrine IV/IO repeated 3–5 minutes **or**
  a single dose of vasopressin IV/IO may be substituted for the first or second epinephrine.
- Consider atropine 1 mg IV/IO if rate is slow.
- Repeat every 3–5 minutes for three doses.
- Intermittently assess for return of pulse or presence of shockable rhythm.

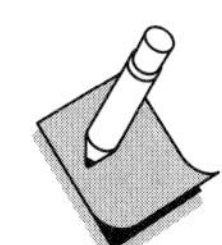

A single dose of vasopressin may be substituted for the first or second dose of epinephrine.

Asystole

Asystole is generally considered a preterminal rhythm. Survival from asystole is extremely poor.

Treatment

- Consider similar reversible causes as for PEA (see page 40).
- Treatment is as for PEA.

Cardiac Arrest Medications (See Table 1.10)

Route of administration:

- The **most rapidly available route** should be used.
- Central venous access?
  - Provides the fastest drug delivery to the central circulation, but
  - **Not** preferred because of required delay in CPR and/or defibrillation during line placement
  - Use if no other access available.
- Peripherally administered drugs should be followed by 20 mL flush and elevation of extremity.
- Endotracheal administration

TABLE 1.10. Medications for Cardiac Arrest

DRUG	DOSE (IV/IO)	MECHANISM
Epinephrine	Adult: 1 mg Pediatric: 0.01 mg/kg	α,β-Adrenergic receptor agonist → ↑ coronary and cerebral perfusion pressures.
Vasopressin	Adult: 40 U	Nonadrenergic peripheral vasoconstrictor
Atropine	Adult: 1 mg Pediatric: 0.02 mg/kg (minimum 0.1mg, maximum 0.5–1mg)	Parasympatholytic
Amiodarone	Adult: 300 mg, repeat at 150 mg. Pediatric: 5 mg/kg, repeat up to 15 mg/kg (maximum 300 mg).	Class III antidysrhythmic (blocks K^+ channels)
Lidocaine	Adult: 1–1.5 mg/kg, repeat at 0.5–0.75 mg/kg every 5–10 minutes PRN (maximum 4 mg/kg). Pediatric: 1 mg/kg every 5–10 minutes PRN (maximum 100 mg).	Class Ib antidysrhythmic (blocks fast Na^+ channels)
Magnesium	Adult: 1–2 g Pediatric: 25–50 mg/kg (maximum 2 g)	↑ Mg levels → improved QT intervals.

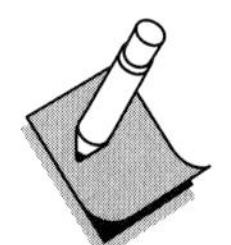

*Central venous access provides the fastest drug delivery to the central circulation, but is **not** preferred because of required delays in CPR to obtain access.*

- May be used for lidocaine, epinephrine, atropine, and naloxone (LEAN)
- Achieves lower serum drug levels compared to IV routes
- Use 2–2.5 times the IV dose (10 × the IV dose in pediatrics), dilute in 10 mL NS, administer directly in ET tube and follow with 5 breaths.

EPINEPHRINE

First-line medication for cardiac arrest.

MECHANISM OF ACTION

- α- and β-adrenergic receptor stimulation → increased coronary and cerebral perfusion pressures during CPR.
- Negative effects: Increased myocardial work and myocardial oxygen consumption

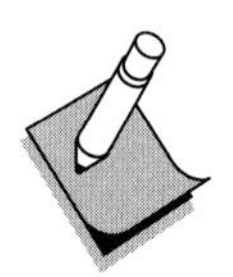

Epinephrine has been shown to increase coronary and cerebral perfusion pressures during CPR.

DOSE

- Adult: 1 mg IV/IO every 3–5 minutes
  - ET tube dose: 2–2.5 mg
- Pediatric: 0.01 mg/kg IV/IO (maximum dose: 1 mg) every 3–5 minutes
  - ET tube dose: 0.1 mg/kg
- Higher doses have **not** been shown to improve survival.

VASOPRESSIN

Has not shown any survival benefit over epinephrine

MECHANISM OF ACTION

- Nonadrenergic peripheral vasoconstrictor
- Coronary and renal vasoconstriction

Vasopressin is a nonadrenergic peripheral vasoconstrictor.

DOSE

- Adult: 40 U IV/IO to replace either the first or second dose of epinephrine
- Following the administration of vasopression, continue to give epinephrine every 3–5 min as indicated.
- Pediatrics: Not recommended

ATROPINE

Second-line for the treatment of slow-arrest rhythms (PEA and asystole)

MECHANISM OF ACTION

- Competitive antagonism of muscarinic acetylcholine receptors (parasympatholytic) → ↑ HR, ↑ SVR, ↑ BP

DOSE

- Adults: 1 mg IV, repeated every 3–5 minute to maximum of 3 mg as needed
- Pediatrics: 0.02 mg/kg IV/IO (minimum: 0.1 mg, maximum: 0.5–1 mg)

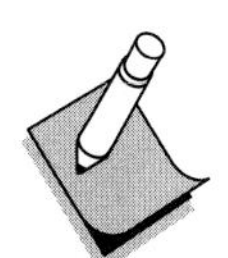

Doses of atropine below the minimum recommended may produce paradoxical bradycardia in children!

COMPLICATIONS

- Small doses (< 0.1 mg) may produce paradoxical bradycardia in pediatric patients.

AMIODARONE

Amiodarone is used in the treatment of VT and VFib. It has many other nonarrest indications for the treatment of tachydysrhythmias.

MECHANISM OF ACTION

- A class III antidysrhythmic
- K^+ channel blockade → prolongation of repolarization (phase 3).
- Has multiple other effects (sodium/calcium channel effects, β-blockade)

DOSE

- Adult: 300 mg IV/IO, followed by 150 mg IV/IO in 3–5 minutes for unstable tachydysrhythmias; 150 mg for stable tachydysrhythmias, repeated every 10 minutes as needed
- Pediatric: 5 mg/kg IV/IO, repeat up to 15 mg/kg to maximum of 300 mg

COMPLICATIONS

- Hypotension, bradycardia, prolonged QT interval

> ***Resuscitation drugs that may be administered via ET tube—***
>
> ***LEAN***
>
> **L**idocaine
> **E**pinephrine
> **A**tropine
> **N**aloxone

LIDOCAINE

Used in the treatment of VT and VFib as an alternative to amiodarone

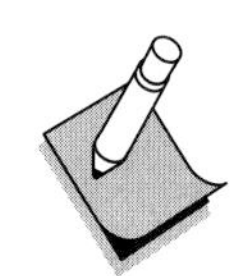

Excessive administration of lidocaine may produce neurological symptoms and seizures.

MECHANISM OF ACTION

- Class Ib antidysrhythmic
- Blocks fast sodium channels → stabilization of membranes

DOSE

- Adult: 1–1.5 mg/kg IV/IO, may be repeated at 0.5–0.75 mg/kg every 5–10 minutes if needed to max of 3 mg/kg
- Pediatric: 1 mg/kg IV/IO to maximum dose of 100 mg

COMPLICATIONS

- Hypotension, bradycardia with block, *seizures*

MAGNESIUM

Used in the treatment of VT or VFib associated with torsades de pointes and prolonged QT

Magnesium treats:
Torsades de pointes
Preeclampsia
Severe asthma

MECHANISM OF ACTION

- Improves serum magnesium levels → improved QT intervals

DOSE

- Adult: 1–2 g diluted in 10 mL D_5W IV/IO
- Pediatric: 25–50 mg/kg IV/IO (maximum: 2 g)

COMPLICATIONS

- Hypermagnesemia can cause decreased reflexes and at high levels decreased respiratory drive, heart block, and asystole.

FIBRINOLYSIS

Administration of tissue plasminogen activator (tPA) may be considered in patients with PEA due to suspected acute PE or MI. It is not indicated in undifferentiated PEA.

DOSE

- Adults: 100 mg IV over 15 minutes

MECHANISM OF ACTION

- Converts plasminogen → plasmin thereby activating fibrinolysis

GLUCOSE

May be a critical intervention in the pediatric population

DOSE

- 0.5–1 g/kg IV/IO (**2–4 mL/kg $D_{25}W$** in pediatrics, $D_{10}W$ in neonates)

INTERVENTIONS THAT ARE NOT HELPFUL

Cardiac pacing is not recommended in the treatment of asystole.

The following interventions have not been shown to be helpful and are therefore **not** recommended in the treatment of cardiac arrest:

- Norepinephrine
- Procainamide
- Cardiac pacing in the treatment of asystole

PERMANENT PACEMAKERS

Generally agreed upon indications (class I) for **permanent** pacemaker placement include:

- High-grade AV block (third-degree and second-degree type II) with
  - Asystole > 3 seconds
  - Escape rate < 40 bpm
  - Following ablation or heart surgery
  - Neuromuscular disease
- Any symptomatic second- or third-degree AV block
- Second-degree AV block with wide QRS (indicating BBB)
- Symptomatic sinus node dysfunction or chronotropic incompetence

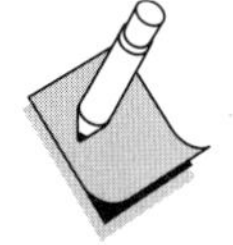

VVI pacemaker = ventricular paced, ventricular sensed, inhibited (response to sensing).

Individual pacer function is determined by a 3–5 letter code, employed by the North American Society of Pacing and Eletrophysiology (see Table 1.11).

TABLE 1.11. Interpretation of Pacemaker Codes

1st letter	2nd letter	3rd letter	4th letter	5th letter
CHAMBER PACED	**CHAMBER SENSED**	**RESPONSE TO SENSING**	**PROGRAMMABLE FUNCTIONS**	**ANTITACHYCARDIA FEATURES**
V = ventricle	**V** = ventricle	**T** = triggered	**P** = programmable rate, output, or both	**P** = antitachycardia pacing
A = atrium	**A** = atrium	**I** = inhibited	**M** = multiprogrammability of rate, output, sensitivity, etc.	**S** = shock
D = dual	**D** = dual	**D** = dual	**C** = communication function (telemetry)	**D** = dual
O = none	**O** = none	**O** = none	**R** = rate modulation	**O** = none
			O = none	

Pacemaker Malfunction

Causes

- **Failure to pace**
  - Failure of pacemaker to output signal
    - Wire fracture/displacement
    - Battery depletion
  - Failure of myocardium to capture signal
    - Wire fracture/displacement
    - Elevated myocardial threshold from fibrosis, metabolic derangement, ischemia, hypoxia
- **Undersensing**
  - Failure of pacemaker to sense native impulses → paced beats in addition to native beats.
  - Causes similar to "failure to pace"
- **Oversensing**
  - Unexpected pacemaker sensing of extracardiac "false" impulses with pacer in inhibit ("I") mode → no paced beat.
  - False impulses may include pectoralis muscle contraction, electrocautery, digital cell phones.
- Inappropriate pacemaker rate ("runaway pacemaker")
  - Rare
  - Dual chamber pacemaker in synchronous AV pacing mode
  - PVC → retrograde atrial depolarization → sensed by atrial lead → paced ventricular impulse → retrograde atrial depolarization, etc.

Symptoms/Exam

- With exception of runaway pacemaker, symptoms are similar to those that prompted pacemaker placement.
- Syncope or near syncope
- Dyspnea
- Palpitations

Diagnosis

- Evaluation of rhythm strip or ECG (see Table 1.12)
- CXR for wire fracture/displacement
  - Usually close to generator or within the heart
- Pacemaker function/battery assessment via cardiologist

TABLE 1.12. ECG Findings in Pacemaker Malfunction

ECG Finding	Pacemaker Malfunction
Absence of pacer spikes when indicated	Failure to output signal
Pacer spikes, but no depolarization	Failure to capture signal
Pacer spikes despite native beats	Undersensing native beats
External motion or interference pattern with absence of pacer spikes	Oversensing

TREATMENT

- Depends on underlying malfunction
- Often requires reprogramming of functions by cardiologist
- Magnet placement
  - Converts pacer to fixed rate
  - Turns off "inhibit" function
- For runaway pacemaker
  - Terminate with a magnet
  - Definitive therapy requires reprogramming the atrial refractory period.

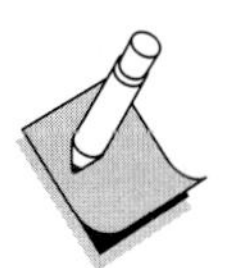

Placing a magnet over the pacemaker generator converts the pacemaker to a fixed-rate pacing mode and turns off the "inhibit" function.

Pacemaker Syndrome

Most commonly seen with VVI pacemakers as a result of atrial contractions against a closed AV valve

PATHOPHYSIOLOGY

- Atrial contractions against closed AV valve →
  - ↑ Atrial pressures → pulmonary and hepatic congestion
  - ↓ Ventricular filling (lack of "atrial kick") → decreased cardiac output (by 20–50%)

SYMPTOMS/EXAM

- Varied and vague
- Light-headedness, syncope, or near-syncope
- Sense of pulsations in neck or abdomen
- Fatigue
- Heart failure
- Chest pain
- Palpitations
- Neck and/or abdominal pulsations

Pacemaker syndrome occurs due to loss of AV synchrony, most commonly with VVI pacemakers.

DIAGNOSIS/TREATMENT

- Diagnosis is primarily clinical.
- Interrogate pacer to rule out malfunction and reprogram setting.

COMPLICATIONS

- Increased risk of atrial fibrillation, thromboembolic events, and heart failure.

> A 58-year-old male presents to the ED complaining of recurrent ICD firing. On the monitor, you see a narrow complex tachycardia at a rate of 150 bpm, which is temporarily converted to sinus rhythm with ICD firing. The patient is hemodynamically stable during the tachydysrhythmia, but has considerable discomfort with each firing. How do you prevent the inappropriate ICD firing in this patient?
>
> Preventing the underlying tachydysrhythmia and/or ICD reprogramming is the definitive treatment, but placing a ring magnet over the generator site will temporarily inactivate the ICD.

IMPLANTED CARDIAC DEFIBRILLATORS (ICD)

ICDs are placed in patients at high risk for sudden cardiac death from VT and VFib. They are programmed to analyze the cardiac rhythm, perform anti-tachycardia pacing, generate an electrical charge, and deliver an electrical shock. All new generation ICDs have ventricular pacing abilities.

Evaluation of a Delivered Shock

Patient-reported shocks may be appropriate (underlying VT or VFib), inappropriate, or phantom (patients think they got shocked but didn't). Only interrogation of the device or monitoring during an event can differentiate appropriate from inappropriate shocks.

Appropriate shocks may result from associated:

- Electrolyte abnormalities
- Myocardial ischemia
- Medications (proarrythmic drugs or med noncomplicance)

Inappropriate shocks may be a result of:

- Nonsustained VT
- SVT inappropriately sensed as VT
- Oversensing T waves as QRS complexes
- External interference sensed as impulses
- Broken/displaced ventricular lead

Diagnosis

- Interrogation of the device
- External cardiac monitoring during ICD event
- ECG and labs to evaluate for ischemia or electrolyte abnormalities
- CXR to evaluate leads
- All patients with repetitive shock warrant diagnostic evaluation.
- Stable patient with isolated shock may warrant less extensive evaluation.

Treatment

- Identify and treat contributing conditions.
- Inappropriate shocks may be prevented with magnet deactivation of the ICD.
  - Second-generation ICDs
    - Deactivate by placing ring magnet over generator for 30 seconds.
    - Reactivate by placing magnet over generator for another 30 seconds.
  - Third-generation ICDs
    - Presence of magnet deactivates ICD (removal reactivates it).
- Reprogramming, as indicated, by cardiologist

Implanated Cardiac Defibrillator Failure

Causes

May be due to the following:

- **Component failure**
  - Lead fracture/displacement
  - Battery depletion
  - Interference with pacemakers

- **Inadvertent inactivation**
  - Any strong magnetic force can cause temporary or permanent (depending on device) failure.
- **Resistant VT or VFib**
  - Device functioning, but rhythm resistant to internal defibrillation

SYMPTOMS/EXAM

- May range from asymptomatic (found on device checkup) to cardiac arrest

TREATMENT

- Definitive is reprogramming or replacement of device.
- No risk from ICD for CPR providers
- If external defibrillation is needed for VT/VFib
  - Use standard paddles, but place them ≥10 cm away from generator.

> A 17-month-old boy is brought in by his parents after 3 days of nonbloody diarrhea. The child has had 6–8 soiled diapers a day, although in the 4 hours prior to presentation the diaper has not required changing. On presentation the child is noted to be clinging to his mother but not crying. His mucous membranes are noted to be dry, and his eyes appear sunken. His HR is 120 and his SBP is 80 mmHg. What is the initial indicator of moderate volume loss in the pediatric patient? What is the most appropriate first treatment?
>
> This child has lost a moderate volume of fluid. Because infants and young children are fairly HR dependent for their cardiac output, tachycardia is the initial indicator of moderate volume loss. The initial treatment should be a normal saline bolus at 10–20 mL/kg.

VOLUME ASSESSMENT

Neonates

Newborns have very poor cardiac reserve and as a result progress rapidly to circulatory collapse in the setting of even moderate volume loss. Volume loss is associated with the following symptoms:

SYMPTOMS/EXAM

- **Tachycardia:** Any increase of HR above the normal range of 120–160 bpm
- **Respiratory distress:** Nasal flaring or grunting. This is a sign of increasing stress and may be seen when volume loss is >5%.
- **Lethargy:** Seen in moderate to severe volume loss (10–15%)
- **BP drop:** Is the final sign of severe volume loss (> 15%) in a neonate and is often precipitous.
- When volume loss has occurred over a period of days
  - Changes in skin turgor are manifested by "doughiness" of the skin.
  - Decreased frequency of wet diapers
  - Sunken eyes and fontanelle
  - Dry mucous membranes and lack of tears

Neonates may present with respiratory distress as a sign of volume loss.

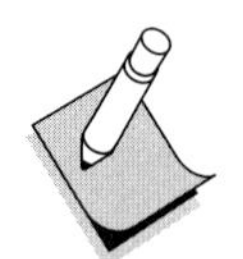

Pediatric hypotension = systolic blood pressure <70 mmHg + (2 × age in years).

Pediatrics

Volume assessment in children is made difficult by the normal variation of vital signs seen with increasing age. Thus, some knowledge of normal vital signs is important (see Table 1.13).

After the neonatal stage, cardiac reserve becomes substantially better. As a result, even significant volume loss may be well compensated for by increasing HRs. However, after a point, this compensation will fail, and blood pressure and HR will both fall precipitously.

SYMPTOMS/EXAM

- **Mild volume loss** (1–5%)
  - Increased thirst
  - Normal examination
- **Moderate volume loss** (5–10%)
  - Tachycardia
  - Irritability
  - Delayed capillary refill
  - Sunken eyes and fontanelle
  - Dry mucous membranes and decreased tears
- **Severe volume loss** (>15%)
  - Marked tachycardia, weak pulse, hypotension
  - Lethargy and somnolence
  - Very delayed capillary refill, cold and mottled.
  - Parched mucous membranes and no tears
  - Very sunken eyes and fontanelle

ADULT

Adults have more or less the same cardiac reserve as older children. However, adults have less vascular tone. As a result, BP changes with far less volume loss are seen in this group of patients. Volume loss can be estimated more precisely in adults than in children since physical findings are more predictable with increasing amounts of loss. The American College of Surgeons Advanced Trauma Life Support course suggests a means of correlating blood loss in trauma with patient appearance and vital signs (see Table 1.14). It is likely that signs and symptoms are similar regardless of the actual mechanism of volume loss.

SYMPTOMS/EXAM

- Tachycardia
- Tachypnea

TABLE 1.13. Normal Vital Signs for Pediatric Patients

AGE	HR (BPM)	RR (BREATHS/MIN)	SYSTOLIC BP (MMHG)
Neonates, 0–28 days	120–160	30–50	> 60
Infants, 1–12 months	100–120	20–30	70–95
Children, 1–8 years	80–100	20–30	80–110

TABLE 1.14. Guidelines for Correlating Volume Loss With Patient Appearance

Hemorrhage Class	Estimated Volume Loss	Signs/Symptoms
I	<15% (750 mL)	No change in VS or patient demeanor
II	15–30% (750–1500 mL)	↑ HR ↑ RR ↓ Pulse pressure Cool, clammy skin Anxiety, agitation
III	30–40% (1500–2000 mL)	Further ↑ in HR and RR ↓ BP Impaired peripheral circulation Confusion, agitation
IV	>40% (>2000 mL)	Marked ↑ in HR and RR Circulatory collapse Confusion, lethargy

- Narrow pulse pressure
- Cool and clammy skin, diminished turgor (late and not as commonly seen as in children)
- Mental status changes: Anxiety, agitation, confusion, lethargy
- Hypotension (late)
- Dry mucous membranes
- Decreased urine output

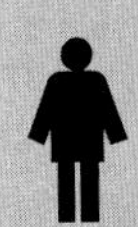

A 45-year-old male is brought to the ED by ambulance after a 2-day history of abdominal pain and bloody diarrhea. Upon presentation he is lethargic and has a HR of 140 bpm and a BP of 90/60. What is the best indicator for shock in this patient?

Diminished end organ perfusion is the single best indicator of shock. Clinical markers include mental status changes, decreased urine output, and increased base deficit or lactate production.

SHOCK

Shock occurs when there is inadequate tissue oxygenation to meet demand. Shock may be thought of as belonging to one of four categories: **hypovolemic, cardiogenic, obstructive, or distributive**. Some emergency physicians like to add a fifth category, dissociative shock, in which the ability to use O_2 is impaired (carbon monoxide or cyanide poisoning).

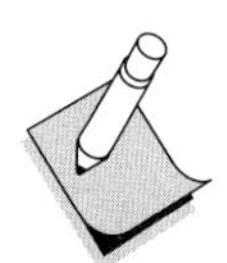

A "normal" blood pressure does not exclude the diagnosis of shock.

Symptoms/Exam

- Vary somewhat with underlying etiology (eg, fever with sepsis, elevated JVP with cardiogenic shock)
- Ill appearance, mottling of skin, pallor
- Abnormal VS: Classically, hypotension, HR > 100, and RR > 22
- Changes in mental status
- Decreased urine output: < 0.5–1 mL/kg/hr

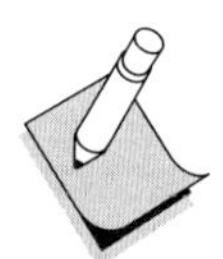

Laboratory evidence for inadequate tissue oxygenation:
Base deficit more negative than –5mEq/L.
Serum lactate > 4 mmol/L.
Multiorgan dysfunction.

Diagnosis

- Based on presence of inadequate tissue oxygenation
- Suspected based on clinical findings (above) and confirmed by laboratory studies
- **Base deficit**
  - The amount of strong base needed to normalize pH of 1 L of blood
  - Indirectly calculated from arterial pH and
  - Abnormal if more negative than –5mEq/L
- **Lactic acidosis:** Serum lactate > 4 mmol/L
- **Multiorgan dysfunction**
  - Elevated renal or hepatic function tests
  - Respiratory failure
- Stress hormone release →
  - **Mild hyperglycemia**
  - **Mild hypokalemia**

Treatment

- Ensure adequate ventilation and oxygenation.
- Improve work of breathing.
  - Intubation or noninvasive ventilation as needed
- Maximize intravascular volume: Fluids, blood, pressors
- Treat underlying cause.

Hypovolemic Shock

Hypovolemic shock occurs when one of either intravascular or total body volume is depleted. The former is seen with acute hemorrhage (**hemorrhagic shock**) while the latter is seen in cases where there is an imbalance between intake and output (**nonhemorrhagic hypovolemic shock**).

Hemorrhagic Shock

Causes

Causes include:

- External bleeding, usually due to trauma
- Internal bleeding including AAA, GI sources, blunt trauma, fractures, arterial or venous injury, ectopic pregnancy

In acute hemorrhagic shock, the initial hemoglobin may be deceptively normal.

Diagnosis

- Diagnosis is mostly clinical.
- Labs may be normal at presentation.
- With time and volume resuscitation hemoglobin and hematocrit will fall.

Treatment

- Ensure adequate oxygenation and ventilation.
- **Volume resuscitation**
  - **NS or Ringer's lactate** boluses through large peripheral intravenous lines, central lines, or intraosseous lines.
    - 1–2 L in adults
    - 10–20 cc/kg in neonates, infants, and young children
  - **Blood products** if no response to two fluid boluses, ongoing hemorrhage, or if impending cardiovascular collapse
    - When time is critical, the use of O-negative blood is standard (O-positive in men is also acceptable).
    - Two units PRBC in adults
    - 10–15 mL/kg PRBC in neonates, infants, and young children
- **Hemorrhage control**
  - Control source of bleeding.
  - Fix hereditary or acquired bleeding diatheses:
    - Platelets when platelet count is <50,000/μL
    - Fresh frozen plasma (FFP), prothrombin complex concentrate, or recombinant factor VIIa for patients on warfarin with an elevated INR
    - FFP and/or cryoprecipitate and specific factors for hemophiliacs

Indications for PRBC tranfusion in hemorrhagic shock:

No response to two fluid boluses

Ongoing hemorrhage

Impending CV collapse

Nonhemorrhagic Hypovolemic Shock

Nonhemorrhagic hypovolemic shock arises when volume intake is insufficient to make up for volume losses. Laboratory analyses are almost always abnormal in these cases since they generally occur over a period of time.

Causes

Causes include:

- Inadequate intake
- Excessive output: Respiratory, renal diuresis, GI losses, skin losses
- Metabolic derangement (inborn error of metabolism)

Diagnosis

- Hematocrit and hemoglobin levels are high due to hemoconcentration.
- BUN rises in relation to creatinine secondary to decreased tubular flow.
- Sodium is usually elevated secondary to free water loss.
  - In DKA and hyperosmolar states, sodium may be factitiously low.

Treatment

- Ensure adequate ventilation and oxygenation.
- **Immediate isotonic intravascular volume resuscitation**
  - NS or Ringer's lactate boluses
    - 1–2 L in adults
    - 20 cc/kg over 5–20 minutes in neonates and pediatrics
- **Restore total body water and sodium.**
  - Adults: 0.45 NS with or without 5% dextrose at a rate of 100–200 cc/hr
  - **Pediatrics**
    - **Deficit fluids:** Percent fluid loss x weight (kg) = L deficit. (ie, 10% loss in 20 kg child = 2 L fluid deficit). Replace one-half the deficit over first 8 hours and remainder over next 16 hours.

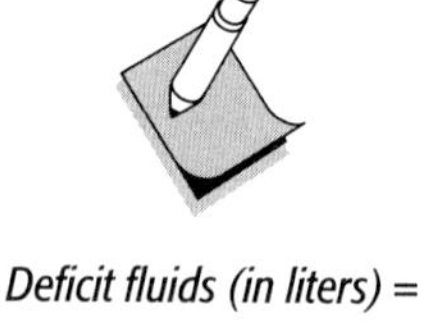

Deficit fluids (in liters) = % fluid loss × weight in kg.

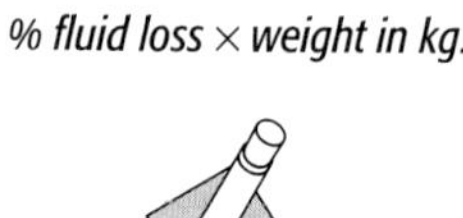

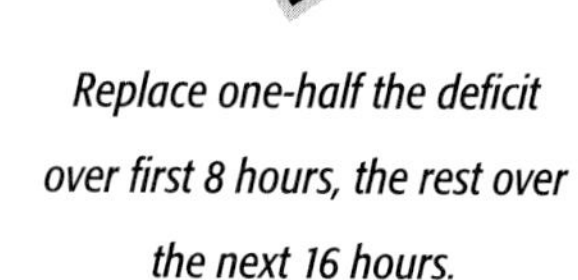

Replace one-half the deficit over first 8 hours, the rest over the next 16 hours.

TABLE 1.15. Calculating Maintenance Fluids

PATIENT WEIGHT	DAILY MAINTENANCE FLUIDS
For the first 0–10 kg	100 mL/kg/day
For the next 10–20 kg	50 mL/kg/day
From 20–70 kg	20 mL/kg/day
Add up total mL and divide by 24 to obtain hourly rate.	

 - **Maintenance fluids**: Calculate maintenance fluids (see Table 1.15) and add to deficit replacement.
 - **Solution:** Use D5.25 NS (D5$^1/_4$ NS) for infants and D5.45 NS (D5$^1/_2$ NS) in children.
- Treatment of the underlying cause should be simultaneous.

A 22-year-old previously healthy male presents to the ED complaining of flulike symptoms and progressive shortness of breath. On examination he appears ill with BP 80/50, HR 120, RR 30 and T 38.0°C. He has evidence of poor perfusion, bilateral rales, and jugular venous distention. Bedside cardiac ultrasound shows diffuse hypokinesis. What is the best initial management of this patient?

This patient is in cardiogenic shock from acute myocarditis. The goal of treatment is to improve myocardial contractility and pump function. Ensuring adequate ventilation and oxygenation is the first step in management, followed by the initiation of dopamine or dobutamine (if SBP > 90 mmHg) to improve pump function.

Cardiogenic Shock

Occurs when a primary cardiac disorder results in a decrease in cardiac output to a level that is insufficient to meet tissue demands for oxygen.

Cardiac output is determined by HR and stroke volume.

$$\text{CO (L/min)} = \text{HR (beats/min)} \times \text{SV (L/beat)}$$

Stroke volume is itself determined by the interrelation of preload, afterload, and contractility. Problems in any of the determinants of CO may cause cardiogenic shock.

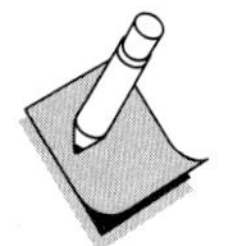

Acute MI is the most common cause of cardiogenic shock.

ETIOLOGY

Etiologies include:

- Classically thought of as pump failure from **myocardial injury** or dysfunction: Myocarditis, cardiomyopathy, ischemia, infarct, contusion
- Arrhythmias

- Valvular disease
- Ventricular septal defect

DIAGNOSIS

- For most causes essential tools will include **ECG** and **echocardiography.**

Clinical cardiogenic shock will occur if 40% of the left ventricle loses contractile function.

TREATMENT

- Will depend on underlying cause
  - Goal is to improve myocardial contractility and pump function.
- Ensure adequate ventilation and oxygenation.
- Decrease work of breathing.
- Inotropes for depressed LV function
  - Dobutamine
    - Primarily a β_1-adrenergic agonist → improved myocardial contractility and augments diastolic coronary blood flow.
  - Dopamine
    - At moderate doses (5–10 μg/kg/min) has α- and β_1-adrenergic effects.
- Intra-aortic balloon pump as bridge to revascularization or valvular repair

Obstructive Shock

Obstructive shock occurs when an extra cardiac obstruction impedes cardiac filling or emptying.

ETIOLOGIES

Etiologies include:

- Cardiac tamponade
- PE
- Tension pneumothorax

TREATMENT

- Relieve obstruction to flow.

Distributive Shock

In distributive shock impaired tissue oxygenation results from a combination of vasodilation with peripheral pooling, capillary leak, and relative cardiac dysfunction.

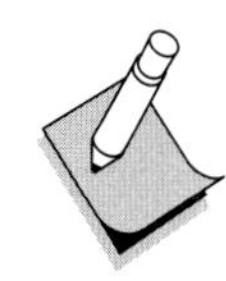

Four causes of distributive shock:
Sepsis/SIRS
Anaphylaxis
Rewarming (severe hypothermia)
Neurogenic shock

There are four major causes of distributive shock: **Sepsis or systemic inflammatory response syndrome (SIRS), anaphylaxis, rewarming in severe hypothermia,** and **neurogenic shock**. Toxic shock syndrome (TSS) is a variant of septic shock and is discussed briefly.

SEPSIS AND SIRS

Sepsis and SIRS are the result of a complicated cascade of cytokines and other immuno and inflammatory modulators.

CAUSES

Triggers include

- Infection (sepsis)
  - Equal frequency between Gram-negative and Gram-positive organisms
- Trauma

- Pancreatitis
- Ingestions
- Burns

DIAGNOSIS

- Based on clinical criteria (see Table 1.16)

TREATMENT

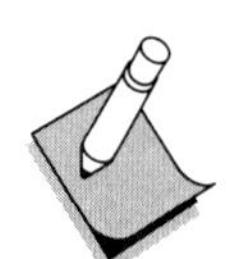

Early goal-directed therapy: Administer fluids to CVP of 8–12 cm H_2O. Begin norepinephrine if MAP remains <65 mmHg. Transfuse PRBCs to Hgb > 10 g/dL if $ScvO_2$ <70%. Begin dobutamine if $ScvO_2$ remains <70%.

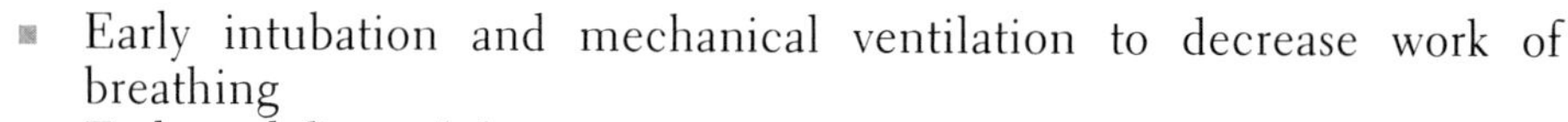

- Early intubation and mechanical ventilation to decrease work of breathing
- Early goal-directed therapy to:
  - **Maximize blood pressure** through use of fluids and/or pressor agents
  - **Improve tissue oxygenation** through cardiac output and oxygen carrying capacity
- For patients with an SBP < 90 mmHg
  - Insert **central line** and administer fluids to **CVP of 8–12 cm H_2O.**
  - If mean arterial pressure remains < 65 mmHg → begin **norepinephrine.**
    - Stimulates α- and β-adrenergic receptors, increasing peripheral vascular tone
    - Alternative agent = dopamine
- Now measure the central venous oxygen saturation($ScvO_2$).
  - If <70% → **transfuse PRBCs** to Hgb concentration of >10 g/dl.
  - If $ScvO_2$ remains <70% → begin **dobutamine.**
    - Stimulates →β_1-adrenergic receptors, increases cardiac contractility and HR with mild dilation of the peripheral vascular bed
- Early broad spectrum antibiotics
  - Empiric (source unknown)coverage for nonneutropenic patient:
    - Neonates: Ampicillin + cefotaxime
    - Child: Vancomycin + cefotaxime
    - Adult: Vancomycin + imipenem
- Low-dose corticosteroids if refractory hypotension to treat relative adrenal suppression

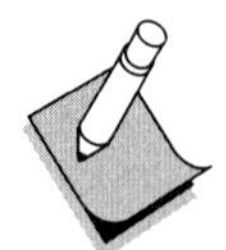

Low-dose corticosteroids are used to treat relative adrenal insufficiency in refractory sepsis.

TABLE 1.16 Clinical Criteria for Diagnosis of SIRS and Sepsis

Systemic inflammatory response syndrome (SIRS)
Two or more of the following: HR > 90 bpm Temperature < 36°C or > 38°C RR > 20 breaths/min or PaCO2 < 32 mmHg WBC ct < 4000 cells/ mm^3 or > 12000 cells/ mm^3 or > 10% immature neutrophils
Sepsis SIRS associated with a source of infection
Severe sepsis Sepsis associated with organ dysfunction, hypoperfusion, or hypotension

COMPLICATIONS

- Multisystem organ dysfunction
- Pulmonary failure or adult respiratory distress syndrome (ARDS)

TOXIC SHOCK SYNDROME

CAUSES

Inflammatory cascade similar to that seen in sepsis, triggered by exotoxin release

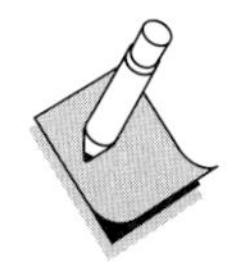

*TSS results from **colonization** with exotoxin-producing S. aureus. STSS results from **infection** with exotoxin-producing group A streptococcus.*

Two distinct syndromes:

Staphylococcal toxic shock syndrome (TSS)

- Due to colonization with exotoxin-producing strain of *Staphylococcus aureus*
- Traditionally associated with tampon use

Streptococcal toxic shock syndrome (STSS)

- Typically due to **infection** with exotoxin-producing strain of group A streptococcus (GAS)

DIAGNOSIS

- Based on established clinical criteria (see Table 1.17)

TREATMENT

- Treatment strategy is the same as for patients with sepsis.
- Major difference is antibiotic usage to cover MRSA as well as group A streptococcus.
  - Nafcillin, clindamycin, and vancomycin concomitantly

> A 55-year-old male is brought to the ED by EMS after collapsing at home shortly after sustaining a bee sting to his R hand. On EMS arrival, the patient is unresponsive and without palpable pulses, but breathing. IM epinephrine is administered, and patient is rapidly transported to ED. On-arrival VS: BP 60/40, HR 130s, RR 20. What is the most appropriate first step in the treatment of this patient?
>
> This patient is in anaphylactic shock with profound hypotension and needs immediate intravenous epinephrine. Other adjunctive therapies include intravenous fluid administration, diphenhydramine, cimetadine, and steroids.

ANAPHYLAXIS AND ANAPHYLACTOID REACTIONS

Caused by the widespread release of inflammatory mediators, specifically histamine, leukotriene C4, and prostaglandin D2, leading to widespread peripheral vasodilation and capillary leakage

PATHOPHYSIOLOGY

- **Anaphylaxis**
  - The initial exposure gives rise to IgE antibodies on the surface of mast cells and basophils.
  - Subsequent exposure results in antigen-antibody binding → cellular degranulation and widespread release of inflammatory mediators.

TABLE 1.17. CDC Criteria for the Diagnosis of TSS and STSS

CDC Criteria for TSS
Fever > 38.9°C (102°F).
Rash (Diffuse, blanching, erythematous with desquamation occurring approximately 1–2 wks later)
Hypotension with SBP < 90 mmHg
Evidence of involvement of ≥3 organ systems (GI, muscular, mucus membranes, renal, hepatic, CNS, hematologic)
Absence of serologic evidence of: Rocky Mountain spotted fever Leptospirosis Measles Hepatitis B Antinuclear antibody Positive VDRL Monospot
CDC Criteria for STSS
Isolation of group A streptococcus (CSF, surgical wound, throat, blood)
Hypotension with SBP < 90 mmHg.
Involvement ≥ 2 organ systems

- Patients on β-blockers are at risk for refractory hypotension and prolonged symptoms.
- **Anaphylactoid reaction**
  - Antigen → direct mast cell degranulation without IgE involvement.
  - Presents in a similar manner but usually not as severe

Anaphylaxis: Mast cell degranulation from IgE response.
Anaphylactoid reaction: Direct mast cell degranulation (no IgE).

SYMPTOMS/EXAM

- Early or mild: Lump in throat, dizziness, nausea and vomiting, skin warmth and flushing
- Hypotension
- Tachycardia
- Stridor, angioedema
- Respiratory distress, bronchospasm
- Urticaria

TREATMENT

- Airway management
- **Epinephrine**

- **Less severe symptoms**
  - Adults: 0.3–0.5 mg of 1:1000 solution **IM** q 5–10 minutes
  - Pediatrics: .01 mg/kg, max 0.3 mg of 1:1000 solution **IM** q 5–10 minutes
- **Severe symptoms**
  - Adults: 1 mL of 1:10,000 solution (0.1 mg) **IV** over 5 minutes (may dilute in 10 mL to 1:100,000 solution); repeat PRN
  - Pediatrics: .01 mg/kg of 1:10,000 solution **IV over 1–2 minutes**; repeat PRN

- Crystalloid boluses via large-bore IVs
  - 1–2 liters in an adult
  - 20 cc/kg in children and infants
- **Histamine blockade**
  - Diphenhydramine (H_1 blocker)
  - Cimetidine (H_2 blocker)
    - Other H_2 blockers are not as efficacious in anaphylaxis as cimetidine.
- **β_2-Receptor agonists** for bronchospasm
  - Aerosolized albuterol
  - Ipratropium and magnesium may be used as well.
- **Corticosteroids** to reduce inflammation, stabilize mast cells and basophils, and prevent rebound phenomenon
  - Methylprednisolone
- **Glucagon**
  - For refractory hypotension in patients on β-blockers
  - 1 mg IV every 5 minutes until hypotension resolved
- Admission, if hypotension present

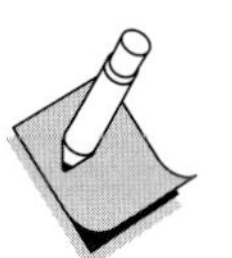

IM administration of epinephrine has shown more consistent absorption over subcutaneous dosing in the treatment of anaphylaxis.

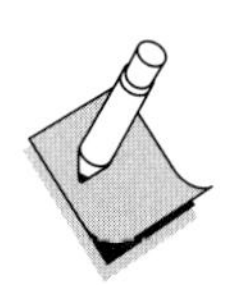

Refractory hypotension from anaphylaxis in patient on β-blockers? Administer glucagon.

REWARMING SHOCK

When a profoundly hypothermic patient is externally rewarmed, vasodilation in the skin occurs. With the distribution of a large portion of plasma volume to the skin there may be ensuing hypotension. In addition to causing vasodilation, external rewarming may result in further cooling of the core ("afterdrop"), which may worsen the patient's cardiac output.

TREATMENT

- Administration of crystalloid boluses (warmed)
- Use core rewarming techniques in patients with severe hypothermia.
- Use of vasoactive pressor agents: Rarely needed.
  - Phenylephrine
  - Norepinephrine
  - Dopamine

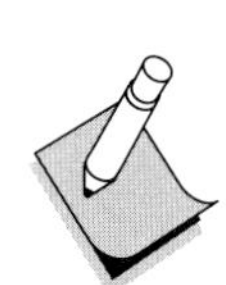

Neurogenic shock is seen with spinal cord injury above T6.

NEUROGENIC SHOCK

Neurogenic shock occurs when an acute spinal cord injury above the level of T6 disrupts the autonomic system, preventing tachycardia and peripheral vasoconstriction.

SYMPTOMS/EXAM

- Acute traumatic injury
- Neurological deficits correlating to a spinal cord level above T6
- No evidence of hemorrhage
- **Hypotension with relative bradycardia**

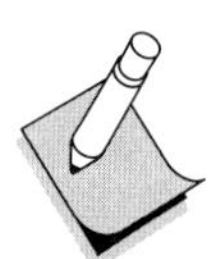

*Shock in a trauma patient should **always** be presumed to be secondary to hemorrhage.*

DIAGNOSIS

- Best diagnosed with a careful exam
- Radiographic studies (X-ray, CT, MRI) may also help in establishing the diagnosis.

TREATMENT

- Crystalloid bolus
- Atropine
- Vasopressor agents to maintain SBP > 90–100 mmHg
  - Norepinephrine
  - Phenylephrine
  - Dopamine
- Monitor urine output as a measure of adequate perfusion.

FLUID RESUSCITATION

There are myriad options for fluid resuscitation available to the emergency physician. They can be categorized as crystalloids, colloids, and blood products.

Crystalloids

Isotonic electrolyte solutions, including normal saline (0.9% NaCl) and Ringer's lactate (NaCl, $CaCl_2$, KCl, Na-lactate)

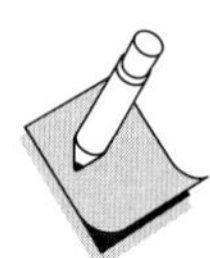

One-third of the volume of infused crystalloid remains intravascular after 20 minutes.

CHARACTERISTICS

- Do not aid in O_2 transport.
- Are hypooncotic → one-third of the volume infused remains in the intravascular space after 20 minutes

CLINICAL INDICATIONS

- Clinically significant hypovolemia
- Regardless of the cause of hypovolemia, crystalloids should always be the first type of fluid given.

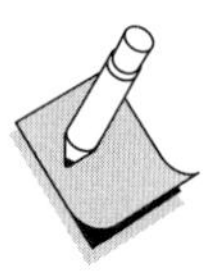

There is no proven benefit of colloids over crytalloids in volume resuscitation.

Colloids

Colloid solutions contain large-molecular-weight particles of high osmolarity that cause fluid to move into the intravascular space. They do not augment O_2 transport.

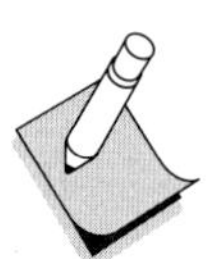

Albumin has the potential for infectious complications.

AVAILABLE PRODUCTS

- Albumin
  - Bovine or human protein
  - Twenty-five percent solution administered in 50-mL or 100-mL aliquots
  - 100 mL felt to be equivalent to 1 L of crystalloid
  - Potential for infectious complications

- Dextrans
  - Highly branched polysaccharides
  - Various formulations available
  - May interfere with hemostasis
  - Maximum dosage 20 mL/kg
- Gelatins
  - Modified derivatives of bovine collagen
  - Various formulations available
  - Dilutional coagulopathy seen with higher volumes
- Polystarches
  - Pentastarch and hexastarch most commonly used
  - Limited usefulness secondary to dilutional coagulopathy and possible platelet inhibition

Clinical Indications

- Colloid solutions are never indicated as primary therapy for volume resuscitation.
  - Possible negative impact on mortality for sepsis
- Indicated for the treatment of spontaneous bacterial peritonitis and for patients receiving large volume paracentesis

Blood Products

Packed Red Blood Cells (PRBCs)

Packed red blood cells have the additional benefit of augmenting O_2 transport. Typically, begin by administering 2 units in adults or 15 mL/kg in children. One unit of PRBCs is sufficient to raise Hgb by 1.0 g/dL.

RBC storage:

- All products are packaged with anticoagulant preservative of citrate, phosphate, dextrose, and adenine.
- Storage results in RBC changes.
  - ↓ Levels of 2,3 DPG
  - Leakage of potassium
  - Spherical and rigid shape of cells

Available Products

- Typed and cross-matched is preferred over type-specific, which is preferred over O negative.
- Women of child-bearing age or younger should not receive Rh-positive blood until testing indicates they are Rh-positive.
- Adult unit = 350 mL, HCT 57%
- Pediatric unit = 60 mL, HCT 72%
- Leukocyte-poor PRBCs will:
  - Prevent febrile nonhemolytic reactions
  - Prevent sensitization to patients eligible for bone marrow transplant
  - Prevent platelet alloimmunization in some cases
  - Minimize risk of virus (CMV, HIV) transmission

Clinical Indications

- Any cause of acute hemorrhage that does not respond to crystalloid
- Known ongoing hemorrhage
- Symptomatic anemia (ischemia, organ dysfunction, hypoxia)

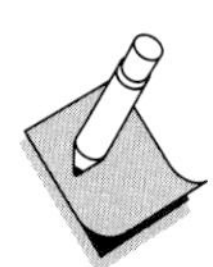

The most common transfusion reaction = febrile transfusion reaction.

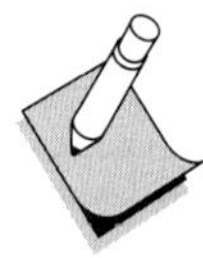

The most serious transfusion reaction = hemolytic transfusion reaction.

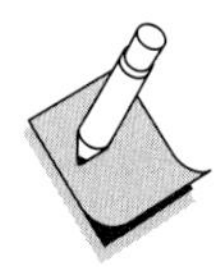

Patient receiving blood transfusion may develop urticaria or hives, but anaphylaxis is rare.

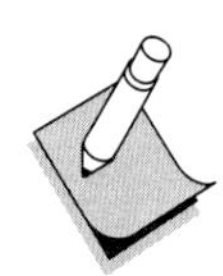

Graft versus host disease is an extremely rare but usually fatal complication of a transfusion. Give irradiated blood products to immunocompromised patients.

COMPLICATIONS

- **In massive transfusion** (>10 units of PRBCs)
  - Coagulopathy
    - Routine transfusion of platelets and FPP is discouraged. Transfuse platelets and FFP based on clinical evidence of abnormal bleeding and abnormal laboratory values.
  - Hypothermia
  - Hypocalcemia (from binding to citrate preservative)
    - Treat symptomatic hypocalcemia with calcium gluconate.
- **Febrile transfusion reaction**
  - Most common transfusion reaction
  - Characterized by fevers/chills, malaise
  - Treatment is symptomatic.
- **Hemolytic transfusion reaction**
  - Most serious transfusion reaction, typically due to clerical error
  - ABO incompatibility → lysis of transfused RBCs → hemoglobinemia and hemoglobinuria.
  - Characterized by immediate fevers/chills, headache, N/V, dark urine, hypotension
  - Treatment includes stopping the transfusion, immediate vigorous crystalloid infusion, and diuretic therapy to maintain urine output at 1–2 mL/kg/hr.
- **Allergic reaction**
  - Urticaria or hives (rarely anaphylaxis)
  - Treatment is symptomatic.
- **Transfusion-related acute lung injury (TRALI)**
  - Indistinguishable from acute respiratory distress syndrome
  - Treatment is supportive. Stop transfusion.
  - No evidence for use of steroids, antihistamines, or diuretics
- **Delayed transfusion reaction**
  - May occur within 3–4 weeks after transfusion as a primary or amnestic response to RBC antigen
  - Characterized by fall in hemoglobin and rise in bilirubin
  - Treatment is supportive.
- **Transfusion-associated graft versus host disease**
  - Occurs in immunocompromised patients from infusion of immunocompetent T lymphocytes, effectively resulting in an unintentional bone marrow transplant; carries 80% mortality
  - Characterized by rash, elevated LFTs, pancytopenia
  - Prevention is key: Use irradiated blood products in immunocompromised patients.
- **Transmitted viral infection**
  - Hepatitis B (1:60,000 units transfused) > hepatitis C (1:1.6 million) > HIV (1:2 million).
  - May transmit CMV, EBV, parvovirus

PLATELETS

One unit of platelets is sufficient to raise platelet count by 10,000/μL. Crossmatching is **not** necessary (though Rh matching is recommended). The normal dosage is 4–6 units of platelets (200 mL volume) per transfusion.

RESUSCITATION

Clinical Indications

- Significant hemorrhage or major procedure with platelets < 50,000/μL
- Life-threatening hemorrhage and abnormal platelet level or function
- Platelets < 10,000/μL for bleeding prophylaxis, except in ITP, TTP, HIT

One unit of platelets will raise the platelet count by 10,000 μL.

Fresh Frozen Plasma (FFP)

One unit of FFP contains 1 U/mL of each clotting factors in addition to 1–2 mg/mL of fibrinogen. It **must be ABO compatible** and is typically dosed as 4–6 units (200–250 mL volume per unit) in adults or 15 mL/kg in children.

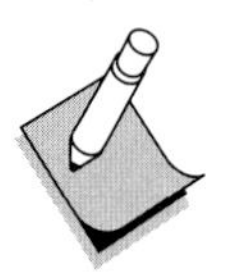

FFP contains fibrinogen and all clotting factors.

Clinical Indications

- Significant hemorrhage secondary to coagulopathy (dilutional-infusion/transfusion-related or warfarin-induced)
- Significant hemorrhages include external or internal bleeds.
- **Not** indicated as primary intravascular volume expander

Cryoprecipitate

Cryoprecipitate contains concentrated factors VIII and XIII, fibrinogen, and von Willebrand factor. Standard dosage is 6–10 units (10–40 mL volume per unit). Does not require ABO matching.

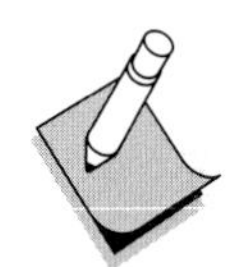

Cryoprecipitate contains factors VIII, XIII, fibrinogen, and von Willebrand factor.

Clinical Indications

- Significant hemorrhage in the setting of low fibrinogen states
- May be used to treat bleeding in hemophilia or von Willebrand disease, although specific factor replacement is preferred over cryoprecipitate

CHAPTER 2

Cardiovascular Emergencies

Gregory W. Burcham, MD, FACEP and Jonathan Claud, MD

Conduction Blocks

RIGHT BUNDLE BRANCH BLOCK (RBBB)

RBBB results from failure of conduction of the R bundle. R ventricular activation occurs via conduction through the L ventricle and is therefore delayed and slowed.

CAUSES

RBBB may occur in a healthy heart but is typically caused by right-sided heart strain:

- Pulmonary hypertension
- Atrial septal defect
- Ischemia
- COPD
- Massive pulmonary embolism (PE)

RBBB can occur in a healthy heart.

ECG FINDINGS (SEE FIGURE 2.1)

- Characterized by terminal slurring of QRS complex
- QRS duration ≥ 0.12 sec
- Terminal R in V_1 (rR′, rSR′)
- Large S wave in V_6
- Appropriately discordant T waves—T waves deflected opposite the terminal deflection of the QRS

Law of Appropriate Discordance: *The T waves should be deflected opposite the terminal deflection of the QRS.*

TREATMENT

- Treat underlying condition.

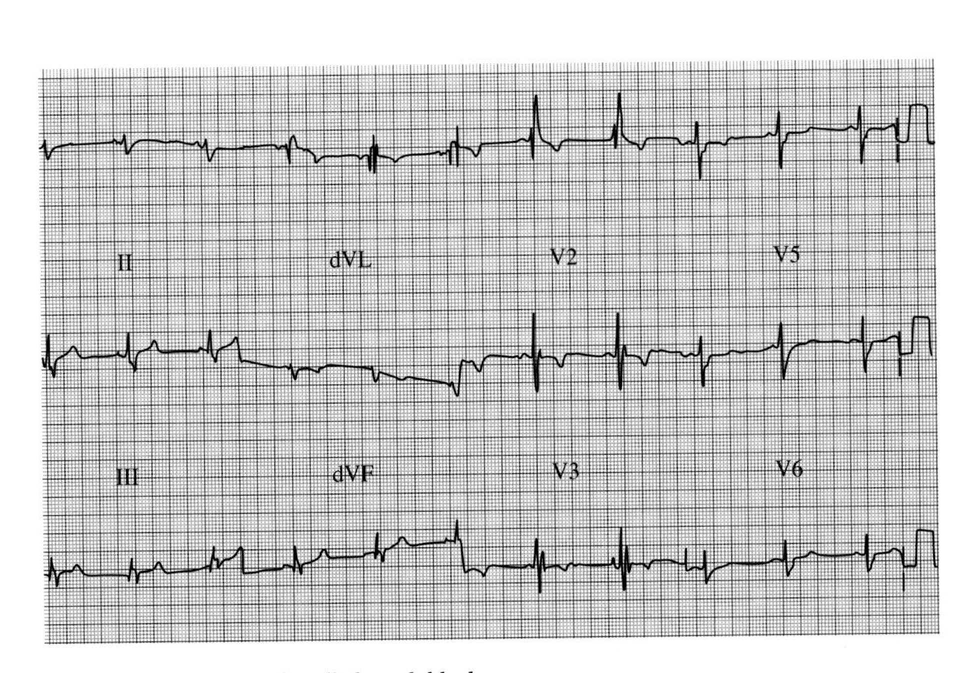

FIGURE 2.1. Right bundle branch block.

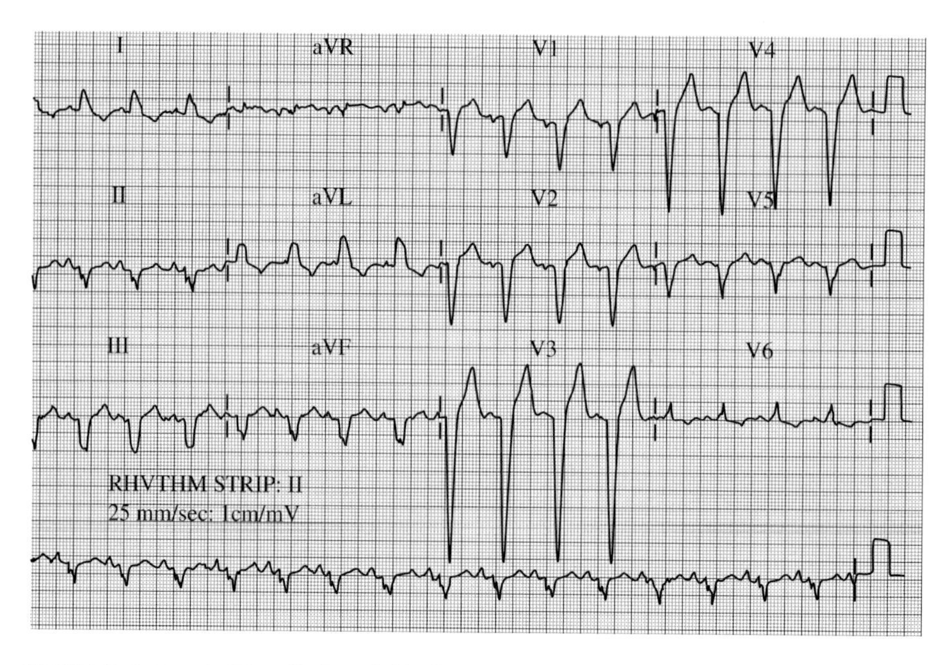

FIGURE 2.2. Left bundle branch block.

LEFT BUNDLE BRANCH BLOCK (LBBB)

In LBBB, both the left anterior and posterior fascicles are blocked and electrical conduction to the L ventricle is delayed (after R ventricular conduction) and slowed.

CAUSES

LBBB does **not** occur in a healthy heart. Causes include:

- Chronic hypertension
- Valvular disease
- Ischemia
- Cardiomyopathy
- Myocarditis
- Congenital heart disease
- Following heart surgery

ECG FINDINGS (SEE FIGURE 2.2)

- Characterized by symmetric slurring through entire QRS complex
- QRS duration ≥ 0.12 seconds
- QS or rS in V_1
- Monophasic R in V_6
- Appropriately discordant T waves

LEFT ANTERIOR FASCICULAR BLOCK (LAFB)

LAFB results from failure of conduction of the left anterior fascicle of the left bundle.

CAUSES

Causes are similar to LBBB.

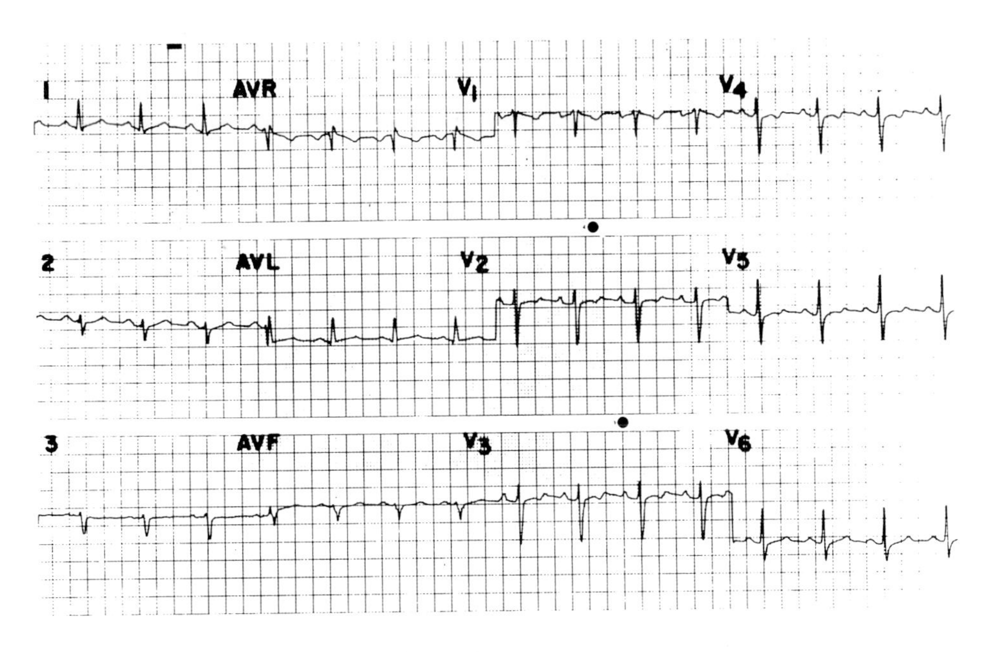

FIGURE 2.3. **Left anterior fascicular block.**

(Reproduced, with permission, from Tintinalli JE, Kelen GD, Stapczynski JS. *Emergency Medicine: A Comprehensive Study Guide,* 6th ed. New York: McGraw-Hill, 2004:195.)

ECG FINDINGS (SEE FIGURE 2.3)

- Normal QRS duration
- Leftward QRS axis of $> -30°$
- Small Q wave in Lead I and S wave in Lead III (Q_1S_3)

TREATMENT

- Treat underlying condition.

LEFT POSTERIOR FASCICULAR BLOCK (LPFB)

LPFB results from damage to the L posterior fascicle of the L bundle.

CAUSES

Causes are similar to LBBB.

ECG FINDINGS (SEE FIGURE 2.4)

- Normal QRS duration
- Right axis deviation
- S wave in Lead I and Q wave in Lead III (S_1Q_3)

TREATMENT

- Treat underlying condition.

LAFB = Q_1S_3

LPFB = S_1Q_3

BIFASCICULAR BLOCK

Bifascicular block occurs when any two of the three major infranodal pathways (R bundle branch, L anterior fascicle, L posterior fascicle) are blocked.

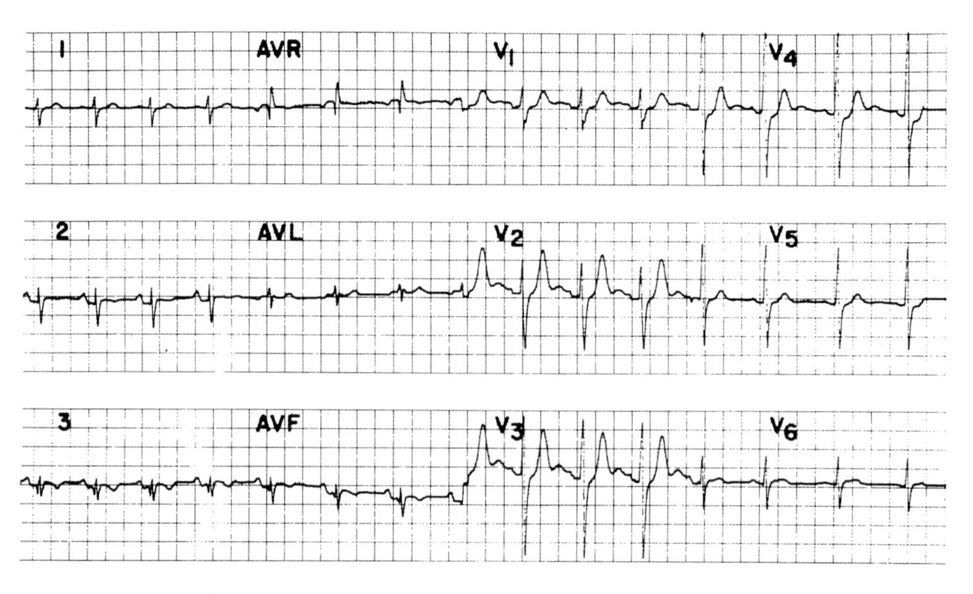

FIGURE 2.4. Left posterior fascicular block.

(Reproduced, with permission, from Tintinalli JE, Kelen GD, Stapczynski JS. *Emergency Medicine: A Comprehensive Study Guide*, 6th ed. New York: McGraw-Hill, 2004:195.)

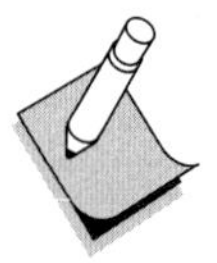

Bifascicular blocks:

- *LBBB*
- *RBBB + LAFB*
- *RBBB + LPFB*

ECG FINDINGS

- LBBB *or*
- RBBB + LAFB *or* LPFB

TREATMENT

- Transvenous pacing if
  - Symptomatic bradycardia
  - Acute MI (extensive damage to conducting system)

Trifascicular blocks:

- *Bifascicular block + first-degree AV block*
- *Alternating RBBB & LBBB*

TRIFASCICULAR BLOCK

Trifascicular block occurs when any combination of three fascicular blocks are found concomitantly.

ECG FINDINGS

- Bifascicular block + first-degree AV block *or*
- Alternating RBBB and LBBB

TREATMENT

- Transvenous pacing if
  - Symptomatic bradycardia
  - In the setting of an acute myocardial infarction (AMI))(extensive damage to conducting system)

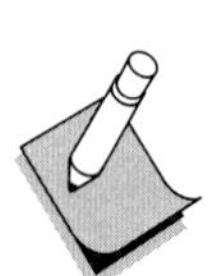

Trifascicular block in the setting of MI necessitates permanent pacemaker insertion.

Ventricular Hypertrophy

RIGHT VENTRICULAR HYPERTROPHY (RVH)

Prominent right-sided forces cause the pattern of RVH on surface ECG.

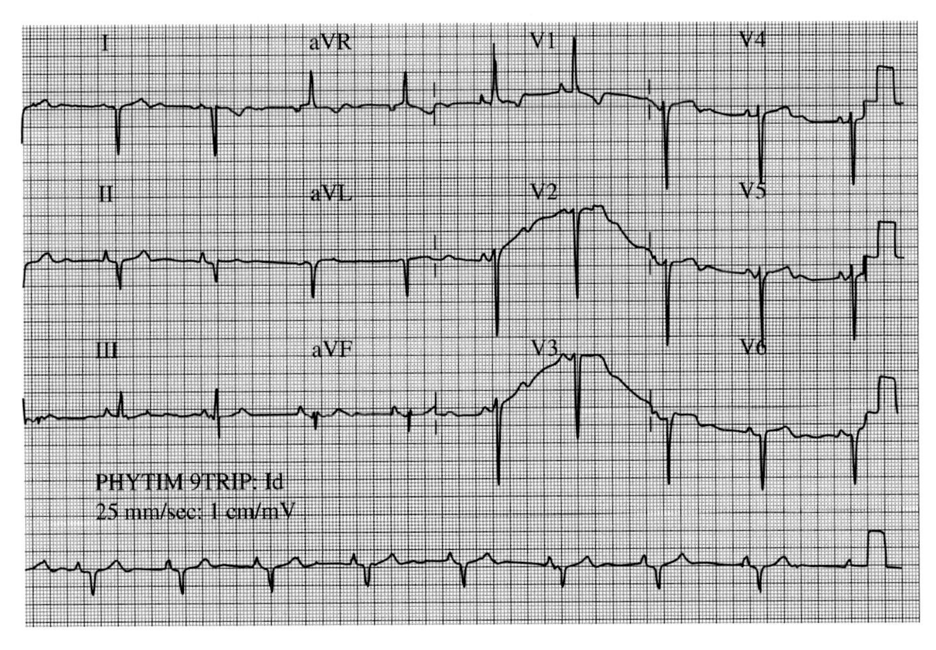

FIGURE 2.5. Right ventricular hypertrophy.

CAUSES

- Mitral stenosis
- Pulmonary hypertension
- Chronic PE
- Left to right shunts

ECG FINDINGS (SEE FIGURE 2.5)

- Right axis deviation
- Tall R wave in V_1 (R wave > S wave)
- Deep S wave in V_6
- Inverted T waves in R precordial leads (R ventricular strain)

LEFT VENTRICULAR HYPERTROPHY (LVH)

Prominent L-sided forces cause characteristic ECG changes.

CAUSES

- Chronic hyptertension (HTN)
- Chronic CAD and ischemia
- Aortic valve disease
- Congenital heart disease
- Hypertrophic cardiomyopathy

ECG FINDINGS (SOKOLOW AND LYON CRITERIA) (SEE FIGURE 2.6)

- S in V_1 + R in V_5 (or V_6) ≥ 35 mm
- R in aVL ≥ 11 mm
- May see T-wave strain pattern

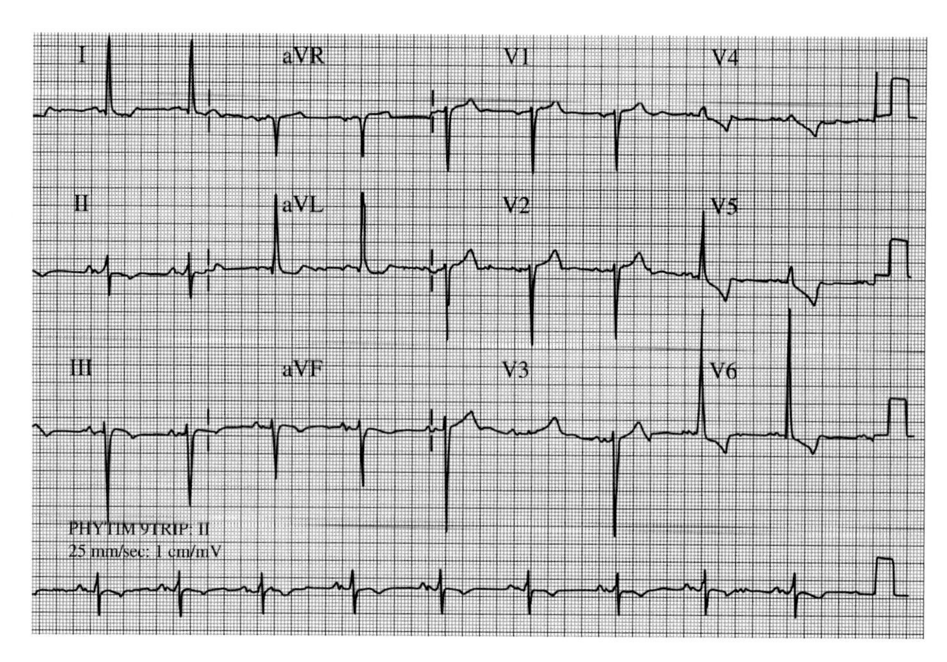

FIGURE 2.6. Left ventricular hypertrophy.

Electrolyte Disturbances

HYPERKALEMIA

Hyperkalemia alters membrane polarization. The degree of ECG changes depends somewhat on the rapidity of onset (slowly developing hyperkalemia → ECG findings at higher K^+ concentrations).

ECG FINDINGS (SEE FIGURE 2.7)

- K^+ = 6.5–7.5 ng/dL: Tall peaked T waves (earliest), PR prolongation
- K^+ = 7.5–8.0 ng/dL: P wave flattens, QRS widens
- K^+ > 9.0 ng/dL: Sine wave pattern of QRS

Tall, peaked T waves are the earliest ECG finding in hyperkalemia.

HYPOKALEMIA

Hypokalemia alters membrane polarization.

ECG FINDINGS (SEE FIGURE 2.8)

- Flattening of the T wave (earliest sign)
- Prominent U waves following T waves
- ST depression at low levels

HYPERCALCEMIA

ECG FINDINGS (SEE FIGURE 2.9)

- Shortened QT intervals (classic finding)
- Depressed and shortened ST segments
- Widened T waves

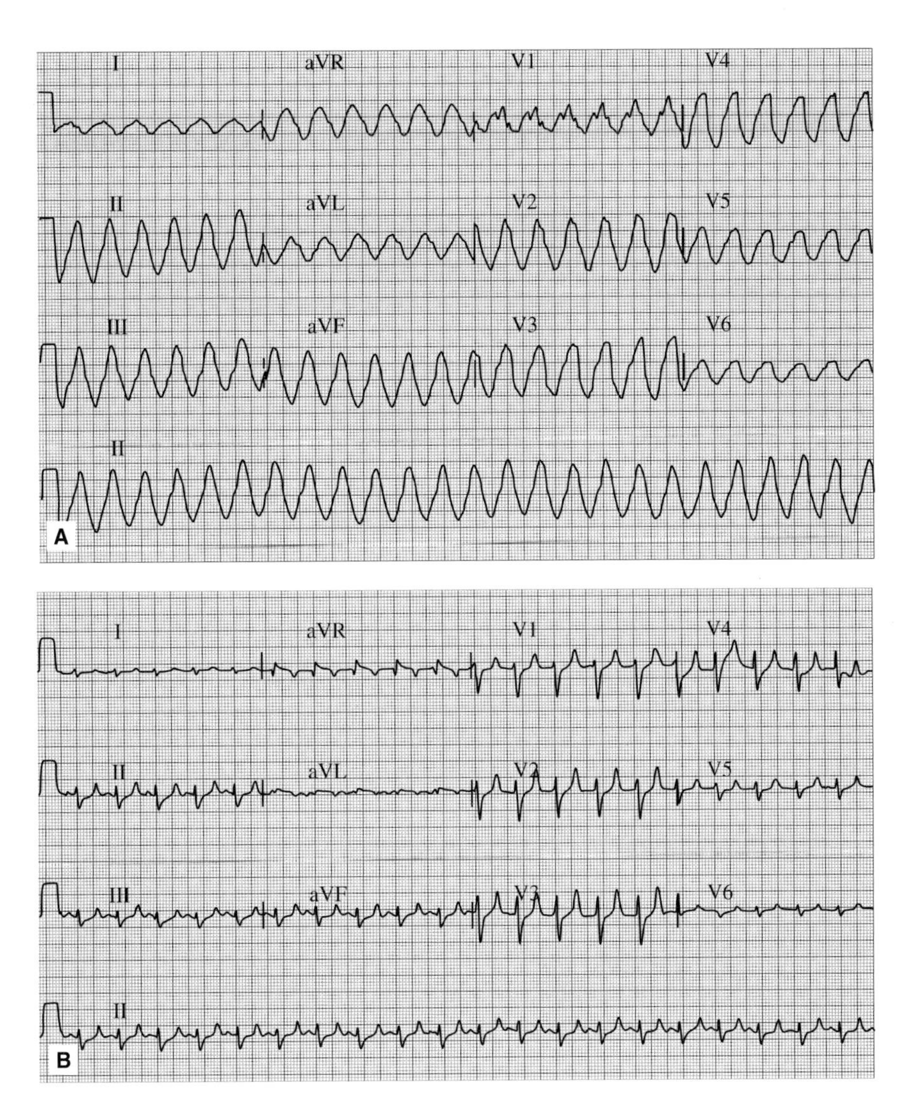

FIGURE 2.7. Hyperkalemia.

A. ECG showing sine wave complexes in severe hyperkalemia ([K^+] = 9.2ng/dL]). B. ECG after treatment. Note peaked T waves and flattened P waves.

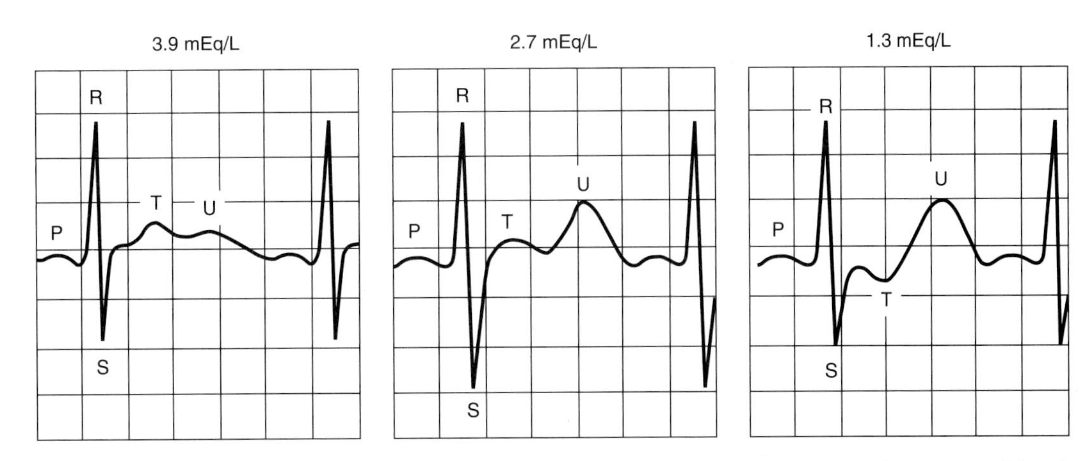

FIGURE 2.8. Hypokalemia: ECG changes with hypokalemia. Note progressive flattening of T waves and development of prominent U waves and ST-segment depression.

(Reproduced, with permission, from Morgan GE, Mikhail MS, Murray MJ, *Clinical Anesthesiology*, 4th ed. New York: McGraw-Hill, 2006: 679.)

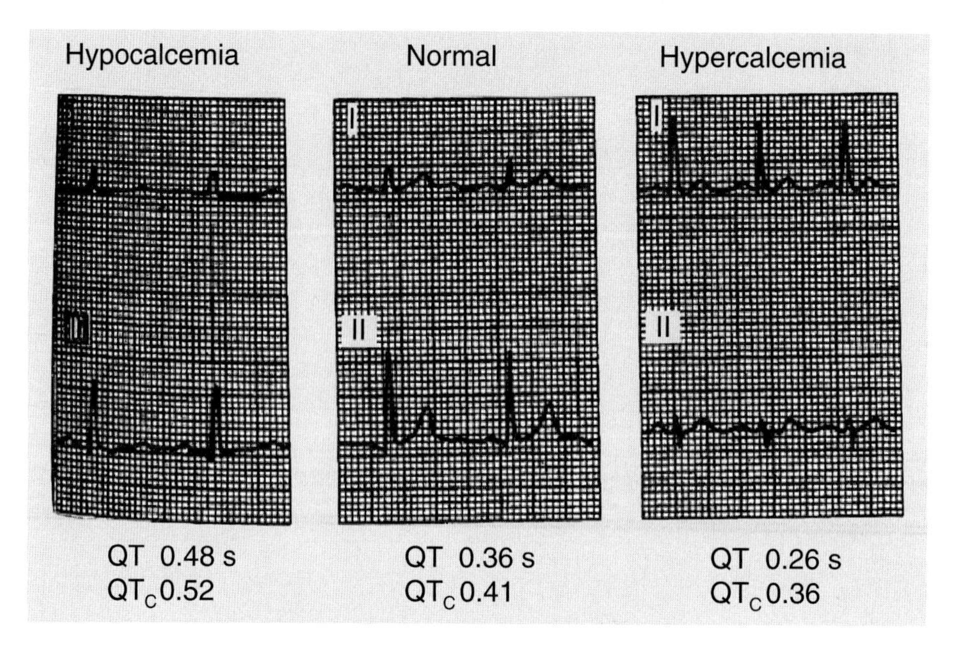

FIGURE 2.9. ECG findings in hypercalcemia and hypocalcemia.

(Reproduced, with permission, from Kasper DL, Braunwald E, Fauci AS, et al. *Harrison's Principles of Internal Medicine*, 16th ed. New York: McGraw-Hill, 2005:1319.)

HYPOCALCEMIA

ECG FINDINGS (SEE FIGURE 2.9)

- Hallmark = QT prolongation
  - Due to lengthening of the ST segment
  - Occurs with $Ca^{+} < 6.0$ mg/dL

Digitalis Effect

This should be differentiated from **digitalis toxicity**.

ECG FINDINGS

- Depressed (scooped or sagging) ST segments
- Shortened QT intervals
- Flattened T waves
- Prominent U waves

Hypothermia

The heart becomes very irritable in the hypothermic (core temperature < 35°C) patient.

ECG FINDINGS (SEE FIGURE 2.10)

- Cardiac conduction abnormalities
  - Typical progression from sinus bradycardia to atrial fibrillation to ventricular fibrillation
- **Osborn (or J) waves** at end of QRS complex
  - Characteristic but *can* be seen in other heart conditions

See Table 2.1 for summary of ECG essentials.

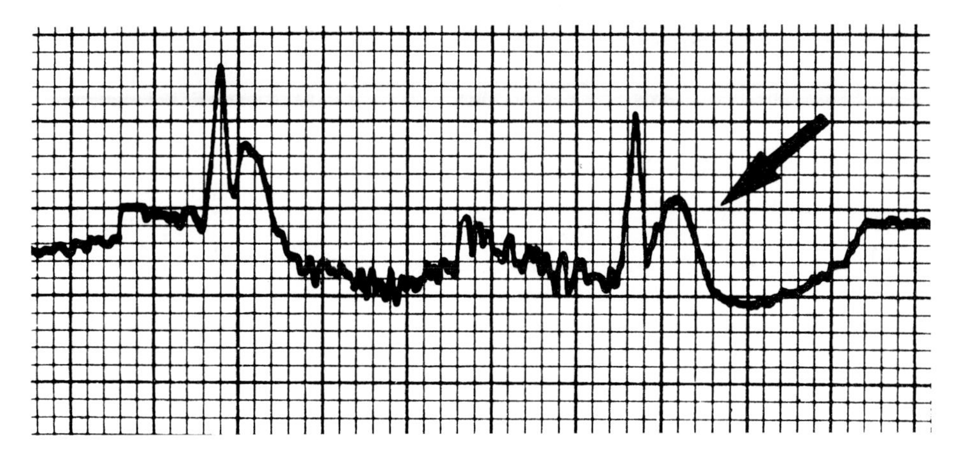

FIGURE 2.10. Osborn wave or J wave, indicating hypothermia.

(Reproduced, with permission, from Tintinalli JE, Kelen GD, Stapczynski JS. *Emergency Medicine: A Comprehensive Study Guide*, 6th ed. New York: McGraw-Hill, 2004:1180.)

The charge nurse calls for you to examine a patient who was given sublingual nitroglycerin 2 minutes earlier. The 49-year-old male presented with acute onset of chest pain with shortness of breath and diaphoresis. His BP is now 80/50 after the administration of the nitro (initial BP 110/70). Review of the initial ECG reveals ST elevation in II, III, aVF and in lead V_4 on the R-sided ECG (V_4R). What is the most appropriate initial therapy for his hypotension?

The ST elevation in lead V_4R indicates RV extension of his inferior MI. These patients are often very preload dependent, so nitroglycerin will exacerbate the situation. Start a normal saline bolus to increase preload. Multiple fluid boluses may be required.

ACUTE CORONARY SYNDROME (ACS)

ACS represents a spectrum of ischemic heart disease from stable angina to non-ST segment MI (NSTEMI) and ST segment elevation myocardial infarction (STEMI).

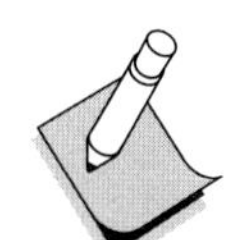

Coronary heart disease is the number one cause of death in the United States, with over 500,000 victims annually.

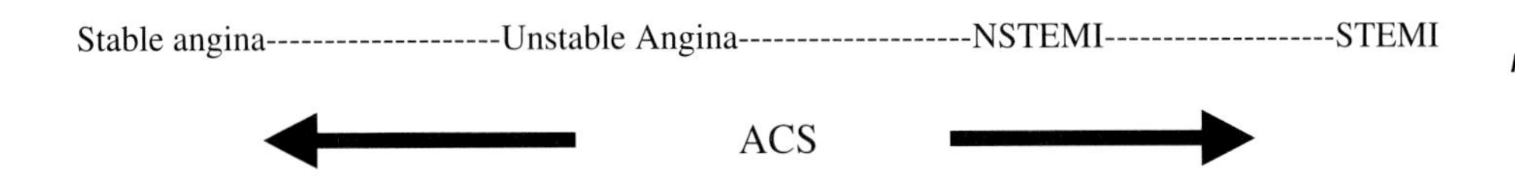

Stable Angina

Stable angina represents the beginning of ACS, when a fixed coronary plaque prevents sufficient blood supply through coronary artery at times of increased O_2 demand. This results in ischemic symptoms, but does not cause infarction.

Stable angina is resolved by alleviating the increased O_2 demand (eg, resting, blood transfusion) or increasing the blood supply through vasodilators such as nitroglycerin. Symptoms usually last only a **few minutes** after cessation of activity or use of nitroglycerin.

TABLE 2.1. Summary of ECG Essentials

	Axis	QRS	Characteristic ECG Findings
RBBB	Right or vertical	Wide	rR′ or rSR′ in V_1 *and* Large S wave in V_6
LBBB	Left	Wide	QS or rS in V_1 *and* Monophasic R in V_6
LAFB	Left (> –30°)	Normal	Q in I, S in III (Q_1S_3)
LPFB	Right	Normal	S in I, Q in III (S_1Q_3)
RVH	Right	Normal	R wave > S wave in V_1 *and* Deep S wave in V_6
LVH	Left or horizontal	Normal	S in V_1 + R in V_5 (or V_6) ≥ 35 mm *and* R in aVL ≥ 11 mm
Hyperkalemia	Any	Normal or wide	Peaked T waves → PR prolongation → P waves flattening → Widened QRS → sine wave
Hypokalemia	Any	Normal	Flattened T waves Prominent U waves
Hypercalcemia	Any	Normal	Shortened QT intervals
Hypocalcemia	Any	Normal	QT prolongation
Digitalis Effect	Any	Normal	Depressed (scooped or sagging) ST segments Shortened QT intervals Flattened T waves Prominent U waves
Hypothermia	Any	Normal or wide	Osborn J waves

It is divided into four classes by the Canadian Cardiovascular Society:

- **Class I**: Angina with strenuous physical activity
- **Class II**: Slight limitation of normal physical activity
- **Class III**: Severe limitation of normal physical activity
- **Class IV**: Inability to perform physical activity

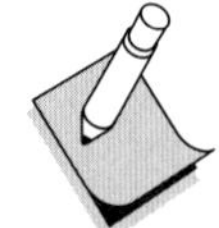

UA = new-onset angina, angina with ↑ frequency or duration, angina with minimal exertion/rest

Unstable Angina (UA)

UA is angina occurring with minimal exertion/rest, new-onset angina (within last 2 months), or an increasing frequency or duration of previously stable angina.

UA is part of the continuum of ACS and overlaps with NSTEMI. A patient experiencing severe UA has a prognosis and risk profile similar to that of a patient with a mild NSTEMI.

Patients with severe UA have a prognosis similar to patients with mild NSTEMI.

Short-term, high-risk factors for death or nonfatal MI in patients with unstable angina include:

- Rest pain > 20 minutes
- CHF or pulmonary edema
- Rest pain with dynamic ECG changes
- Chest pain with new or worsening mitral regurgitation (MR) murmur
- Chest pain with hypotension

CARDIOVASCULAR EMERGENCIES

Myocardial Infarction (MI)

MI encompasses both NSTEMI and STEMI. It is defined as myocardial cell death and necrosis as diagnosed by a rise and fall of cardiac enzymes (in association with appropriate clinical presentation) or by pathologic findings of prior MI (eg, new Q waves on ECG).

PATHOPHYSIOLOGY

ACS results from insufficient O_2 supply to meet cardiac muscle demands:

- Progressive fixed atherosclerotic lesions within the coronary arteries → ↓ luminal diameter and ↓ coronary blood flow
- Acute coronary artery plaque disruption → exposed thrombogenic endothelium → platelet aggregation and thrombus formation
- Coronary artery vasospasm
- Less common: dissection of the coronary arteries, microemboli, excess demand states, vasculitis, vasospasm

Risk factors:

- Smoking
- HTN
- Diabetes
- Dyslipidemia
- Family history
- Advanced age
- Male gender
- Cocaine use
- SLE
- Obesity
- Postmenopausal state

SYMPTOMS

- Classic symptoms include chest pain or pressure (may radiate to the arm, back, chest, or jaw), shortness of breath, sweating, nausea, and impending sense of doom.
- Beware of atypical presentations (more common in diabetics, the elderly, and women).
  - Fatigue or generalized weakness
  - Shortness of breath without chest pain
  - Epigastric abdominal pain or "indigestion"
    - Consider a cardiac etiology in any patient with GERD-type symptoms on the boards even if symptoms abate with antacids.
  - Mental status change

Maintaining a high index of suspicion for MI is essential as the initial ECG is diagnostic for MI < 50% of the time and may be normal in up to 5% of cases.

TABLE 2.2. Regional ECG Findings in the Setting of MI

REGION OF ST ELEVATION	REGION OF INFARCT	AFFECTED VESSEL	SPECIAL CONSIDERATIONS
II, III, aVF Reciprocal changes in aVL	Inferior	Right coronary artery–posterior descending branch	Anticipate RV or posterior infarct.
V_3, V_4 Reciprocal changes in II, III, aVF	Anterior	Left anterior descending–diagonal branch	Anticipate BBB, LV dysfunction, complete heart block.
V_1, V_2	Septal	Left anterior descending–septal branch	Anticipate BBB.
V_5, V_6, and I, aVL	Lateral	Left circumflex–circumflex or diagonal branch	Anticipate LV dysfunction with CHF.
On *R-sided ECG*: V_4R (See Figure 2.11.)	Right ventricle	Right coronary artery–proximal branches	Anticipate hypotension with clear lungs. Preload dependent.
Posterior ECG: precordial leads *Anterior ECG:* ST **depression** in V_1, V_2 with prominent R waves; tall, upright T wave in V_1 instead of normally inverted T wave; helpful to obtain additional posterior ECG leads V_8 and V_9	Posterior	Left circumflex–posterior circumflex *or* right coronary artery–posterior descending	Rarely occurs in isolation, usually with inferior or lateral MI Anticipate LV dysfunction.

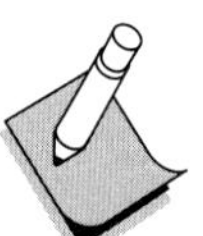

Always get an R-sided ECG to look for RV infarct in inferior wall MI.
Patients with RV infarct are preload dependent.

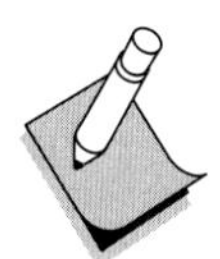

ST depression in V_1, V_2 with prominent R waves? Suspect posterior MI!

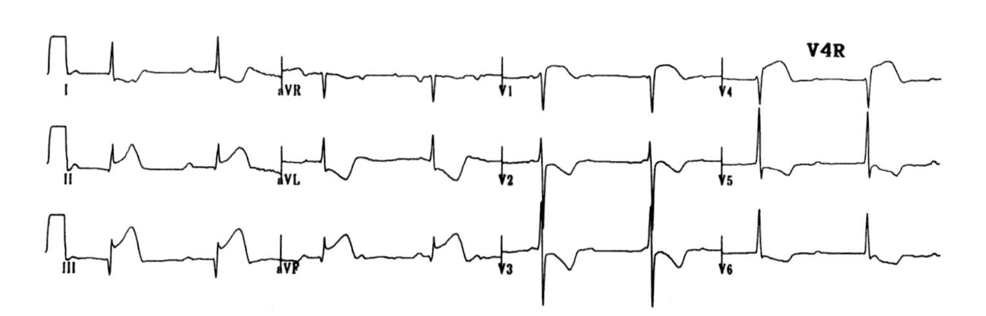

FIGURE 2.11. Right-sided ECG in patient with inferior MI.

(Reproduced, with permission, from Fuster V, Alexander RW, O'Rourke, RA. *Hurst's The Heart*, 12th ed. New York: McGraw-Hill, 2008:300.)

EXAM

- Findings are often nonspecific and may include pallor, diaphoresis, and tachypnea.
- Listen for new heart murmur (mitral regurgitation).
- 15% of patient with proven MI have reproducible chest pain on exam.
- Look for signs that increase risk for heart disease or suggest an alternate diagnosis.

DIFFERENTIAL

- PE, aortic dissection, pericarditis, tension pneumothorax, musculoskeletal pain, gastroesophageal reflux (a diagnosis of exclusion, rarely the correct answer on boards), esophageal rupture

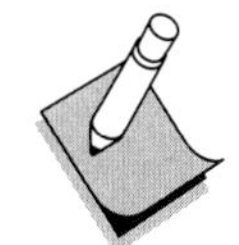

ECG findings suggestive of MI:

- *Hyperacute T waves*
- *ST segment elevation*
- *Reciprocal ST segment depression*
- *T-wave inversions in regional distribution*
- *New LBBB*

DIAGNOSIS

ECG Findings Suggestive of MI

- **Hyperacute T waves**
  - Earliest ECG finding
  - Transient
  - Differential includes hyperkalemia, LVH, pericarditis
- **ST segment elevation**
  - **"Domed" or upwardly concave**
  - Occurring in **regional distribution**
  - **Dynamic**—waxing and waning with time
  - May be associated with evolving Q waves (infarct)
- **Reciprocal ST segment depression**
  - Changes in region electrically opposite that of injury
  - Indicates a larger area of injury, lower ejection fraction, and ↑ mortality
- **T-wave inversions in regional distribution**
  - May occur before or after ST elevation
  - **Wellen's T waves**—deep symmetric or biphasic T wave inversions in the anterior precordial leads suggest LAD lesion
  - Differential includes LVH, BBB, pacer, myocarditis, and pericarditis
- **New LBBB**
- **In presence of preexisting LBBB or ventricular-paced rhythm:**
  - ST segment elevation > 5 mm
  - ST segment depression > 1 mm in lead V_1, V_2, or V_3
  - ST segment elevation *with concordance*
    - An LBBB follows the **Law of Appropriate Discordance**: It is **appropriate** for the ST segment elevation/depression to be **discordant** with the direction of the primary QRS vector.

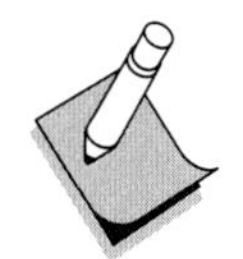

Hyperacute T waves are the earliest ECG finding of STEMI.

Differential Diagnosis of ST Elevation on ECG:

- Left ventricular (LV) aneurysm
  - History of prior MI
  - ECG with anterior (usually) Q waves and ST elevation
  - ST without dynamic or reciprocal changes
  - Can be visualized on echocardiography
- Early repolarization (see Figure 2.12)
  - Characterized by no more than 3 mm of J-point elevation in the precordial leads with an upwardly concave morphology
  - Rarely seen in leads V_1 and V_2

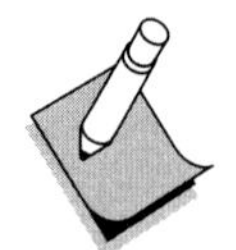

*A normal ECG does **not** rule out ACS.*

The initial ECG is nondiagnostic in the majority of patients with MI.

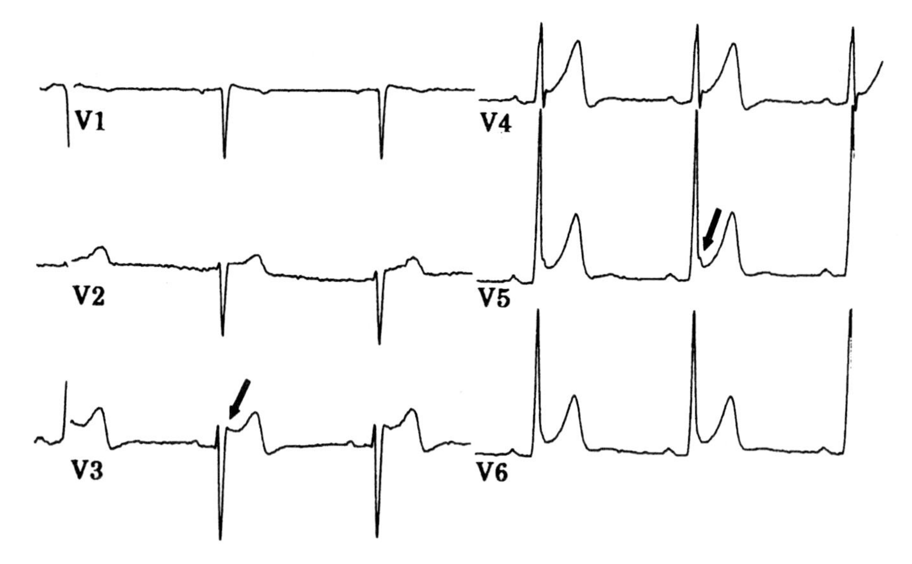

FIGURE 2.12. Early repolarization ECG findings.

(Reproduced, with permission, from Fuster V, Alexander RW, O'Rourke, RA. *Hurst's The Heart*, 12th ed. New York: McGraw-Hill, 2008:303.)

- Left ventricular hypertrophy (see Figure 2.6)
  - May mimic or obscure ACS
  - Characterized by a large S wave in V_1, V_2, and tall R wave in V_5, V_6
  - "Strain" pattern with asymmetrically inverted T waves in inferior and lateral leads may also be present.
- Pericarditis
  - Diffuse ST elevations in multiple regions
  - PR depression

Serum Markers

- May be normal early despite ongoing ischemia
- Become elevated in NSTEMI and STEMI (see Table 2.3)
- **Myoglobin**
  - Early rise but poor specificity
  - Rises in 1–2 hours
  - Peaks in 4–6 hours
  - Normalizes in 24 hours
- **CK-MB**
  - Not as sensitive or specific as troponin
  - Rises in 3–4 hours
  - Peaks in 12–24 hours
  - Normalizes in 1–2 days
  - May also be elevated in pericarditis, myocarditis, and skeletal muscle disease

TABLE 2.3. Timeline for Serum Markers in the Evaluation of ACS

Marker	Rises	Peaks	Normalizes
Myoglobin	1–2 hr	4–6 hr	24 hr
CK-MB	3–4 hr	12–24 hr	1–2 d
Troponin	3–6 hr	12–24 hr	7–10 d

- **Troponin I**
  - Most sensitive and specific but delayed rise
  - Rises in 3–6 hours
  - Peaks at 12–24 hours
  - Normalizes in 7–10 days
  - Unlike troponin T, is **not** elevated in skeletal muscle disease or renal failure

Cardiac Testing

- **Cardiac catheterization** is definitive.
- **Echocardiogram** can identify regional wall motion abnormalities, but cannot differentiate ischemia from acute or chronic infarction and **cannot reliably** detect subendocardial ischemia.
- **Perfusion imaging** during symptoms
  - IV radionuclide (eg, thallium 201, technetium 99m-sestamibi) is taken up by myocardium.
  - Uptake is proportional to blood flow, so areas with poor perfusion are demonstrated.
- Stress testing is **contraindicated** in the presence of MI or unstable angina.
- **Electron beam CT (EBCT)** is a new technology that shows calcium plaques in arteries and may be a good screening tool for presence of CAD.

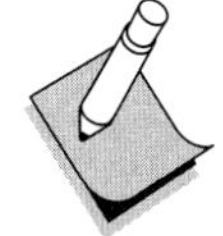

Echocardiogram cannot reliably detect subendocardial ischemia.

Risk Stratification

See Table 2.4.

TABLE 2.4. Risk Stratification

	High Likelihood	Intermediate Likelihood	Low Likelihood
History	Chest or left arm pain or discomfort typical of prior angina Known history of CAD or MI	Chest or left arm pain or discomfort Age > 70 Male Diabetes	Probable ischemic symptoms without any high or intermediate likelihood features Recent cocaine use
Examination	Transient mitral regurgitation Decreased BP Diaphoresis Rales/pulmonary edema	Extracardiac vascular disease	Chest discomfort reproduced by palpation
ECG	New ST-segment deviation (≥ 0.05 mV) or T-wave inversion (≥ 0.2 mV) while having symptoms	Stable chronic changes (Q waves, abnormal ST segments or T waves)	Normal or T-wave flattening or inversion in leads with dominant R waves
Cardiac Markers	Elevated	Normal	Normal

CARDIOVASCULAR EMERGENCIES

TABLE 2.5. ED Core Measures for ACS (From Time-of-Arrival to ED)

ASA on arrival
ECG interpreted within 10 min
If STEMI: ▪ Door to needle (fibrinolytics) < 30 min *or* ▪ activation of catheter team < 30 min and ▪ door to catheterization < 90 min
β Blockers within 24 h

TREATMENT

UA requires more aggressive treatment than stable angina, and is **similar to** treatment for **NSTEMI**:

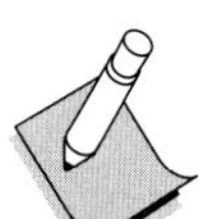

In patients who present to the ED with chest pain, the ECG should be interpreted by the physician ***within 10 minutes*** of patient's arrival.

Goals of care (ED core measures) from time of arrival to ED (see Table 2.5)

- ASA given on arrival (unless contraindicated)
- ECG interpreted by physician within 10 minutes
- If STEMI:
  - Door to needle (if fibrinolytics utilized) < 30 minutes
    or
  - Activation of catheterization team < 30 minutes **and** door to catheterization time < 90 minutes
- β-Blockers within 24 hours

Medications

- **O_2**
  - May reduce the area of ischemia
  - Uncertain benefit in the literature, but easy and safe (even in the COPD patient)
- **Aspirin**
  - Antiplatelet agent—irreversibly inhibits platelet cyclooxygenase activity, thereby inhibiting the formation of thromboxane A_2
  - Onset of action is *minutes*.
  - ↓ Long-term mortality (to the same degree as thrombolytics!)
  - Use with caution with active peptic ulcer disease (consider rectal administration).
- **Clopidogrel (Plavix) or ticlodipine (Ticlid)**
  - Antiplatelet agent—irreversibly inhibits platelet aggregation via adenosine diphosphate receptor antagonism
  - Onset of action is *hours*.
  - Indicated in patients with aspirin allergy
  - Do not use in patients who may require a surgical intervention (CABG) within the next 5 days.
- **Nitroglycerin**
  - Sublingual X 3, then IV if symptoms persist
  - Dilates coronary arteries and relaxes vascular smooth muscle, resulting in decreased preload/afterload and decreased myocardial **O_2** demand

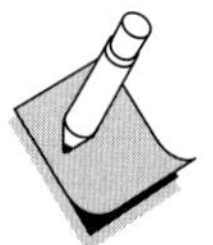

Aspirin is the most cost-effective treatment available for patients with ACS. It independently reduces mortality of patients with MI.

- May ↓ infarct size and mortality in MI
- Titrate to 10% (if normotensive) **or** 30% (if hypertensive) BP reduction (**not** to chest pain resolution).
- Contraindications:
  - SBP < 100 mmHg
  - Presence of RV infarction or severe aortic stenosis
  - Use of medications for erectile dysfunction in prior 24 hours (48 hours with tadalafil [Cialis])—may cause cardiovascular collapse
- Commonly causes a headache

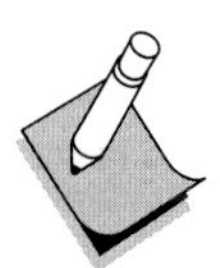

Always ask the patient about use of Viagra or other phosphodiesterase inhibitors before administering nitroglycerin.

- **β-Blockers**
  - Give *as early as possible.*
  - Blocks sympathetic stimulation, reducing heart rate
  - ↓ Myocardial O_2 consumption
  - ↓ Incidence of ventricular fibrillation
  - Relative contraindications include:
    - SBP < 100 mmHg
    - HR < 60
    - Left ventricular failure with pulmonary edema
    - Second- and third-degree heart block
    - Severe reactive airway disease
  - ↓ Long-term mortality by 23%
- **Morphine**
  - Blocks sympathetic activity and relieves anxiety, decreasing myocardial O_2 consumption
  - Mild vasodilator, decreasing preload
  - Analgesic for intractable chest pain
  - No proven ↓ in mortality
  - Contraindicated in patients with SBP < 100 mmHg

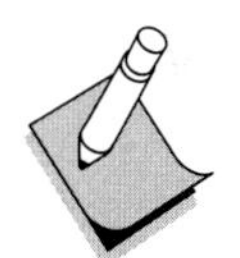

Morphine has not been shown to ↓ mortality in ACS.

- **Heparin**
  - Antithrombotic agent—binds antithrombin III → inactivates thrombin and activated factor X, decreasing clot formation and propagation
  - Synergistic effect with aspirin to ↓ mortality in patients with MI or severe unstable angina
- **Low-molecular-weight heparin**
  - Similar mechanism to heparin
  - Longer half-life and more reliable effect allows for subcutaneous dosing.
  - Preferred over unfractionated heparin in UA and NSTEMI

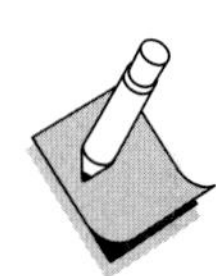

Low-molecular-weight heparin is preferred over unfractionated heparin in unstable angina and NSTEMI.

- **Glycoprotein (GP) inhibitors IIb/IIIa**
  - Abciximab (ReoPro), eptifibatide (Integrilin), and tirofiban (Aggrastat)
  - Blocks final common pathway of platelet aggregation by inhibiting the GP IIb/IIIa receptor on platelets
  - Used primarily for patients with ACS in whom percutaneous coronary intervention (PCI) is planned
  - Contraindications:
    - Active internal bleeding
    - Bleeding disorder < 30 days prior
    - Platelet count < 150,000/mm^3
    - History of intracranial hemorrhage, AVM, aneurysm, or stroke < 30 days prior
    - Major surgical procedure or trauma < 30 days prior

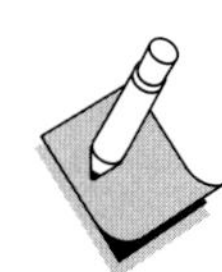

GP IIb/IIIa inhibitors are used for patients with ACS who are undergoing PCI.

- **Angiotensin converting enzyme (ACE) inhibitors**
  - Less commonly initiated in ED
  - Reduce adverse LV remodeling
  - Decrease incidence of CHF, sudden death, and subsequent MIs
  - Proven mortality benefit for MI patients with EF < 40% when administered orally *within 24 hours*

- IV ACE after MI may cause hypotension, so administer orally.
- Contraindications:
  - Pregnancy
  - History of angioedema
  - SBP < 100 mmHg
  - Renal failure
  - Hyperkalemia
- Angiotensin receptor blockers (ARBs) may be used in patients with ACE inhibitor intolerance.

- **HMG coenzyme A reductase inhibitors (statins)**
  - Less commonly initiated in ED
  - ↓ Incidence of recurrent angina and subsequent MIs
- **Calcium channel blocker**
  - Indicated for the treatment of coronary vasospasm only
  - Otherwise, has been shown to increase mortality

Reperfusion Therapy: Percutaneous Coronary Intervention (PCI) Versus Thrombolytic Therapy

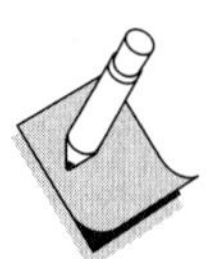

Administration of a β-blocker in MI → ↓ incidence of VFib and has a significant impact on long-term mortality.

- PCI consists of catheterization with angioplasty and stent placement.
- Thrombolytics bind plasminogen, which then degrades fibrin, "busting clots." The primary risk of thrombolytic therapy is bleeding (including intracranial hemorrhage).
  - Alteplase (tPa)—front-loaded or accelerated
  - Reteplase (rPA)
  - Tenecteplase (TNK)
- Indications for reperfusion therapy include 1–2 mm ST elevation in regional distribution or new LBBB (see Table 2.6).
- PCI is generally preferred in the setting of STEMI if
  - Transfer to a PCI facility can be accomplished within 2 hours. However, the goal is always a door to balloon time < 90 minutes.
  - Presentation >3 hours after onset of symptoms
  - Uncertain diagnosis
  - Complications (CHF, unstable)
  - Contraindications to thrombolytics (see Table 2.7)
- Most effective PCI centers perform >200 PCIs per year.
- Commonly seen rhythm following reperfusion = accelerated idioventricular rhythm (AIVR)—benign and rarely requires treatment (see Figure 2.13)

See Table 2.8 for a summary of agents used in the treatment of ACS.

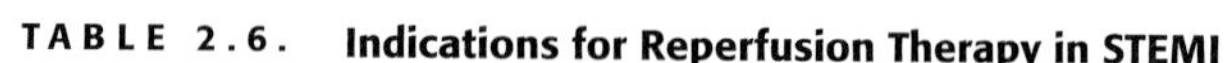

TABLE 2.6. Indications for Reperfusion Therapy in STEMI

Indications for Thrombolytic Therapy or PCI in AMI
1 mm ST elevation in two contiguous limb leads
2 mm ST elevation in two contiguous precordial leads
New LBBB

TABLE 2.7. Contraindications to Fibrinolytic Therapy in Acute Myocardial Infarction

Absolute contraindications
Previous hemorrhagic stroke at any time
Bland CVA in past year
Known intracranial neoplasm
Active internal bleeding (excluding menses)
Suspected aortic dissection or pericarditis
Relative contraindications
Severe uncontrolled blood pressure (> 180/100 mmHg)
History of chronic severe hypertension
History of prior CVA or known intracranial pathology not covered in contraindications
Current use of anticoagulants with known INR > 2–3
Known bleeding diathesis
Recent trauma (past 2 wk)
Prolonged CPR (>10 min)
Major surgery (<3 wk)
Noncompressible vascular punctures (including subclavian and internal jugular central lines)
Recent internal bleeding (2–4 wk)
Prior streptokinase (should not receive streptokinase)
Pregnancy
Active peptic ulcer disease
Other medical conditions likely to increase risk of bleeding

(Reproduced, with permission, from Tintinalli JE, Kelen GD, Stapczynski JS. *Emergency Medicine: A Comprehensive Study Guide*, 6th ed. New York: McGraw-Hill, 2004:353.)

COMPLICATIONS

Divided into early and late complications (see Table 2.9)

SPECIAL GROUPS IN ACUTE CORONARY SYNDROME (ACS)

Women

- Prolonged atypical prodromal symptoms: fatigue, shortness of breath, anxiety, ingestion
- Delay in seeking care
- Physicians tend to minimize their symptoms.

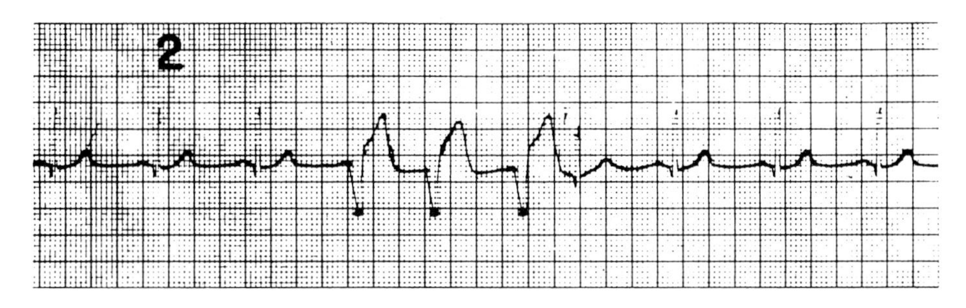

FIGURE 2.13. Accelerated idioventricular rhythms.

(Reproduced, with permission, from Tintinalli JE, Kelen GD, Stapczynski JS. *Emergency Medicine: A Comprehensive Study Guide*, 6th ed. New York: McGraw-Hill, 2004:189.)

TABLE 2.8. Agents Used in the Treatment of Acute Coronary Syndrome

Agent	Effect/Benefits	Contraindications
O_2	Uncertain	None
Aspirin	Antiplatelet agent Onset = **minutes** Reduces long-term mortality	Allergy
Clopidogrel Ticlodipine	Antiplatelet agent Patient with aspirin allergy Onset = **hours**	Expected CABG within 5 d
Nitroglycerin	Dilates coronary arteries Relaxes vascular smooth muscle ↓ Preload and afterload ↓ Myocardial O_2 demand May ↓ infarct size and ↓ mortality	SBP < 100 mmHg RV infarct Use of erectile dysfunction meds Severe AS
β-Blockers	↓ Sympathetic stimulation ↓ Myocardial O_2 demand ↓ VFib ↓ Long-term mortality	SBP < 100 mmHg HR < 60 bpm Pulmonary edema 2nd-, 3rd-degree heart block Reactive airway disease
Morphine	↓ Sympathetic activity ↓ Preload ↓ Myocardial O_2 demand No proven ↓ in mortality	SBP < 100 mmHg
Heparin	Antithrombotic agent Synergistic effect with ASA LMW preferred in unstable angina or NSTEMI	
Glycoprotein IIb/IIIa inhibitors	Blocks platelet aggregation Benefit in patients undergoing PCI	Active internal bleeding Bleeding < 30 d Platelet count < 150,000 History of intracranial hemorrhage, AVM, aneurysm Stroke < 30 d Major surgery or trauma < 30 d
Thrombolytics	Used in STEMI < 12 h from onset Bind plasminogen, which degrades fibrin "Clot busting"	See Table 2.7.
Primary coronary intervention	Preferred over lytics in STEMI if: Door to cath < 90 minutes > 3 h since onset Uncertain diagnosis	PCI not available
ACE inhibitors	LV remodeling ↓ CHF, sudden death and subsequent MI ↓ Mortality if EF < 40%	Pregnancy History of angioedema SBP < 100 mmHg Renal failure Hyperkalemia

TABLE 2.9. **Complications of Myocardial Infarction**

	Clinical Features	Treatment
Early Complications		
Congestive heart failure	Ranging from mild congestion (Killip II MI) to pulmonary edema (Killip III MI) (15–40% mortality)	Standard MI therapy Diuresis Reperfusion
Cardiogenic shock	Pulmonary congestion and peripheral hypoperfusion (Killip IV MI; 80% mortality)	Reperfusion Inotropes Balloon pump
Bradydysrhythmias and AV block	Inferior MI: AV nodal, proximal to HIS bundle Stable and transient Anterior MI: Infranodal at lower HIS bundle, poor prognosis Respond poorly to therapy	Observation Transvenous pacing if: Symptomatic bradycardia, 2nd-degree AVB type II, new bifascicular block with Ist-degree AV block, bilateral BBB
Tachydysrhythmias	Occur in majority of patients	ACLS
Left ventricular free wall rupture	Rapid decline to PEA, pericardial effusion on ultrasound	Pericardiocentesis and surgical repair
Rupture of inter-ventricular septum	Rapid decline with new, harsh, systolic murmur	Surgical repair
Papillary muscle rupture	Day 3–5 after inferior MI. Acute pulmonary edema with new systolic murmur.	Surgical repair
Infarct pericarditis (different from Dressler's syndrome)	Transmural infarct ECG abnormalities often masked by evolutionary changes	Supportive care
Late Complications		
LV thrombus	Stroke or emboli	Anticoagulation
Pleuropericarditis (Dressler's syndrome)	2–10 weeks post-MI Fever, leukocytosis, friction rub, pericardial or pleural effusion	NSAIDs and steroids
LV aneurysm	Following large MI (anterior most common) CHF, dysrhythmias, thromboemboli, persistent ST-elevation on ECG	Anticoagulation, surgery

- More likely to have DM and HTN, less likely to be smokers
- Older than men at time of first MI
- Worse prognosis because of delayed and less aggressive care

Cocaine-associated

- Greatest risk within first hour after use
- Arterial vasoconstriction, sympathetic stimulation, increased platelet aggregation, accelerated atherosclerosis and thrombosis
- Only one-third of cocaine-associated MI have significant CAD on cardiac catheterization
- Atypical symptoms: dyspnea, diaphoresis, nausea
- ECG changes more atypical
- 6% of all cocaine chest pain patients rule in by cardiac markers
- Treat with O_2, NTG, ASA, benzodiazepines. Beware of using β-blockers (including labetalol) because of unopposed α adrenergic effects.
- Complications are extremely rare if they do not present within 12 hours of presentation.

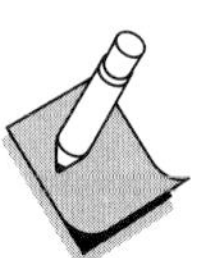

Ischemic heart disease is the most common cause of heart failure in the United States.

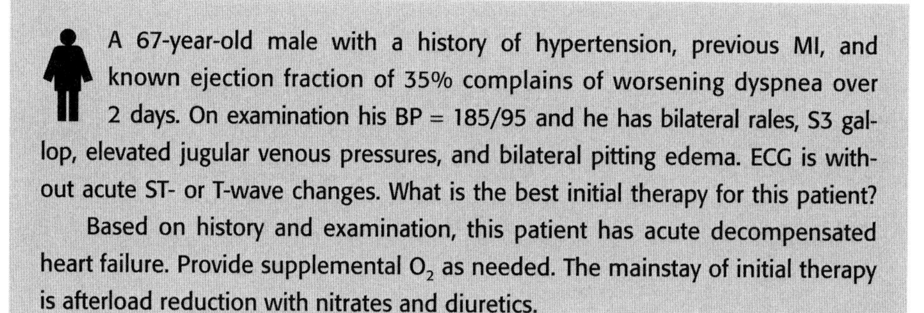

A 67-year-old male with a history of hypertension, previous MI, and known ejection fraction of 35% complains of worsening dyspnea over 2 days. On examination his BP = 185/95 and he has bilateral rales, S3 gallop, elevated jugular venous pressures, and bilateral pitting edema. ECG is without acute ST- or T-wave changes. What is the best initial therapy for this patient?

Based on history and examination, this patient has acute decompensated heart failure. Provide supplemental O_2 as needed. The mainstay of initial therapy is afterload reduction with nitrates and diuretics.

HEART FAILURE

Heart failure is the inability of the myocardium to adequately meet the demands of the body.

CAUSES

Common causes are listed in Table 2.10.

Systolic Versus Diastolic Dysfunction

Systolic dysfunction:

- Usually from ischemic heart disease and myocardial cell death
- Impaired contractility
- Ejection fraction (EF) < 40%
- Output is dependent on resistance to emptying the ventricle (afterload).

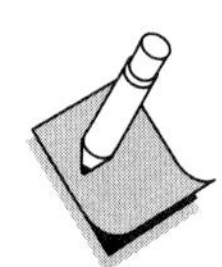

With diastolic dysfunction, cardiac output is dependent on ventricular filling (preload).

Diastolic dysfunction:

- Usually from chronic HTN and left ventricular hypertrophy
- **Impaired relaxation and ventricular filling**
- Normal ejection fraction
- Output is dependent on filling of the ventricle (preload)

With systolic dysfunction, cardiac output is dependent on resistance to emptying the ventricle (afterload).

Other terms used to describe heart failure are based on clinical presentation:

- Left-sided vs R-sided heart failure
- High output heart failure

TABLE 2.10. Common Causes of Heart Failure

Common Causes of Heart Failure
Ischemic heart disease–most common
Cardiomyopathy
Congenital heart disease
Valvular disease
Hypertension
Myocarditis
Constrictive pericarditis
Tamponade
Pulmonary disease (from pulmonary HTN)
High-output states (thyrotoxicosis, anemia, beriberi, Paget disease, arteriovenous fistula)

- Acute heart failure vs chronic heart failure
- Cor pulmonale: enlargement of the right ventricle from underlying lung disease

PATHOPHYSIOLOGY

What determines ideal myocyte contraction?

- **Preload**—the force (volume) stretching the myocytes **before** contraction
- **Afterload**—the force needed to overcome both the volume of blood in the ventricle and the peripheral vascular resistance **during** contraction
- **Contractility** of myocytes

Underlying disease process → myocyte cell death and/or hypertrophy.

- Predominance of cell death → ↓ contractility and low EF → neurohormonal response with ↑ aldosterone, renin, and circulating catecholamines → fluid retention (above ideal preload) and ↑ afterload.
- Predominance of cell hypertrophy → stiff, less compliant heart → poor ventricular filling with a preserved EF.
- Often both are present simultaneously.

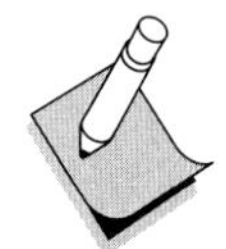

Ideal myocyte contraction is determined by preload, afterload, and contractility.

Decompensated Heart Failure and Pulmonary Edema

CAUSES

Triggers of acute decompensation include:

- ACS
- Dysrhythmia
- Acute HTN
- Acute valvular dysfunction
- Severe high output state: Anemia, thyrotoxicosis, acute AV shunt
- Myocarditis
- PE
- Increased metabolic demand: Infection, exertion

- Medication: Effect or noncompliance
- Sodium load (diet)
- Volume overload, often iatrogenic

Decompensation may be acute or gradual in onset, depending on the underlying trigger. Cardiogenic pulmonary edema occurs when a rapid elevation of pulmonary capillary hydrostatic pressure forces fluid from the intravascular space into the alveolar space.

SYMPTOMS

- Fatigue, weakness, memory problems
- Mild dyspnea to marked respiratory distress (depending on severity)
- Left heart failure
  - Dyspnea
  - Orthopnea
  - Paroxysmal nocturnal dyspnea
- Right heart failure
  - Dyspnea
  - Abdominal distention or pain
  - Leg swelling

EXAM

- Diaphoresis, tachycardia, HTN: From sympathetic activation
- Tachypnea, rales, and/or "cardiac" wheezes
- S3 and S4 gallop
- Underlying or associated right heart failure
  - Hepatic enlargement
  - Peripheral edema
  - Jugular venous distention
  - Hepatojugular reflex
- End stage = severe hypoxia and ventilatory failure with mental status change and terminal dysrhythmias
- Look for evidence of underlying cause/event: infection, PE, valvular disease.

DIFFERENTIAL

- Noncardiogenic pulmonary edema in which capillary membrane *permeability* is compromised (infection, ARDS, drug reaction)
- Pneumonia, asthma, COPD, PE

DIAGNOSIS

BNP < 100 pg/mL makes heart failure unlikely.

- **ECG**
  - Look for LVH, ischemia, dysrhythmias.
- **Upright chest radiograph (CXR)**
  - CXR findings may lag clinical findings!
  - **Progression of CXR changes**
    - Vascular congestion (cephalization of vessels) →
    - Interstitial edema (Kerley B lines, haziness) →
    - Alveolar infiltrates (butterfly pattern, effusions)
  - Normal heart size? Suspect noncardiogenic pulmonary edema or acute valve failure.
- Labs
  - To identify underlying causes: renal failure, anemia, MI, hyperkalemia
- **B-type natriuretic peptide (BNP)**
  - Released in response to ventricular myocyte stretch
  - Level ↑ with severity of CHF

- BNP < 100 pg/dL makes heart failure unlikely.
- BNP > 500 pg/dL makes heart failure highly probable.
- Should be compared to patient's baseline values
- Can be elevated in the elderly, renal failure, PE, or cor pulmonale
- Tends to be lower in obese patients

- **Echocardiogram**
  - Assesses systolic, diastolic, and valvular function

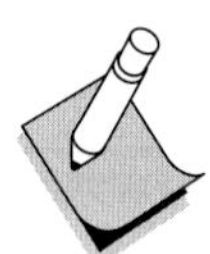

The echocardiogram is the most helpful study to assess cardiac function in heart failure.

TREATMENT

- Aggressiveness of treatment depends on severity of presentation.
- Supportive therapy, as needed
- Supplemental O_2
- **Noninvasive positive pressure ventilation**
  - BiPAP or CPAP
  - Benefits: ↑ Oxygenation, ↓ work of breathing, ↓ preload and afterload
- **Nitroglycerin (NTG)**
  - Sublingual, then IV if needed
  - ↓ Preload by venodilation
  - ↓ Afterload (at high doses) via arterial vasodilation
  - Direct coronary vasodilator (good in ischemia)
  - May not be tolerated if patient is hypotensive
- **Morphine sulfate**
  - ↓ Myocardial O_2 consumption by ↓ catecholamines
  - ↓ Preload from mild vasodilator effect
  - ↓ Pain and anxiety
  - May ↑ mortality
- **Furosemide**
  - For patients with evidence of fluid retention that usually develops over days; not for use in rapid decompensation as these patients are volume neutral or even dehydrated
  - Rapid symptom relief from venodilator effect
  - Delayed effects = ↓ preload and pulmonary congestion by reducing volume

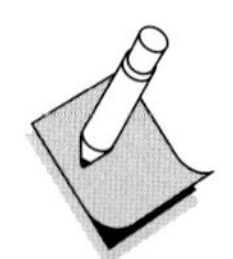

Furosemide may provide rapid symptoms relief from venodilator effects.

- **Nitroprusside**
  - For persistent hypertension, not relieved with NTG
  - More potent arterial vasodilator than NTG, ↓ afterload
  - ↓ Preload via venodilator effect
  - May dilate normal coronaries more than diseased → coronary steal syndrome

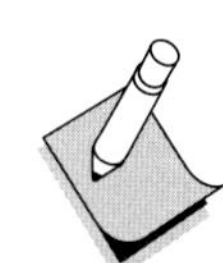

Nitroprusside may dilate normal coronaries more than diseased coronaries, causing a coronary steal syndrome.

- **Nesiritide**
  - For acute decompensated heart failure without cardiogenic shock
  - Antagonizes renin-aldosterone system and sympathetic nervous system →
    - Diuresis
    - ↓ Preload via venodilation
    - ↓ Afterload via vasodilation
  - May ↑ mortality
- **Treatment of cardiogenic shock**
  - Suspect if hypotension **and** poor perfusion are present
  - Correct any underlying hypovolemia *first* with judicious fluid challenge (to maximize preload).
  - Dopamine/dobutamine
    - Both are + inotropes and + chronotropes.
    - Dobutamine may exacerbate hypotension (vasodilator effect).
  - Norepinephrine
    - If persistent hypotension despite above measures
    - ↑ Systemic vascular resistance

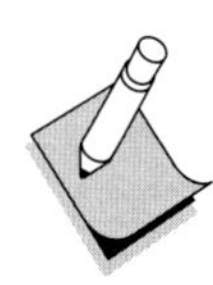

Norepinephrine will ↑ HR and myocardial O_2 demand.

TABLE 2.11. Medications for Decompensated Heart Failure and Pulmonary Edema

Medication	Beneficial Effects	Deleterious Effects
Nitroglycerin	↓ Preload ↓ Afterload (high doses) Coronary vasodilation	Severe hypotension with: Viagra use Aortic stenosis Hypertrophic cardiomyopathy RV infarct
Morphine	↓ Catecholamines ↓ Preload (mild) ↓ Anxiety, pain	CNS and respiratory depression
Furosemide	Immediate venodilator effect (↓ preload) Delayed diuresis	Hypotension from hypovolemia Hypokalemia
Nitroprusside	↓ Afterload ↓ Preload Coronary vasodilation	Coronary steal Hypotension
Nesiritide	Diuresis ↓ Preload ↓ Afterload	Hypotension Renal failure ?Increased mortality

        - ↑ BP and coronary perfusion pressure
        - Will ↑ HR and myocardial O_2 demand
    - Intra-aortic balloon pump as bridge to revascularization or valvular repair (contraindicated in acute aortic regurgitation)
- **Treat any precipitating events**
    - Blood pressure control
    - Correct dysrhythmias (rate control or conversion)
    - Treat infection, ischemia, etc.
- **Avoid**
    - Nitrates in patients taking erectile dysfunction drugs.
    - Nitrates in severe aortic stenosis, RV infarct, and diastolic dysfunction (need preload!)
    - Excessive diuresis in patients with acute pulmonary edema or preload dependent states (may actually need the intravascular volume)

Table 2.11 summarizes the medications for decompensated heart failure and pulmonary edema.

Complications

- Dysrhythmias and sudden death
- Intracardiac thrombus and embolism
- Progression of disease

Stable Chronic Heart Failure

Symptoms

- The New York Heart Association (NYHA) classifies heart failure based on severity of symptoms (see Table 2.12). These classifications have prognostic and treatment implications.

TABLE 2.12. NYHA Functional Classification for Chronic Heart Failure

CLASS	FUNCTIONAL ABILITY
Class I (Mild)	No limitation of ordinary physical activity
Class II (Mild)	Mild dyspnea, fatigue, or palpitations with ordinary physical activity
Class III (Moderate)	Symptoms with less than ordinary physical activity
Class IV (Severe)	Marked symptoms at rest

TREATMENT

- Lifestyle modification
- Treat underlying etiology when possible.
- Aggressive blood pressure and heart rate control (key component in isolated diastolic dysfunction)
- **ACE inhibitors**
  - ↓ Mortality and hospitalizations
  - Beneficial effects on LV remodeling
  - Complications include cough, angioedema, and renal failure.
- **Angiotensin receptor blockers**
  - If ACE inhibitor not tolerated
- **Hydralazine with nitrates**
  - If ACE inhibitors not tolerated
- **β-Blockers**
  - ↓ Mortality and improves symptoms
  - Allows for ↑ filling time in diastolic dysfunction
  - Do **not** start during acute decompensation of systolic function.
- **Diuretics**
  - For patients with evidence of fluid retention
- **Digoxin**
  - For refractory cases of systolic dysfunction
- If class IV symptoms:
  - Spironolactone
  - Mechanical assist device
  - Heart transplant
  - Inotrope infusion

PERICARDIAL DISEASE

Pericarditis

The pericardium may become inflamed for a variety of reasons. The resulting clinical presentation is sometimes confused with acute myocardial infarction. The **vast majority** of cases are **idiopathic**. Identified causes include:

- Infectious
  - Viral (eg, coxsackie, adenovirus)
  - Bacterial: Less common
  - TB
  - Fungal
  - Parasitic
  - Rickettsia

- Medications
  - Procainamide
  - Hydralazine
  - INH
- Systemic diseases
  - SLE
  - Scleroderma
  - Rheumatic fever
- Post MI (2–10 weeks): Dressler syndrome
- Malignancy
- Uremia
- Posttraumatic

The chest pain of pericarditis is characteristically exacerbated by deep inspiration and relieved by leaning forward.

PATHOPHYSIOLOGY

- Inflammation of pericardium → pericardial thickening and effusion

SYMPTOMS

- Substernal chest pain
  - Exacerbated by deep inspiration
  - Relieved by **leaning forward**
  - Radiation to the trapezius sometimes seen
- Fatigue
- Intermittent fever

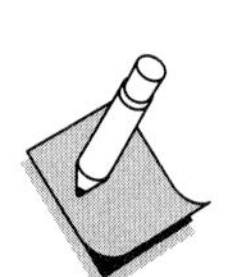

Hallmark of pericarditis = pericardial friction rub

EXAM

- **Pericardial friction rub** = classic finding
  - Auscultate with patient leaning forward.
  - Biphasic and "scratchy," best at left sternal border

DIFFERENTIAL

- Myocarditis
- Acute coronary syndrome
  - PR depression is seen in atrial infarction.
  - If ST elevation present, look for regional distribution and reciprocal T wave inversions (not seen in pericarditis).

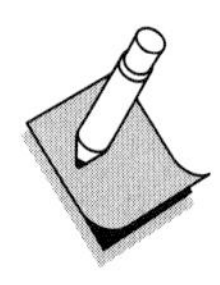

PR depression is specific for pericarditis.

DIAGNOSIS

- Suspect in any patient presenting with chest pain and fever (although fever is not a necessary finding)

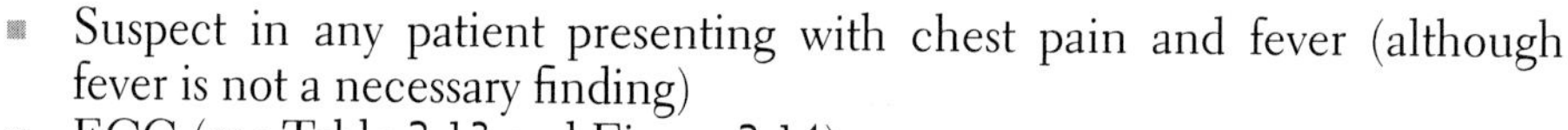

- ECG (see Table 2.13 and Figure 2.14)
  - Stage 1 (first hours to days): PR depression and diffuse (except aVR, V_1) ST elevation with concave up segments
  - Stage 2: ST and PR segments normalize, T waves flatten
  - Stage 3: Diffuse T-wave inversions
  - Stage 4: Returns to normal
- CXR: Usually nonspecific, but may show cardiomegaly if a pericardial effusion is present
- Echocardiogram: To evaluate for pericardial effusion and tamponade (see below)
- Laboratory studies: Expect leukocytosis, ↑ESR, ↑cardiac enzymes, ↑ BUN/Cr (if uremic etiology)

TABLE 2.13. **Progression of ECG Changes in Acute Pericarditis**

ECG in Acute Pericarditis	
Stage 1	PR depression and diffuse ST elevation
Stage 2	ST and PR normalize, T waves flatten
Stage 3	Diffuse T-wave inversion
Stage 4	Returns to normal

Treatment

- Treat underlying etiology.
- ASA or NSAIDs for anti-inflammatory effects and pain control
- Narcotics for intractable pain
- Steroids in patients with ongoing symptoms after infectious etiology excluded
- Mild cases attributed to viral origin can usually be managed as outpatients.

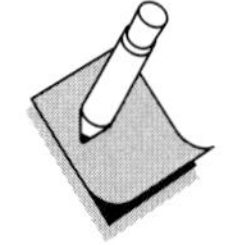

Steroids are used in chronic pericarditis and in patients who cannot tolerate NSAIDs.

Complications

- Pericardial tamponade
- **Constrictive pericarditis**
  - Fibrotic change reduces diastolic filling.
  - Kussmaul's sign: increase in JVP during inspiration
  - "Dip and plateau" LV filling (or diastolic) tracing

Pericardial Effusion and Tamponade

While cardiac tamponade results from a pericardial effusion, **not all effusions** cause tamponade. An effusion that develops slowly allows for the pericardium to stretch and the LV volume to increase in response to the fluid, decreasing the likelihood of tamponade.

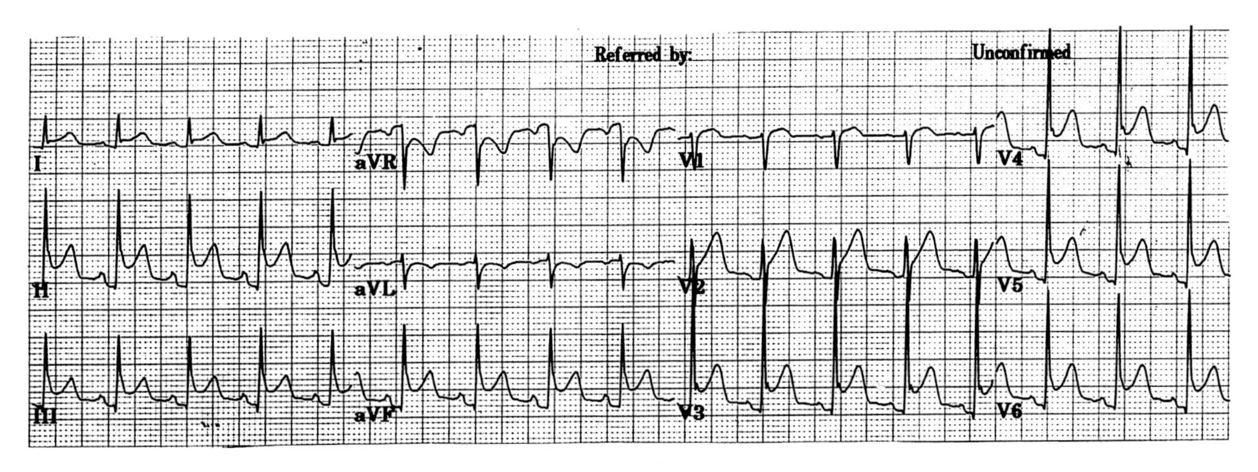

FIGURE 2.14. **Pericarditis with ST elevation in multiple regions.**

(Reproduced, with permission, from Fuster V, Alexander RW, O'Rourke, RA. *Hurst's The Heart,* 12th ed. New York: McGraw-Hill, 2008:303.)

ETIOLGIES

Most common etiologies of pericardial effusion:

- Trauma
- Pericarditis
- Renal failure

SYMPTOMS/EXAM

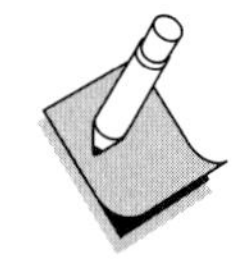

Beck's triad (tamponade):

Hypotension

JVD

Muffled heart sounds

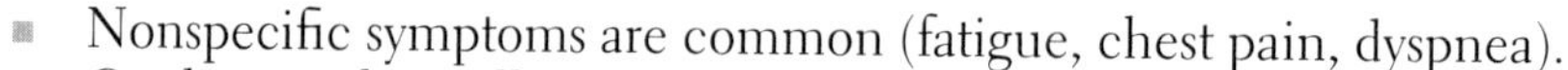

- Nonspecific symptoms are common (fatigue, chest pain, dyspnea).
- Cardiovascular collapse may occur if rapidly developing (eg, traumatic effusion).
- **Beck's triad** is classic for tamponade.
  - Hypotension
  - Jugular venous distention (JVD)
  - Muffled heart sounds
- Pericardial friction rub
- Tachycardia
- Narrowed pulse pressure
- **Kussmaul's sign** = ↑ in jugular venous pressure during inspiration
- Pulsus paradoxus = inspiratory reduction in systolic pressure of > 10 mmHg

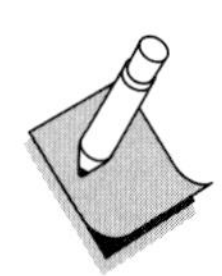

Kussmaul's sign—may also be seen with restrictive cardiomyopathy and constrictive pericarditis.

DIAGNOSIS

- Suspect based on history and physical examination
- ECG
  - Low QRS voltage = nonspecific
  - **Electrical alternans** = variation of height of the QRS complexes as a result of the heart swinging within the pericardial effusion
- Echocardiogram—diagnostic study of choice
  - Tamponade physiology represented by **R ventricular collapse during diastole**
  - Sniff test → lack of proximal IVC collapse with quick breath in through nose ("sniff")
  - Magnitude of the effusion can be evaluated.

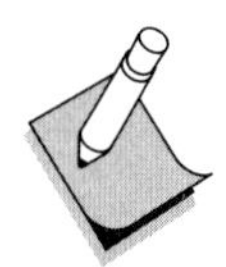

Electrical alternans = tamponade until proven otherwise.

TREATMENT

- No tamponade physiology
  - Supplemental O_2
  - Volume resuscitation to improve left ventricular filling pressures
  - Immediate cardiothoracic surgery or cardiology consult
  - Prepare for pericardiocentesis.
- Pericardial tamponade → immediate pericardiocentesis

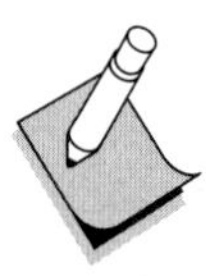

ECHO confirmation of tamponade = RV collapse during diastole.

> A 25-year-old male presents with flu-like symptoms, chest pain, and worsening shortness of breath. He has no past medical history, but recently returned from a 2-week camping trip to Central America. On examination, the patient has bilateral rales, S3, and jugular venous distention. His ECG shows tachycardia and nonspecific T-wave changes. Echocardiogram shows diffuse hypokinesis. What is the most likely etiologic agent in this patient?
>
> This patient likely has myocarditis from the parasite *Trypanasoma cruzi*. Chagas disease, which results from infection with *Trypanasoma cruzi,* is the most common etiology of myocarditis worldwide. It is especially common in Latin America.

MYOCARDITIS

Myocarditis is characterized by inflammation of the myocardium.

A number of **infectious agents** have been implicated (see Table 2.14).

- Viral agents are the most common etiology in the United States.
- *Trypanasoma cruzi* is the most common etiology worldwide.
  - Chagas disease, from the bite of the kissing bug
  - Common in Latin America

Myocarditis may also result from **autoimmune diseases, chemical exposure, or drugs**.

- Kawasaki's, sarcoidosis, SLE
- Penicillins, sulfonamides, cocaine

PATHOPHYSIOLOGY

- Direct invasion or inflammatory response to agent → myocardial damage.
- Often associated with pericarditis.

SYMPTOMS

- Flu-like symptoms: Fever, fatigue, myalgias, vomiting, diarrhea
- Retrosternal chest pain
- Dyspnea
- Palpitations
- Syncope or near syncope

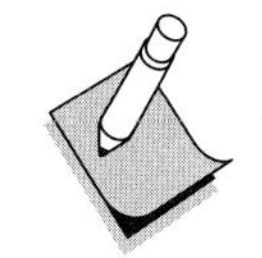

Flu-like symptoms and new CHF? Suspect myocarditis.

EXAM

- Sinus tachycardia beyond what would be expected from fever
- Rales
- Peripheral edema
- Jugular venous distention

DIAGNOSIS

- Suspect in any patient presenting with flu-like symptoms and CHF
- ECG
  - Tachycardia
  - Nonspecific ST-T changes
  - AV block or other conduction abnormalities
  - Low QRS voltages

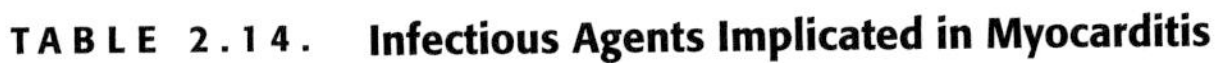

TABLE 2.14. Infectious Agents Implicated in Myocarditis

VIRAL	BACTERIAL	PARASITIC
Coxsackie B virus	β-Hemolytic strep (rheumatic fever)	*Trypanasoma cruzi* (Chagas disease)
Adenovirus	*Mycoplasma pneumoniae*	*Trichinella spiralis* (trichonosis)
Echovirus	*Corynebacterium diphtheria* (diphtheria)	
	Borrelia burgdorferi (Lyme disease)	

- CXR: Usually normal, but may show cardiomegaly or pulmonary edema
- ECG: Dilated chambers and diffuse or focal hypokinesis
- CBC: Mild elevation of WBC count
- Elevated ESR
- Elevated cardiac enzymes
- Biopsy: May be helpful but can miss areas of involvement (false-negative)

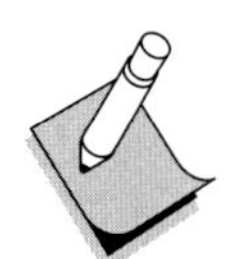

ACE inhibitors play an important role in the treatment of myocarditis.

TREATMENT

- Address infectious etiology, if identified.
- Supportive care
- Bed rest
- IVIG and ASA for Kawasaki's in children
- Diuresis for CHF
- **ACE inhibitors** help reduce myocardial inflammation.

COMPLICATIONS

- Sudden death
- Emboli
- Dysrhythmias
- Dilated cardiomyopathy

> A 32-year-old female presents to the ED with 2 days of progressive shortness of breath. She is 3 weeks postpartum after an uneventful pregnancy and vaginal delivery. On examination, the patient is in mild respiratory distress, has bilateral rales, jugular venous distention, and is tachycardic to a rate of 120 bpm. Bedside echocardiogram shows dilated chambers and poor systolic function. What is the treatment of choice for this patient?
>
> The patient likely has a peripartum dilated cardiomyopathy. ACE inhibitors are essential in the treatment of dilated cardiomyopathies. If they are not tolerated (or if the patient were still pregnant) a combination of hydralazine and nitrates should be started.

CARDIOMYOPATHIES

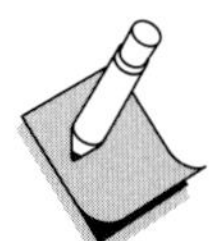

Four types of cardiomyopathy:
Dilated
Hypertrophic
Restrictive
Arrhythmogenic right ventricular dysplasia

Cardiomyopathies encompass a group of pathologies that alter the structure of the heart itself, impairing normal cardiac function. Based on the World Health Organization classification, there are four types of cardiomyopathy:

- Dilated
- Hypertrophic
- Restrictive
- Arrhythmogenic right ventricular dysplasia

Extrinsic causes of cardiomyopathy include hypertension, valvular disease, ischemia, systemic disease, and inflammation.

Dilated Cardiomyopathy

Dilated cardiomyopathy is a spectrum of disorders resulting in depressed myocardial systolic function and pump failure. **All four chambers are dilated.**

CAUSES

The vast majority of cases are **idiopathic**, but known causes include:

- Peripartum
  - Most common in first two months postpartum but can occur between last month of pregnancy and first six months postpartum
  - More common in older multiparous women and twin gestations
  - 50% will have complete resolution.
- Heavy alcohol use
- Heavy cocaine use
- Viral myocarditis
- Amyloidosis: Can also cause restrictive cardiomyopathy
- CAD
- Hypothyroidism and hyperthyroidism

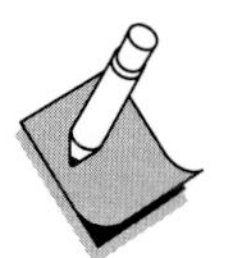

Amyloidosis can cause a dilated or a restrictive cardiomyopathy.

PATHOPHYSIOLOGY

- Myocardial cell death and fibrosis → cardiac chamber dilatation and systolic dysfunction

SYMPTOMS

- Dyspnea
- Fatigue
- Palpitations
- Lower extremity swelling

EXAM

- Rales
- Laterally displaced point of maximal impulse (PMI)
- Jugular venous distention
- Peripheral edema

DIAGNOSIS

- ECG is nonspecific, but may include
  - Left atrial enlargement
  - Left ventricular hypertrophy
  - Conduction abnormalities
  - Atrial fibrillation
- CXR
  - "Globular" enlarged heart
  - Pulmonary edema
- Echocardiogram demonstrates four-chamber enlargement and impaired LV function.

TREATMENT

- Supportive therapy
- ACE inhibitors
  - Provide afterload reduction
  - Reduce morbidity and mortality
  - Alternative (if ACE inhibitor contraindicated) = combination of hydralazine and nitrates
- β-Blockers: Improve survival
- Diuretics and digitalis: Improve symptoms, but not survival
- AICD placement
- Anticoagulation
- Severe cases require transplantation.

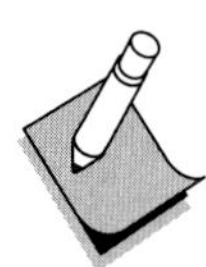

Diuresis and digoxin improve symptoms in dilated cardiomyopathy, but do not improve survival.

COMPLICATIONS

- Sequelae of CHF
- Dysrhythmias
- Pulmonary and peripheral embolization from mural thrombus
- Sudden death

Restrictive Cardiomyopathy

Restrictive cardiomyopathy is characterized by heart muscle disease that results in restricted ventricular filling while systolic function remains normal.

Systemic disorders associated with restrictive cardiomyopathy include amyloidosis, sarcoidosis, hemochromatosis, and tropical endomyocardial fibrosis (most common cause worldwide).

PATHOPHYSIOLOGY

- Fibrotic process reduces the size of the left ventricle → reduced filling of L ventricle → ↑ diastolic pressures and ↓ diastolic volumes.

R-sided heart failure symptoms (JVD, hepatomegaly) predominate in restrictive cardiomyopathy.

SYMPTOMS

- R-sided heart failure symptoms may predominate
- Dyspnea
- Fatigue
- Lower extremity swelling

EXAM

- **Kussmaul's sign:** Increase in jugular venous pressure during inspiration
- Rales
- Jugular venous distention
- Hepatomegaly
- Edema

DIFFERENTIAL

- It is important to exclude **constrictive pericarditis** and diastolic LV dysfunction (eg, HTN) as these are both treatable.

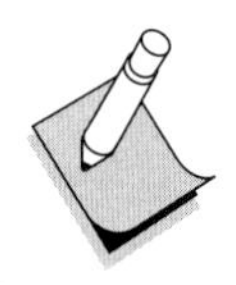

Consider restrictive cardiomyopathy in the patient presenting with CHF without cardiomegaly or systolic dysfunction.

DIAGNOSIS

- ECG: Nonspecific, decreased voltages, conduction abnormalities
- CXR: Mild (if any) cardiomegaly
- Echocardiogram: Normal left ventricular size and systolic function, dilated atria
- Characteristic **"dip and plateau"** (also seen with constrictive pericarditis) of LV pressures on catheterization
- Biopsy is definitive.

TREATMENT

- Limited treatment modalities
- Diuretics
- Treat underlying disease process, if present.

COMPLICATIONS

- CHF

A 17-year-old male presents to the ED after passing out during basketball practice. He has no symptoms now, but his mom insisted he come in because his cousin died while playing basketball 2 years ago. On examination, there is a systolic murmur that worsens with standing. What is the most likely diagnosis?

Hypertrophic cardiomyopathy. Syncope is an independent predictor of sudden cardiac death in patients with HCM. This patient requires hospitalization for further monitoring and evaluation.

Hypertrophic Cardiomyopathy (HCM)

HCM was previously referred to as idiopathic hypertrophic subaortic stenosis (IHSS). This is often an autosomal dominant disorder, so always ask about sudden death or early cardiac disorders in family members. It is characterized by asymmetric thickening of the LV septal wall.

Pathophysiology

- Decreased diastolic filling (diastolic dysfunction) from reduced compliance
- Obstruction of the LV outflow tract
- Overall cardiac function is usually normal.

Symptoms

- Dyspnea
- **Exertional syncope** or sudden cardiac death
- Chest pain
- Palpitations and decreased exercise tolerance

Murmur of hypertrophic cardiomyopathy

↓ LV filling (standing, valsalva) = ↑ murmur.

↑ LV filling (squatting, leg elevation) = ↓ murmur.

This is the opposite of aortic stenosis!

Exam

- Loud crescendo-decrescendo systolic murmur heard best at the left lower sternal border.
- Murmur increases with ↓ LV filling (standing, valsalva) by increasing obstruction of LV outflow tract.
- Murmur decreases with ↑ LV filling (squatting, leg elevation, or Trendelenburg) by lessening obstruction.
- Paradoxically split S2
- Bifid arterial pulse

Differential

- Aortic stenosis, pulmonary stenosis, VSD, mitral regurgitation

Diagnosis

- Suspect in any young person with exertional syncope, family history of sudden death or characteristic murmur
- ECG: Left atrial enlargement and LVH, **septal Q waves**
- CXR: Mild cardiomegaly
- Echo: Confirmatory: Left ventricular hypertrophy, asymmetric septal hypertrophy

Treatment

- Counsel avoidance of exertion.
- Endocarditis prophylaxis

- β-Blockers and calcium channel blockers to decrease obstruction
- Treat atrial fibrillation (consider anticoagulation).
- **Avoid:** Positive inotropes or nitrates, which will worsen obstruction.
- Admit for monitoring if syncope, near-syncope, or presence of dysrhythmia.
- Surgery

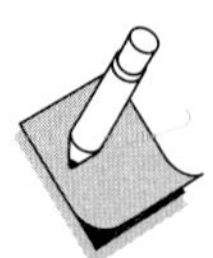

β-Blockers and/or calcium channel blockers are the mainstay of therapy for hypertrophic cardiomyopathy.

COMPLICATIONS

- Dysrhythmias (atrial fibrillation, PVCs most common)
- Exertional syncope
- Sudden cardiac death

Arrythmogenic Right Ventricular Dysplasia

As the name implies, this cardiomyopathy is characterized by right ventricular dysplasia and ventricular dysrhythmias. It is an autosomal dominant disorder common in regions of Italy.

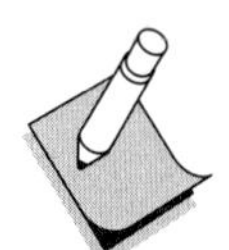

Unlike other cardiomyopathies, the physical exam is typically normal in arrhythmogenic right ventricular dysplasia.

PATHOPHYSIOLOGY

- Replacement of right ventricle myocardium with fibrofatty tissue
- Overall cardiac function is normal.

SYMPTOMS/EXAM

- Sudden cardiac death or ventricular dysrhythmias
- Normal examination

DIAGNOSIS

- ECG: May see **RBBB pattern**
- CXR: Normal
- Echo: Right ventricular enlargement and dysfunction
- Biopsy is confirmatory.

TREATMENT

- Antidysrhythmics and/or AICD to prevent sudden death

A 24-year-old female with a history of injection drug use presents with complaint of fever and chills with generalized malaise over the last 2 days. On examination, she is afebrile, but you find tender nodules on the tip of her second and third fingers. What is the most appropriate management for this patient?

This patient likely has *Staphylococcus aureus* infective endocarditis. Her fingertip lesions are referred to as Osler's nodes, one of the immunologic manifestations of endocarditis. The most appropriate management is to obtain blood cultures, administer vancomycin, and admit the patient.

INFECTIVE ENDOCARDITIS

Infective endocarditis is an infection of the endocardium that typically involves the valves and adjacent structure. A wide range of infecting organisms has been identified. Of the organisms, *Staphylococcus aureus* is considered to be the most virulent, with a rapid destruction of affected valves.

Risk factors for endocarditis include:

- Congenital heart disease
- Rheumatic heart disease
- Injection drug use (IDU)
- Prosthetic valves
- Mitral valve prolapse with regurgitation
- Presence of a cardiac pacemaker

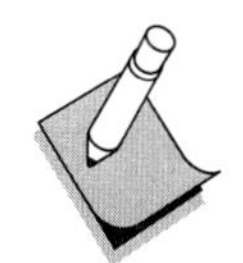

***R-sided endocarditis**–think IVDA, acute/fulminant course, S. aureus.*

***L-sided endocarditis**–think native valve disease, indolent course, Streptococci.*

PATHOPHYSIOLOGY

- The presence of a foreign body or the disruption of normal flow through the valves → turbulence → platelet aggregation and fibrinogenesis.
- These sterile vegetations are subsequently colonized by bacteria leading to infection and valvular destruction (see Table 2.15).

SYMPTOMS

- Fever (most common): But absence of fever does not rule out endocarditis
- Malaise, weakness
- Body aches, back pain
- Dyspnea

EXAM

- Fever (most common)
- Regurgitation murmur
- Vascular phenomena
  - Septic pulmonary emboli (R-sided disease)
  - CNS emboli (L-sided disease) → hemiplegia, aphasia
  - Janeway lesions—nontender erythematous macules on palms, soles, or fingers

TABLE 2.15. Etiologies of Endocarditis

PREDISPOSING FACTORS	LOCATION	USUAL PATHOGENS
Prosthetic valve < 60 days (early)	Replaced valve	*Staphylococcus* sp.[a] *Enterobacteriaceae* Diphtheroids Fungi
IDU	Tricuspid valve most often	*Staphylococcus aureus*
Native valve	Mitral > aortic >> tricuspid	Streptococci (viridans or others)[a] Staphylococci Enterococci
Prosthetic valve > 60 days (late)	Replaced valve	Same as native valve
Pacemaker, implantable defibrillator	Infection of pacemaker pocket, leads	*Staphylococcus aureus* *Staphylococcus epidermidis*

[a]Most common organism

  - Conjunctival or splinter hemorrhages
  - Petechiae
- Immunologic phenomena:
  - Glomerulonephritis
  - Osler's nodes: Tender nodules on fingertips
  - Roth's spots: Retinal hemorrhages with central clearing
  - Rheumatoid factor

DIAGNOSIS

- Presumptive diagnosis based on predisposing condition and presence of fever
- Duke criteria (see Table 2.16)

TREATMENT

- Antibiotics: Empiric therapy, awaiting culture results
  - Native valves: Penicillin G + nafcillin + gentamicin
  - Injection drug use: Vancomycin
  - Prosthetic valves: Vancomycin + gentamicin + rifampin
- Surgical valve repair or replacement as needed

COMPLICATIONS

- Valvular destruction with resulting CHF
- Septic emboli and sequelae
  - CNS abscesses, mycotic aneurysm, meningitis
  - Septic pulmonary emboli
  - Paraspinal abscesses

Prophylaxis for Endocarditis

The following populations need antibiotics prior to procedures (* = high-risk groups):

- *Prosthetic heart valve
- *Complex congenital heart disease
- *Previous bacterial endocarditis
- Other congenital heart diseases (unrepaired)

TABLE 2.16. Duke Criteria for Establishing the Diagnosis of Endocarditis

Major criteria	Positive blood cultures (≥ 2 separated by site and time) Major echo findings (vegetations, abscess, new regurgitation, dehiscence of prosthetic valve)
Minor criteria	Predisposing conditions Fever Embolic disease Immunologic phenomena Single positive blood culture Nonmajor echo findings
Diagnosis requires: Two major criteria **or** one major + three minor criteria, **or** five minor criteria	

TABLE 2.17. **Antibiotic Recommendation for Endocarditis Prophylaxis**

Prophylaxis for Dental, Oral, Respiratory, and Esophageal Procedures	
Standard	Amoxicillin
Penicillin allergy	Clindamycin **or** Cephalexin **or** Azithromycin
Prophylaxis for Genitourinary and Gastrointestinal (Nonesophageal) Procedures	
Moderate-risk patients	Amoxicillin PO
Moderate-risk patients allergic to penicillin	Vancomycin IV
High-risk patients	Ampicillin + gentamicin IV
High-risk patients allergic to penicillin	Vancomycin + gentamicin IV

- Hypertrophic cardiomyopathy
- Acquired valvular heart disease
- Mitral valve prolapse with murmur

Recommended antibiotics for prophylaxis are listed in Table 2.17. An equivalent intravenous antibiotic should be chosen for patients unable to take the oral recommendations. No prophylaxis is needed for clean procedures (laceration repairs, Foley catheter placement, intubation).

A 45-year-old male presents to the ED with chest pain and severe shortness of breath. Clinically and radiographically, there is evidence of pulmonary edema. He reports a history of IDU and "angina." On cardiac auscultation, there is a loud holosystolic murmur heard throughout the lower precordium with radiation to the apex. The murmur does not change intensity with inspiration or with passive leg elevation. This presentation and murmur is most consistent with what valvular lesion?

This patient is presenting with acute mitral regurgitation. The likely causes include infective endocarditis or acute coronary syndrome, which may be differentiated by ECG. In either case the treatment is aggressive afterload reduction with nitroprusside, dobutamine (if hypotensive), and immediate valve replacement.

VALVULAR EMERGENCIES

The most common **congenital** valvular lesion is a bicuspid aortic valve.

The most common **acquired** valvular lesion is secondary to rheumatic heart disease.

Table 2.18 summarizes the causes and exam findings for common valvular lesions.

CARDIOVASCULAR EMERGENCIES

TABLE 2.18. Valvular Lesions With Associated Physical Findings

Valvular Lesion	Common Etiologies	Murmur	Physical Findings
Aortic stenosis	Calcific valve degeneration Bicuspid aortic valve (< 65 yrs)	Crescendo-decrescendo **systolic** Radiating → neck	Paradoxically split S2 Narrowed pulse pressure Diminished and slow-rising carotid pulse
Aortic regurgitation	**Acute** Endocarditis Aortic dissection **Chronic** Rheumatic heart disease Bicuspid aortic valve	Blowing **diastolic** Heard best at left sternal border	**Acute** Pulmonary edema and CV collapse **Chronic** Widened pulse pressure Rapid ↑ and ↓ of carotid pulse Nail pulsations To-and-fro murmur over femoral artery Soft mid-diastolic rumble
Mitral stenosis	Rheumatic heart disease	**Diastolic** Heard best at apex	Loud S1
Mitral regurgitation	**Acute** Endocarditis ACS **Chronic** Rheumatic heart disease	Loud **holosystolic** Heard best at apex Radiating → base	**Acute** Pulmonary edema and CV collapse **Chronic** LV heave
Mitral valve prolapse	Unknown, likely congenital	Late **systolic** Heard best at left lateral heart border	Early to mid **systolic click**

Aortic Stenosis (AS)

The most common causes are calcific valve degeneration (patients over 65 years), congenital bicuspid valve (younger patients), and rheumatic heart disease (less common). Rheumatic aortic stenosis should be suspected if there is concomitant mitral valve disease.

PATHOPHYSIOLOGY

- Blood flow from the left ventricle is hindered → LVH, ↓ cardiac output, and eventual dilated cardiomyopathy with hypertrophy
- There are usually no signs or symptoms until the aortic outflow tract is reduced by at least 75% (to <1 cm).
- Survival is 2–5 years from onset of symptoms without definitive treatment.

SYMPTOMS

- The **classic triad** of symptomatic aortic stenosis is dyspnea on exertion (CHF), chest pain, and syncope.
- Sudden death from dysrhythmias or acute onset of failure may occur.

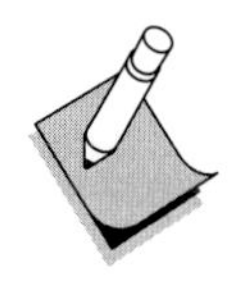

Classic triad of symptomatic aortic stenosis:

Dyspnea, chest pain, and syncope

EXAM

- Crescendo-decrescendo systolic murmur radiating to the neck
- Paradoxically split S2
- Narrowed pulse pressure due to drop in systolic BP
- Low amplitude (**parvus**) and slow rising (**tardus**) carotid pulse
- Brachioradial delay
- Pulmonary edema if severe AS

DIAGNOSIS

- **ECG:** LVH with strain, left bundle branch block
- **CXR:** LVH, pulmonary congestion (if CHF is present)
- **Echocardiography:** Confirms the diagnosis, allows measurement of valve area

TREATMENT

- Treat CHF with gentle diuresis.
- Rule out ACS in acute presentations.
- Hydrate gently for hypotension.
- **Avoid**
  - Preload or afterload reducers (**no nitroglycerin**)
  - Negative inotropes
  - These may cause acute decompensation and severe hypotension.
- Prophylaxis for endocarditis
- Definitive treatment is valve replacement.

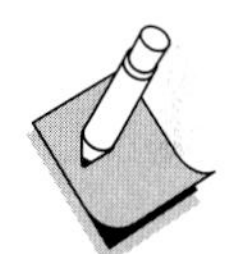

Avoid nitrates in the treatment of aortic stenosis since they may lead to severe hypotension refractory to therapy.

Aortic Regurgitation (Aortic Insufficiency)

Aortic regurgitation (AR) may be acute or chronic. It is important to make this differentiation as acute aortic regurgitation is a surgical emergency requiring immediate valve replacement.

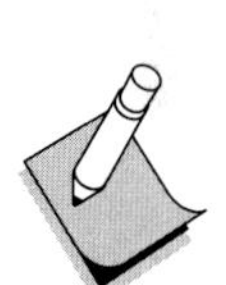

Acute aortic regurgitation? Consider endocarditis, aortic dissection, and trauma.

ETIOLOGIES

- Acute aortic regurgitation
  - Infective endocarditis
  - Aortic dissection with proximal extension
  - Trauma
- Chronic aortic regurgitation
  - Rheumatic heart disease
  - Bicuspid aortic valve
  - Dilation of the aortic root (Marfan, ankylosing spondylitis, rheumatoid arthritis)

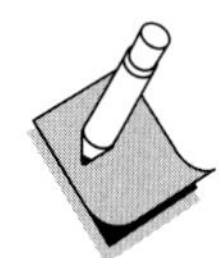

Acute aortic regurgitation is a surgical emergency.

PATHOPHYSIOLOGY

- Acute aortic valve failure → rapid rise in LV diastolic pressure → acute pulmonary edema and cardiogenic shock
- Chronic aortic valve failure → compensatory LVH, gradual left ventricular dilation → gradual onset of heart failure symptoms

ACUTE AORTIC REGURGITATION

SYMPTOMS

- Abrupt onset of dyspnea, tachypnea
- Recent intravenous drug use or fever, if endocarditis
- Chest pain and presence of risk factors, if aortic dissection

EXAM

- Pulmonary edema and cardiovascular collapse
- High-pitched blowing diastolic murmur heard best at left sternal border
- **Normal pulse pressure**

DIAGNOSIS

- Suspect based on history and physical examination
- CXR: Pulmonary edema
- Echocardiography confirms diagnosis

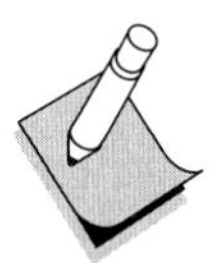

Aggressive afterload reduction is key to stabilizing the patient with acute aortic regurgitation. Intra-aortic balloon pump is contraindicated.

TREATMENT

- Standard treatment for pulmonary edema
- Nitroprusside for afterload reduction
- Dobutamine (in addition to nitroprusside) if hypotensive
- Immediate valve replacement
- Antibiotics: If endocarditis suspected
- **Avoid:** Intra-aortic balloon pump (may worsen regurgitation and is contraindicated in aortic dissection)

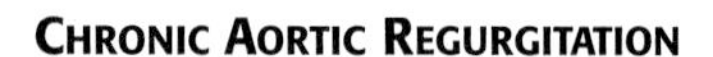

CHRONIC AORTIC REGURGITATION

SYMPTOMS

- Gradual onset of dyspnea on exertion, orthopnea, nocturnal dyspnea

EXAM

- Congestive heart failure
- High-pitched blowing diastolic murmur heard best at left sternal border
- Widened pulse pressure (opposite of AS)
- **Austin Flint murmur** (soft mid-diastolic rumble)
- **"Water hammer" pulse** (rapid rise and fall)
- **Quincke's sign** (pulsations of nailbeds)
- **Duroziez's murmur** (to-and-fro murmur over femoral artery)

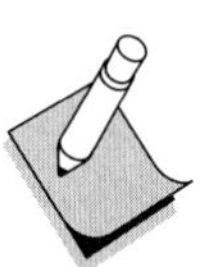

Chronic aortic regurgitation is associated with many CV exam findings, including CHF, widened pulse pressure, pulsations of nailbeds, "water hammer" pulse, and a to-and-fro femoral artery murmur.

DIAGNOSIS

- Suspect diagnosis based on history and physical examination.
- ECG: LVH, left atrial enlargement
- CXR: Congestive heart failure
- Echocardiography confirms diagnosis.

TREATMENT

- Afterload reducers, nitrates, digoxin, and surgical referral for elective valve replacement
- Prophylaxis for endocarditis

Mitral Stenosis

Mitral valve stenosis most commonly results from **rheumatic heart disease**. Other causes include atrial myxoma, congenital abnormalities, and calcific valve degeneration. Atrial fibrillation is the most commonly associated complication.

Pathophysiology

- Mitral valve narrowing → increasing pressures across the mitral valve → left atrial hypertrophy and eventual dilation with left heart failure.
- Increased pulmonary venous pressure → hemoptysis.

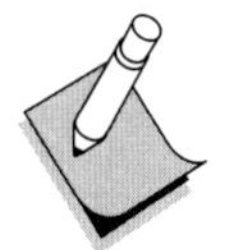

Left atrial overload in mitral stenosis → hemoptysis and atrial fibrillation.

Symptoms

- Exertional dyspnea, orthopnea
- Fatigue
- Palpitations (from atrial fibrillation)
- Hemoptysis

Exam

- Opening snap, then diastolic murmur heard best at the apex
- Loud S1
- Pulmonary edema if severe disease

Diagnosis

- Suspect diagnosis based on symptoms and examination.
- ECG: Left atrial enlargement, possibly atrial fibrillation
- CXR: Often normal, may see left atrial enlargement, CHF
- Echocardiogram is confirmative.

Treatment

- Treat atrial fibrillation (consider anticoagulation).
- Anticoagulate if systemic embolization occurs.
- Prophylaxis for endocarditis
- Elective valve replacement

Complications

- Atrial fibrillation (very common)
- Massive **pulmonary hemorrhage**
- Pulmonary HTN and right heart failure
- Systemic emboli from left atrial thrombus

A 67-year-old man presents to the ED with sudden onset of chest pain and shortness of breath. He is 5 days status-post inferior wall myocardial infarction. On examination the patient has pulmonary edema and a loud holosystolic murmur heard best at the left lateral sternal border, with radiation to the base. What is the most appropriate initial management?

Based on the presentation following recent MI, this patient likely has acute mitral valve regurgitation from papillary muscle rupture. This is a surgical emergency that requires immediate valve replacement. Nitroprusside and dobutamine can be used together to help improvement forward flow. Intra-aortic balloon pump may also be used as a bridge to surgery.

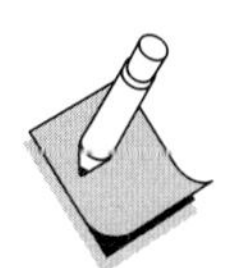

Acute mitral regurgitation is a surgical emergency.

Mitral Regurgitation

Mitral valve regurgitation (MR) may be acute or chronic. As with aortic regurgitation, it is important to make this differentiation as acute MR is a surgical emergency requiring **immediate** valve replacement.

ETIOLOGIES

- Acute mitral regurgitation
  - Endocarditis
  - Myocardial infarction
  - Trauma
- Chronic mitral regurgitation
  - Rheumatic heart disease is most common.
  - Other causes include mitral valve prolapse, connective tissue disorders.

PATHOPHYSIOLOGY

- Acute injury or dysfunction of the valve, papillary muscle, or chordae tendinae → acute valve failure → acute left atrial overload and pulmonary edema.
- Chronic valve failure → compensatory dilation of left atrium and gradual onset of CHF.

ACUTE MITRAL REGURGITATION

SYMPTOMS

- Abrupt onset of dyspnea, tachypnea
- Cardiogenic shock
- Chest pain
- Symptoms of underlying disease process (endocarditis, MI, trauma)

EXAM

- Loud holosystolic murmur heard best at the apex, with radiation to the base
- Left ventricular heave
- Pulmonary edema

DIAGNOSIS

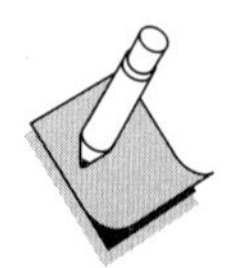

Acute mitral regurgitation? Treat with nitroprusside, dobutamine (if hypotensive), and intra-aortic balloon pump until OR is available.

- ECG: *Absence* of left atrial enlargement and LVH
- CXR: Normal cardiac silhouette, pulmonary edema

TREATMENT

- Standard treatment for pulmonary edema
- Nitroprusside for afterload reduction
- Dobutamine (in addition to nitroprusside) if hypotensive
- Intra-aortic balloon pump as bridge to surgery
- **Immediate** valve replacement
- Treat underlying disease process.

COMPLICATIONS

- Acute pulmonary edema
- Cardiogenic shock

Chronic Mitral Regurgitation

Symptoms

- Often asymptomatic
- Gradual progression of dyspnea
- Palpitations (from atrial fibrillation)

Exam

- Holosystolic murmur heard best at the apex with radiation to the base
- S3 heart sound

Diagnosis

- ECG: Left atrial enlargement, LVH, atrial fibrillation (common)
- CXR: CHF in advanced cases

Treatment

- Treat CHF and atrial fibrillation (consider anticoagulation).
- Anticoagulate if systemic embolization occurs.
- Endocarditis prophylaxis
- Valve replacement

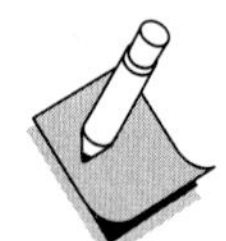

Atrial fibrillation and systemic emboli are common in chronic mitral regurgitation.

Complications

- Atrial fibrillation (very common)
- Systemic emboli from left atrial thrombus
- Endocarditis

Mitral Valve Prolapse

This is one of the most common valvular disorders. The prototypical patient is a young, thin female. The exact etiology is unknown, but is likely congenital. Associated with anxiety, eating disorders, panic attacks.

Pathophysiology

- Myxomatous proliferation of valve leaflet → abnormal stretching of valve leaflets during systole.

Symptoms

- Usually asymptomatic
- Atypical chest pain
- Palpitations
- Lightheadedness
- Dyspnea

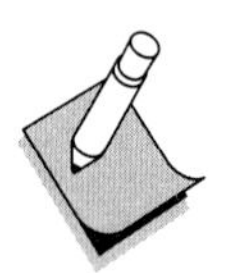

In mitral valve prolapse, decreasing the LV volume will accentuate the click and move it closer to S1.

Exam

- Early to midsystolic click with high-pitched late systolic murmur heard best at left lateral heart border.
  - Decreasing the LV volume (standing, Valsalva maneuver) → earlier and greater prolapse → accentuates the click and moves it closer to S1.

DIAGNOSIS

- ECG: Nonspecific ST-T wave changes, paroxysmal supraventricular tachycardia (PSVT)
- CXR: No specific findings
- Echo: Confirmatory

TREATMENT

- No treatment if asymptomatic
- Prophylaxis for endocarditis if regurgitation or thickened valve leaflets
- β-Blockers may help with atypical chest pain.

COMPLICATIONS

- Stroke
- Endocarditis
- Tachydysrhythmias (atrial and ventricular)
  - PSVT (most common dysrhythmia)
  - Increased incidence of WPW, PACs, PVCs
  - VT possible
- Sudden death
  - Risk factors include syncope/near syncope, murmur, inferolateral ST-T changes, PVCs

Risk factors for sudden death in MVP include syncope, murmur on exam, inferolateral ST-T changes, and PVCs.

Tricuspid Regurgitation

CAUSES

The most common causes are right ventricular dilation (from pulmonary HTN), endocarditis, and rheumatic heart disease.

SYMPTOMS

- Fatigue
- Dyspnea
- Lower extremity swelling

EXAM

- Holosystolic murmur at left lower sternal border

DIAGNOSIS

- ECG: Right atrial and ventricular enlargement, atrial fibrillation (in the majority of cases)
- Echo is confirmatory.

TREATMENT

- Treat atrial fibrillation.
- Endocarditis prophylaxis

Prosthetic Valve Complications

Prosthetic heart valves may be mechanical or bioprosthetic (porcine or bovine). Mechanical valves have a metallic sound on auscultation and require lifelong anticoagulation. Complications include paravalvular leak, valve thrombosis, endocarditis, and systemic embolization.

VALVE FAILURE

Ranges from gradually worsening paravalvular leak to abrupt mechanical valve failure

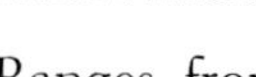

SYMPTOMS/EXAM

- Vary with location and rapidity of valve failure
- Findings of severe anemia (due to hemolysis)
- Findings consistent with aortic/mitral regurgitation (acute or chronic)
- Muted mechanical valve sounds, if mechanical valve failure

TREATMENT

- Standard treatment for aortic/mitral regurgitation
- Valve replacement

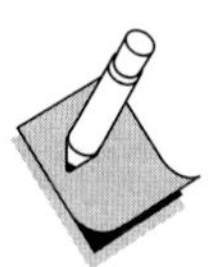

*Mechanical valve failure → CHF, muted valve sounds **with** presence of regurgitation murmur.*

*Valve thrombosis → CHF, muted mechanical valve sounds **without** regurgitation murmur.*

VALVE THROMBOSIS

Thrombus is more likely to form on a mechanical valve and can cause systemic embolization or valve thrombosis.

SYMPTOMS/EXAM

- If sudden, acute onset of hypotension, CHF
- Muted mechanical valve sounds
- May have a more gradual course

TREATMENT

- Anticoagulation
- Valve replacement

ARTERIAL CIRCULATORY DISORDERS

Arterial Aneurysms

Aneurysms can occur anywhere in the arterial system but are most common in the abdominal aorta. Of those occurring in the peripheral arteries, popliteal artery aneurysm is the most common (bilateral in >50%).

Arteries are composed of three layers: Tunica intima (inner layer), tunica media, and tunica adventitia (outer layer).

- A **true aneurysm** involves all three layers of vessel wall.
- A **false aneurysm** or **pseudoaneurysm** communicates with the vessel lumen, but is contained only by adventitia or surrounding soft tissues.

PATHOPHYSIOLOGY

- Weakening of the media (cystic medial degeneration) → dilatation of the vessel wall → true aneurysm.
- Trauma to vessel wall → leakage of blood contained by adventitia or surrounding soft tissue → pseudoaneurysm.
- Aneurysms naturally enlarge over time.

Symptoms are caused by rupture (unlikely with peripheral artery aneurysms), impingement of adjacent structures, thrombosis, or embolism.

ABDOMINAL AORTIC ANEURYSM

Abdominal aortic aneurysms (AAAs) are most commonly *true* aneurysms and involve the *infrarenal* aorta. At this level an aortic diameter >3 cm = AAA.

The primary risk factors for AAA development include:

- Increasing age
- Family history
- Atherosclerotic risk factors

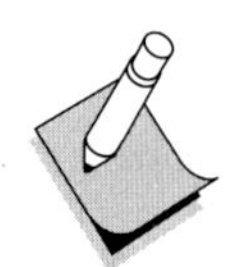

An AAA of any size can rupture, but those >5 cm are more likely to rupture.

Other predisposing factors include infection, trauma, connective tissue disease, and arteritis.

An AAA of any size **can** rupture, but the likelihood ↑ with increasing size. The most common location of rupture is to the retroperitoneum. Rupture is associated with an 80–90% overall mortality (many patients do not even reach the hospital).

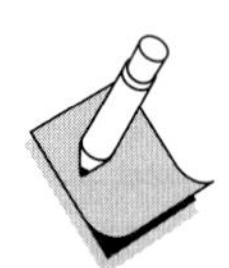

The most common location of AAA rupture = retroperitoneum.

SYMPTOMS

- Most aneurysms are asymptomatic when discovered and become symptomatic when **expanding or ruptured**.
- Acute pain in abdomen, back, or flank
- Nausea and vomiting
- Syncope or near syncope

EXAM

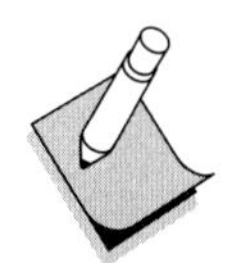

Cullen's sign = periumbilical ecchymosis.

Grey-Turner's sign = flank ecchymosis.

- Vital signs may be surprisingly normal.
  - Hypotension and shock if rupture with significant blood loss
- Abdominal tenderness, distension, or pulsatile abdominal mass
- Evidence for retroperitoneal hematoma
  - Periumbilical ecchymosis (**Cullen's sign**)
  - Flank ecchymosis (**Grey-Turner's sign**)
- Massive GI bleed if rupture into GI tract (aortoenteric fistula)
- High-output heart failure if rupture into vena cava (aortocaval fistula)

DIAGNOSIS

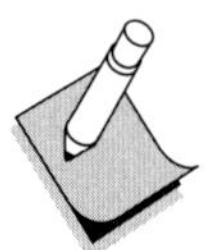

Triad of abdominal pain, hypotension, pulsatile abdominal mass = AAA until proven otherwise, although triad is rare.

- The diagnosis should be suspected in any patient >50 years old presenting with abdominal pain, flank pain, or hypotension.
- Abdominal X-ray
  - May see curvilinear calcified outline of enlarged aorta
- **Ultrasound** (see Figure 2.15)
  - 100% sensitive when aorta is visualized
  - Modality of choice in the unstable patient
  - May not be able to identify rupture, site of leak, or retroperitoneal hematoma
- **CT** (see Figure 2.16)
  - Highly sensitive
  - Requires stable patient for transport
  - Better than ultrasound at detecting rupture and retroperitoneal blood
- **MRI or aortography** are rarely indicated in the ED.

TREATMENT

- Ruptured aneurysms require immediate surgical intervention with operative or endovascular repair.
  - There is no such thing as a stable rupture!
  - 50% operative mortality
- Fluid and blood resuscitation: **To SBP 90–100 mmHg**.
- Thoracotomy with cross clamping of aorta: If severe hemodynamic compromise or cardiac arrest

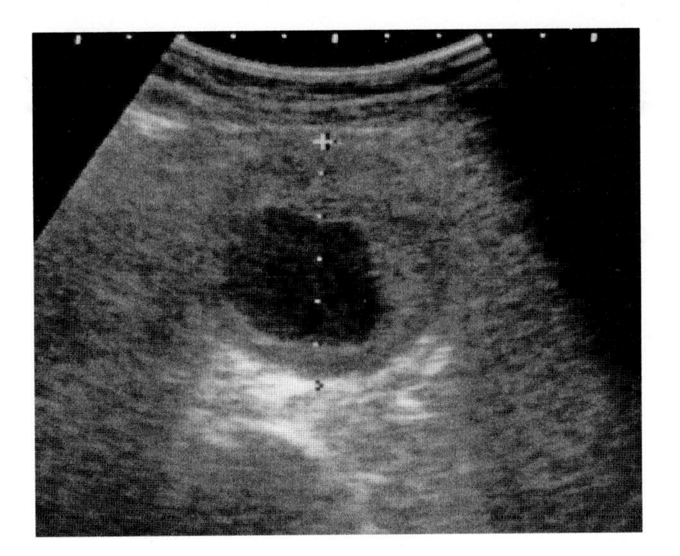

FIGURE 2.15. Transabdominal ultrasound showing 6-cm AAA.

- Asymptomatic aneurysms can be scheduled for repair based on aneurysm size and patient comorbidities.
- Endovascular repair with stent graft is increasingly used.

COMPLICATIONS

- Rupture
- **Atheroembolism:** *Microemboli* from atherosclerotic aneurysms
  - Lodge in *distal* small vessels
  - **"Blue toe syndrome"** is classic presentation.
  - Can also occur from nonaneurysmal atherosclerotic plaques

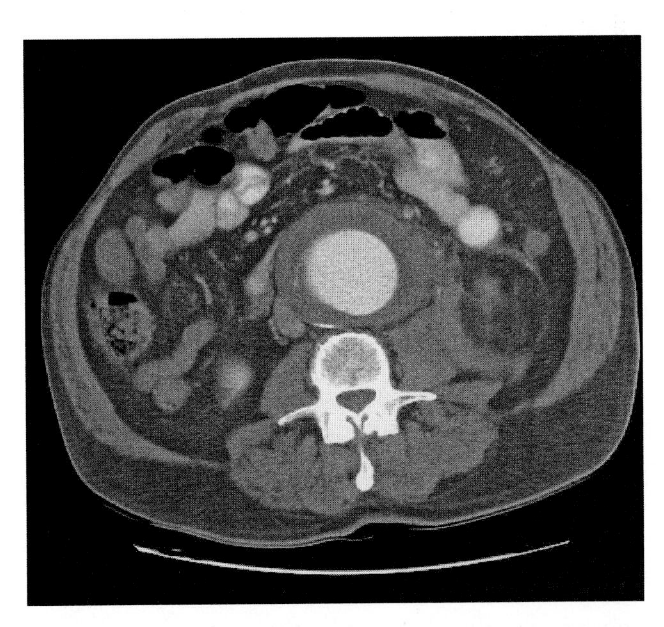

FIGURE 2.16. Contrast-enhanced abdominal CT showing large AAA with rupture.

(Courtesy of Matthew J. Fleishman, MD, Radiology Imaging Associates. Englewood, Colorado.)

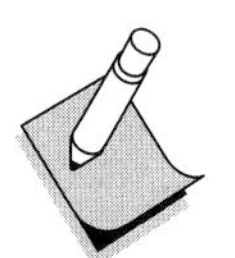

Endoleak = leak outside of graft lumen, but within existing aneurysm sac.

- **Graft complications**
  - Graft infection
  - Secondary aortoenteric fistula
  - **Endoleak:** Leak outside of graft lumen, but within existing aneurysm sac (continued risk for AAA rupture!)

THORACIC AORTIC ANEURYSM

Often an incidental finding on chest radiography. A **thoracic aorta diameter of >4.5 cm** is considered aneurysmal. Risk factors are similar to those for AAA. Risk of rupture is high when diameter ≥6 cm.

SYMPTOMS/EXAM

- Typically asymptomatic unless expanding, ruptured, or compressing adjacent structure
- Chest or back pain
- Congestive heart failure if associated aortic insufficiency
- Pericardial effusion if aortic valve involvement
- Hoarseness: Compression of recurrent laryngeal nerve
- Cough, wheezing with compression of trachea
- If ruptured: Hypotension and shock

DIFFERENTIAL

- Includes ACS, PE, aortic dissection, pneumothorax, esophageal rupture

DIAGNOSIS

- CXR: May appear normal, but often shows wide mediastinum, enlarged aortic knob
- CT is confirmative.
- Use TEE in the unstable patient.

TREATMENT

- Resuscitation and **immediate** surgical consult for repair if unstable patient
- Aggressive BP control as with aortic dissection
- Asymptomatic aneurysms can be scheduled for repair based on aneurysm size and patient comorbidities.

> A 55-year-old male with a history of poorly controlled HTN presents after a syncopal event while lifting weights at the gym. He complains of severe, sharp, left-chest pain and is diaphoretic and apprehensive. His initial BP is 88/55 and HR is 122. Exam reveals equal breath sounds, prominent JVD, distant heart tones, and weak radial pulses. What is the best initial imaging study?
>
> Bedside cardiac ultrasound. This patient is too unstable for CT. Ultrasound will demonstrate pericardial effusion and tamponade from proximal aortic dissection, indicating the need for emergent surgery.

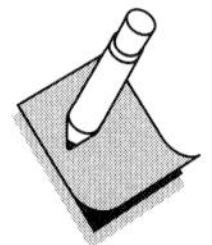

Proximal aortic dissections = surgical management. Distal aortic dissection = medical management.

Aortic Dissection

Aortic dissections are classified by their location (see Figure 2.17). Location has important implications for management as proximal (ascending) dissections are managed surgically and distal dissections are typically managed medically.

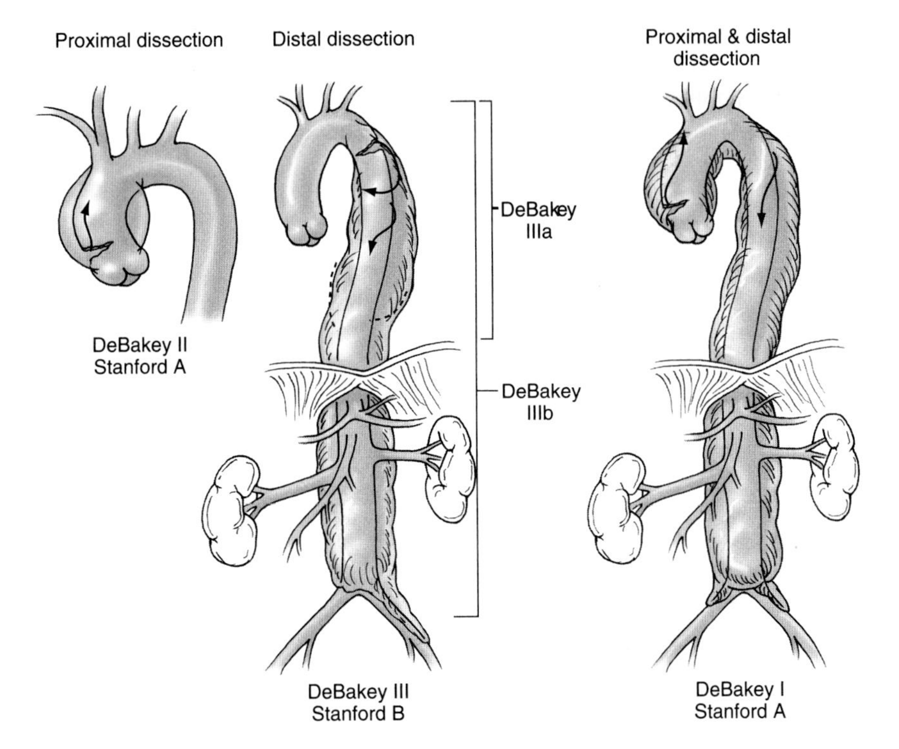

FIGURE 2.17. DeBakey and Stanford classifications of aortic dissection.

(Reproduced, with permission, from Brunicardi FC. *Schwartz's Principles of Surgery*, 8th ed, New York: McGraw-Hill 2005:704.)

The most common predisposing risk factor (see Table 2.19) for aortic dissection = uncontrolled HTN.

PATHOPHYSIOLOGY

- Disruption of intima of aortic wall → blood travels (dissects) into media, creating false lumen.
- Dissection can propagate down/up the aorta through the false lumen:
  - Proximally into aortic root → right coronary artery involvement, tamponade, aortic regurgitation
  - Into carotid artery → stroke symptoms

TABLE 2.19. Risk Factors for Aortic Dissection

Uncontrolled hypertension
Advancing age
Connective tissue disease (eg, Marfan syndrome)
Congenital heart disease (eg, bicuspid aortic valve)
Giant cell arteritis
Annuloaortic ectasia
Family history
Stimulant abuse
Iatrogenic (catheterization or surgery)

- Involving spinal cord artery → paresis
- Involving other major branches → limb or organ ischemia
- May ultimately empty back into true lumen of aorta, or rupture through adventitia

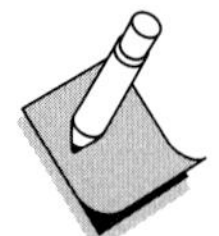

Pain (chest, neck, or back) is present in the vast majority of patients with aortic dissection.

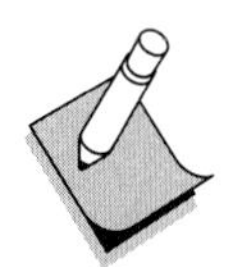

Patient with chest pain and stroke symptoms? Consider aortic dissection!

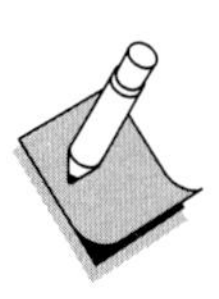

A new aortic regurgitation murmur in a patient with acute chest pain is highly suggestive of proximal aortic dissection.

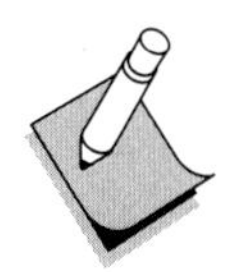

Asymmetric pulses (or BP) will occur only if the subclavian artery is involved.

SYMPTOMS

- Severe chest, neck, or back pain
  - **Present in >90% of patients**
  - Classically described as "ripping" or "tearing" but actually more commonly described as sharp (64%)
  - Abrupt and maximal in onset (85%)
  - Anterior chest pain more common (73%) than posterior chest pain (36%) or back pain (53%), although this varies depending on whether it is a Type A dissection (anterior chest pain more common) or Type B dissection (back pain more common)
- May migrate as dissection progresses
  - Dissection into distal aorta = abdominal or flank pain
- Nausea, vomiting, diaphoresis
- Syncope (5–10% of patients)
- Neurologic symptoms (5%): If carotid or spinal artery involvement
  - Mental status change, stroke symptoms, paresis

EXAM

- May be surprisingly normal
- Hypertension: Common unless tamponade or rupture present
  - Normal or low BP does **not** exclude dissection.
- If subclavian artery involved: Asymmetric pulses (or BPs). This is a relatively rare finding (15%).
- If proximal dissection, may find
  - Shock and hypoperfusion (tamponade)
  - New murmur of aortic regurgitation ± CHF
- If involving carotid or spinal arteries, may find
  - AMS, stroke symptoms, paresis

DIFFERENTIAL

- Includes acute coronary syndrome, PE, pneumothorax, ruptured aneurysm, esophageal perforation

DIAGNOSIS

- Suspect diagnosis in any patient presenting with chest pain, especially patient with history of uncontrolled HTN (or other risk factors), shock, or associated neurologic symptoms.
- **ECG**
  - To exclude coronary artery involvement (inferior ischemia indicating RCA involvement)
  - LVH is common finding (26%).
  - Small portion (<5%) of acute aortic dissection will have new Q waves or ST segment changes.
- **CXR** (vast majority, >85%) will have some abnormality (See Figure 2.18)
  - Widened mediastinum (62%)
  - Loss of aortic knob (50%)
  - Pleural capping
  - Aortic shadow extending >5 mm from aortic calcification (14%)

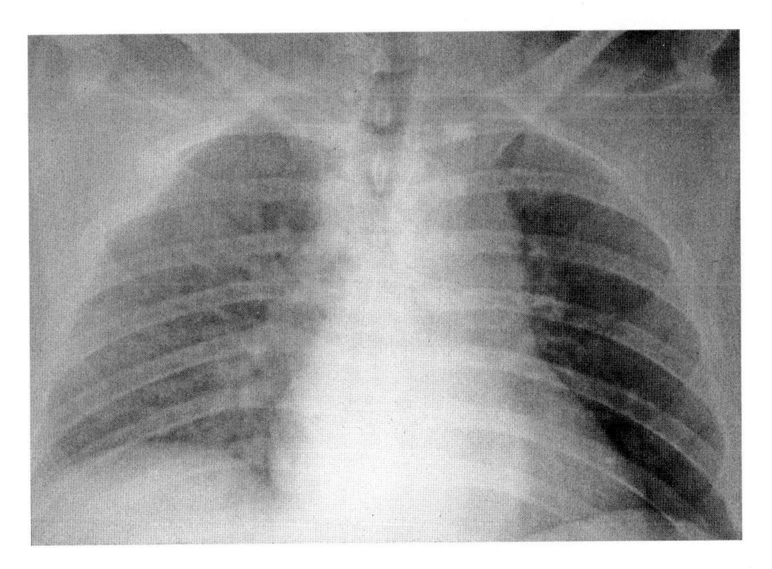

FIGURE 2.18. AP chest radiograph showing widened mediastinum and loss of aortic knob in patient with aortic dissection.

(Courtesy of Matthew J. Fleishman, MD, Radiology Imaging Associates. Englewood, Colorado.)

- **Ultrasound**
  - Poor sensitivity overall
  - Used to confirm diagnosis of tamponade in unstable patient
- **Transesophageal echocardiography**
  - If diagnosis in question in unstable patient
- **CT angiograph** (see Figure 2.19)
  - To confirm diagnosis in stable patients
  - High sensitivity and specificity
  - Entire aorta and branches visualized

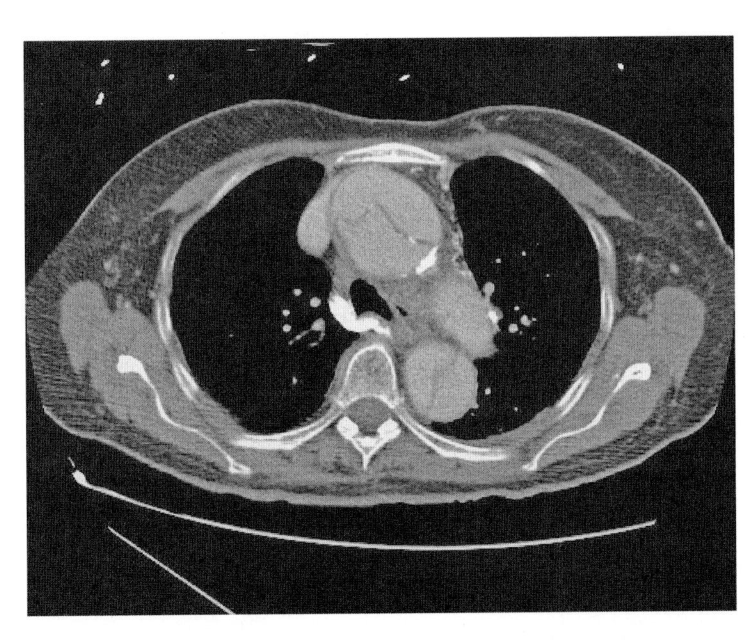

FIGURE 2.19. Contrast-enhanced chest CT showing type A aortic dissection.

(Courtesy of Matthew J. Fleishman, MD, Radiology Imaging Associates, Englewood, Colorado.)

- **MRI**
  - Good visualization, but limited utility in the ED
- **Aortography**
  - The classic "gold standard," but largely supplanted by CT angiography

TREATMENT

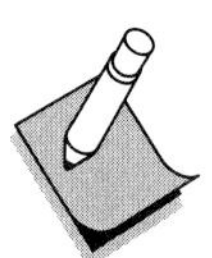

Initial drug of choice in aortic dissection is IV esmolol (or labetalol) → decrease shearing forces.

- Goal (after resuscitation) is to **decrease shearing forces** by reducing BP and the rate of rise of the arterial pulse (dP/dT).
- **If hypotension present:**
  - Intravenous fluids, pressors
  - Consider pericardiocentesis, if tamponade.
- **If systolic BP > 120:**
  - **Start with IV β-blockers** (*esmolol* or labetalol drip).
  - Add IV nitroprusside, if needed.
  - Goal is systolic BP 100–120.
  - **Avoid**: Nifedipine.
- Type A: Surgical repair
- Type B: Admit to ICU for medical management.
  - Indications for OR: Rupture limb or organ ischemia, progression of dissection, uncontrolled HTN

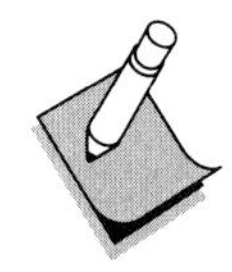

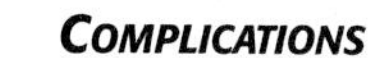

Inferior MI is the most common injury pattern seen in aortic dissection due to involvement of the RCA.

COMPLICATIONS

- Free rupture through adventitia, nearly always fatal
- Aortic regurgitation and CHF in proximal dissection
- MI if coronary arteries involved
- Tamponade if dissection ruptures into pericardium
- CVA or paresis if carotid or spinal arteries involved
- Limb or organ ischemia

Occlusive Arterial Disease

ACUTE ARTERIAL THROMBOEMBOLISM

Arterial thromboembolism is a limb-threatening emergency that requires rapid diagnosis and intervention. It often occurs in patients **without** chronic atherosclerotic disease. Because such patients lack extensive collateral arterial circulation, severe ischemia results.

Common sources of emboli are cardiac in origin.

PATHOPHYSIOLOGY

- Thrombus forms in region of turbulent flow → embolus to distal artery.
- Common sources of thrombus:
  - **LV mural thrombus** following MI (most common)
  - **Left atrial thrombus** from mitral valve disease and atrial fibrillation
  - Mechanical valve
  - Mural thrombus from large arterial aneurysms
- Most common sites of embolism:
  - Bifurcation of common femoral artery (#1)
  - Popliteal artery

The most common site of acute arterial embolism = bifurcation of common femoral artery.

SYMPTOMS/EXAM

- Pain
- Pallor
- Paresthesias (indicates limb-threatening ischemia)
- Pulselessness

- Paralysis (indicates limb-threatening ischemia)
- Presence of light touch sensation indicates tissue viability.

> ***The five Ps of acute arterial occlusion:***
>
> **P**ain
> **P**allor
> **P**aresthesias
> **P**ulselessness
> **P**aralysis

DIFFERENTIAL

- **Atheroembolism:** *Microemboli* from proximal atherosclerotic plaques or aneurysms
  - Lodge in *distal* small vessels
  - "**Blue toe syndrome**" is classic presentation
  - Arterial pulses are maintained
- Acute thrombotic occlusion (thrombosis-in-situ)
- Arterial vasospasm
- **Raynaud's disease:**
  - Vasospasm of **distal small arteries**
  - Characteristic bilateral **triphasic response to cold or emotion:** Fingers become white, blue, then red
  - Resolves spontaneously, benign course
- Vasculitis

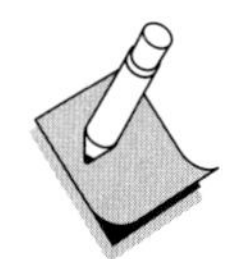

Normal doppler arterial signal is triphasic.

DIAGNOSIS

- Clinical diagnosis based on history and examination
- Doppler ultrasonography
  - Normal doppler arterial signal is **triphasic**.
- Angiography is confirmative.
  - Abrupt cutoff in disease-free artery

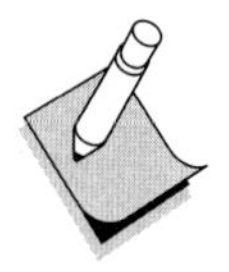

In acute arterial occlusion, surgical embolectomy must occur within 4–6 hours.

TREATMENT

- Immediate heparinization
- Surgical embolectomy
  - The likelihood of return to normal limb function is minimal after 4–6 hours of occlusion.

ACUTE THROMBOTIC OCCLUSION (THROMBOSIS-IN-SITU)

Acute thrombotic occlusion is associated with advanced atherosclerotic disease the vast majority of the time. Because these patients have developed collateral circulation, the obstruction is less commonly limb-threatening.

PATHOPHYSIOLOGY

- Plaque rupture or endothelial erosion → thrombus formation → distal ischemia.
- Degree of ischemia is determined by extent of collateral flow, duration of obstruction, extent of obstruction.
- Other less common causes include trauma, vasculitis.

SYMPTOMS/EXAM

- Limb ischemia as described above.
- Symptoms are often less dramatic and less intense because of collateral arterial flow.

DIFFERENTIAL

- Most important diagnosis to exclude is arterial thromboembolism.
- Other diagnoses include atheroembolism, arterial vasospasm, vasculitis.

DIAGNOSIS

- Suspect based on clinical presentation
- Doppler ultrasound: Will confirm a **decreased ankle brachial index** (ABI) in the affected extremity:
  - Divide systolic BP in the ankle by systolic BP in the radial artery.
    - Normal >0.9
    - Moderate arterial insufficiency = 0.5–0.7
    - Severe arterial insufficiency <0.5
- **Arteriogram** is definitive.
  - Shows abrupt cutoff at branch point in atherosclerotic artery
- **Duplex ultrasonography** is reasonably accurate alternative.

Most patients with acute arterial thrombosis have collateral circulation and therefore will not need immediate surgical intervention.

TREATMENT

- Depends on degree of collateral flow and location of thrombus.
- Patients with limb-threatening ischemia need aggressive therapy.
- Options include:
  - Heparinization alone
  - Catheter-directed thrombolysis
    - Reperfusion with this modality frequently takes hours.
    - **Not** a good choice for limb-threatening ischemia
  - Percutaneous thrombectomy
  - Surgical thrombectomy or vascular bypass
- The likelihood of return to normal limb function is minimal after 4–6 hours of complete ischemia.

CHRONIC LIMB ISCHEMIA

The vast majority of chronic limb ischemia is due to atherosclerotic arterial disease. Another less common cause is thromboangiitis obliterans (Buerger disease), an inflammatory disease of young, typically male, smokers.

Phlebitis migrans = segmental inflammation of the neurovascular bundle in patients with Buerger disease.

PATHOPHYSIOLOGY

- Peripheral vascular atherosclerotic lesions reduce arterial luminal diameter and blood flow → tissues ischemia when blood flow does not meet O_2 demand.
- **Buerger disease:** Segmental acute and chronic inflammation in smaller arteries of arms and leg (infrapopliteal in legs) → tissue ischemia.
  - Eventual fibrous encasement of neurovascular bundle → visible tender, dark nodules = *phlebitis migrans*.

SYMPTOMS

- Claudication: Fatigue, pain, or weakness in involved extremity or digit
  - Exertional symptoms become rest symptoms as disease progresses.
- Painful ulcerations
- **Leriche syndrome**: Triad of bilateral hip claudication, erectile dysfunction, absent femoral pulses = aortoiliac occlusive disease
- Raynaud's-like response to cold: Associated with Buerger disease.

EXAM

- Atrophy of skin and soft tissues
- Hair loss, cool pale skin
- Ulcers: Typically at end of digits, less commonly at pressure points

Diagnosis

- Suspect based on history and examination
- Ankle brachial index ≤ 0.9
- **Arteriogram** is definitive.
  - Shows diffuse atherosclerosis, irregular cutoff, collaterals

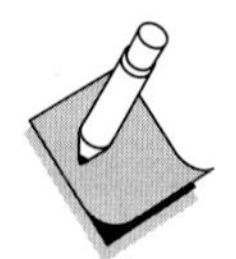

ABI < 0.9 is seen in claudication.

Treatment

- Risk-factor modification
- Antithrombotic therapy (aspirin, clopidogrel, warfarin)
- Immediate surgical intervention if limb-threatening ischemia
  - Stents or arterial bypass surgery
- Wound care for ulcerations
- Cessation of smoking = only effective therapy for Buerger's

Diabetic patients may have a paradoxically normal ABI due to calcification and noncompressibility in the dorsalis pedis and posterior tibial arteries.

A 65-year-old male with a history of HTN treated with lisonopril and atenolol presents with a 6-hour history of headache, vomiting, and progressive confusion. Initial BP is 220/130, and remains on repeat measurement. Emergent head CT shows no hemorrhage. What is the goal for managing this patient's blood pressure?

Reduce MAP by 25% within 30–60 minutes with a titratable agent such as nitroprusside. Do not use oral agents because precise BP control is harder to achieve.

HYPERTENSION

HTN is defined as a SPB > 140 or a DBP > 90. HTN the is a major risk factor stroke, heart disease, renal failure, vascular disease, and retinal disease.

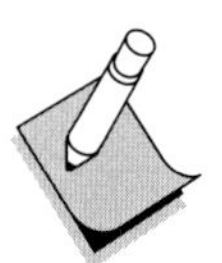

Hypertension = SBP > 140 or DBP > 90.

The Joint National Committee on Prevention, Detection, Evaluation, and Treatment of High Blood Pressure has stratified BP into categories (see Table 2.20).

Etiology

- **Essential (primary) hypertension** comprises >90% of all cases of HTN. Although no specific cause has been identified, most cases have a common end pathway of activation of the renin-angiotensin system.
- **Secondary hypertension:** Underlying cause has been identified (see Table 2.21).

In the ED, HTN can be classified as transient HTN, mild HTN, hypertensive urgency (a historical term), or hypertensive emergency.

TABLE 2.20. Classification of Blood Pressure for Adults

Category	Systolic		Diastolic
Normal	< 120	and	< 80
Prehypertension	120–139	or	80–89
Stage 1 HTN	140–159	or	90–99
Stage 2 HTN	≥ 160	or	100

TABLE 2.21. Causes of Secondary Hypertension

CATEGORY	EXAMPLES
Renovascular	Renal artery stenosis Fibromuscular dysplasia
Renal parenchymal	Glomerulonephritis Chronic pyelonephritis
Hormonal	Estrogens 1° hyperaldosteronism Glucocorticoids
Illicit drug intoxication/withdrawal	Cocaine intoxication Alcohol withdrawal
Circulating catecholamines	Pheochromocytoma Tyramine Clonidine withdrawal
Coarctation	
Hypercalcemia	

Mild Hypertension

Patients with persistent (not transient) mild elevations of BP without any evidence for end-organ damage

Symptoms/Exam

- Patient is typically asymptomatic.
- Retinal: A-V nicking, narrowing of arterial diameter
- Cardiac: S4 gallop, signs of LVH
- Use appropriately sized cuff.
  - Too large → falsely low reading.
  - Too small → falsely elevated reading.
- Coarctation: Upper extremity hypertension, systolic murmur (best over back), delayed femoral pulses
- Renovascular disease: Flank bruits
- Pheochromocytoma: Palpitations, apprehension, malaise, tachycardia, diaphoresis

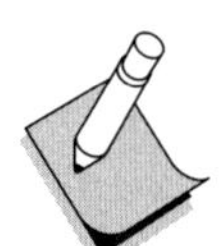

Coarctation → upper extremity HTN, systolic murmur, delayed femoral pulses.

Treatment

- Identify and correct underlying secondary causes.
- Lifestyle and dietary changes: Mild sodium restriction, weight loss (if needed), decreased cholesterol and fat intake, exercise, smoking cessation
- Initiation of antihypertensive therapy if:
  - Stage 2 HTN
  - Two or more risk factors (see Table 2.22) for complications

Hypertensive Urgency

A historical term indicating a persistent and marked elevation of blood pressure in a patient at risk for end-organ damage, but **without** acute organ injury

TABLE 2.22. **Risk Factors for Complications From HTN**

Risk Factors for Complications from HTN
African American
Male
Early age of onset
DPB >115
Smoking
Diabetes
Hypercholesterolemia
Obesity
Alcoholism
Evidence of end-organ dysfunction

It is a subjective determination, and there is no evidence-based data to guide management.

SYMPTOMS/EXAM

- Often asymptomatic, but with history of CAD, CHF, or renal insufficiency indicating at-risk patient
- BP often markedly elevated

DIAGNOSIS

- Exclude acute end-organ damage with exam, creatinine, UA, ECG

TREATMENT

- Treat any secondary causes of HTN.
- Begin empiric *oral* antihypertensive agents with goal of lowering blood pressure over period of 24–48 hours.

Hypertensive Emergency

Hypertensive emergency is defined as HTN with evidence for *acute end-organ dysfunction*. The absolute BP is not as important as the presence of dysfunction. The heart, brain, and kidneys are the organs most frequently affected (see Table 2.23).

TABLE 2.23. **Types of Hypertensive Emergencies**

Types of Hypertensive Emergencies
Myocardial ischemia
Pulmonary edema
Acute aortic dissection
Hypertensive encephalopathy
Eclampsia
Acute renal failure
Uncontrolled bleeding

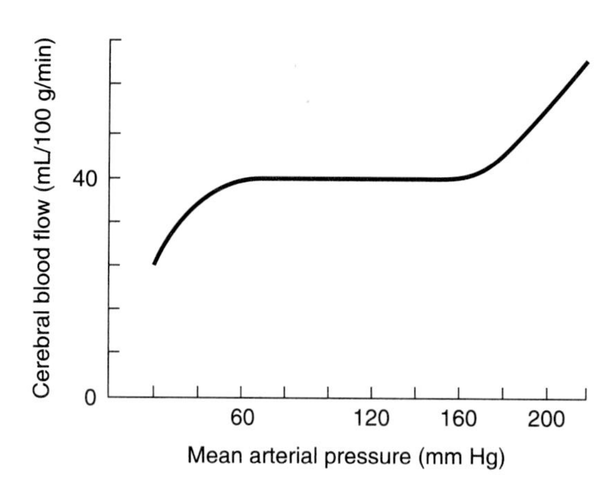

FIGURE 2.20. The normal cerebral autoregulation curve.

(Reproduced, with permission, from Morgan GE, Mikhail MS, Murray MJ, *Clinical Anesthesiology*, 4th ed. New York: McGraw-Hill, 2006:616.)

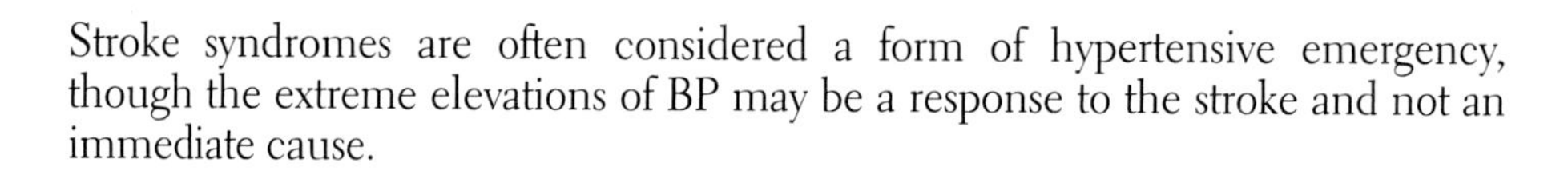

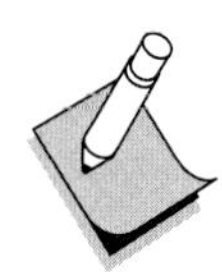

Hypertensive emergency = HTN with acute end-organ dysfunction.

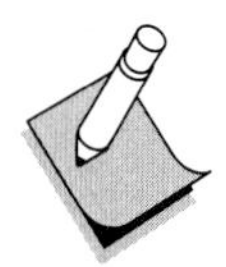

$MAP = P_{diastolic} + 1/3(P_{systolic} - P_{diastolic})$

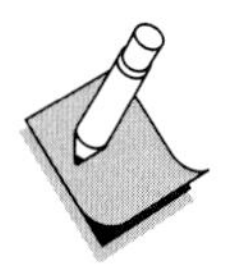

Cerebral autoregulation is effective between a MAP of 60–160 mmHg.

Stroke syndromes are often considered a form of hypertensive emergency, though the extreme elevations of BP may be a response to the stroke and not an immediate cause.

Accelerated hypertension (malignant hypertension) is a term that reflects progressive end-organ damage.

PATHOPHYSIOLOGY

- In the heart, an abrupt, severe elevation of BP → acute left ventricular failure or increase myocardial O_2 demand → ischemia and pulmonary edema.
- In the brain, an abrupt rise in BP that exceeds the upper limits of cerebral autoregulation (typically MAP > 160, see Figure 2.20) → hypertensive encephalopathy.
- Chronic hypertension shifts the cerebral autoregulation curve to the **right**, which has important implications during treatment.
- In the kidney a sustained elevation of blood pressure → ↓ renal perfusion, ischemia, and renal impairment.
- Other presentations include uncontrolled bleeding, eclampsia, aortic dissection.

SYMPTOMS

- Chest pain, dyspnea, nausea if myocardial ischemia
- Dyspnea, cough, pink-tinged sputum if pulmonary edema
- Tearing pain in chest or upper back if aortic dissection
- Severe headache, nausea, vomiting, confusion, visual changes if hypertensive encephalopathy

EXAM

- Blood pressure is often markedly elevated, exceptions being eclampsia and aortic dissection with tamponade.
- Evidence of end-organ damage may include:
  - S3, new murmur, unequal pulses
  - Rales, wheezing, hypoxia, respiratory distress
  - Decreased mental status, seizures, focal deficits
  - Papilledema, retinal hemorrhages

DIAGNOSIS

- Clinical exam or studies showing evidence of end-organ damage

TREATMENT

Hypertensive emergency mandates immediate treatment, with a goal to **reduce MAP by 25% in 30–60 minutes or reduction of diastolic pressure to about 110 mmHg**. Reduction beyond this goal puts the patient at risk for end-organ ischemia due to relative hypotension. This is especially true for the patient with chronic HTN in whom the cerebral autoregulation curve has shifted to the right. An exception to this is in the treatment of aortic dissection, where a lower MAP is necessary to eliminate shear forces. A short-acting, titratable IV agent is preferred (see Table 2.24). Oral agents should **not** be used.

- Sodium nitroprusside
  - Drug of choice for most emergencies
  - Arteriolar and venodilator
  - Cerebral vasodilator (careful in stroke syndromes)
  - Dilates normal coronary arteries > diseased → **coronary steal**
  - Cyanide is a metabolite, so long-term use is limited.
  - Contraindicated in pregnancy
- Fenoldopam
  - Peripheral dopamine-1 receptor agonist
  - Improves renal function acutely

In hypertensive emergencies, reduction of MAP > 25% puts the patient at risk for end-organ ischemia due to relative hypotension.

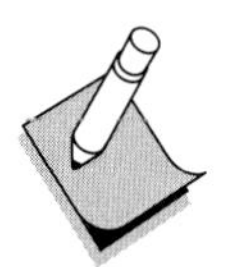

Sodium nitroprusside is a cerebral vasodilator and should be used carefully in stroke syndromes.

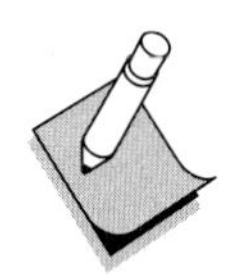

Nicardipene ↓ cerebral vasospasm, and therefore is a good agent for stroke syndromes.

TABLE 2.24. Antihypertensive Agents for Hypertensive Emergencies

CONDITION	AGENT OF CHOICE
Accelerated hypertension, hypertensive encephalopathy, or acute renal failure	Sodium nitroprusside Labetalol Nicardipene
Myocardial ischemia	Nitroglycerin Labetalol
Pulmonary edema	Nitroglycerin Sodium nitroprusside Fenoldopam
Aortic dissection	Esmolol or labetalol (first) Sodium nitroprusside
Catecholamine crisis	Benzodiazepine sedation Labetalol Phentolamine
Eclampsia	Magnesium Labetalol Nicardipine Hydralazine

- **Nicardipene**
  - Calcium channel blocker
  - ↓ Peripheral vascular resistance
  - ↓ Cerebral vasospasm (good for **stroke syndromes**)
- **Nitroglycerin**
  - Venous >> arteriolar dilation
- **Labetalol**
  - α_1-, β-Adrenergic blocker
  - Much more β-blockade than α-blockade
  - Effective as single agent
- **Esmolol**
  - β_1-Adrenergic blocker
  - Very short acting
  - Often used with nitroprusside to blunt tachycardia
- **Hydralazine**
  - Direct arteriolar vasodilator (watch for reflex tachycardia)
- **Phentolamine**
  - Pure α-blocker

CARDIOVASCULAR TESTING

The following summary briefly reviews some of the common modalities used to further delineate primary cardiovascular disorders. It is not a comprehensive source but rather covers key points pertinent to the ED physician's management of patients with cardiovascular diseases.

ECHOCARDIOGRAM

- Transthoracic echo (TTE)
  - Evaluates ventricular size and function
  - Identifies valvular pathology
  - Detects effusions and tamponade physiology
  - Stress echo identifies areas of hypokinesis, akinesis, or dyskinesis during exercise or pharmacologic stress tests.
- Transesophageal echo (TEE)
  - Due to placement in the esophagus, more detailed studies can be obtained.
  - Identifies mural thrombi prior to cardioversion
  - Higher sensitivity than TTE in detecting aortic dissection
  - More invasive and technically more difficult than TTE

HOLTER MONITORING

- Ambulatory ECG monitor that records dysrhythmias and other pathologies
- Correlated with patient's diary of symptoms
- An event recorder allows the patient to activate the recorder at the onset of symptoms.

TILT-TABLE TESTING

- Used to evaluate patients with suspected vasovagal syncope
- Goal is to provoke syncope while patient is monitored.
  - As table tilts, blood pools in LE venous system.
  - Venous return ↓
  - Myocardial contraction ↑ to compensate

- Ventricular mechanoreceptors are stimulated.
- Vagal tone ↑ and sympathetic tone ↓.
- Syncope occurs.

Tilt-table testing is primarily used in the evaluation and treatment of vasovagal syncope.

MYOCARDIAL PERFUSION IMAGING

- Radionuclide testing
  - Thallium or technetium-99m marker is infused during ACS symptoms or at maximal exertion.
  - Marker is taken up by myocardium in proportion to blood flow, so areas of poor perfusion are demonstrated.
    - A perfusion defect both at rest and during stress (irreversible defect) = old infarction.
    - A perfusion defect that occurs only during stress (reversible) = myocardial ischemia.
  - Technetium-99m has the advantage of allowing for delayed imaging (up to 3 hours) compared to immediate imaging required with Thallium.

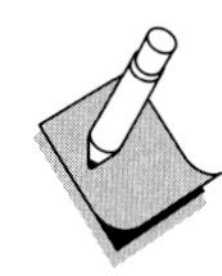

Myocardial perfusion defects present both at rest and during stress = old infarction.

GRADED EXERCISE STRESS TESTING

- Bruce protocol: Exercise pace and/or incline of treadmill increases every 3 minutes.
  - ECG response: ST segment abnormalities are evaluated by
    - Time of onset of abnormality
    - Time of resolution
    - Magnitude of depression or elevation
  - Vital signs: Peak heart rate, blood pressure
  - Higher risk of CAD if
    - Cannot complete 6 minutes of exercise
    - Ischemia in first 3 minutes
    - Drop in SBP
    - ST depression in multiple leads
    - Exercise-induced angina
- Value of test depends on pretest probability of CAD: Low-risk patients commonly have false-positive tests.
- Should not be done in the setting of unstable angina, MI, severe HTN, uncontrolled dysrhythmias, severe aortic stenosis

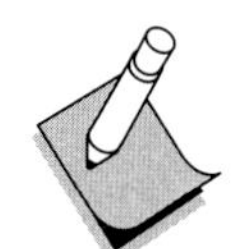

Exercise stress testing should not be performed in the setting of unstable angina, severe HTN, or severe aortic stenosis.

PHARMACOLOGIC STRESS TESTING

- Variety of agents used for patients who cannot complete exercise stress test for a variety of reasons
- Inotropic agents
  - Dobutamine: ↑ HR without exercise
  - Concurrent echo examined for evidence of LV hypokinesis.
- Vasodilators: Persantine, adenosine
  - These agents decrease flow to the coronary arteries, exposing areas of decreased uptake on thallium scan.

ELECTRON BEAM CT

- New technology that allows for calculating the degree of calcium build-up in the coronary arteries (calcium score)
- High calcium score = high likelihood of CAD.
- May be a good screening tool to **exclude CAD** in the ED patient

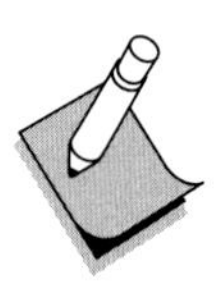

In patients who present with syncope, the following factors increase the risk of dysrhythmia or sudden death:

1. *Age > 45 years old*
2. *History of ventricular dysrhythmias*
3. *History of CHF*
4. *Abnormal ECG*

SYNCOPE

Syncope is defined as a transient loss of consciousness and postural tone with subsequent spontaneous recovery. It results from transient cerebral hypoperfusion from a variety of causes (see Table 2.25). It is most commonly benign but is associated with life-threatening conditions. A post-ictal period is notably absent, differentiating syncope from seizure.

SYMPTOMS/EXAM

- Transient loss of consciousness
- Complete recovery without intervention
- Other symptoms and exam findings vary with underlying etiology.
- Table 2.26 lists the classic presentations of syncope.

DIFFERENTIAL

- It may be difficult to differentiate syncope from seizure.
  - A history of seizures makes a seizure more likely.
  - In rare instances, true syncope leads to seizure.
  - Both may be associated with extremity movement and urinary incontinence.
  - A classic aura, post-ictal confusion, and muscle pain indicate seizure.

TABLE 2.25. Causes of Syncope

Acutely life-threatening vascular catastrophe Aortic dissection, ruptured AAA, ruptured ectopic, subarachnoid hemorrhage, tamponade, PE, severe hemorrhage (GI, retroperitoneal etc.)
Obstruction to cardiac flow Aortic stenosis, hypertrophic cardiomyopathy, congenital heart disease, myxoma
Primary dysrhythmia Vast majority occur with underlying structural heart disease (congenital or acquired) or ischemia. Exception to above is familial disorders (eg, congenital long QT syndrome, Brugada syndrome).
Neurocardiogenic or reflex-mediated Abnormal autonomic response to stimulus → vagal hyperactivity and symptoms. Classic vasovagal, carotid sinus syndrome, cough, micturition
Medication-induced
Orthostatic
Neurologic Transient ischemic attack, subclavian steal, migraine
Psychiatric (hyperventilation)

TABLE 2.26. Classic Presentations of Syncope

PRESENTATION	SUSPECTED DIAGNOSIS
17-year-old male, syncope during running	Hypertrophic cardiomyopathy
29-year-old female, syncope and abdominal pain	Ectopic pregnancy
68-year-old male, syncope and abdominal or flank pain	Abdominal aortic aneurysm
34-year-old female, sudden severe headache and syncope	Subarachnoid hemorrhage
72-year-old male with history of MI and CHF, syncope at home	Dysrhythmia
40-year-old female, syncope while standing in line, prodrome of nausea, sweating, warmth	Vasovagal
78-year-old female with cancer, sudden onset of SOB and syncope	PE

DIAGNOSIS

- A complete history and exam are critical to guide the ordering of tests.
- ECG should be done in all cases to screen for underlying cardiovascular disease, dysrhythmias, presence of familial disorder (eg, Brugada syndrome; see Figure 2.21) or electrolyte abnormalities.
- Echocardiography: To screen for underlying cardiovascular disease if diagnosis remains unclear
- Patients at high risk for cardiac etiology:
  - Age > 45
  - History of ventricular dysrhythmias

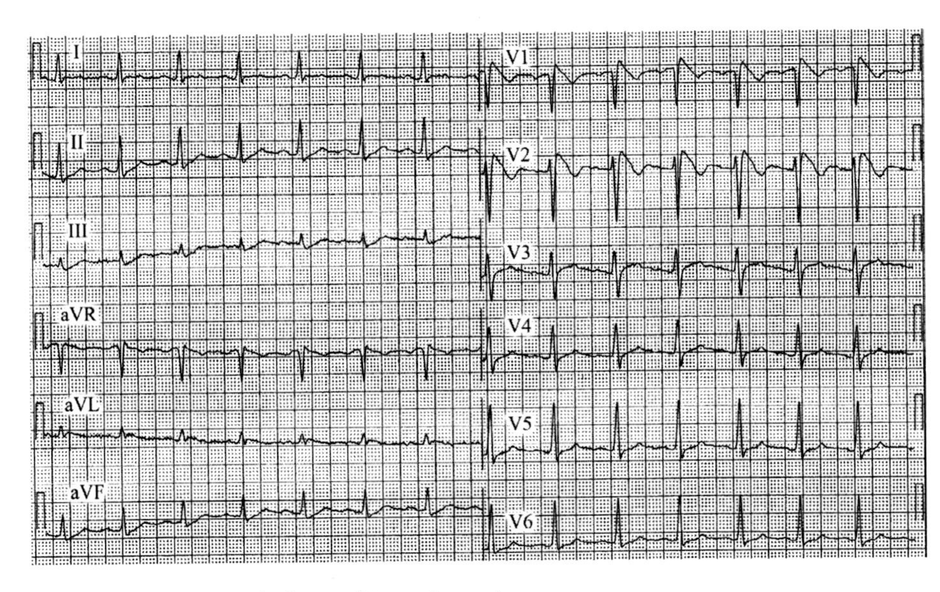

FIGURE 2.21. Typical ECG of Brugada syndrome.

(Reproduced, with permission, from Fuster V, Alexander RW, O'Rourke, RA. *Hurst's The Heart*, 12th ed. New York: McGraw-Hill, 2008:1837.)

- History of congestive heart failure
- Abnormal ECG
- Syncope in supine position
- Exertional syncope
- Syncope associated with chest pain
- Patient at low risk for cardiac etiology
  - Young patient, normal physical examination, normal ECG
  - Clinical presentation suggestive of vasovagal syncope

Goals of Care (ED core measures) for syncope: ECG for every patient >60 years old with a discharge diagnosis of syncope from ED

TREATMENT

- Resuscitation, as needed
- Identifying and treating the underlying etiology is the mainstay of treatment.
- Admit for monitoring and echocardiogram: If no identifiable cause in high-risk patient (one-third of patients).

VENOUS CIRCULATORY DISORDERS

Deep Venous Thrombosis

Deep venous thrombosis (DVT) can occur anywhere in the deep venous system, but is most common in the deep veins of the legs.

In the legs, the deep venous system constitutes a network of veins that extend from the calf veins to the femoral (which is, in fact, a deep vein, although it is often called the "superficial femoral vein") and iliac veins. The superficial veins in the legs include the greater and short saphenous veins and the perforator veins.

There are many clinical factors that increase the susceptibility to DVT formation (see Table 2.27).

Virchow's triad: Damage to vessel wall, venostasis, hypercoagulable state.

PATHOPHYSIOLOGY

- Damage to the vessel wall, venostasis, or hypercoagulable state (Virchow's triad) → thrombus formation.
- Once formed, thrombus can propagate or embolize proximally.
- Massive thrombus can cause vasospasm of adjacent artery.

TABLE 2.27. Clinical Risk Factors for Deep Venous Thrombosis

T	Trauma, travel
H	Hypercoagulable, hormone replacement
R	Recreational drugs (intravenous drugs)
O	Old (age > 60 y)
M	Malignancy
B	Birth control pill, blood group A
O	Obesity, obstetrics
S	Surgery, smoking
I	Immobilization
S	Sickness

(Reproduced, with permission, from Tintinalli JE, Kelen GD, Stapczynski JS. *Emergency Medicine: A Comprehensive Study Guide*, 6th ed. New York: McGraw-Hill, 2004:409.)

SYMPTOMS/EXAM

- Symptoms and physical examination are often nonspecific.
- Unilateral limb swelling, pain
- Tender palpable cord
- Erythema and warmth
- Distended collateral veins
- Homan's sign (pain in calf or posterior knee with passive dorsiflexion of foot) is unreliable.
- **Phlegmasia cerulean dolens (painful blue leg)** = massive iliofemoral thrombosis causing acute, massive edema, severe pain, and cyanosis.
- **Phlegmasia alba dolens (painful white leg)** = massive iliofemoral thrombosis causing arterial spasm and a swollen, pale leg.

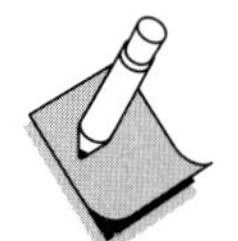

Phlegmasia cerulean dolens (painful blue leg) = massive thrombosis with venous insufficiency.

Phlegmasia alba dolens (painful white leg) = massive thrombosis with arterial spasm.

DIFFERENTIAL

- **Superficial thrombophlebitis**
- Cellulitis
- Lymphedema
- Musculoskeletal injury
- Baker's cyst

DIAGNOSIS

- The diagnosis should be considered in **all** patients presenting with symptoms/exam that raise concerns for DVT, especially in presence of risk factors.

Risk Stratification

- **Well's criteria** (see Table 2.28)
- Initial step in establishing diagnosis
- Estimates the pretest likelihood of DVT
- Score < 2 indicates a **low or moderate pretest risk** for DVT.

TABLE 2.28. Well's Pretest Probability for Predicting DVT

CRITERIA	SCORE
Active cancer	1
Paralysis/immobilization	1
Bedridden 3 days/surgery in last 12 weeks	1
Tender along deep vein (localized)	1
Entire leg swollen	1
Unilateral calf swelling (>3 cm)	1
Pitting edema, 1 leg	1
Collateral superficial nonvaricose vein	1
Previous documented DVT	1
Alternative diagnosis likely	–2
Score < 2 = low or moderate risk for DVT	
Score ≥ 2 = high risk for DVT	

TABLE 2.29. Clinical Evaluation for Deep Venous Thrombosis

Low or moderate pretest risk
If D-dimer normal → no DVT present.
If D-dimer elevated → obtain extremity ultrasound to exclude DVT.
High pretest risk
Obtain extremity ultrasound to exclude DVT.
If ultrasound negative but D-dimer elevated → plan repeat ultrasound in 5–7 days.
If ultrasound and D-dimer both negative → no DVT present.
Suspected pelvic vein or vena caval thrombosis
Obtain CT with contrast or MR venography.

D-dimer measured by ELISA is more accurate than the latex agglutination method.

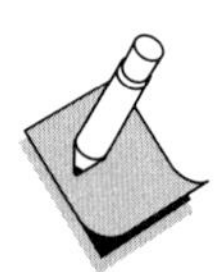

LMW heparin requires dose adjustment in renal failure.

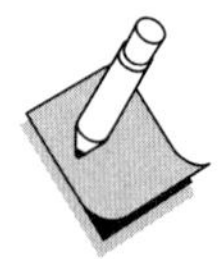

*Thrombolysis is **not** more effective than heparin for preventing PE in DVT.*

- Score ≥ 2 indicates a **high pretest risk** for DVT.
- **D-dimer**
  - Fibrin breakdown product
    - Indicates presence of a clot (somewhere) within **past 72 hours**
    - Elevated levels may be seen in sepsis, pregnancy, trauma, MI, liver disease, cancer (and more).
  - ELISA (quantitative) is more accurate than latex agglutination (qualitative).
- **Duplex ultrasound** = study of choice
  - Ultrasound with color Doppler flow evaluation
  - Highly sensitive for proximal DVT of leg, but
  - May not identify calf vein or iliac vein thrombosis
- **Venography:** Gold standard, but rarely used (invasive, radiation, cost)
- **MRI**
  - Highly sensitive for DVT
  - Useful for DVT in iliac vein or vena cava where ultrasound cannot be used
- A clinical diagnosis is established using a combination of the above modalities (see Table 2.29).

Treatment

- **Immediate anticoagulation** with LMW heparin
  - Requires dose adjustment in renal failure
  - Does not prevent investigation for hypercoagulable state
  - If heparin contraindicated (eg, heparin-induced thrombocytopenia), use thrombin inhibitor, such as lepirudin **or danoparoid**.
- **Long-term anticoagulation:** Warfarin, first dose in the ED
- **Thrombolysis** is **not** more effective than heparin for preventing PE, but
  - May accelerate clot lysis and **reduce complications of venous insufficiency** in massive thrombosis
  - Contraindications: As with myocardial infarction
- **IVF filter** indications include:
  - Contraindication to or complication of anticoagulation (bleeding, heparin-induced thrombocytopenia)
  - Propagation of DVT despite adequate anticoagulation with warfarin and heparin
  - Presence of free-floating nonadherent iliofemoral thrombus >5 cm
  - Massive clot burden
- Many possible clinical scenarios exist in the treatment of DVT (see Table 2.30).

TABLE 2.30. Clinical Considerations in the Treatment of DVT

Proximal DVT Immediate anticoagulation with heparin and warfarin until INR therapeutic
Massive DVT Vascular surgery consult for thrombectomy Consider thrombolysis Consider IVC filter placement
Isolated calf vein thrombosis These veins have a low risk for embolization **but** At least 25% will propagate proximally, where they **may** embolize Options include anticoagulation (for high-risk patients) **or** ASA and follow-up ultrasound in 3–7 days
Proximal greater saphenous vein clot Too close to the deep system for comfort! Anticoagulate
Recurrent DVT on adequate warfarin Add heparin Indication for IVC filter placement
Propagation of DVT on adequate warfarin and heparin Indication for IVC filter placement

Complications

- PE
- Chronic venous insufficiency
- SVC syndrome (upper extremity clot)
- From therapy: Heparin-induced thrombocytopenia, warfarin skin necrosis, bleeding
- Post-phlebitic syndrome

A 40-year-old female 1 week status post mastectomy presents with mild R-sided pleuritic chest pain and dyspnea. Her initial BP is 124/72, HR is 122, O_2 saturation is 90% on room air, and temperature is 101°F. Exam reveals equal breath sounds with no rales or rhonchi. There is no redness or swelling over the chest wall. There is no swelling in the legs. What is the study of choice in this patient?

CT angiogram of chest to evaluate for PE. Because this patient has a high pretest probability for PE, a D-dimer is not indicated. CT can also detect abscess or pneumonia in this patient.

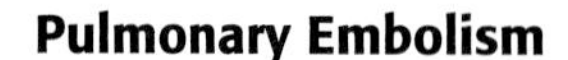

Pulmonary Embolism

By far the most common source of PE is thrombus in the lower extremity deep venous system. Risk factors are therefore identical to DVT (see Table 2.27). Other possible emboli include fat, amniotic fluid, and tumor.

Symptoms in PE are sudden onset only half the time!

PATHOPHYSIOLOGY

- Thrombus formed in venous system → embolizes to lung → acute obstruction of the pulmonary arterial system and pulmonary ischemia/infarction.
- Large emboli → obstruction of right ventricular outflow and circulatory collapse.

SYMPTOMS

- Nonspecific
- Shortness of breath: Most common complaint
- Chest pain: Classically pleuritic (but not always)
- Cough and/or hemoptysis
- Syncope and acute cardiovascular collapse may occur.

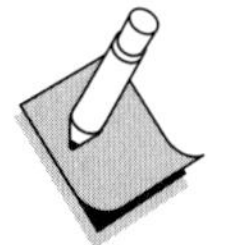

Most common ECG in PE = tachycardia and nonspecific ST-T changes. Classic ECG finding = $S_1Q_3T_3$.

EXAM

- Tachypnea: Most common finding
- Tachycardia
- Clear lungs (but may hear rales/wheezes)
- Hypoxia
- Fever (<102°F)
- Evidence of acute R heart failure, hypotension: If massive

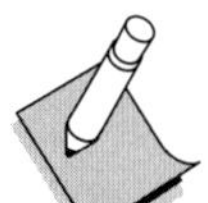

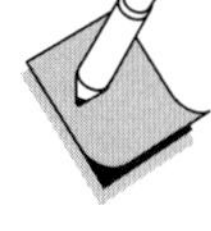

A-a gradient at sea level: $150-(PO_2 + PCO_2/0.8)$

DIAGNOSIS

Diagnosis should be suspected in any patient presenting with dyspnea and/or chest pain, especially in the presence of risk factors.

Multiple tools are available to risk stratify patients for PE; diagnostic evaluation should be based on individual risk assessment. Recent studies suggest that the Wells clinical prediction rule is a useful risk stratification tool (see Table 2.31).

Normal A-a gradient = Age/4 + 4.

- **ECG:** Abnormal in most, but not diagnostic
  - Tachycardia and nonspecific ST-T changes most common.
  - **Any** evidence of R heart strain: Classic is S wave in lead I, Q wave in lead III and T-wave inversion in lead III ($S_1Q_3T_3$ pattern)
- **ABG:** May demonstrate respiratory alkalosis, hypoxemia, and a widened A-a gradient; a normal ABG does not *exclude* PE
- **CXR:** Abnormal in most, but nonspecific (eg, effusion, atelectasis)
  - **Hampton's hump** = pleural-based, wedge-shaped density indicating infarcted lung.
  - **Westermark's sign** = ↓ vessel markings distal to embolus (oligemia) (**rarely** seen).
- **D-dimer:** Described in the section "Deep Venous Thrombosis," page 132.
  - Test virtually excludes PE in a low-risk (low clinical suspicion) patient.
- **CT angiography** (see Figure 2.22): Study of choice where available
  - High sensitivity and specificity
  - Preferred over V/Q scan in pregnancy due to *lower* fetal radiation exposure

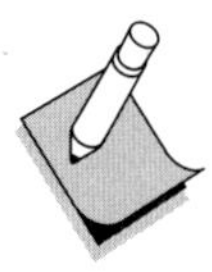

A negative D-dimer virtually excludes PE in a low clinical suspicion patient.

TABLE 2.31. **Wells Clinical Prediction Rule for PE**

CLINICAL FEATURE	POINTS
Clinical symptoms of DVT	3
Other diagnosis less likely than PE	3
Heart rate > 100 bpm	1.5
Immobilization or surgery within past 4 weeks	1.5
Previous DVT or PE	1.5
Hemoptysis	1
Malignancy	1
High risk for PE: > 6 points **Moderate risk for PE: 2–6 points** **Low risk for PE: < 2 points** Note: Newer studies are dichotomizing patients into low (≤4 points) or high (>4 points) risk.	

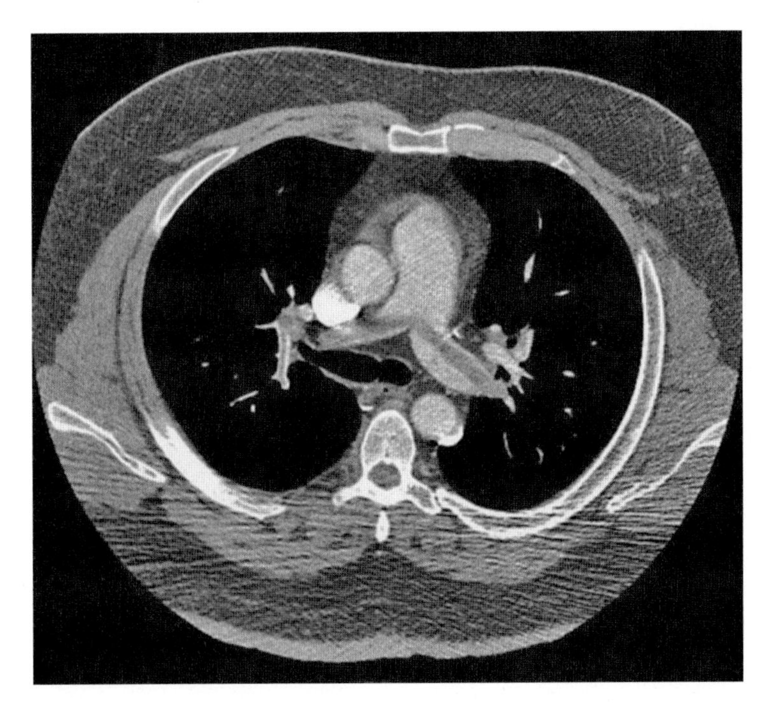

FIGURE 2.22. **Contrast-enhanced helical chest CT, showing large filling defect in both pulmonary arteries from a saddle pulmonary embolus.**

(Courtesy of Matthew J. Fleishman, MD, Radiology Imaging Associates. Englewood, Colorado.)

- **V/Q scan**
  - Matches inhaled radionuclide distribution (ventilation) to pulmonary vasculature radionuclide (perfusion).
    - *Normal* perfusion = no PE.
    - High probability = definite PE.
    - Low probability with low clinical suspicion = no PE.
    - All others need further imaging.
  - Indications include renal failure, contrast allergy.
  - Less useful if underlying lung disease or abnormal CXR
  - Insensitive
- **Pulmonary arteriography:** Classic gold standard, but mostly supplanted by chest CT
- **Duplex ultrasound**
  - Presumptive PE if + for DVT in correct clinical setting (negative test **not** helpful in excluding PE)

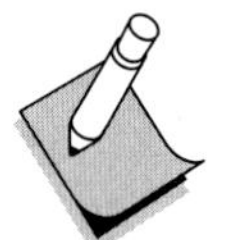

Indications for thrombolysis in PE = clinical evidence of massive PE.

TREATMENT

- **Immediate anticoagulation** with unfractionated heparin infusion or LMW heparin
  - If heparin is contraindicated use thrombin inhibitor, such as lepirudin or danoparoid.
- **Thrombolysis** should be used if there is clinical evidence of massive PE (hypotension, cardiac arrest, evidence of R heart strain).
  - tPA is preferred agent (100 mg over 2 hours).
  - Contraindications similar to thrombolytics in MI (see Table 2.7).
  - No evidence that mortality is lowered, but will improve R heart function.
- **Embolectomy**
  - Procedure of last resort in critically ill patient when thrombolysis is contraindicated
- **IVC Filter**
  - To prevent recurrent PE in patient with contraindications to anticoagulation or with recurrent PE on anticoagulation

COMPLICATIONS

- Cardiac arrest and death
- Development of pulmonary hypertension

Venous Insufficiency

Chronic elevation of venous pressure can compromise the integrity of valves in the deep and perforating veins in the leg. This results in edema, varicose veins, and chronic changes in the skin and soft tissues.

CAUSES

- DVT: Most common
- Trauma
- Others: Varicose veins, pelvic vein obstruction, AV fistula

EXAM

- Edema is the earliest finding.
- Later signs: Stasis dermatitis, varicosities, ulceration

DIFFERENTIAL

- CHF
- Renal disease
- Lymphedema
- Arterial insufficiency

TREATMENT

- Treat underlying condition.
- Elevation
- Avoid prolonged dependency.
- Compression garments
- Wound care for skin breakdown/ulceration
  - Unna's boot, wet-to-dry dressing, wound vacuums
  - Debridement and skin grafting
- Antibiotics: If infection is present

CHAPTER 3

Trauma

Hagop M. Afarian, MD, MS

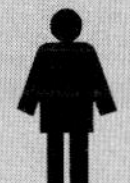

A 40-year-old female is brought in by ambulance after sustaining a high-speed rollover MVC. She has signs of injury to the head, chest, and abdomen. What are the first steps in assessing this patient?

ABCDE—assess **A**irway, **B**reathing, **C**irculation, and **D**isability (mental status). **E**xpose patient completely, then cover to prevent hypothermia.

INITIAL TRAUMA—STABILIZATION AND RESUSCITATION

EXAM/DIAGNOSIS

As with any critically ill patient, the initial assessment of a trauma patient begins with ABCs. Further assessment and treatment should be directed to specific complaints or injuries. In a patient with multiple injuries, the ABCDE approach described by the Advanced Trauma Life Support (ATLS) guidelines provide a methodical approach to patient assessment and treatment.

Head injury and thoracic vascular injury are the two most common causes of death in trauma patients.

Primary Survey

- **A**irway, with C-spine stabilization
- **B**reathing and ventilation
- **C**irculation and control of bleeding
- Neurologic **D**isability (mental status)
- **E**xposure of patient

AIRWAY

- O_2 delivery: High-flow O_2 via a nonrebreather is preferred for patients with potentially serious injuries.
- Airway devices/maneuvers (jaw thrust, nasopharyngeal airway, etc.)
- Intubation for:
  - Altered mental status due to head injury or intoxication
  - Airway compromise due to trauma to the face or neck
  - Significant chest trauma (ie, flail chest)
  - Profound hypotension
  - Maintain C-spine immobilization during intubation.

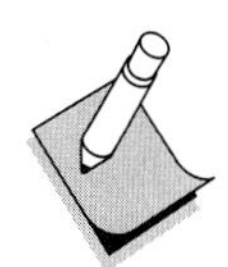

A trauma patient with a normal RR and O_2 saturation may require intubation for immobilization if agitated to allow imaging or to protect the airway from anticipated swelling due to face or neck trauma or burns.

BREATHING

- Listen to breath sounds to assess symmetry and an appropriate volume of air movement.
- Look for adequate chest rise and fall.
- A chest X-ray should be obtained in patients with chest pain, evidence of chest trauma, hypotension, or altered mental status.

CIRCULATION

- Assess circulation by measuring HR and BP grossly with cap refill and peripheral pulses followed by a manual BP.
- There are four classes of hemorrhage (see Table 3.1). Hypotension in patients with a normal HR is still hypotension and requires both treatment and an aggressive search for blood loss or other cause.

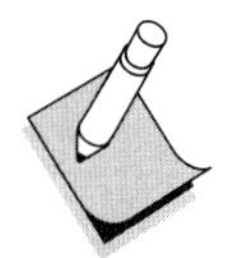

Class II hemorrhage: Tachycardia
Class III hemorrhage: Tachycardia and hypotension

TABLE 3.1. Classes of Hemorrhage

	CLASS I	CLASS II	CLASS III	CLASS IV
BP	Normal	Normal	**Decreased**	Decreased
HR	<100	**100–120**	120–140	>140
Volume blood loss	<750 mL	750–1500 mL	1500–2000 mL	>2000 mL
Percent blood loss	<15%	15–30%	30–40%	>40%

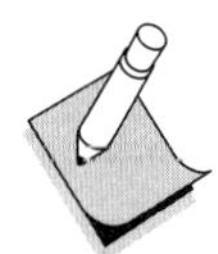

An easy way to remember the maximum GCS score is to remember 4, 5, 6 moving down from the eyes (max. 4) to the mouth (max. 5) to the arms (max. 6).

- Following trauma, patients can elicit any of the five types of shock:
  - Hypovolemic (hemorrhage)
  - Distributive (brain/spinal cord injury)
  - Cardiogenic (direct myocardial injury)
  - Obstructive (tension pneumothorax or cardiac tamponade)
  - Dissociative (inhalation of carbon monoxide or cyanide)
- Treat hypotension with an initial challenge of 1–2 L of isotonic fluid.

DISABILITY

- Perform a rapid neurologic evaluation to assess patient's level of consciousness.
- The Glasgow Coma Scale (GCS) is a 3–15 score of mental status that measures three attributes: Eye opening, verbal response, and best motor response (see Table 3.2).
- AVPU (**A**lert; responds to **V**ocal stimuli; responds to **P**ainful stimuli; **U**nresponsive) is a simpler method of describing level of consciousness.
- Assessment of extremity motor and sensation is part of the secondary survey.

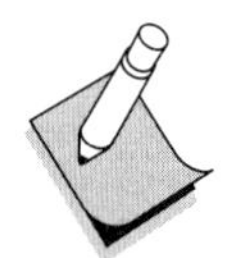

GCS was designed for use specifically in the setting of trauma.

EXPOSURE/ENVIRONMENT

- Undress the patient to look for additional injuries to torso and extremities.
- Cover the patient in a warm blanket or external warming device to prevent hypothermia. Check a core temperature in patients who may be cold or hot.

TABLE 3.2. The Glasgow Coma Scale

EYE OPENING	SCORE	VERBAL RESPONSE	SCORE	MOTOR RESPONSE	SCORE
Spontaneous	4	Oriented	5	Follows commands	6
To voice	3	Confused	4	Localizes pain	5
To painful stimuli	2	Inappropriate words	3	Withdraws from pain	4
Never	1	Unintelligible sounds	2	Flexor response	3
		None	1	Extensor response	2
				None	1

Secondary Survey

- The secondary survey includes a directed history and a detailed physical examination.
- A Focused Assessment with Sonography for Trauma (FAST) exam is a quick tool that can be used during a secondary survey to evaluate for intra-abdominal/pelvic and cardiac injuries.
- A FAST exam showing free fluid in the abdomen in a hypotensive victim of blunt trauma suggests that the patient has intra-abdominal hemorrhage and suggests the need for immediate exploratory laparotomy.

TREATMENT

- Any patient with concern for circulatory compromise needs to have two large-bore IVs for fluid resuscitation.
- In the setting of hypovolemia, administer an initial 1–2 L of crystalloid.
- If the patient remains hypotensive, transfuse with O-negative blood or type-specific blood if available.
- This treatment should be provided concurrent with efforts to identify and treat sources of hemorrhage as well as other possible causes of hypotension including cardiac, chest, and spinal injury.

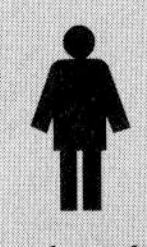

A young man arrives in the ED following isolated head trauma with loss of consciousness (LOC). His mental status has returned to baseline, but he has been vomiting and complains of persistent headache. What should you do next?

This patient has a moderate risk for intracranial injury based on his presenting symptoms. Administer antiemetics and obtain a head CT with or without C-spine imaging.

HEAD TRAUMA

The brain is contained within a fixed volume (the skull). After trauma, bleeding and swelling can cause an increase in increased intracranial pressure (ICP), which can lead to herniation of the brain, most commonly along the falx cerebelli (uncal herniation). The goal of the emergency physician is to support oxygenation and BP to prevent secondary brain injury and to identify head injuries that require intervention or observation (see Table 3.3).

SYMPTOMS

Symptoms depend on severity of injury and range from mild focal headache to loss of consciousness, amnesia, vomiting, or headache.

EXAM

- Varies with severity of injury
- Calculate GCS (Table 3.2).
- Review vital signs—ICP may cause the **Cushing reflex**: Hypertension, bradycardia, and irregular respirations.
- Pupillary exam
  - A single fixed and dilated pupil may be a sign of ipsilateral uncal herniation (but in awake patients, is usually indicative of ocular trauma).
  - Bilateral fixed and dilated pupils may indicate complete uncal herniation, poor brain perfusion, or stimulant use.

TABLE 3.3. **Categorization of Traumatic Brain Injury (TBI)**

TBI SEVERITY	MILD TBI			MODERATE TBI	SEVERE TBI
GCS	14–15			9–13	< 9
Risk for injury	**Low**	**Moderate**	**High**	High	High
	No LOC No/mild HA Normal exam	LOC Amnesia Vomiting Diffuse HA	Skull fracture Neuro deficit High-risk patient		
Head CT required? Incidence of surgical intervention	No 0.1%	Yes 1–3%	Yes Up to 10%	Yes 8%	Yes
Mortality				20%	60%

- Motor exam: To assess for focal neurologic deficits or posturing
  - **Decorticate posturing**: Abnormal flexion of the upper extremities ("clutch the cortex"), extension of lower extremities
  - **Decerebrate posturing**: Extension/adduction and internal rotation of arms and legs with flexion of wrist, fingers, feet (plantar), and toes
- Brainstem exam: Via evaluation of respiratory pattern, papillary size, and eye movements
  - **Oculocephalic response** (pontine gaze centers): "Doll's eyes" response with eyes moving in direction opposite of head turning (once C-spine is cleared) indicates intact brainstem function in the comatose patient.
  - **Oculovestibular response**: Instillation of 30 mL ice-cold saline into the ear; nystagmus with fast component away from indicates intact brainstem function.

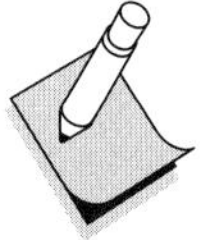

Cushing reflex: Hypertension, bradycardia, and irregular respirations

TRAUMA

DIAGNOSIS

- CT scan without contrast is the diagnostic test of choice. CT anyone with a change in mental status. Have a low threshold for head CT in patients who are elderly or have coagulopathy, vomiting, or have persistent headaches.
- For children < 2 years old, head CT is appropriate in the presence of:
  - Focal neurologic abnormality
  - Altered mental status
  - Any scalp trauma (laceration/ecchymosis/contusion/abrasion)
  - Vomiting

TREATMENT

- Patients with findings or suspicion of head injury warrant aggressive management to prevent secondary brain injury.
- Ensure adequate oxygenation and ventilation.
- Intubate if GCS ≤ 8 or presence of intracranial injury by CT.
- Elevate head of bed to 30°.
- Aggressively treat hypotension with fluids or blood transfusion to maintain SBP ≥ 90 mmHg.

- Seizure prophylaxis with phenytoin to prevent early posttraumatic seizures; indications include severe head injury, intracranial injury by CT, presence of skull fracture
- Antiemetics for nausea/vomiting
- Antibiotics if penetrating injury
- If evidence for herniation or clinical deterioration:
  - Hyperventilate to P_{CO_2} of 30–35 mmHg
  - Mannitol 0.25–1 g/kg IV bolus to produce osmotic diuresis
  - Emergent burr hole
- Patients with a GCS of ≤8 usually require invasive monitoring of ICP (either a bolt with pressure monitor placed into the subdural space or a ventriculostomy). Ventriculostomy has the added benefit of allowing drainage of CSF to decrease ICP.

Intracranial Hemorrhage

Cerebral Contusion

- Usually frontal/temporal lobes
- Contusion may be at side opposite to injury—"contrecoup."

Traumatic Subarachnoid

- Caused by disruption of subarachnoid vessels (see Figure 3.1)
- Most common intracranial bleed in moderate to severe TBI (see Table 3.4)
  - Typically see HA, photophobia, and/or meningeal signs

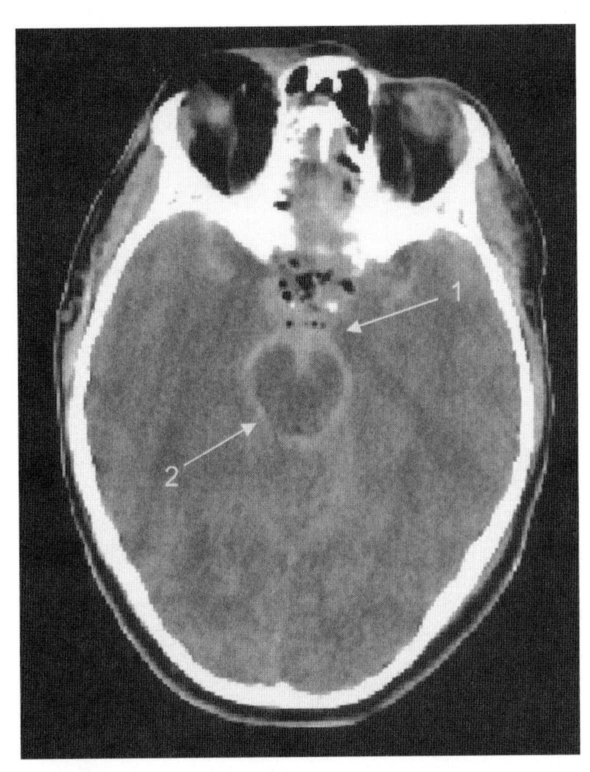

FIGURE 3.1. Subarachnoid hemorrhage. Non-contrast head CT showing blood surrounding the brainstem at the level of the midbrain (1, 2).

(Reproduced, with permission, from Tintinalli JE, Kelen GD, Stapczynski JS. *Emergency Medicine: A Comprehensive Study Guide*, 6th ed. New York: McGraw-Hill, 2004:1567.)

TABLE 3.4. Intracranial Hematomas

	Type of Patient	Anatomic Location	CT Findings	Common Cause	Classic Symptoms
Epidural	Most common in young adults, rare in the elderly	Potential space between skull and dura mater	Biconvex, football-shaped hematoma	Skull fracture with tear of the middle meningeal artery	Immediate LOC with a "lucid" period prior to deterioration (only occurs in about 20% of patients)
Subdural	More risk for the elderly and alcoholics	Space between dura mater and arachnoid	Crescent- or sickle-shaped hematoma	Acceleration–deceleration with tearing of the bridging veins	Acute: Rapid LOC–lucid period possible Chronic: Altered MS and behavior with gradual decrease in consciousness
Subarachnoid	Any age group following blunt trauma	Subarachnoid	Blood in the basilar cisterns and hemispheric sulci and fissures	Acceleration–deceleration with tearing of the subarachnoid vessels	Mild to moderate TBI with meningeal signs and symptoms
Contusion/ intracerebral hematoma	Any age group following blunt trauma	Usually anterior temporal or posterior frontal lobe	May be normal initially with delayed bleed	Severe or penetrating trauma; shaken-baby syndrome	Symptoms range from normal to unconscious

(Reproduced, with permission, from Tintinalli JE, Kelen GD, Stapczynski JS. *Emergency Medicine: A Comprehensive Study Guide*, 6th ed. New York: McGraw-Hill, 2004:1568.)
Abbreviations: LOC = loss of consciousness; MS = mental state; TBI = traumatic brain injury.

EPIDURAL HEMATOMA

- Usually associated with skull fracture after blunt trauma (see Figure 3.2)
- Classically an injury to the **middle meningeal artery**, but epidurals may occur in other locations
- Arterial bleeding results in rapid expansion.
- CT shows biconvex opacity usually at temporo/temporoparietal area.
- Classically presents with lucid interval after initial LOC followed by recurrence of unconsciousness from expanding hematoma
- A surgical emergency: Evacuation is required unless very small.

SUBDURAL HEMATOMA

- Caused by tearing of bridging veins (see Figure 3.3)
- Common in the elderly and alcoholics because of atrophy and increased intracranial space, leading to increased movement of the brain and shearing forces on bridging veins; may be associated with minor or no known trauma
- Crescent-shaped hematoma on CT: Bright if acute, dark if chronic (>14 days)
- Surgical intervention usually required for acute (<24 hours) and subacute (<2 weeks) bleeds, and any bleed associated with a change in mental status or significant midline shift

Basilar Skull Fracture

Most commonly through the petrous portion of temporal bone

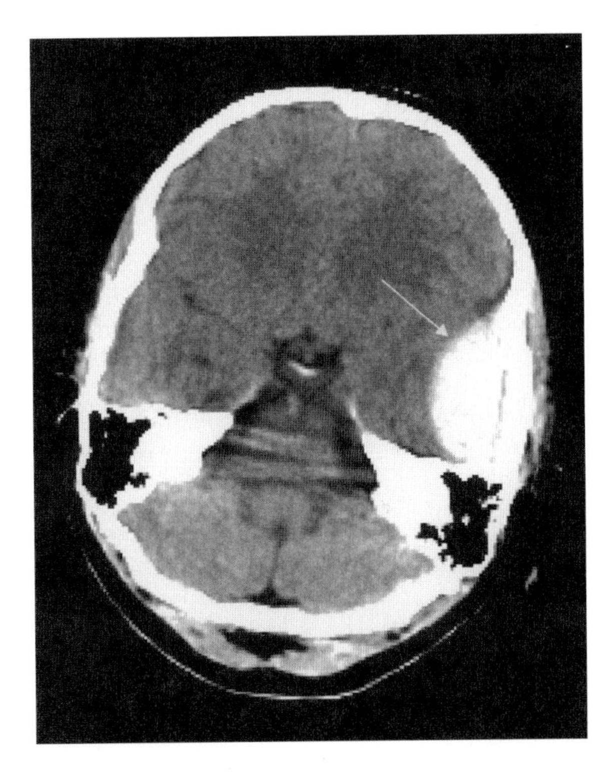

FIGURE 3.2. Epidural hematoma.

(Reproduced, with permission, from Tintinalli JE, Kelen GD, Stapczynski JS. *Emergency Medicine: A Comprehensive Study Guide*, 6th ed. New York: McGraw-Hill, 2004:1567.)

TRAUMA

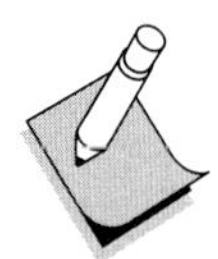

In patients who have very low GCS but no findings on CT, consider diffuse axonal injury (DAI) resulting from shearing of axonal fibers.

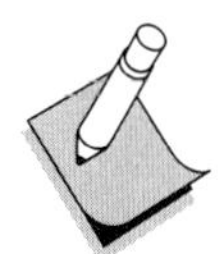

CPP = MAP–ICP

Ideal CPP > 60 mmHg

Ideal MAP > 80 mmHg

Ideal ICP < 15 mmHg

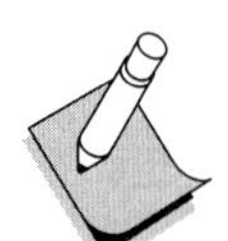

Nimodipine is used for treatment of SAH from spontaneous ruptured aneurysm but not for traumatic head injury.

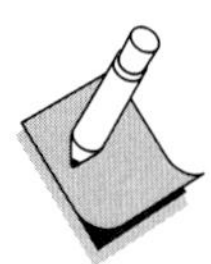

GSWs to the head result in cavitation injury three to four times the bullet's diameter.

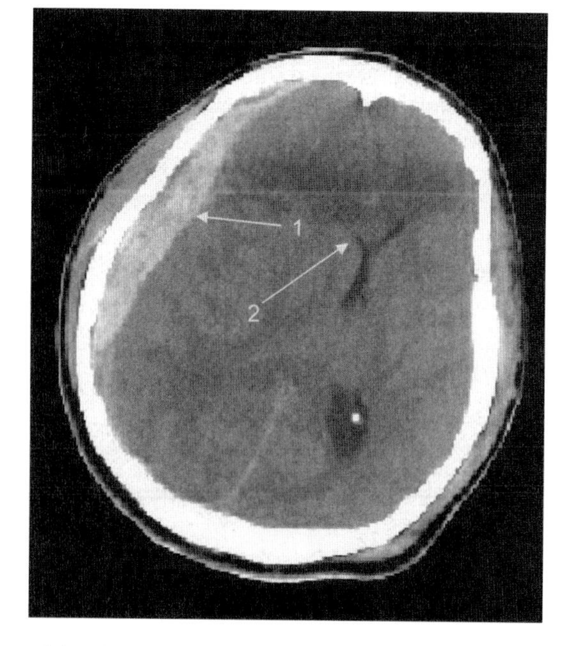

FIGURE 3.3. Subdural hematoma. Non-contrast head CT showing right subdural hematoma (1) with collapse of the right ventricle and midline shift (2).

(Reproduced, with permission, from Tintinalli JE, Kelen GD, Stapczynski JS. *Emergency Medicine: A Comprehensive Study Guide*, 6th ed. New York: McGraw-Hill, 2004:1568.)

SYMPTOMS/EXAM

- Vertigo
- Hearing difficulties
- CSF otorrhea or rhinorrhea
- Mastoid ecchymosis (Battle's sign)
- Periorbital ecchymosis (raccoon eyes)
- Hemotympanum
- Seventh nerve palsy

TREATMENT/COMPLICATIONS

- Generally, patients with basilar skull fractures do not require treatment other than pain medications, antiemetics, and observation.
- Consider discharge for adults with simple linear fractures who are neurologically intact.
- Meningitis may occur following basilar skull fracture, and requires antibiotics and neurosurgical consultation. There is no consensus on the use of prophylactic antibiotics.

Fracture of Skull Convexity

EXAM

- Evaluate for lacerations, exposed, fractured, or depressed bone.
- Overlying hematomas or lacerations may indicate underlying fracture.
- Look for pneumocephalus on CT.

TREATMENT

- Operative repair is required for fractures depressed beyond one full thickness of the skull because of increased likelihood of direct compression of the brain.
- Antibiotics should be given to patients with open skull fractures.

Concussion

Mechanisms

- Any blunt trauma to the head: Sporting injuries (boxing, football, soccer, basketball, baseball) commonly lead to concussions

Symptoms

- Brief LOC/cognitive and memory dysfunction/personality change
- Dizziness/balance disturbance
- Headache/photophobia/tinnitus
- Nausea/vomiting

Treatment

- Supportive care and close monitoring (usually at home)
- Patients will usually completely recover, although 30–80% have symptoms 3 months out, and 15% have symptoms at 1 year (postconcussion syndrome).
- **Patients should not return to contact sports until complete resolution of symptoms.** An initial head injury may predispose patients to worse outcomes following a second head injury.

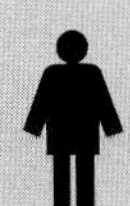

A 71-year-old male presents with bilateral arm weakness after a ground-level fall. He denies neck pain and moves his neck without pain. What's the diagnosis and mechanism of injury?

Central cord syndrome, resulting from hyperextension injury with buckling of the ligamentum flavum against the central cord. X-rays are often normal. MRI is confirmative.

SPINAL FRACTURES

Acute spinal injuries are classified into four categories according to mechanism of injury:

- Flexion fractures (eg, wedge, flexion teardrop, clay shoveler's)
- Vertical compression fractures (eg, burst, Jefferson)
- Flexion-rotation (eg, unilateral facet)
- Extension (eg, hangman's)

Mechanisms

- Motor vehicle crashes
- Sports, falls, diving in shallow water
- Judicial hanging with knot in front (causing hyperextension)
- Abrupt flexion during lifting (clay shoveler's fracture)

Cervical Spinal Fractures

Symptoms/Exam

- Individuals with C-spine fractures typically complain of posterior midline neck pain and pain with movement of the neck.
- The exam varies with the fracture location and degree of associated spinal cord injury.

DIAGNOSIS

Although posterior neck tenderness is one of the NEXUS criteria, posterior neck pain is not.

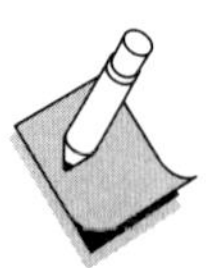

The NEXUS criteria can be divided into two groups:

1. *Criteria suggesting injury: Tenderness, neurologic deficit.*
2. *Criteria that impede exam: AMS, intoxication, distracting injury.*

- The decision to image the C-spine is based on the mechanism of injury, pain, tenderness, neurologic findings, and the alertness of the patient.
- The **National Emergency X-Radiography Utilization Study (NEXUS)** has identified five criteria that have 99.6% sensitivity of detecting clinically significant C-spine injury.
- According to NEXUS, spinal imaging is not required if patient has all of the following:
  - No posterior midline cervical spine tenderness
  - No focal neurologic deficits
  - No evidence of intoxication
  - Normal level of alertness
  - No painful distracting injuries
- A C-spine series consists of AP, lateral, swimmer's, and odontoid views. Obliques may be included.
  - Up to 80% of C-spine injuries can be detected by the lateral C-spine film.
  - The C7-T1 junction must be included as 20% of injuries occur at C7.
- Swelling of the prevertebral soft tissue suggests injury; a measurement > 7 mm at C2 and 21 mm at C6 are abnormal.
- On a lateral C-spine X-ray, three imaginary lines are identified (see Figure 3.4). Disruption to any line suggests injury.
  - Anterior contour line: Formed by anterior margin of vertebral body
  - Posterior contour line: Formed by posterior margin of vertebral body
  - Spinolaminar line: Connects the bases of the spinous processes and extends to the posterior aspect of the foramen magnum

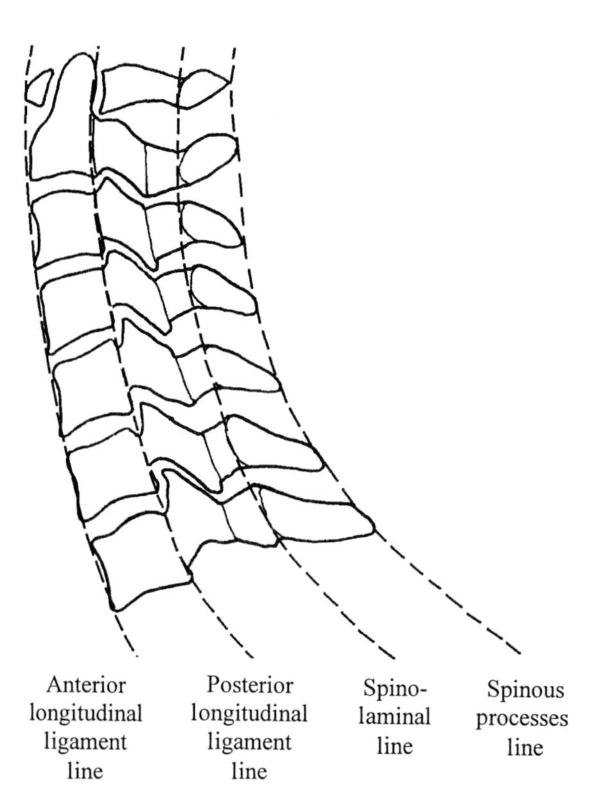

FIGURE 3.4. Diagram of lines on lateral C-spine.

(Reproduced, with permission, from Tintinalli JE, Kelen GD, Stapczynski JS. *Emergency Medicine: A Comprehensive Study Guide*, 6th ed. New York: McGraw-Hill, 2004:1703.)

- CT scan should be obtained in all patients with abnormal or inadequate C-spine X-rays or high clinical suspicion for injury.
- Injuries are divided into unstable fractures (see Table 3.5 and Figures 3.5–3.8) and stable fractures (see Table 3.6) based on radiographic imaging.
- If ligamentous injury is suspected and plain film and CT imaging is negative, MRI is indicated; flexion-extension views are limited by muscle spasm and pain and therefore have little utility in the immediate post-injury period.
- Odontoid fractures are classified as:
  - Type I: Avulsion of the tip (stable)
  - Type II: Fracture at junction of odontoid and body of C2 (most common)
  - Type III: Fracture at base of dens

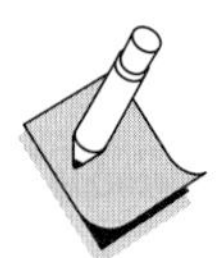

Abnormal soft-tissue findings on a lateral C-spine: Remember 6 at 2 and 22 at 6, and adjust up and down by 1 to get 7 mm and 21 mm.

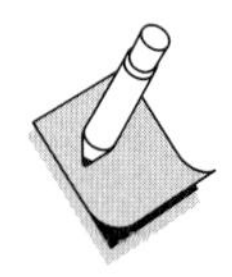

Most common fracture level is C5. Most common subluxation is C5 on C6.

THORACOLUMBAR FRACTURES

The thoracic spine (to approximately T11) is more rigid than the cervical and lumbar spine due to its articulation with the rib cage but its canal is narrow. Injury to the thoracic spine is therefore less common, but is often associated with spinal cord injury.

SYMPTOMS/EXAM

- Individuals with thoracolumbar fractures typically complain of pain in the region of injury.
- The exam varies with the fracture location and degree of associated spinal cord injury.

TABLE 3.5. Unstable Fractures of the C-Spine

TYPE	IMAGE	MECHANISM	CLINICAL STORY	NOTES
Jefferson fracture (C1 burst fx)	Figure 3.5	Axial load with vertical compression	Football player spearing another player	Seen on odontoid view
Bilateral facet dislocation	Figure 3.6	Flexion	Although called locked facets the injury is unstable	Anterior displacement > 50% diameter of vertebral body.
Odontoid type II/III	Figure 3.7	Flexion	Severe high cervical pain or pain radiating to the occiput	Usually due to major forces Consider other C-spine and bodily injuries.
Atlantoaxial or atlanto-occipital dislocations		Flexion or extension		Atlanto-occipital dissociation usually results in death.
Hangman's fracture (bilateral C2 pedicle fx)	Figure 3.8	Extension; C2 displaced anteriorly on C3	Judicial hanging with ball of noose in front	Not common with suicide hangings
Teardrop fracture		Flexion or extension (an avulsion fracture)		The teardrop is the anteroinferior portion of the vertebral body.

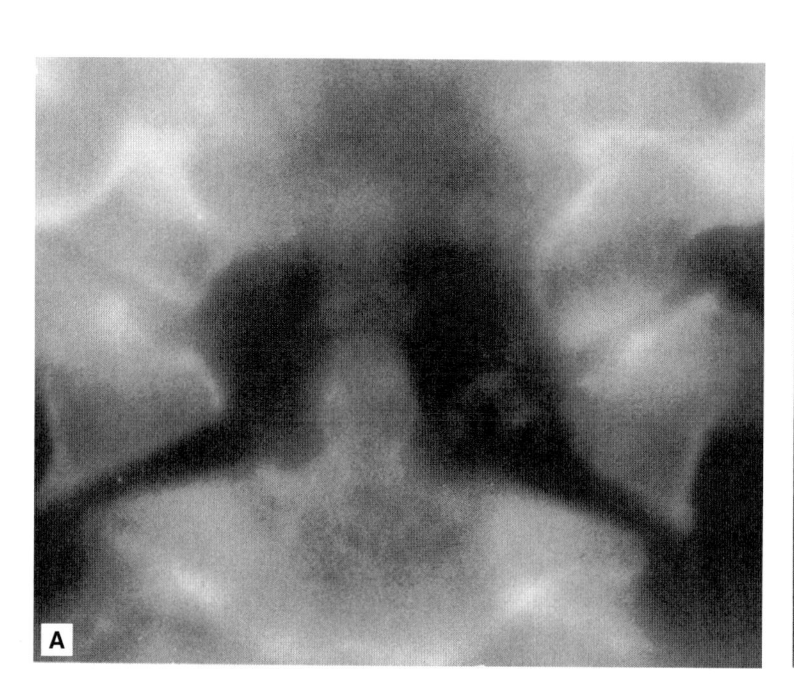

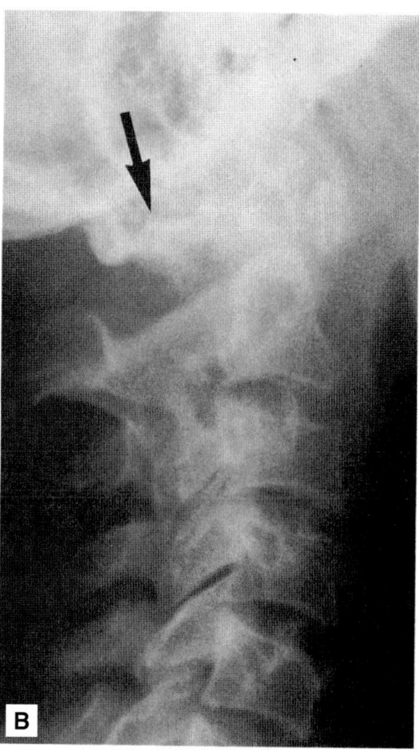

FIGURE 3.5. Jefferson Fracture. Odontoid view showing fragment from C1 to the right of the odontoid (A) and lateral view showing fracture of the posterior arch of C1 (B).

(Reproduced, with permission, from Hall JB, Schmidt GA, Wood LD. *Principles of Critical Care*, 3rd ed. New York: McGraw-Hill, 2005:1410.)

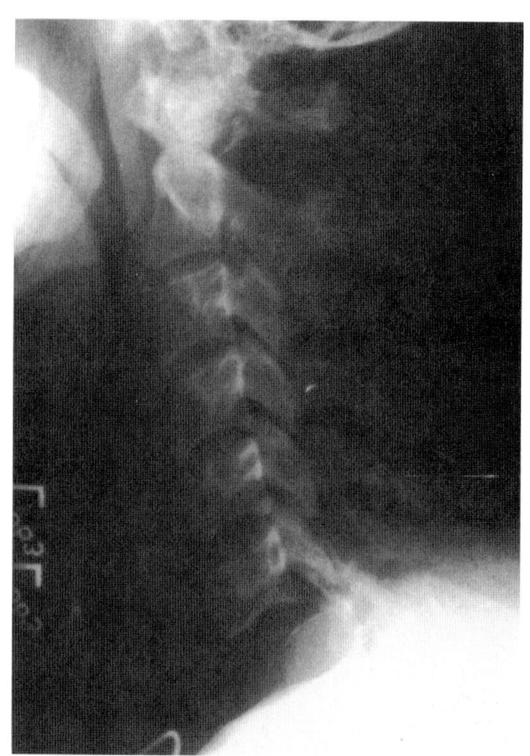

FIGURE 3.6. Bilateral facet dislocation.

(Reproduced, with permission, from Tintinalli JE, Kelen GD, Stapczynski JS. *Emergency Medicine: A Comprehensive Study Guide*, 6th ed. New York: McGraw-Hill, 2004:1708.)

DIAGNOSIS

- Suspect based on clinical presentation and/or plain radiographs
- CT scan is confirmative and can fully define the injury.
- Injuries are divided into major fractures (see Table 3.7) and minor fractures (transverse process, spinous process, and pars interarticularis) based on radiographic imaging.

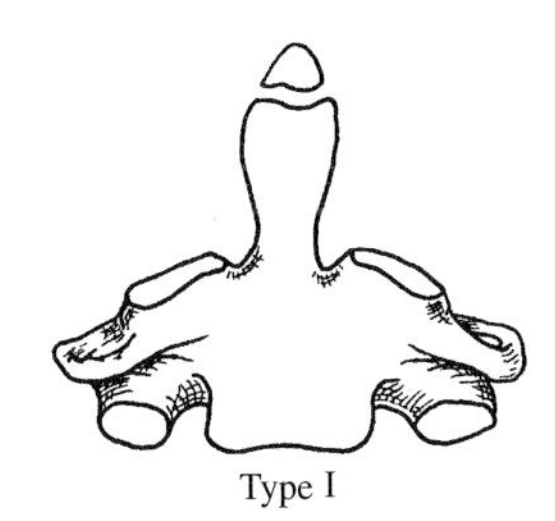

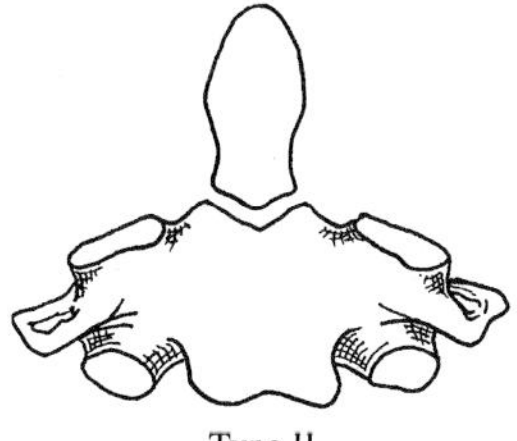

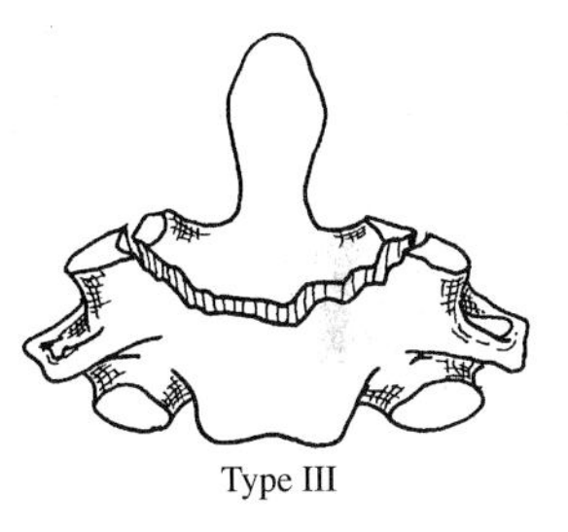

FIGURE 3.7. Odontoid fractures.

(Reproduced, with permission, from Tintinalli JE, Kelen GD, Stapczynski JS. *Emergency Medicine: A Comprehensive Study Guide*, 6th ed. New York: McGraw-Hill, 2004:1704.)

Spinal Cord Injuries

Spinal cord injuries may be complete (total loss of function below lesion) or incomplete.

INCOMPLETE SPINAL CORD INJURIES

The most common incomplete lesions include:

- Central cord syndrome
- Brown-Séquard syndrome
- Anterior cord syndrome

Central Cord Syndrome (Fair Prognosis)

- The most common incomplete spinal cord lesion
- Caused by a hyperextension injury on a congenitally narrow cord or preexisting cervical spondylosis (older patients), resulting in buckling of the ligamentus flavum and compression of the central cord.
- **Symptoms/exam:** Weakness and numbness **greater in the arms than the legs** (patients may have complete quadriplegia); bowel and bladder control remain in all but the most severe cases.
- Although function usually returns, most patients do not regain fine motor control in upper extremities.

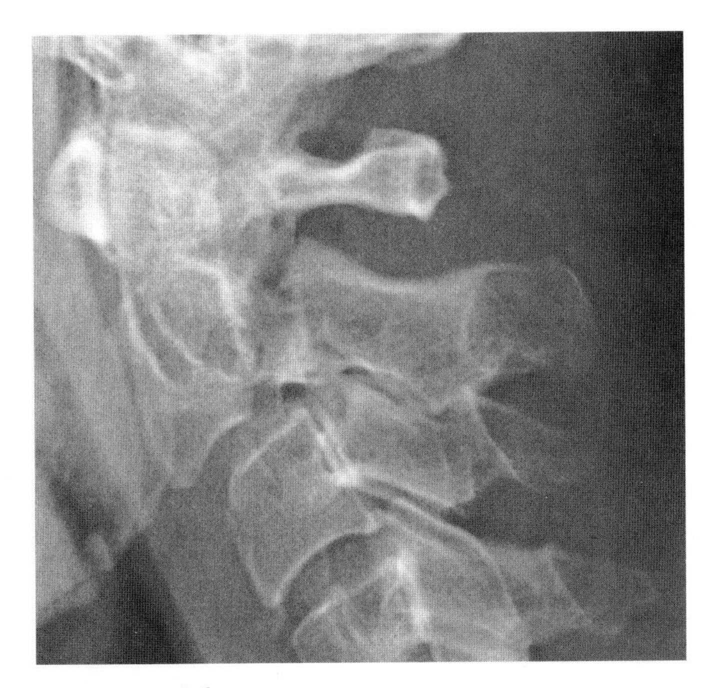

FIGURE 3.8. Hangman's fracture.

(Reproduced, with permission, from Tintinalli JE, Kelen GD, Stapczynski JS. *Emergency Medicine: A Comprehensive Study Guide*, 6th ed. New York: McGraw-Hill, 2004:1707.)

Unstable C-spine fractures—

Jefferson Bit Off A Hangman's Thumb
Jefferson fracture
Bilateral facet dislocation
Odontoid type II/III
Atlantoaxial or atlanto-occipital dislocations
Hangman's fracture
Teardrop fracture

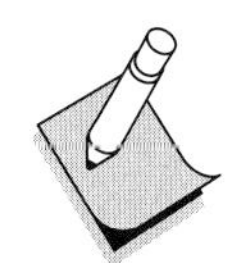

Instability increases with multicolumn injuries.

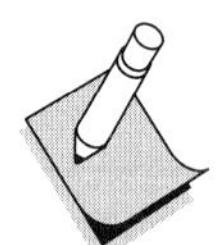

Markers of unstable C-spine injury include damage to anterior 20% of vertebral body and loss of >50% of body height.

TABLE 3.6. Stable Fractures of the C-Spine

Type	Mechanism	Notes
Wedge fracture	Flexion	Multiple wedge fxs or loss of >50% of vertebral body height may be unstable
Transverse process fracture	Flexion	
Clay shoveler's fracture (spinous process avulsion)	Flexion against contracted posterior muscles	Most commonly at C7
Unilateral facet	Flexion and rotation	Anterior displacement <50% of width
Burst fracture	Vertical compression	Can be unstable if fragments enter canal
Isolated fractures of articular pillar and vertebral body	Vertical compression	"Double-outline" sign

Anterior Cord Syndrome (Poor Prognosis)

- Caused by flexion or extension with vascular injury of the anterior spinal artery or bony fragment injury
- Symptoms/exam: Include **paralysis and loss of pain and temperature sensation** but preserved position, crude touch, and vibration

TABLE 3.7. Major (Unstable) Thoracolumbar Spine Fractures

Fracture	Mechanism	Radiographic Findings
Wedge compression fracture	Flexion injury	Loss of anterior vertebral body height Neurologic deficit uncommon
Chance fracture	Flexion around an anterior axis usually associated with lap belt	Horizontal fracture through the vertebral body and all posterior elements
Burst fracture	Vertical compression	Loss of anterior and posterior height
Flexion-distraction fracture	Flexion with compression of anterior elements and distraction of posterior elements	"Fanning"—increased posterior interspinous space
Translational fracture	Shear	Shift of one or more vertebral body causing complete disruption

Brown-Séquard Syndrome

- **Hemisection of the cord** usually associated with penetrating trauma
- **Symptoms/exam:** Typically see ipsilateral paralysis, loss of proprioception and vibratory sensation, and contralateral loss of pain and temperature sensation

SPINAL SHOCK

MECHANISMS

- Due to a partial or complete injury at or above T6 resulting in a transient reflex depression of all cord function below the level of injury
- Reflex function below the level of injury spontaneously returns (typically within 24–48 hours), at which time degree of cord injury can be fully determined

SYMPTOMS/EXAM

- Flaccid paralysis, including bowel and bladder, priapism
- Bulbocavernosus reflex (anal sphincter contraction in response to squeezing penile glans or pulling on the Foley) returns first.

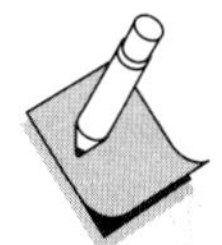

Hemorrhagic shock: Patient is cold, clammy, pale, tachycardic.
Neurogenic shock: Patient is warm, vasodilated, bradycardic.

NEUROGENIC SHOCK

Diagnosis of exclusion in the trauma victim

MECHANISMS

Results from loss of sympathetic outflow in spinal cord injury, leading to unopposed vagal tone

SYMPTOMS/EXAM

Hypotension, bradycardia, peripheral vasodilation

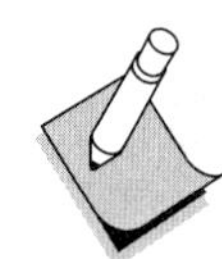

SCIWORA is defined by neurologic deficits with negative X-ray and CT. MRI is often positive. Occurs mostly in children < 8 years old and in older adults.

Spinal Cord Injury Without Radiographic Abnormality (SCIWORA)

- Trauma patients with neurologic deficits consistent with a spinal cord injury but with **negative plain films and CT**
- SCIWORA is thought to be common in children, but also occurs in older patients.
- Central cord syndrome, which results from buckling of the ligamentum flavum during hyperextension, is the classic form of SCIWORA in adults (mainly the elderly).
- MRI in patients with SCIWORA will often show spinal cord injury.

DIAGNOSIS

Any patient exhibiting signs of neurologic dysfunction following trauma, with or without vertebral fracture, needs MRI with possible MRA for evaluation of extent of cord and vascular damage.

C3, C4, C5 keep the diaphragm alive (via the phrenic nerve).

TREATMENT

- Spinal injury at or above C5 usually requires intubation because of weakness of the diaphragm.

- Patients with C-spine fractures, ligamentous instability, or neurologic deficits consistent with a C-spine injury should be immobilized.
- Neurosurgical consultation is appropriate.
- Volume and pressors may be necessary for hypotension secondary to neurogenic shock, but be sure to rapidly evaluate for other causes of hypotension (ie, hemorrhage).
- While it remains controversial, **high-dose methylprednisolone** has become the standard of care in the United States for blunt (not penetrating) injury to the spinal cord.
  - First dose must be given within 8 hours of injury.
  - 30 mg/kg IV over 15 minutes
  - 45-minute pause
  - Then 5.4 mg/kg/hour for 23 hours
- Worsening neurologic function following spinal cord injury is usually an indication for surgical intervention.

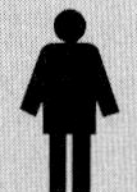

A 60-year-old female is brought into the ED after MVC with hypotension, dyspnea, and tracheal deviation to the right. Lung sounds are absent over the left chest. What should be your first step?

This patient clinically has a tension pneumothorax. Do not wait for X-ray confirmation. Perform immediate decompression by placing a 14-g angiocatheter in the L second intercostal space at the midclavicular line.

BLUNT CHEST TRAUMA

Simple Pneumothorax

The accumulation of air within the pleural space, most commonly a result of trauma, though may occur spontaneously

Symptoms/Exam

- Chest pain and shortness of breath are the most common presenting complaints.
- Decreased or abnormal breath sounds, hyperresonance on the ipsilateral lung may be present

Diagnosis

- Upright CXR: Findings that suggest pneumothorax include: Absent lung markings in the periphery of the lung field, mediastinal shift, subcutaneous emphysema, or a low lateral diaphragm on the side of the injury (deep sulcus sign) all suggest pneumothorax (see Figure 3.9).
- An expiratory film may allow visualization of a small pneumothorax not seen on initial CXR.
- CT may pick up occult pneumothorax (one not seen on upright CXR).

Treatment

- Small pneumothorax (<1 cm from chest wall and only in upper third of chest in adults) may be treated with **100% O_2 via NRB mask** and repeat CXR.
- Large pneumothorax should receive a chest tube (24F or smaller if no hemothorax).

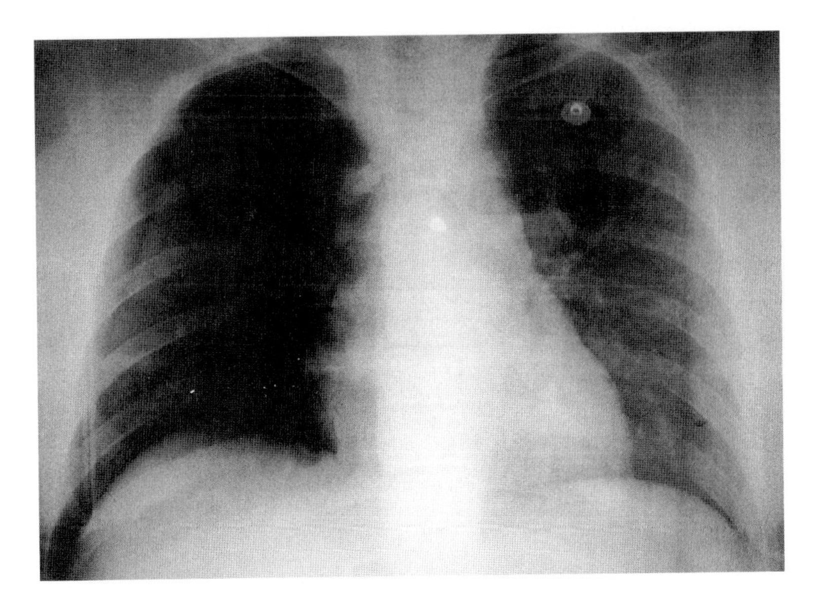

FIGURE 3.9. Right-sided pneumothorax.

(Reproduced, with permission, from Stone CK, Humphries, RL. *Current Emergency Diagnosis and Treatment*, 5th ed. New York: McGraw-Hill, 2004:232.)

- If a patient with an untreated pneumothorax requires intubation, consider chest tube placement prior to or immediately following intubation or monitor carefully for signs of pneumothorax enlargement.
- If the lung does not reexpand after chest tube placement and there is no mechanical malfunction, consider the possibility of a large tear in lung parenchyma or a bronchial injury.
- If placement of a second chest tube doesn't reinflate the lung then surgical intervention is needed either via bronchoscopy or thoracotomy.
- Stable asymptomatic patients with isolated chest injury and negative CXRs for pneumothorax at 6 hours apart may be discharged.

Tension Pneumothorax

Mechanisms

- Caused by a one-way communication from lung parenchyma into pleural space, allowing air into the space but not out (see Figure 3.10)
- Progressive increase in air in the pleural space increases pressure of the hemithorax, causing shifting of the mediastinum, compression of the vena cava, **obstruction of venous return**, and decreased cardiac output.

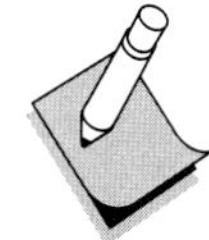

Findings of hypotension with distended neck veins may also occur with cardiac tamponade. The lung exam and response to thoracostomy should differentiate the two.

Symptoms/Exam

- Shortness of breath
- **Hypotension**
- Distended neck veins
- Diminished/absent breath sounds on affected side
- Tracheal deviation to opposite side
- Hyperexpansion of chest wall on affected side

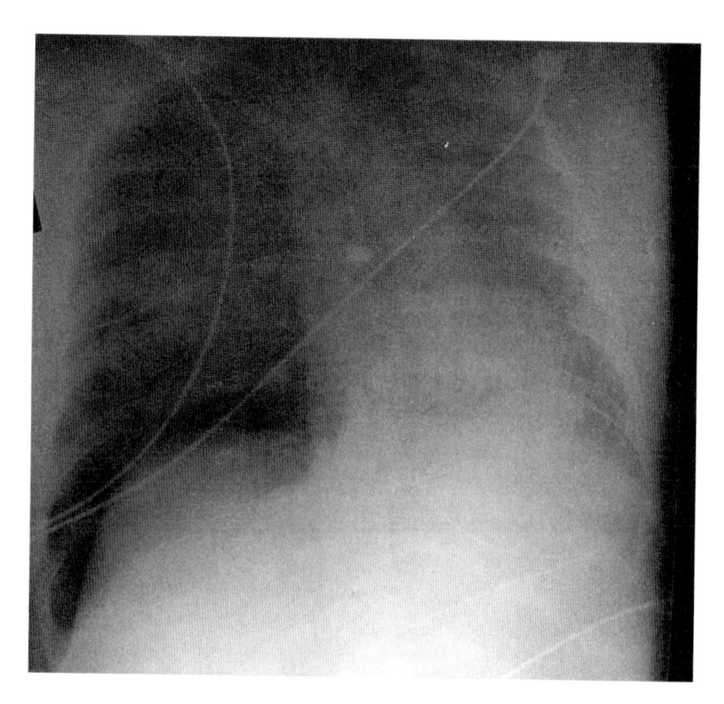

FIGURE 3.10. Tension pneumothorax.

(Reproduced, with permission, from Stone CK, Humphries, RL. *Current Emergency Diagnosis and Treatment*, 5th ed. New York: McGraw-Hill, 2004:455.)

Serious/symptomatic pneumothorax:

- *Tension pneumothorax*
- *Pneumothorax > 40% of a hemithorax (2.5 cm from chest wall in adults)*
- *Concurrent with hemorrhagic shock or preexisting cardiopulmonary disease*

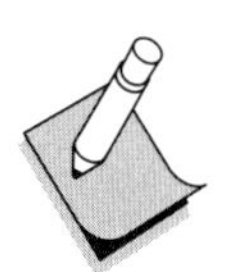

Lung opacification after trauma:

- *Massive hemothorax*
- *Diaphragmatic rupture with herniation*
- *Lung collapse*

DIAGNOSIS/TREATMENT

- Diagnosis is clinical.
- Immediate placement of a 14-g angiocatheter into the second intercostal space at the midclavicular line should yield a rush of air and decompression of the pneumothorax.
- All patients require subsequent chest tube placement.

Hemothorax

MECHANISMS

- Results from traumatic injury to the chest with bleeding from lung parenchyma, intercostal arteries, internal mammary artery, and less commonly, hilar and great vessels
- An associated pneumothorax is present in 25% of cases.

SYMPTOMS/EXAM

- Diminished or absent breath sounds
- Dullness to percussion (pneumothorax will have resonant percussion)
- Hypotension

DIAGNOSIS

- Upright CXR will reveal blunting of the costophrenic angle when >250 mL blood present.
- Supine films typically just show haziness even with >1000 mL of blood present.
- White-out of one hemithorax implies a massive hemothorax, usually associated with mediastinal shift away from the hemothorax.

TREATMENT

- Large-bore chest tube (36–40Fr): Smaller chest tubes will clot.
- Massive hemothorax is defined as an initial output of >1500 mL of blood.
- Initial chest tube output of >1200–1500 mL (>20 mL/kg) or persistent output of >200 mL/hour (>7 mL/kg/hour) or 600 mL/6 hours indicates need for thoracotomy.
- Persistent hypotension in the setting of hemothorax is also an indication for surgical intervention even if chest tube output does not cross the above threshold.
- Consider autotransfusion in the setting of massive hemothorax, but be wary of contamination from occult GI injury.

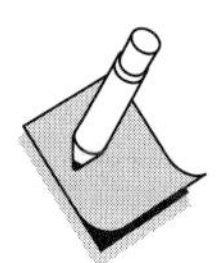

In patients with traumatic hemothorax, initial chest tube output of >1500 mL or subsequent output of >200 mL/hour are indications for operative repair.

COMPLICATIONS

- Undrained or insufficiently drained blood from the pleural space can get infected or can cause late pleural fibrosis limiting lung expansion. Get the blood out.
- Chest tubes can also introduce infection into the chest: Meticulous sterile technique should be used.
- Left lung opacification may be due to traumatic diaphragmatic hernia or **right main-stem intubation** with left lung collapse.
- Shift of the mediastinum away from the opacification and the presence of an NG tube going and staying below the diaphragm support the diagnosis of hemothorax.

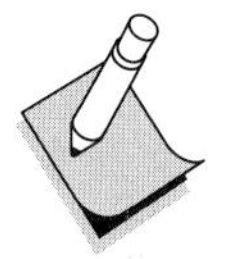

Pediatric bony structures are more pliable than adults. As a result, children are less likely to have fractures but more likely to have underlying contusion/injury following blunt trauma.

Rib Fractures

SYMPTOMS/EXAM

Posttrauma chest pain

DIAGNOSIS

- Assume rib fractures in any chest trauma patient with localized pain and tenderness over the ribs or pain with deep inspiration, even if not seen on CXR.
- >50% of rib fractures are not evident on CXR.
- Most common chest injury in adults (usually ribs 4–9)

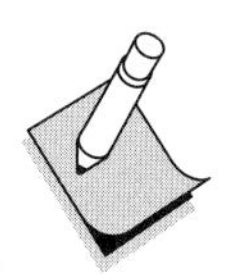

Consider admission in patients with multiple rib fractures or with single rib fractures and age >50 years or underlying lung disease.

TREATMENT

- Consider admission for pain control (opioids, rib block, epidural) and for observation/workup for other injuries, especially in individuals >50 years old, smokers, and those with multiple rib fractures.
- All patients need to maintain lung volumes (ie, 10 deep breaths every hour while awake) to prevent atelectasis and pneumonia.

COMPLICATIONS

- First and second rib fractures require a lot of force and are associated with other significant injuries and with poor outcomes in 15–30% of cases. These fractures can be associated with vascular, bronchial, and myocardial injuries.
- Two or more rib fractures are associated with higher incidence of internal injuries. These patients are also at higher risk for fat emboli and aspiration pneumonitis (from diminished cough), which can take 24–48 hours to elucidate on CXR.
- If a hypotensive patient has fractures of ribs 9–11 consider liver and/or spleen injuries.

The greater the number of rib fractures, the greater the morbidity and mortality.

TRAUMA

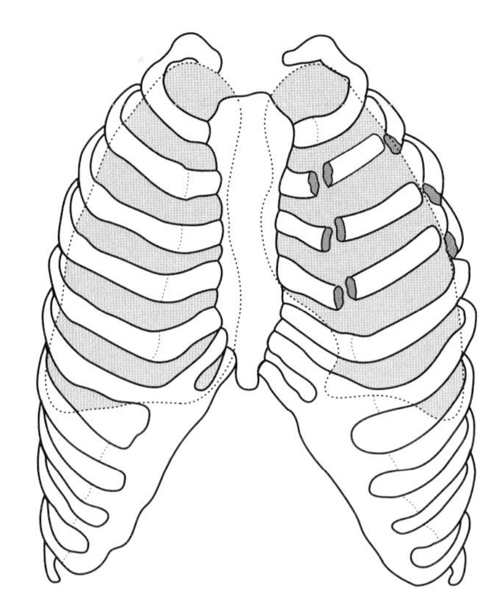

FIGURE 3.11. Diagram of flail chest.

(Reproduced, with permission, from Doherty GM. *Current Surgical Diagnosis and Treatment*, 12th ed. New York: McGraw-Hill, 2005:214.)

Flail Chest

Flail chest is defined by the presence of fractures in more than one location on each of three or more adjacent ribs causing a free floating segment of ribs and an unstable chest (see Figure 3.11).

SYMPTOMS/EXAM

- Flail segment may move discordant with the rest of the chest (in with inspiration and out with expiration).
- Significant flail chest is often associated with tachypnea and hypoxia.

DIAGNOSIS

- CXR or CT scan may reveal multiple rib fractures.
- Flail may only be minimally apparent immediately after injury and becomes more apparent as lung compliance worsens, necessitating greater inspiratory effort.

TREATMENT

- Primary treatment is analgesia, coughing and chest physiotherapy, and preventing fluid overload and consequent lung edema. These measures maximize tidal volumes and help prevent hypoxia and PNA.
- Do not wrap the chest as this inhibits chest expansion.
- **Intubation and ventilation** may be needed in patients with shock, three or more associated injuries, head injury, underlying pulmonary disease, eight or more rib fractures, age >65 years, or Pao_2 <80 mmHg on supplemental O_2.
- Early ventilatory support can help reduce mortality of severe flail chest from 69% down to 7%.

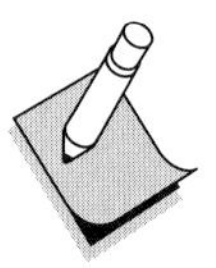

*In patients with flail chest, underlying **lung contusion** is the main cause of hypoxemia.*

COMPLICATIONS

Anticipate patient fatigue because of decreased mechanical efficiency causing increased work of breathing.

Sternal Fracture

Typically seen in victims of head-on MVCs, either from anterior chest striking steering wheel or from diagonal part of seat belt restraining upper sternum.

Symptoms/Exam

- Anterior chest pain, often pleuritic
- Point tenderness
- Palpable deformity

Diagnosis

- A sternal fracture is usually evident on a **lateral CXR**, but only if you are looking for it. The PA or AP film is often normal.
- The incidence of blunt myocardial injury (BMI) with sternal fractures is 1.5–6%.
- Mortality of MVC patients with sternal fractures is 0.7%.
- Patients with sternal fracture, nl vitals, and nl EKG should be on cardiac monitor for 4–6 hours and may need repeat EKG in 6 hours to rule out blunt myocardial injury, although recent evidence shows that sternal fractures are not strongly associated with significant BMI.

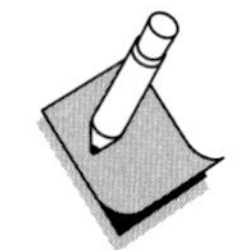

Restrained passengers are much more likely to have sternal fractures than unrestrained occupants.

Treatment

Pain control

Pulmonary Contusion

Mechanisms

- Compression-decompression injury of lung parenchyma
- The uninjured lung may also develop edema in response to the reflex shunting of blood flow.

Symptoms/Exam

- Hemoptysis is present in up to 50% of pulmonary contusions.
- Other findings include dyspnea, tachypnea, tachycardia.
- Chest wall bruising or tenderness

Diagnosis

- CXR may show contusions (opaque patches of lung) **within minutes to six hours**.
- Appearance on CXR is usually milder than actual extent of damage, which may be better visualized on CT.

Treatment

- Respiratory support to prevent hypoxia
- Percent of involved lung may help determine when mechanical ventilation is needed: Unlikely for <18% (one lobe), consider in patients with >28% contusion.
- Severe pulmonary contusions may require high-frequency oscillation (kinetic therapy), turning the patient to place uninjured lung in dependant position to match perfusion and ventilation, and pressure-controlled inverse-ratio ventilation.

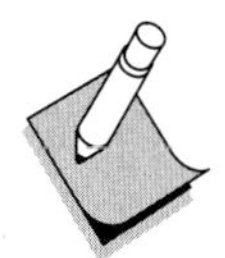

Pulmonary contusions are the most common significant chest injury in children, due to chest wall elasticity.

COMPLICATIONS

Mortality of isolated pulmonary contusion is up to 16% and greater with concurrent extrathoracic injury.

Pneumomediastinum

Pneumomediastinum is air within the mediastinum. It may occur in the absence of trauma following a ruptured alveoli, but in relationship to trauma its presence implies injury to air containing structures in mediastinum such as larynx, trachea, major bronchi, pharynx, or esophagus.

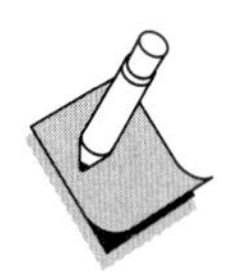

Consider tracheal injury in patients with blunt neck trauma and subcutaneous emphysema. Tracheal laceration warrants surgical evaluation and tracheal transections require repair.

SYMPTOMS/EXAM

- Often asymptomatic
- Findings include SQ emphysema of neck and crunching sound over heart during systole (**Hamman's sign**).
- Can be seen on CXR but better visualized by chest CT
- Further testing to **exclude esophageal injury** (such as a barium swallow) may be necessary in patients with a history of penetrating trauma, vomiting, or other mechanism that might implicate the esophagus.

Cardiac Contusion/Blunt Myocardial Injury (BMI)

BMI injuries include:

- Wall rupture: 90% die on scene
- Septal rupture
- Valvular injuries (aortic most common)
- Contusion is the most common injury, usually affecting the anterior surfaces of the heart (**right ventricle**).
- Coronary artery laceration or thrombosis
- Pericardial injury

SYMPTOMS/EXAM

- Vary with severity of injury
- Chest pain
- Tachycardia not explained by injury or blood loss
- Dysrhythmias (AFib, PACs, PVCs, blocks)

DIAGNOSIS

- There are no good screening tests for BMI and $<3\%$ develop significant cardiac complications.
- Patients with suspected BMI can be safely discharged if initial EKG is normal and they have been observed for 4–6 hours on cardiac monitor without arrhythmia.
- A negative 4- to 6-hours postinjury troponin can help further exclude BMI.

TREATMENT

- Patients with BMI should be on supplemental O_2 to keep $PaO_2 > 80$ mmHg.
- Treat hypotension with fluids and pressors as needed.
- Complete recovery usually occurs within 3–6 weeks.

COMPLICATIONS

Patients may develop posttraumatic pericarditis, ventricular septal defect, valvular defect, ventricular aneurysm, pericardial tamponade.

Aortic Injury/Traumatic Rupture of the Aorta (TRA)

MECHANISMS

- Consider in the setting of high-speed deceleration and lateral impact MVCs
- Consider in presence of multiple rib fractures or flail chest (although one-third of blunt aortic injuries have no obvious external thoracic injury)

SYMPTOMS/EXAM

- Retrosternal or interscapular pain
- Dysphagia
- Shortness of breath
- Stridor or hoarseness in the absence of laryngeal injury
- Harsh murmur over precordium or space between the scapula
- Signs of superior vena cava syndrome
- Hypotension

DIAGNOSIS

- Compare BP in upper versus lower extremities (upper extremity hypertension suggests acute coarctation syndrome).
- CXR (10% of initial CXR in patients with TRA are completely normal) (see Table 3.8)
  - **Widened mediastinum** (see Figure 3.12)
    - Defined by a width >8 cm on a supine AP film
    - Sensitivities are estimated at 50–92%.
    - Specificity is estimated at 10%. Often the mediastinum will be wide in patients who do not have TRA.
  - Esophageal deviation
  - Loss of distinct aortic knob
  - Loss of paraspinal stripe/displacement of right paraspinous interface
  - Widening of the right paratracheal stripe
  - Loss of clear space between aortic knob and left pulmonary artery (apical cap)
  - Displacement of left main stem bronchus 40° below horizontal

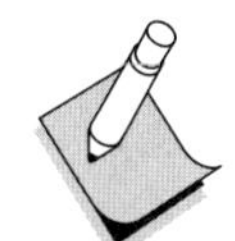

Dissection of the descending aorta (Stanford type B or Debakey type III) is usually managed medically. Traumatic rupture of the aorta is almost always treated surgically, regardless of location.

TABLE 3.8. CXR Findings Suggesting Aortic Injury

Widened mediastinum
Esophageal deviation
Loss of distinct aortic knob
Loss of paraspinal stripe/displacement of right paraspinous interface
Widening of the right paratracheal stripe
Loss of clear space between aortic knob and left pulmonary artery (apical cap)
Displacement of left main stem bronchus 40° below horizontal

Half of all patients with TRA who reach the hospital and survive for 1 hour die within 24 hours, and 75% die within 7 days.

TRAUMA

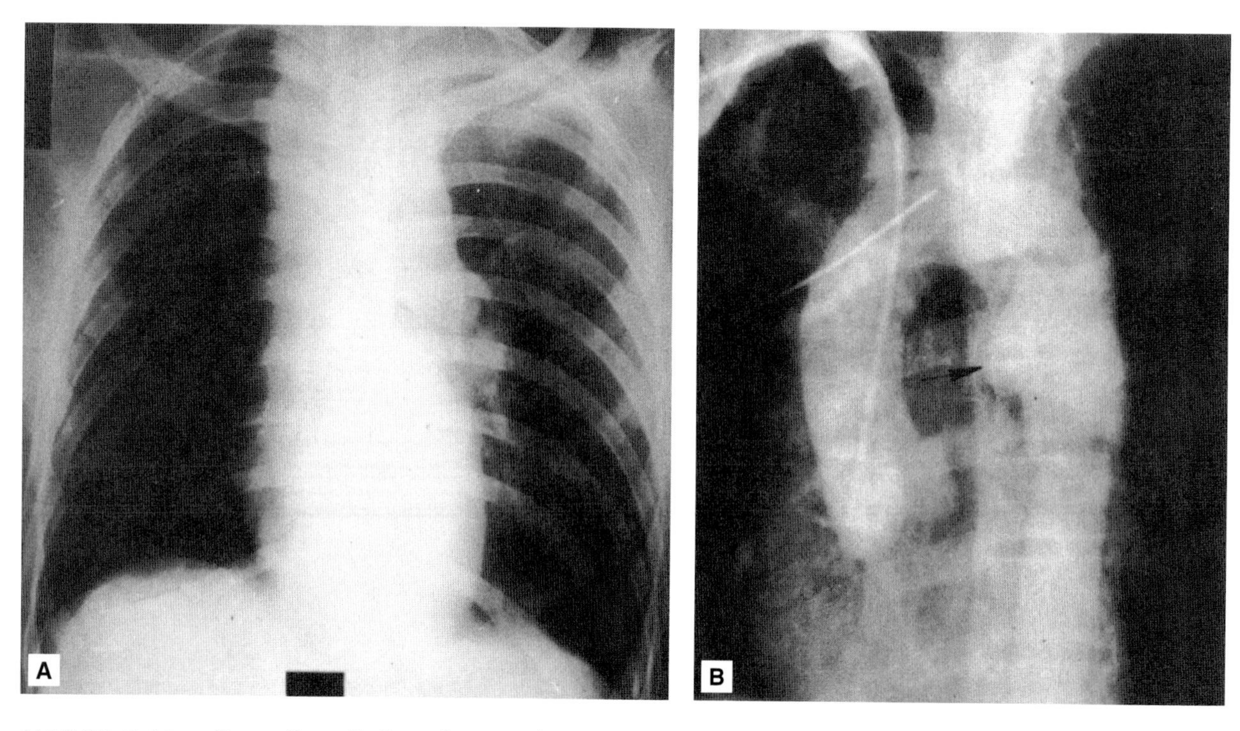

FIGURE 3.12. Traumatic aortic disruption. Anterior-posterior view showing wide mediastinum (A). Lateral view with contrast showing defect in the anterior aspect of the descending aorta (B).

(Reproduced, with permission, from Fuster V, Alexander RW, O'Rourke RA. *Hurst's The Heart*, 12th ed. New York: McGraw-Hill, 2008:2207.)

TRAUMA

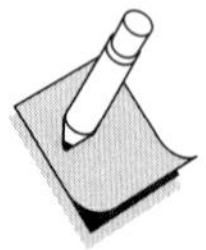

Ninety percent of blunt aortic injuries occur at the isthmus of the aorta, between left subclavian artery and ligamentum arteriosum. The second most common great vessel injury is to the innominate artery.

- CT with contrast is a good test for stable patients.
- Transesophageal echocardiogram can be performed at the bedside in unstable patients.

TREATMENT

- Use β-blockade to control blood pressure (keep SBP < 120 mmHg and replace fluids carefully, to prevent worsening tear/rupture).
- Instruct patient not to valsalva.
- **Operative repair** is almost always necessary, but there is no clear consensus as to the optimal timing (immediate or delayed) or method (open vs intravascular).

PENETRATING CHEST TRAUMA

Open Pneumothorax (Sucking Chest Wound)

MECHANISMS

- Open communication between outer chest wall and pleural space with air moving in and out
- Usually resulting from a large chest stab wound or GSW

Symptoms of descending aortic injury include paraplegia (vertebral artery deficits), mesenteric and LE ischemia, and anuria.

SYMPTOMS/EXAM

- Shortness of breath
- Decreased breath sounds

- Sucking chest wound
- Subcutaneous emphysema
- Auscultation should reveal diminished breath sounds.

DIAGNOSIS

- The presence of air movement or bubbles at the site of a chest wound identifies an open pneumothorax.

TREATMENT

- Place a three-sided dressing to allow air to exit and not enter the pleural space while preparing for placement of a chest tube.
- A dressing that completely occludes the wound may cause a tension PTX.
- Do not insert a chest tube through the wound because it may push foreign material into the chest and may also preferentially follow the tract into the lung parenchyma or across the diaphragm.

Heart

SYMPTOMS/EXAM

- Consider cardiac injury in patients with:
  - GSW anywhere above the umbilicus
  - Stab wound to the left chest, the right chest medial to the midclavicular line, or upper abdomen
- Look for signs of tamponade such as Beck's triad and pulsus paradoxus (a reduction in SBP of >10 mmHg on inspiration).

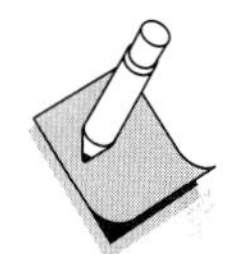

Beck's triad:

- *Hypotension*
- *JVD*
- *Muffled heart sounds*

DIAGNOSIS

- A globular cardiac silhouette on CXR may indicate tamponade, but most cases of tamponade have a normal CXR.
- The cardiac view of the fast exam is a quick way to detect pericardial blood. A subxyphoid view may be necessary in patients with concurrent pneumothorax.

TREATMENT

- Traditionally, fluids are given to maximize cardiac output.
- Thoracotomy should be performed for traumatic effusion/tamponade in the setting of shock. Removing only 5–10 mL of blood can increase stroke volume by 25–50%.

TRAUMA

Great Vessels

EXAM

Bruits on auscultation of the chest may indicate vascular injury.

DIAGNOSIS

- Foreign body (eg, bullet) within the chest that appears "fuzzy" on CXR may indicate vascular injury. Blurring of the borders of the foreign body may occur because of movement with cardiac pulsations.
- Never probe a chest wound or remove an impaled FB because you may dislodge a clot and cause massive hemorrhage.

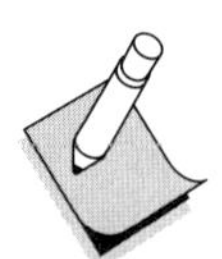

Unilateral absence of radial pulse following chest trauma implies subclavian artery occlusion/disruption.

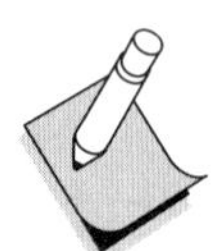

Evaluate possible esophageal injury with a contrast esophagram. Consider endoscopy in patients with a high likelihood of injury.

TRAUMA

TREATMENT

In penetrating chest trauma, ED thoracotomy is indicated if:

- Patient loses signs of life in the ED or immediately before arrival (especially with narrow PEA).
- SBP < 50 mmHg not responsive to fluids/blood
- Severe shock with signs of tamponade

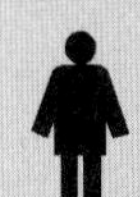

A 14-year-old male presents to the ED after falling forward onto the handle bars of his bike. CT scan of the abdomen is negative. The patient complains of persistent pain. What injuries should you be worried about?

Pancreas and duodenal injuries are classic for this mechanism. An occult diaphragmatic rupture should also be considered.

BLUNT ABDOMINAL TRAUMA

Diaphragmatic Injury

Diaphragmatic injury occurs in 1–6% of patients with multisystem trauma. Only 22% of patients have diaphragmatic injury diagnosed at the time of injury.

MECHANISMS

- Blunt trauma accounts for the majority of diaphragmatic injuries and typically results in a 5- to 15-cm defect in left posterolateral area.
- The **left diaphragm** is injured three times more often than the right, due to protection from the liver.
- Tension viscerothorax, when the herniated abdominal contents shift the mediastinum compressing the other lung, may occur.

SYMPTOMS/EXAM

- Findings result from presence of abdominal contents in chest.
- Shortness of breath
- Abdominal pain radiating to the ipsilateral shoulder, worse when supine
- Absent breath sounds or positive bowel sounds in the chest
- Visceral obstruction (obstructive phase) will eventually develop, at which time patients will have clear signs of bowel strangulation or respiratory compromise.

DIAGNOSIS

- None of the imaging modalities is sensitive for diaphragm injury. CXR has only 40–50% accuracy.
- Initial CXR usually shows blurring of left hemidiaphragm, LLL atelectasis.
- CXR showing coiling of a nasogastric tube in the chest is diagnostic.
- CT, MRI, and contrast studies aid in the diagnosis.

TREATMENT/COMPLICATIONS

- **Missed injuries tend not to heal** because of the negative intrathoracic pressure promoting upward herniation of abdominal contents. For this reason, surgical repair is required for even small diaphragmatic injuries.

- Diaphragmatic injuries **misinterpreted as a hemothorax** may be treated inappropriately with tube thoracostomy. CXR following NG tube placement will usually show the location of the stomach.
- An association has been identified between diaphragmatic injuries and aortic injuries and pelvic fractures. Consider them when you see diaphragmatic injuries.

*The three abdominal injuries in blunt trauma that are difficult to diagnose with CT imaging are **diaphragm, pancreas, and bowel.***

Hollow Viscus

MECHANISMS

- Injuries can range from bowel contusions to lacerations/rupture.
- Signs of hemoperitoneum can result if there are tears of the mesentery.
- Small-bowel injuries, which may be caused by compression of bowel between seat belt and spine, are particularly hard to find on CT, but may be suggested on physical exam by abdominal wall contusion (seat belt sign).
- Approximately one-third of patients with a seat-belt sign will have intra-abdominal injuries.
- The jejunum is the most commonly injured section of bowel.

SYMPTOMS

- Unlike solid organ injuries, which present with signs of blood loss, hollow viscus injuries tend to cause peritoneal signs due to bacterial contamination or irritation from gastric contents.
- On initial exam, peritoneal signs may be absent.

DIAGNOSIS

- Although only present occasionally, on CXR look for free air under the diaphragm indicating hollow viscus injury.
- CT is the preferred modality for evaluating bowel injuries.

TREATMENT

Bowel perforations should undergo laparotomy, while contusions can be observed.

TRAUMA

Solid Organs

In blunt trauma, the **spleen is the most often injured organ** and two-thirds of the time the only injured organ. The liver is the second most commonly injured organ. Renal injuries are less common.

DIAGNOSIS

- CT with IV contrast is confirmative.
- Lipase and amylase levels are neither sensitive nor specific for pancreatic injury (injured may be normal, uninjured high); however, they can be used in conjunction with other tests and trended.

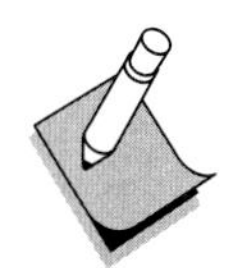

Management of solid organ injury is based on hemodynamic status, not grade.

TREATMENT

- The majority of liver and splenic injuries are treated expectantly rather than surgically.
- Surgery for splenic injuries grade III or higher and in patients <55 years

- High-grade liver injuries have a higher likelihood of requiring surgical intervention; however, these can be managed nonoperatively as long as the patient is hemodynamically stable.
- Interventional radiology is taking on an increasingly greater role in the treatment of solid organ injury, using embolization to help delay or prevent surgical intervention.

PENETRATING ABDOMINAL TRAUMA

Seventy percent of anterior stab wounds penetrate peritoneum, and 50% of those cause organ damage. A lower chest stab wound has a 15% chance of causing intra-abdominal injury.

The most commonly injured organs in penetrating trauma are:

- Stab wound: Liver first, then small bowel (both have large surface areas)
- Gunshot wound: Small bowel, then colon, then liver

TREATMENT

- Penetrating trauma with peritonitis requires immediate surgery.
- Stab wounds to the abdomen may be evaluated using **local wound exploration** (a surgical procedure).
- Digital probing or injection of contrast is not recommended.
- Triple contrast CT scans (CT with PO, IV, and rectal contrast) can be used to evaluate a penetrating abdominal injury, especially if direct exploration is not possible or is inconclusive.
- Observation with serial exams without imaging is an acceptable method of evaluating penetrating abdominal trauma with a low likelihood of significant injury.

Studies in Abdominal Trauma

FOCUSED ASSESSMENT WITH SONOGRAPHY FOR TRAUMA

- Four views:
  - Hepatorenal (Morison's) space (see Figure 3.13)
  - Splenorenal space
  - Pelvis (Pouch of Douglas or rectovesicular pouch)
  - Pericardium (see Figure 3.14)
- In hypotensive victims of blunt trauma, a positive FAST suggests intra-abdominal hemorrhage and the need for exploratory laparotomy.
- In patients who are not hypotensive, a positive FAST may serve as a triage tool to expedite diagnostic evaluation and surgical consultation.
- In general, a FAST exam does not determine where the injury lies, only that there is an injury. The location of fluid does not correlate with the injured organ.
- FAST exams do not exclude intra-abdominal injury. Observe or CT scan patients with suspected injuries who have a negative FAST exam.
- False-positive FAST exams may be found in patients who have cirrhosis and in females who may have a small amount of physiologic free fluid in the pouch of Douglas.

Positive DPL:

10 cc of blood on initial draw

> 100,000 RBC/μL after putting 1 L of NS into abdomen

DIAGNOSTIC PERITONEAL LAVAGE (DPL)

- DPL can be performed at the bedside with an open or a closed technique.
- DPL in patients with pelvic fractures should be done open and above the umbilicus to prevent false-positives due to pelvic hematomas.

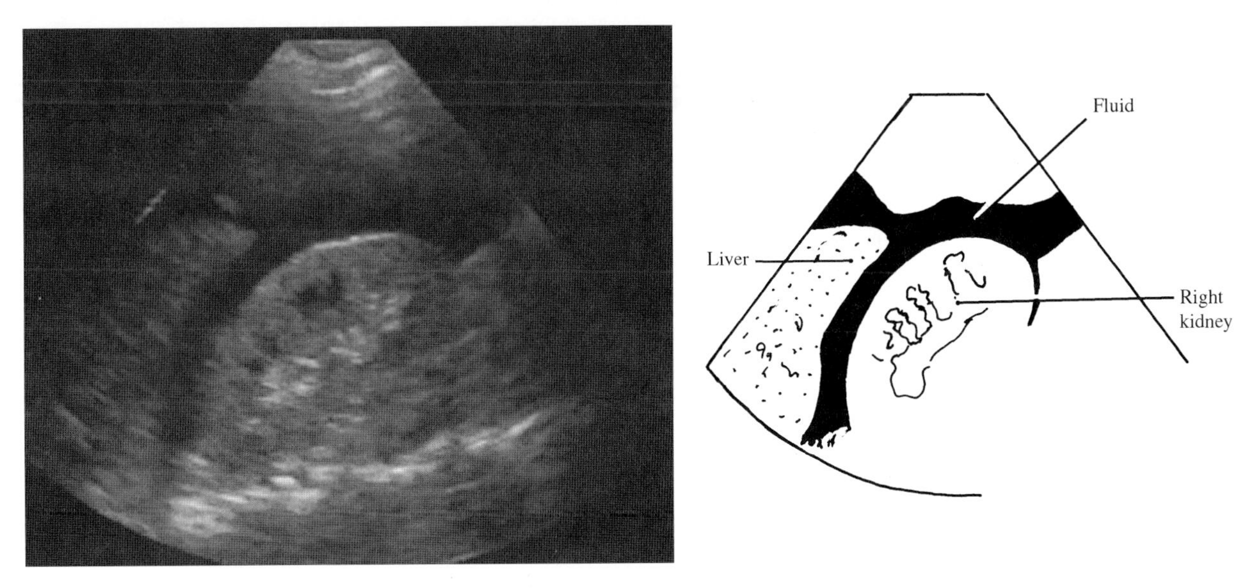

FIGURE 3.13. Positive FAST exam with fluid stripe in hepatorenal space.

(Courtesy of Michael J. Lambert, MD, RDMS as reproduced, with permission, from Knoop KJ, Stack LB, Storrow AB. *Atlas of Emergency Medicine*, 2nd ed. New York: McGraw-Hill, 2002:616.)

- Major complications (bowel injury, bleeding, infection) have a 1% incidence.
- A positive test is defined as drawing back 10 mL of blood initially or 100,000 RBC/μL (5000 RBC/μL for GSW and lower chest wounds) after instilling 1 L of NS and allowing it to drain by gravity.
- DPL has been largely replaced by CT and ultrasound in the evaluation of blunt abdominal trauma.

Indications for Laparotomy

Blunt

- Abdominal injury (free fluid by FAST or blood by DPL) with hypotension
- Evisceration through the abdominal wall

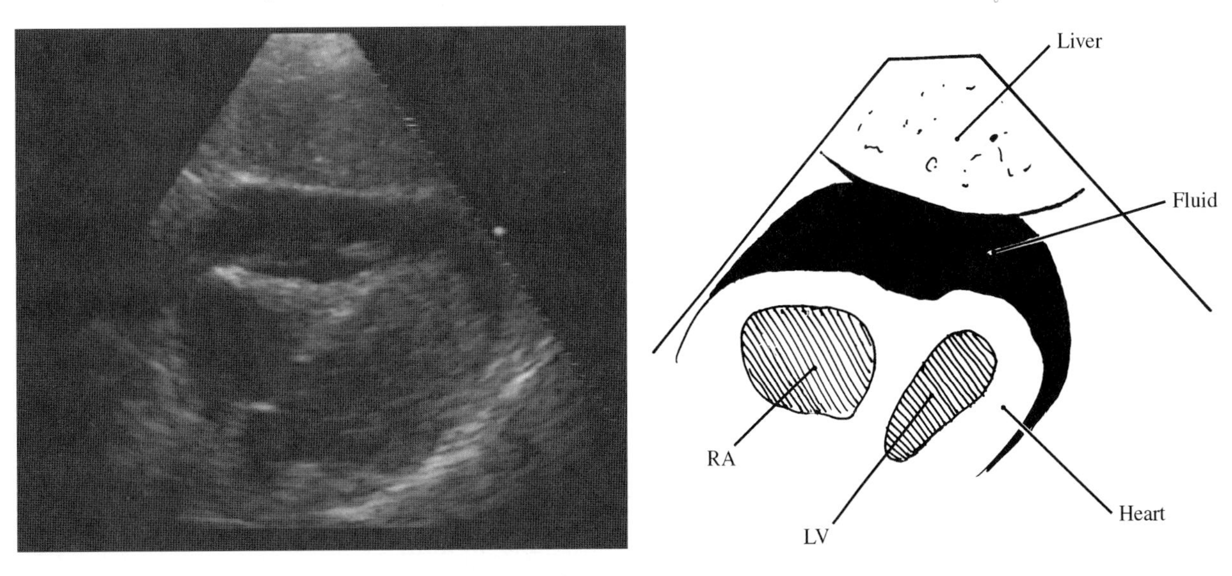

FIGURE 3.14. Positive FAST exam with pericardial fluid.

(Courtesy of Paul R. Sierzenski, MD, RDMS, FAAEM as reproduced, with permission, from Knoop KJ, Stack LB, Storrow AB. *Atlas of Emergency Medicine*, 2nd ed. New York: McGraw-Hill, 2002:614.)

- Peritonitis
- Free air under diaphragm on CXR or on CT
- Injury to pancreas, diaphragm, aorta, bowel, or kidney with urine leaking outside of Gerota's fascia
- Persistent blood from NGT, rectum, or vagina

PENETRATING

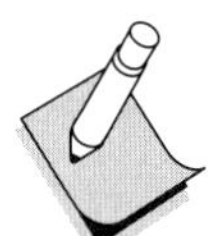

Initial Hgb may not reveal significant bleeding as it takes hours for volume to be replaced by extracellular fluid. Serial values will show a trend.

- Injury with hypotension
- Tenderness not related to the abdominal wall wound (peritonitis)
- Evisceration of abdominal contents through wound
- Positive DPL
- Any GSW to abdomen which entered was believed to have entered peritoneum by evaluation of projectile trajectory
- Local wound exploration that reveals violation of abdominal wall
- Foreign body in abdomen
- Diaphragmatic injury
- Blood from NGT, rectum, or vagina

TRAUMA IN PREGNANCY

MECHANISMS

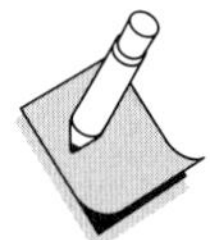

Consider abuse in injured pregnant patients, particularly those with abdominal injury who report a fall.

- MVCs account for half of trauma in pregnancy. Failure to wear a **seat belt** and placement of the lap belt over the pregnant abdomen increase the risk of fetal death.
- **Abuse** during pregnancy is also common with the abdomen being the most common site of injury. Pregnant women injured by a partner often say that an accidental fall was the cause of the injury.

SYMPTOMS/EXAM

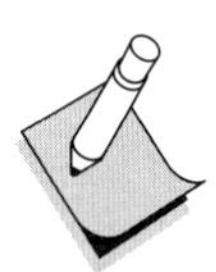

Fetal viability: 24 weeks gestation, dome of uterus above umbilicus

- Changes in normal vital signs in pregnant patients may complicate the evaluation of the injured pregnant patient:
  - Baseline heart rate increases by 10–15 bpm.
  - Baseline BP decreases in the first and second trimesters.
  - In the third trimester, supine hypotension may occur due to **uterine compression of the inferior vena cava**. Positioning the patient in the **left lateral decubitus position** may improve venous return.
- The normal fetal heart rate is **120–160 bpm**. An abnormal rate suggests fetal distress.
- The presence of vaginal discharge mandates a pelvic exam to access for rupture of membranes (ferning, pH > 7).
- Continuous fetal monitoring should be initiated in patients beyond 24 weeks of gestation. Abnormal rates and decelerations after a uterine contraction indicate fetal distress and may also be a marker of occult maternal distress.

DIAGNOSIS

A P_{CO_2} of 40 mmHg during the latter half of pregnancy suggests hypoventilation.

- Changes in normal laboratory values during pregnancy complicate interpretation in the trauma patient:
  - Baseline hematocrit is decreased to 32–34%.
  - Baseline P_{CO_2} is decreased to 30 mmHg.
  - Baseline serum bicarbonate is decreased to 21 mEq/L.
- **Ultrasound** is the initial modality of choice both for evaluating for intra-abdominal bleeding and for assessing gestational age and fetal viability.

- Shield the fetus whenever possible to prevent radiation exposure.
- Because of concerns about radiation exposure, CT of the abdomen is probably inappropriate in stable patients who can be admitted for observation.
- Rh-negative women should receive Rh immunoglobulin.
- The **Kleihauer-Betke test** quantifies the volume of fetomaternal hemorrhage in order to determine the need for larger volumes of Rh immunoglobulin.

TREATMENT

- Emergent C-section is indicated if the fetus is viable and shows signs of distress, uterine rupture, or premature labor with fetal malpresentation.
- Management of an unstable mother with a fetus showing signs of distress should **focus on resuscitating the mother** and stabilizing or repairing her injuries. Emergent C-section should be considered if there is evidence of fetal distress and the mother can tolerate the procedure.
- **Absence of fetal heart tones indicates fetal death.** Emergent C-section is inappropriate in this setting (spontaneous labor usually occurs within one week).

PELVIC FRACTURES

Pelvic fractures may be divided into major ring fractures, acetabular fractures, and avulsion/single bone fractures (see Table 3.9).

Major ring fractures:

Result from the following forces:

- Lateral compression force → horizontal fractures.
- Anteroposterior compression force → vertical fractures.
- Vertical shear force (eg, fall onto feet with weight of upper body transmitted through spine pushing down between hips) → vertical fractures with vertical displacement.

Acetabular fractures:

Acetabular fractures typically occur via head-on injury with knee hitting dashboard, causing or lateral compression. Sciatic injury may occur.

TABLE 3.9. Classification of Major Pelvic Fractures

Type	Incidence[a]	Mechanism	Radiographic Findings
Lateral compression	45–50%	T-bone MVC or pedestrian struck on side	Transverse pubic ramus fracture Sacral compression fracture Iliac wing fracture
Anteroposterior compression (open book)	25%	Head on MVC	Pubic symphysis or SI joint disruption
Vertical shear	5%	Fall/jump from height	Fracture fragments/symphysis displaced vertically

[a]The remaining 20–25% result in a combination of the above types.

TRAUMA

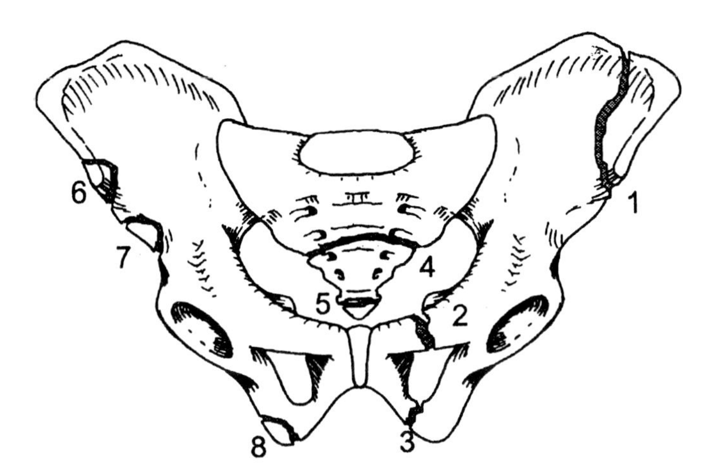

FIGURE 3.15. Avulsion fractures of the pelvis. 1. Iliac wing fracture (Duverney fracture). 2. Superior pubic ramus fracture. 3. Inferior pubic ramus fracture. 4. Transverse sacral fracture. 5. Coccyx fracture. 6. Anterior superior iliac spine avulsion. 7. Anterior inferior iliac spine avulsion. 8. Ischial tuberosity avulsion.

(Reproduced, with permission, from Tintinalli JE, Kelen GD, Stapczynski JS. *Emergency Medicine: A Comprehensive Study Guide*, 6th ed. New York: McGraw-Hill, 2004:1718.)

Avulsion and single-bone fractures:

Occur as a result of direct trauma from falls or from forceful muscle contraction (see Figure 3.15)

Three types of pelvic fractures:
Lateral compression (most common)
AP compression
Vertical shear

SYMPTOMS

- Pain and tenderness of pelvis: Worse with ambulation
- Perineal/pelvic edema/ecchymosis/lacerations/deformities
- Hematomas above inguinal ligament or over scrotum (Destot sign)

EXAM

- Medial or posterior compression of pelvis at iliac crests or posterior compression at symphysis pubis can demonstrate instability. If instability exists, minimize further movement of the pelvis.
- Rectal and perineal exam
  - Evaluate perineum for lacerations to exclude open pelvic fracture, which if present require antibiotics and operative repair.
  - Palpate rectum for hematoma, tenderness, or bony prominence (Earle sign).
  - Evaluate sphincter tone to assess for neurologic deficit.
  - Evaluate for gross blood, suggesting rectal injury.
  - Palpate prostate for superior or posterior displacement suggesting intraperitoneal or urologic injury. Abnormal prostate position or blood at the urethral meatus requires **urethrogram prior to Foley placement** to assess for urethral injury.

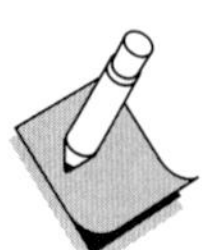

One-third of all pelvic fractures involve individual bones but not the ring.

DIAGNOSIS

- Initial AP plain film of pelvis will show most fractures.
- Displacement of ring fractures may be better defined with inlet view (superior-inferior) and outlet view (anterior-posterior).

- Oblique (Judet) views better define acetabulum fractures.
- When one part of the pelvic ring has been fractured, always look for a second fracture or opening. Double ring fractures are unstable.

TREATMENT

- Nondisplaced fractures can be treated with bed rest while displaced fractures require ORIF.
- Hip dislocations should be reduced as soon as possible in attempt to restore blood supply to femoral head. Fragments of acetabulum may prohibit reduction.
- Bleeding into the retroperitoneal space commonly results from injury to venous plexus and small veins and may be life-threatening.
- Patients with pubic symphysis widening should be treated with pneumatic antishock garment, pelvic binder (such as bed sheets wrapped around the pelvis), or external fixation to minimize the volume of the pelvis which will help control bleeding.
- In patients with hemorrhagic shock, angiography can help control bleeding through transarterial embolization. This may not stop the bleeding because **often the bleeding is venous**. Indications for embolization include:
  - Persistent hypovolemia/hypotension after treatment of other sources of bleeding
  - 4 units PRBC/24 hours or 6 units PRBC/48 hours
  - Large pelvic hematoma on CT

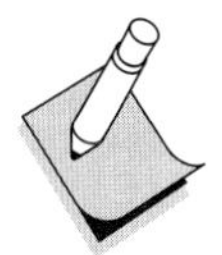

Perform a bimanual vaginal exam on all women with pelvic fractures. Vaginal lacerations are most commonly seen with anterior pelvic fractures and usually require operative repair.

HIP DISLOCATION

Hip dislocations may be **anterior** (due to an anterior and a medial force applied to the abducted leg), **central** (direct impact through acetabulum) or **posterior** (posterior force through a flexed knee).

Posterior Hip Dislocation

Typically result from a head-on MVC with the knee hitting the dashboard and the body moving forward over a fixed femur; often associated with posterior wall/lip fractures of the acetabulum (see Figure 3.16)

EXAM/DIAGNOSIS

- Extremity is shortened, internally rotated, and adducted.
- X-ray is confirmative.

TREATMENT/COMPLICATIONS

- Closed reduction under conscious sedation
- Sciatic nerve injury may occur.

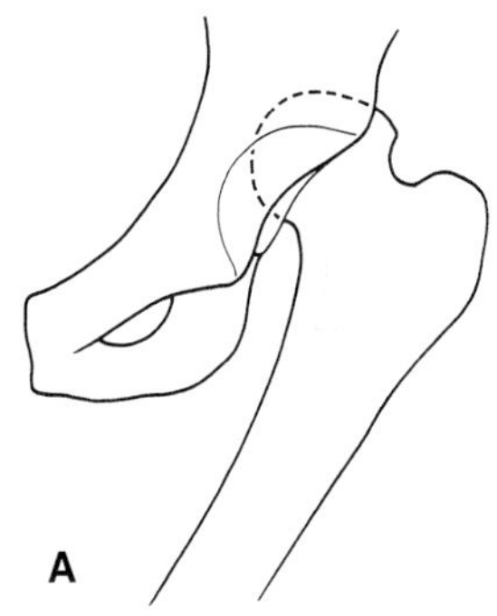

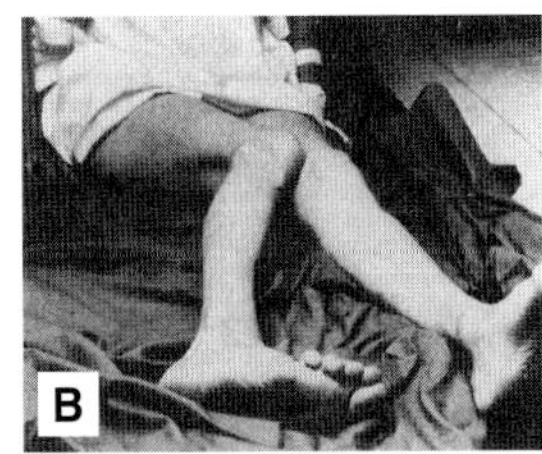

FIGURE 3.16. Posterior hip dislocation.

(Reproduced, with permission, from Tintinalli JE, Kelen GD, Stapczynski JS. *Emergency Medicine: A Comprehensive Study Guide*, 6th ed. New York: McGraw-Hill, 2004:1724.)

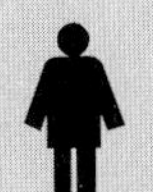

A 30-year-old male arrives in the ED after a 10-foot fall with perineal/pelvic pain and inability to void. Rectal examination reveals a high-riding prostate. What is the most appropriate next step?

Obtain a retrograde urethrogram to rule out the presence of a urethral injury. This should always follow more critical resuscitative procedures, but must be done prior to Foley placement.

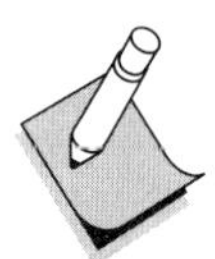

Isolated microscopic hematuria does not mandate further imaging. Exceptions include:
- *Rapid deceleration injuries where renal pedicles can be damaged with minimal to no hematuria*
- *Hematuria in a patient with even transient hypotension*
- *Hematuria following penetrating trauma to the flank*

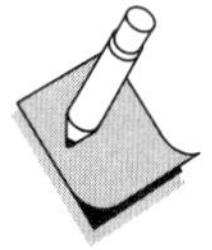

Degree of hematuria does not always correlate with the degree of injury.

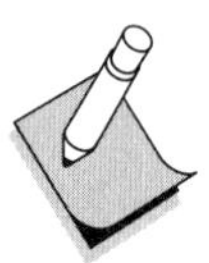

IVP or cystogram in patients who have received oral contrast may be difficult to interpret due to a background of abdominal contrast.

Bladder

Mechanisms

- Usually due to blunt trauma, often associated with pelvic fracture
- Bladder contusion: Hematoma causes bladder to change shape and shift superiorly.
- **Intraperitoneal bladder rupture:** Laceration of the dome of the bladder with communication into peritoneum (see Figure 3.17)
- **Extraperitoneal bladder rupture**: Laceration at bladder neck (no communication to peritoneum)

Symptoms/Exam

- Abdominal pain and tenderness
- Gross hematuria
- Inability to void
- Peritonitis (if intraperitoneal rupture)

Diagnosis

- Retrograde cystogram (plain film or CT)–300 mL (5 mL/kg in children) of contrast is instilled into bladder via a Foley catheter.
  - Intraperitoneal rupture: Contrast will leak into cul-de-sac posterior to bladder.
  - Extraperitoneal rupture: Contrast will extravasate into surrounding tissue in a flame pattern.

Treatment

- **Surgery necessary only for intraperitoneal rupture** and penetrating injuries.
- Catheter placement for incomplete lacerations or extraperitoneal rupture.
- No intervention necessary for contusions.

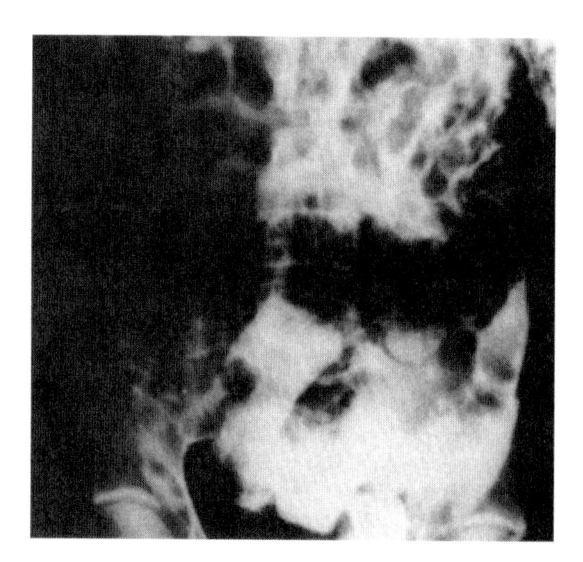

FIGURE 3.17. Intraperitoneal bladder rupture seen on retrograde cystogram with contrast surrounding loops of bowel.

(Reproduced, with permission, from Tanagho EA, McAninch JW. *Smith's General Urology*, 17th ed. New York: McGraw-Hill, 2008:290.)

Kidney

Mechanisms

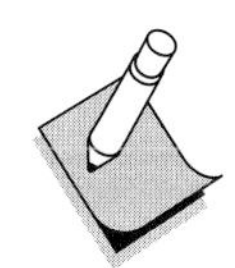

Considerable blunt force is necessary to damage the kidneys because they are so well protected.

- Renal contusions (92%)
- Renal lacerations (5%)
  - Minor: Cortical
  - Major: Involves medulla and/or collecting system
- Pedicle injury (2%): Injuries to the renal vasculature, may result in renal artery thrombosis and loss of kidney
- Renal ruptures (1%): Expanding perirenal hematoma

Diagnosis

- CT with IV contrast
- Retrograde pyelogram specifically for renal pelvis
- Angiogram or venogram used for suspected renal pedicle injuries, such as when a contrast CT or IVP demonstrates no contrast in the kidney

Treatment

- Isolated contusions, minor lacerations < 1 cm, and nonexpanding hematomas may be sent home.
- Absolute indication for surgery is renal injury with retroperitoneal bleeding and hemodynamic instability.
- Surgery is also indicated for the following:
  - Uncontrolled renal hemorrhage
  - Most penetrating injuries
  - Multiple kidney lacerations
  - Ruptured kidney
  - Avulsed major renal vessel or vascular injury: In patients with pedicle injuries, surgical intervention should occur within 12 hours to prevent kidney loss.
  - Extensive extravasation of contrast on imaging
- Most patients with kidney injuries who do not need surgery should be admitted for observation.

Complications

Renovascular hypertension (1%)

Ureter

Ureteral injury is usually due to penetrating trauma.

Symptoms/Exam

- Hematuria (rarely present with complete tears)
- Flank pain and mass

Diagnosis

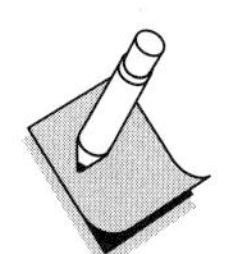

All ureteral injuries require intervention either surgical or IR.

- CT with IV contrast
- Retrograde pyelogram

Treatment

Repair or stenting

Urethral

MECHANISMS

- Posterior urethral injuries typically result from pelvic fractures.
- Anterior urethral injuries: Direct blow to the urethra, instrumentation, and penile fractures

SYMPTOMS/EXAM

- Posterior urethral injuries: Perineal hematoma and high-riding prostate on rectal exam
- Anterior urethral injuries: "Butterfly" perineal hematoma
- In females, urethral injuries are often associated with vaginal bleeding.

DIAGNOSIS

Retrograde urethrogram (RUG) should always be performed before placing a Foley in the setting of meatal blood or a high-riding prostate and suspected pelvic fracture (see Figure 3.18).

TREATMENT

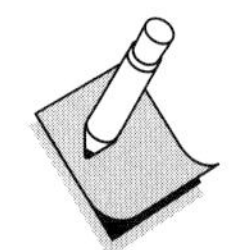

Blood at urethral meatus mandates RUG before Foley placement.

- Contusions heal with or without catheter placement.
- Partial lacerations are managed with a catheter placed by urologist.
- Complete lacerations are managed surgically.
- It is not inappropriate to conservatively manage urethral injuries with suprapubic cystostomy.
- A Foley should only be placed when the path of the urethra is still intact, and is best placed by a urologist under direct visualization via cystoscopy.

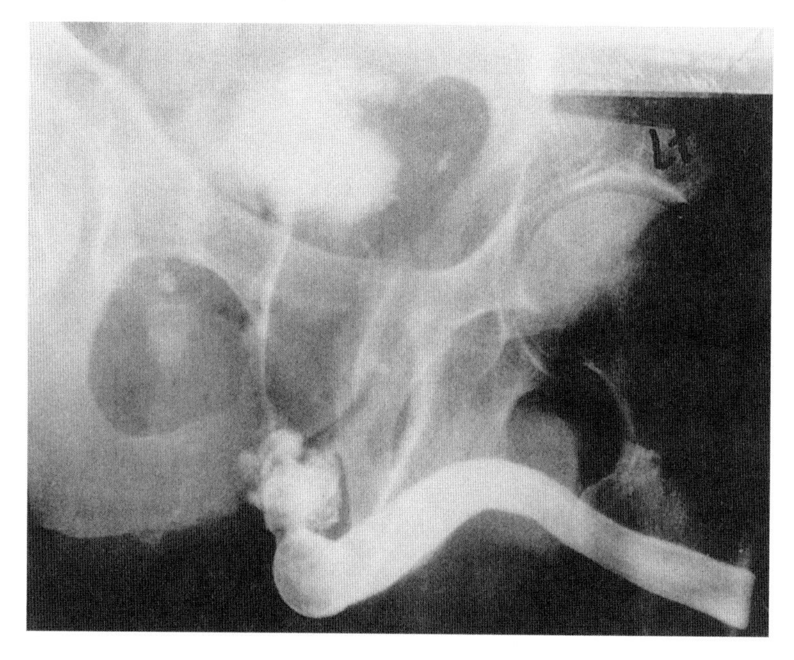

FIGURE 3.18. Retrograde urethrogram positive for urethral injury.

(Reproduced, with permission, from Tintinalli JE, Kelen GD, Stapczynski JS. *Emergency Medicine: A Comprehensive Study Guide*, 6th ed. New York: McGraw-Hill, 2004:1221.)

External Genitourinary Trauma

Penile Fracture

Results from traumatic rupture of corpus cavernosum. Most commonly caused by blunt trauma to erect penis, usually during sexual intercourse with penis striking perineum, pubic symphysis, desk, etc. May also result from manipulation to achieve detumescence.

Symptoms/Exam

Patients report cracking sound, pain, detumescence, and hematoma.

Treatment

- Treated surgically with immediate hematoma evacuation and **repair of tunica albuginea**.
- Amputations must be reattached within 8–12 hours.
- Skin lacerations can be repaired with 4–0 absorbable suture. Skin avulsions usually require grafting.
- 10% will be permanently deformed.

Testicular Trauma

Trauma to the testicles may result in hematoma, contusion, laceration, fracture, or dislocation.

Diagnosis

Color Doppler ultrasound of testis will help determine severity of injury, by assessing blood flow and hematoma formation.

Treatment

- Laceration, disruption, and dislocation of testis mandate operative repair.
- All other injuries can be managed with ice, rest, and pain control.

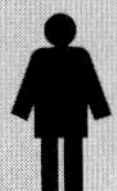

A stable patient has sustained a stab wound to the neck. What should be your first consideration in determining extent of injury? Visual inspection to determine if the platysma has been violated.

NECK TRAUMA

Laryngotracheal Injuries

Mechanisms

- Neck hyperextension/hyperflexion or rotation
- Direct impact (handle bars, clothes lines, seat belts, assault)

Symptoms

- Hoarseness
- Shortness of breath
- Hemoptysis

EXAM

- Dysphonia
- Stridor
- Tenderness
- SQ emphysema
- Loss of anatomic landmarks

DIAGNOSIS

- CXR, PA and lateral soft-tissue neck films, and C-spine films, or CT of neck
- Look for SQ emphysema, narrowing of subglottic airway, and hyoid bone fractures.
- Follow up suspected injuries with laryngoscopy and bronchoscopy.

Intubation of patients with laryngotracheal injuries may create a "false lumen" and loss of airway.

TREATMENT

- Early intubation versus tracheostomy, ideally in the operating room by the most experienced personnel, being careful to prevent creation of a false lumen
- **Cricothyroidotomy may worsen the injury.**

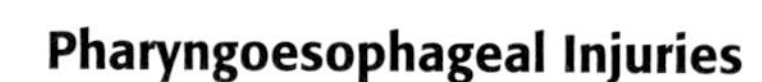

Pharyngoesophageal Injuries

SYMPTOMS/EXAM

Often asymptomatic initially, but may lead to life-threatening mediastinal infections. May also see:

- Hematemesis
- Odynophagia
- SQ emphysema
- Blood in saliva or nasogastric tube

DIAGNOSIS

- Plain film CXR and neck films may show pneumomediastinum or retropharyngeal air.
- Sensitivity of endoscopy or esophagography alone are poor; these tests together have improved sensitivity.

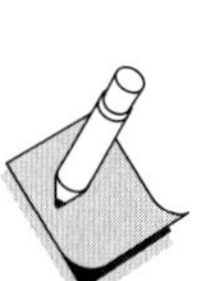

Esophageal injuries are rare but are the most commonly missed injuries of the neck.

TREATMENT

- Broad spectrum ABX with anaerobic coverage
- NPO: Do not place NGT blindly.
- Surgical repair is required for full-thickness injuries.

Vascular Injuries

Vessels may develop pseudoaneurysm and dissection with secondary thrombosis leading to occlusion or emboli via the following mechanisms:

- Hyperextension: Artery compressed against C-spine
- Hyperflexion: Artery compressed between C-spine and mandible
- Direct impact: Including seatbelt across lateral neck
- Intraoral trauma
- Basilar skull fractures damaging intracranial portion

SYMPTOMS/EXAM

- Pulsatile hematoma
- Bruits

- Pulse deficit
- Horner syndrome (ptosis, myosis, anhydrosis)
- TIA/CVA
- Motor or sensory deficits
- Airway compromise

DIAGNOSIS

Diagnosis is made by angiography although contrast CT scan or MRA may assist in determining need for angiography.

TREATMENT

- Anticoagulation
- Surgical intervention if neurologic deficit

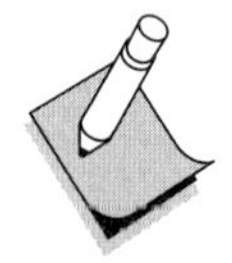

To remember the zones, remember the neck goes from clavicles to base of skull split into thirds at the cricoid and angle of mandible, and that you go up from bottom to top.

Penetrating Neck Trauma

In regard to penetrating trauma, the neck is anatomically divided into zones that have both anatomic (Table 3.10) and management implications. Trauma to any zone may injure spinal cord, vertebral arteries, and carotids.

SYMPTOMS/EXAM

- Findings that suggest major injury (**hard signs**) include expanding hematoma, severe active bleeding, vascular bruit/thrill, cerebral ischemia, airway obstruction, and decreased/absent radial pulse.
- Unfortunately, lack of physical findings does not rule out injury.

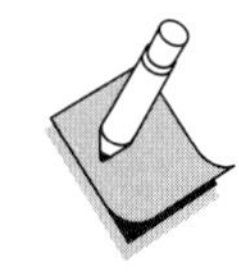

Penetrating neck trauma
Zone I: Angiography, esophageal, and tracheal evaluation
Zone II: Surgery if hard signs, otherwise angiography
Zone III: Angiography

TREATMENT

- Consider early intubation in patients with suspected arterial injury as expanding hematomas can quickly lead to airway compromise.
- Neck wounds with **intact platysma** can be closed.
- Violation of the platysma indicates a possibility of significant neck injury and requires surgical consult.
- Do not probe neck wounds beyond the level of the platysma because of the risk of dislodging a clot.
- Zones I and III can be difficult to evaluate surgically and therefore angiography or CT angiography is usually indicated for these injuries.
- Zone I injuries should also undergo esophageal evaluation.
- Zone II injuries with hard signs of injury are typically explored surgically.
- Zone II injuries without hard signs may be evaluated with angiography and esophageal imaging/visualization.

TABLE 3.10. Zones of the Neck

Zones	Landmarks	Involved Structures	
Zone I	Clavicles to cricoid cartilage	Thoracic vessels, superior mediastinum, lungs, thoracic duct, thyroid	Trachea esophagus
Zone II	Cricoid cartilage to angle of mandible	Jugular veins, larynx	
Zone III	Angle of mandible to base of skull	Pharynx	

- With open venous injuries, prevent venous air embolism with direct pressure and Trendelenburg position.

SOFT-TISSUE TRAUMA

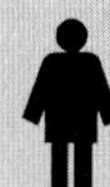

A 24-year-old male presents with severe pain in his left calf after leg run was over by a car. The calf appears tense. The X-ray is normal. What diagnosis should be considered? Compartment syndrome.

Compartment Syndrome

Occurs when a compartment pressure gets high enough to prevent adequate perfusion

MECHANISMS

- Constriction around the compartment
  - Cast or external wrapping
  - Prolonged compression
  - Deep circumferential burns
- Swelling within the compartment
  - Hemorrhage
  - **Fractures** (tibia, forearm, supracondylar)
  - Crush injury
  - Drug or medication injections
  - Ischemic and/or reperfusion injury

ANATOMY

Compartment syndrome is most commonly associated with long-bone fractures of the tibia, but may result from isolated soft-tissue injuries and involve any extremity compartment.

- Two arm compartments: Anterior, posterior
- Two forearm compartments: Dorsal, volar
- Four hand compartments: Thenar, hypothenar, central, interossei
- Three gluteal compartments: Gluteus maximus, gluteus medius and minimus, and tensor fascia latae.
- Three thigh compartments: Anterior, medial, posterior
- Four leg compartments: Anterior, lateral, superficial posterior, and deep posterior.
- Four foot compartments: Medial, lateral, central, interosseous

PATHOPHYSIOLOGY

- Normal compartment pressure is 0–10 mmHg. At 20 mmHg capillary blood flow is affected, and at >30–40 mmHg muscles and nerves can undergo ischemic necrosis.
- Nerves are the first structure to be affected by compartment syndrome.
- Even at elevated compartment pressures arteries and arterioles are often not affected and therefore loss of pulse is a late finding.

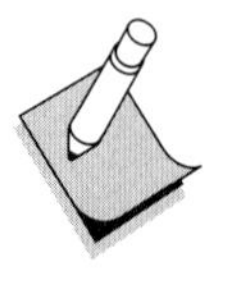

__Loss of pulse is a late finding__ in compartment syndrome. Do not exclude the diagnosis based on the presence of a pulse.

SYMPTOMS/EXAM

- Tense compartment/extremity
- Pain out of proportion to injury or physical findings
- Pain with passive stretch of muscle

- Paresthesias with decreased sensation
- Paresis
- Distal pulses, perfusion, and capillary refill are unreliable (arterial insufficiency is a late finding).

Pain out of proportion to exam:

- *Compartment syndrome*
- *Mesenteric ischemia*
- *Necrotizing fasciitis*

DIAGNOSIS

- Primarily a clinical diagnosis
- Measurement of tissue pressures is confirmatory and defines the involved compartments. Measurements should be made within 5 cm of a fracture.

TREATMENT

- Always remove any external wrapping or compressive force.
- <15 mmHg: No treatment is needed.
- 20–30 mmHg: Maintain close observation and repeat measurements.
- >30 mmHg: Consider fasciotomy.
- An elevated pressure on its own may not require fasciotomy. In an observational study of consecutive patients with lower extremity fractures who did not have compartment syndrome and did well without fasciotomy, a large portion of patients had initial pressures > 30 mmHg.
- With strong clinical suspicion fasciotomy may be required even when compartment pressures are normal as this is a clinical diagnosis.
- Some cases (ie, compartment syndromes of the hand) may be treated with **hyperbaric O_2** and **limb elevation**.
- **Avoid fasciotomy following snake bites**. Extremity snake bites may cause increased compartment pressure, but animal studies show worse outcomes with fasciotomy.

Rhabdomyolysis

Rhabdomyolysis is a syndrome characterized by injury to skeletal muscle followed by release of intracellular contents.

CAUSES

Most common causes in adults include:

- Alcohol and drug abuse
- Toxin ingestion
- Trauma (typically crush injury)
- Infection (most frequently *Legionella*)
- Prolonged immobility
- Heat-related injury
- Strenuous physical activity (especially when poorly conditioned, older age, excessive heat/humidity, or inadequate fluid intake)
- Myoglobin (released from dying muscle) has a toxic effect on the kidneys and may cause renal failure in extreme cases.

SYMPTOMS/EXAM

- Myalgias
- Weakness
- Fever
- Dark/brown urine
- Occasional altered mental status (urea-induced encephalopathy)

DIAGNOSIS

- Elevated creatine phosphokinase (>5 times normal) is the most sensitive marker.
- Myoglobinuria is pathognomonic, but is rapidly cleared.
  - UA with blood on urine dipstick, but minimal RBCs on microscopic evaluation
- Electrolyte abnormalities include hypocalcemia (most common), hyperphosphatemia, hyperkalemia.

TREATMENT

- Mainstay of therapy is aggressive **hydration** with crystalloid that does not contain potassium.
- Intravenous **bicarbonate** to urine pH > 6.5 to enhance renal myoglobin clearance (uncertain benefit)
- Consider mannitol to maintain urine output.
- All cases require admission to follow and treat metabolic abnormalities.

COMPLICATIONS

- Acute renal failure
- DIC
- Metabolic abnormalities (especially hyperkalemia)
- Compartment syndrome
- Peripheral neuropathy

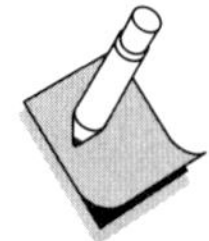

In rhabdomyolysis, hydration and alkalinization of urine (pH > 6.5) prevent renal failure by preventing precipitation of myoglobin in the urine.

Peripheral Vascular Injuries

MECHANISMS

- Occlusive (complete loss of distal perfusion)
  - Transection (most common vascular injury)
  - Thrombosis
  - Reversible spasm
- Nonocclusive (some perfusion remains)
  - Intimal flap
  - AV fistula
  - Pseudoaneurysm

Cases in which you give intravenous bicarbonate:
- *Rhabdomyolysis*
- *Salicylate toxicity*
- *Tricyclic antidepressant toxicity*
- *Hyperkalemia with acidosis*
- *Severe acidosis*

SYMPTOMS/EXAM

- **Hard findings (90% chance of injury)**
  - Pulsatile bleeding
  - Audible bruit
  - Palpable thrill
  - Expanding/pulsatile hematoma
  - Cyanosis
  - Decreased temperature
- Soft findings (up to 35% chance of injury; most do not require emergent repair)
  - Diminished pulse/BP when compared with uninjured extremity
  - Isolated peripheral nerve injury (next to vasculature)
  - Large nonpulsatile hematoma

DIAGNOSIS

- Doppler of pulse may reveal complete loss, or change from triphasic to biphasic/monophasic sound.
- Ankle-brachial index (ABI) or arterial pressure index (API)
- Measure SBP using Doppler with cuff inflated proximal to injury, and compare to uninjured side.
- If ratio of injured SBP/uninjured SBP < 0.9, then further testing with arteriography or ultrasonography is indicated. If ratio is 0.9–0.99 then observe/reassess in 12–24 hours.
- Knee dislocations have a high risk of popliteal injury and in the past have had routine angiography. Current thinking suggests, however, that these may be closely evaluated with less invasive techniques as long as there is no discrepancy in blood pressures between injured and uninjured legs (ankle-ankle index).

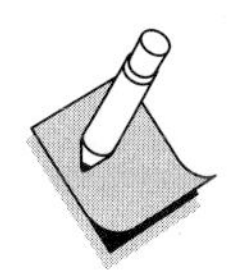

In the setting of nerve injury, always consider vascular injury as ***nerves and vessels usually travel together.***

TREATMENT

- Direct pressure to stop bleeding.
- Blind clamping and tourniquets are not recommended.
- Hypotensive resuscitation (controversial): Keep SBP around 90 mmHg prior to surgical repair to prevent dislodging clot and persistent bleeding.
- Major arterial injuries must be repaired within 6 hours.
- Minor arterial injuries (intact distal circulation, no active hemorrhage, and <5 mm intimal flap or pseudoaneurysm on angio) can be closely observed. Be cautious with children and vasculopaths.
- Major venous injuries usually require repair.

COMPLICATIONS

- As with compartment syndrome, ischemic muscle contracture resulting from nerve and muscle damage may occur.
- Prolonged ischemia may require amputation.

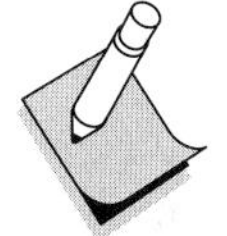

Knee dislocations have a high risk for popliteal injury.

Amputation/Replantation

TREATMENT

- To protect amputated body part:
  - Wash with sterile saline (do not scrub or use antiseptics).
  - Wrap in saline-soaked gauze and place in plastic bag and then on ice (**do not place directly on ice**).
- Amputated appendages can tolerate 6–8 hours of warm ischemia and 12–24 hours of cold ischemia at 4°C.
- Penis may be reimplanted up to 6 hours after amputation
- Other than great toe, toes are not usually reimplanted.
- Fingertip amputations fit into three categories:
  - Zone I: Proximal two-thirds of nail bed intact
  - Zone II: Exposed bone
  - Zone III: Amputation of entire nail bed
- Try to save thumb and index finger. Always attempt reimplantation in children.
- For fingertip amputations with wounds < 1 cm^2, healing by secondary intention should be adequate.
- Rongeur exposed bone and suture to provide soft-tissue coverage. **Do not leave bone exposed.**

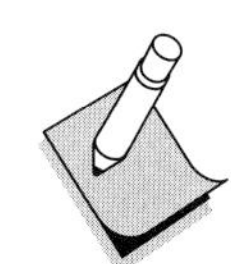

Cooling extends the duration of viability of the amputated part.

TRAUMA

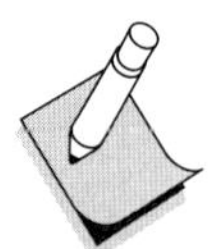

The more proximal the amputation, the less ischemia time it can tolerate.

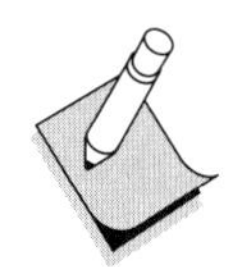

5 mm of healthy nail bed is required for nail adherence.

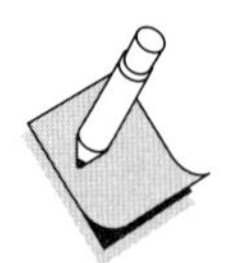

High-pressure injection injuries require immediate surgical consultation.

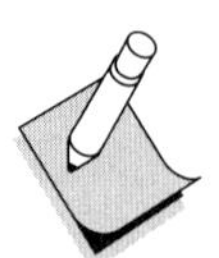

Thermal injury below vocal cords only occurs with steam inhalation.

TRAUMA

High-Pressure Injection Injuries

- Tend to have a benign appearance but high morbidity.
- Must be referred to hand specialist or plastic surgeon immediately for debridement.
- Give prophylactic Abx, update Td, and elevate and splint extremity.
- Plain film X-ray may show widespread radiopaque material and air.
- Do not perform a digital block as this may increase compartment pressure.

BURNS

Thermal Burns

Burns are described according to depth, with superficial burns involving only the epidermis, partial-thickness burns involving both the epidermis and part of the dermis, full-thickness burns destroying the entire epidermis and dermis, and subdermal burns involving the subdermal tissues (see Table 3.11).

Symptoms/Exam

- Evaluation of burns involves five main components:
  - Evaluation of airway and breathing
  - Consideration of possible carbon monoxide and cyanide exposure
  - Estimation of involved TBSA
  - Determination of depth of burned skin (see Table 3.12)
  - Evaluate for involvement of critical parts and for circumferential burns.
- Signs of inhalational injury:
  - Fire in enclosed space
  - Facial burns or singed nasal hair
  - Carbonaceous sputum, soot in mouth or nose
  - Hoarseness, stridor, expiratory wheezing
- To estimate involved TBSA in adults, the Rule of Nines is commonly used (see Figure 3.19):
  - 9 for each upper extremity
  - 18 for each lower extremity
  - 18 each for front and back of torso
  - 9 for the head
  - 1 for perineum

TABLE 3.11. Burn Classifications

New Terminology	Old Terminology	Depth
Superficial	First-degree	Epidermal layer only
Partial-thickness Superficial	Second-degree	Epidermis and superficial dermis
Deep		Epidermis to deep dermis, including hair follicles and sweat/sebaceous glands
Full-thickness	Third-degree	Epidermis and dermis (all structures)
Subdermal	Fourth-degree	Subdermal structures (muscles, nerves, bone)

TABLE 3.12. Burn Clinical Findings and Prognosis

Type	Clinical Findings	Prognosis
Superficial	Similar to sunburn: red, painful, tender, no blistering	Heals without scarring in 1 wk
Superficial partial-thickness	Red, painful, blistering, blanching	Hair follicles and sweat glands are retained. Usually heals with minimal scarring in 2–3 wk
Deep partial-thickness	Red to pale white-yellow, blistering with rupture, no blanching. Decreased two-point discrimination but can feel pressure	Healing can take 3–8 wk with scarring, and contracture.
Full-thickness	Charred, white/black, painless, and leathery	Surgical grafting is required unless <1 cm diameter.
Subdermal	Severe burns	Life and limb threatening

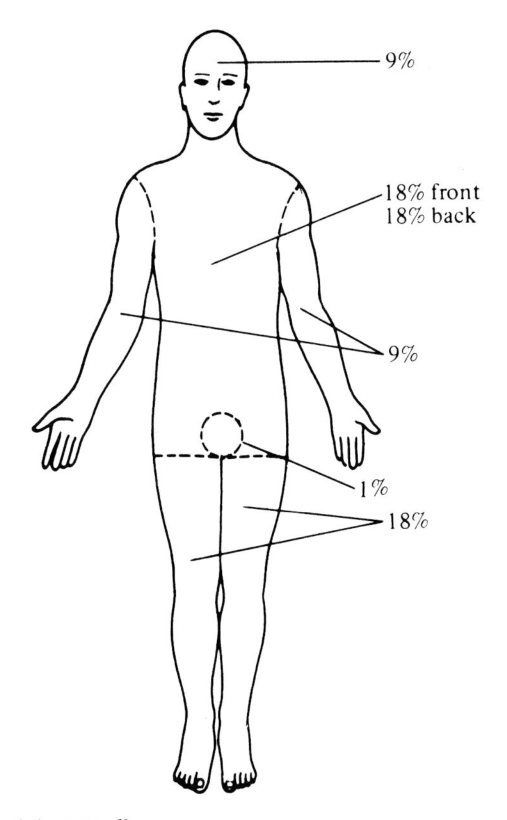

FIGURE 3.19. Adult TBSA diagram.

(Reproduced, with permission, from Tintinalli JE, Kelen GD, Stapczynski JS. *Emergency Medicine: A Comprehensive Study Guide*, 6th ed. New York: McGraw-Hill, 2004:1221.)

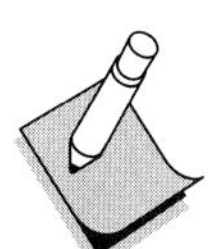

Area of the patient's palm is approximately 1% TBSA, which is useful when evaluating children.

- Estimation of burn depth may be difficult on initial evaluation.
- For this reason, burns should be reevaluated in 24 hours as usually true depth and extent of tissue damage are not initially apparent.

TREATMENT

- Treatment for inhalational injury:
  - Humidified 100% O_2
  - Intubation for:
    - Full-thickness face or perioral burns
    - Circumferential neck burns
    - Supraglottic edema and inflammation on bronchoscopy
    - Tachypnea, hypoxia, or AMS
- The Parkland Formula provides a guide for fluid resuscitation for patients with significant burns:

  4 mL × %burn × weight (kg) = fluid requirement (mL) over first 24 hrs

  - Use only area of second- and third-degree burns to determine TBSA for resuscitation.
  - Give half over first 8 hours. Multiply by 3 mL instead of 4 mL in children and add maintenance fluids. The Parkland Formula is merely a guide, and adequate fluid must be given to maintain urine output.
- **Circumferential burns** to extremities run the risk of circulatory compromise due to pressure from burn/swelling. Circumferential burns to the torso may interfere with breathing via constriction. Consider early escharotomy for both.
- Blisters that are large or across joints should be ruptured, while smaller immobile ones may be left alone.
- Silvadene to body but not to face because of scarring risk. Use topical agent like bacitracin to face.
- Keep wounds out of sun to prevent scarring, and follow up in 24 hours.

DISPOSITION

- Major: Burn center (see Table 3.13)
- Moderate: Hospitalization

TRAUMA

TABLE 3.13. Criteria for Transfer to Burn Unit

Partial-thickness burns greater than 10% total body surface area (BSA)
Burns that involve the face, hand, feet, genitalia, perineum, or major joints
Third-degree burns in any age group
Electrical burns, including lightning injury
Chemical burns
Inhalation injury
Burn injury in patients with preexisting medical disorders that could complicate management, prolong recovery, or affect mortality
Any patients with burns and concomitant trauma (such as fractures) in which the burn injury poses the greatest risk of morbidity or mortality
Burned children in hospitals without qualified personnel or equipment for the care of children
Burn injury in patients who will require special social, emotional, or long-term rehabilitative intervention

(Reproduced, with permission, from Tintinalli JE, Kelen GD, Stapczynski JS. *Emergency Medicine: A Comprehensive Study Guide,* 6th ed. New York: McGraw-Hill, 2004:1222.)

- Partial-thickness 15–25% in 10- to 50-year-olds
- Partial-thickness 10–20% in <10- or >50–years old
- Full-thickness 2–10%

- Minor: Outpatient
  - Partial thickness <15% in 10- to 50-year-olds
  - Partial thickness <10% in <10- or >50-year-olds
  - Full thickness < 2%

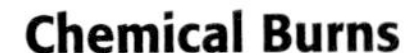

Chemical Burns

The classes of burning chemicals include acids, alkalis, oxidizing agents, corrosives, reducing agents, desiccants, vesicants, protoplasmic poisons (see Table 3.14).

- **Acids cause coagulative necrosis,** creating a tough eschar preventing deep penetration of burn.
- **Alkalis cause liquefactive necrosis**, a poor barrier, so burns travel much deeper. For this reason, alkali burns tend to be worse than acid burns.
- **Cement** contains lime, which is converted with water to the alkali calcium hydroxide.

Common alkalis ("lyes") include drain and toilet cleaners, detergents, cement, and paint removers. Treat with copious irrigation.

TREATMENT

- The first line in chemical-burn therapy is ample irrigation to remove the offending agent, except with
  - Dry powder (lime): Brush away before hydration.
  - Sodium metals: Use oil, not water.
  - Phenol (carbolic acid)
- Be careful of heat production when chemicals react with water or their neutralizing agents.
- Lacrimators (tear gas and pepper spray) irritate mucosa (eye, nose, and mouth) and are treated with copious water irrigation.
- Airbag deployment utilizes an exothermic reaction that can cause burns (sodium azide) and keratitis (sodium hydroxide). These are treated with thorough irrigation with water.

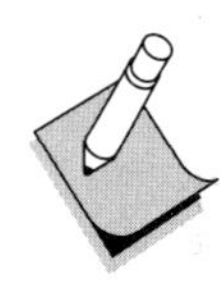

***Glass etching** => **hydrofluoric acid burn** => treat with **calcium gluconate**. The skin often looks normal and pain may not begin for hours after exposure.*

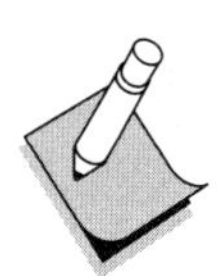

The primary treatment for almost all chemical exposures except metals, dry powder lime, and phenol is water irrigation.

BALLISTICS

Bullets cause injury by crush (permanent cavitation) and by temporary cavitation (tissue stretch).

Characteristics that determine injury pattern:

- Bullet mass: Determines depth of penetration and diameter of crush injury.
- Bullet construction: Increased deformity or fragmentation (hollow point bullets and lead bullets without a cap) yields great crush injury.
- Bullet yaw (tilt off long axis): Greater yaw yields greater crush injury.
- Bullet velocity: Higher velocity yields greater **cavitation**.
  - Shorter gun barrels produce lower velocity because the expanding gases are released into the atmosphere sooner.
  - As a result, **handguns fire low-velocity bullets** and do not produce significant cavitation.

Chemical burns to the eyes are emergencies and require immediate and copious irrigation to restore ocular pH to 7.3–7.7.

TABLE 3.14. Chemical Burns

	Where Found	Damage	Treatment	Special
Acids				
Acetic acid	Hair wave neutralizer	Partial-thickness burns to scalp	Water irrigation	Oral abx for **persistent bacteria on the scalp**
Carbolic acid (Phenol)	Industrial and medicinal	Painless white/brown coagulum—**may prevent penetration of water irrigation**	Polyethylene glycol and industrial methylated spirits or isopropyl alcohol	**Penetrates more deeply when dilute than when concentrated**
Chromic acid	Industrial chromium plating and glass cleaning	Chronic penetrating ulcerating lesions	Water irrigation and surgical excision to **prevent systemic toxicity**	**High systemic toxicity following skin absorption**
Formic acid	Industrial and agricultural	Coagulative necrosis	Water irrigation	Acidosis, hemolysis, hemoglobinuria
Hydrochloric/ sulfuric acid	Toilet bowl/ drain cleaners Battery acid Bleach Industrial	Dark brown or black burns	Water irrigation	
Hydrofluoric acid	High-octane fuel, etching, semiconductors, rust remover	Deep painful burns with possible blue-gray skin and erythema	Irrigation **Calcium gluconate (topical/IM/SQ/ intra-arterial)** **Treat until pain is gone.**	**Concentration effect not duration effect** Ca↓, Mg↓, K↑, myocardial instability **Pain parallels extent of injury.**
Methacrylic acid	Nail cosmetics	Dermal burns	Water irrigation	Preschoolers
Nitric acid	Metal work, fertilizers	Yellowish burns	Water irrigation	
Oxalic acid	Leather and blueprint		Water irrigation and IV calcium	Binds Ca, inhibits muscle contraction
Alkalis				
Lyes Ammonium Barium Ca, Li KOH, NaOh	Drain cleaners, detergents, paint removers	Deep burns	Prolonged water irrigation	**Ingestion can cause airway occlusion and/or esophageal trauma.**

TRAUMA

TABLE 3.14. Chemical Burns (*Continued*)

	WHERE FOUND	DAMAGE	TREATMENT	SPECIAL
Lime (calcium oxide)	Cement	Exothermic rxn when neutralized with water	Profuse water via strong stream to prevent burn	First, brush away dry particles.
Metals	Agricultural	Molten metal burns	**Mineral oil and excision—no water**	**Metal can ignite when in contact with air or water.**
Hydrocarbons	Gasoline and tar	Fat-dissolving corrosive injury	Decontamination Polysorbate to remove tar	Frostbite and dehydration from skin contact
Vesicants	DMSO Cantharides Mustard gas	Deep penetration, blisters, ulcers	Water irrigation or adsorbent powder	Anoxic necrosis
Alkyl mercury	Disinfectant Fungicide Wood preservative	Erythema and blistering	Debride and drain blisters Water irrigation	**Blisters contain mercury.**
White phosphorus	Explosives Insecticides	Deep and superficial	Water irrigation Copper sulfate	**May ignite when dry, keep wet**

- Tissue type: Inelastic tissue (brain, liver, spleen, and bone) is more prone to cavitation injury. By contrast, highly elastic tissue such as muscle may be injured by crush but not by cavitation.

Shotgun pellets tend to produce less damage owing to small size and spherical shape, unless fired at close range. At close range the pellets clump together and cause much deeper tissue penetration.

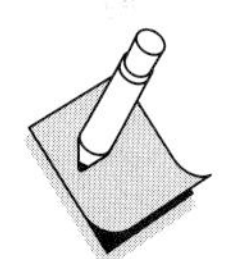

Determinant of injury:
Crush—mass, deformation, yaw
Cavitation—velocity, tissue elasticity

EXAM

- Determination of entrance and exit sites is prone to error and has potential legal implications.

TREATMENT/COMPLICATIONS

- To preserve evidence in GS victims do not:
  - Cut through bullet holes on clothing
  - Cut through bullet holes on skin unless medically necessary
  - Handle bullets/fragments with metal instruments so as not to disturb/cause markings
  - Describe wounds as entrance or exit
- **Bullets can embolize.**
  - If bullets are not found in their expected location, further workup is warranted.
  - In general embolized bullets must be removed.

Handguns fire low-velocity bullets.

TRAUMA

Bullets are not sterilized by the heat of firing, and they can track in skin/clothing/FBs.

- Bullets lodged within the spinal canal may migrate and cause further damage. Consult Neurosurgery. Removal should be considered.
- Lead poisoning is not usually a concern since bullets usually become encapsulated in fibrous tissue. However, bullets resting in synovial fluid (intra-articular, disk space, and bursa) may dissolve and release lead into the body. Bullets must be removed from joints to prevent mechanical and lead damage to joints and lead poisoning.

CHAPTER 4

Orthopedics

Kim Fredericksen, MD

EVALUATION OF ORTHOPEDIC INJURIES

All open fractures require emergent orthopedic consultation because of high risk of infection.

DEFINITIONS OF FRACTURES AND THE ORTHOPAEDIC TRAUMA ASSOCIATION (OTA) CLASSIFICATION SYSTEM

- **Closed fractures:** Break in the bone or cartilage with skin intact
- **Open fractures:** Any fracture where there is a traumatic wound allowing the outside to communicate with the bone
  - **High risk of infection**
  - Treatment includes prophylactic antibiotics, tetanus prophylaxis, irrigation and debridement, and emergent orthopedic consultation.

Components of OTA classification system of fractures (see Figure 4.1):

1. **Bone:** Describes the bone(s) that is/are involved, eg, radius.
2. **Segmental location:** Describes the location of the fracture relative to the bone, eg, physis (see Chapter 5, Pediatrics, for Salter-Harris classification system), proximal, diaphyseal, distal
3. **Type:** Describes the complexity of the fracture, eg, simple, wedge, complex, articular
4. **Group:** Describes the orientation of the fracture line, eg, hairline, greenstick, torus, nightstick, linear, transverse, oblique, segmental, spiral, crush
5. **Subgroup:** Describes further the relative orientation of the fracture line, eg, displacement, separation, shortening, angulation, rotation

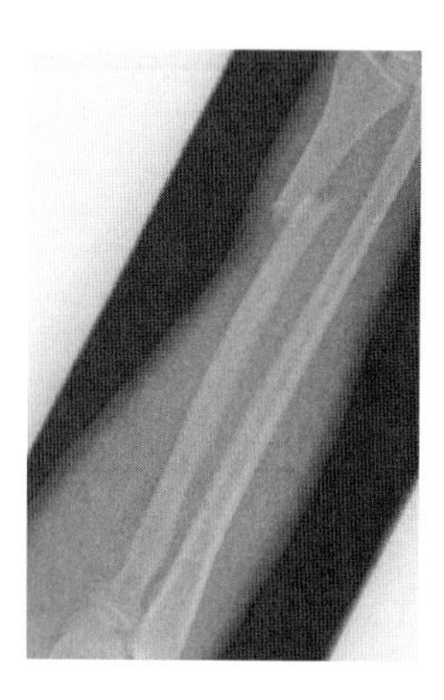

FIGURE 4.1. The AP view of the forearm shows a simple, transverse distal radial shaft fracture with approximately 90% displacement.

ASSESSMENT OF NEUROVASCULAR STRUCTURES

See Table 4.1 for common injuries and their associated neurovascular complications.

Neurovascular evaluation–

PMS
Pulse
Motor
Sensation

MANAGEMENT OF ORTHOPEDIC INJURIES

- Analgesia
- Reduction if necessary
  - Reassess neurovascular status.
- Splints
  - Shoulder immobilizer
  - Sling
  - Long-arm gutter
  - Sugar-tong
  - Short-arm gutter
  - Thumb spica
  - Knee immobilizer
  - Posterior ankle mold
  - Ankle stirrup
- Orthopedic consultation or referral

COMPLICATIONS OF ORTHOPEDIC INJURIES

- Malunion or nonunion
- Avascular necrosis
  - Hip dislocation
  - Scaphoid fracture

TABLE 4.1. Common Injuries and Associated Neurovascular Complications

Types of Fractures or Dislocations	Neurovascular Complications
Anterior shoulder dislocation Musculocutaneous nerve injury	Axillary nerve and artery injury
Extension supracondylar fracture Posterior elbow dislocation	Brachial artery injury Ulnar and median nerve injury Radial nerve injury for supracondylar fracture
Knee dislocation	Popliteal artery injury Peroneal and tibial nerve injury
Humeral shaft injury	Radial nerve injury
Medial epicondylar fracture	Ulnar nerve injury
Lateral tibial plateau fracture	Peroneal nerve injury

  - Talus fracture
  - Proximal humerus fracture
- Infection
- Vascular injury or hemorrhage
- Nerve injury: Pain, paresthesias, weakness, or paralysis
- Soft-tissue or organ injury
- **Compartment syndrome**
- Fat emboli syndrome
  - Most common after **long bone and pelvic fractures**
  - See petechiae, altered mental status, hypoxia.
- Volkmann ischemic contracture
  - Flexion contracture of hand/wrist due to untreated forearm compartment syndrome and resultant muscle ischemia.
- Reflex sympathetic dystrophy (complex regional pain syndrome)

The 5 Ps of compartment syndrome:

Pain (most common symptom)
Paresthesias
Pallor
Paralysis
Pulselessness (**late finding!**)

INJURIES TO THE UPPER EXTREMITIES

A football player snags his index finger in another player's jersey and finds it difficult to catch the football for the rest of the game. When you immobilize the PIP and MCP joints in extension, he is no longer able to flex the DIP joint. What is injured and how is it treated?

The football player has a flexor digitorum profundus (FDP) tendon avulsion, or "**jersey finger**," which is treated by splinting the finger in a comfortable position and referral to orthopedics as soon as possible.

Digits

Amputated Digits

- Require immediate hand surgery consultation
- Wrap in sterile gauze soaked in normal saline (NS) and surround with plastic bag, then place bag with digit(s) in ice water.

- Absolute contraindications to reimplantation: Unstable patient or severe crush injury

FRACTURES OF DIGITS

- Fractures of digits are most often stable and nondisplaced. Treat with buddy taping.
- Unstable fractures and intra-articular fractures of digits should be reduced and splinted and will often require internal fixation.

FLEXOR TENDON INJURIES

MECHANISM

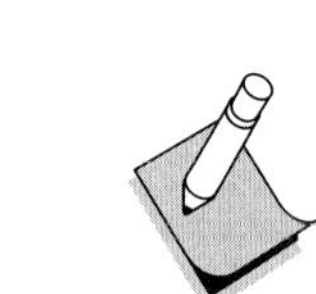

If the FDS is cut, the patient can still flex both the DIP and PIP joint.

- These injuries are most commonly associated with lacerations of the flexor digitorum superficialis (FDS) and flexor digitorum profundus (FDP) and can cause loss of flexion of the PIP and DIP joint. However, if only the FDS is cut, patients can still flex both joints.
- Closed injuries are associated with **rheumatoid arthritis** and **athletic injury**.
- Classic athletic injury occurs when a football player grabs another player's jersey (thus the term "**jersey finger**"), avulsing the profundus tendon from its bony insertion.

TREATMENT

- Both open and closed injuries usually require surgical repair.

COMPLICATIONS

- Laceration injuries may cause damage to the digital arteries and nerves.

MALLET FINGER

MECHANISM

Forced flexion of the DIP ("jammed finger"), leading to rupture of the extensor tendon at its insertion at the base of the distal phalanx or bony avulsion of the tendon insertion site.

DIAGNOSIS

- Unable to extend DIP: X-ray may reveal avulsion fracture (see Figure 4.2).
- Splint DIP in strict extension for 6 to 8 weeks (with a Stack-type splint): Watch for development of pressure sores!

COMPLICATIONS

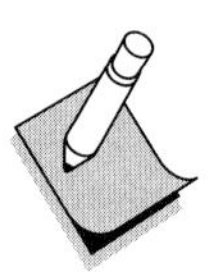

*An untreated mallet finger can result in a **swan-neck deformity.***

- If untreated, a swan neck deformity (hyperextension of PIP, flexion of DIP) may result.

BOUTONNIERE DEFORMITY

MECHANISM

- Forced flexion at PIP, causing tear of the central portion of the extensor tendon at the PIP joint

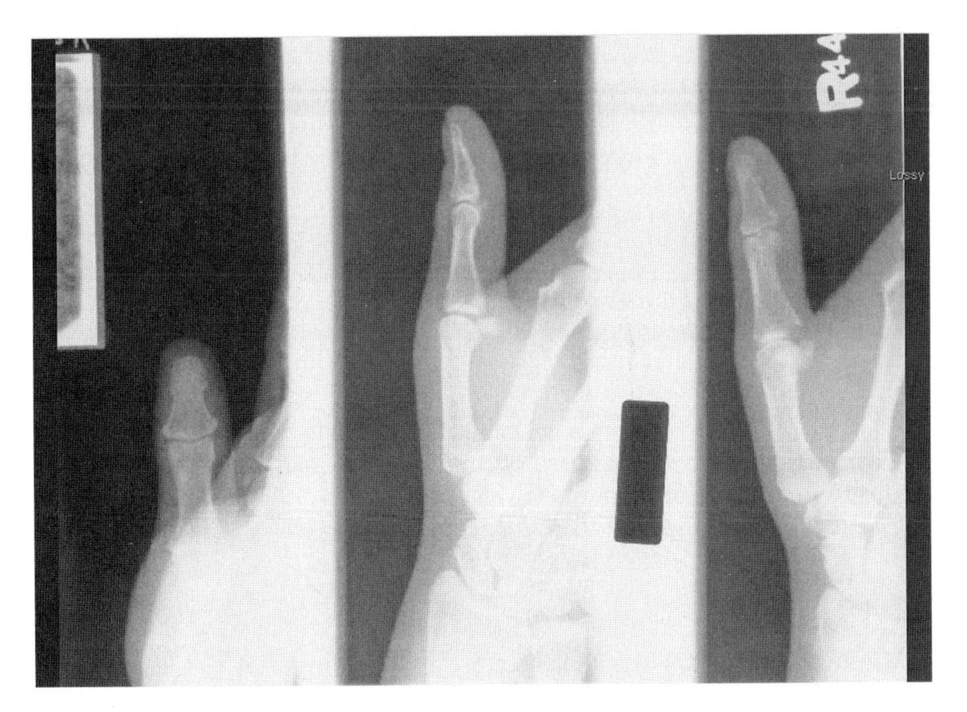

FIGURE 4.2. **Gamekeeper's thumb. An avulsion fracture off the medial base of the proximal phalanx due to the pull of the ulnar collateral ligament.**

DIAGNOSIS

- Unable to fully extend PIP with the wrist and metacarpophalangeal (MCP) joints fully flexed

TREATMENT

- Treat by splinting PIP in extension for 4–6 weeks.

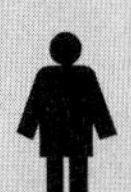

A 19-year-old man presents to a university health clinic with a swollen and tender hand over the fourth and fifth metatarsal and a laceration over the fifth knuckle. What fracture is most likely?

A **boxer's** fracture, and the laceration is probably due to a tooth. Do not suture these lacerations. See Table 4.5 for acceptable degrees of angulation for metacarpal fractures.

Hand Injuries

RUPTURE OF THE ULNAR COLLATERAL LIGAMENT

Also known as **gamekeeper's thumb** and **skier's thumb**

MECHANISM

Valgus force on thumb leads to tear of ulnar collateral ligament. It may also occur with avulsion of tendon insertion site at the base of the proximal phalanx (see Figure 4.2). 30% are associated with fractures.

Diagnosis

- Swelling and tenderness over the ulnar side of the MP joint of the thumb.
- Pinch strength is markedly reduced and causes pain.
- Stress testing may differentiate incomplete (<30° laxity) versus complete (≥30°–45° laxity) tears.

Treatment

- Incomplete tear: Thumb spica, follow-up with hand surgeon
- Complete tear: Surgical repair

Bennett's Fracture

- **Intra-articular** fracture at base of thumb metacarpal with associated **subluxation or dislocation** at the CMC joint
- Treat with thumb spica, orthopedic consult.

Rolando's Fracture

- **Comminuted intra-articular** fracture of the thumb at the base of the metacarpal
- Treat with thumb spica, orthopedic consult.
- Prognosis is worse than with Bennett's fracture.

Metacarpal Neck Fracture (Boxer's Fracture)

A boxer's fracture with angulation >40° may result in functional impairment and must be reduced.

Mechanism

Usually dominant hand involved from an altercation involving direct impaction forces. A fracture of the fifth metacarpal neck is referred to as a boxer's fracture.

Diagnosis

X-ray reveals fracture of metacarpal neck with volar angulation.

Treatment

- Fractures without significant angulation (see Figure 4.3) may be treated with an ulnar gutter splint.
- Fracture with unacceptable degrees of angulation or with rotational deformity require orthopedic evaluation for closed/open reduction.

Carpal bones (starting at articulation with radius)–

Some **L**overs **T**ry **P**ositions **T**hat **T**hey **C**an't **H**andle
Scaphoid
Lunate
Triquetrum
Pisiform
Trapezium
Trapezoid
Capitate
Hamate

Wrist Injuries

Scaphoid Fracture

Most common carpal fracture

Mechanism

Fall on outstretched hand (FOOSH)

Diagnosis

Suspect diagnosis if **snuff box tenderness** is present. Wrist and scaphoid X-rays should be obtained, but may be negative in the setting of acute fracture.

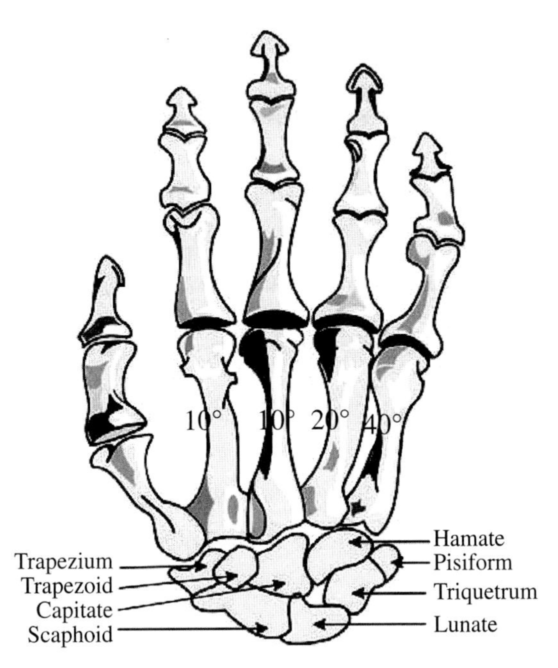

FIGURE 4.3. Acceptable degrees of angulation for metacarpal neck fractures. Correct all rotational deformities.

(Reproduced, with permission, from familypracticenotebook.com.)

Treatment

Thumb spica splint, orthopedics referral

Complications

Avascular necrosis: The more proximal the fracture, the greater likelihood of avascular necrosis and the longer the fracture needs to be immobilized.

Triquetral Fracture

Fracture of the triquetrum is the **second most common carpal fracture**. It is usually a dorsal chip fracture but can also occur through the body of the triquetrum (which is associated with perilunate and lunate dislocations).

Mechanism

Direct blow to the bone or impingement of the ulnar styloid with dorsiflexion and ulnar deviation.

Diagnosis

Tenderness distal to ulnar styloid

Treatment

Volar splint

Lunate Fracture

Lunate fracture is the third most common carpal fracture. It usually occurs in association with other injuries (rare to have isolated lunate fracture)!

Mechanism

FOOSH

Diagnosis

Suspect diagnosis if there is tenderness over middorsum of the wrist, worse with axial compression of the middle finger. X-rays are often negative in acute injury.

Treatment

Thumb spica, referral

Complications

Kienbock's disease (avascular necrosis of the lunate)

Scapholunate Dissociation

The most common carpal ligamentous wrist injury, typically resulting from an acute tear of the scapholunate ligament

Mechanism

FOOSH is most common, though may result from chronic overuse

Diagnosis

- **Signet ring sign** on AP radiograph: Loss of ligamentous support results in rotary subluxation and palmar tilt of the scaphoid, causing the circular cortex to appear as a ring.
- **Terry Thomas sign** (widening of the scapholunate joint space) on AP X-ray (see Figure 4.4): Terry Thomas was a comedian with a large space between his two front teeth. The space between the scaphoid and lunate is normally the same as between the other carpal bones (<2 mm).

Treatment

Radial gutter splint and orthopedic consultation

Complications

May be associated with lunate and perilunate dislocations

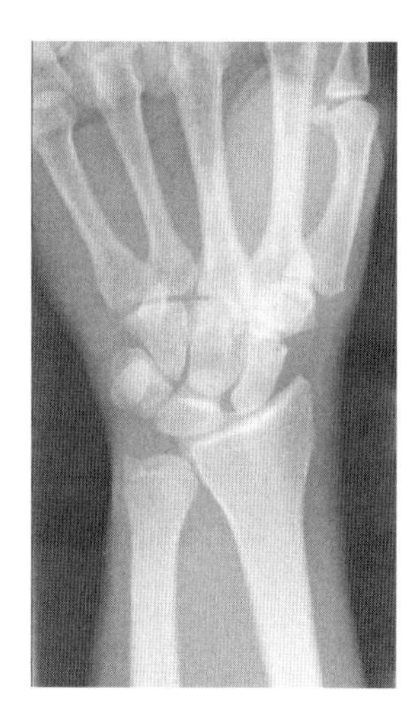

FIGURE 4.4. Scapholunate dissociation.

Lunate Dislocation

Mechanism

FOOSH (of significant force, eg, fall from height) with wrist hyperextension and disruption of carpal ligaments

Diagnosis

X-ray findings include the **spilled teacup sign** (lateral view) and **piece-of-pie sign** (AP view)(lunate normally has a quadrangular shape on AP X-ray but when dislocated, it looks triangular; see Figure 4.5).

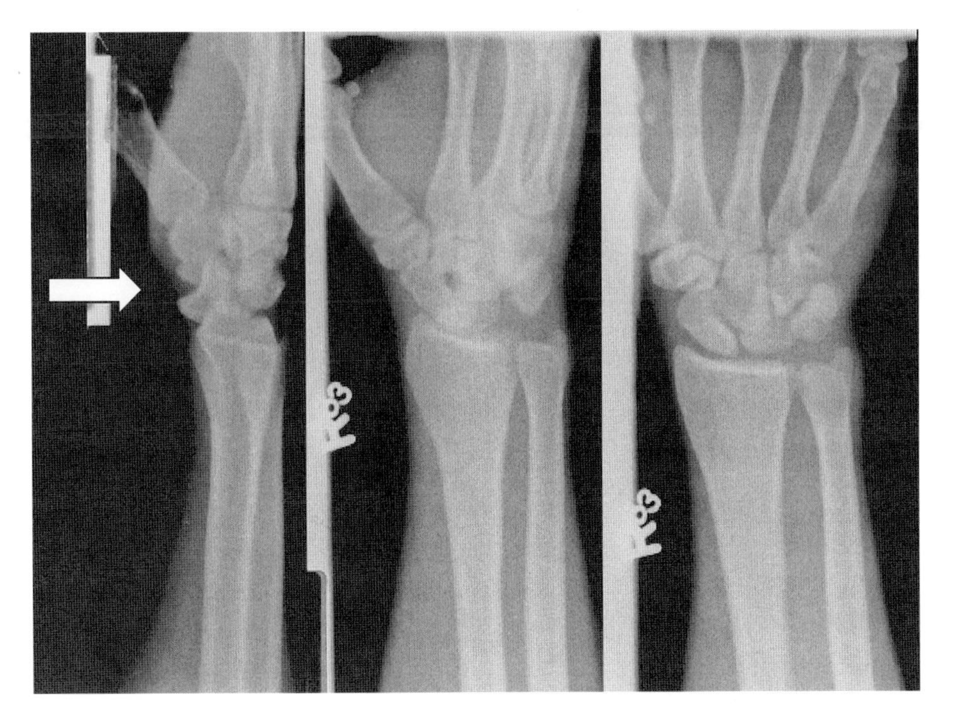

FIGURE 4.5. **Lunate dislocation. "Piece-of-pie-shaped" lunate on the frontal view is a clue but the "spilled teacup" (see arrow) on lateral view is diagnostic. Normally the axis of the lunate should line up with that of the distal radius and the capitate on the lateral view.**

TREATMENT

Reduction by orthopedist

COMPLICATIONS

Median nerve injuries, acute carpal tunnel syndrome, early arthritis, avascular necrosis

PERILUNATE CARPAL DISLOCATION

Most common carpal dislocation

MECHANISM

FOOSH (again, significant forces involved) with wrist hyperextension and disruption of carpal ligaments.

DIAGNOSIS

Teacup is upright but the capitate does not sit on top of the lunate (capitate is most frequently found **dorsally** displaced sitting on top of radius; see Figure 4.6).

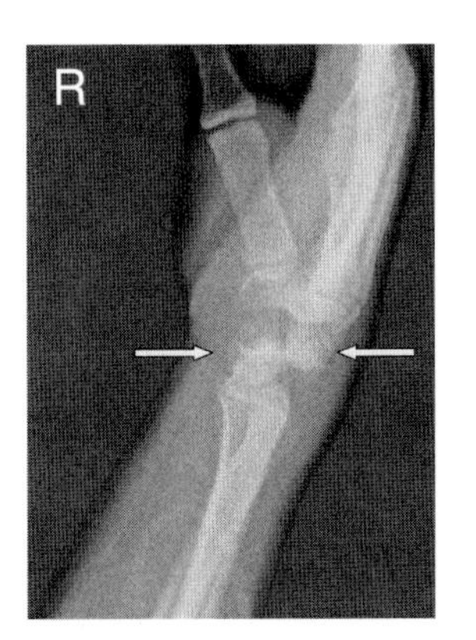

FIGURE 4.6. **Perilunate dislocation. The "teacup" (lunate) is upright but the capitate is positioned posterior to the lunate.**

TREATMENT

Reduction and orthopedic consultation

COMPLICATIONS

Same as lunate dislocations

Forearm Injuries

COLLES FRACTURE

MECHANISM

FOOSH.

DIAGNOSIS

X-ray shows fracture of distal radius with dorsal displacement (“**dinner fork deformity**”).

TREATMENT

- Closed reduction should be performed if fracture fragment has any dorsal angulation (distal radius is normally tilted 15° volarly). Goals of reduction are to restore volar tilt, inclincation, and length to radius.
- Sugar-tong splint, orthopedic follow-up.

COMPLICATIONS

Early arthritis (if intra-articular), malunion, median nerve injury, 60% associated with ulnar styloid fracture

SMITH FRACTURE (REVERSE COLLES FRACTURE)

DIAGNOSIS

Distal radius with volar displacement (“**garden spade deformity**”) of the distal fragment (see Figure 4.7)

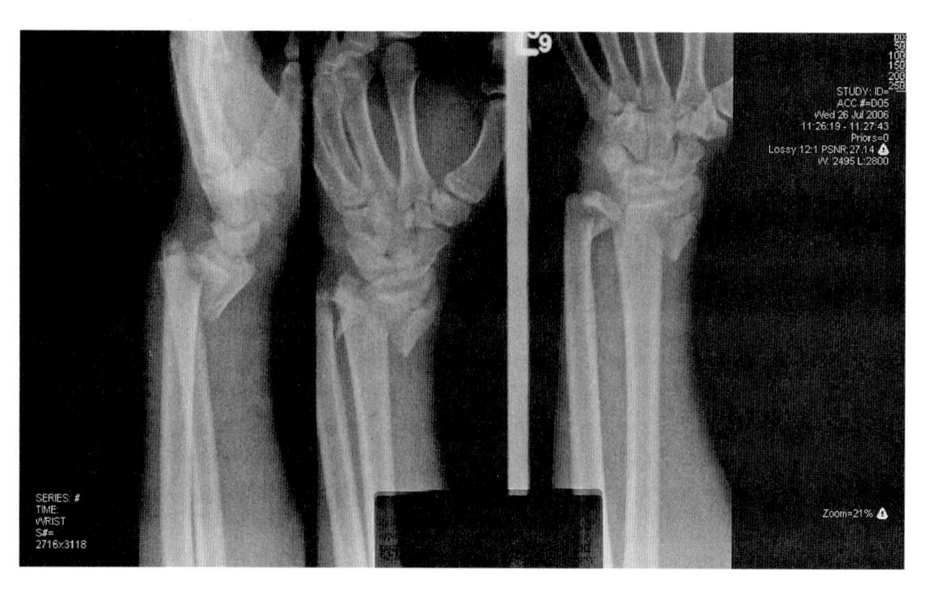

FIGURE 4.7. Smith fracture.

Treatment

Closed reduction, long arm or sugar-tong splint, orthopedic follow-up

Complications

Median nerve injury

Barton Fracture

Dorsal or volar rim fractures of the distal radius

Diagnosis

X-ray reveals intra-articular fracture of the volar or dorsal rim of the radius, which may be comminuted on the AP view.

Treatment

Long arm sugar-tong splint, close orthopedic follow-up. Typically these fractures require ORIF, especially if the fracture involves more than 50% of the articular surface.

Complications

Early arthritis

Nightstick Fracture

This isolated ulnar fracture typically results from a direct blow to the forearm.

Diagnosis

X-ray shows midshaft ulnar fracture. Always examine the proximal radius to exclude a Monteggia fracture.

Treatment

- Long arm splint for simple nightstick fractures
- If displaced >50% or angulated >10°, obtain orthopedic referral for possible ORIF.

Essex-Lopresti Fracture

- A radial head fracture with dislocation of the distal radial/ulnar joint and disruption of the interosseous membrane
- Treat with splint and referral to orthopedics for ORIF.

Galeazzi Fracture

Mechanism

FOOSH in force pronation or direct blow.

Diagnosis

- Suspect if patient has pain and swelling to both wrist and elbow
- X-rays show distal radial shaft fracture and distal radioulnar joint injury (eg, widening of joint space).

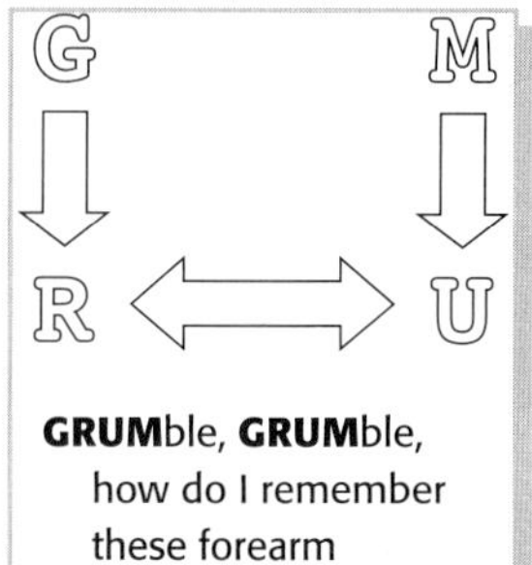

GRUMble, **GRUM**ble, how do I remember these forearm fractures?
Galeazzi = **R**adial fracture and radioulnar dislocation.
Monteggia = **U**lnar fracture with radial dislocation.

TREATMENT

Sugar-tong splint, referral to orthopedics for ORIF. Because this is an unstable fracture, closed reduction is usually unsuccessful.

COMPLICATIONS

Ulnar nerve injury, compartment syndrome

MONTEGGIA FRACTURE

Ulna fracture (usually proximal shaft) with radial head dislocation (see Figure 4.8)

MECHANISM

FOOSH

DIAGNOSIS

- Suspect if patient has significant pain and swelling to the elbow
- X-ray shows proximal ulnar shaft fracture with radial head dislocation.

TREATMENT

Reduction, long arm splint, ORIF

COMPLICATIONS

Radial nerve injury, compartment syndrome

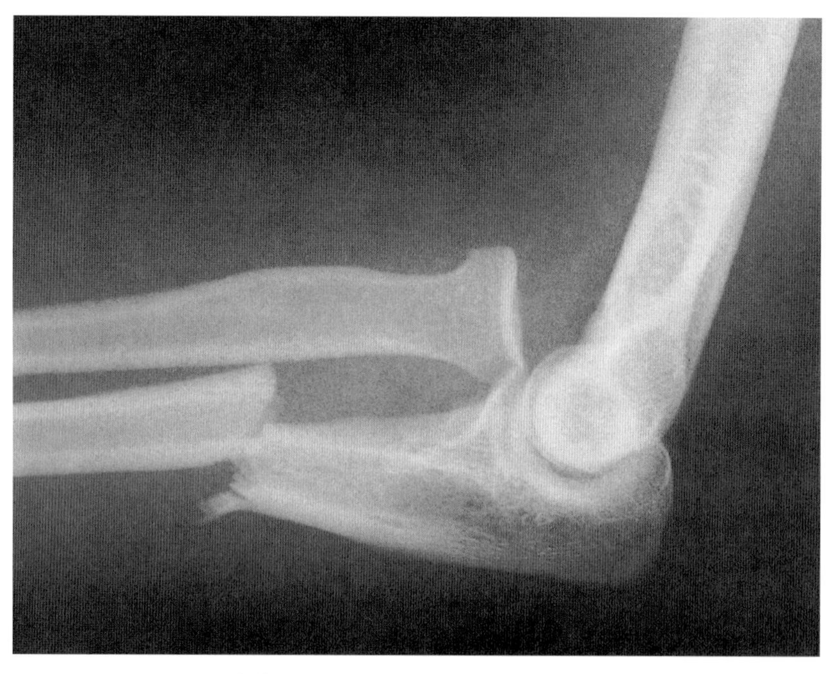

FIGURE 4.8. Monteggia fracture.

(Reproduced, with permission, from Knoop KJ, Stack LB, Storrow AB. *Atlas of Emergency Medicine*, 2nd ed. New York, McGraw-Hill, 2002:297.)

Elbow Injuries

OLECRANON FRACTURES

- For a nondisplaced olecranon fracture, stabilize with a posterior splint. For an olecranon fracture with >2 mm displacement, obtain orthopedic consult for ORIF.
- Ulnar nerve injuries are sometimes seen.

DISTAL HUMERUS CONDYLAR FRACTURES

DIAGNOSIS

Distal humerus condylar fracture usually involves both the articular (trochlea, capitellum) and the nonarticular (epicondyle) surfaces. Lateral condylar fractures are much more common than medial, which are limited to children.

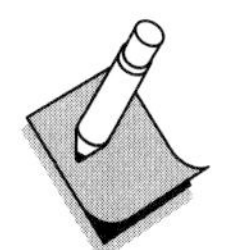

In all views, the axis of the proximal radius should pass through the center of the capitellum if it is not dislocated.

TREATMENT

- For nondisplaced condylar fractures, stabilize with a posterior arm splint.
- Condylar fractures with >3 mm displacement will need surgical fixation.

COMPLICATIONS

Nonunion, ulnar nerve palsy, avascular necrosis, compartment syndrome

ELBOW ARTICULAR SURFACE FRACTURES

DIAGNOSIS

Trochlea and capitellum fractures

TREATMENT

- For nondisplaced articular surface fractures, stabilize with a posterior arm splint.
- Articular surface fractures with even minimal displacement require orthopedic consult.

COMPLICATIONS

Associated with posterior elbow dislocation

DISTAL HUMERUS EPICONDYLAR FRACTURES

MEDIAL EPICONDYLAR FRACTURE

- Common in children and adolescents
- Occurs from repeated valgus stress (**little leaguer's elbow**), posterior elbow dislocation, or a direct trauma

TREATMENT

- Nondisplaced medial epicondylar fractures can be stabilized with a posterior splint with the elbow in 90° flexion and the forearm in pronation.
- Fractures with >3–5 mm displacement or intra-articular fractures require orthopedic consult.

COMPLICATIONS

60% of epicondylar fractures will have an associated ulnar nerve injury.

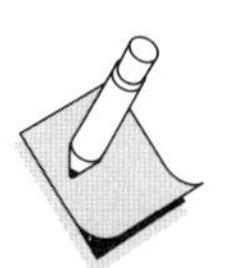

*Elbow fractures (particularly of the radial head) can be occult on radiograph so look for a **posterior** fat pad sign, which is always **pathologic**. A large anterior fat pad (**sail sign**) can also sometimes be pathologic.*

LATERAL EPICONDYLAR FRACTURE

- Very rare!

TREATMENT

Nondisplaced fractures can be stabilized with a posterior splint with the elbow in 90° flexion and the forearm in supination.

A six-year-old presents after falling off the jungle gym at school. The patient is diagnosed with a supracondylar fracture. The boy's arm is splinted with pulse, motor, and sensation intact. The patient is sent home and given instructions to follow up with orthopedics in 48–72 hours. When Mom presents to the orthopedist, she states that he has been crying almost nonstop since the accident. What complication might have occurred?

Always consider compartment syndrome with supracondylar fractures and any fracture involving the forearm. If untreated, forearm ischemia can lead to Volkmann's ischemic contracture.

DISTAL HUMERUS SUPRACONDYLAR FRACTURE

Accounts for 60% of elbow fractures in children

MECHANISM

The vast majority are due to FOOSH with hyperextension of elbow.

DIAGNOSIS

X-ray shows presence of posterior fat pad sign and anterior displacement of the anterior humeral line (see Figure 4.9).

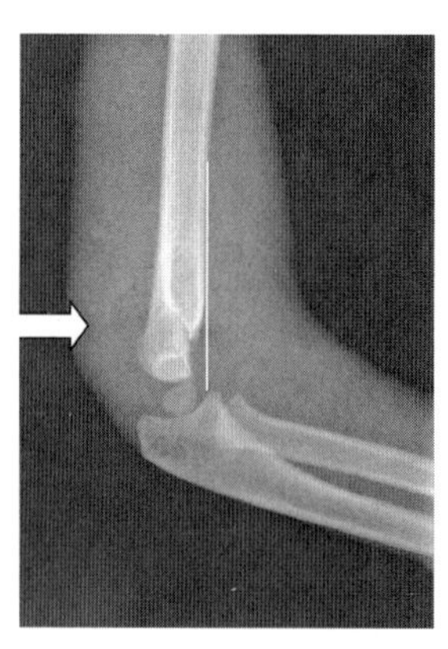

FIGURE 4.9. Supracondylar fracture of the humerus. Note displaced fat pads (arrow) signifying joint effusion. A line along the anterior cortex of the humerus should pass through the middle third of the capitellum on a true lateral view for a normal elbow.

TREATMENT

- Nondisplaced supracondylar fractures can be immobilized in posterior splint.
- Displaced fractures require urgent orthopedic reduction and pinning.

COMPLICATIONS

Complications include injuries to the brachial artery, median nerve (anterior interosseous nerve), compartment syndrome and **Volkmann's ischemic contracture**, and can also result in radial and ulnar nerve injury.

POSTERIOR ELBOW DISLOCATION

By far the most common elbow dislocation; typically results from FOOSH

DIAGNOSIS

- Posterior prominence of the olecranon with swelling and 45° of joint flexion
- Exam with posterior prominence of the olecranon with swelling and 45° of joint flexion
- X-ray shows a posteriorly displaced radius and ulna.

TREATMENT

Reduction

COMPLICATIONS

Elbow fractures in 30–60% of cases; brachial artery injury

ANTERIOR ELBOW DISLOCATION

DIAGNOSIS

Elbow is usually in full extension with forearm supinated.

TREATMENT

Reduction

COMPLICATIONS

- Avulsion of triceps is common.
- Very high incidence of vascular impairment especially brachial artery

Humerus Injuries

HUMERAL SHAFT FRACTURE

TREATMENT

- Nondisplaced humeral shaft fractures require stabilization with sugar-tong and sling and swathe.
- Displaced humeral shaft fractures or fractures with neurovascular compromise need orthopedic consult.

Radial nerve injury causes weakness of the extensors of the wrist and digits and numbness of the dorsoradial aspect of the hand.

COMPLICATIONS

Adhesive capsulitis of the shoulder, delayed union, radial nerve injuries, brachial artery injuries; less commonly ulnar and median nerve injuries

PROXIMAL HUMERUS FRACTURE

- Neer classification
  - Based on the number of displaced segments of the proximal humerus
  - Significant fragment displacement is >1 cm separation or greater than 45° of angulation between fragments.
  - 85% are classified as two-part nondisplaced (surgical neck).

TREATMENT

- Proximal humeral fractures with no significantly displaced segments are treated with immobilization and early range of motion.
- Fractures with any displaced segments need to be referred to orthopedics for operative management.

COMPLICATIONS

Brachial plexus injury, axillary nerve or artery injuries, posterior shoulder dislocation, adhesive capsulitis, avascular necrosis of the humeral head

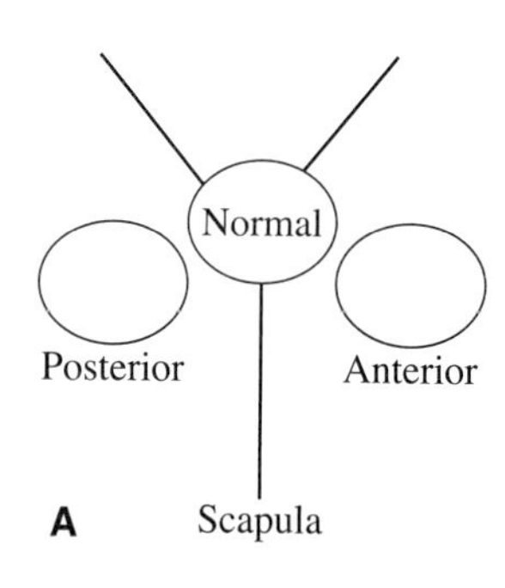

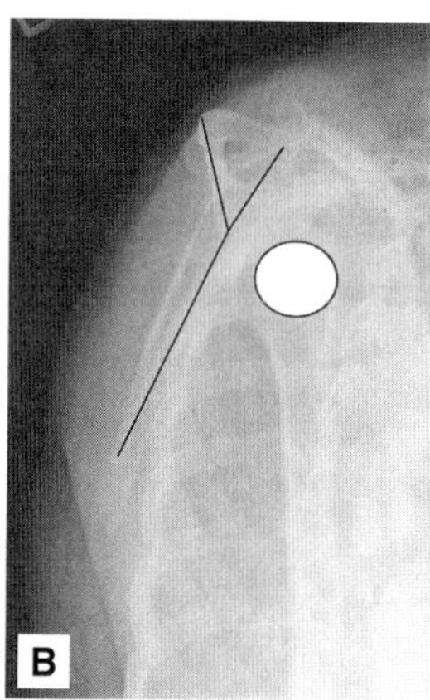

FIGURE 4.10. On the scapular Y-view shoulder radiograph for an anterior dislocation, the humeral head will often appear anterior to the glenoid [as pictured in (A) and for a posterior dislocation the humeral head will usually appear posterior (B)].

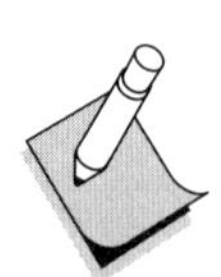

The Kocher and Hippocratic techniques for reducing anterior shoulder dislocations have unacceptably high complication rates.

> ***Bankart lesions—***
>
> **TUBS**
> **T**raumatic
> **U**nilateral
> **B**ankart
> **S**urgery

Shoulder Injuries

ANTERIOR SHOULDER DISLOCATION

DIAGNOSIS

There are four distinct types of anterior shoulder dislocation:

- **Subcoracoid (most common anterior shoulder dislocation > 90%)**
- Subglenoid
- Subclavicular
- Intrathoracic

DIAGNOSIS

- Clinical: Outer round contour of shoulder is flattened. Displaced humeral head is palpated inferiorly. Arm is **abducted and slightly externally rotated.**
- Two-view X-ray of the shoulder, including AP view and axillary or Y view (see Figure 4.10), shows dislocation.

TREATMENT

Reduction methods for anterior dislocations:

- Stimson or hanging weight
- Scapular manipulation
- Traction-countertraction
- External rotation (Hennepin technique)
- Milch (forward elevation)
- Kocher (external rotation, forward elevation, followed by internal rotation) and Hippocratic (foot in the axilla for counter-traction) techniques are **not recommended** because of unacceptable high complication rates.
- Recheck pulse, motor, sensation, and apply Velpeau dressing or shoulder immobilizer.
- Orthopedic follow-up

COMPLICATIONS

- Axillary nerve injuries. Loss of sensation at "badge" area of shoulder.
- **Bankart lesions**: A tear of the anteroinferior glenoid labrum (often diagnosed on MRI, but may have bony component). If present, high incidence of instability and may require surgery.
- **Hill-Sachs deformity:** A defect on the posterolateral aspect of the humeral head (impaction fracture; see Figure 4.11).

POSTERIOR SHOULDER DISLOCATION

Requires significant direct force to the anterior shoulder classically from a **seizure** or **high-speed injury**

DIAGNOSIS

- Clinical: Arm is usually **adducted** and slightly **internally rotated**. The coracoid process is prominent anteriorly.
- On AP X-ray the proximal humerus may look like a **lightbulb or drumstick** (due to internal rotation). The humeral head is displaced posteriorly in the Y or axillary view.

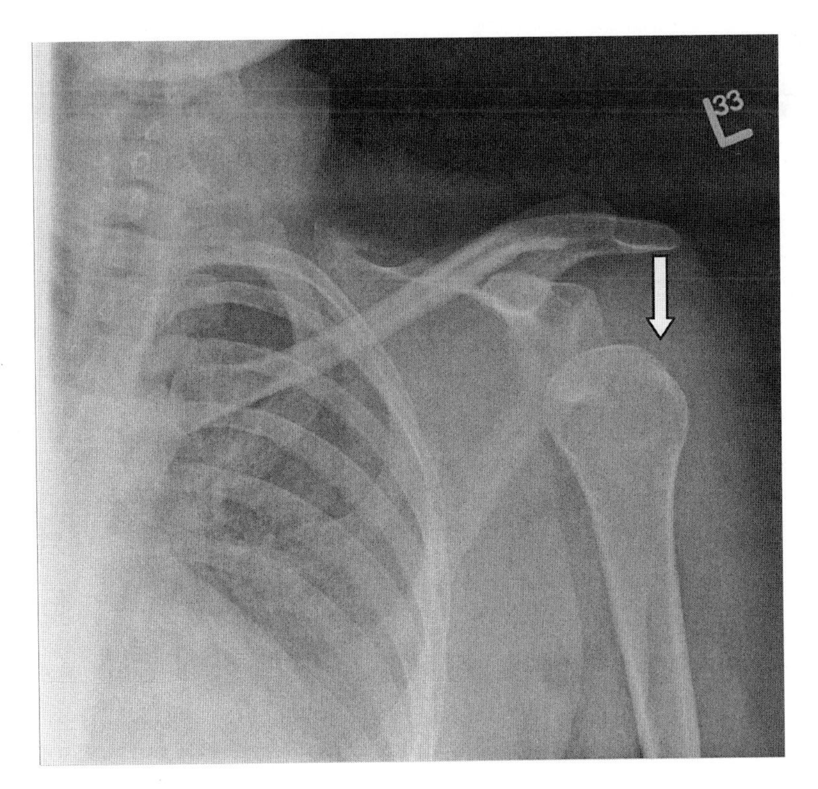

FIGURE 4.11. Anterior shoulder dislocation with a small Hill-Sachs deformity (arrow).

TREATMENT

Traction and reduction of humeral head **anteriorly**

COMPLICATIONS

Often associated with humerus fractures

INFERIOR SHOULDER DISLOCATION (LUXATIO ERECTA)

- The **rarest** of shoulder dislocations (<2%)
- Always indicative of serious injury
- Results from **hyperabduction** of the shoulder

DIAGNOSIS

Arm is held in a fixed position up over head (180° of elevation). X-ray is confirmative (see Figure 4.12).

TREATMENT

Reduction by traction-countertraction

COMPLICATIONS

- Almost always accompanied by disruption of the rotator cuff and tear through the inferior capsule
- High incidence of neurovascular compromise, including axillary nerve, brachial plexus, and axillary artery injuries
- Fractures of the proximal humerus

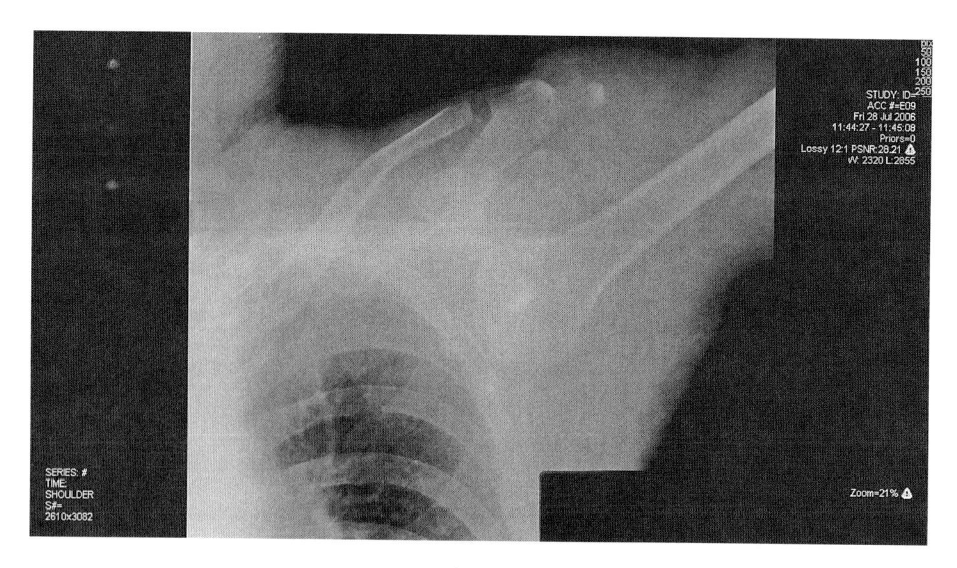

FIGURE 4.12. Inferior shoulder dislocation (luxatio erecta).

ROTATOR CUFF INJURIES

Continuum of injury: Mechanical impingement → rotator cuff tendonitis → rotator cuff tear.

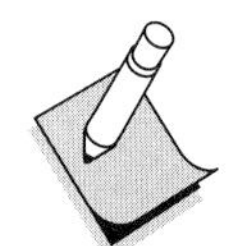

*Most common **elbow** dislocation = **posterior** dislocation.*

*Most common **shoulder** dislocation = **anterior** dislocation.*

MECHANISM

Impingement of subacromial space by humeral head due to repeated elevation of arms above shoulders

DIAGNOSIS

- Shoulder pain (initially only with activity) and eventual loss of motion
- All have pain between 60° to 120° of shoulder abduction (**painful arc**).
- **Rotator cuff tendonitis:** Preserved strength of rotator cuff **SITS** muscles (supraspinatus, infraspinatus, teres minor, subscapularis) especially after **lidocaine injection**
- **Rotator cuff tear:** Most are acute injuries to a tendon weakened from chronic impingement. Weakness of SITS muscles. Positive **drop arm test**, which is the inability to hold the arm in 90° abduction. MRI can be diagnostic.

> ***Most common types of dislocations–***
>
> **PEAS**
> **P**osterior for
> **E**lbow
> **A**nterior for
> **S**houlder

TREATMENT

Physical therapy, steroid injection, surgery if rotator cuff tear

ACROMIOCLAVICULAR (AC) SEPARATION

AC separation usually results from a fall with a direct blow downward on the outer shoulder (snowboarders, football players).

DIAGNOSIS

The diagnosis can usually be made clinically by reproducing the pain with palpation of the AC joint.

TREATMENT

Depends on the degree of separation (see Table 4.2)

TABLE 4.2. Types of Acromioclavicular Separation

Type of AC Separation	Description	Treatment
1	Sprain of the AC ligament Radiograph is normal.	Sling, 1–2 weeks
2	Disruption of AC ligament with coracoclavicular (CC) ligament sprain Distance between acromion and clavicle is increased by ≤ **half clavicle width**.	Sling and orthopedic referral; rehab
3	Both AC and CC are disrupted. Distance between acromion and clavicle is increased by **full width** of clavicle.	Sling and orthopedic referral; surgical fixation controversial
4	Clavicle displaced ***posteriorly***	For Types 4–6, sling and orthopedic referral with likely surgical fixation
5	Clavicle displaced far ***superiorly and anteriorly***	
6	Clavicle displaced ***inferiorly***	

Clavicular Fractures

Diagnosis

Classified by segment (distal third, middle third, or medial third)

Treatment/Complications

- **Distal third (group 2):** Immobilization with sling; may require surgery if associated with rupture of coracoclavicular ligament to avoid nonunion
- **Middle third (group 1 = 80% of clavicle fractures):** Reduction, immobilization with sling
- **Medial third (group 3):** Immobilization with sling; may be associated with intrathoracic injuries and can be life-threatening if there is injury to underlying vascular structures

Sternoclavicular Dislocations

- Very uncommon; usually result of MVC or sport injuries where the shoulder is forcefully rolled forward
- Anterior dislocations are far more common.

Diagnosis

- Patient typically has severe pain that is exacerbated by shoulder movement.
  - X-rays are usually not helpful. CT is the most helpful imaging study.
  - **First-degree dislocation:** Sprain, mild pain/swelling
  - **Second-degree dislocation:** Subluxation of clavicle with complete tear of sternoclavicular ligament and sprain of costoclavicular ligament
  - **Third-degree dislocation:** Complete rupture with clavicle dislocation

TREATMENT

- **First-degree dislocation:** Arm sling
- **Second-degree dislocation:** Figure-of-eight clavicular strap or sling
- **Third-degree dislocation:**
  - Anterior: Reduction attempt and sling
  - Posterior: Neurovascular assessment, with possible need for emergent orthopedic and thoracic surgery consults and rapid reduction

COMPLICATIONS

With third-degree posterior dislocations, there is a 25% chance of life-threatening injuries to esophagus, trachea, or great vessels.

SCAPULAR FRACTURES

Require a significant amount of blunt force and are **frequently associated with intrathoracic injuries**

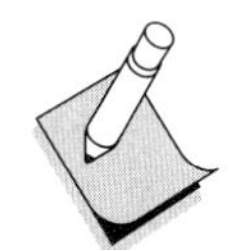

Scapula fractures** are often associated with **very serious intrathoracic injuries.

DIAGNOSIS

Shoulder **and CXRs**

TREATMENT

- Most are treated with sling and immobilization.
- ORIF is required for severely displaced or angulated fractures.

COMPLICATIONS

Rib fractures, pneumothorax, hemothorax, pulmonary contusion, clavicular fractures, shoulder dislocation with associated rotator cuff tears, neurovascular injuries, vertebral compression fractures

INJURIES TO THE LOWER EXTREMITIES

Knee and Lower Leg Injuries

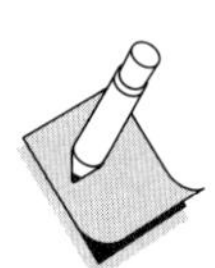

Always check for an intact extensor mechanism if a patient has a patella fracture.

PATELLA FRACTURE

Transverse fractures are most common and may result from blunt trauma or from the pull of the quadriceps muscle (quadriceps avulsion fracture).

DIFFERENTIAL

Bipartite patella is a normal variant and can be differentiated from a true fracture by its smooth cortical margins. If in doubt, x-ray the other knee as this condition is usually bilateral.

DIAGNOSIS

- Patellar tenderness and swelling: With a transverse fracture, the patient may be unable to extend the knee.
- X-rays of the knee: AP, lateral and sunrise views should be obtained.

TREATMENT

- Nondisplaced patella fractures require immobilization in full extension and advanced weight bearing as tolerated, with orthopedic referral.
- Patella fractures with >3 mm displacement or loss of extensor function mandate orthopedic referral for surgical intervention.

PATELLA DISLOCATION

The patella usually displaces laterally over the lateral femoral condyle, as a result of twisting of the knee with the leg held in a fixed position. This is common in adolescent females.

TREATMENT

ED reduction is accomplished by placing the knee in full extension, the hip in some flexion, and pushing on the patella in a medial direction up and over the lateral condyle. Procedural sedation aids reduction. Once reduced, immobilize in full extension.

Ottawa Knee Rules

Obtain radiographs if at least one of the following is true:

- *Age >55*
- *Fibular head tenderness*
- *Isolated tenderness of patella*
- *Inability to flex knee to 90°*
- *Inability to bear weight in the ED for four steps after injury*

> A 30-year-old female is complaining of knee pain after a motor vehicle collision. Exam shows a grossly deformed knee with lateral and rotational displacement. What else do you need to evaluate in this patient and how will you do so?
>
> The patient has a knee dislocation. It is important to check pulses, motor, and sensation, especially investigating for injury to the popliteal artery (7–42% dislocations) and peroneal nerve injury (25–35%). Perform arteriography or check ABI (ankle brachial index); < 0.8 is an indication for arteriogram. For evaluation of the peroneal nerve, check sensation of the dorsum of the foot, and strength of dorsiflexion.

KNEE DISLOCATION

Five types of knee dislocations (anterior and posterior are most common):

- Anterior dislocation
- Posterior dislocation
- Medial dislocation
- Lateral dislocation
- Rotational dislocation

TREATMENT

- **Immediate** reduction
- Evaluate for neurovascular injury: Check ABIs or obtain arteriogram; test peroneal and tibial nerves.
- Posterior splint with immobilization in 15° of flexion
- Obtain orthopedics +/– vascular surgery consultation.

COMPLICATIONS

- **Peroneal nerve injury** (foot drop)
- **Popliteal artery injury** especially with anterior and posterior dislocations
- Less commonly, tibial nerve injury, ligamentous and meniscal injury

Tibial Plateau Fracture

- **Most common fracture of the knee**
- Most involve the lateral plateau.

Mechanism

Impact that drives the femoral condyles into the tibial plateau, such as fall from height or impact with automobile bumper

Diagnosis

Maintain a high index of suspicion. X-rays (AP, lateral, and oblique views) often reveal the fracture, but sometimes only show an effusion. CT is sometimes needed to diagnose the fracture.

Treatment

- Nondisplaced fractures can be treated with knee-immobilizer and non-weight bearing.
- Displaced fractures require ORIF.

Complications

Popliteal and anterior tibial artery injuries can occur. Associated ligamentous injuries are present in one-third of cases. Early arthritis can occur if the fracture is intra-articular.

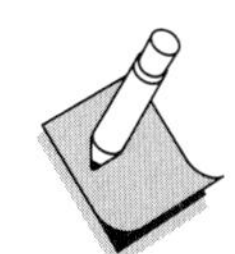

*Arthrocentesis may be performed to relieve some of the pressure associated with a large joint effusion. If **lipohemarthrosis** is present, this is indicative of an **intra-articular knee fracture**.*

Rupture of Extensor Mechanism of the Knee

Causes

- Quadriceps tendon rupture (>40 years old)
- Patellar tendon rupture (<40 years old)
- Patella fracture
- Avulsion of the tibial tuberosity

Mechanism

Forceful contraction of quadriceps muscle or fall on a flexed knee

Diagnosis

- Knee pain and swelling with inability to extend knee
- May have high-riding patella with patellar tendon rupture

Treatment

Orthopedics consult for surgical repair

Chondromalacia Patella (Patellofemoral Syndrome)

This is an overuse syndrome of the articular cartilage of the patella that stems from malalignment of the patellofemoral tracking complex. It is the **most common cause of knee pain** (frequently seen in female athletes) and is often bilateral.

Symptoms/Exam

- Anterior knee pain worsens after prolonged sitting, climbing stairs, or squatting. Sticking or buckling of the knee may occur. There is usually no history of trauma.

- Exam reveals genu valgum (knock-knee) and atrophied quadriceps muscles (particularly the vastus medialis obliquus).

DIAGNOSIS

- **Patella compression test:** Pain and crepitus occur with compression of the patella into the femoral groove when the knee is extended and quadriceps muscle tightened.
- **Apprehension test:** The quadriceps contracts involuntarily as the patella is pushed laterally in anticipation of pain.
- **Increased Q angle:** The angle between two lines drawn from (1) the anterior superior iliac spine to the center of the patella and (2) the center of the patella through the tibial tubercle. Q angle > 20° is abnormal.

TREATMENT

NSAIDs and quadriceps-strengthening exercises

PATELLAR TENDINITIS (JUMPER'S KNEE)

SYMPTOMS/EXAM

Anterior knee pain; night pain; pain with sitting, standing up, squatting, kneeling, climbing stairs

DIAGNOSIS

- **Tenderness to palpation over patellar tendon:** There is normal range of motion but can be painful at full extension and with resisted extension.
- X-rays are usually normal but may show hyperostosis at the upper and lower pole of the patella.

TREATMENT

Heat, NSAIDs, quadriceps-strengthening exercises

Ligamentous and Meniscal Injuries of the Knee

ANTERIOR CRUCIATE LIGAMENT (ACL) INJURY

The most common knee ligamentous injury, it results from **high-speed, traumatic twisting movements (especially if accompanied by a valgus stress)** and can occur from a noncontact injury.

SYMPTOMS/EXAM

- A "**pop**" is frequently heard at the time of injury.
- Hemarthrosis is common (75% of all knee hemarthroses are caused by ACL tears).

DIAGNOSIS

Positive **Lachman's test** (most sensitive) and **anterior drawer sign** are suggestive (see Table 4.3). MRI or arthroscopy is diagnostic.

TREATMENT

Rest, ice, elevate, NSAIDs, immobilization, orthopedics referral, physical therapy

TABLE 4.3. Physical Examination of the Knee

Test	Maneuver	Abnormality
Valgus stress	Instability with valgus stress in 30° flexion	Tear of the MCL
Varus stress	Instability with varus stress in 30° of flexion	Tear of the LCL
Anterior drawer sign	Instability with anterior stress with knee in 90° of flexion	Tear of the ACL
Lachman's test	Instability with anterior stress in 15–30° of flexion; more sensitive than drawer signs	Tear of the ACL
Posterior drawer sign	Instability with posterior stress in 90° of flexion	Tear of the PCL
McMurray's test	Pain as the knee is brought from full flexion to 90° flexion while the leg is externally rotated with compression over the medial joint line **and/or** when the leg is internally rotated with compression over the lateral joint line	Medial joint line pain = medial meniscus injury. Lateral joint pain = lateral meniscus injury.
Ege's test	In squatting position, pain, and/or click on maximum rotation of knee	External rotation = medial meniscus tear. Internal rotation = lateral meniscus tear.

COMPLICATIONS

If resulting from lateral blow to knee is often associated with **medial collateral ligament tear and lateral meniscus injury (terrible triad)**

POSTERIOR CRUCIATE LIGAMENT (PCL) INJURY

Far less common than ACL tears and usually occurs in combination with other injuries

DIAGNOSIS

Positive posterior drawer test is suggestive. MRI or arthroscopy is diagnostic.

TREATMENT

Rest, ice, elevate, NSAIDs, immobilization, orthopedics referral, physical therapy

MEDIAL COLLATERAL LIGAMENT (MCL) AND LATERAL COLLATERAL LIGAMENT (LCL) INJURIES

DIAGNOSIS

Positive varus (medial) stress test for LCL injury or valgus (lateral) stress test for MCL injury are suggestive. MRI or arthroscopy is diagnostic.

Treatment

Rest, ice, elevate, NSAIDs, immobilization, orthopedics referral, physical therapy

Medial and Lateral Meniscus Injuries

Medial meniscus is injured twice as often. Injury usually results from quickly changing directions, squatting, or twisting knee.

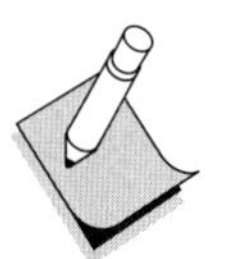

The Lachman's test is better than the anterior drawer test for detecting ACL injuries. Diagnoses for meniscal and ligamentous injuries are improved when tests are used in combination.

Symptoms/Exam

Pain and swelling (acute injury), clicking, or locking of the knee

Diagnosis

Positive **McMurray's** and Ege's tests are suggestive. MRI or arthroscopy is diagnostic.

Treatment

Rest, ice, elevate, NSAIDs, orthopedics referral

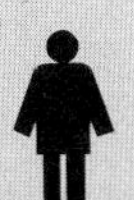

Match the Mechanism to the Injury:

1. While downhill skiing, a skier catches the edge of one ski, causing his skis to go in different directions. A twisting fall ensues, causing a tearing sensation in the knee.
2. While running downfield during a soccer match, a defender plants her foot to decelerate and change directions, causing a pop in her knee. A large effusion is seen shortly afterward.
3. While bending down to pick up a heavy box with his right knee externally rotated, a man feels a pop in his knee. He has had problems with his knee locking since the incident.
4. The patient's knee hit the dashboard in an MVC. No fracture is found, but patient is complaining of knee pain.

   a. PCL injury
   b. ACL injury
   c. LCL injury
   d. MCL injury
   e. Lateral meniscus injury
   f. Medial meniscus injury

Answers:

1. d
2. b
3. f
4. a

Ankle Injuries

Lateral Ligamentous Ankle Injury

- Ankle inversions with lateral ankle sprains are far more common than medial injuries (>90%).
- The anterior talofibular ligament is the most commonly injured ligament, followed by the calcaneofibular ligament and the posterior talofibular ligament.

Mechanism

Inversion with internal rotation of a plantar-flexed foot

Diagnosis

- Abnormal **anterior drawer test** (ankle plantar flexed 10° from neutral, knee slightly flexed, one hand on base of tibia, other hand cups the heel, instability when pulling anteriorly) with anterior talofibular ligament rupture
- Abnormal **talar tilt test** (>5° rotation with inversion) with presence of both anterior talofibular **and** calcaneofibular ligament ruptures

Medial Ligamentous Ankle Injury

Far less common because the **medial deltoid** ligament is much stronger

Mechanism

Eversion and external rotation of foot

Diagnosis

Significant tenderness and swelling at the level of and distal to the medial malleolus.

Complication

Sometimes associated with a proximal fibula fracture, ie, Maisonneuve fracture

Distal Tibiofibular Syndesmotic Ligament Injuries

Mechanism

Dorsiflexion and eversion of foot with an axial load

Diagnosis

Positive **squeeze test** in which the examiner firmly grasps the patient's lower leg and "squeezes" the distal tibia and fibula together, causing pain if the injury is present

Ankle Sprains

First-Degree Ankle Sprain

Diagnosis

- Able to bear weight
- No joint instability

- Full range of motion
- Normal function
- Minimal swelling
- Only mild localized tenderness

Treatment

Rest, ice, compression, elevation, elastic bandage, follow-up in 1 week if not improved

Second-Degree Ankle Sprain

Diagnosis

- Pain with exam
- Abnormal function
- Moderate swelling

Treatment

Rest, ice, compression, elevation, elastic bandage, follow-up in 1 week if not improved

Third-Degree Ankle Sprain

Diagnosis

- Inability to bear weight
- Joint instability
- Severe pain
- Egg-shaped swelling
- Marked functional impairment
- Abnormal stress test

Treatment

If ankle is unstable, consider posterior mold and urgent orthopedic referral. If ankle is stable but patient is unable to bear weight, rest, ice, compression, elevation, crutches, apply ankle brace, and follow up in 1 week with orthopedics.

Achilles Tendon Rupture

Commonly seen in deconditioned athletes, eg, "weekend warriors," patients with rheumatoid arthritis, lupus, and recent **fluoroquinolone use**

Mechanism

Forceful plantar flexion against resistance

Symptoms/Exam

Often hear a "pop" during the acute injury; tenderness and a possibly a defect 2–6 cm above the insertion site to the calcaneus

Diagnosis

Abnormal **Thompson's test** (position the patient prone with both feet extending past the edge of the table, squeeze the calf and if tendon is intact, the foot should be plantar flexed).

Treatment

Apply posterior splint in plantar flexion and orthopedic consult. Early surgical repair leads to a better outcome.

Complications

Twenty-five percent are initially misdiagnosed as ankle sprains

Peroneal Tendon Subluxation/Dislocation

Most often associated with **skiing injuries**

Mechanism

Forced dorsiflexion with peroneal muscle contraction

Diagnosis

There is swelling posteriorly over lateral malleolus **in absence of** tenderness over anterior talofibular ligament; **often mistaken for ankle sprains!**

On exam with foot dorsiflexed and everted, there is anterior tendon subluxation. Fifty percent have a small avulsion fracture of lateral ridge of distal fibula.

Treatment

Splint in midplantar flexion, orthopedic referral for possible surgical repair

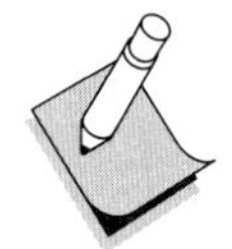

Ottawa ankle and midfoot Rules

Get ankle films if there is malleolar pain and any of the following:

1. *Tenderness on the posterior edge, tip, or distal 6 cm of lateral or medial malleolus*
2. *Inability to complete four steps (or two steps on bad ankle), now and at the scene of the injury*

Get foot films as well if midfoot pain and any of the following:

1. *Navicular tenderness*
2. *Base of fifth metatarsal tenderness*
3. *Inability to complete four steps*

Maisonneuve Fracture

Ankle-eversion injury with forces causing disruption of the tibiofibular syndesmosis

Diagnosis

Rupture of the deltoid ligament or avulsion fracture of medial malleolus, along with fracture of the proximal fibula

Treatment

Often requires ORIF to stabilize the tibiofibular syndesmosis

Foot Injuries

Calcaneus Fracture

Most commonly fractured tarsal bone

Mechanism

Usually severe axial load caused by a fall from a significant height

Diagnosis

Bohler's angle < 20° (angle between a line formed from the posterior tuberosity of the calcaneus and the apex of the posterior facet and a line between the

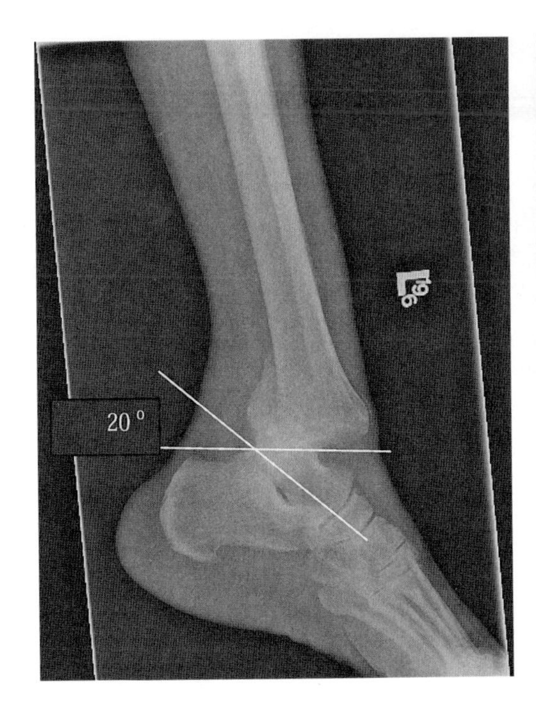

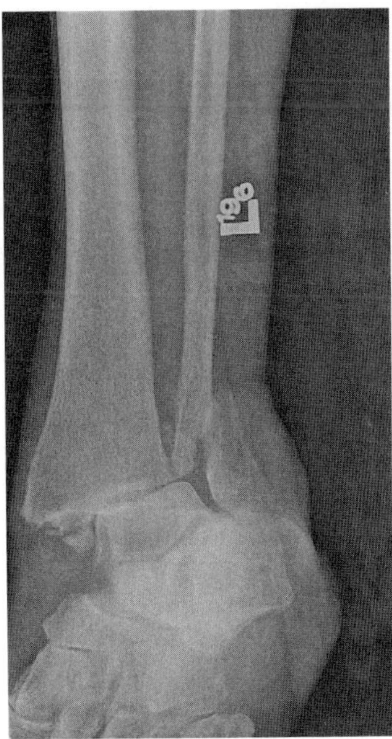

FIGURE 4.13. Trimalleolar fracture/dislocation. Although the calcaneus is posteriorly displaced, there is no calcaneal fracture as signified with Bohler's angle of 20°.

apex of the posterior facet and anterior process of the calcaneus). A Bohler's angle of 20°–40° is normal. CT scan may be needed to determine if injury is extensive enough to require surgery.

Treatment

Posterior splint, non-weight-bearing; orthopedic consult

Complications

- Comminuted fractures have high rates of **compartment syndrome.**
- Associated **lumbar vertebrae compression fractures** (10–15%)
- Chronic pain and disability

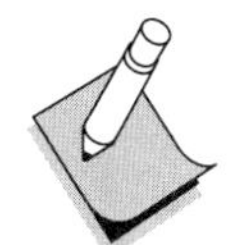

Lover's triad:*

Calcaneal fractures

Lumbar compression fractures

Forearm fractures

**Lover jumps out window to flee from husband*

Talus Fracture

The talar neck is the most common location.

Treatment

- Minor avulsion fractures can be treated with a posterior splint and crutches.
- Major fractures of the neck and body require orthopedic consultation as these fractures often require ORIF.

Complications

High rates of **avascular necrosis** and chronic arthritis

Lisfranc (Tarsometatarsal) Fracture

Lisfranc joint is a six-bone tarsometatarsal complex made up of the proximal most medial (1–3) metatarsals and their adjoining tarsal bones.

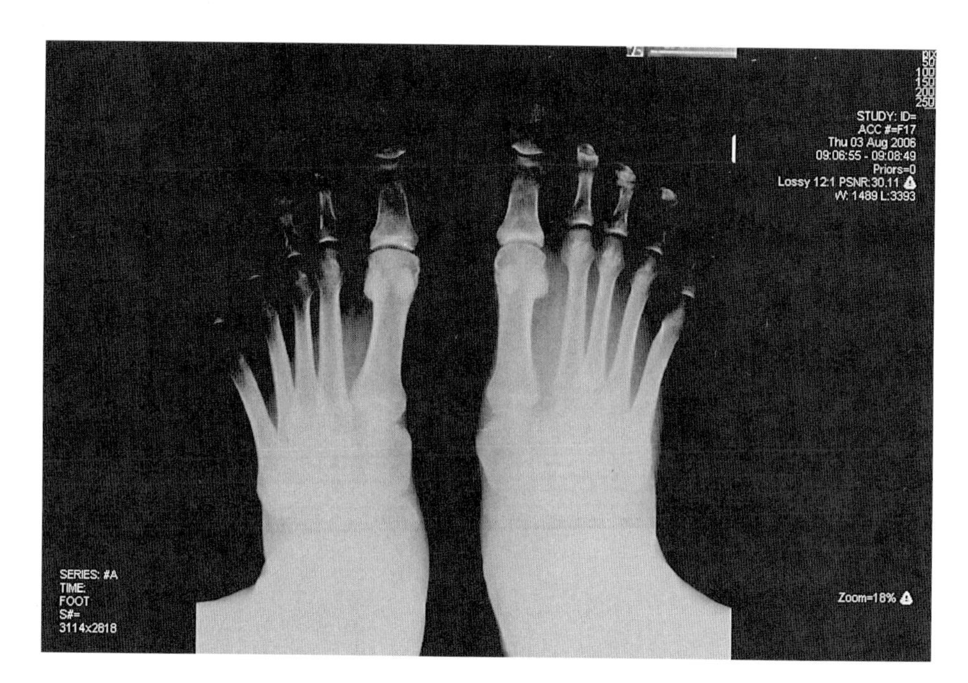

FIGURE 4.14. Lisfranc fracture. The space between the base of the first and second metatarsal is widened, which indicates disruption of the tarsometatarsal joint.

*Midpart (navicular, cuboid, cuneiforms). Separated from hindpart by **Chopart's** joint. Separated from forepart by **Lisfranc's** joint.*

MECHANISM

Can be quite varied (axial load, crush injury, or rotational stress); may occur with relatively minor trauma

DIAGNOSIS

- **Plantar ecchymosis sign** is a bruise over the plantar aspect of the midfoot.
- Gap > 1 mm between the bases of the first and second metatarsal (see Figure 4.14).
- **Fleck sign** is an avulsion fracture of the base of the second metatarsal on the medial side. It is pathognomonic of a Lisfranc fracture.

TREATMENT

Emergent orthopedic referral

COMPLICATIONS

Frequently associated with dorsal pedis artery injury, early arthritis, and chronic pain

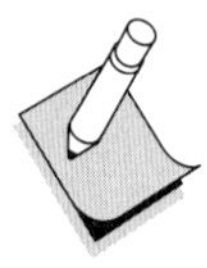

A fracture of the base of the second metatarsal on the medial side is pathognomonic of a Lisfranc fracture.

JONES FRACTURE

DIAGNOSIS

Jones fracture is a transverse fracture through the **metaphyseal-diaphyseal junction** of the fifth metatarsal. The fracture line will be at least 1.5 cm distal to the base of the fifth metatarsal (see Figure 4.15).

TREATMENT

Cast/splint, non-weight-bearing, and orthopedic referral for ORIF evaluation

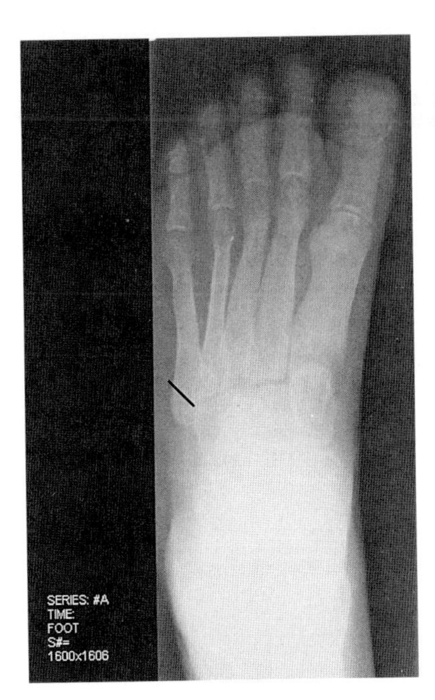

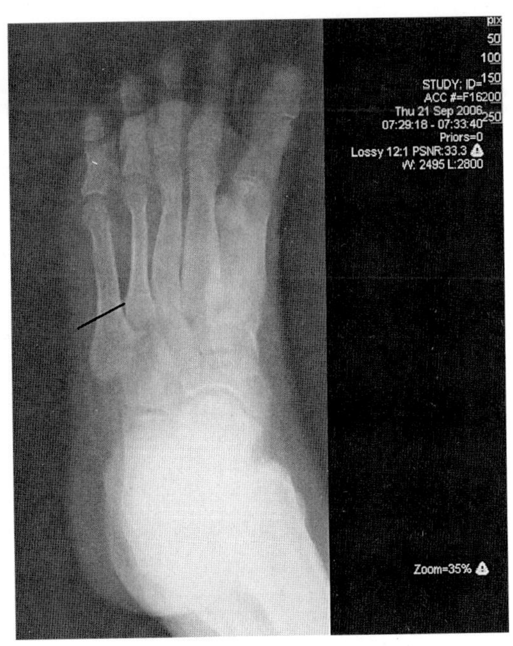

FIGURE 4.15. **Jones and pseudo-Jones fracture. The lines indicate the general appearance of the location of fracture sites, with a pseudo-Jones as a very proximal avulsion-type fracture (left) and a Jones as a proximal shaft fracture (right).**

COMPLICATIONS

Frequent nonunion or malunion

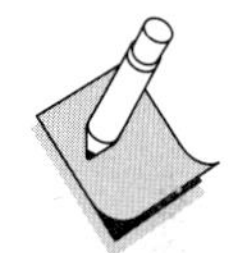

The Jones fracture is frequently complicated by nonunion or malunion.

Pseudo-Jones Fracture

More common than the Jones fracture

DIAGNOSIS

Avulsion fracture of the base of the fifth metatarsal (see Figure 4.15)

TREATMENT

Ankle stirrup splint, hard post-op shoe, or rocker walker

See Table 4.4 for indications for emergent and urgent (<72 hours) orthopedic referral in ankle and foot injuries.

OSTEOMYELITIS

Osteomyelitis is an inflammatory condition of the bone usually caused by infection.

- Hematogenous spread from bacteremia; occurs mainly in children
  - Neonate: *Staphylococcus aureus*, *Enterobacter* species, group A and B *Streptococcus*
  - Children (4 months to adult): *S. aureus*, group A *Streptococcus*, *Haemo-philus influenzae*, and *Enterobacter* species
  - Adult: *S. aureus*

TABLE 4.4. Indications for Emergent Ankle or Foot Orthopedic Intervention and Injuries for Orthopedic Referral

ORTHOPEDIC EMERGENCIES	ORTHOPEDIST REFERRAL (<72 HOURS)
Major talar neck and body fractures	Extra-articular calcaneal fractures
Intra-articular calcaneus fractures	First metatarsal fracture
All open fractures	Displaced metatarsal shaft
All fracture dislocations	Unstable ligamentous injuries
Maisonneuve fractures with neurovascular compromise	Stable unimalleolar fracture
Bimalleolar and trimalleolar fractures with neurovascular compromise	Peroneal dislocations
Lisfranc injuries	Maisonneuve, bimalleolar, and trimalleolar fractures with good reduction, no neurovascular compromise, and ensured orthopedic follow-up
Compartment syndromes	Jones fracture

- Direct or contiguous spread from nearby soft tissue infection
  - *S. **aureus***, *Enterobacter* species, and *Pseudomonas*
  - Puncture through sole of shoe: *S. aureus* is most common; ***Pseudomonas*** is the most characteristic
  - Sickle cell disease: *S. aureus* is most common; ***Salmonella*** is the most characteristic
- Often trauma related
- Vertebral osteomyelitis is more common in patients >45 years old.

SYMPTOMS/EXAM

- Can be relatively nonspecific
- Fever
- Fatigue
- Local swelling, erythema, and tenderness

DIAGNOSIS

- Clinical suspicion; two of four criteria required:
  - Purulent material on aspiration of affected bone
  - Positive culture of bone tissue or blood
  - Localized bony tenderness with overlying soft-tissue erythema or edema
  - Positive radiological imaging study
- X-ray may reveal periosteal elevation or soft-tissue edema. Later, bony lucencies may be apparent. Most often, no X-ray abnormalities early in the course of disease.

- CT, MRI, and radionuclide bone scan are more sensitive than X-ray for early detection.

TREATMENT

- Early antibiotics
  - Penicillinase-resistant synthetic penicillin (PRSP) and third-generation cephalosporin
  - If MRSA is suspected, use vancomycin or clindamycin instead of PRSP.
  - If sickle cell–related, start a fluoroquinolone to cover *Salmonella*. Do not use fluoroquinolones in children—use third generation cephalosporin.
  - If puncture through the sole of a shoe, cover *Pseudomonas* with ceftazidime or ciprofloxacin.
- Antibiotic bead implants
- Hyperbaric oxygen
- Surgical debridement of wound or removal of bone may be necessary

COMPLICATIONS

Sepsis, bone abscess, pathological fracture, nonhealing wound

DISORDERS OF THE SPINE

Low Back Pain

The causes of low back pain are varied and often impossible to pinpoint in the emergency department. It is more important to determine if an emergency exists that requires neurosurgical intervention or a condition, eg, osteomyelitis that requires specific treatment. Patients at high risk for a serious cause of back pain include injection drug users, the elderly, immunocompromised, and those with a history of cancer or recent trauma.

SYMPTOMS

Symptoms that indicate a potential neurosurgical emergency include:

- Fever
- Severe pain, which may be radicular
- Neurological impairment
- Bladder or bowel retention or incontinence

EXAM

- Fever
- Findings that indicate a neurosurgical emergency, including:
- Motor weakness
- Loss of perianal/perineal sensation
- Loss of deep tendon reflexes
- **Straight leg raise test (SLR):** A positive SLR is back pain that radiates ***past*** the knee at an elevation < 60°. **A positive contralateral SLR is *highly specific* for sciatica.**
- Decreased rectal tone

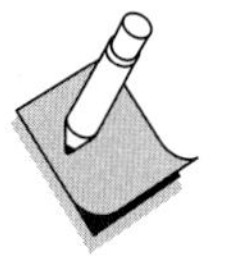

A straight leg raise test is positive when it elicits back pain that radiates past the knee at an elevation < 60°. ***A positive contralateral straight leg raise is* highly *specific for sciatica.***

DIFFERENTIAL

- Back strain
- Herniated disc
- Osteomyelitis

- Epidural abscess
- Aortic aneurysm
- Kidney stone/infection
- Cancer
- Fracture
- Spinal stenosis

DIAGNOSIS

- History and exam are critical!
- Lumbosacral X-rays are generally overused but should be considered if
  - Patient's age >55
  - Trauma with vertebral tenderness
  - Pain lasting longer than 1 month
  - History of IDU
  - Suspicion for cancer or infection such as fever or weight loss
- CT scan and MRI are more sensitive for infection and cancer.
- MRI better for herniated discs and neurological impairment

TREATMENT

- Treat underlying cause.
- If musculoskeletal in origin:
  - Ice in first 24–72 hours; afterward, heat may be helpful.
  - Pain medication
  - Muscle relaxants
  - Activity as tolerated: **Neither complete bedrest nor active physical therapy that causes pain is helpful.**
- Neurosurgical or spine specialist consultation if any neurological impairment

COMPLICATIONS

Chronic pain, neurological impairment, disability, opiate addiction

Cauda Equina Syndrome

Usually stems from a herniated disc that protrudes midline and compresses the nerve roots of the cauda equine; can also be caused by tumor and infection

SYMPTOMS

- Back pain
- Leg weakness
- Numbness
- **Bladder and/or bowel retention** (**followed by incontinence**)

EXAM

- Loss of sensation in the "saddle distribution"
- Loss of rectal tone
- Loss of bulbocavernosus reflex
- Loss of deep tendon reflexes
- Distended bladder

DIAGNOSIS

- Clinical suspicion
- MRI or CT myelogram

Treatment

- Emergent spine consultation

Complications

- Permanent loss of bladder/bowel function
- Leg weakness

JOINT ABNORMALITIES

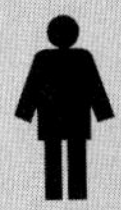

A 26-year-old male comes into the ED with a fever; a swollen, painful right knee and left elbow; and a vesiculopustular lesions on his fingers. He had been treated for an STD two weeks earlier. What is his diagnosis? Gonococcal arthritis.

Arthritis

Arthritis is joint damage as a result of degeneration (eg, osteoarthritis), inflammation (eg, rheumatoid arthritis, gout), or infection. It is characteristically divided into mono-articular, symmetric oligo-/polyarticular, and asymmetric oligo-/polyarticular causes (see Tables 4.5, 4.6, and 4.7).

A monoarticular arthritis should be presumed to be septic until proven otherwise.

Symptoms/Exam

- Swollen, tender joint(s)
- Associated symptoms: Depending on etiology, look for urethritis, eye pain/discharge, rash

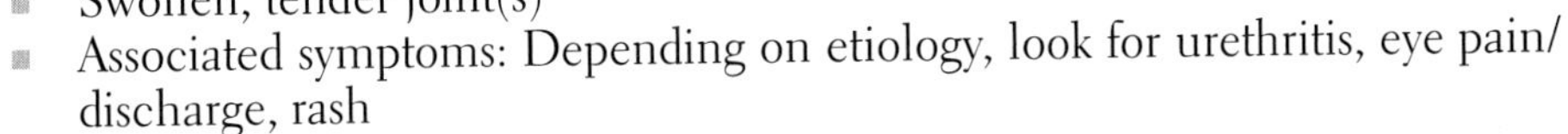

TABLE 4.5. Causes of Monoarticular Arthritis

Condition	Joints Involved	Unique Features	Treatment
Septic	Knee; unique sites in IVDU patients include sacroiliac, sternoclavicular, and intervertebral joints	*S. aureus* is most common organism.	Antibiotics starting with vancomycin
Gout	First MTP, knee	Needle-shaped; negatively birefringent crystals; yellow when parallel and blue when perpendicular to polarizing light	NSAIDs, steroid injection, colchicine. **Do not use allopurinol for acute attacks.**
Pseudogout (chondrocalcinosis)	Knee, first MTP, wrist	Rhomboid-shaped; positively birefringent crystals; blue when parallel and yellow when perpendicular to polarizing light	NSAIDs, steroid injection
Osteoarthritis	Hip, knee	Older age group, weight-bearing joints	Rest, NSAIDs, joint replacement surgery
Trauma	Knee	Hemarthrosis associated with intra-articular fractures and ligamentous injury	Compression dressing and aspiration if necessary for symptomatic relief

TABLE 4.6. Causes of Symmetric Polyarthritis

CONDITION	JOINTS INVOLVED	UNIQUE FEATURES	TREATMENT
Rheumatoid	Hand (MCP and PIP joints), wrist	Women in their 20s and 30s; associated with HLA-DR4 haplotype; early morning stiffness; sparing of DIP joints; multisystem involvement common	NSAIDs, immunosuppressants, antimalarials, gold, methotrexate
Systemic lupus	All. Usually PIP and MCP joints of the hand	Women 15–40 years old; can be migratory; associated with rash: malar, discoid, or photosensitivity	NSAIDs, immunosuppressants
Rheumatic fever	Large joints (knees, ankles, elbows, wrists)	Migratory	NSAIDs, immunosuppressants
Viral	All joints		

Reiter syndrome: Can't see (conjunctivitis), can't pee (urethritis), can't bend my knee (arthritis)

- Fever, most commonly with septic arthritis
- Characterized by number of joints (mono, poly, oligo), symmetry, migratory

DIFFERENTIAL

- Bursitis
- Tendonitis
- Fracture
- Cellulitis

TABLE 4.7. Causes of Asymmetrical Polyarthritis

CONDITION	JOINTS INVOLVED	UNIQUE FEATURES	TREATMENT
Reiter syndrome (reactive arthritis)	Weight-bearing joints (sacroiliac, hip, knee)	Males 15–30 years old; **triad: conjunctivitis, urethritis, arthritis;** 80–90% are HLA-B27 positive; often preceded 2–6 wks by viral illness, diarrhea, or infection with *Chlamydia* or *Ureaplasma*	NSAIDs; **antibiotics not helpful**
Gonococcal	Wrist, hand, ankle	Young sexually active adults; often associated with a vesiculopustular lesions on the fingers; can be migratory; **synovial fluid cultures often negative**	Penicillin
Henoch-Schönlein purpura	Ankle, knee	Children 4–12 years old; **triad: migratory arthritis, palpable purpuric rash on lower extremities, abdominal pain**	NSAIDs
Lyme	Knee	Migratory; occurs **months** after the initial infection	Antibiotics (doxycycline, amoxicillin, Penicillin G, ceftriaxone)

TABLE 4.8. Features of Synovial Fluid

TYPE	WBC/μL	CLARITY	COLOR
Noninflammatory	< 2000	Transparent	Clear
Inflammatory	2000–75,000	Cloudy	Yellow
Infectious	> 80,000	Cloudy	Yellow

DIAGNOSIS

- **Joint aspiration is the key!**
- Send joint fluid for cell count, crystals, Gram stain, and culture.
- Considerable overlap of WBC count exists between inflammatory and infectious etiologies of arthritis. In particular, gout and pseudogout can have WBC counts > 70,000 (see Table 4.8).
- Peripheral WBC, ESR, and CRP are neither sensitive nor specific but should be obtained, as they can help with monitoring effectiveness of treatment.
- X-ray may be helpful to diagnose trauma, tumor, avascular necrosis, or osteomyelitis.

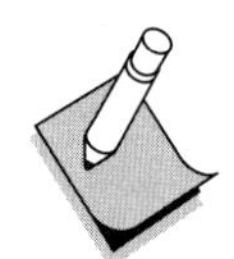

Do not use allopurinol for acute gout attacks.

Sacroiliitis

Sacroiliitis is an inflammation of one or both of the sacroiliac joints.

Causes include

- Spondylarthropathies, eg, ankylosing spondylarthritis
- Trauma or overuse
- Infection, eg, injection drug use
- Pregnancy
- Degenerative arthritis

SYMPTOMS

- Generally vague
- Low-grade fever
- Pain in lower back, thighs, or buttocks, especially in the morning or after prolonged rest
- Limp
- Decreased range of motion

EXAM

- Tender sacroiliac joint
- Lumbar X-ray: If patient has ankylosing spondylitis, will see **bamboo spine**—the squaring off of the vertebral bodies.
- Positive **stork test**: The examiner stands behind the patient with his thumbs over the most posterior portion of the patient's superior iliac spine. The patient then flexes their hip and knee on one side to a minimum of 90° (like a stork) while standing straight with the other leg. A normal test is when the thumb on the side of the bent knee moves caudad in relation to the thumb with the straight leg. Cranial movement of the thumb suggests sacroiliac dysfunction. Test both sides.

Differential

Septic hip, psoas abscess, sciatic, herniated disc, pyelonephritis, ankylosing spondylitis

Diagnosis

- X-rays show symmetric erosion and sclerosis of the SI joint.
- MRI of SI joint
- Aspiration and blood cultures if infection suspected

Treatment

Depends on underlying cause (eg, anti-inflammatory agents for inflammatory causes, antibiotics if infection suspected)

Complications

May be a part of a larger inflammatory arthritis, ie, ankylosing spondylitis, which is a seronegative spondyloarthropathy typically found in young males with prolonged (>3 months) back pain

RHABDOMYOLYSIS

Breakdown of muscle that leads to a cascade of events, including: hypovolemia (fluid build-up in injured myocytes); hyperkalemia (from release of the intracellular stores in the injured myocytes); and renal failure (from clogging of glomeruli with myoglobin and toxic effects of myocyte breakdown products); accounts for about 10% of all cases of acute renal failure

Symptoms/Exam

- Symptoms are often very subtle; must maintain a high index of suspicion.
- Only half of patients complain of muscle pain.
- Only a small fraction of patients complain of dark urine.
- Tender or focal muscle swelling is rare. If present, must consider compartment syndrome!

Etiology

- Trauma (most common)
- Ischemia
- Polymyositis
- Toxins/drugs
- Excessive muscle activity
- Seizures
- Burns
- Sepsis
- Viral illness

Diagnosis

- CK > 5–10x above normal. However, if CK levels > 2–3x normal, repeat CK level—it peaks about 24 hours from initial insult.
- Urine dipstick test is **positive for blood (globin) but there are no RBCs** in the urine microscopic exam.
- LDH and AST are elevated.
- Check serum for elevated potassium, phosphate, creatinine. Serum calcium may be low.

- Monitor platelets, PT/PTT for early DIC.
- Measure compartment pressures if compartment syndrome is suspected.

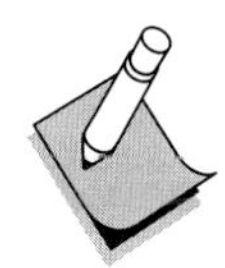

Suspect rhabdomyolysis when the urine dipstick test is positive for blood but there are no RBCs in the urine microscopic exam.

TREATMENT

- **Aggressive IV hydration:** Administer isotonic fluid at a rate of 500 cc/hour to produce a urine output of 2 cc/kg/hour.
- **Urinary alkalinization** to a pH of 6.5 or above with D5W with 2–3 amps of $NaHCO_3$ to help solubilize the myoglobin and promote excretion; **be careful of worsening hypocalcemia**
- Diuretics (eg, mannitol) if patient is oliguric
- Treat associated hyperkalemia if present.
- Admit to telemetry unit for continued treatment and monitoring of fluids, electrolytes, and renal function.

COMPLICATIONS

- Renal failure
- Electrolyte abnormalities: Hyperkalemia, hypocalcemia
- Fluid overload
- DIC
- Compartment syndrome

OVERUSE SYNDROMES

Bursitis

Bursitis refers to any inflammation over any one of the body's >100 bursae. It is usually caused by overuse or local trauma and can be complicated by the presence of infection. *Staphylococcus* and *Streptococcus* species account for the vast majority of associated infections.

SYMPTOMS/EXAM

- Swelling, tenderness over superficially located bursa, usually located near a large joint (elbow, knee, shoulder, hip)
- Common areas: **Prepatellar** (housemaid's knee, pauper's knee), **olecranon** (student's elbow), **subacromial, trochanteric**
- Redness, warmth, and fever may signify an infection or associated cellulitis.

DIFFERENTIAL

Cellulitis, tendonitis, abscess, arthritis

DIAGNOSIS

- Characteristic history and exam
- Aspiration of the bursa may be necessary to establish diagnosis or presence of infection.

TREATMENT

- Ice, rest, elevation, compression
- Steroid injection may be helpful but presence of infection must first be eliminated.
- Complete drainage via aspiration and oral antibiotics covering staphylococcal and streptococcal species are usually adequate to treat an infected bursitis.

Carpal Tunnel Syndrome

A compressive neuropathy of the median nerve at the level of the carpal tunnel in the volar aspect of the wrist

- Most common peripheral compressive neuropathy
- Lifetime risk of acquiring carpal tunnel syndrome is 10%.
- More common in females than males
- Often found in patients with repetitive strain of the hands and wrists, eg, typists, musicians, etc.
- Patients often have associated trauma, obesity, TB, renal failure, hypothyroidism, or diabetes.

Symptoms

- Gradual onset and progression
- Usually bilateral but may begin first in dominant hand
- Early, paresthesias in median nerve distribution (palmar aspect of first three digits and radial half of the fourth digit)
- Late, persistent pain present, atrophy of thenar muscles

Exam

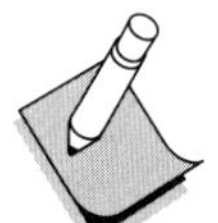

Positive Durkin's compression test, Phalen's sign, Tinel's sign, and Flick sign are all indicative of carpal tunnel syndrome.

- **Durkin's compression test**: Reproduction of symptoms with compression of carpal tunnel for 30 seconds
- **Phalen's sign**: Reproduction of symptoms with hyperflexion of wrist at 90° for 1 minute
- **Tinel's sign**: Pins-and-needles sensation in the median nerve distribution with tapping on the carpal tunnel
- **Flick sign**: Shaking or "flicking" the hands provides relief of symptoms during episodes
- Weakness of resisted thumb abduction
- Thenar atrophy may be present late in disease.
- Decreased sensation in median nerve distribution

Differential

Brachial plexus compressive neuropathy, peripheral neuropathy of other causes

Diagnosis

- Usually a clinical diagnosis
- Electromyography (EMG) and nerve conduction studies establish severity of disease.

Treatment

- NSAIDs
- Volar splint in neutral position
- Local steroid injection
- Surgery for release of the transverse carpal ligament

Complications

Chronic pain, weakness, paresthesias, and disability

Plantar Fasciitis

Plantar fasciitis is a common cause of plantar heel pain that occurs where the plantar fascia arises from the medial calcaneal tuberosity. Inflammation in both the bone and plantar fascia occurs from chronic degeneration in the fascia fibers that arise from the bone.

SYMPTOMS/EXAM

- Pain worse upon awakening or after prolonged rest
- Pain localized to the heel or arch of the foot and, occasionally, over the Achilles tendon
- Flat feet
- Point tenderness over the plantar medial calcaneal tuberosity (anterior medial aspect of the calcaneus)

DIFFERENTIAL

Calcaneal stress fracture/tumor, fat pad atrophy, sciatica, tarsal tunnel syndrome, rupture of the plantar fascia

DIAGNOSIS

- Clinical diagnosis (characteristic pain after rest and localized heel tenderness)
- X-ray may reveal calcaneal spur.

TREATMENT

- Heel pads
- Arch supports
- Night splints to stretch plantar fascia and hold the Achilles tendon to length
- Achilles and plantar stretching exercises
- Corticosteroid injection and surgery rarely needed

SOFT-TISSUE INFECTIONS

Felon

Felon is infection of the fingertip pulp. The fingertip is separated into small closed spaces by vertical septae. Infection can easily spread along these compartments and cause an abscess. *S. aureus* is the most common agent.

SYMPTOMS/EXAM

- Swollen, tender fingertip, usually thumb or index finger
- Fever
- Previous finger trauma or splinter

DIAGNOSIS

- Clinical diagnosis
- X-ray if foreign body, fracture, or osteomyelitis suspected

TREATMENT

- If early, warm soaks and antibiotics may be sufficient.
- Incision and drainage are usually required with midlateral or midline longitudinal incision through the fingerpad. Probe very gently with a blunt instrument to avoid injury to nearby tendons and neurovascular bundle; loose packing.

- Culture if MRSA prevalent in the area.
- Antibiotics to cover MRSA and *Eikenella corrodens* if patient is immunosuppressed

COMPLICATIONS

Osteomyelitis, tenosynovitis, septic joint

Paronychia

Paronychia is a soft-tissue infection along the border of the fingernail or paronychium that results from the breakdown of the skin and entry of bacteria or fungi into the nail fold.

- Most common hand infection
- Acute: Caused by minor trauma and infiltration mainly by *S. aureus*. *Streptococcus*, *Pseudomonas*, and anaerobic and Gram-negative species are other possible causes.
- Chronic: Primarily caused by *Candida albicans*. Patients often have a history of chronically moist hands, eg, bartenders, housekeepers, marine workers. Indinavir treatment is the most frequent cause of chronic paronychia in HIV patients.

SYMPTOMS/EXAM

- Acute: Swollen, tender, erythematous lateral nail fold usually after minor trauma, most commonly nail biting
- Chronic: Symptoms > 6 weeks. It can be episodic. There is usually no fluctuance. Patient may have thickened and discolored nail plates. Patients often have a history of working with chemicals in moist environments with hands, eg, bartenders, housekeepers, marine workers.

DIFFERENTIAL

Herpetic whitlow (clear vesicles on an erythematous base), skin cancers, warts, chancres, granulomas

DIAGNOSIS

- Clinical diagnosis of acute paronychia is sufficient.
- KOH prep may be helpful to distinguish chronic cases caused by *C. albicans*.
- Tzanck smear or viral culture if herpetic whitlow suspected

TREATMENT

- Acute: If early, warm soaks and antibiotics may suffice. If an abscess has developed, drainage can usually be accomplished by elevating the paronychium with a blunt instrument. More advanced abscesses must be incised with a No. 11 blade and drained. Occasionally, a portion of the nail plate must be removed. Antibiotics are indicated for 5–7 days to cover Gram-positive organisms.
- Chronic:
  - Avoid water and irritating substances; topical antifungals for persistent cases.
  - **Do not incise the lesion if herpetic whitlow is suspected.**

COMPLICATIONS

Osteomyelitis, bacteremia

Flexor Tenosynovitis

The flexor tendons of the fingers are covered by a double layer of synovium to promote gliding of the tendon underneath. Infection of these flexor tendon sheaths presents a true surgical hand emergency. It is usually associated with penetrating trauma, although the patient may not recall the injury. *Staphylococcus* is the most common cause identified; however, the infection can be polymicrobic, including anaerobic organisms.

SYMPTOMS/EXAM (KANAVEL'S CARDINAL SIGNS)

- Flexed posture of the involved digit
- Fusiform swelling of the finger
- Tenderness over the flexor tendon sheath
- Pain with passive extension

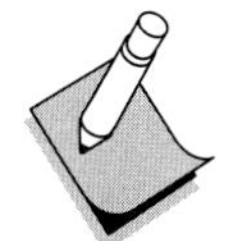

Kanavel's cardinal signs of flexor tenosynovitis:

1. *Flexed posture of the involved digit*
2. *Fusiform swelling of the entire digit*
3. *Tenderness over the flexor tendon sheath*
4. *Pain with passive extension*

DIFFERENTIAL

Cellulitis, subcutaneous abscess

DIAGNOSIS

- Clinical diagnosis
- X-ray may reveal air or a foreign body.

TREATMENT

- Hand should be immobilized and elevated.
- IV antibiotics with ampicillin/sulbactam, first-generation cephalosporin or vancomycin
- Hand surgeon consultation for possible surgical drainage

COMPLICATIONS

- Osteomyelitis
- Septic arthritis
- Loss of digit
- Chronic stiffness

CHAPTER 5

Pediatrics

Aaron E. Chen, MD and Hardin A. Pantle, MD

Colic

Infants with colic have persistent crying without a clear cause. To meet traditional definitions of colic, the infant must cry **at least 3 hours a day, at least 3 days a week, for at least 3 weeks**. Roughly 15% of infants have colic at some time, occurring between the ages of 2 and 16 weeks, with a peak incidence at 6 weeks of age.

Colic: Crying at least 3 hours a day, at least 3 days a week, for at least 3 weeks.

SYMPTOMS/EXAM

The physical exam is normal for colicky infants. During episodes of crying, infants may flex their legs up to their abdomen, arch their backs, and have abdominal distention. A careful physical examination is required to rule out other causes of persistent crying (see below).

DIFFERENTIAL

Because crying is nonspecific, the differential diagnosis for colic is extensive (see Table 5.1). Infants with colic should have a history of appropriate weight gain and growth.

DIAGNOSIS

Diagnosis is based on careful history and physical examination. A urinalysis and culture may be useful for ruling out a UTI, with other laboratory studies sent depending upon the clinical suspicion of possible etiologies.

Differential diagnosis of colic—

CAN'T FART
- **C**orneal abrasion, congenital abnormality
- **A**nal fissure
- **IN**tussusception, i**N**fection
- **T**ourniquet (around digit or penis)
- **F**ormula intolerance, **F**oreign body in eye
- **A**buse
- **R**ecent immunization
- **T**esticular torsion

TABLE 5.1. Differential Diagnosis of Colic

Differential Diagnosis of Colic
Gastroesophageal reflux
Formula intolerance
Infection (UTI, otitis media, meningitis)
Intussusception
Child abuse (occult fractures, occult subdural hemorrhage)
Corneal abrasion
Congenital abnormality (heart disease, metabolic disorder)
Foreign body in eye (most commonly an eye lash)
Anal fissure
Testicular torsion
Hair tourniquet (hair or thread wrapped tightly around digit or penis)
Recent immunization (most commonly after DTP)

Treatment

Once the diagnosis is made, treatment involves reassuring the parents that colic is normal and will resolve spontaneously without intervention. Pharmacologic therapies are not generally effective. Simethicone, while generally safe, is no more effective than placebo. Dicyclomine (an anticholinergic) may improve symptoms of colic, but is contraindicated in infants under the age of 6 months due to possible side effects of sedation, apnea, coma, and seizures. Other interventions that may provide some benefit in symptoms include changes in feeding technique, gentle motion (such as driving a car), and tight swaddling.

Complications

- Child abuse
- Disruption in breastfeeding
- Increased risk of maternal depression

Neonatal Jaundice

Healthy, full-term infants normally develop some degree of physiologic jaundice in the first 4 days of life due to the metabolism of red blood cells (see Figure 5.1). Elevated serum bilirubin can damage the infant's brain, causing irreversible **kernicterus**. Kernicterus is rare, but is a known and preventable cause of cerebral palsy.

Newborns are at high risk for developing jaundice for multiple reasons.

- Prematurity (immature hepatic conjugation system)
- Breastfeeding (mild dehydration in interval before mother starts to produce milk)
- Increased bilirubin load delivered to liver
  - High fetal RBC volume (polycythemia)
  - Decreased fetal RBC survival (cephalohematoma provides an additional source of RBC breakdown usually from forceps or vacuum-assisted delivery)

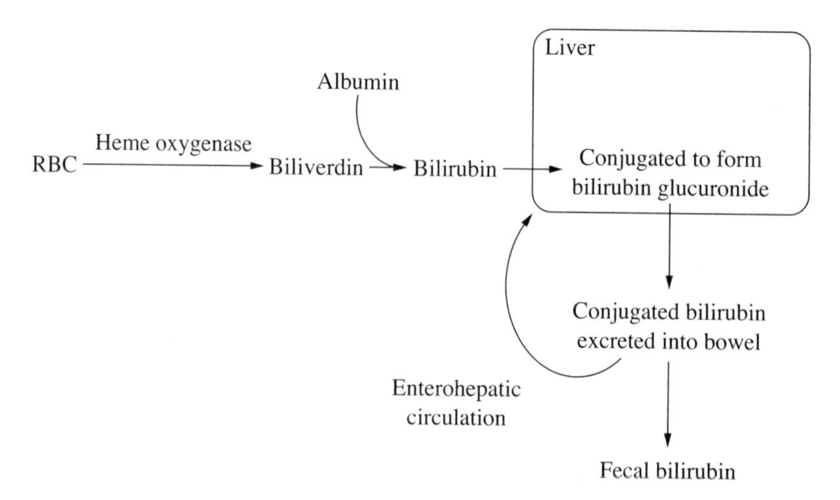

FIGURE 5.1. Summary of red blood cell (RBC) metabolism.

TABLE 5.2. Clinical Jaundice and Serum Bilirubin Levels

Face/eyes	7–8 mg/dL
Shoulder/torso	8–10 mg/dL
Lower body	10–12 mg/dL
Generalized	>12 mg/dL

    - Immune-mediated (Rh or ABO incompatibility)
    - Congenital RBC abnormalities (spherocytosis, G6PD, thalassemia)
    - Inborn errors of metabolism (Gilbert syndrome, galactosemia)
    - Increased enterohepatic circulation
- Decreased ability to excrete conjugated bilirubin (biliary atresia, hepatitis)
- Sepsis
- Hypothyroidism

SYMPTOMS/EXAM

As serum bilirubin levels increase, jaundice will become more detectable, starting at the infant's head and progressing toward the feet (see Table 5.2). Estimates of bilirubin levels based on physical examination, however, are unreliable.

Symptoms of bilirubin toxicity include:

- Extensor rigidity
- Tremor
- Loss of suck reflex
- Lethargy
- Seizures

DIAGNOSIS/TREATMENT

Diagnosis and treatment options are based upon the serum bilirubin level. Serum bilirubin levels should be interpreted relative to the infant's age in hours, not days. **Hyperbilirubinemia is always abnormal if present in the first 24 hours of life.**

- Additional lab studies that may be indicated include maternal and infant blood types, Coomb's test, infant CBC, reticulocyte count, and peripheral blood smear.
- Consider phototherapy if total bilirubin is > 5 × the birth weight in kilograms (usually 15–20 mg/dL).
- Consider exchange transfusion if total bilirubin is > 10 × the birth weight in kilograms (usually 25–30 mg/dL)

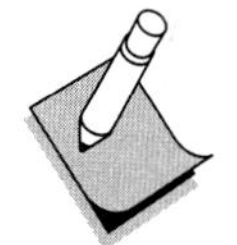

Unconjugated bilirubin = indirect bilirubin. Conjugated bilirubin = direct bilirubin. Total bilirubin = indirect bilirubin + direct bilirubin.

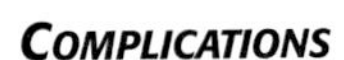

COMPLICATIONS

Kernicterus

Diarrhea

Diarrhea is a nonspecific symptom most often caused by inflammation or infection of the bowels (enteritis). In the United States, diarrheal diseases are responsible for nearly 10% of all pediatric hospitalizations. Worldwide, diarrheal diseases continue to cause significant morbidity and mortality.

Symptoms/Exam

The term "diarrhea" describes an increased frequency of loose bowel movements. Important history includes the presence of blood or mucus in the stool, as well as ill contacts. Typically, viral enteritis is associated with non-bloody diarrhea, without mucus (<5 PMN/hpf on microscopic examination of the stool). Diarrheal diseases caused by viruses usually last around 5 days, and occur most frequently in the late winter or spring. Bacterial enteritis may present with severe abdominal pain, tenesmus, bloody/mucoid stool, fever, and possibly altered mental status.

Differential

See Table 5.3.

Perform a careful physical examination to evaluate for the presence of intra-abdominal emergencies, such as intussusception, as well as extra-abdominal infections (such as otitis media or pneumonia).

Diagnosis

- Based on history and physical examination
- Stool guaiac and fecal leukocytes may support a class of infection.
- Lab studies are not routinely needed unless a child is moderately to severely ill or the diagnosis is unclear.

TABLE 5.3. Differential Diagnosis of Diarrhea

Infection—viral	*Rotavirus* *Enterovirus* Norwalk virus
Infection—bacterial	*Salmonella* *Shigella* *Escherichia coli* Other: *Campylobacter, Yersinia, Vibrio cholera, Staphylococcus aureus, Bacillus cereus*
Infectious colitis	*Clostridium difficile* colitis; typically associated with antecedent antibiotics
Inflammatory bowel disease	Crohn disease or ulcerative colitis
Intussusception	Classically associated with bloody diarrhea, intermittent crying, and lethargy
Hemolytic uremic syndrome	Preceding infection with *E. coli*
Other infections	UTI, otitis media, pneumonia
Malabsorption	Cystic fibrosis, celiac disease
Other	Overflow with chronic constipation, endocrine, drugs

- Urine may be sent to rule out a UTI.
- Diarrhea may lead to severe dehydration, as well as a non–anion gap metabolic acidosis due to loss of bicarbonate in the stool.

TREATMENT

- Oral rehydration therapy is often effective, but can be labor intensive and time consuming.
- IV fluids of either normal saline or lactated ringers in boluses of 20 cc/kg may be required to treat severe dehydration or if the child is unable to tolerate oral intake.

A full-term infant vomits after her initial feeding, and subsequently develops bilious emesis after each feeding. Physical examination reveals a lethargic infant with absent bowel sounds. Plain abdominal radiographs reveal a paucity of air in the distal bowel. What is the most likely diagnosis and management?

Malrotation with volvulus. Management should include IV fluid resuscitation, NG tube placement, and emergent surgical consultation.

Vomiting

Vomiting is a nonspecific sign that may be caused by a wide variety of conditions. All of the conditions described in Table 5.3 may have associated vomiting. The etiology of vomiting can usually be clarified by determining whether the emesis is bilious, the time course of the symptoms, the associated symptoms, and the age of the child. In general, vomiting is caused by:

- Infection (GI or elsewhere)
- GI inflammation
- GI obstruction
- CNS process
- Metabolic process

Isolated vomiting is potentially ominous, and careful consideration must be given to possible increased intracranial pressure (ICP).

SYMPTOMS/EXAM

Vary widely based upon the etiology and extent of vomiting

DIFFERENTIAL

See Table 5.4.

In general, a bowel obstruction distal to the ligament of Treitz will present with bilious emesis. An obstruction proximal to the ampulla of Vater will present with nonbilious emesis.

DIAGNOSIS

Diagnosis is based on a careful history and physical examination. Ancillary studies, such as barium enema, abdominal or chest radiographs, abdominal or head CT scans, lumbar puncture, urine analysis, or blood work, may be necessary.

TABLE 5.4. Differential Diagnosis of Vomiting

Infection	GI infections: Viral or bacterial Meningitis, pneumonia, UTI, otitis media
GI inflammation	Inflammatory bowel disease, pancreatitis, celiac disease
GI obstruction	Malrotation with volvulus, intussusception, atresia or stenosis of GI tract, pyloric stenosis, incarcerated hernia, appendicitis
CNS process	Subdural hematoma, increased ICP
Metabolic process	Inborn errors of metabolism, DKA, diabetic gastroparesis
Other processes	Posttussive emesis, eating disorders, psychological conditions, emotional distress

TREATMENT

Stabilization and diagnosis are paramount, with specific treatment directed toward the underlying condition.

CARDIOLOGY

Murmurs

COMMON NONPATHOLOGIC MURMURS

Characteristics of pathologic murmurs:

- Grade III or higher
- Radiation to back
- Maximal at apex
- Any diastolic murmur
- Associated sounds (eg, clicks, gallops)

A 4-day-old infant born via uncomplicated vaginal delivery presents to the ED with tachypnea and mild cyanosis. Cardiac exam reveals no heart murmur but a single second heart sound and increased precordial activity. Pulse oximetry reveals an O_2 saturation of 85%. What are the differential considerations and next step in diagnosis?

Cyanotic congenital heart disease, likely hypoplastic left heart. Hyperoxia test and urgent echocardiogram.

Congenital Heart Disease

Incidence of CHD estimated at ~4–10 in 1000 live births. Most common congenital heart defect is bicuspid aortic valve. Closure of the ductus arteriosus occurs 10–15 hours after birth functionally, and fibroses usually around 2–3 weeks (ligamentum arteriosum); pulmonary vascular resistance declines over the first week of life.

SYMPTOMS

Infants and children can present to the ED with undiagnosed CHD at any time. Both the age at presentation and type of presentation (presence/absence cyanosis, presence/absence of increased pulmonary blood flow, presence/absence of CHF) can give important clues to the underlying type of CHD. **In infants, symptoms are most often elicited during feedings.** Poor feedings, weak cry, coughing, wheezing, and poor growth or weight gain are also associated with CHD.

CHD in infants often presents with sweating during feeding or poor feeding.

EXAM

Look for presence of typical murmurs and check pulse, blood pressure, and differential O_2 saturation in all four extremities, comparing bilateral upper to lower extremities.

DIFFERENTIAL

Sepsis, inborn errors of metabolism, endocrine disorders, and drug ingestion. Patients with known CHD usually present for exacerbation of their underlying condition, for which an evaluation of their underlying anatomy is often needed (evaluation of shunt patency, etc.).

DIAGNOSIS

- The **hyperoxia test** is often helpful in testing for presence of a shunt as cause of cyanosis (ability to increase P_{O_2} above 150 mm Hg on 100% O_2 suggests pulmonary cause of cyanosis rather than CHD).
- Other useful tests include ECG, CXR, and blood gas (see Figure 5.2).
- Further testing (eg, echocardiogram, MRI) depends on suspected diagnosis

TREATMENT

Depends on underlying disorder

TETRALOGY OF FALLOT (TOF)

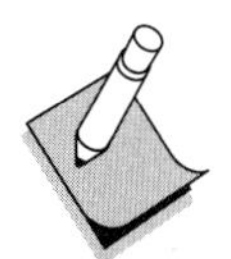

The most common cyanotic CHD; the tetrad—R ventricular outflow tract obstruction, overriding aorta, VSD, right ventricular hypertrophy (RVH). These defects result in decreased pulmonary blood flow and varying degrees of R → L shunting. Cyanosis can present at any time during infancy, depending on severity of R → L shunting.

TOF tetrad: RV outflow tract obstruction, Overriding aorta, VSD, RVH

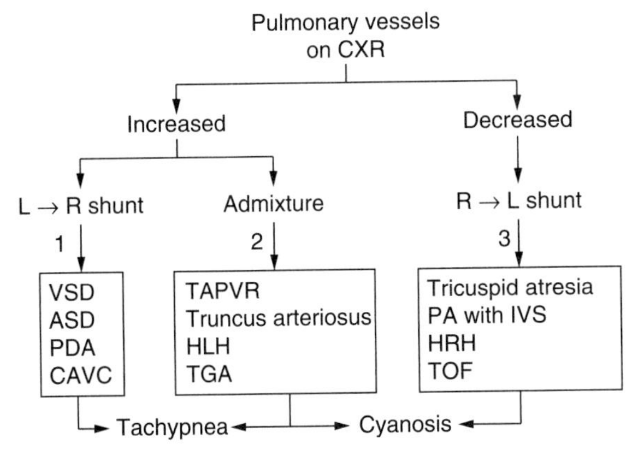

CAVC: complete atrioventricular canal
TAPVR: total anomalous pulmonary venous return
HLH: hypoplastic left heart
TGA: transposition of the great arteries
PA with IVS: pulmonary atresia with intact ventricular septum
HRH: hypoplastic right heart
TOF: tetralogy of fallot

FIGURE 5.2. Classification system for congenital heart disease lesions based on CXR findings and associated symptomatology.

(Reproduced, with permission, from Le T, Lam W, Rabizadeh S, Schroeder A, Vera K. *First Aid for the Pediatric Boards*, New York: McGraw-Hill, 2006:63.)

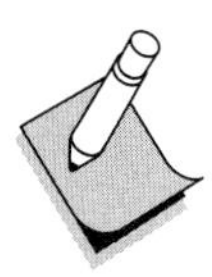

First maneuver in treatment of tet spell: Squating or knee-to-chest position.

Hypercyanotic spells ("**tet spells**") are often associated with crying or feeding (thought to be due to acute worsening of pulmonary outflow tract obstruction causing increased R → L shunting). Maneuvers that increase systemic vascular resistance (such as squatting) often help counteract this by decreasing the gradient for this R → L shunting.

DIAGNOSIS

- CXR may show a "**boot-shaped" heart**.
- Physical exam reveals a single loud S2 and a harsh systolic murmur (**pulmonic stenosis**).
- Echocardiogram reveals the anatomy.

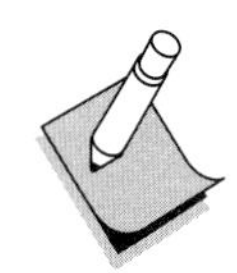

Boot-shaped heart on CXR = TOF

TREATMENT

- Acute cyanosis (tet spell): place patient in squatting or knee-to-chest position, administer O_2 and morphine. Patients unresponsive to these measures should receive IVF (to increase pulmonary blood flow), sodium bicarbonate (to treat acidosis) and vasopressors (to increase SVR).
- Definitive treatment is complete surgical repair.
  - Palliative shunts such as Blalock-Taussig (anastomosis of subclavian artery to pulmonary artery) shunt are aimed at increasing pulmonary blood flow.

HYPOPLASTIC LEFT HEART (HLH) SYNDROME

Hypoplasia of the left ventricle is associated with hypoplasia of the aorta; a patent PDA is essential for systemic blood flow. As the PDA closes, infants present with a shocklike state as blood flow to the systemic circulation is cut off.

TREATMENT

- Initial management focuses on maneuvers to keep the PDA open—"relative hypoxia" (avoidance of high FiO_2), prevention of acidosis, and prostaglandin infusion.
- Three-stage surgical repair: Norwood → Glenn → completion Fontan.

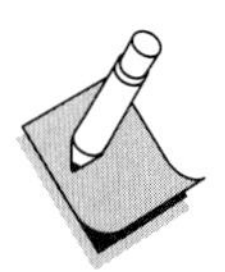

Egg on a string-shaped heart of CXR = TGA

TRANSPOSITION OF THE GREAT ARTERIES (TGA)

Essentially, pulmonary and systemic system running in parallel with VSD, ASD, or PDA allowing mixing of blood.

DIAGNOSIS

- Auscultation reveals single S2 and no murmur.
- CXR reveals "**egg on a string**" due to narrow upper mediastinum from abnormally positioned great vessels.
- Echocardiogram reveals the anatomy.

TREATMENT

- Prostaglandin infusion to keep the PDA open until palliative atrial septoplasty (to create large ASD) can be performed)
- Definitive surgical treatment with arterial or atrial level switch (Mustard or Senning procedure)

TRUNCUS ARTERIOSUS

Single arterial trunk from ventricles becomes aorta and pulmonary arteries. VSD is always present. Pulmonary overcirculation can lead to CHF.

VENTRICULAR SEPTAL DEFECT (VSD)

A defect (hole) in the ventricular septum

Symptoms/Exam

- Small defects are usually asymptomatic early on but associated with loud, harsh holosystolic murmur at LLSB.
- Larger defects usually manifest with tachypnea (due to pulmonary overcirculation/edema), fatigue, sweating during feeds, and poor weight gain.
- Progression from L → R shunting to more ominous R → L shunting is termed **Eisenmenger syndrome** due to progression to a high pulmonary vascular resistance from long-term pulmonary overcirculation.

Treatment

- Heart failure is treated with digoxin +/– diuretics.
- Definitive treatment with patch closure if not responsive to medical therapy or no spontaneous closure over time.

Atrial Septal Defect (ASD)

Fixed split S2, loud S1; may be associated with atrial dysrhythmias

Patent Ductus Arteriosus (PDA)

Persistence of ductus arteriosus past 1 week of life is considered abnormal.

Symptoms/Exam

Bounding pulses from aortic to pulmonary artery diastolic runoff; continuous **"machinery-like" heart murmur**, radiating to the back

Treatment

Indomethacin in premature infants; often surgical closure required

Coarctation of the Aorta

Localized narrowing of the aortic lumen, typically just distal to the origin of the L subclavian artery

Symptoms/Exam

Symptoms depend on the degree and location of narrowing. Key clinical findings include upper extremity hypertension and decreased lower extremity pulses, blood pressure, and O_2 saturations.

Treatment

Definitive surgical repair

Chest Pain

Unlike adults, chest pain in children is generally benign. Little workup, other than attention to vital signs, is needed unless significant historical or physical exam findings are present.

Dysrhythmias

Bradycardia

Bradycardia is usually secondary to systemic or noncardiac causes in children. In the infant, hypoxia is a common cause. Other causes include hypothermia, hypothyroidism, elevated ICP.

HEART BLOCK

Heart block is most commonly seen postoperatively following cardiac surgery. Other causes include rheumatic heart disease, myocarditis, lupus, and Kawasaki's disease.

SUPRAVENTRICULAR TACHYCARDIA (SVT)

SVT is the most common significant arrhythmia in pediatrics. Most children with SVT have a structurally normal heart. Treatment consists of vagal maneuvers or adenosine, and possible cardioversion if unstable.

PROLONGED QT SYNDROME

Prolonged QT syndrome can be cause of syncope and/or sudden death. Bazett's formula: QT interval divided by the square root of the RR interval. It can be associated with deafness (**Jervell and Lange-Nielson syndrome**) or without deafness (**Romano-Ward syndrome**). Corrected QTc is usually >0.46 ms but varies with age. Treatment is with β-blockers and occasionally placement of pacemaker or ICD device.

DERMATOLOGY

Diaper Dermatitis

The most common etiologies of diaper rash are shown in Table 5.5.

Seborrhea

- Inflammation due to increased production of sebaceous glands
- Peak incidence—2 weeks of age
- Typically resolves spontaneously by 1 year of age

SYMPTOMS/EXAM

Greasy scale accumulation on the face, scalp ("cradle cap"), and sometimes diaper area (see Figure 5.3)

DIAGNOSIS

Clinical diagnosis

TABLE 5.5. Common Etiologies of Diaper Dermatitis

	CHARACTERISTICS	TREATMENT
Contact dermatitis	Spares deep skin folds	Increase frequency of diaper changes; keep skin clean, dry
Candida albicans	Affects deepest skin folds; may have satellite lesions	Topical antifungal
Seborrhea	Greasy scale; may have satellite lesions	Topical steroid
Impetigo	Yellow crusting	Oral antibiotic

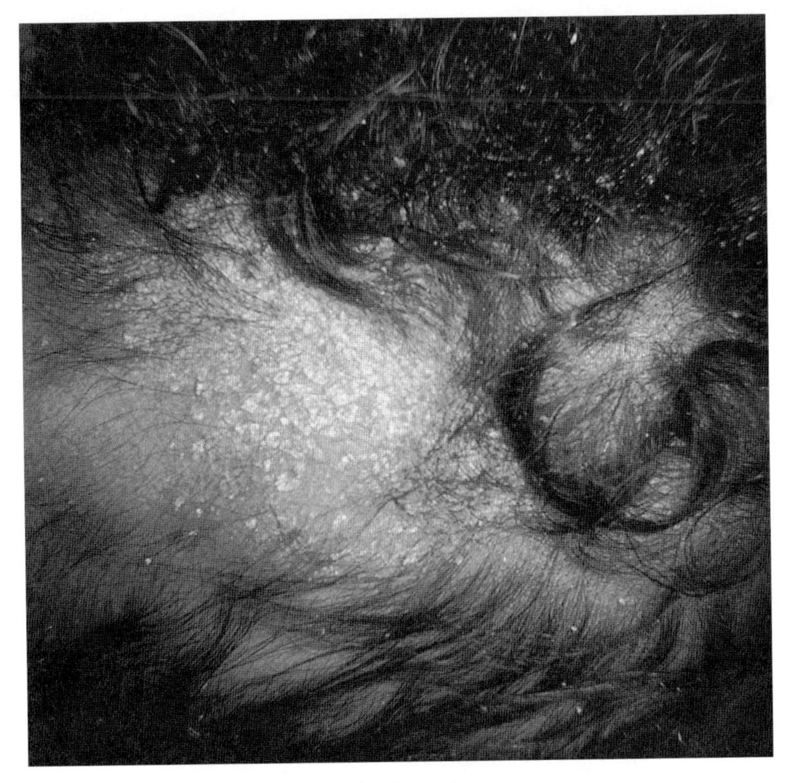

FIGURE 5.3. Seborrhea. (See also color insert.)

(Reproduced, with permission, from Shah BR, Lucchesi M. *Atlas of Pediatric Emergency Medicine*. McGraw-Hill, 2006:295.)

Treatment

- Scalp: Mineral oil, followed by antidandruff shampoo
- Other areas: Topical steroids

Eczema

- Chronic, recurrent skin lesions associated with other allergic conditions (asthma, seasonal allergies)
- Etiology is unclear, but numerous triggers for eczema flares have been identified including local skin trauma, foods, environmental allergens, and emotional distress.
- 60–80% of patients will have resolution of eczema by adulthood.

Symptoms/Exam

- Pruritic, scaly, erythematous lesions (see Figure 5.4)
- Typical distribution:
  - Infants: Face
  - Children (<12 years old): Extensor surfaces
  - Adolescents: Flexor surfaces

Diagnosis

Clinical diagnosis

Treatment

- Skin moisturizers
- Topical steroids

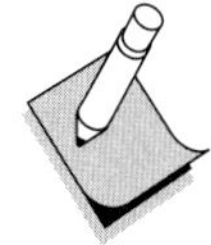

If it doesn't itch, it's probably not eczema.

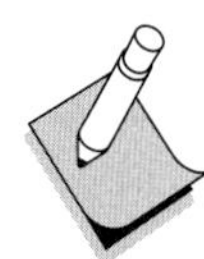

Eczema herpeticum: Eczema superinfected with herpes simplex virus

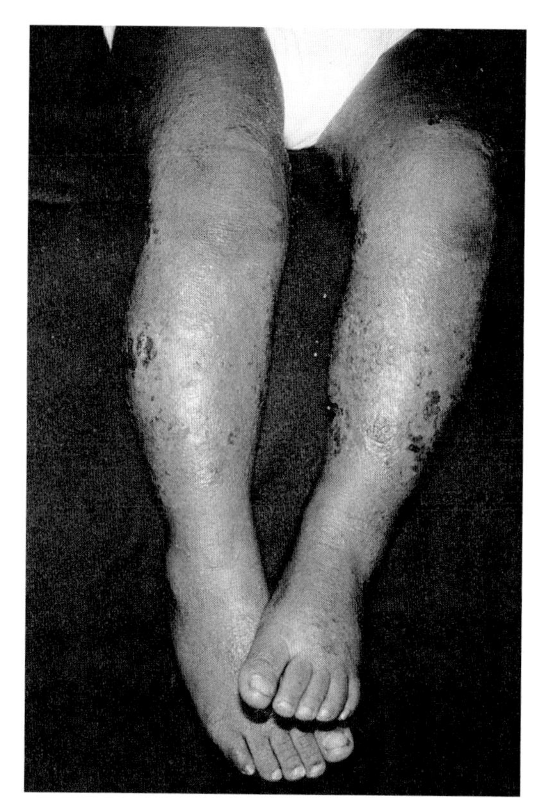

FIGURE 5.4. **Eczema.**

(Reproduced, with permission, from Shah BR, Lucchesi M. *Atlas of Pediatric Emergency Medicine*. New York: McGraw-Hill, 2006:303.)

- Systemic antihistamines for pruritis
- Oral antibiotics if superimposed skin infection

COMPLICATIONS

Complications include increased risk for bacterial or viral skin infections. Superinfection with herpes simplex virus (eczema herpeticum) can be life threatening.

Molluscum Contagiosum

- Poxvirus
- Self-limited skin lesions, typically lasting weeks to months
- Peak incidence: School-age children
- Transmission: Direct contact

SYMPTOMS/EXAM

- **Small, flesh-colored papules that have a centrally depressed area (umbilicated papule,** see Figure 5.5).
- Painless, and usually asymptomatic
- Typically affect face, torso, and extremities (sparing palms, soles, and scalp)
- No systemic symptoms

DIAGNOSIS

Clinical diagnosis is based on the morphology of the lesions.

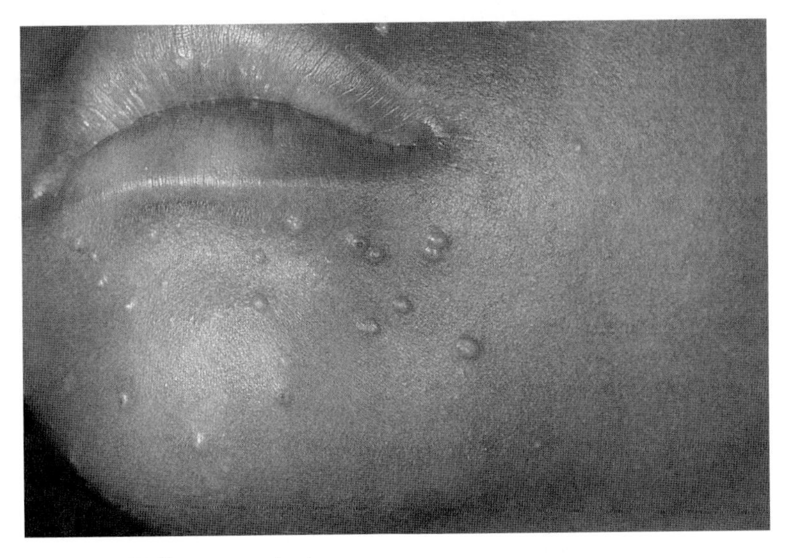

FIGURE 5.5. Molluscum contagiosum.

(Reproduced, with permission, from Shah BR, Lucchesi M. *Atlas of Pediatric Emergency Medicine*. New York: McGraw-Hill, 2006:342.)

TREATMENT

Generally no treatment is indicated because the lesions are self-limited and resolve without scarring.

Pityriasis Rosea

- Etiology is unknown, but possibly a viral agent (human herpes virus: HHV-7).
- Highest incidence is in adolescents.

SYMPTOMS/EXAM

- **Herald patch** precedes other symptoms in 50% of patients. The herald patch is a scaly, erythematous, oval lesion typically on the torso.
- 1–2 weeks after appearance of herald patch there is a development of generalized rash, with oval, pink macules aligned along the skin dermatomes of the torso ("**Christmas tree**" distribution; see Figure 5.6).
- Typically, palms and soles are spared.
- Rash may last up to several months.

DIFFERENTIAL

- 2° syphilis (especially if palms and soles are involved)
- Acute drug reaction
- Reaction to recent immunization
- Herald patch may resemble tinea corporis.

DIAGNOSIS

Clinical diagnosis

TREATMENT

- No treatment is known to shorten length of rash.
- Symptomatic treatment for pruritis: Skin moisturizers, oral antihistamines, possibly topical steroids

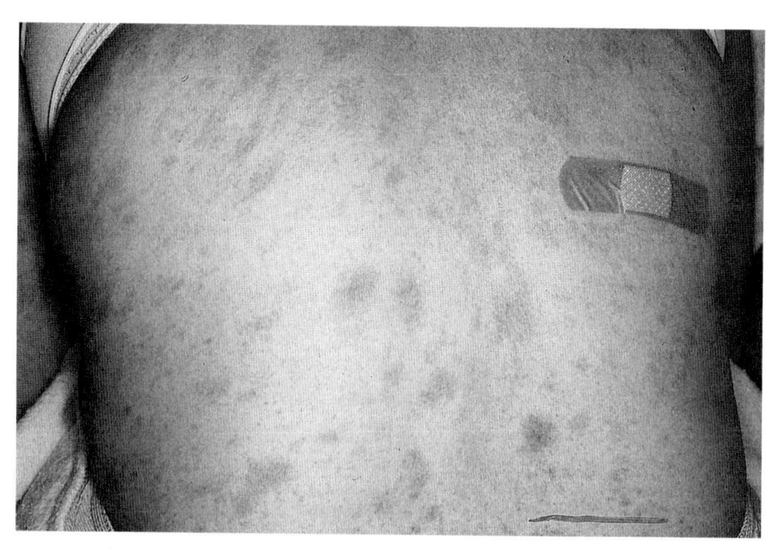

FIGURE 5.6. Pityriasis rosea.

(Reproduced, with permission, from Wolff K, Johnson RA, Suurmond D. *Fitzpatrick's Color Atlas & Synopsis of Clinical Dermatology*, 5th ed. New York: McGraw-Hill, 2005:119.)

COMPLICATIONS

Hyperpigmentation can occur (especially in patients with dark skin color) due to chronic skin inflammation.

Exanthems and Enanthems

- **Exanthem**: An eruption on a skin surface
- **Enanthem**: An eruption on a mucous membrane

MEASLES (RUBEOLA)

- Viral infection (RNA virus)
- Incidence of infection reduced by 98% after vaccination introduced in 1963
- Transmitted by respiratory droplets
- Incubation 10–12 days between exposure and onset of symptoms

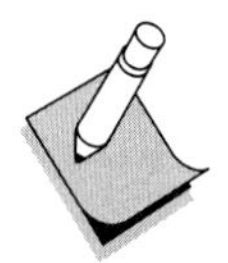

Measles (rubeola): Fever and rash with cough, conjuctivitis, coryza, and Koplik spots

SYMPTOMS/EXAM

- High fever (up to 104°F).
- Cough, conjunctivitis, coryza (nasal congestion)
- Exanthem: Erythematous, nonblanching, maculopapular rash that starts at the hairline, then spreads down face, to trunk/extremities (see Figure 5.7).
- Enanthem: **Koplik spots** (pinpoint-sized white spots with red background which appear on the buccal mucosa opposite molars; see Figure 5.8).
- Rash may coalesce into salmon-colored patches, then disappear typically within 1 week of onset.

DIAGNOSIS

- Clinical diagnosis may be challenging, particularly since many physicians rarely see patients with the diagnosis.

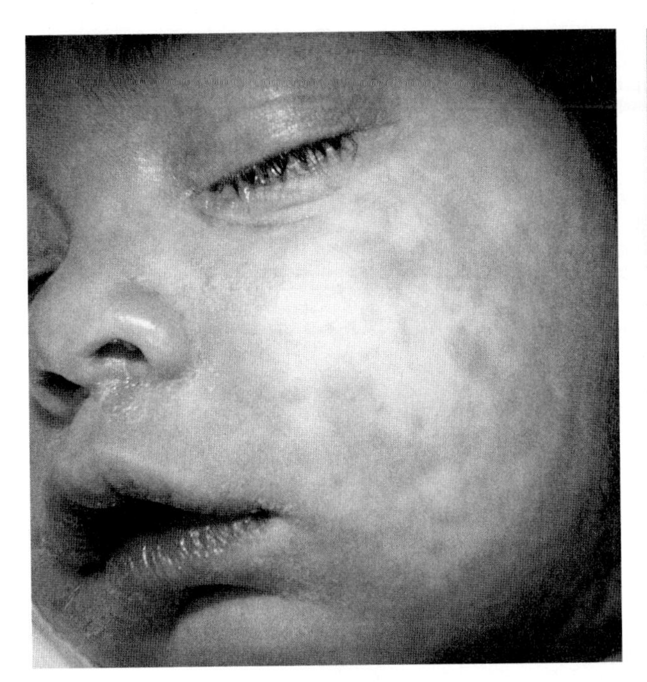

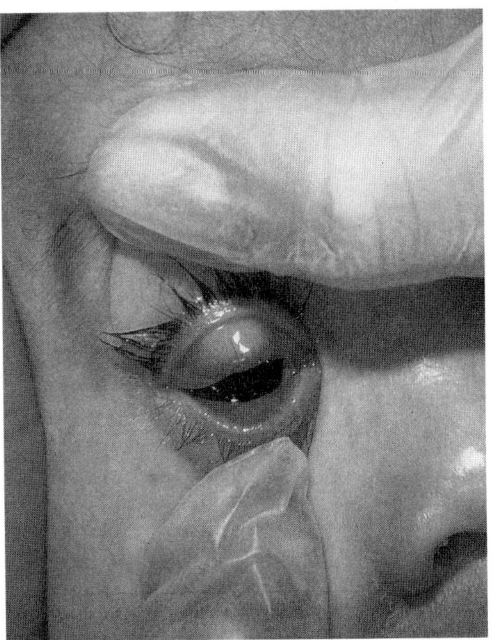

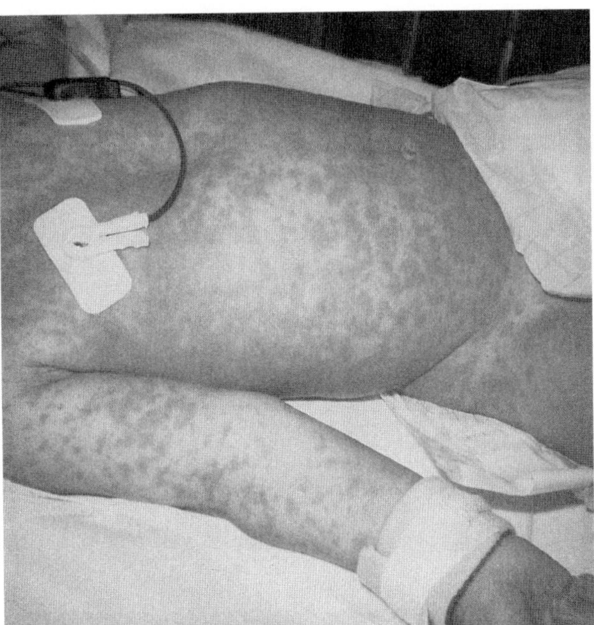

FIGURE 5.7. Measles (rubeolla). (See also color insert.)

(Reproduced, with permission, from Shah BR, Lucchesi M. *Atlas of Pediatric Emergency Medicine*. New York: McGraw-Hill, 2006:135.)

- Lab studies can confirm clinical suspicion.
  - Presence of IgM to measles is diagnostic.
  - Rise in antibody titers during course of illness
  - Viral cultures can also be performed.

TREATMENT

- Supportive care: Antipyretics, prevent of dehydration
- Treat 2° bacterial infections with antibiotics.
- Respiratory isolation

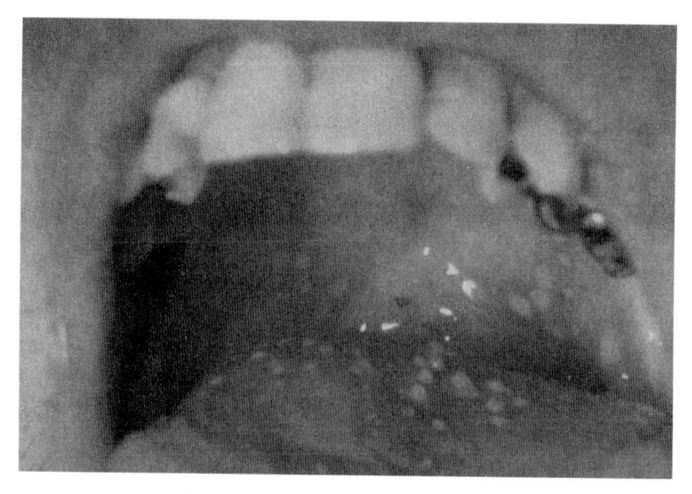

FIGURE 5.8. Measles (rubeolla). (See also color insert.)

(Reproduced, with permission, Kane K S-M, Ryder JB, Jonson RA, et al. *Color Atlas & Synopsis of Pediatric Dermatology*. New York: McGraw-Hill, 2002:585.)

- Immunize close contacts who are unvaccinated. (Note MMR vaccine is contraindicated in patients who are pregnant or who have significant immunosuppression. Patients who cannot receive MMR should receive immunoglobulin.)
- Report disease to state health authorities.

COMPLICATIONS

- Acute purulent otitis media is the most common complication.
- Pneumonia is most common reason for admission.
- Encephalitis (1/1000 cases)
- Death (2/1000 cases in United States)
- Measles infection during pregnancy may cause spontaneous abortion.

RUBELLA (GERMAN MEASLES)

- Viral infection (RNA virus)
- Immunity conferred by MMR vaccination
- Transmitted by respiratory droplets
- Typically mild illness, except for congenital infection, which can cause major birth defects

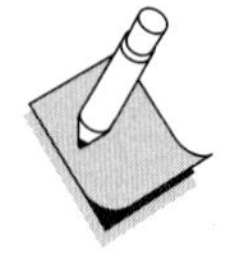

Rubella (German measles): Rash with tender postauricular lymphadenopathy

SYMPTOMS/EXAM

- Low-grade fever
- Exanthem: Erythematous papular rash begins on face, spreads to trunk (see Figure 5.9).
- Tender lymphadenopathy is common and usually involves the postauricular, suboccipital, and posterior cervical chains.

DIAGNOSIS

- Clinical diagnosis
- Serum testing can confirm diagnosis.

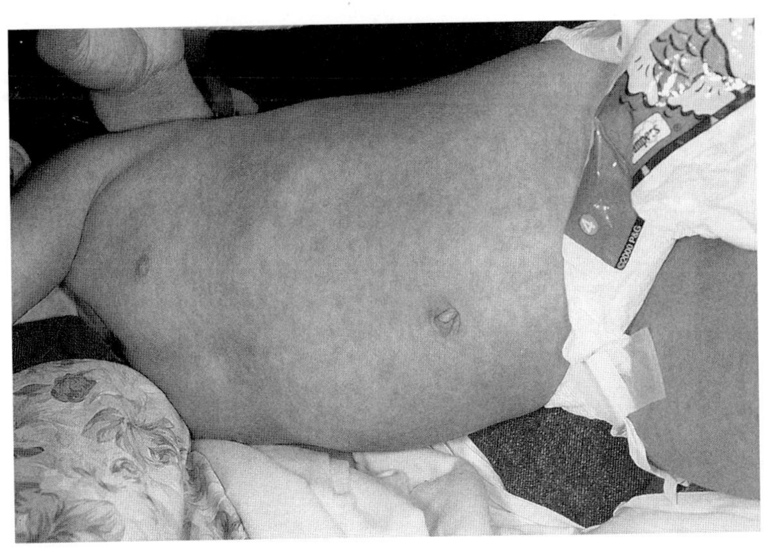

FIGURE 5.9. Rubella (German measles). (See also color insert.)

(Reproduced, with permission, from Shah BR, Lucchesi M. *Atlas of Pediatric Emergency Medicine*. New York: McGraw-Hill, 2006:137.)

TREATMENT

Supportive

COMPLICATIONS

- Noncongenital infection may lead to arthritis or arthralgia (particularly in young women).
- Congenital infection is a major concern, and can lead to fetal viremia and major birth defects.

ROSEOLA INFANTUM (EXANTHEM SUBITUM)

- Viral infection caused by human herpes virus (HHV-6)
- Peak incidence in spring and fall
- Affected children typically 6 months to 3 years of age
- Transmitted by respiratory droplets

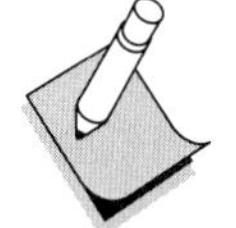

Roseola Infantum: Onset of rash with resolution of fever

SYMPTOMS/EXAM

- High fever lasting 3–4 days (increased risk of febrile seizure)
- Exanthem: Pale pink macules, typically located on the neck; rash usually appears as the fever resolves, with rash persisting 1–2 days (see Figure 5.10)

DIFFERENTIAL

Can mimic other very serious infections, including pneumococcal sepsis or meningitis

DIAGNOSIS

Clinical diagnosis

TREATMENT

Supportive care

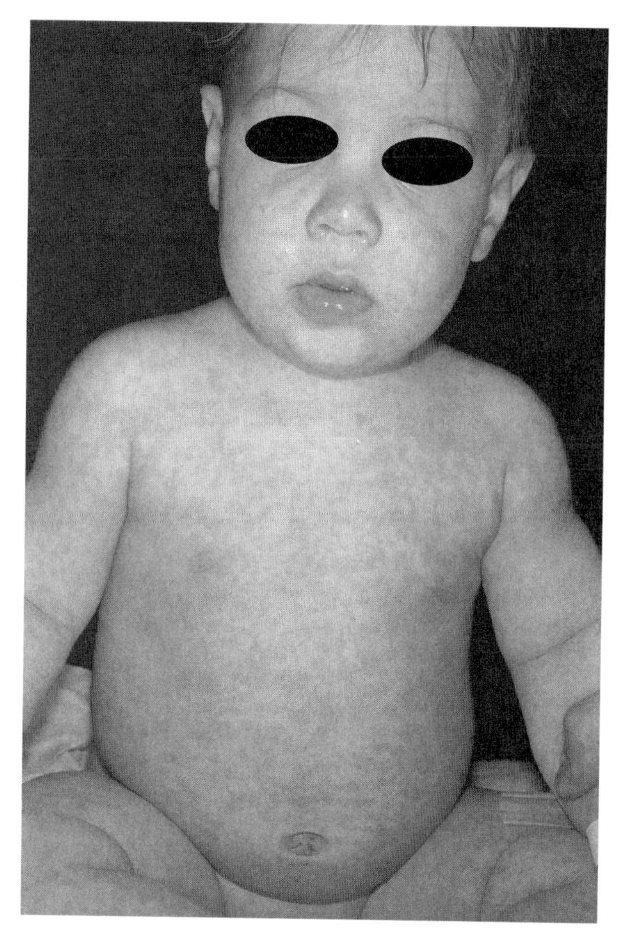

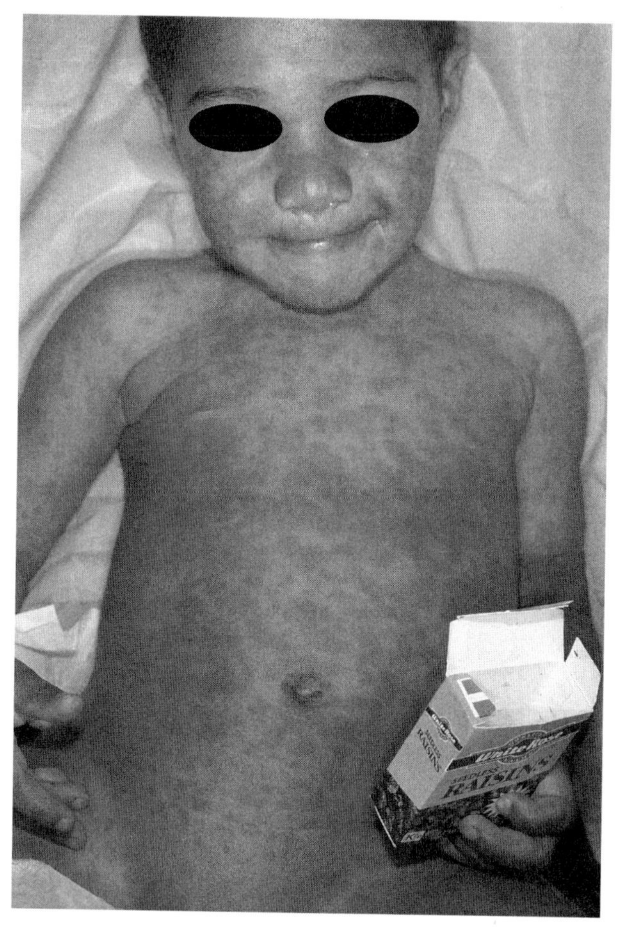

FIGURE 5.10. Roseola. (See also color insert.)

(Reproduced, with permission, from Shah BR, Lucchesi M. *Atlas of Pediatric Emergency Medicine*. New York: McGraw-Hill, 2006:137.)

COMPLICATIONS

Complications are very rare, but hepatitis or encephalitis can occur.

COXSACKIE A-16 VIRUS (HAND-FOOT-MOUTH DISEASE)

- Peak U.S. incidence: Summer
- Fecal-oral and respiratory transmission
- Typically affects children <5 years of age

SYMPTOMS/EXAM

- Fever
- Painful vesicles/ulcers on tongue and palate
- Vesicles on palms and soles

DIFFERENTIAL

Other viral infections: Varicella, herpes, herpangina (which is typically caused by other serotypes of Coxsackie virus)

DIAGNOSIS

Clinical diagnosis

TREATMENT

Supportive

COMPLICATIONS

- Myocarditis may develop in 2% of patients who have hand-foot-mouth disease.
- Meningoencephalitis is a rare complication.
- Dehydration from decreased oral intake

ERYTHEMA INFECTIOSUM (FIFTH DISEASE)

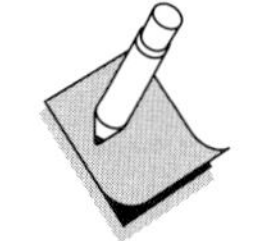

Erythema infectiousum (fifth disease): "Slapped cheeks" appearance

- Etiology: Infection with parvovirus B19.
- Peak incidence: 4–15 years of age, most common during winter and spring
- Transmission: Respiratory droplets

SYMPTOMS/EXAM

- Prodrome (lasts 2–3 days): Mild coryza, headache, fever
- Facial rash (bright red) develops 7 days later: **"slapped cheeks"** appearance (see Figure 5.11)

DIAGNOSIS

Clinical diagnosis

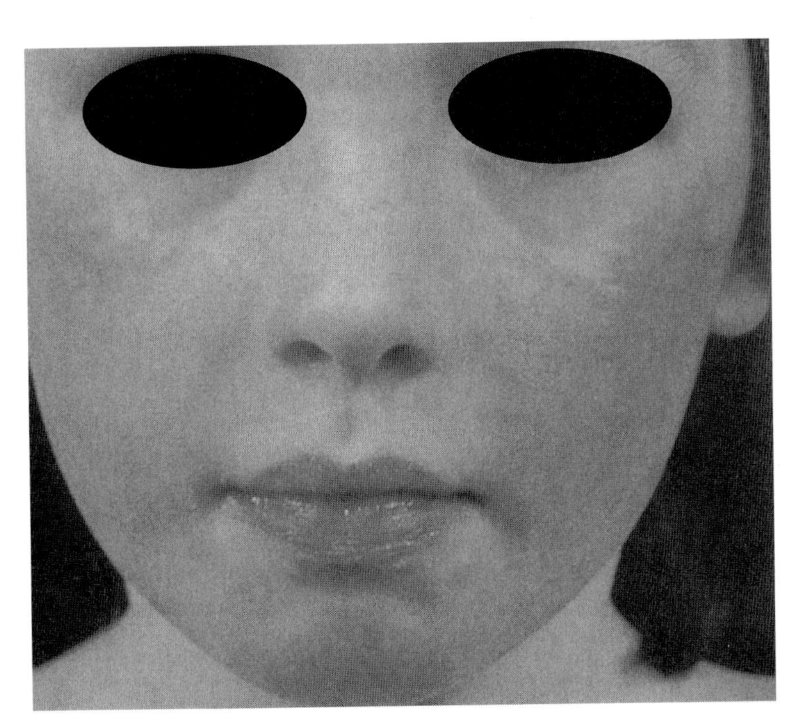

FIGURE 5.11. Erythema infectiosum. (See also color insert.)

(Reproduced, with permission, from Kane KS-M, Ryder JB, Jonson RA, et al. *Color Atlas & Synopsis of Pediatric Dermatology*. New York: McGraw-Hill, 2002:579.)

TREATMENT

Symptomatic care only

COMPLICATIONS

Aplastic anemia may develop in patients who have an underlying hemoglobinopathy (such as sickle cell disease). Anemia may be severe, requiring RBC transfusion.

VARICELLA ZOSTER VIRUS (VZV)

- A herpes virus
- 1° infection: Varicella (chickenpox)
  - Highest incidence in late winter, early spring
  - Historically affected children <10 years of age
  - Transmission via direct contact or airborne droplets
- Reactivation of previous VZV infection: Zoster (shingles, Herpes zoster)
  - Highest incidence in immunocompromised and elderly.

SYMPTOMS/EXAM

Chickenpox

- Fever precedes rash by 1–2 days.
- Rash typically starts at hairline, with initial formation of macules, which progress to fluid-filled vesicles (**"dew drops on a rose petal"**). Crops of lesions typically appear at the same time with vesicles in various stages of healing on body (as opposed to smallpox, which has all lesions in the same stage of healing) (see Figure 5.12).

Zoster

Rash in **dermatomal distribution**, typically on trunk or face

DIAGNOSIS

Clinical diagnosis

TREATMENT

Chickenpox

- In healthy children <12 years of age, chickenpox is usually a self-limited illness, requiring supportive care (oral antihistamines to treat itching, and antipyretics).
- **Avoid aspirin due to the risk of Reye's syndrome.**
- Children >12 years of age are at higher risk for severe disease, and should receive oral acyclovir.
- Immunocompromised patients should receive IV acyclovir and VZIG.

Zoster

Treat with oral acyclovir if within 72 hours of eruption onset.

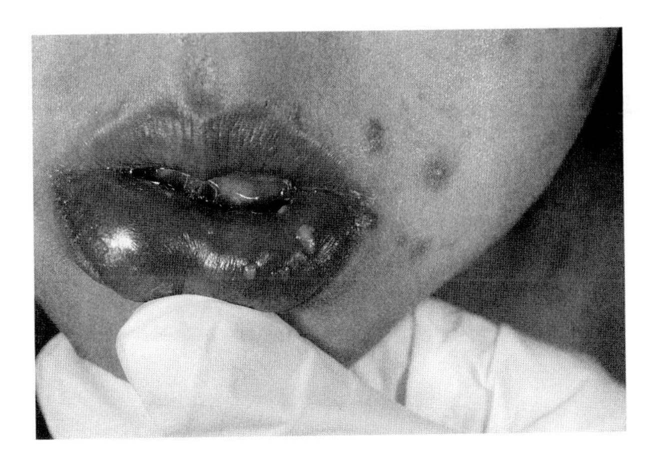

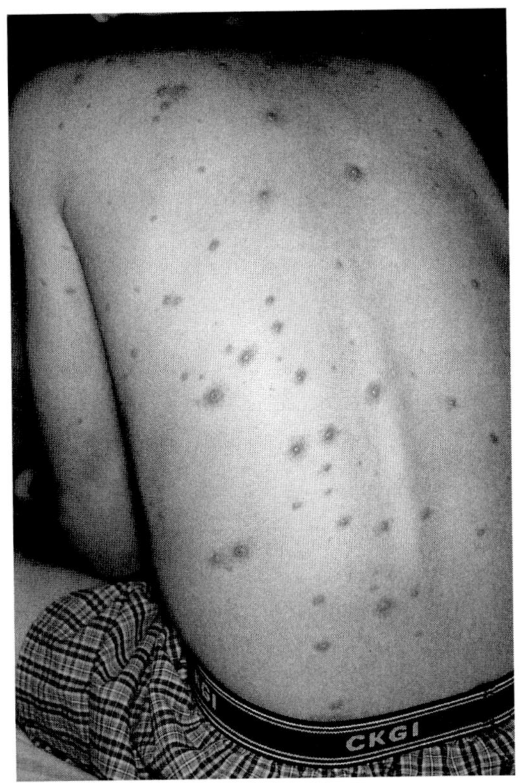

FIGURE 5.12. Varicella.

(Reproduced, with permission, from Shah BR, Lucchesi M. *Atlas of Pediatric Emergency Medicine*. New York: McGraw-Hill, 2006:119.)

COMPLICATIONS

Chickenpox

- Bacterial skin infections are most common complication.
- Children who are immunocompromised are at higher risk for disseminated disease, potentially resulting in meningoencephalitis, pneumonia, hepatitis.

- **Maternal infection during first or second trimester can result in congenital varicella, leading to fetal scarring, limb atrophy, and CNS abnormalities.**
- **Maternal varicella infection at delivery is associated with up to 30% fetal mortality.**

Zoster

- Postherpetic neuralgia (uncommon in children)

SCARLET FEVER

- Caused by group A β-hemolytic streptococcus, which produces an erythrogenic toxin
- Streptococcal infection is typically located in the throat (strep throat), but can also occur from skin infections such as impetigo.

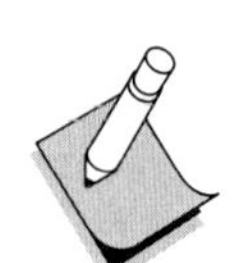

Scarlet fever: Strawberry tongue, sandpaper rash, Pastia's lines

SYMPTOMS/EXAM

- Typically sore throat and fever are present for 1–2 days before the appearance of the rash.
- Enanthem: "**Strawberry tongue**"
- Exanthem: Erythematous, coarse, sandpaper texture rash located typically on the torso and face with sparing of the circumoral area (see Figure 5.13). Desquamation occurs after the rash fades. "**Pastia's lines**" is linear nonblanching erythema of the skin fold in joints.

DIFFERENTIAL

- Toxic shock syndrome
- 2° syphilis
- Infectious mononucleosis

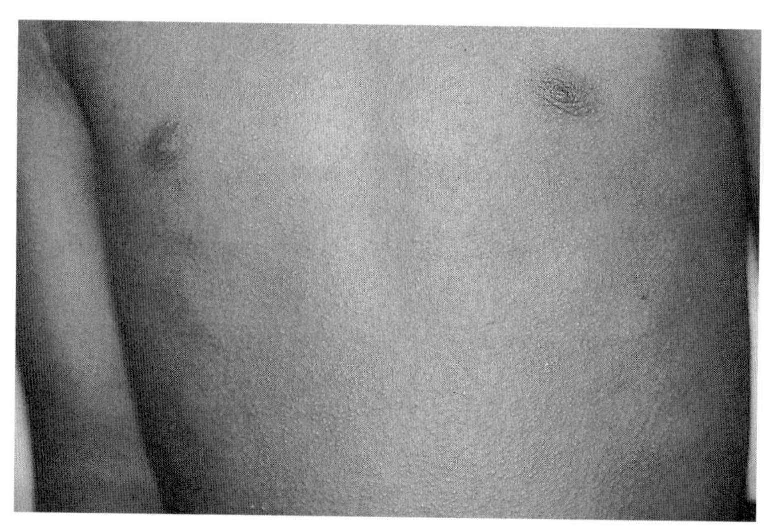

FIGURE 5.13. Scarlet fever.

(Reproduced, with permission, from Wolff K et al. *Fitzpatrick's Dermatology in General Medicine*, 7th ed. New York: McGraw-Hill, 2008:1718.)

Diagnosis

Clinical suspicion, confirmed by throat culture positive for strep, or a rising antistreptolysin-O (ASO) titer.

Treatment

Penicillin or erythromycin for 10 days

Complications

- Rheumatic fever (can be prevented by treating scarlet fever with antibiotics)
- Glomerulonephritis (**not prevented** by treating scarlet fever with antibiotics)

Staphylococcal Scalded Skin Syndrome

- Occurs as a result of (usually) clinically inappent colonization with an exotoxin-producing strain of S. *aureus*
- Typically affects children < 5 years of age

Symptoms/Exam

- Exanthem: Generalized, tender erythema
- Skin exfoliates; **Nikolsky's sign**: Pressure on affected skin leads to blister formation

Differential

- Toxic epidermal necrolysis
- Stevens-Johnson syndrome
- Bullous impetigo

Diagnosis

Clinical diagnosis

Treatment

- Antibiotics (to treat staph infection)
- IV fluid resuscitation
- Isolation

Complications

- Dehydration
- 2° bacterial infection can occur.

Toxic Shock Syndrome (TSS)

Toxic shock syndrome is triggered by exotoxin release due to inflammatory cascade similar to that seen in sepsis.

Two distinct syndromes:

Staphylococcal toxic shock syndrome (TSS)

- Due to colonization with exotoxin-producing strain of *Staphylococcus aureus*
- Traditionally associated with tampon use

Streptococcal toxic shock syndrome (STSS)

- Typically due to **infection** with exotoxin-producing strain of group A streptococcus (GAS).

DIAGNOSIS

- Based on established clinical criteria (see Table 1.17)

TREATMENT

- Treatment strategy is the same as for patients with sepsis.
- Major difference is antibiotic usage to cover MRSA as well as group A streptococcus.
- Nafcillin, clindamycin, and vancomycin concomitantly

ROCKY MOUNTAIN SPOTTED FEVER (RMSF)

- Rickettsial infection caused by the Gram-negative, obligate intracellular *Rickettsia rickettsii*
- Transmitted via tick bite
- RMSF occurs throughout the United States (**not only in the Rocky Mountain area**).
- Peak season: April–October
- Peak incidence: 5–9 years of age

RMSF Triad (present in 60% of cases):

1. Fever

2. Rash

3. Headache

SYMPTOMS/EXAM

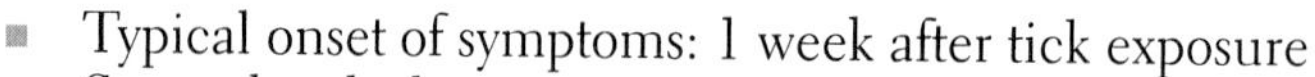

- Typical onset of symptoms: 1 week after tick exposure
- Severe headache
- Exanthem: Appears 3–5 days after onset of other symptoms. Initially, presents as blanching, erythematous macules located on the wrists and ankles. Rash spreads to palms, soles, and torso. Rash then typically becomes nonblanching purpura or petechiae (see Figure 5.14).
- May develop hypotension, CNS involvement, abdominal pain, renal failure, and ARDS

DIFFERENTIAL

Extensive, including:

- Meningococcal disease
- Ehrlichiosis
- 2° syphilis
- Henoch-Schönlein purpura
- Kawasaki disease
- Drug reactions
- Toxic shock syndrome
- Viral infections (enterovirus, influenza)

Treatment of RMSF should be based on clinical suspicion. Do not exclude the diagnosis of RMSF because of lack of rash or tick exposure.

DIAGNOSIS

Clinical suspicion, confirmed by antibody testing

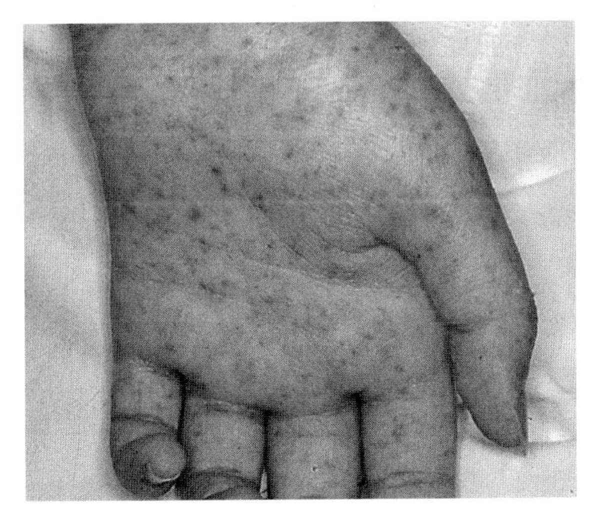

FIGURE 5.14. Rocky Mountain spotted fever.

(Reproduced, with permission, from Weinberg S, Prose NS, Kristal L., *Color Atlas of Pediatric Dermatology*, 4th ed. New York: McGraw-Hill, 2008:56.)

Treatment

- Prevent tick exposure.
- Prompt removal of ticks (RMSF unlikely if tick attached <12 hours)
- Treatment of suspected RMSF should begin based on clinical suspicion alone (prior to confirmatory testing). Doxycycline can be used in children of all ages.

Complications

- Mortality up to 25% if treatment delayed by >5 days after the onset of symptoms
- Severe cases can result in gangrene, with loss of digits or extremities.

Meningococcal Disease

- *Neisseria meningitidis:* Gram-negative diplococcus that can cause meningitis or bacteremia
- Infections occur year round, with peak incidence in winter and spring.
- Peak incidence < 4 years of age, with a second peak between the ages of 15 and 18 years.
- Transmission is via airborne droplets.

Symptoms/Exam

- Severe illness, with sudden onset and rapid progression of symptoms
- Exanthem: Maculopapular rash typically progressing to petechiae
- Fever
- Hypotension
- In patients with meningitis, nuchal rigidity and altered mental status are usually present.

DIAGNOSIS

- Culture of organism from sterile body fluid (blood, CSF)
- Gram stain demonstrating Gram-negative diplococci supports the presumptive diagnosis of infection.
- DIC may be present.

TREATMENT

- Antibiotics (penicillins or cephalosporins): Give early!
- Chemoprophylaxis for close contacts (rifampin or ceftriaxone for children; ciprofloxacin for adults)
- Report diagnosis to local health department.

COMPLICATIONS

- Fatality rate 10% for all ages (fatality rate up to 25% in adolescents): Give early!
- Bilateral sensorineural deafness is the most common complication from meningitis caused by N. *meningitidis.*
- Myocarditis
- Pericarditis
- Pneumonia

ENDOCRINE AND METABOLIC DISORDERS

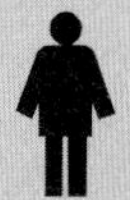

A 3-week-old male infant presents to the ED with a history of poor feeding, poor weight gain since birth, lethargy, irritability, and occasional vomiting. Laboratory evaluation shows an Na of 128, a K of 7, and glucose of 52. What is the likely diagnosis?

Congenital adrenal hyperplasia.

Congenital Adrenal Hyperplasia

The ED physician may be the first to diagnose this condition. Urgent recognition of the condition can be life saving.

Females will usually present with ambiguous genitalia due to virilization; males have normal genital development and usually present with salt wasting during infancy and precocious puberty during childhood.

SYMPTOMS/EXAM

- When the defect primarily involves the adrenal system, children present with more gradual onset of malaise, anorexia, and weight loss.
- **Ambiguous genitalia**
- **Acute salt-wasting crisis**
- **Precocious virilization** in older children

DIAGNOSIS

- Electrolytes and blood glucose testing reveal hyponatremia, hyperkalemia, and hypoglycemia
- ACTH stimulation testing confirms the diagnosis of adrenal insufficiency.
- Specific enzyme testing should reveal the specific enzymatic deficiency.

TREATMENT

- Initial management is focused on fluid resuscitation with isotonic saline.
- Mineralocorticoid replacement is usually reserved for long-term management, whereas glucocorticoid replacement is usually done in both the acute and chronic setting.
- Salt wasting during infancy can be a true life-threatening emergency and urgent diagnosis and hospital admission are warranted.

Diabetes

Most children with diabetes have type 1/IDDM (insulin-dependent diabetes mellitus). An increasing number of type 2/NIDDM (noninsulin-dependent diabetes mellitus) are being seen, thought to be due to the increasing epidemic of obesity. Most cases of new-onset diabetes, even if not in DKA, are admitted to the hospital for initiation of therapy and education.

DIABETIC KETOACIDOSIS (DKA)

SYMPTOMS/EXAM

- Signs of DKA include Kussmaul respirations, tachypnea, acetone breath, vomiting, abdominal pain (sometimes mimicking an acute abdomen) and altered mental status.
- **Cerebral edema** is the most feared complication; early manifestations include headache, lethargy, and altered mental status, eventually progressing to obtundation, seizures, and posturing.

DIAGNOSIS

- Increased anion gap metabolic acidosis
- Elevated glucose
- Elevated osmolarity
- Elevated ketones
- Additional labs to consider: Triglycerides, HgbA1C, antiislet cell and anti-insulin and anti-GAD antibodies, urinalysis, and ECG

TREATMENT

- **Judicious rehydration**. Use normal saline bolus of 20 cc/kg in most cases (10 cc/kg if signs of altered mental status present). Cornerstone of management is insulin replacement usually by continuous infusion and IVF with replacement of potassium. **Do not bolus insulin to start treatment**.
- Avoid overaggressive rehydration or lowering serum glucose too quickly; both can lead to cerebral edema.

COMPLICATIONS

Cerebral edema from overaggressive rehydration. Risk factors include low $Paco_2$ and high BUN on presentation, treatment with bicarbonate and intubation with hyperventilation to a $Paco_2$ lower than 22.

Inborn Errors of Metabolism

ORGANIC ACIDURIAS

Characterized by ketoacidosis and abnormal urinary excretion of organic acids; include MMA (methylmalonic acidemia), PPA (propionic acidemia), and IVA (isovaleric acidemia)

SYMPTOMS/EXAM

Symptoms are often detected on newborn screening. Infants may present with lethargy, vomiting, and poor feeding and growth.

DIAGNOSIS

Suspected cases should have plasma amino acids and urine organic acids sent.

- Anion gap metabolic acidosis
- Hypoglycemia
- Ketosis
- Mild hyperammonemia

TREATMENT

- Avoidance of protein
- Intravenous infusion of high dextrose-containing solution (such as D10) with addition of bicarbonate if acidotic
- IV carnitine (detoxifying agent)

UREA CYCLE DEFECTS

Characterized by hyperammonemia without significant acidosis. The most common form is OTC (ornithine transcarbamylase) deficiency.

SYMPTOMS/EXAM

Irritability and/or lethargy

DIAGNOSIS

- Elevated ammonium level
- Urine organic acid screen

TREATMENT

Protein restriction

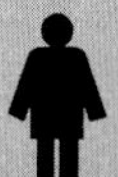

A 6-month-old infant presents in the morning to the ED with mild lethargy. The mother states that he has had a minor URI recently and has not fed since late last night. Laboratory evaluation reveals a glucose of 39; UA shows absent glucose and absent ketones. What is the likely diagnosis?

Fatty acid oxidation defect.

FATTY OXIDATION DISORDERS

Most common manifestation is nonketotic hypoglycemia, which usually occurs during a period of fasting or stress.

DIAGNOSIS

- Hypoglycemia
- Urinalysis, if obtained concomitantly, will show a lack of ketones, which is inappropriate in the setting of hypoglycemia.

TREATMENT

- Supportive
- Intravenous infusion of dextrose containing solution

GLYCOGEN STORAGE DISEASES

- Von-Gierke, Pompe, Forbes, Andersen, McArdle, and Hers Tarui
- Often have problems with hypoglycemia
- Many forms cause deposition in cardiac tissue leading to cardiomyopathy.

LYSOSOMAL STORAGE DISEASE

Mucopolysaccharidoses

- Hurler's, Hunter's, Sanfilippo, Morquio, Maroteaux-Lamy, and Sly
- Characterized by deposition in multiple organ systems causing characteristic coarse facial features, visceromegaly, and short stature
- Patients have a significantly increased risk of upper airway obstruction that often makes airway management and intubation challenging.

Lipodoses

- Gaucher, Niemann-Pick, Tay-Sachs, metachromatic leukodystrophy, Fabry, and Krabbe
- Characterized by various degrees of neurologic (hypotonia, optic atrophy), bony, and liver/spleen involvement (hepatosplenomegaly)

GASTROENTEROLOGY

Congenital Disorders

TRACHEOESOPHAGEAL FISTULA (TEF)

Tracheoesophageal fistula is the most common cause of esophageal obstruction in neonates. During embryonic development, the trachea and esophagus normally separate and develop in linear fashion. When a TEF is present, there is an abnormal communication between the trachea and the esophagus. The most common type of TEF (90%) results in the proximal esophagus terminating in a blind pouch, while the distal esophagus communicates with the trachea (see Figure 5.15).

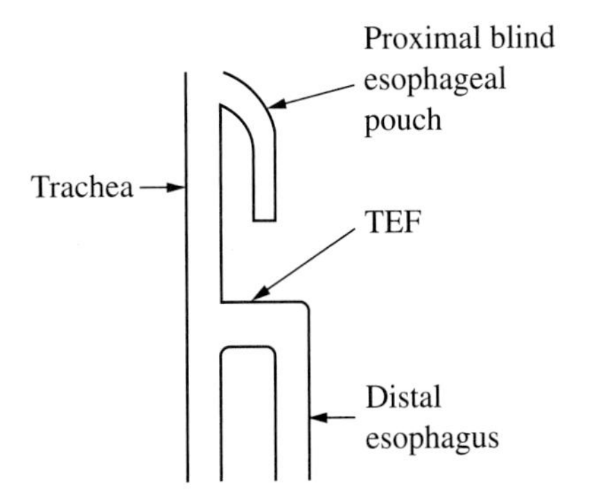

FIGURE 5.15. Most common type of TEF.

SYMPTOMS

- Respiratory distress
- Drooling, with difficulty handling oral secretions
- Nonbilious vomiting immediately after/during feeding

EXAM

Physical exam may be normal, or there may be associated abnormalities, including the **VATER complex**.

> ***The VATER complex:***
>
> **V**ertebral anomalies
> **A**nus (imperforate)
> **T**EF
> **R**enal defects

DIFFERENTIAL

Extensive differential diagnosis, including sepsis, gastroesophageal reflux, choanal atresia

DIAGNOSIS

Inability to pass an NGT into the stomach. The blind proximal esophageal pouch can often be demonstrated on plain radiographs by injecting a small amount of air into the catheter when the chest radiograph is taken. Surgical exploration confirms the diagnosis.

TREATMENT

- Fluid resuscitation
- Antibiotics to cover possible sepsis
- Surgical correction

COMPLICATIONS

Chemical pneumonitis can occur if gastric contents reflux into the distal esophagus, enter the TEF, and go into the lungs. Dehydration may also occur.

MALROTATION WITH VOLVULUS

During the first 3 months of gestation, there is normally a 270 degree counterclockwise rotation of the midgut, with subsequent fixation of the small bowel in the left upper quadrant (ligament of Treitz) and right lower quadrant. When malrotation occurs, the small bowel is not anchored in the LUQ or RLQ. Bands of tissue (Ladd's bands) form between the cecum and duodenum, potentially causing duodenal obstruction. Worse, the narrow vascular pedicle of the SMA is prone to clockwise volvulus of the midgut. Of patients with malrotation, 33% present with symptoms within the first week of life, 50% present within the first month, and 85% present within the first year. A number of congenital anomalies may be associated with malrotation, including:

- Diaphragmatic hernia
- Abdominal wall defects
- Duodenal atresia
- Hirschsprung disease
- Intussusception

SYMPTOMS/EXAM

Symptoms depend upon the degree of bowel obstruction. Most common presentation is that of intermittent duodenal obstruction at the site of the Ladd bands. Patients with intermittent duodenal obstruction typically will have:

- Abdominal pain
- Bilious emesis
- Abdominal distention
- Hematochezia

Bilious emesis in a neonate is malrotation until proven otherwise.

DIAGNOSIS

- Based on clinical suspicion
- Abdominal radiograph (AXR): No gas beyond the duodenum. The classical AXR for duodenal obstruction is the "double bubble" sign of air fluid level in the stomach and proximal duodenum.
- Upper GI series: Obstruction at the level of the duodenum, with ligament of Treitz present to the right of the vertebral column and a "corkscrew" appearance of the jejunum in the right upper quadrant (RUQ).
- Barium enema shows a mobile cecum present in the RUQ.

Classic AXR for duodenal obstruction: Double bubble sign.

TREATMENT

- IV fluid resuscitation
- IV antibiotics
- NGT to decompress proximal bowel
- Emergent surgical consultation

COMPLICATIONS

- Recurrent volvulus in 5–10%
- Short-gut syndrome if large portion of bowel resected

MECKEL'S DIVERTICULUM

Meckel's diverticulum is a short, blind pouch extending from the ileum, usually within 100 cm of the ileocecal valve. It may be lined with ectopic mucosa, such as gastric mucosa, which may ulcerate and bleed, leading to painless lower GI bleeding in children. In children, roughly 50% of lower GI bleeding is due to a Meckel's diverticulum. Fifty percent of cases will present by 1 year of age; 70% of cases by 2 years of age.

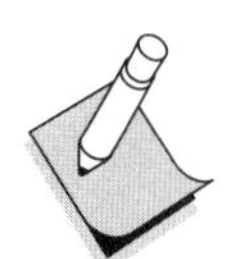

Rule of 2s for Meckel's diverticulum:
***2%** prevalence, **2**:1 male to female ratio, **2 feet** proximal to ileocecal valve and half of those symptomatic are under **2 years** old.*

SYMPTOMS/EXAM

- May be asymptomatic
- If the diverticulum ulcerates, the child may present with massive lower GI bleeding.

DIAGNOSIS

A labeled Technetium-99m scan (**Meckel scan**) may demonstrate the presence of ectopic gastric mucosa within the Meckel's diverticulum.

TREATMENT

If symptomatic, surgical excision is indicated.

COMPLICATIONS

- Massive lower GI bleeding, with resulting anemia and hemorrhagic shock
- Meckel's diverticulum can act as the lead point for intussusception.
- Perforation and peritonitis

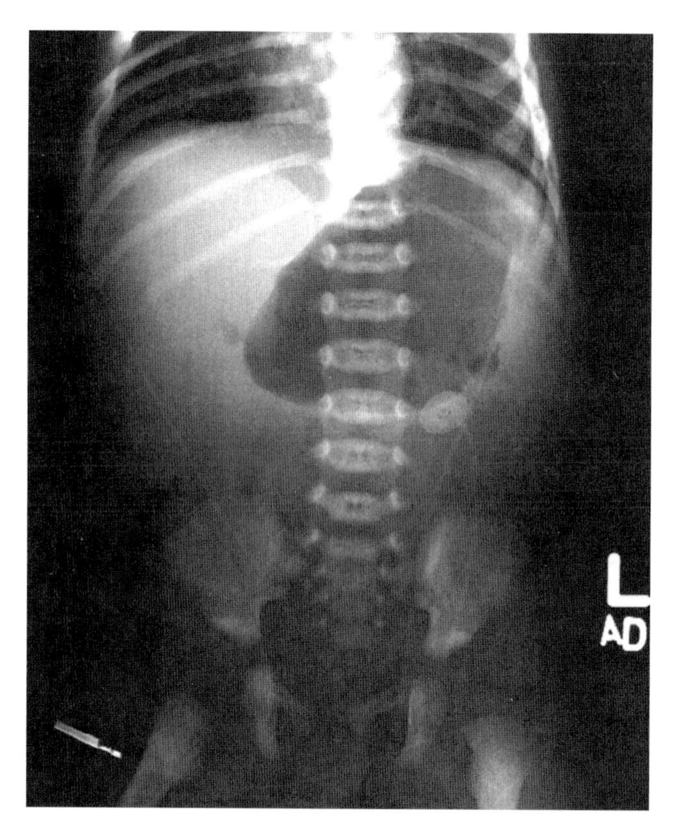

FIGURE 5.16. Malrotation with volvulus.

(Reproduced, with permission, from Brunicardi FC, Andersen DK, Billiar TR, et al. *Schwartz's Principles of Surgery*, 8th ed. New York; McGraw-Hill, 2005:1489.)

HIRSCHSPRUNG DISEASE

Patients with Hirschsprung disease have a segment of bowel that lacks normal ganglion cell innervation in the myenteric and submucosal tissue. The affected area always begins at the internal anal sphincter, and extends proximally for a variable distance. Eighty percent of patients have involvement only of the rectosigmoid bowel. Affected bowel rarely extends proximally past the splenic flexure. Ganglion cells normally oppose the tonic contractions of the bowel. Portions of bowel without ganglion cells have unopposed contraction, potentially leading to obstruction of the large bowel. Normally innervated bowel proximal to the obstruction becomes dilated. Males are affected more frequently than females (4:1).

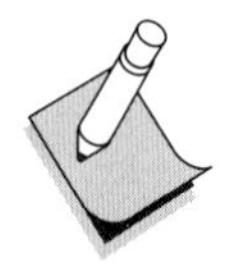

Toxic megacolon is the most feared complication of Hirschsprung disease and typically occurs in patients < 2 years old.

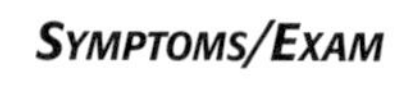

SYMPTOMS/EXAM

- Wide spectrum of disease, depending upon the length of involved bowel
- Symptoms typically develop in the first few days to weeks of life.
- The diagnosis should be considered in neonates who have delayed passage of meconium or failure to pass meconium.
- Hirschsprung disease may cause typical symptoms of colonic obstruction.
- Enterocolitis (toxic megacolon) is the most feared complication of Hirschsprung disease, and typically occurs in patients <2 years old.
- Older patients, who typically have a shorter segment of affected bowel, may present with abdominal distention, constipation, and failure to thrive.

DIAGNOSIS

- Barium enema may demonstrate a **cone-shaped transition zone** between the dilated proximal bowel and the abnormally contracted distal bowel.
- Anorectal manometry
- Rectal suction biopsy (gold standard)

TREATMENT

- Patients who are suspected of having Hirschsprung disease with enterocolitis or who have evidence of colonic obstruction should receive:
  - IV fluid
  - IV antibiotics
  - NG tube
  - Rectal tube
  - Emergent surgical consultation

COMPLICATIONS

- Failure to thrive
- Constipation
- Enterocolitis

Acquired Disorders

PYLORIC STENOSIS

Pyloric stenosis is the most common cause of gastric obstruction in infants. Typically, infants present with symptoms at 3–4 weeks of life, but may occur anytime up to 5 months of age. Because neonates do not develop symptoms until they are at least a week old, this condition is not thought to be truly congenital. The etiology of pyloric stenosis is unknown, but the end result is hypertrophy of the pyloric muscle with resulting gastric outlet obstruction. The incidence is roughly 1 in 500 live births, with males affected more than females (4:1). Caucasians are affected more than other groups, with an increased incidence in families.

SYMPTOMS

- **Nonbilious, projectile vomiting** that typically occurs after feedings
- Affected infants have a vigorous suck and appear hungry.

EXAM

Up to 90% of affected infants have a palpable mass ("**olive**") in the RUQ, although this finding may be difficult to elicit in an agitated infant.

DIAGNOSIS

- If the RUQ mass is detected, no imaging is indicated and surgical consultation should be obtained.
- If the diagnosis is less certain, an ultrasound should be obtained. Pyloric stenosis is confirmed if the ultrasound reveals a pylorus >4 mm thick and longer than 16 mm.
- If ultrasound is not available, an upper GI series will reveal a narrowed pylorus ("**tram-track sign**").

- If the infant has been vomiting for a few days, serum chemistries will reveal the classic hyponatremic, hypochloremic, hypokalemic metabolic alkalosis.

Treatment

- IV fluid resuscitation
- Electrolyte repletion
- Surgical consultation

Complications

- Weight loss
- Dehydration
- Electrolyte abnormalities

Necrotizing Enterocolitis (NEC)

NEC occurs due to bacterial overgrowth in the bowel, with translocation of bacteria into the bowel wall and the production of bacterial endotoxin and gas. A combination of factors is thought to predispose an infant to NEC, including:

- Prematurity
- Ischemia, with perfusion-reperfusion injury to the bowel
- Infection
- Introduction of parenteral feeding
- Reduced immune response

Infants typically develop NEC in the first few days of life, but NEC can appear as late as 1 month of age. The terminal ileum is affected most commonly, followed by the colon.

Symptoms/Exam

- Abdominal distention
- Nonbilious emesis
- Grossly bloody or guaiac positive stools
- Sepsis (lethargy, temperature instability, apnea, bradycardia)
- Abdominal wall erythema and firm loops of bowel (if bowel necrosis develops)

Diagnosis

- AXR radiograph may demonstrate **pneumatosis intestinalis** (gas in the wall of the bowel) or portal venous air (see Figure 5.17).
- Pneumoperitoneum may be present if perforation has occured.
- Labs: May see evidence of DIC (thrombocytopenia, elevated INR), hyponatremia, and metabolic acidosis

Treatment

- NPO
- IV fluid resuscitation
- IV antibiotics
- NG tube
- Surgical consultation; emergent bowel resection is required only if bowel is necrotic or perforated.

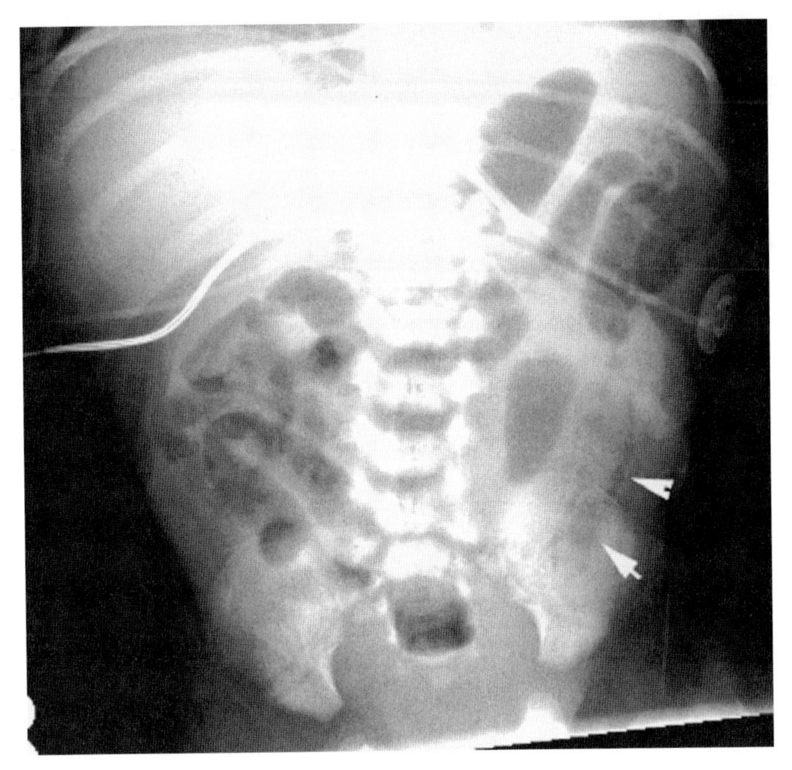

FIGURE 5.17. Necrotizing enterocolitis.

(Reproduced, with permission, from Brunicardi FC et al (eds). *Schwartz's Principles of Surgery*, 8th ed. New York: McGraw-Hill, 2005:1493.)

Complications

- Intestinal perforation
- Infants who recover from NEC may have bowel strictures, and postoperatively may develop short gut syndrome.

Intussusception

- Occurs when a proximal portion of bowel telescopes into a more distal portion, typically with the ileum inserting through the ileocecal valve
- Most common cause of bowel obstruction in infants between the ages of 3 and 12 months
- Peak incidence of intussusception is between the ages of 5 and 9 months, although intussusception may occur anytime from birth through childhood. In children >2 years old, an abnormal lead point such as a tumor, Meckel's diverticulum, or polyp is much more likely.
- Males are affected more frequently than females.

Symptoms

Classic triad:

- 85%, colicky abdominal pain
- 75%, vomiting
- 40%, rectal bleeding ("**currant jelly stools**" is a late finding due to sloughing of the bowel mucosa). Most cases of intussusception are diagnosed prior to bowel necrosis.

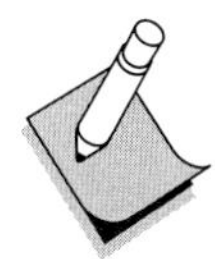

Currant jelly stools is a late finding of intussusception

EXAM

- Variable physical exam, ranging from well-appearing and asymptomatic to toxic and lethargic
- "**Dance's sign,**" which is reduced bowel gas in the RLQ may be appreciated (see Figure 5.18).

DIAGNOSIS

- AXR: Reduced bowel gas in the RLQ (radiographic "**Dance's sign**")
- Ultrasound is noninvasive and easily obtained.
- Contrast enema: May be therapeutic as well as diagnostic. The traditional teaching is for the surgeon to be present in the radiology suite when the enema is administered in case surgical intervention is required. Barium enemas are contraindicated if there is evidence of perforation or peritonitis; air- or water-soluble contrast may be used. Enemas may successfully reduce intussusception for 70–95% of patients. Air-contrast enema has become the method of choice because of the reduced risk of complications and higher success rate.

TREATMENT

- NG tube, IV fluids if dehydrated, NPO, and IV antibiotics
- Air contrast enema
- Surgical intervention is indicated if the contrast enema fails to reduce the intussusception or if intussusception recurs.

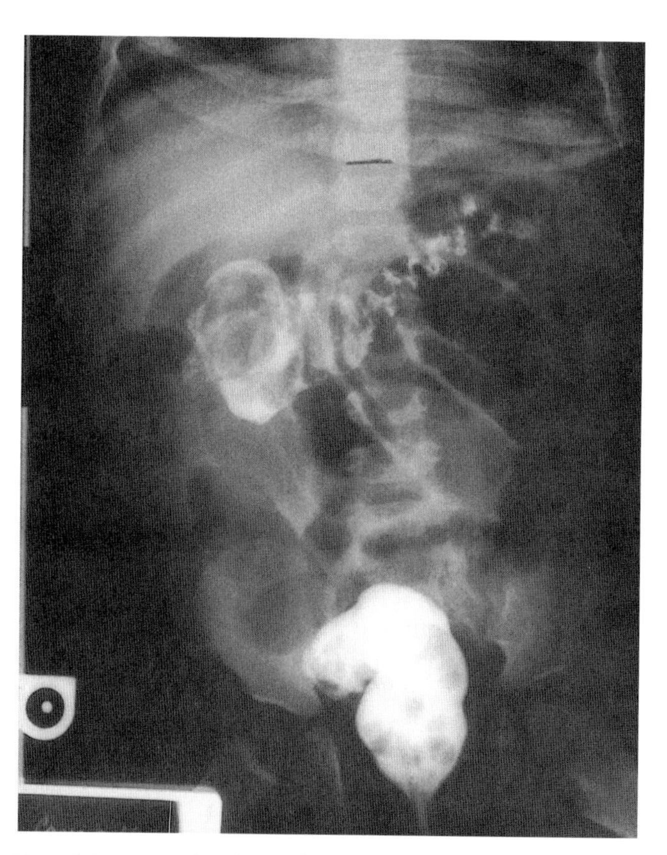

FIGURE 5.18. Intussusception (Dance's sign).

(Reproduced, with permission, from Shah BR, Lucchesi M. *Atlas of Pediatric Emergency Medicine*. New York: McGraw-Hill, 2006:431.)

COMPLICATIONS

- Bowel perforation
- Peritonitis

GENITOURINARY

Wilm's Tumor

The most common renal tumor in children, with a peak incidence at 3–4 years of age (98% occur before age seven). It may be congenital or acquired.

SYMPTOMS/EXAM

- Abdominal mass, with or without abdominal pain
- Hematuria (25%)
- Hypertension (25%)
- Congenital **W**ilm's tumor is associated with **A**niridia, **GU** anomalies, and mental **R**etardation (WAGR syndrome).

DIAGNOSIS

- CT abdomen and chest

TREATMENT

- Surgical excision
- Adjuvant chemotherapy, sometimes with addition of radiation

COMPLICATIONS

- Metastatic spread of tumor
- Recurrent disease after treatment

Urinary Tract Infection

The term UTI includes lower tract infections of the urethra and bladder (urethritis or cystitis), and upper tract infections of the kidney (pyelonephritis). Most UTIs are due to ascending infection of enteric bacteria, although occasionally a child with bacteremia may directly seed the kidney, resulting in pyelonephritis. Infants are most likely to become infected by group B streptococcus. UTIs in all other pediatric age groups are most commonly caused by *E. coli*. The overall incidence of UTIs before puberty is 3% of girls, and 1% of boys. **There is a higher incidence of UTI in Caucasians, infants, and uncircumcised males.**

SYMPTOMS/EXAM

- Depends upon the age of the child and severity of infection
- Among infants, the presentation may be subtle, with poor feeding, dehydration, and increased crying. Fever may be present, particularly in infants with pyelonephritis.
- In older children:
  - Dysuria and frequency, fever and flank pain if development of pyelonephritis

Diagnosis

The diagnosis of UTI depends upon obtaining an appropriate sample. **In children under the age of two, the bladder should be catheterized.**

- + Nitrite
- Moderate (or greater) leukocyte esterase
- + Gram stain for bacteria
- >10 WBC/hpf
- If there is a clinical suspicion for UTI, a urine culture should be obtained.

Treatment

- Septic children or infants: Admit for IV antibiotics
- Mild infection (cystitis): Consider oral antibiotics with close follow-up
- Children <3 years old with the first UTI should receive radiographic evaluation for vesicoureteral reflux, and for structural abnormalities of the kidneys and ureters.
  - Renal ultrasound
  - Voiding cystourethrogram (VCUG)
  - Patients with reflux or pyelonephritis should have a nuclear medicine study with dimercaptosuccinate (DMSA) to evaluate for renal scarring.
  - Children with reflux should receive prophylactic antibiotics, and have close follow-up with a pediatric urologist. Surgery may be required to correct VUR.

Complications

- Reflux is present in up to 50% of infants who have a UTI.
- Children with reflux are at risk for renal damage, resulting in chronic renal insufficiency, and an increased risk of hypertension.

Hydrocele

A hydrocele is a collection of fluid around the testicle. There are three categories of hydroceles:

1. **1° hydrocele**: Infants born with excess fluid in scrotum—typically resolves spontaneously by 1 year of age; not significant
2. **2° hydrocele**: Reactive fluid collection within scrotum due to infection, trauma, testicular torsion, or tumor
3. **Communicating hydrocele**: Fluid collection due to the presence of an indirect inguinal hernia, which allows fluid to communicate between the peritoneum and scrotum

Symptoms/Exam

- **1° hydrocele**: Nontender fluid collection in scrotum, typically transilluminates
- **2° hydrocele**: Hydrocele may be an incidental finding in the setting of infection, trauma, testicular torsion, or tumor.
- **Communicating hydrocele (indirect hernia)**: Typically nontender, with size of hydrocele increasing during the course of the day, and resolving after the child has been lying flat (gravity draws fluid back into peritoneum)

Differential

- Incarcerated inguinal hernia
- Testicular torsion

- Infection (epididymitis, orchitis)
- Testicular trauma
- Testicular tumor

DIAGNOSIS

A scrotal mass that transilluminates does not rule out an incarcerated inguinal hernia.

Hydroceles can usually be diagnosed clinically. Occasionally, a testicular ultrasound may be required to rule out other diagnostic possibilities. If there is clinical concern for incarcerated inguinal hernia, a pediatric surgeon should be emergently consulted.

TREATMENT

- **1° hydrocele**: Observation only. If a 1° hydrocele persists beyond 2 years of age, consider referral to a pediatric surgeon for a possible communicating hydrocele.
- **2° hydrocele**: Management of the underlying process
- **Indirect hernia**: Referral to a pediatric surgeon for evaluation of a presumed indirect inguinal hernia

COMPLICATIONS

- **2° hydrocele**: Progression of underlying process
- **Indirect hernia**: Incarceration of bowel loop

Hemolytic Uremic Syndrome

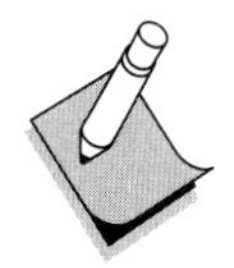

HUS triad:

1. *Microangiopathic hemolytic anemia*
2. *Thrombocytopenia*
3. *Renal insufficiency*

HUS is the leading cause of renal failure in children in the United States. 90% of patients with HUS have diarrhea, most often caused by **enterohemorrhagic *E. coli* of the 0157:H7 serotype** (produces a shiga toxin causing hemorrhagic colitis). Peak age is 9 months to 4 years.

SYMPTOMS/EXAM

- Prodrome of a abdominal pain, bloody diarrhea
- HUS develops 2–14 days after start of diarrhea
- Pallor with petechial or purpural rash
- Decreased urinary output
- CNS symptoms (minority of patient): stroke, seizures, coma

DIAGNOSIS

- Anemia, thrombocytopenia
- Elevated creatinine, possible hyperkalemia
- Elevated indirect bilirubin (due to hemolysis)
- Hematuria often present
- Stool culture confirms presence of 0157:H7 *E. coli*.

TREATMENT

- **Avoid antibiotics and antidiarrheal agents in children who have hemorrhagic diarrhea** (both agents may increase subsequent risk of developing HUS).

- Supportive care
- Consider PRBC transfusion if hemoglobin < 6 g/dL.
- Avoid platelet transfusion unless active bleeding or a surgical procedure is required.
- Plasma exchange, if CNS symptoms

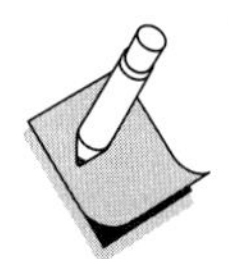

Avoid antibiotics and antidiarrheal agents in children who have hemorrhagic diarrhea; they increase risk of HUS!

Complications

- About 40–50% of children with HUS develop renal failure and require dialysis (with up to 70% of those who require dialysis eventually recovering normal renal function).
- About 15–20% have seizure or coma.
- Mortality 3–5%

IMMUNOLOGY

Juvenile Rheumatoid Arthritis

The term JRA encompasses a variety of conditions (see Table 5.6), which all share the common feature of joint pain lasting longer than 6 weeks. Affected joints are painful, swollen, stiff, warm to the touch, often have reduced range of motion, and may be erythematous. The etiology of JRA is unknown, with possible connections to antecedent viral infections or related to host immune characteristics.

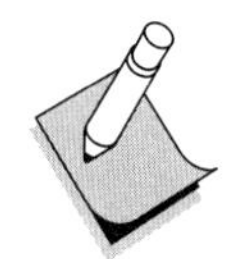

JRA is the most common form of arthritis in children.

Symptoms/Exam

Variable, often with at least some of the following:

- Warm, swollen joint
- Morning stiffness that improves with activity
- Increased pain after periods of rest
- Low-grade fever
- Fatigue
- Anorexia and weight loss

Systemic onset JRA typically includes some combination of the following symptoms:

- Daily, spiking fever
- Rash (transient macules on torso, proximal extremities)

TABLE 5.6. Types of JRA

	Number of Joints	Systemic Symptoms	Age at Onset	Sex	ANA
Polyarticular onset	Usually ≥5	Mild or symmetric	Early–late moderate childhood	♀ > ♂	Positive 25%
Pauciarticular onset	<5; mostly knees, ankles, elbows	Iridocyclitis (anterior uveitis)	Early childhood	♀ > ♂	Positive 60%
Systemic onset	Variable	See text	Any age	♂ > ♀	Negative

- Hepatosplenomegaly
- Lymphadenopathy
- Pleuritis or pericarditis
- Rarely: Myocarditis, hepatitis, DIC

Differential

- Infection: Septic arthritis, osteomyelitis, Lyme disease
- Malignancy: Either systemic (such as leukemia) or bone
- Trauma
- Orthopedic conditions: Slipped capital femoral epiphysis (SCFE), Osgood-Schlatter disease, Legg-Calvé-Perthe's disease
- Avascular necrosis

Diagnosis

Diagnosis of JRA requires eliminating alternative etiologies. Serum or synovial fluid analysis may support the diagnosis of JRA, but no studies are pathognomonic.

- Anemia
- Leukocytosis
- Thrombocytosis
- Elevated ESR, c-reactive protein (CRP)
- Synovial fluid: WBC 10,000–100,000/mm^3, low glucose

Treatment

- Treatment options are limited.
- NSAIDs are most often prescribed.
- Rest, physical therapy, and occupational therapy may also be important.
- For patients with pauciarticular disease, regular slitlamp examinations are important to detect the onset of iridocyclitis (anterior uveitis) and begin specific therapy before vision is compromised.
- Adjunctive therapies, including systemic steroids, hydroxychloroquine, methotrexate, and oral gold should generally not be prescribed through the ED without the involvement of a pediatric rheumatologist.

Complications

- Deformity of limbs and joints in a minority of patients with JRA
- Growth disturbances of limbs
- Recurrent arthritis
- Blindness may develop in patients with iridocyclitis if treatment is not started promptly.

Henoch-Schönlein Purpura

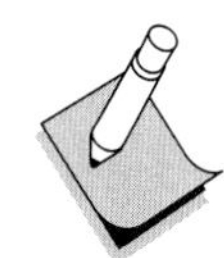

Triad of symptoms for HSP: Purpura, abdominal pain, arthritis

- HSP is an **acute, systemic vasculitis**, primarily affecting venules and arterioles.
- Etiology is unknown, but may be due to the host response to an infection (such as strep pharyngitis, varicella, or mycoplasma).
- Typically affects children 3–7 years of age, with males affected more frequently than females (2:1)
- Symptoms typically last 4–6 weeks, with 50% of patients having recurrent symptoms usually within weeks of the initial diagnosis.

SYMPTOMS/EXAM

- Rash: Palpable purpura, usually starting on lower extremities and progressing toward the torso (see Figure 5.19)
- Crampy abdominal pain
- Arthritis, usually periarticular and most often affecting the knees
- Hematuria
- Additional symptoms can include: Nonpitting edema of the extremities and face, melena, hematemesis, fever, hepatomegaly, headache, seizures

DIFFERENTIAL

- Abdominal pain can mimic acute appendicitis.
- Rash: Consider meningococcal sepsis, bleeding disorder or drug reaction.
- Arthritis: JRA or SLE

DIAGNOSIS

- Lab tests supporting the diagnosis of HSP include
  - Elevated WBC
  - Anemia
  - Elevated ESR
  - Hematuria
- Abdominal CT may reveal the "thumbprinting" of submucosal hemorrhage.

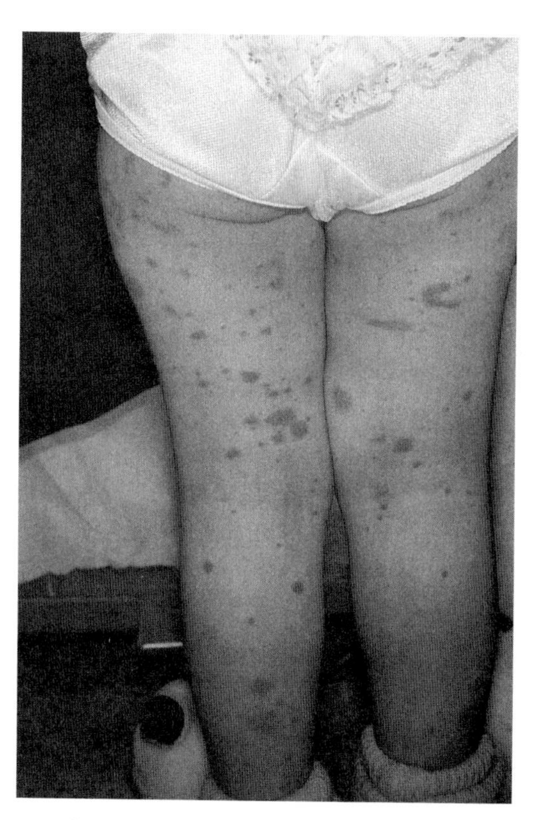

FIGURE 5.19. Henoch-Schönlein purpura. (See also color insert.)

(Reproduced, with permission, from Shah BR, Lucchesi M. *Atlas of Pediatric Emergency Medicine*. New York: McGraw-Hill, 2006:109.)

TREATMENT

- Treatment is mostly supportive, and can include IVF if dehydrated.
- Most patients diagnosed with HSP in the ED can be discharged to home with follow-up through their PMD.
- Patients who have severe abdominal pain or GI bleeding should be admitted.
- Steroids may reduce incidence of intussusception.
- No known therapy is available to prevent renal complications.

COMPLICATIONS

- Intussusception due to lead point caused by edema or hemorrhage into bowel wall
- Nephrotic syndrome with chronic renal disease
- Uncommon complications include: Bowel perforation, pancreatitis, hypertension.

Kawasaki Syndrome

- Kawasaki syndrome is a self-limited, acute vasculitis that affects arterioles, venules, and capillaries throughout the body.
- **It is the leading cause of acquired heart disease in children in the United States.**
- Peak incidence is between the ages of 18 and 24 months, with the majority of patinets <4 years old and boys affected more frequently than girls.
- Etiology is unknown, but may involve either an infectious agent or the host immune response to infection.

SYMPTOMS/EXAM

There are three phases to Kawasaki syndrome (see Table 5.7).

DIFFERENTIAL

- Infections (viral, bacterial, or rickettsial)
- Toxic shock syndrome
- Stevens Johnson syndrome
- Rheumatologic conditions, such as JRA

DIAGNOSIS

Based on a series of criteria (see Table 5.8). Kawasaki syndrome should be entertained, however, for children who have a prolonged, unexplained fever that does not respond to antibiotics—not all patients who have Kawasaki syndrome may actually meet the diagnostic criteria.

TREATMENT

- Hospitalize.
- If Kawasaki syndrome is confidently diagnosed, start IVIG (intravenous gamma globulin) and high-dose aspirin.

TABLE 5.7. Phases of Kawasaki Syndrome

Acute Phase (1–2 wk)

- Fever
- Lymphadenopathy (usually anterior cervical)
- Conjunctivitis (bilateral, painless, without exudate)
- Oropharynx: Cracked lips, **"strawberry tongue"** (prominent papillae on tongue), pharyngeal erythema
- Rash on perineum, often progressing to torso
- Erythema/edema of hands and feet
- Vasculitis may affect virtually any organ system: Pneumonitis, myocarditis, enteritis, meatitis, hepatitis, uveitis.

Subacute Phase (2–4 wk)

- Thrombocytosis (platelets up to 500,000–1,000,000/mm^3)
- Resolution of fever
- Desquamation of hands and feet

Convalescent Phase (>2 mo)

- Scarring and calcification of affected coronary arteries

Complications

- **Aneurysms of coronary arteries** develop in 20% of patients who are untreated. Patients at highest risk are male, <1 year old, and with the greatest degree of inflammation.
- Hydrops of gallbladder
- Mortality <1% for children in the United States.

Rheumatic Fever

- Mediated by the host immune response to a preceding group A strep infection
- Affected patients are typically school age
- Symptoms develop 2–3 weeks after a strep infection, with target organs including heart, joints, CNS, and skin.

TABLE 5.8. Diagnostic Criteria for Kawasaki Syndrome

Fever = 5 days, **and** four out of five of the following criteria:

1. Bilateral conjunctivitis
2. Oropharyngeal changes (fissuring of lips, "strawberry tongue," erythema of lips of pharynx)
3. Changes to skin on hands/feet (erythema → desquamation)
4. Rash on torso
5. Cervical lymphadenopathy (at least one lymph node greater in size than 1.5 cm)

And no other diagnosis to explain symptoms.

SYMPTOMS/EXAM

Variable, depending upon which organ systems are affected

- Carditis causing damage to mitral or aortic valves, resulting in valvular insufficiency
  - Mitral regurgitation murmur: Holosystolic at apex
  - Aortic regurgitation murmur: Diastolic at base
- Arthritis, typically affecting >5 joints
- Sydenham's chorea due to CNS involvement
- Erythema marginatum (serpiginous, evanescent rash that typically spares the face)
- Subcutaneous nodules (pea-sized bumps on the extensor surfaces of extremities)

DIFFERENTIAL

- JRA
- Septic arthritis
- Kawasaki syndrome
- Myocarditis/pericarditis
- SLE
- Serum sickness
- Henoch-Schönlein purpura

> ***JONES criteria for diagnosis of rheumatic Fever–***
>
> **J**oints
> **O**h, no—carditis!
> **N**odules
> **E**rythema marginatum
> **S**ydenham's chorea

DIAGNOSIS

The JONES criteria (see Table 5.9) are used to confirm the diagnosis.

- Routine labs should include CBC, ESR, antistreptolysin titers (ASO), ECG, CXR, cardiac ECHO.

TABLE 5.9. 1992 JONES Criteria

1. Evidence of preceding group A streptococcus infection: ▪ Elevated or rising ASO titer, or ▪ +Throat culture, or ▪ +Rapid antigen test
AND
2. Either two major manifestations, or one major and two minor manifestations: *Major manifestations:* ▪ Carditis ▪ Polyarthritis ▪ Sydenham's chorea ▪ Erythema marginatum ▪ Subcutaneous nodules *Minor manifestations:* ▪ Arthralgia ▪ Fever ▪ Elevated ESR or CRP ▪ Prolonged PR interval on ECG

Treatment

- Primary prevention of rheumatic fever: Treat strep pharyngitis with antibiotics within 9 days of symptom onset.
- Secondary treatment once rheumatic fever is diagnosed
  - High-dose aspirin
  - Antibiotics to treat residual strep infection

Complications

- Damage to heart valves
- Recurrent episodes of acute rheumatic fever

INFECTIOUS DISEASES

Fever in Children <3 Years Old

In general, fever is defined as a rectal temp 38.0°C (100.4°F). Oral and axillary temps are typically 0.6°C (1.0°F) and 1.1°C (2.0°F) lower than rectal temps, respectively. Serious bacterial infection (SBI) includes bacteremia, meningitis, urinary tract infection, bacterial pneumonia, or bacterial gastroenteritis. In general, the workup for fever is determined by age at presentation in conjunction with other factors such as underlying medical conditions (eg, cancer, immunosuppression) and coexisting factors (eg, immunization status).

Low-risk criteria have been proposed for febrile infants <8 weeks (see Table 5.10).

TABLE 5.10. Rochester Criteria and Philadelphia Protocol Low-Risk Criteria

Rochester Criteria	Philadelphia Protocol
Infant appears generally well. Infant has been previously well. ▪ Born at term (> 37 wk gestation) ▪ No antibiotics perinatal ▪ No unexplained hyperbilirubinemia ▪ No previous antimicrobial therapy ▪ No previous hospitalization ▪ No chronic or underlying illness ▪ Not hospitalized longer than mother No evidence of skin, soft tissue, bone, joint, or ear infection Laboratory values: ▪ WBC 5000–15,000/mm³ ▪ Absolute band count ≤ 15,000/mm³ ▪ WBC ≤ 10/hpf on microscopic exam of spun urine ▪ WBC ≤ 5/hpf on microscopic exam of a stool smear (for infants with diarrhea)	Infants >28 days old Infant Observation Score ≤10 No recognizable bacterial infection on exam Laboratory values: ▪ WBC < 15,000/mm³ ▪ Band-to-neutrophil ratio <0.2 ▪ WBC ≤ 10/hpf on microscopic exam of spun urine ▪ WBC ≤ 8/hpf and Gram negative stain in a nonbloody CSF specimen No evidence of a discrete infiltrate on CXR as determined by an attending physician Stool smear negative for blood and few or no WBCs (for infants with diarrhea)

FEVER 0 TO 28 DAYS

Most common causative organisms of SBI in this age range are reflective of maternal vaginal flora: Group B streptococcus, enteric Gram-negative bacilli (especially *E. coli*), *Listeria monocytogenes*, herpes virus.

Remember—full sepsis w/u, empiric antibiotics, and admission for all febrile infants 0 to 28 days old

SYMPTOMS/EXAM

- Workup in this age range is based on the premise that SBI can be present in the absence of significant historical or physical exam findings other than fever.

DIAGNOSIS

- All patients should have a CBC with differential, blood culture, catheter UA, urine culture, and LP.
- CXR should be considered in those with any respiratory symptoms.
- Stool for WBC and culture should be considered for those with diarrhea.
- Consider testing for HSV if any signs suggestive of disseminated HSV (vesicular rash, bloody LP not attributable to traumatic LP, significantly elevated transaminases), or if mom has history of HSV (especially if vaginal delivery with active lesions).

TREATMENT

- Empiric intravenous antibiotics with ampicillin plus cefotaxime (gentamicin is an alternative) and hospitalization
- IV acyclovir should be started immediately for those in whom HSV is suspected.

FEVER 29 TO 90 DAYS

Most common causative organisms in this age range are: Pneumococci, meningococci, *Hemophilus influenza*.

SYMPTOMS/EXAM

Improved developmental skills and maturing immune system allow more reliance on physical exam findings; nonetheless, infants with SBI in this range can still present with overall "well appearance."

DIAGNOSIS

Well-appearing infants without focus for infection usually only need a limited workup to include CBC with differential, blood culture, catheter UA, and urine culture.

TREATMENT

- Infants at "low risk" of SBI with WBC 5000–15,000/mm^3, band/neutrophil ratio <0.2, normal UA, and reliable caretaker can be discharged home for close outpatient follow-up.
- Infants not meeting low-risk criteria should have lumbar puncture done to complete the sepsis workup with strong consideration of empiric antibiotic coverage (ceftriaxone as single agent) and hospital admission.

FEVER 3 MONTHS TO 3 YEARS

Children with commonly recognized viral syndromes (eg, bronchiolitis, stomatitis, croup) in this age range are unlikely to have SBIs.

Symptoms/Exam

- Physical exam findings and historical clues are usually more reliable in pinpointing the diagnosis in this age range. The ED workup and treatment are usually directed toward clinically recognizable syndromes (eg, pneumonia, cellulitis, scarlet fever).
- Immunization status is extremely important to note.

Diagnosis

- Children with focal infections, eg, otitis media, cellulitis, should have workup and treatment directed as appropriate.
- Children without focal findings or helpful historical clues should have further workup:
  - CBC with differential
  - Blood culture for those with WBC <5000 or >15,000
  - UA and urine culture for females <2 years, circumcised males <6 months or uncircumcised males <12 months
  - Consider LP for those with signs of meningitis (nuchal rigidity, + Kernig's, or + Brudzinski's signs) or excessive irritability (especially if paradoxical) or toxic appearance
  - CXR for those with physical exam findings suggestive of pneumonia (mild hypoxia or tachypnea out of proportion to fever may be only clues)

Treatment

- Therapy directed at the likely causative organisms
- Patients who are well appearing but do not have a focus for infection can generally be followed as outpatients. Those with an elevated WBC >15,000 or incomplete immunization status should usually be given a single dose of IM ceftriaxone with close follow-up pending culture results.

Pediatric Exanthems

Measles

Measles is caused by an RNA virus in the Paramyxoviridae family. Humans are only known natural hosts.

TABLE 5.11. Buzzwords for Pediatric Exanthems

Buzzwords	Disease
"Cough, coryza, conjunctivitis"; Koplik's spots	Measles
"Slapped cheek rash"; aplastic crisis	Fifth disease; parvovirus B19
Tender postauricular lymphadenopathy	Rubella
Onset of rash occurs with resolution of fevers	Roseola; HHV-6
"Dewdrops on a rose petal"	Varicella
Macules, papules, vesicles on hands and feet, and posterior oropharynx	Hand-foot-mouth disease; coxsackievirus

SYMPTOMS/EXAM

- Usually ill appearing with high fevers (up to 104°F) and malaise
- Rapid progression to coryza, cough, and conjunctivitis
- Maculopapular rash characteristically starts on upper body and progresses downward, becoming coalescent (see Figure 5.7).
- Associated enanthem: Fine white spots on erythematous background (**Koplik's spots**) appear on buccal mucosa (see Figure 5.8).

DIAGNOSIS

- Clinical diagnosis
- Confirmation is suggested by testing serum for IgM antibody (detectable for 1 month after rash onset) or viral cultures of urine, blood, throat, or nasopharyngeal specimens.

TREATMENT

- Supportive care is indicated. Vitamin A supplementation in select cases may be associated with decreased morbidity and mortality.

COMPLICATIONS

- Most common bacterial complication is acute purulent otitis media.
- Bronchopneumonia, croup, diarrhea, acute encephalitis, and SSPE (subacute sclerosing panencephalitis)

RUBELLA

Rubella is also known as German measles. Caused by a togavirus, it is an important cause of congenital infection.

SYMPTOMS

Typically associated with a rash that begins on the face and spreads downward on the body (see Figure 5.9)

EXAM

- **Tender lymphadenopathy** is common.
- Low-grade fevers < 39.0°C are common during the first few days.

DIAGNOSIS

- Clinical diagnosis
- Serologic confirmation only in select cases (eg, pregnant adolescent patient)

TREATMENT

Supportive care and antipyretics

ERYTHEMA INFECTIOSUM (FIFTH DISEASE)

Causative agent is parvovirus B19

SYMPTOMS/EXAM

- Characteristic "**slapped cheek**" rash, with progression to a lacy maculopapular rash (often pruritic) starting on the upper extremities and then generalizing (see Figure 5.11)
- Usually afebrile
- Arthralgias and arthritis occur in only 10% of children but commonly occur in adults.

DIAGNOSIS

- Clinical diagnosis
- Serologic confirmation only in select cases

TREATMENT

Supportive care

COMPLICATIONS

Aplastic crisis can occur in patients with chronic hemolytic anemias, sickle cell disease, or HIV infection.

ROSEOLA INFANTUM (EXANTHEM SUBITUM)

Caused by HHV-6 (human herpesvirus 6)

SYMPTOMS/EXAM

- Rapid onset of high fever (often up to 104.9°F) in an otherwise well-appearing child with few symptoms
- After 2–4 days of fever, the child becomes afebrile.
- Rash usually appears after fever resolves.
- Typical rash consisting of discrete, small, blanching maculopapules appears starting on the trunk and spreading to the periphery (see Figure 5.10).

TREATMENT

Supportive care and antipyretics

VARICELLA CHICKENPOX

Varicella chickenpox is a herpes virus infection. The reactivation syndrome is known as zoster (shingles, herpes zoster).

SYMPTOMS/EXAM

- Low-grade fevers <39°F for the first few days, but may be afebrile
- Characteristic pruritic rash starts on the trunk and spreads to extremities. The rash begins as papules, which evolve into vesicles on an erythematous base ("**dewdrops on a rose petal**") and pustules over the course of 6–8 hours, with new crops occurring every 2–4 days (see Figure 5.12).

DIAGNOSIS

Clinical diagnosis, although varicella virus can be recovered from vesicular lesions

TREATMENT

- Primarily supportive, with antihistamines
- Oral acyclovir can be considered for young infants <6 months, children on oral/inhaled steroids, children presenting within 24 hours of onset of rash or high fevers.
- Immunosuppressed children require IV acyclovir and hospitalization.

COMPLICATIONS

Rare but may include encephalitis, pneumonia, hepatitis, bacterial superinfection, Reye's syndrome, and group A streptococcal sepsis or necrotizing fasciitis

Other Common Pediatric Infections Presenting to the ED

HAND-FOOT-MOUTH DISEASE

- Causative agent is coxsackievirus A16
- Transmission by fecal-oral route
- Peak incidence summer and early fall

SYMPTOMS/EXAM

Brief prodrome of low-grade fever, pharyngitis, and malaise followed in 24–48 hours by oral ulcers (usually posterior pharyngeal) and erythematous macular and/or vesicular rash occurring predominantly on the palms and soles

DIAGNOSIS

Clinical diagnosis; termed herpangina if only oral lesions are present

TREATMENT

Supportive care

MUMPS

Caused by an RNA virus in the Paramyxoviridae family; humans are only known natural hosts

SYMPTOMS/EXAM

- Painful swelling of one or more salivary glands (parotid most commonly)
- Fever
- Weakness and fatigue

DIAGNOSIS

- Clinical diagnosis
- Diagnosis is confirmed by viral culture of throat washing, saliva, spinal fluid, or urine, or by serologic testing (IgM antibody, or acute and convalescent sera for IgG)

TREATMENT

Supportive

COMPLICATIONS

Rare, but include orchtis pancreatitis, encephalitis, meningitis

PINWORMS

- Caused by *Enterobius vermicularis* (a nematode/roundworm)
- Humans only natural hosts; passed on as fomites, eg, from inorganic material such as clothing and fecal-oral route

SYMPTOMS/EXAM

Anal and/or vulvar pruritis

DIAGNOSIS

- **Tape test** (application of transparent adhesive tape to perianal skin, exam under microscope for eggs, highest yield with three consecutive specimens taken on first awakening in the morning)
- Occasionally direct visualization of worms, usually 2–3 hours after child goes to sleep

TREATMENT

- Children >2 years of age: Mebendazole single dose, repeated in 2 weeks
- All family members and close contacts should be treated empirically.

SCABIES

Caused by *Sarcoptes scabiei* mite

SYMPTOMS/EXAM

- Intense pruritis with erythematous, papular rash (especially in finger webs, wrists, axillae) caused by burrowing of adult female mites in the upper layers of epidermis
- Younger children and infants differ from older children and adults in that the rash is often vesicular and can affect areas usually spared in older children (eg, head, neck, palms, soles) due to a hypersensitivity reaction to the parasite.

DIAGNOSIS

- Clinical; mite is not visible to naked eye
- Can be confirmed by microscopic identification of the mite or eggs (mineral oil scrapings of burrows placed on a slide and examined under low power)

TREATMENT

- Topical 5% permethrin cream applied from neck down, washed off in 8–12 hours; reapplication in 7 days recommended
- Decontamination of bedding, clothing, bath towels, and similar items is needed as well.

HEAD LICE

Caused by head louse (*Pediculosis humanus capitis*)

SYMPTOMS/EXAM

Patients typically present with pruritis. Nits (eggs) are typically found close to the scalp, firmly adherent to hair.

DIFFERENTIAL

Clinical diagnosis

DIAGNOSIS

Clinical diagnosis

TREATMENT

- Initial therapy with over the counter 1% permethrin, applied to scalp and hair for 10 minutes after washing and towel drying. Second application 1 week later is often recommended.
- For treatment failure, malathion (0.5%) is recommended for children ≥6 years, applied to dry hair as 8- to 10-hour application; lindane 1% shampoo can also be used in older children as second line but carries risk of potential CNS toxicity that has occasionally led to seizures and death

NEUROLOGY

Febrile Seizures

Febrile seizures may occur in the setting of fever, but are not due to a 1° infection or disturbance of the brain (see Table 5.12).

- Febrile seizures are common, with 2–4% of children affected between the ages of 3 months to 5 years.
- Peak incidence is 2 years of age.
- Children who have very high fevers or who have a family history of febrile seizures are at greatest risk for developing febrile seizures.
- A careful, detailed history is essential, including a history of recent illness, trauma, medication exposure, or immunizations.

TABLE 5.12. Types of Febrile Seizures

	NUMBER OF SEIZURES	DURATION	TYPE OF SEIZURE
Simple febrile seizure	One	<15 min	Generalized tonic-clonic
Complex febrile seizure	>1 in 24 hours	>15 min	Focal

SYMPTOMS/EXAM

- May be postictal
- Febrile seizures usually occur early in the course of a febrile illness, so no specific signs or symptoms of infection may be found. Sometimes patients may have a clear source of infection, such as URI, pharyngitis, or otitis media.
- Signs not consistent with febrile seizures include: Bulging fontanelle, petechiae, meningismus, and unusually large head circumference (in infants).

Have a low threshold for performing an LP to exclude meningitis, particularly in younger children or those already taking antibiotics.

DIFFERENTIAL

- CNS infection (meningitis, encephalitis)
- Head trauma
- Medication exposure (intentional or accidental)
- Hypoglycemia
- Dehydration leading to electrolyte abnormalities
- Other infections associated with seizures (*Shigella*, roseola)

DIAGNOSIS

The diagnosis of febrile seizures is a clinical one, with additional studies used to exclude other causes of seizures. Serum glucose should be checked in all children suspected of having a febrile seizure. If the history supports possible dehydration, serum electrolytes should also be checked. Additional serum studies, blood cultures, and urine studies should be sent if there is concern for SBI. Routine CT or MRI of the brain is not indicated to rule in febrile seizures, but may be useful if there is concern for other causes of seizure. Routine EEG is not indicated.

TREATMENT

Actively seizing:

- Stabilize airway.
- Lorazepam 0.05–0.1 mg/kg IV (max dose 2 mg)

Postictal:

- Observe for 2–4 hours, and discharge when mental status normal.
- Reassure parents about benign nature of febrile seizure.
- Educate parents: Up to 15% of children will have a recurrent febrile seizure within 24 hours of the initial seizure.
- Follow-up with pediatrician
- Consider admission if child required lorazepam, diagnosis is unclear, social situation for child is unstable, or follow-up is not available.

COMPLICATIONS

- 33% of children will have recurrent febrile seizures.
- 75% of recurrent febrile seizures occur <1 year after initial febrile seizure.
- Epilepsy (recurrent seizures not associated with fever) rarely develops in children with febrile seizures: <2% of children who have a febrile seizure will develop epilepsy. Children with complex febrile seizures are at greater risk for developing epilepsy.

Neonatal Seizures

Neonatal seizures are rarely idiopathic, and usually signify serious neurologic disease. Additionally, persistent or prolonged seizures may damage the developing brain. Incidence of neonatal seizures is 0.5% in term infants, but can be up to 20% in premature infants.

Neonatal seizures usually signify serious neurological disease. They rarely present with generalized tonic-clonic movement.

Symptoms/Exam

Generalized tonic-clonic seizures are uncommon in infants. Neonatal seizures may present with autonomic dysfunction (tachycardia, apnea), or repetitive movements of the eyes, mouth, face, or extremities.

Differential

Tremor, myoclonus, or agitation from maternal narcotic withdrawal may mimic seizure activity. Causes of neonatal seizures include:

- Hypoglycemia
- Encephalopathy (hypoxic-ischemic)
- Intracranial hemorrhage
- Infection (especially CNS)
- Metabolic (electrolyte disturbances or in-born errors of metabolism)

Diagnosis

Extensive efforts should be directed toward identifying the underlying cause of the neonatal seizure.

- Serum glucose
- Serum electrolytes, including sodium, calcium, magnesium
- Arterial blood gas, lactate, ammonia
- Lumbar puncture
- Head CT
- Urine studies
- Cultures of blood, urine, CSF
- EEG to confirm seizure activity
- If etiology still unclear, consider evaluation for in-born errors of metabolism.

Treatment

Actively seizing:

- Stabilize airway.
- Lorazepam 0.05–0.1 mg/kg IV (max dose 2 mg)
- Phenobarbital 10–20 mg/kg IVPB
- Specific treatment directed at etiology of seizure
- Admission to hospital

Complications

- Depend on etiology of seizure
- Overall mortality 15%
- High incidence of mental retardation and cerebral palsy

Causes of Seizures in Children—

TIMED IT

Trauma
Infection (meningitis)
Metabolic (hypoglycemia, hyponatremia, hypernatremia, hypocalcemia)
Epilepsy (medication noncompliance common)
Drugs (lead, cocaine, aspirin, carbon monoxide)
In-born errors of metabolism
Tumor

Pediatric Seizures

Seizures occur due to an involuntary discharge of cortical neurons. Types of seizures are listed in Table 5.13. The diagnosis of epilepsy requires the child to have >1 seizure. About 1% of children <20 years of age develop epilepsy.

SYMPTOMS/EXAM

- May be postictal
- May be incontinent or tongue biting
- Examine closely for evidence of trauma, infection, or focal neurological deficit.

DIAGNOSIS

- Based on a detailed history of the event
- Workup may include:
  - Serum glucose
  - Serum electrolytes (sodium, calcium, magnesium), CBC
  - Therapeutic drug levels if child is taking antiepileptic drugs
  - Lumbar puncture if concern for meningitis or subarachnoid bleed
  - Head CT if partial seizure, focal neurological deficit, or presence of trauma

TREATMENT

Actively seizing:

- Stabilize airway.
- Lorazepam 0.05–0.1 mg/kg IV (max dose 2 mg)
- Phenytoin (10–15 mg/kg IV) or phenobarbital (10–20 mg/kg IV) may be necessary if seizures persist in spite of benzodiazepines.
- Admission to hospital if first focal seizure or focal neurological deficit
- Consider discharge to home if first generalized seizure (and normal ED evaluation)
- Follow-up with pediatrician and pediatric neurologist
- If patient is discharged, the decision to start antiepileptic drugs should be made in consultation with a pediatric neurologist.

TABLE 5.13. Classification of Pediatric Seizures

SEIZURE TYPE	CLINICAL CHARACTERISTICS
Partial seizures (focal seizures)	
Partial simple	No loss of consciousness
Complex partial	Loss of consciousness
Partial evolving to generalized	Focal symptoms progressing to generalized seizure
Generalized seizures	
Absence seizure	Nonconvulsive, last <15 sec
Myoclonic	Minor symmetric motor spasms
Tonic	Increased tone
Clonic	Rhythmic spasms
Tonic-clonic	Alternating increased muscle tone with muscle spasm
Atonic	Loss of muscle tone

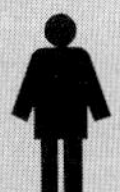

A 12-year-old obese African-American male begins to limp for 3 days. He has no fever and there is no associated trauma. What is a likely diagnosis?

SCFE (slipped capital femoral epiphysis).

Nursemaid's Elbow

- Most common elbow injury in children <5 years of age
- Proximal end of the radial head is held in place by the overlying annular ligament. It is fairly straight and does not become flared and nodular until approximately 5–6 years of age, allowing it to slip out of place.
- The typical mechanism of injury is when the child's arm is pulled in an extended, pronated position.

Symptoms/Exam

- The child usually cries immediately after the injury and refuses to use the arm.
- Injured arm is held in a characteristic position—slightly flexed at the elbow and pronated ("**thumb rotated in toward the body**").
- Usually well appearing, other than refusal to use the arm
- May be diffusely tender along the entire arm, but should not have any visible deformity or swelling

Diagnosis

Clinical history and exam are usually sufficient. Radiographs are indicated only if history is unclear or the exam suggests another injury.

Treatment

Place your thumb over the radial head, supinate the forearm, then flex the elbow. A palpable click is usually felt with successful reduction. With successful reduction, the child will begin to use the affected arm within a few minutes.

Limp

In the ED evaluation of a child with limping, careful history taking and physical examination are key. X-rays are usually needed, often of the entire affected extremity; other ancillary studies may include blood cultures, CBC with differential, ESR, CRP. The differential diagnosis can often be narrowed based on age, history of trauma, and/or likelihood of infectious causes. Four of the more common causes are listed below; other causes include nutritional deficiencies (eg, rickets), fractures (eg, toddler's fractures, avulsion fractures, stress fractures), sprains/contusions, JRA, osteomyelitis, and neoplasms (Ewing's sarcoma, osteogenic sarcoma, leukemia).

Legg-Calvé-Perthes

- Also known as avascular necrosis of the femoral head (specifically the capital femoral epiphysis)
- Typical age is 2–12 years, primarily in boys
- Bilateral in 15%
- Unknown cause, other than association with sickle cell disease

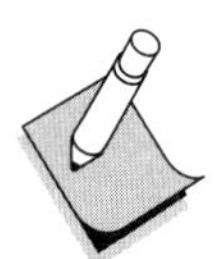

Young children often have difficulty localizing pain. Beware when children point to their knee, as the true pathology may actually be in the hip!

SYMPTOMS/EXAM

- Limp
- Pain is usually in the groin or inner thigh; younger children can have difficulty localizing the pain and may point to their knee.
- Restricted motion of the hip, especially of internal rotation and abduction

DIAGNOSIS

AP and frog-leg lateral radiographs of the pelvis/hips

TREATMENT

- Goal is to prevent subluxation of femoral head out of acetabulum.
- Children <6 years of age without significant subluxation and at least 40–45 degrees of abduction can be observed.
- Children >6 years old usually require containment with brace or surgery.

OSGOOD-SCHLATTER

- Also known as osteochondritis of the tibial tuberosity
- Overuse injury
- Typical patient is a physically active teenage boy.
- Results from repeated stress at the insertion of the patellar tendon onto the tibial tuberosity

SYMPTOMS/EXAM

- Tenderness at the insertion of the patellar tendon onto the tibial tubercle
- Pain with climbing, jumping, or kneeling
- Pain with resisted knee extension

DIAGNOSIS

Knee radiographs are usually normal, but may show soft-tissue swelling, irregularity, or prominence of tibial tubercle, and/or ossification anterior to the tibial tubercle.

TREATMENT

Treatment includes restriction of activity, ice after activity, NSAIDs. In severe cases, immobilization may be necessary.

Think of the femoral head as an ice cream cone (the epiphyseal portion is the "ice cream"; metaphyseal and diaphyseal portion is the "cone"). The "ice cream" usually stays within the socket (acetabulum) and the "cone" usually slips laterally and anteriorly.

SLIPPED CAPITAL FEMORAL EPIPHYSIS (SCFE)

- SCFE is displacement of the epiphyseal portion of the femoral head from the metaphyseal/diaphyseal portion (through the physis). The epiphyseal portion stays within the acetabulum, but is usually rotated medially and posteriorly in relation to the metaphyseal portion.
- Typical patient is an obese, African-American, adolescent male.
- Other risk factors include hypothyroidism, growth hormone deficiency, renal osteodystrophy.

SYMPTOMS/EXAM

- Limp
- Hip/groin pain common, but also may complain of pain localized to the knee
- Painful range of motion of hip, especially with internal rotation

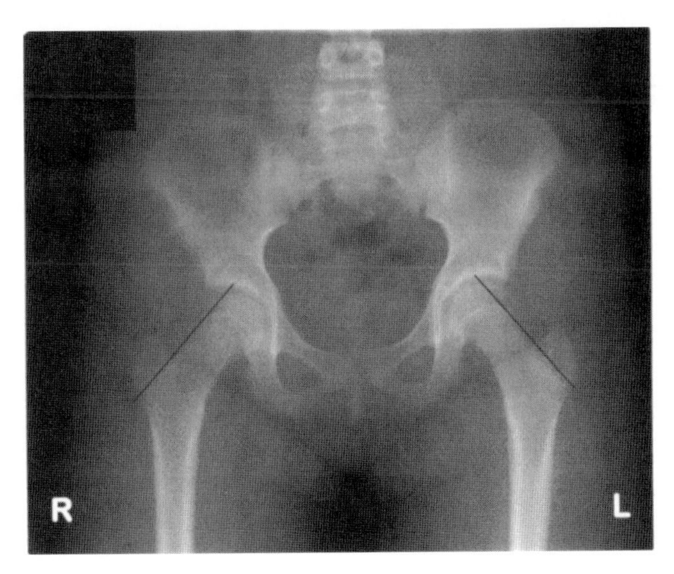

FIGURE 5.20. Klein line.

(Reproduced, with permission, from Stead LG, Stead SM, Kaufman MS. *First Aid for the Pediatric Clerkship*. New York: McGraw-Hill, 2004:336.)

Diagnosis

- AP and frog-leg lateral radiographs of the pelvis
- **Bloomberg's sign** (widening or blurring of the epiphyseal plate)
- **Klein line** (line drawn along the superior border of the femoral neck) should intersect the femoral head (see Figure 5.20); if not, suspect a SCFE.
- In subtle cases, MRI may be helpful.

Toxic Synovitis

- Also known as transient synovitis
- Thought to be a self-limited, reactive arthritis that follows a viral infection
- Most commonly involves the hip joint
- Typical age range: 3–10 years

Symptoms/Exam

- Limp
- Usually well appearing, nontoxic, and afebrile.

Diagnosis

- Diagnosis of exclusion: It must be differentiated from other causes of arthritis, the most important of which is septic arthritis.
- Laboratory evaluation usually shows a normal or minimally elevated WBC and ESR.
- Radiographs may show signs of an effusion but are usually normal.
- In equivocal cases, aspiration of the joint in question (usually by ultrasound guidance) is necessary to further evaluate for possibility of septic arthritis (signs suggestive of septic arthritis include WBC >50,000, Gram-positive stain, or culture for bacterial organisms).
- Lyme arthritis should be considered in endemic areas. Diagnosis is usually made by initial ELISA testing with confirmatory Western blot assay.

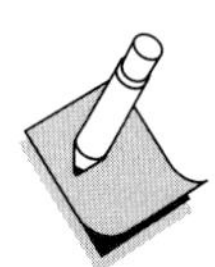

Salter-Harris type II is the most common form of a physeal fracture (75%).

TREATMENT

- Supportive; NSAIDs for pain control
- If Lyme arthritis, treat with oral doxycycline (if (8 years age) or amoxicillin (if < 8 years age) for 21–28 days.

Fractures

SALTER-HARRIS FRACTURES

The Salter-Harris classification is used for physeal injuries only (see Figure 5.21). Type II fractures are the most common and, along with Type I, have the best prognosis as the growth plate is not affected. Tenderness over a physis, even with normal radiographs, should be treated as a Salter-Harris I fracture.

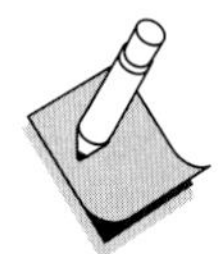

Children with normal initial radiographs may still have a Salter I fracture; the presence of pain and tenderness over a growth plate should prompt splinting and orthopedic follow-up.

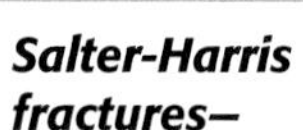

Salter-Harris fractures–

SALTR

S (I) = **S**lipped epiphysis
A (II) = fracture **A**bove physis
L (III) = fracture be**L**ow physis
T (IV) = fracture **T**hrough physis
R (V) = w**R**ecked physis

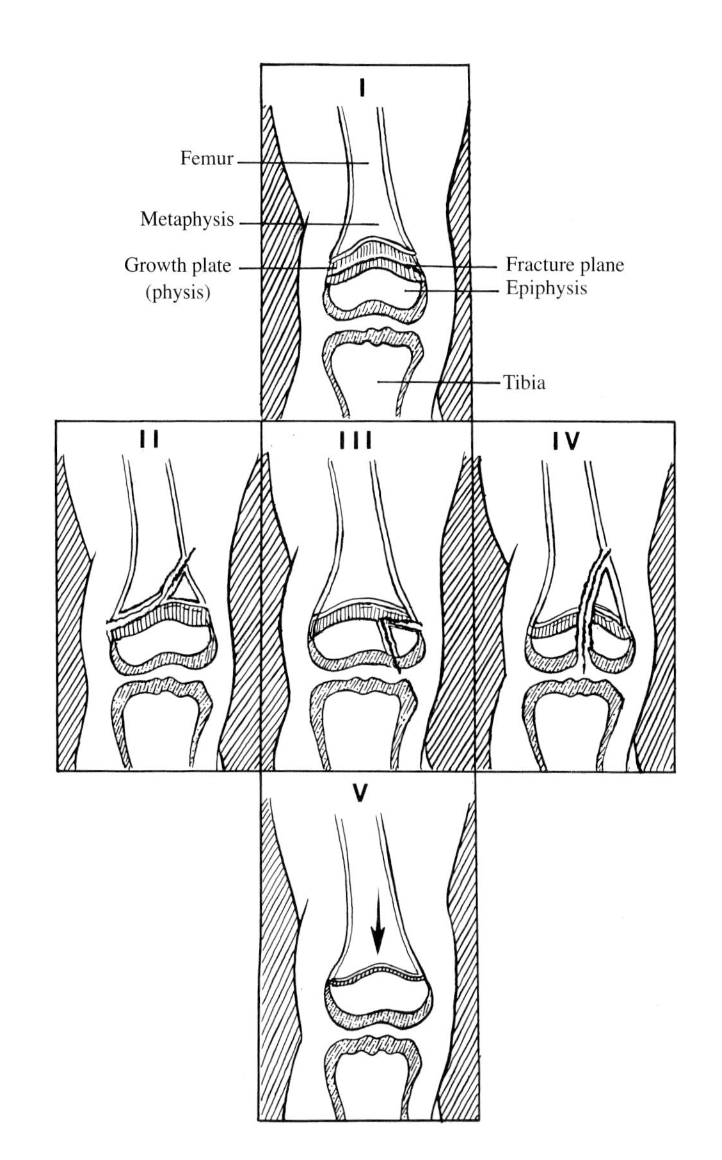

FIGURE 5.21. Salter-Harris classification of fractures.

(Reproduced, with permission, from Knoop KJ, Stack LB, Storrow AB. *Atlas of Emergency Medicine*, 2nd ed. New York: McGraw-Hill, 2002:467.)

GREENSTICK, TORUS, AND BOWING FRACTURES

These fracture patterns occur almost exclusively in children due to the pliability of bone (see Figure 5.22). Torus fractures are also known as compression or buckle fractures. Bowing fractures are also known as plastic deformation fractures.

DIAGNOSIS

- **Torus fracture**: Mechanism is usually **axial compression**, such as occurs with a fall on an outstretched arm. **Most common site is the distal radius**.
- **Greenstick fracture:** Mechanism is usually **axial compression with twisting**, such as occurs with falling backward on a supinated or pronated forearm. XRs show an intact bony cortex on one side with a fracture through the cortex on the opposite side.
- **Bowing fracture:** Mechanism is usually from **longitudinal compression**. Clinically, the patient will have a deformity suggesting a fracture. XRs show a bowing deformity without an obvious break in the bony cortex. Comparison views with the opposite extremity are extremely helpful and often necessary.

TREATMENT

- **Torus fractures** are treated with simple casting for 2–4 weeks.
- **Greenstick fractures** may require reduction of the rotational or angular deformity in addition to casting.
- **Bowing fractures** should be referred to an orthopedic surgeon for evaluation because remodeling is minimal and these fractures are commonly associated with long-term cosmetic and functional deficits.

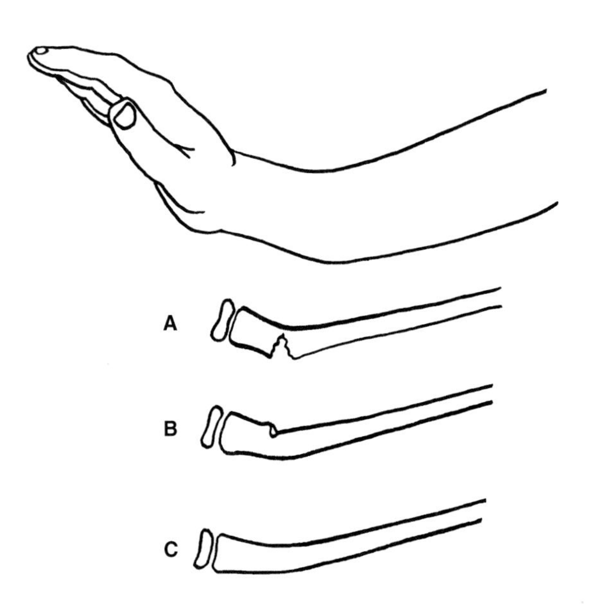

FIGURE 5.22. Pediatric fractures. A: Greenstick fracture. B: Torus fracture. C: Plastic deformation (bowing fracture).

(Reproduced, with permission, from Skinner HB. *Current Orthopedics*, 4th ed. New York: McGraw-Hill, 2006:636.)

Causes of apnea and bradycardia in infants–

HAS CRASH
Hypoglycemia
Aspiration
Sepsis (infections: Respiratory syncytial virus [RSV], pertussis)
Cardiac arrhythmias
Reflux
Anemia
Seizures
Hydrocephalus

PULMONARY

Apnea of Prematurity and Acute Life-Threatening Event

Apnea is defined as 20 seconds of no respirations, or by a shorter period accompanied by cyanosis. Apnea of prematurity generally resolves shortly after birth, but premature infants are at risk for recurrent episodes of apnea and bradycardia. These episodes are called apparent life-threatening events (ALTE). Clinically, the history is crucial for determining the severity of an event and the degree of evaluation required.

SYMPTOMS/EXAM

- In the ED, all symptoms may be gone and the infant may appear normal.
- Cyanosis, pallor, loss of consciousness, or loss of muscle tone all suggest a potentially lethal event.

DIAGNOSIS

- An accurate history is essential.
- Supporting data including serum glucose, electrolytes, CBC, and an ECG may be helpful.
- CT head, CXR, UA, and cultures of blood and urine may also be useful.

TREATMENT

- Supportive, with specific therapy directed toward the cause of the event.
- In general, infants with an ALTE should be admitted to a monitored bed.

A 2-year-old boy becomes upset after his parents take away a favorite toy. He cries vigorously, then becomes limp, cyanotic, and his parents describe seizure-like activity. Upon arrival in the ED, he is alert with normal vital signs and a normal physical exam. What is the appropriate ED workup?

Reassurance and education.

Breath Holding

Breath holding is a behavioral response to being emotionally upset. It typically occurs in children between the ages of 6 months and 5 years with the peak incidence at 2 years of age.

SYMPTOMS

- Loss of consciousness
- May have associated pallor or cyanosis
- May have associated clonic jerks
- No postictal period

EXAM

Normal vital signs and normal physical exam.

DIFFERENTIAL

- Seizures
- Syncope

DIAGNOSIS

Clinical diagnosis based mainly upon history

TREATMENT

Reassure parents, and educate them not to reinforce child's behavior.

Obstructive Lung Disease

BRONCHOPULMONARY DYSPLASIA (BPD)

BPD is associated with prematurity and very low birth weight. Typically these infants will have a history of an O_2 requirement. The precise pathophysiology of BPD is unknown, but the condition is the end result of numerous pulmonary insults during the neonatal period (eg, infections, meconium aspiration, prolonged ventilator support). Infants with BPD will usually present to the ED with acute deterioration of respiratory function from some additional insult.

SYMPTOMS/EXAM

- Respiratory distress
- Tachypnea
- Hypoxia is common.

DIAGNOSIS

- Clinical diagnosis
- Viral infections are the most common trigger of an acute exacerbation, especially RSV (see Table 5.14).

TABLE 5.14. Causes of Acute Respiratory Distress in Infants with BPD

Causes
Respiratory infection
Sepsis
Aspiration
▪ Gastroesophageal reflux
▪ Incoordinate sucking or swallowing
Bronchospasm
Pulmonary edema or congestive heart failure
Dehydration
▪ Gastroenteritis
▪ Diuretic therapy
Anemia

(Reproduced, with permission, from Tintinalli JE, Kelen GD, Stapczynski JS. *Emergency Medicine: A Comprehensive Study Guide,* 6th ed. New York: McGraw-Hill, 2004:769.)

Treatment

- O_2, inhaled bronchodilators, and corticosteroids
- Some patients may also respond to diuretics.
- IV fluids for patients who are dehydrated
- Admit if hypoxic, there is a concurrent infection (such as RSV or pneumonia), or if respiratory distress persists despite treatment.

Complications

- Apnea, hypercarbia, or hypoxemia
- Dehydration
- Cor pulmonale

Cystic Fibrosis

Cystic fibrosis is the most common lethal congenital condition in the United States, occurring in roughly 1 in 2500 Caucasians. The incidence in other ethnic groups is 1 in 17,000. Although there are hundreds of different mutations leading to CF, the most common is DeltaF508. The gene product affected by all of these mutations is the CFTR protein, which regulates chloride transport across cell membranes. Patients with CF have a reduction in chloride transport back into epithelial cells, resulting in thick secretions. As a result, CF patients develop respiratory disease similar to early-onset COPD, with additional deficiencies in the pancreatic exocrine function, male infertility, and abnormally elevated levels of chloride in sweat.

Symptoms

- Frequent lung and sinus infections
- Failure to thrive due to malabsorption of fats
- Increased incidence of rectal prolapse
- Meconium ileus in infants
- Fatty stools

Exam

- Increased AP diameter of the chest
- Small size for age

Diagnosis

- CF is generally not diagnosed in the ED setting.
- Sweat chloride testing
- Serum electrolytes reveal low chloride and sodium levels.

Treatment

- Antibiotics
- Inhaled bronchodilators
- Steroids

Complications

- Respiratory failure
- Hemoptysis
- Dehydration, particularly during warm weather or exertion
- Electrolyte abnormalities: Low serum chloride, low serum sodium, elevated serum bicarbonate

A 6-year-old boy with a history of asthma presents to the ED in severe respiratory distress. In the ED, he has already received inhaled bronchodilators, steroids, and magnesium, without any significant improvement. His RR is 45, O_2 saturation is 89% on a 100% FiO_2 albuterol neb. What additional medication should he receive?

Epinephrine 1:1000, subcutaneously or intramuscularly, at a dose of 0.01 mg/kg (maximum single dose of 0.3 mg).

ASTHMA

(See also Chapter 10, "Thoracic and Respiratory Emergencies.")
Asthma falls into the spectrum of atopic disease that includes eczema and seasonal/food allergies. Patients with asthma have chronic inflammation of the airways. Acute flares of asthma result from the **triad** of airway inflammation (often with mucus plugging), bronchial hyperresponsiveness, and intermittent reversible airway obstruction. **Triggers** of asthma flares include viral URIs, cold weather, exercise, cigarette smoking, and other allergens (eg, dust mites, cockroaches).

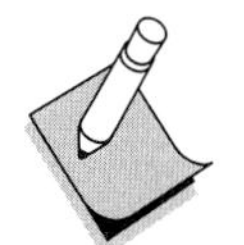

Asthma triad: Airway inflammation (often with mucous plugging), bronchial hyperresponsiveness, and intermittent reversible airway obstruction

SYMPTOMS/EXAM

- Episodes of wheezing with respiratory distress
- Persistent cough: 30% of children with asthma have cough-variant asthma and may not wheeze.

DIFFERENTIAL

Wheezing does not always mean asthma! Other causes of wheezing include GERD, CHF, foreign body aspiration, pneumonia, bronchiolitis.

DIAGNOSIS

- Mainly a clinical diagnosis
- Peak expiratory flow rate (PEFR), CXR, and ABG may be helpful (see Chapter 10).

TREATMENT

- O_2 as needed, to correct hypoxemia
- Inhaled β-agonists (albuterol)
- Inhaled anticholinergics (ipratropium)
- Oral or IV steroids
- Epinephrine SQ/IM for severe exacerbations
- Adjunctive therapies include ketamine and heliox.

Infectious Disorders

BACTERIAL TRACHEITIS

- Bacterial superinfection of the trachea causing rapid and severe respiratory symptoms
- **Median age is 4 years old** but wide age range

- Causative organisms include *Moraxella catarrhalis*, streptococcal species (especially pyogenes), MRSA as emerging etiology, *Klebsiella, Pseudomonas*

SYMPTOMS/EXAM

- Typically preceded by a viral URI for a few days
- Fever
- Rapid and severe inspiratory and expiratory stridor with toxic apperance Stridor (inspiratory and expiratory)
- Cough or raspy, hoarse voice

DIFFERENTIAL

- Epiglottitis
- Croup
- Foreign body in airway
- Viral URI
- Fever

DIAGNOSIS

- High index of suspicion based on clinical grounds
- Soft-tissue neck X-rays demonstrate subglottic narrowing with a rough-appearing tracheal lining.
- Bronchoscopy confirms diagnosis.

TREATMENT

- Antibiotics, eg, penicillinase-resistant penicillin, third-generation cephalosporin, clindamycin.
- Typically requires emergent intubation in the OR.

COMPLICATIONS

Airway compromise and respiratory collapse.

Bronchiolitis: Up to 75% of cases caused by RSV

BRONCHIOLITIS

- Bronchiolitis is a lower respiratory tract viral infection, most commonly caused by RSV.
- Other etiologies include adenovirus, parainfluenza, rhinovirus, influenza, and mycoplasma.
- Affected children are usually < 1–2 years old, with the most severely affected infants < 6 months old.
- The peak incidence is winter to spring.
- Symptoms may last 3–10 days.

SYMPTOMS/EXAM

- Wheezing
- Respiratory distress (retractions, nasal flaring)
- Tachypnea (often leading to decreased oral intake and dehydration)
- Hypoxemia
- Rhinorrhea, fever, and pharyngitis
- Apnea may occur in infants.

DIFFERENTIAL

- Pneumonia
- Asthma exacerbation
- Viral infections, such as URI or croup
- Aspirated foreign body

DIAGNOSIS

- Rapid antigen testing of nasopharyngeal sample
- CXR may show patchy atelectasis.

RSV bronchiolitis often gets worse in the second or third day of the illness. Symptoms are often worse at night.

TREATMENT

- Supplemental O_2
- Racemic epinephrine nebulizer may be effective.
- Antibiotics, if there is concern of 2° bacterial infection (acute otitis media, pneumonia, UTI)
- Steroids are generally not indicated unless the child has an underlying condition such as asthma or BPD.

COMPLICATIONS

- Apnea or respiratory failure
- Dehydration
- Rarely 2° bacterial infections

CROUP

- Croup is a viral infection of the upper airway which is most commonly caused by parainfluenza virus. Other etiologies include influenza, RSV, and adenoviruses.
- Affected children are 6 months to 3 years. Peak prevalence in the ages of 1–2 years.
- Peak incidence is fall to winter.
- Symptoms may last 3–7 days.

SYMPTOMS/EXAM

- Stridor with retractions and tachypnea, usually worse at night
- Prodrome of cough, coryza prior to onset of stridor
- Barking cough (sounds like the bark of a seal)
- Fever

DIFFERENTIAL

- Other causes of stridor include: Foreign body aspiration, hemangiomas, papillomas, subglottic stenosis.
- Epiglottitis
- Retropharyngeal abscess

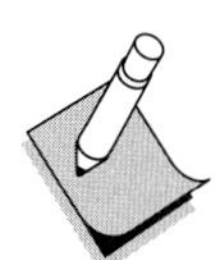

*Neck radiographs in croup may show the classical "**steeple sign**" due to symmetric narrowing of the trachea.*

DIAGNOSIS

- Clinical diagnosis
- Soft tissue neck X-ray may reveal classical "**steeple sign**" due to symmetric narrow of the supraglottic airway (see Figure 5.23). It may also help to exclude other causes of stridor.
- CXR to exclude pneumonia or aspirated foreign body

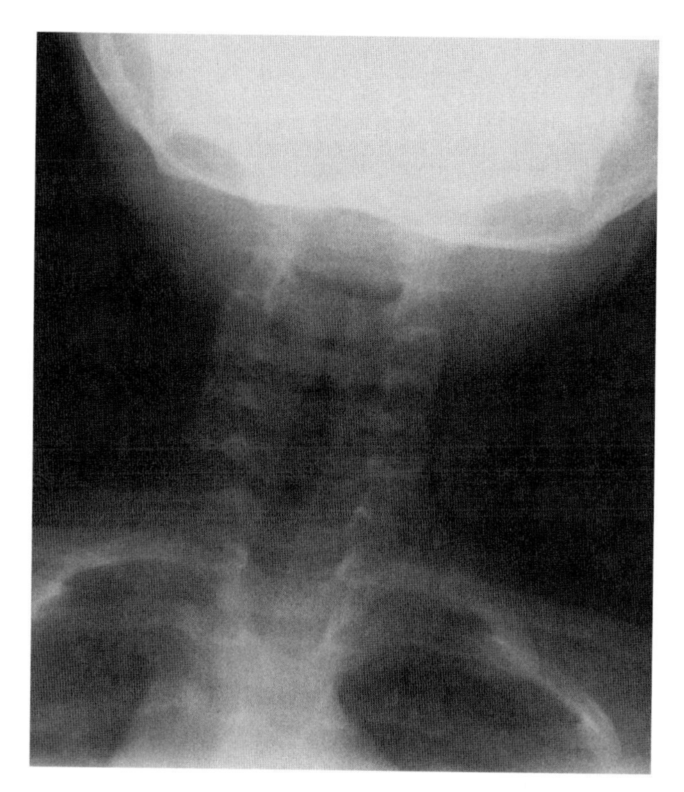

FIGURE 5.23. Steeple sign of croup.

(Reproduced, with permission, from Shah BR, Lucchesi M. *Atlas of Pediatric Emergency Medicine*. New York: McGraw-Hill, 2006:241.)

TREATMENT

- Supplemental humidified O_2 and cool mist is commonly used but has not been shown to improve outcomes.
- Steroids in the form of one dose of dexamethasone lead to faster recovery. Oral route has been shown to be as effective as IM injections.
- Epinephrine nebs (if patient has stridor at rest or stridor with significant respiratory distress)

COMPLICATIONS

- Upper airway obstruction
- Dehydration

PERTUSSIS

Known as **"whooping cough,"** this lower respiratory tract infection is caused by *Bordetella pertussis* (Gram-negative coccobacillus).

SYMPTOMS/EXAM

Clinically, pertussis is an illness lasting longer than 2 weeks, with paroxysms of coughing (spasms or fits of multiple coughs in a row), followed by an inspiratory whoop and often with associated posttussive emesis. There are three stages to the illness:

1. Catarrhal stage (7–10 days)—similar to URI
   - Coryza
   - Cough
   - Conjunctivitis
2. Paroxysmal stage (1–4 weeks)
   - Spasmodic fits of coughing, with inspiratory whoop
   - Physical exam may be normal between paroxysms
   - Fever uncommon
3. Convalescent stage (several months)
   - Decreasing frequency and severity of paroxysms

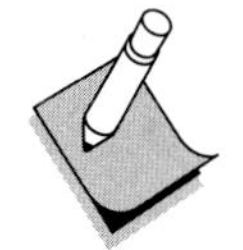

Antibiotic treatment for pertussis begun after paroxysmal stage has begun does not ameliorate course of disease, but does help decrease bacterial shedding and spread of disease

DIFFERENTIAL

- Pneumonia
- Cough-variant asthma
- Aspirated foreign body

DIAGNOSIS

- Nasopharyngeal aspirate may be sent for testing to confirm clinical suspicion of pertussis.
- WBC may be elevated (20,000–50,000/mm^2), with a lymphocytosis.
- CXR to rule out other etiologies

TREATMENT

- Erythromycin estolate, clarithromycin, or azithromycin
- Prevention through immunization (DTaP = diphtheria, tetanus, acellular pertussis)

COMPLICATIONS

- Pneumonia
- Seizures, encephalitis
- Children <6 months are at highest risk for complications.

PNEUMONIA

Pneumonia is a lower respiratory tract infection caused by viruses, bacteria, or atypical agents. The **etiology varies with the age of the child**, with viruses more common than bacteria for all ages. Viruses causing pneumonia include RSV, parainfluenza, influenza, adenoviruses, rhinoviruses, enteroviruses, varicella, measles, CMV, HSV, EBV, and rubella. Bacterial pneumonia in newborns is most commonly caused by group B streptococcus, with older infants and children affected by *Streptococcus pneumoniae* more than any other bacterial agent. Rarely, *S. aureus* or *H. influenzae* may cause bacterial pneumonia in children. Atypical agents, such as *Mycoplasma pneumoniae* or *Chlamydia pneumoniae*, are associated with pneumonia in older children and teenagers.

SYMPTOMS/EXAM

Symptoms are variable and depend upon the age of the child and severity of illness. Young infants may have no respiratory symptoms, but may present only with fever and dehydration. The classical presentation of pneumonia describes a patient infected with *S. pneumoniae*, and includes the sudden onset of fever, chills, dyspnea with tachypnea, and a productive cough.

- **Rust-colored sputum**: *S. pneumoniae*
- **Bullous myringitis**: *M. pneumoniae*
- Rales: Alveolar fluid
- Bronchial breath sounds: Consolidation
- Dullness to percussion/decreased breath sounds: Pleural effusion
- Wheezing/rhonchi: Bronchial congestion

DIAGNOSIS

- Mainly still a clinical diagnosis
- CXR helpful for confirmation
  - Bacterial pneumonia classically presents with focal or unilobar infiltrates.
  - Strep pneumonia is associated with round infiltrates.
- Elevated WBC > 15,000 cells/mL.
- Elevated CRP is associated with bacterial pneumonia.

TREATMENT

- Antibiotics: Traditionally penicillins or cephalosporins are prescribed. Macrolides (erythromycin, clarithromycin or azithromycin) should be given if there is concern of an atypical pneumonia. Fluoroquinolones (such as levofloxacin or gatifloxacin) are also effective for older patients and patients with cystic fibrosis.
- Any child discharged with the diagnosis of pneumonia should be reevaluated in 24–48 hours to ensure appropriate response to therapy.

COMPLICATIONS

- Bacteremia, with risk of developing 2° infections, such as meningitis or septic arthritis
- Empyema
- Respiratory failure
- Apnea, particularly in infants

SUDDEN INFANT DEATH SYNDROME

- SIDS is the unexplained death of an infant under the age of 1 year.
- Peak incidence is ages 2–5 months.
- 90% of all cases occur in infants before the age of 6 months.

SYMPTOMS/EXAM

Infant is typically found lifeless in crib.

DIFFERENTIAL

The etiology of SIDS is unclear. Some evidence suggests SIDS may be related to apnea, accidental suffocation, or an immature ability to respond to noxious stimuli (such as rising serum CO_2 and falling serum O_2). Fewer than 5% of cases are thought to be due to child abuse.

RISK FACTORS

- Sleeping in prone position
- Mother who smokes (during pregnancy or postnatally)

- Infants sleeping on excessively soft surface or with objects that may accidentally occlude airway (such as pillows, toys, loose bedding) are particularly susceptible.
- Excessive ambient heat
- Prematurity
- Male sex
- Infant with history of ALTE (although <10% of infants who die from SIDS have a history of ALTE)
- Possibly a family history of SIDS (such as sibling who died from SIDS), may increase risk; consider child abuse if >2 siblings with SIDS.

TREATMENT

- Support for family
- No known treatment other than prevention
  - "**Back to sleep**" is the recommendation that infants sleep on their backs. Since the introduction of this campaign, the incidence of SIDS has decreased by >40%.
  - Encourage maternal smoking cessation.

CHAPTER 6

Toxicology

Jennie A. Buchanan, MD, Carrie D. Mendoza, MD,
Sean H. Rhyee, MD, MPH, and Jason Hoppe, DO

DIFFERENTIAL DIAGNOSIS BY CHIEF COMPLAINT

Although the poisoned patient may present with varied symptoms and complaints, the chief presenting complaint or symptom may suggest a diagnosis (see Table 6.1).

TOXIDROMES

Recognition of grouped symptoms and findings consistent with a toxidrome (see Table 6.2) can guide diagnosis and treatment in the poisoned patient.

TABLE 6.1. Primary Considerations for Presenting Chief Complaint in the Poisoned Patient

CHIEF COMPLAINT	COMMON CAUSES
Coma	Alcohols Antipsychotics Antiseizure medications Carbon monoxide Muscle relaxants Opiates Sedative/hypnotics
Delirium	Anticholinergics/cholinergics Muscle relaxants Sympathomimetics Withdrawal syndromes
Seizure	Isonaizid Anticholinergics/cholinergics Antidepressants Mushrooms (*Gyrometra* sp.) Sympathomimetics Toxic alcohols Withdrawal syndromes
Hepatic injury	Acetaminophen Carbon tetrachloride Ethanol Mushrooms *(Amanita phalloides)*
Renal injury	Ethylene glycol Heavy metal salts (mercury) Mushrooms (*Cortinarius orellanus)* Rhabdomyolysis (cocaine, amphetamines)

TABLE 6.2. Toxidromes

TOXIDROME	COMMON AGENTS	PRESENTATION	TREATMENT
Anticholinergic (see also p. 331–332)	Antihistamines Jimsonweed (scopolamine) Deadly nightshade (atropine)	Altered mentation Dry, flushed skin Mydriasis Hyperthermia Seizures Tachycardia Urinary retention	Benzodiazepines Physostigmine (rarely indicated)
Cholinergic (see also p. 332–333)	Organophosphates Carbamates Sarin	Altered mentation Bradycardia Bronchospasm ↑ Secretions Miosis N/V, defecation Seizures Urination	Atropine 2-PAM (for organophophates)
Sympathomimetic (see also p. 379–381)	Ephedrine Ma Huang Cocaine Amphetamines	Agitation Diaphoresis Hallucinations HTN Hyperthermia Mydriasis Muscular rigidity Tachycardia	Benzodiazepines Sodium bicarbonate (for wide complex dysrhythmias)
Opioid (see also p. 366–367)	Morphine Heroin Dextromethorphan	CNS depression Bradycardia Hypothermia Miosis Respiratory depression	Naloxone

PRINCIPLES OF GASTROINTESTINAL DECONTAMINATION

Gastrointestinal (GI) decontamination refers to therapies that may decrease the amount of poison absorbed from the GI tract lumen.

The following methods of GI decontamination are available:

- Induced emesis
- Gastric lavage
- Activated charcoal
- Whole-bowel irrigation

Induced Emesis

Induced emesis utilizes syrup of ipecac to induce vomiting, theoretically emptying the stomach and reducing absorption of an ingested agent. Syrup of ipecac induces vomiting by activation of both local and central emetic sensory receptors.

Induced emesis has largely been abandoned in clinical practice. The most recent policy statements released by both the American Academy of Pediatrics (2003) and the American Association of Poison Control Centers (2005) discourage the use of syrup of ipecac in the out-of-hospital setting.

Dose

- Suggested doses are 30 mL for adults, 15 mL for children 1–12 years old. If no vomiting occurs by 30 minutes, the initial dose may be repeated.
- Children 6–12 months old should receive a single, 10-mL dose.

Indications

- Ingestion of a substance with high toxic potential **and:**
  - Within 1 hour of ingestion
  - No other forms of GI decontamination are available or effective for the given substance.
  - Potential benefits outweigh risks.

Contraindications

- Substances not meeting above indications
- Spontaneous emesis
- Diminished level of consciousness/unprotected airway reflexes
- Ingestion of hydrocarbons or caustic agents
- Foreign body ingestion
- Patient requires therapy by PO route, such as activated charcoal.

Gastric Lavage

Gastric lavage (GL) attempts to directly remove stomach contents by means of an orogastric tube.

Indications

- Ingestion of a substance with high toxic potential **and:**
  - Within 1 hour of ingestion
  - Ingested substance is not bound by activated charcoal or has no effective antidote.
  - Potential benefits outweigh risks.

Contraindications

- Substance not meeting above indications
- Spontaneous emesis
- Diminished level of consciousness/unprotected airway reflexes (intubate first)
- Ingestion of hydrocarbons or caustic agents
- Foreign body ingestion
- Patient is at high risk for esophageal or gastric injury (GI hemorrhage, recent surgery, etc.).

Technique

- Recommended tube size is 36–40 French for adults, 22–28 French for children.
- Secure airway via intubation, if necessary.
- Position patient in left-lateral decubitus position, with head lowered below level of feet.

- Confirm tube placement following insertion.
- Aspirate any available stomach contents.
- Lavage with 250 mL (10–15 mL/kg in children) aliquots of warm water or saline.
- Continue until fluid is clear and a minimum of 2L has been used.
- Instill activated charcoal through same tube, if indicated.

COMPLICATIONS

- The primary risks are vomiting, aspiration, and esophageal injury or perforation.

Activated Charcoal

Activated charcoal (AC) is ingested by the patient in order to adsorb poisons within the GI tract lumen.

DOSE

- The recommended dose of AC is a 10:1 ratio relative to the ingested poison (ie, ingestion of 1 g of poison requires 10 g of AC). Hence, the common ED practice of administering 50 to 100 g (1 g/kg) of AC to an overdose patient may be inadequate for larger ingestions.

INDICATIONS

- Patient presents within 1 to 2 hours after ingestion.
- Patient has ingested a potentially dangerous amount of a poison adsorbed by charcoal.

CONTRAINDICATIONS

- Ingested substance is poorly adsorbed by AC (eg, iron, lithium, heavy metals, toxic alcohols).
- Diminished level of consciousness/unprotected airway reflexes (AC can be given by naso- or orogastric tube following intubation)
- Patient presents over 2 hours after ingestion.
- Ingestion of caustic agents
- Cases where endoscopy will be required

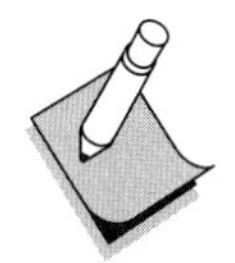

*Substances that do **not** adsorb to activated charcoal: Metals (eg, iron, lead, lithium), caustics, hydrocarbons, alcohols*

RISKS

- The primary risk of single-dose AC is vomiting.
- Constipation and diarrhea
- Bowel obstruction does not occur from single-dose AC.
- Repeated doses of cathartics given with charcoal may cause dehydration or electrolyte abnormalities.

Whole-Bowel Irrigation

Whole-bowel irrigation (WBI) flushes the GI tract to decrease the transit time of luminal contents, thereby limiting absorption.

DOSE

- Polyethylene glycol (PEG) solution is administered at a rate of 1–2 L/hour. This rate of administration usually requires a naso- or orogastric tube. End-points for therapy are the appearance of clear rectal effluent or a total irrigation volume of 10 L.

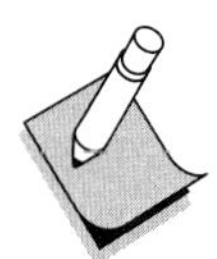

Common indications for whole-bowel irrigation: Drug packets, sustained-release formula, metals

Endpoints for whole-bowel irrigation: Clear rectal effluent or total irrigation volume of 10 L

TOXICOLOGY

Indications

- Removal of ingested drug packets (eg, body stuffers)
- Large ingestion of a sustained-release drug
- Potentially toxic ingestion that cannot be treated with activated charcoal (eg, lithium, lead, iron)

Contraindications

- Diminished level of consciousness/unprotected airway reflexes (intubate first)
- Decreased GI motility or bowel obstruction
- Significant GI hemorrhage
- Persistent emesis

Complications

- The primary risk associated with WBI is vomiting.
- Patient discomfort: Bloating, cramping, and flatulence
- WBI with balanced PEG solutions does not generally cause electrolyte abnormalities.

PRINCIPLES OF ENHANCED ELIMINATION

The goal of enhanced elimination is to increase the clearance of a poison from the body *after* it has been systemically absorbed. The following methods of enhanced elimination are available (see Table 6.3):

- Multiple-dose activated charcoal
- Urinary alkalinization
- Hemodialysis

TABLE 6.3. Enhanced Elimination: Drug Characteristics and Examples

Technique	Drug Characteristic	Examples
Multiple-dose activated charcoal	Enterohepatic circulation	Phenobarbital Carbamazepine Theophylline Aspirin
Urinary alkalinization	Weak organic acid with renal excretion	Aspirin Phenobarbital Formic acid
Hemodialysis	Low molecular weight, low plasma protein binding, small volume of distribution, poor endogenous clearance	Lithium Aspirin Alcohols
	OR Acidosis caused by toxin	Metformin

Multiple-Dose Activated Charcoal

Uses repeated doses of activated charcoal (every 2–4 hours) to increase poison clearance. MDAC exerts its effects through disruption of enterohepatic circulation or direct adsorption across the GI mucosal surface.

Single-dose activated charcoal is used to decrease poison absorption. Multiple-dose activated charcoal is used to increase poison elimination.

Indications

- Drugs that have enterohepatic circulation and can possibly be treated with MDAC include:
  - Phenobarbital
  - Carbamazepine (Tegretol)
  - Theophylline
  - Aspirin
  - Dapsone

Contraindications

- MDAC is contraindicated in the same settings as AC.

Risks

- The risks associated with MDAC are similar to those with AC; however, there is a greater risk of bowel obstruction with MDAC.

TOXICOLOGY

Urinary Alkalinization

Urinary alkalinization attempts to increase renal elimination of a drug by increasing urine pH. Urinary acidification to increase the clearance of weak bases is not recommended due to the risk of renal injury.

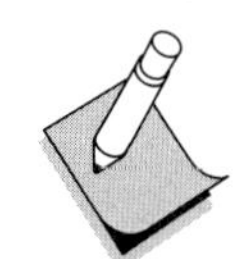

Urinary alkalinization will not occur unless hypokalemia is corrected.

Dose

- Alkalinization is accomplished via a sodium bicarbonate ($NaHCO_3$) infusion. The most common method uses 150 mEq of $NaHCO_3$ (3 amps) in 1 L D_5W, infused at 1.5 to 2 × the normal IV fluid maintenance rate.

Indications

- Urinary alkalinization only affects the clearance of drugs that are weak organic acids.
  - Aspirin (most common use for alkalinization)
  - Phenobarbital
  - Formic acid

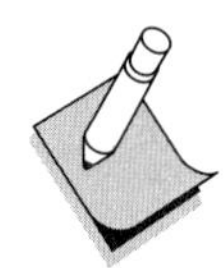

Urinary alkalinization is used for weak organic acids: Aspirin, phenobarbital, formic acid (methanol metabolite).

Contraindications

- Poisoning with agents that are not weak organic acids and are not primarily cleared by the kidneys
- Patients who cannot tolerate excess sodium/water loading (eg, CHF, renal failure)

Risks

Can precipitate hypokalemia and decrease ionized calcium levels

Hemodialysis

Hemodialysis (HD) directly removes toxins from a patient's plasma, using the same technology applied to renal failure.

Indications

- For HD to be useful in a poisoned patient, the ingested poison should have the following characteristics:
  - Low molecular weight
  - Low plasma protein-binding
  - Small volume of distribution
  - Poor endogenous clearance
- HD can also treat severe acidosis caused by a toxin, even if the toxin itself is not readily dialyzable.

Contraindications

- Toxins that do not satisfy the conditions listed above.

Risks

- HD requires central venous access, with all the usual accompanying risks (bleeding, pneumothorax, etc.).
- HD must be used cautiously in patients that are hemodynamically unstable.

ECG PRINCIPLES IN TOXICOLOGY

The ECG is used as a screening tool in the evaluation of the patient with a suspected ingestion/overdose. Specific ECG findings may be associated with ingestion of certain classes of drugs (see Table 6.4).

A 35-year-old male presents to the ED with a complaint of abdominal pain, nausea and blurry vision. He has a history of ETOH abuse and reports ingesting "something from the garage" earlier in the day. On examination, he appears inebriated and tachypnic. His labs reveal an osmolal gap and a wide-anion-gap metabolic acidosis. What is the most appropriate initial treatment?

This patient has likely ingested methanol, based on his presentation of inebriation with visual changes ("blind drunk") and wide-anion-gap acidosis. Initial therapies include administration of fomepizole or ethanol (via drip) to decreased formation of formic acid (the toxic metabolite) and urinary alkalinization to increase its clearance. Visual changes are an indication for treatment with hemodialysis.

ALCOHOLS

The alcohol ingestions most commonly seen in the ED include ethanol, methanol, ethylene glycol, and isopropyl alcohol.

Alcohols are primarily metabolized in the liver via alcohol dehydrogenase (ADH) using NAD as a cofactor. In the case of methanol and ethylene glycol it is a metabolite (**not** the parent compound) that causes severe toxicity, making ADH blockade a key factor in the treatment of these ingestions.

Ethanol

Ethanol is the most common poison seen in the ED.

TABLE 6.4. **ECG Findings and Associated Classes of Drugs**

ECG Finding	Associated Classes of Drugs
Bradysrhythmias Sinus bradycardia AV block	β-Blockers Ca^{++} channel blockers Cardiac glycosides Clonidine Other antidysrhythmic agents
Tachydysrhythmias Sinus tachycardia SVT Ventricular tachycardia (VT)	Anticholinergics Sympathomimetics Stimulants
QRS widening	Na^{++} channel blocking drugs: Some anticholinergics Tricyclic antidepressants Sympathomimetics
QTc prolongation Screening tool for conduction abnormality that could degenerate into torsades de points	Antidysrhythmic agents Antipsychotic medications Antidepressants Many others
Ischemic changes	Sympathomimetics Stimulants
Classic toxicology-related ECG findings	**Digoxin** Digitalis effect—seen in both therapeutic use and overdose Digoxin-induced bidirectional VT (rare) **Tricyclic antidepressants** Rightward deviation of the terminal 40 msec of the QRS axis

TOXICOLOGY

SYMPTOMS/EXAM

- Behavioral changes (eg, increased sociability, irritability, aggressiveness, etc.)
- CNS depression ranging from mild sedation to coma
- Ataxia, gait instability

DIFFERENTIAL

- Consider other etiologies of CNS depression, especially with relatively low serum ethanol levels.
- Common conditions associated with ethanol use include hypoglycemia, withdrawal, head trauma, and other toxin/drug overdose.

DIAGNOSIS

- Usually obvious from patient's history and exam
- Serum levels are readily available in most EDs.
- The correlation between serum levels and patient symptoms varies widely due to individual tolerance.

TREATMENT

- Supportive care
- Be careful not to overlook concomitant injuries or medical illness.

COMPLICATIONS

- Chronic alcohol use is associated with a wide variety of illnesses including hypoglycemia, alcoholic ketoacidosis, cirrhosis, pancreatitis, GI bleeding, malnutrition, neurologic disease, trauma.

TOXICOLOGY

Methanol

Methanol is found in windshield wiper fluid, antifreeze, photocopier fluid, and solid fuels (eg, Sterno). Patients may ingest methanol by accident, as a suicide attempt, or as an ethanol substitute.

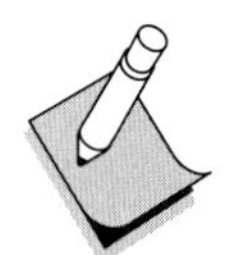

Osmolal gap = measured serum osmolality – calculated serum osmolality (normal = < 10 mOsm/kg).

MECHANISM/TOXICITY

- Methanol itself has minimal toxicity: It causes mild intoxication.
- Metabolized by alcohol dehydrogenase (ADH) to a toxic metabolite, **formic acid**
- Formic acid accumulation → anion gap metabolic acidosis, retinal toxicity.

SYMPTOMS/EXAM

- Intoxication, headache, CNS depression
- Visual changes: Classic description is "looking through a snow field," hyperemic optic discs, blindness.
- Tachycardia, tachypnea
- Abdominal pain, N/V

Calculated serum osmolality = 2(Na) + (BUN/2.8) + (glucose/18) + (ethanol/4.6).

DIFFERENTIAL

- Consider other causes of acute metabolic acidosis.
- The combination of acute onset visual changes with acidosis is highly suggestive of methanol toxicity.

DIAGNOSIS

- Gold standard is direct serum measurement.
- Suspect methanol ingestion if patient has a high osmolal gap, anion gap metabolic acidosis, and a consistent history and exam.
- Metabolism, and therefore toxicity, may be **delayed** with coingestion of alcohol.

"Blind drunk," osmolal gap, and anion gap metabolic acidosis = methanol toxicity.

TREATMENT

- **Antidote = fomepizole** or **ethanol.**
  - Blocks ADH, preventing production of formic acid

- **Folate:** Improves the metabolism of formic acid.
- **Urinary alkalinization:** Improves renal clearance of formic acid.
- Consider **hemodialysis** in cases of severe acidosis, visual changes or a serum level >50 mg/dL; effectively removes both the parent compound and formic acid.

Urinary alkalinization is used to increase renal clearance of formic acid.

COMPLICATIONS

- Permanent visual losses and parkinsonian motor dysfunction may occur.

Ethylene Glycol

Ethylene glycol is mostly available in engine coolants (antifreeze). It is ingested under similar circumstances as methanol.

MECHANISM/TOXICITY

- Ethylene glycol itself has minimal toxicity: It causes mild intoxication.
- Metabolized by ADH to a toxic metabolite, **oxalic acid**
- Oxalic acid accumulation → anion gap metabolic acidosis and direct renal toxicity.

SYMPTOMS/EXAM

- Intoxication, headache, CNS depression, cranial neuropathy (delayed)
- Abdominal pain, N/V
- Acute renal failure

DIAGNOSIS

- Gold standard is direct serum measurement.
- Suspect ethylene glycol ingestion if patient has an osmolal gap, anion gap metabolic acidosis and acute renal failure.
- Presence of **oxalate crystals in the urine** (suggestive of diagnosis, but is not sensitive or specific)
- Some brands of antifreeze contain fluorescent dyes to aid in the identification of coolant leaks and will fluoresce under Woods lamp (UV light); however, the practice of examining a patient's urine under UV light is highly unreliable and should not be used to confirm or rule out ingestion.

Intoxicated patient with osmolal gap, anion gap metabolic acidosis, and acute renal failure = ethylene glycol.

TREATMENT

- **Antidote = fomepizole** or **ethanol.**
  - Blocks ADH, preventing production of formic acid
- **Thiamine** and **pyridoxine** (vitamin B_6) may help convert oxalic acid to nontoxic metabolites.
- Consider **hemodialysis** in cases of severe acidosis (pH <7.3), renal failure or a serum level >50 mg/dL.

Antidote to methanol and ethylene glycol poisoning = fomepizole or ethanol.

COMPLICATIONS

- Renal damage may be irreversible in severe poisonings.

Isopropanol (Isopropyl Alcohol)

Isopropanol is found in rubbing alcohol and some hand sanitizers. It is most often ingested as an ethanol substitute. Intoxication due to isopropanol is more severe than that due to an equivalent amount of ethanol.

Isopropanol intoxication (as compared to ethanol) = "twice as drunk for twice as long."

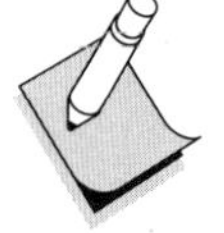

All alcohols will cause an elevated osmolal gap. Only methanol and ethylene glycol metabolism cause an anion gap metabolic acidosis.

Unlike methanol and ethylene glycol, isopropanol is **not** metabolized to an organic acid. It is converted directly to **acetone** by alcohol dehydrogenase.

Mechanism/Toxicity

- Toxicity is primarily due to CNS depression and hemorrhagic gastritis.

Symptoms/Exam

- Intoxication, CNS depression, coma
- Abdominal pain, N/V, hemorrhagic gastritis

Diagnosis

- Isopropanol can be directly measured in serum.
- Ingestion should be suspected in patients who appear intoxicated but have low or undetectable ethanol levels.
- Other clues include an increased osmolal gap and detectable serum acetone.
- Isopropanol does **not** directly cause a metabolic acidosis.

Treatment

- Supportive care only

> A 33-year-old female with a history of depression and chronic pain is brought to the ED via EMS for a suspected overdose. On arrival, her BP is 80/40 with an HR in the 120s. She is lethargic but responds to tactile stimuli. Her ECG shows sinus tachycardia with a QRS duration of 130 msec. What is the best treatment for this patient's hypotension?
>
> Any patient with a suspected ingestion who presents with CNS depression and QRS widening >100 msec should be presumed to have tricyclic antidepressant (TCA) toxicity. TCA-mediated Na^{++} channel blockade may result in life-threatening cardiovascular toxicity, manifesting as hypotension with QRS widening >100 msec. The drug of choice is sodium bicarbonate, given initially in boluses and followed by a continuous infusion.

ANTIDEPRESSANTS

The broad classes of antidepressants are:

- Tricyclic antidepressants (TCAs)
- Selective serotonin reuptake inhibitors (SSRIs)
- Monoamine oxidase inhibitors (MAOIs)
- Newer drugs that act at multiple CNS receptors

Tricyclic Antidepressants

TCAs are associated with life-threatening CNS and cardiovascular toxicity. Safer medications, such as SSRIs, have decreased the use of TCAs for depression, and they are now more commonly used at lower doses for treatment of chronic pain syndromes, migraine prophylaxis, and enuresis.

Examples include:

- Amitriptyline (Elavil)
- Nortriptyline (Aventyl)
- Imipramine (Tofranil)

MECHANISM/TOXICITY

TCAs have seven pharmacologic effects that contribute to toxicity, including:

- Histamine receptor blockade → antihistamine effects.
- Muscarinic receptor inhibition → anticholinergic effects.
- α-Adrenergic receptor blockade
- GABA receptor antagonism → seizures.
- Na^{++}-channel blockade → prolongation of phase 0 (rapid depolarization) → quinidine-like effects.
  - Worsened by acidosis (respiratory or metabolic)
- K^{+}-channel antagonism
- Inhibition of amine uptake

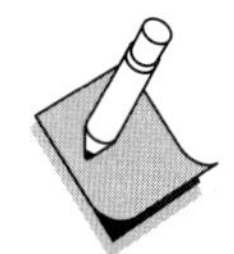

Life-threatening cardiac toxicity results from Na^{++}-channel blockade.

SYMPTOMS/EXAM

Table 6.5 summarizes the clinical findings in TCA poisonings.

- Early poisoning → reflex sinus tachycardia and hypertension.
- Life-threatening toxicity → Na^{++} channel blockade → **hypotension with QRS widening >100 msec**.

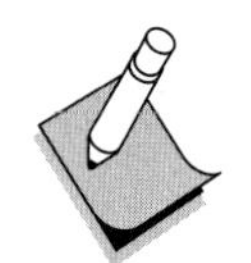

Acidosis worsens Na^{++} channel blockade.

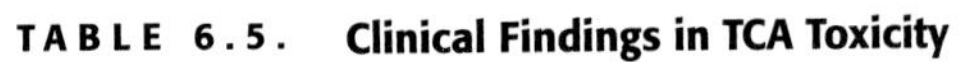

TABLE 6.5. Clinical Findings in TCA Toxicity

PHARMACOLOGIC EFFECT	SYMPTOMS/EXAM
Antihistamine	CNS excitation ↔ coma
Anticholinergic	Dry, flushed skin Mydriasis Hyperthermia Seizures Tachycardia Urinary retention CNS excitation ↔ coma
α-Adrenergic receptor blockade	Reflex tachycardia Orthostatic hypotension Miosis
GABA receptor blockade	Seizures
Na^{++} channel blockade	QRS widening Decreased contractility Hypotension
K^{+} channel antagonism	QT prolongation
Inhibition of amine uptake	Initial hypertension CNS excitation ↔ coma

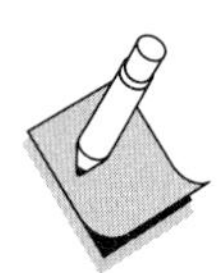

ECG findings consistent with sodium channel blockade: Rightward deviation of the terminal 40 msec of the QRS Prolonged PR interval QRS >100 msec

- **Seizures** are typically self-limited, but are associated with acidosis, which in turn worsens the Na^{++} channel blockade.
- **Rapid deterioration** can occur.

DIFFERENTIAL DIAGNOSIS

- False-positive serum TCA screen may occur with carbamazepine, cyclobenzaprine, diphenhydramine, and phenothizines.
- Antidysrhythmic overdose
- Cocaine toxicity

DIAGNOSIS

- Suspect based on history and presentation.
- ECG findings of Na^{++} channel blockade:
  - Rightward deviation of the terminal 40 msec of the QRS = terminal R in lead aVR of >3 mm and S wave in lead I (see Figure 6.1).
  - Prolongation of PR interval
  - QRS widening
    - QRS >100 msec is associated with increased risk of seizures.
    - QRS >160 msec is associated with increased risk of wide-complex dysrhythmias.
- Plasma TCA level
  - Serious intoxications are generally >1000 ng/mL.
- Urine tox screen for TCAs.
  - False positives include diphenhydramine, carbamazepine.

Sodium bicarbonate is the treatment of choice for TCA-induced dysrhythmias.

TREATMENT

- Supportive care
  - Early intubation to avoid respiratory acidosis
- Gastric lavage and charcoal if early and no CNS depression
- IV fluid boluses for hypotension
- **Sodium bicarbonate,** indications:
  - Rightward deviation of the terminal 40 msec of the QRS
  - QRS >100 msec
  - Ventricular dysrhythmias
  - Hypotension unresponsive to fluids
  - Administer boluses of 1–2 mEq/kg until improvement, then start drip (3 ampules in 1 L of D_5W at maintenance rate).

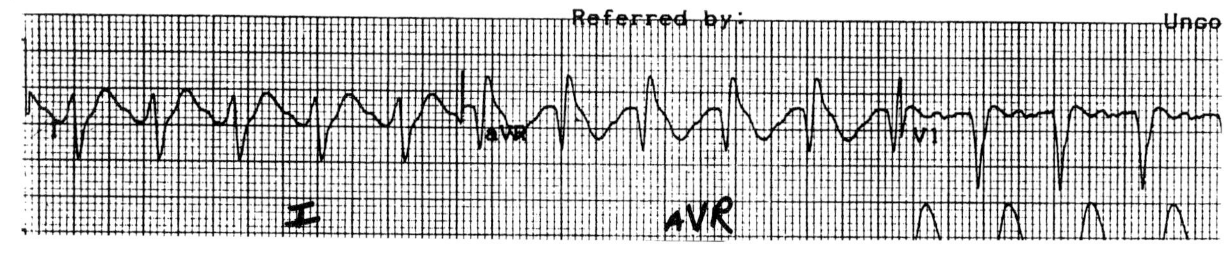

FIGURE 6.1. Sodium channel blockade in TCA toxicity.

(Reproduced, with permission, from Tintinalli JE, Kelen GD, Stapczynski JS. *Emergency Medicine: A Comprehensive Study Guide,* 6th ed. New York: McGraw-Hill, 2004:1031.)

- **Benzodiazepines** for seizures
  - Sodium bicarbonate is **not** indicated for seizures (seizures are not due to Na^{++} channel blockade!).
- **Norepinephrine** for hypotension unresponsive to fluid and sodium bicarbonate
- **Magnesium sulfate** if torsades de pointes
- **Avoid:**
  - Physostigmine (no treatment benefit and may cause seizures)
  - Respiratory and/or metabolic acidosis (worsens Na^{++} channel blockade)
  - Class IA and IC antidysrhythmics (fast Na^{++} channel blockers)
  - Class III antidysrhythmics (K^{++} channel blockers)
  - Phenytoin (no treatment benefit)

COMPLICATIONS

- Aspiration
- Hypoxic brain injury
- Cardiovascular collapse

Selective Serotonin Reuptake Inhibitors

SSRIs are widely used for depression because of their large therapeutic window. Fatal overdoses are rare.

Examples include:

- Fluoxetine (Prozac)
- Citalopram (Celexa)
- Paroxetine (Paxil)

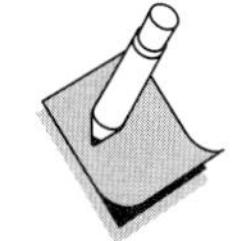

Serotonin syndrome may occur with overdose or routine use.

MECHANISM/TOXICITY

- Inhibition of presynaptic serotonin reuptake → increased CNS serotonin.

SYMPTOMS/EXAM

- N/V, abdominal pain
- Sinus tachycardia
- CNS sedation and tremor
- Less commonly—seizures, more serious cardiovascular toxicity
- **Serotonin syndrome** may occur with overdose or routine use.
  - Autonomic dysfunction → hyperthermia (>38°C), diaphoresis.
  - CNS dysfunction → agitation and/or altered mental status.
  - Neuromuscular dysfunction → nystagmus, myoclonus, hyperreflexia, muscular rigidity (lower extremities predominantly), tremor.

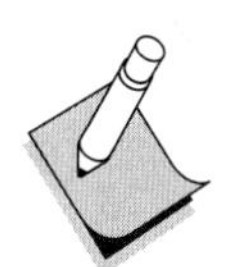

Serotonin syndrome is characterized by increased autonomic, CNS, and neuromuscular activity.

DIAGNOSIS

- Clinical diagnosis is based on history of ingestion, constellation of signs, and symptoms. Typical history includes increasing the dose of an SSRI or more commonly, adding a second serotonergic agent.
- SSRIs are not typically detected on standard toxicology screens.

TREATMENT

- Supportive care
- Activated charcoal if early and no CNS depression

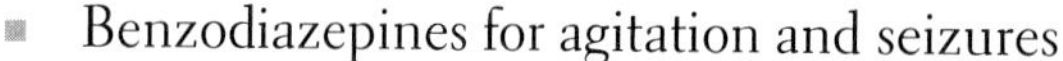

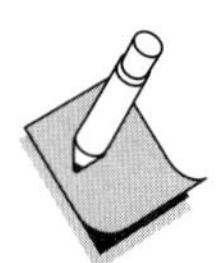

Antidote to SSRIs, used in mild-moderate serotonin syndrome = cyproheptadine.

- Benzodiazepines for agitation and seizures
- Sodium bicarbonate for QRS widening >100 msec
- **Antidote = cyproheptadine** (serotonin antagonist).
  - Oral formulation only
  - Indicated *for serotonin syndrome* in the patient able to take oral medication

Monoamine Oxidase Inhibitors

Rarely used today as first-line agent for depression due to narrow therapeutic window and drug interactions

Examples include:

- Phenelzine (Nardil)
- Tranylcypromaine (Parnate)
- St. John's Wort—an herbal preparation for depression thought to have some monoamine oxidase inhibitor action
- MAOB inhibitors (selegiline, rasagiline) are used to treat Parkinson disease and are much less toxic in overdose.

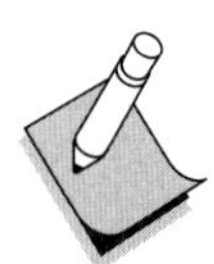

Symptom onset following MAOI overdose is frequently delayed 6–12 hours.

Mechanism/Toxicity

- Inhibition of monoamine oxidase → decreased inactivation of biogenic amines, including epinephrine, norepinephrine, serotonin → excessive circulating catecholamines.
- Monamine oxidase may take weeks to regenerate after discontinuation of MAOIs!

Symptoms/Exam

MAOI overdose symptoms are those of life-threatening excessive sympathetic activity.

- Characterized by **excessive sympathetic activity**
- Symptoms are usually **delayed 6–12 hours** following overdose!
- Agitation, mydriasis
- Tachycardia, hyperthermia, hypertension
- Muscle rigidity, hyperreflexia, myoclonus
- Seizures, coma
- **Tyramine reaction**—after ingestion of tyramine-containing foods (red wine, cheese, etc.)
  - Headache, hypertension, diaphoresis, palpitations, and neuromuscular excitation lasting for several hours

Differential

- Cocaine, amphetamines, PCP, ephedrine

Diagnosis

- Clinical diagnosis based on patient presentation.
- MAOIs are usually not detected on standard toxicology screens.

Treatment

- Supportive care
- Aggressive treatment of hyperthermia
- Activated charcoal, if early
- Benzodiazepines for agitation, rigidity, seizures, tachycardia

TABLE 6.6. Toxicity Related to Newer Antidepressants

Medication	Major Toxicity
Bupropion (Wellbutrin)	Seizures (hallmark of toxicity)
Mirtazapine (Remeron)	Hypotension Serotonin syndrome
Trazadone (Desyrel)	Similar to SSRIs Serotonin syndrome Hypotension
Venlafaxine (Effexor)	CNS sedation Serotonin syndrome

- Sodium nitroprusside or phentolamine, if severely hypertensive
- **Avoid:**
  - β-Blockers (→ unopposed α-adrenergic stimulation)
  - All indirect sympathomimetics (dopamine)

Complications

- Serotonin syndrome
- Sequelae of hypertensive emergency
- Rhabdomyolysis

Newer Antidepressants

Heterogeneous group of newer medications that block dopamine, norepinephrine, and serotonin CNS reuptake to varying degrees.

Common examples and toxicities are listed in Table 6.6.

ANTIBIOTICS AND ANTIRETROVIRALS

Most antibiotics and antivirals are associated with adverse drug effects (eg, allergic reactions) or complications from chronic therapy.

This section is limited to medications that are associated with severe toxicity in overdose.

Isoniazid

Isoniazid is one of the first-line agents used to treat tuberculosis (TB).

Chronic use is associated with peripheral neuropathy, hepatitis, drug-induced systemic lupus erythematosus (SLE).

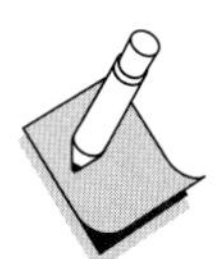

Seizing patient refractory to standard therapy? Consider INH toxicity.

Mechanism/Toxicity

- Reduction of vitamin B_6 in brain → ↓ γ-aminobutyric acid (GABA) production → seizures.

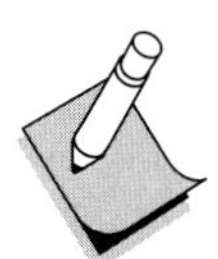

INH is listed as a cause of an anion gap metabolic acidosis because it causes a profound lactic acidosis from seizure activity. It does not cause lactic acidosis when seizures are not present.

Symptoms/Exam

- Nausea and vomiting
- Slurred speech, ataxia, depressed mental status, and seizures
- The classic presentation is persistent seizures and resultant metabolic acidosis.

Diagnosis

- Should be suspected in any patient with seizures who is undergoing treatment for TB or is refractory to standard treatment
- INH levels take too long to be clinically useful in the ED.

Treatment

- Supportive care
- Activated charcoal if early and no CNS depression
- Benzodiazepines for status epilepticus until antidote available
- **Antidote: Pyridoxine (vitamin B_6)** replenishes vitamin B_6 stores to help replete GABA.

Complications

- Chronic large doses of pyridoxine may cause peripheral neuropathy.

Reverse Transcriptase Inhibitors

Reverse transcriptase inhibitors are antiretroviral agents used in the treatment of HIV. Highly active antiretroviral therapy (HAART) refers to a drug regimen combining reverse transcriptase inhibitors with agents from two other antiretroviral classes, protease inhibitors and fusion inhibitors.

Reverse transcriptase inhibitors include didanosine (ddI), stavudine (d4T), lamivudine (3TC), and others.

Mechanism/Toxicity

- Mitochondrial toxicity → lactic acidosis, hepatotoxicity, pancreatitis.

Symptoms/Exam

- Malaise
- Tachypnea
- N/V, abdominal pain

Diagnosis

- Suspect based on clinical presentation.
- Confirmed with laboratory findings (elevated lactate, etc.)
- Muscle or liver biopsy is definitive for diagnosis of mitochondrial toxicity.

Reverse transcriptase inhibitors may cause a profound lactic acidosis due to mitochondrial toxicity.

Treatment

- Discontinue implicated drug(s).
- Supportive care
- If severe lactic acidosis → sodium bicarbonate
- Hemodialysis may be considered.

A 23-year-old male with a history of depression presents to the ED via EMS for altered mentation. On presentation he is agitated and delirious. Physical examination reveals tachycardia, dilated pupils, mild hypertension, fever, dry mucous membranes, and flushed, dry skin. Ingestion of which groups of drugs is suggested by this patient's presenting symptoms?

This patient is presenting with an anticholinergic toxidrome, which may be caused by over-the-counter antihistamines, certain plants, or a variety of prescription medications.

ANTICHOLINERGICS/CHOLINERGICS

Anticholinergics

The anticholinergic toxidrome may result from exposure to medications or plants (see Table 6.7).

Mechanism/Toxicity

- Competitive antagonism of acetylcholine at muscarinic and central nervous system cholinergic receptors

Symptoms/Exam

- Agitation, delirium, hallucinations ↔ coma, seizures.
- Hyperthermia
- Dry, flushed, warm skin
- Mydriasis and blurry vision
- Tachycardia
  - Sinus tachycardia
  - Tachydysrhythmias are unusual, but may occur.
- QRS prolongation and wide complex dysrhythmias may be seen with certain agents (TCAs, diphenhydramine), but is due to other drug effects (Na^{++} channel blockade).

TABLE 6.7. Common Anticholinergic Agents

Prescription Medications
Antipsychotics
Scopolamine
Gastrointestinal antispasmodics
Skeletal muscle relaxants
Over-the-Counter Medications
Antihistamines
Plants
Jimsonweed (*Datura stramonium*)
Deadly nightshade (*Atropa belladonna*)

- Hypertension
- Diminished bowel sounds, decreased defecation
- Urinary retention

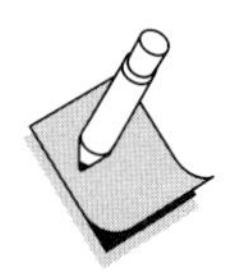

Anticholinergic toxidrome:

Mad as a hatter

Red as a beet

Dry as a bone

Blind as a bat

Hot as a hare

Seizing like a squirrel

Tachy as a pink flamingo

Full as a flask

DIFFERENTIAL

- Encephalitis
- Neuroleptic malignant syndrome
- Sympathomimetic toxicity may have similar presentation, but skin is typically moist (not dry).

DIAGNOSIS

- Clinical diagnosis is based on exposure history and physical exam.
- Labs and imaging as needed to exclude nontoxicologic causes.
- ECG used to screen for TCA toxicity.

TREATMENT

- Supportive care
  - Passive and active cooling measures may be needed.
- Benzodiazepines (for seizures, agitation, hyperthermia)
- Intravenous hydration
- **Antidote = physostigmine.**
  - Indications include tachycardia uncontrolled with standard therapy and agitation uncontrolled with sedatives.
- **Avoid**
  - β-Blockers
  - Sedatives with anticholinergic effects such as diphenhydramine or antipsychotic agents

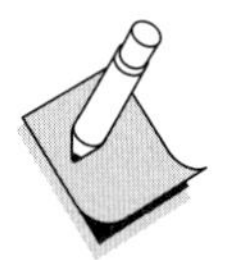

Benzodiazepines are the mainstay of therapy for anticholinergic poisoning.

COMPLICATIONS

- Rhabdomyolysis
  - May be the result of agitation, coma, or hyperthermia
  - Sedate with benzodiazepines to control psychomotor agitation and hyperthermia.
  - Treat with intravenous fluids, follow CK, creatinine, as indicated.

Cholinergics

The cholinergic toxidrome is uncommon, but may result from exposure to cholinergic agents (see Table 6.8).

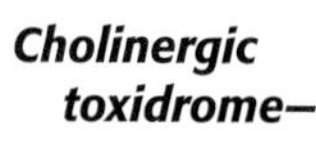

Cholinergic toxidrome–

SLUDGE
Salivation/Sweating
Lacrimation
Urination
Defecation
Gastrointestinal distress
Emesis
plus
"The Killer Bs":
Bradycardia
Bronchorrhea
Bronchospasm

MECHANISM/TOXICITY

- Inhibition of the enzyme acetylcholinesterase → excess acetylcholine at muscarinic and nicotinic receptors.

SYMPTOMS/EXAM

- Altered mental status (delirium to coma), seizures
- Increased secretions → lacrimation, salivation, sweating, bronchorrhea.
- Bronchospasm
- Miotic (constricted) pupils
- Bradycardia (bradydysrhythmias may occur)
- Urinary incontinence
- Hyperactive bowel sounds and bowel incontinence (vomiting/diarrhea)
- Muscle fasciculations

TABLE 6.8. Cholinergic Agents

Some Alzheimer medications Donepezil
Myasthenia gravis medications Pyridostigmine Edrophonium
Insecticides Organophosphate compounds Carbamate compounds
Chemical weapons Nerve agents (sarin)
Glaucoma agents Pilicarpine
Cytocybe and inocybe mushrooms

DIAGNOSIS

- Clinical diagnosis is based on exposure history and physical exam.
- RBC cholinesterase levels may be indicated in chronic exposures.
- ECG used to screen for blocks, dysrhythmias.

TREATMENT

- Supportive care
- **Atropine** (very high doses often needed)
  - Hemodynamically unstable bradycardia
  - Excessive secretions—endpoint is drying of airway secretion.
- **Benzodiazepines** for seizures and agitation
- **Antidotes**
  - **Atropine** (above)
  - **Pralidoxime (2-PAM)** for organophophate poisoning.

Warfarin blocks the synthesis of (vitamin K–dependent) clotting factors II, VII, IX, X.

ANTICOAGULANTS

Warfarin

Warfarin is an oral anticoagulant.

MECHANISM/TOXICITY

- Blocks conversion of vitamin K to its active form, thereby preventing synthesis of vitamin K–dependent clotting factors (II, VII, IX, X)
  - Effect is delayed until preformed stores of vitamin K and clotting factors are depleted (typically ≥15 hours).
  - The duration of action may be up to 6 days.
- Blocks the synthesis of antithrombotic proteins C and S → prothrombotic period before vitamin K–dependent factors are depleted

Onset of effect in overdose is delayed and PT and INR should be monitored for 3–4 days.

TOXICOLOGY

Symptoms/Exam

- Bleeding—may be spontaneous or related to trauma

Differential

- Other "warfarin-like" anticoagulants, heparin/LMWH, ingestion of brodifacoum (rat poison).

Diagnosis

- Usually clear from patient's history and exam.
- PT and INR should be monitored periodically for 3–4 days.

Treatment

- Supportive therapy, including PRBC transfusion as needed
- Activated charcoal—if within 1–2 hours (with airway control as needed)
- **Oral cholestyramine** may enhance elimination.
- Approach depends on INR level and presence of bleeding (see Table 6.9).
- **Vitamin K_1**
  - Will reverse the blockade, but will not activate enough factors to reverse coagulopathy for several hours
  - Can be given prophylactically for those patients not requiring anticoagulation

TABLE 6.9. Guidelines for Treatment of Overanticoagulation with Warfarin

Condition	Treatment
INR < 5, no clinically significant bleeding	Lower or skip dose. Resume when INR therapeutic.
INR 5–9, no clinically significant bleeding	Omit next one or two doses. *or* Skip dose and give vitamin K_1 (1–2mg PO). Resume at lower dose when INR therapeutic.
INR > 9, no clinically significant bleeding	Hold warfarin. Give higher dose of vitamin K_1 (5–10 mg PO). Resume at lower doses when INR therapeutic.
Serious bleeding at any elevation of INR	Hold therapy. Give vitamin K_1 (10 mg slow IV). Give FFP or prothrombin complex concentrate (PCC). Recombinant factor VIIa is an alterative therapy.
Life-threatening bleeding	Hold warfarin. Give FFP, PCC or recombinant factor VIIa. Give vitamin K_1 (10 mg slow IV). Repeat as necessary.

- **Fresh frozen plasma**
  - 10–15mg/kg will restore factor levels to ≥ 30% of normal.
- **Prothrombin complex concentrate and recombinant factor VIIa**
  - Allow for factor replacement and *immediate complete reversal* of anticoagulation

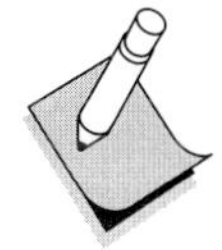

Prothrombin complex concentrates and recombinant factor VIIa are used when immediate and complete reversal of warfarin anticoagulation is desired.

COMPLICATIONS

- Intravenous Vitamin K_1 therapy can rarely cause anaphylaxis.
- Warfarin-induced skin necrosis:
  - Occurs 3–8 days after initiating warfarin therapy in patients with protein C deficiency (transient hypercoagulable state)
  - Thrombosis of cutaneous vessels
  - Prevented by coadministration of heparin during initiation of warfarin therapy
  - Treated with discontinuation of warfarin and initiation of heparin therapy

Heparin

MECHANISM/TOXICITY

- Binds antithrombin III → heparin-antithrombin III complex → inhibits multiple steps (IX_a, X_a, XI_a, XII_a and thrombin) in intrinsic and extrinsic pathways.
- Low-molecular-weight heparins (LMWH) are obtained from heparin, but have a longer half-life, greater bioavailability, and greater activity against factor X_a.

SYMPTOMS/EXAM

- Bleeding may be spontaneous or related to trauma.

DIFFERENTIAL

- Warfarin, other "warfain-like" anticoagulants, ingestion of brodifacoum (rat poison)

DIAGNOSIS

- Usually clear from patient's history and exam
- Elevation of PT/INR and aPTT

TREATMENT

- Stop heparin.
- **Protamine sulfate:**
  - Indicated for severe bleeding complications only (risk of serious anaphylaxis with administration)
  - Reverses the effect of heparin and partially inactivates LMWH
  - Dose is calculated from the dose of heparin given.
  - Onset of action is 30–60 seconds with a duration lasting 2 hours.

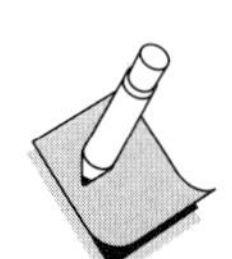

Heparin-induced thrombocytopenia is associated with systemic venous and arterial thrombotic events.

COMPLICATIONS

- **Heparin-induced thrombocytopenia (HIT)**: May occur 5–8 days after initiating therapy or as late as 3 weeks after stopping therapy. Antibodies cause significant drop in platelets (>50%) and skin changes at injection sites. Systemic **venous and arterial *thrombotic* events** can cause a wide variety of end organ damage. This is more common with heparin versus LMWH.

ANTICONVULSANTS

Anticonvulsant medications were developed for the treatment of seizures, but they are also used for treatment of pain (carbamazepine, gabapentin), mood disorders (carbamazepine, valproic acid, lamotragine), and migraines (valproic acid, toperamide).

MECHANISM/TOXICITY

Cardiac toxicity with intravenous phenytoin administration is due to its propylene glycol diluent.

- Slow conduction through Na^+ channels (phenytoin, carbamazepine, toperamide) *or* increase activity in the GABA system (gabapentin, valproic acid, phenobarbital)
- *All* → CNS depression in overdose.
- *Some* → slowed intracardiac conduction in overdose (carbamazepine, toperamide).
- Rapid infusion of phenytoin → myocardial depression and cardiac arrest from **propylene glycol diluent** (not present in fosphenytoin).

DIAGNOSIS

- Clinical laboratories can measure serum levels for many antiepileptics. However, there is substantial intrasubject sensitivity to the effects of these drugs, so levels are not accurate predictors of toxicity.
- An elevated ammonia level is one of the most sensitive indicators of valproic acid toxicity. Results from depletion of carnitine and interference with the urea cycle.

SYMPTOMS/EXAM

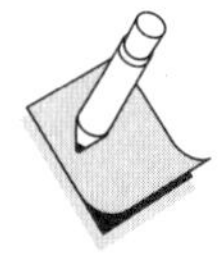

Carbamazepine has a structural similarity to TCA → at high levels can cause similar CNS and cardiac toxicity.

- Carbamazepine
  - Mild/moderate toxicity is characterized by ataxia and nystagmus.
  - Serious ingestions (levels >40 mg/L) present with seizures, respiratory and CNS depression, and dysrhythmias (AV blocks, QRS/QT prolongation).
- Phenytoin
  - Mild to moderate toxicity: nystagmus, ataxia, and dysarthria
  - Severe toxicity (level >40 mg/L): stupor, coma, and respiratory arrest
  - Rapid IV injection → hypotension, bradycardia, and cardiac arrest.
  - Tissue infiltration → "**purple glove syndrome**": edema, pain, ischemia, tissue necrosis, compartment syndrome
- Valproic acid
  - N/V, CNS depression
  - Severe toxicity (levels >850 mg/L): coma, respiratory depression, seizures, metabolic disturbances, cardiac arrest

TREATMENT

Valproic acid toxicity (as compared to phenytoin and carbamazepine) can be treated with hemodialysis.

- Supportive therapy
- Observe asymptomatic patients for at least 6 hours (depending on formulation).
- Activated charcoal
- Hemodialysis is **not** effective in most overdoses; may be considered in massive valproic acid ingestion.
- Charcoal hemoperfusion has been used for carbamazepine and phenytoin poisoning, but it is rarely available and of unproven value.
- Multiple-dose activated charcoal increases the clearance of carbamazepine and phenobarbital.

COMPLICATIONS

- **Hypersensitivity reactions** may occur 1–6 weeks after starting phenytoin therapy, eg, SLE, TEN, erythema multiforme.
- **Gingival hyperplasia** can be seen with chronic phenytoin therapy.
- Chronic ingestion of valproic acid: Hepatic failure

ANTIPARKINSONISM DRUGS

In Parkinson disease, cells in the substantia nigra degenerate, reducing the production of dopamine, an essential neurotransmitter for the control of movement and coordination.

The drugs used in the treatment of Parkinson disease can be divided into two main groups: Dopamine agonists and anticholinergics (see Table 6.10).

Acute overdose of antiparkinsonism drugs is rare.

MECHANISM/TOXICITY

- Dopamine agonists: Excessive activation of dopaminergic neurons. Activation of serotonergic systems may also occur.
- Anticholinergics: Inhibition of central and peripheral muscarinic receptors
- Monoamine oxidase inhibition (selegiline): May become nonselective at high doses → excessive circulating catecholamines.

SYMPTOMS/EXAM

Dopamine Agonism

- Acute toxicity: Anxiety, confusion, agitation, insomnia, tachycardia, hypotension
- Chronic toxicity: Dystonia, hallucinations, hypersexuality, delusions

Anticholinergics

- Anticholinergic toxidrome

TABLE 6.10. Drugs Used in the Treatment of Parkinson Disease

DRUG	MECHANISM OF ACTION
Dopamine Agonists	
Levodopa	Converts to dopamine
Catechol-O-methytransferase (COMT) inhibitors	Extend the duration of effect of levodopa
Selegiline	Selective monoamine oxidase inhibitor, blocks reuptake of dopamine
Bromocriptine	Dopamine receptor agonist
Anticholintergics	
Benztropine (and others)	Inhibit the excess central muscarinic activity caused by dopamine deficiency

TOXICOLOGY

Selegiline

- Limited data, may see classic MAOI toxicity

DIAGNOSIS

- Clinical diagnosis is based on history and examination.
- Selegiline is metabolized to L-methamphetamine, which can be detected on urine toxicology screening.

TREATMENT

- Supportive care
- Cessation of medication
- Sedation with benzodiazepines, as needed

ANTIPSYCHOTICS

Antipsychotics were developed for the treatment of psychoses, but are also commonly used in the treatment of N/V, migraines, and to control the agitated patient.

Therapeutic effects are due to antagonism of mesolimbic dopamine receptors, but variable affinity for other receptors causes a variety of side effects and toxicity in therapeutic use.

They are divided into two major groups (see Table 6.11):

Typical antipsychotics

- The original medications introduced in the 1950s
- Characterized by less receptor specificity → greater incidence of side effects than newer agents

Atypical antipsychotics

- The newer generation medications, first introduced in the 1990s

Acute overdose is common, but toxicity resulting in severe morbidity or mortality is rare.

MECHANISM/TOXICITY

- Nonspecific dopamine receptor antagonism → extrapyramidal symptoms and neuroleptic malignant syndrome.
- α_1-Adrenergic antagonism → orthostatic hypotension and reflex tachycardia.

TABLE 6.11. Common Antipsychotic Agents

TYPICAL ANTIPSYCHOTICS	ATYPICAL ANTIPSYCHOTICS
Haloperidol (Haldol)	Risperidone (Risperdal)
Chlorpromazine (Thorazine)	Quitiapine (Seroquel)
Promethazine (Phenergan)	Olanzapine (Zyprexa)
Proclorperazine (Compazine)	Aripiprazole (Abilify)

- Muscarinic receptor antagonism → anticholinergic symptoms.
- Histamine receptor antagonism → sedation.
- Cardiac K^+ channel blockade → prolonged qTc.

SYMPTOMS/EXAM

- Adverse effects related to nonspecific receptor blockade are common (see Table 6.12).
- Again, typical agents are more likely to have adverse effects than atypical agents.
- Findings in acute overdose are an extension of these adverse effects.

DIAGNOSIS

- Clinical diagnosis is based on history of exposure, physical exam findings.
- ECG is used to monitor prolonged qT_c

TREATMENT

- Supportive therapy
- Continuous monitoring

TOXICOLOGY

TABLE 6.12. Adverse Effects of Antipsychotics

ADVERSE EFFECT	MECHANISM/TOXICITY	SYMPTOMS/EXAM	TREATMENT
Extrapyramidal symptoms	Basal ganglia dopamine receptor antagonism	See Table 6.13.	
Neuroleptic malignant syndrome (NMS)	Anterior hypothalamus and basal ganglia dopamine receptor antagonism	Altered mental status Hyperthermia Muscular rigidity	Stop medication. Benzodiazepines Intubate and paralyze as needed.
Altered mental status	Histamine and muscarinic receptor antagonism	Agitated delirium Somnolence Coma	Benzodiazepines for agitation Support airway as needed.
Hypotension	α_1-Adrenergic receptor antagonism	Mild to moderate hypotension	Intravenous fluids Pressors may be needed.
Tachycardia	α_1-Adrenergic (reflex tachycardia) and muscarinic receptor antagonism	Mild to moderate sinus tachycardia	
Prolonged qTc	K^+ channel blockade	Theoretical concern for torsades de pointes, but rare	Cardiac monitoring Check electrolytes. Treat torsades using standard therapies.
Blood dyscrasias	Adverse drug effect associated with clozaril	Agranulocytosis, leukopenia, neutropenia.	Stop medication.

TABLE 6.13. **Extrapyramidal Symptoms**

Name	Onset/Reversibility	Symptoms/Exam	Treatment
Akathisia	Hours to days Reversible	Anxiety Acute motor restlessness	Stop medication. Benzodiazepines Diphenhydramine
Acute dystonia	Hours to days after exposure Reversible	Sustained muscle contractions → facial grimacing. Torticollis Trismus Laryngospasm Opisthotonos	Stop medication. Benzodiazepines Diphenhydramine
Parkinsonism	Days to months of exposure Usually reversible	Akinesia or bradykinesia Masked facies Muscular rigidity Tremor Gait instability Cognitive impairment	↓ Dose or stop medication. Benztropine
Tardive dyskinesia	Months to years of exposure Usually irreversible	Involuntary, repetitive orofacial, trunk and extremity movements	No specific treatment available

- Activated charcoal: For large ingestions within 1–2 hours (with airway protection as needed)
- Norepinephrine: For hypotension unresponsive to IVF
- Intravenous magnesium sulfate, overdrive pacing, isoproterenol for torsades
- Benzodiazepines: To control agitation and seizures

A 65-year-old male presents to the ED via EMS with weakness and dizziness. He has a history of depression, CHF, and HTN, and is on multiple "heart" medications. Physical examination reveals sinus bradycardia, hypotension, mild temperature depression, and normal mentation. Overdose of which groups of cardiac drugs is suggested by this patient's presentation?

Overdose of β-blockers, calcium channel blockers, clonidine, digoxin and central-acting agents should be suspected in any patient presenting with hypotension and bradycardia.

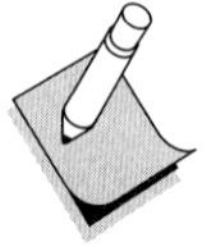

Class IA and IC agents are notorious for prolonging the QRS and/or QT, causing VT or torsades.

CARDIOVASCULAR MEDICATIONS

Antidysrhythmic Agents

Antidysrhythmic agents are classified via Vaughn-Williams into groups based on electrophysiologic properties (see Table 6.14). Toxicity is unique to each class.

TABLE 6.14. **Overview of Antidysrhythmic Agents**

Vaughn-Williams Classification	Mechanism of Action	Examples	Symptoms of Toxicity	Treatment
Class I	Fast Na^+ channel blockers → stabilization of membranes.	**IA:** Procainamide Quinidine Disorpyramide **IB:** Lidocaine Phenytoin **IC:** Flecainide Propafenone	Vary with agent Agitation, confusion Hypotension Ventricular or brady-dysrhythmias	Supportive care Activated charcoal (if early) Sodium bicarbonate for QRS widening
Class II	β-Blockers	See text	See text	See text
Class III	K^+ channel blockers → prolongation of repolorization. Sotalol also has β-blocking activity.	Amiodarone Sotolol	Vary with agent Hypotension and bradycardia QT prolongation → VT, Vfib, torsades. Chronic amiodarone therapy: interstitial pneumonitis, grey or bluish skin changes, corneal microdeposits	Supportive care Activated charcoal (if early) Gastric lavage (if early sotalol) Sodium bicarbonate for QRS widening
Class IV	Calcium channel blockers	See text	See text	See text

β-Blockers

Normal function of β-adrenergic receptors:

- β-1: Heart (increases rate, contractility, conduction), kidney (increased secretion of renin), eye (increased production of aqueous humor)
- β-2: Smooth muscle relaxation
- β-3: Adipose tissue (lipolysis)

Mechanism/Toxicity

- β-Adrenergic receptors blockade

Symptoms/Exam

- Varying degrees of hypotension, bradycardia
  - Patient may present in cardiogenic shock.
- Respiratory depression, apnea
- QRS and QT prolongation
- Bronchospasm (β-2) in susceptible patients, respiratory depression, and apnea

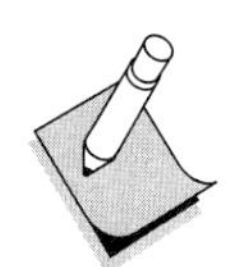

Propranolol, due to its lipophilicity, can cause delirium in the absence of cardiovascular effects.

- AMS and coma
- Seizures with lipophilic agents (eg, propranolol)
- Hypoglycemia (potentially, in children)
- Hyperkalemia

DIFFERENTIAL

- Calcium channel blocker, clonidine, or digoxin toxicity

DIAGNOSIS

- Should be considered in the differential of any patient with bradycardia and hypotension

TREATMENT

- Supportive therapy
- GI decontamination
  - Gastric lavage: If early presentation with a large overdose, given lack of antidote and potential lethality of these agents
  - Activated charcoal: Give in all cases (with patent airway)
  - Whole-bowel irrigation: If large overdose of sustained-release preparation
- Bradycardia and hypotension
  - Treat initially with atropine and vasopressors.
  - **Calcium** supplementation
    - After ruling out digoxin toxicity
    - Increases movement of calcium into the cell
  - **Glucagon**
    - Requires high doses (5–10 mg)
    - Activates adenyl cyclase and increases cyclic AMP, resulting in increased calcium influx into the cell
  - **High-dose insulin** (with glucose to maintain euglycemia)
    - Increases cardiac output via unclear mechanisms
  - Cardiac pacing, intra-aortic balloon pump, and bypass should be considered if these pharmacologic measures fail.

Calcium Channel Blockers

Prescribed for the treatment of hypertension, arrhythmias, and migraines

MECHANISM/TOXICITY

- Blockade of L-type voltage gated Ca^{++} channels → decreased Ca^{++} influx into cells.
  - In cardiac muscle cells → decreased SA node activity, decreased contractility, slowed AV conduction.
  - In smooth muscle cells (peripheral vascular system) → relaxation and vasodilitation.
- Agent specificity:
  - Verapamil: Major effect at sinoatrial and atrioventricular nodes
  - Diltiazem: Intermediate activity at both cardiac and peripheral vasculature
  - Dihydroperidines (eg, nifedipine): Major effect on peripheral vasculature

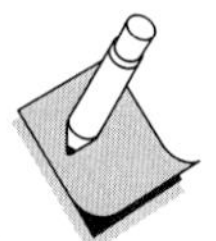

Specificity between peripheral and central cardiovascular effect may be lost in overdose.

Symptoms/Exam

- Varying degrees of hypotension, bradycardia
  - Patient may present in cardiogenic shock.
- Respiratory depression, apnea, QRS and QT prolongation
- AMS, seizures, and coma
  - Fewer CNS effects when compared to β-blockers
- Hyperglycemia (mild)

Hyperglycemia is suggestive of calcium channel blocker overdose in the undifferentiated hypotensive and bradycardic patient.

Differential

- β-Blockers, clonidine, digoxin

Diagnosis

- Should be considered in the differential of any patient with bradycardia, hypotension, and *hyper*glycemia

Treatment

- GI decontamination
  - Gastric lavage: If early presentation with a large overdose, given lack of antidote and potential lethality of these agents
  - Activated charcoal: Give to all patients (with patent airway).
  - Whole-bowel irrigation: Consider if large overdose of sustained release preparations.
- Bradycardia and hypotension
  - Treat initially with atropine and vasopressors.
  - **IV calcium**
    - After ruling out digoxin toxicity
    - Increases movement of Ca^{++} into the cell
  - **Glucagon**
    - Requires high doses (5–10 mg)
    - Activates adenyl cyclase and increases cyclic AMP, resulting in increased calcium influx into the cell
    - May be less successful than with β-blocker toxicity
  - **High-dose insulin** (with glucose to maintain euglycemia)
    - Increases cardiac output via unclear mechanisms
  - Cardiac pacing, intra-aortic balloon pump, and bypass should be considered if these pharmacologic measures fail.

Digoxin

Digoxin is a cardiac glycoside derived from the foxglove plant. It is used to increase the force of myocardial contraction in systolic heart failure and to decrease AV conduction in atrial fibrillation. Digoxin has a narrow therapeutic-toxic window and is eliminated primarily via renal excretion.

Mechanism/Toxicity

- Inactivation of the Na^+K^+ATPase pump on the cardiac cell membrane → increased intracellular Ca^{++} and extracellular K^+.
- Increased automaticity
- Decreases conduction through the AV node via increased vagal tone

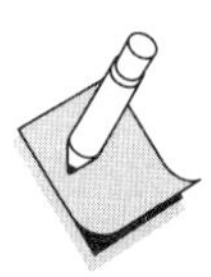

Hyperkalemia in acute digoxin toxicity is a predictor of poor outcome.

Toxicity may be either acute or chronic:

- Acute toxicity
  - Results from an acute ingestion (eg, children or suicidal)
  - Tends to cause severe Na^+K^+ATPase pump malfunction → hyperkalemia
  - Hyperkalemia in acute toxicity is a predictor of poor outcome.
- Chronic toxicity
  - Results from an increase in dose or decrease in renal excretion of digoxin in a patient on chronic therapy
  - Hypokalemia may enhance chronic toxicity → toxicity at lower digoxin levels.
  - Has a higher overall mortality (sicker patient population at baseline)

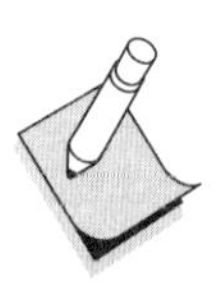

Hypokalemia in a patient on chronic digoxin therapy may lead to toxicity at lower digoxin levels.

SYMPTOMS/EXAM

- Onset of symptoms is often insidious in chronic toxicity
- Nausea/vomiting, anorexia
- Visual disturbances (eg, scotomata, yellow halos around lights)
- Mental status changes
- Headaches, generalized weakness
- **Dysrhythmias:** Virtually *any* dysrhythmia is possible.
  - PVCs (most common ECG finding)
  - Bradycardia
  - Atrial tachycardia with block
  - Slow atrial fibrillation
  - Bidirectional ventricular tachycardia (fairly specific).
  - Acute toxicity → more bradycardia and blocks.
  - Chronic toxicity → ventricular dysrhythmias more common.

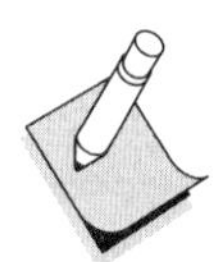

Bidirectional VT is fairly specific for cardiac glycoside toxicity.

DIAGNOSIS

- Usually obvious from patient's history and presentation
- Serum digoxin levels: May not correlate with symptoms and may take 6–12 hours to reach steady state in acute ingestion
- Potassium and renal function monitoring are essential.

TREATMENT

- Supportive therapy
- Activated charcoal (with airway protection, as needed)
- Hyperkalemia: Treat in the normal manner, but **calcium should be avoided**.
- Hypokalemia in chronic toxicity: Replete if <4.0 mEq/dL.
- Bradycardias
  - Treat with atropine and/or pacing.
- Tachydysrhythmias
  - Cardioversion and defibrillation may induce VT/Vfib.
  - Phenytoin and lidocaine are felt to be safest drugs.
    - Phenytoin can increase AV nodal conduction.
- **Antidote = digoxin-specific antibodies** (see Table 6.15 for indications).
  - Acute = 10 vials
  - Chronic = 5 vials

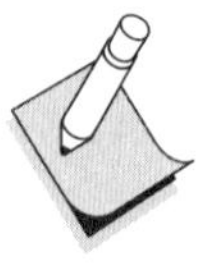

Calcium may precipitate fatal cardiovascular collapse if given in digoxin toxicity.

Angiotensin-Converting Enzyme Inhibitors and Angiotensin Receptor Blockers

Both are prescribed for the treatment of HTN and CHF. ACE-I are also used post-MI and for diabetic nephropathy.

TABLE 6.15. Indications for Digoxin-Specific Antibodies

INDICATIONS FOR DIGOXIN-SPECIFIC ANTIBODIES
Ventricular dysrhythmias
Bradycardia unresponsive to therapy
$K^+ > 5.0$ mEq/dL in acute ingestion
Potentially massive overdose

Complications of chronic use include angioedema, nonproductive cough, renal insufficiency (with renal artery stenosis).

Serious toxicity is not expected in ACE-I or ARB overdose as a single agent.

TOXICOLOGY

Mechanism/Toxicity

- ACE-I: Decreased angiotensin II formation
- ARB: Block the receptor for angiotensin II on the blood vessels, heart, and adrenal cortex
- Blockage of angiotensin II results in decreased aldosterone release (→ decreased sodium and water retention) and vasodilation.

Symptoms/Exam

- Mild hypotension
- Hyperkalemia

Diagnosis

- Usually obvious from patient's history

Treatment

- Supportive care with IV fluids and pressors (if needed) is usually sufficient.

Clonidine

An imidazoline compound prescribed for the treatment of hypertension. It is also used for treatment of pediatric behavioral disorders.

Mechanism/Toxicity

- Central postsynaptic α_2-adrenergic agonist → decreased sympathetic (norepinephrine) outflow → decreased HR and BP.
- Peripherally this postsynaptic α agonism may result in vasoconstriction and paradoxical transient hypertension.

Symptoms/Exam

- Initial, short-lived hypertension progresses to hypotension and bradycardia.
- Hypoventilation with hypoxia
- Mental status changes and coma
- Miosis

DIFFERENTIAL

β-Blockers, calcium channel blockers, digoxin

DIAGNOSIS

- Usually obvious from patient's history
- Should be considered in the differential of any patient with bradycardia and hypotension

TREATMENT

- Supportive care
- Activated charcoal with protected airway if large and recent ingestion
- Bradycardia and hypotension typically respond to IV fluids, but may require atropine and/or vasopressors.
- Naloxone has been reported to reverse some of the sedation, but a mechanism and evidence are lacking.

Other Antihypertensive Agents

Table 6.16 lists other hypertensive agents that may present with acute toxicity in overdose.

These drugs usually will cause symptoms, but they are rarely as life-threatening as a single drug ingestion.

DIAGNOSIS

- Usually obvious from patient's history

TREATMENT

- Supportive care with IV fluids and vasopressors (if needed) is usually sufficient.

TABLE 6.16. Toxicity From Other Hypertensive Agents

ANTIHYPERTENSIVE AGENT	MECHANISM/TOXICITY	SYMPTOMS/EXAM
Hydralazine	Direct acting vasodilator	Hypotension Tachycardia Hypokalemia
Minoxidil	Inhibits Ca^{++} uptake into cells → vasodilation	Hypotension Tachycardia
Methyldopa	Metabolite stimulates central α_2-receptors → ↓ sympathetic output.	Hypotension Miosis Sedation Respiratory depression
Guanethidine Guanadrel	Decreases norepinephrine release from nerve terminals	Hypotension
Doxazocin Prazosin Terazosin	Selective α_1-receptor blocker → ↓ PVR.	Hypotension Tachycardia Dizziness/syncope

A 72-year-old male presents to the ED via EMS for weakness and altered mental status. He has a history of dementia and diabetes. EMS found bottles of metformin and acarbose in the bathroom. Physical examination reveals a finger stick of 48, sinus tachycardia, and sweaty skin. The patient is awake, but confused. Which of the drugs found in his house is likely responsible for his hypoglycemia?

Neither biguanides nor α-Glucosidase inhibitors cause hypoglycemia. Consider insulin, sulfonylureas, or other nontoxicologic causes of hypoglycemia.

DIABETES MEDICATIONS

Sulfonylureas

Agents include

- Glipizide
- Glyburide

MECHANISM/TOXICITY

- ↑ Secretion of preformed insulin from pancreatic β cells → hypoglycemia (primary mechanism).
- Hepatic or renal impairment and drug interactions may be inciting event.

SYMPTOMS/EXAM

- Most agents require 8 hours to reach peak effect.
- Symptoms of hypoglycemia
  - Mental status changes, agitation
  - Headache
  - Focal neurologic deficits or seizures
  - Tachycardia, hypertension
  - Diaphoresis
  - Nausea

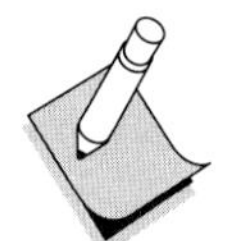

Ingestion of a single sulfonylurea tablet can produce severe hypoglycemia in young children.

DIFFERENTIAL

- Other causes of hypoglycemia including insulin excess, sepsis, hepatic dysfunction.

DIAGNOSIS

- Usually clear from patient's history and exam
- Rapid finger-stick glucose can confirm diagnosis of hypoglycemia.

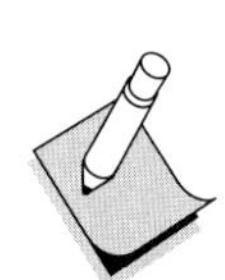

Octreotide inhibits the release of insulin from the pancreas and therefore can be used in sulfonylurea-induced hypoglycemia.

TREATMENT

- Correct hypoglycemia via dextrose administration.
- Activated charcoal if recent ingestion and protected airway
- All patients who become symptomatic should be admitted for 24 hours of observation regardless of response to treatment.
- **Antidote = octreotide.**

TABLE 6.17. Toxicity From Other Hypoglycemic Agents

ANTIHYPERGLYCEMIC CLASS	MECHANISM OF ACTION	SYMPTOMS/EXAM
Biguanides (metformin)	↑ Peripheral glucose use ↓ Hepatic production and intestinal absorption of glucose	Lactic acidosis → N/V, malaise, tachypnea Does NOT cause hypoglycemia
Glinide derivatives	Release of insulin	Hypoglycemia (similar to sulfonylureas)
α-Glucosidase inhibitors	Delays breakdown of complex carbohydrates in small intestines	No reported toxicity in acute overdose
Thiazoladinediones	↑ Insulin sensitivity	No reported toxicity in acute overdose

TOXICOLOGY

- Long-acting synthetic analog of somatostatin, which inhibits the release of insulin from the pancreas
- Decreases dextrose requirements and further episodes of hypoglycemia

- **Antidote = diazoxide.**
  - Antihypertensive/vasodilator, which also inhibits the release of insulin from the pancreas
  - Neither as effective nor as safe as octreotide
  - Reserved for patients who don't respond to octreotide

COMPLICATIONS

- Disulfiram reactions (headache, flushing, N/V) are possible with all sulfonylureas following exposure to alcohol.

Other Antihyperglycemic Agents

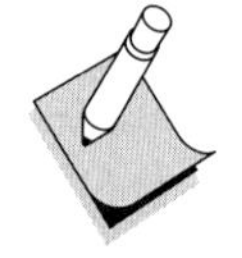

Nonspecific symptoms in patient on metformin? Suspect lactic acidosis.

Table 6.17 lists other diabetic agents that may present with acute toxicity in overdose.

A 25-year-old male presents to the ED via EMS after being found difficult to arouse. He has a history of cocaine binges. Physical examination reveals sinus bradycardia, dry skin, and normal temperature. The patient is alert and oriented after vigorous stimulation. Urine toxicology screen is positive for cocaine metabolites. What is the treatment?

Despite the positive drug screen, this is not cocaine toxicity and there is no immediate treatment necessary. The screen doesn't correlate with toxicity, and this is more likely a "wash out" period following a cocaine binge. The management includes observation and ruling out other serious pathology.

DRUGS OF ABUSE

Cocaine

Natural alkaloid derived from the coca shrub; occasionally still used medicinally as an ester-type topical anesthetic and local vasoconstrictor

Timing and duration of symptoms vary with preparation (see Table 6.18).

Cocaine alkaloid ("crack, free base") is heat stable and is usually smoked. Cocaine hydrochloride cannot be smoked, but is water soluble and may be snorted or injected.

MECHANISM/TOXICITY

Cocaine has multiple mechanisms of action:

- Blocks presynaptic reuptake of biogenic amine neurotransmitters (ie, norepinepherine, serotonin, dopamine) → sympathomimetic effects.
- Na^{++} channel blockade → local anesthesia and IA/IC cardiac antidysrythmic effects.

SYMPTOMS/EXAM

- **Sympathomimetic toxidrome**
  - CNS: Agitations, hallucinations
  - Tachycardia, hypertension
  - Hyperthermia with diaphoretic (**not dry**) skin
  - Mydriasis
  - Muscular rigidity
  - Wide complex tachycardia: From Na^{+} channel blockade.

DIFFERENTIAL

- May be confused with anticholinergic toxidrome (dry skin = anticholinergic, wet skin = sympathomimetic)
- Serotonin syndrome
- Encephalomeningitis
- Thyroid storm
- Ethanol/sedative hypnotic withdrawal

DIAGNOSIS

- Usually clear from history and examination
- Urine screens for metabolite benzoylecgonine
  - Clears in 72 hours
- ECG: Establish rhythm and screen for ischemic changes
- CT of abdomen and pelvis: May be indicated if body packer or stuffer

Sympathomimetic toxidrome:

Agitation
Hyperthermia
Tachycardia
Hypertension
Mydriasis
Diaphoresis

TABLE 6.18. Timing of Symptoms Following Cocaine Use

Route	Onset (Seconds)	Peak (Minutes)	Duration (Minutes)
Inhalation	3–5	1–3	5–15
IV	10–60	3–5	20–60
Oral/intranasal	60–300	15–30	60–90

TREATMENT

- Supportive care
  - Passive and active cooling measures, as needed
  - Intravenous hydration
  - Muscle paralysis may be necessary for heat control.
- **Benzodiazepines:** For sedation, hyperthermia, tachycardia, seizures, muscular rigidity
- **Sodium bicarbonate:** For wide complex dysrhythmias
- Cocaine chest pain
  - Benzodiazepines
  - Aspirin
  - Nitroglycerin (phentolamine if no response)
- **Avoid**
  - β-Blockers due to concern for unopposed α-receptor stimulation

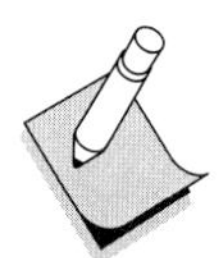

Wide complex dysrhythmia during cocaine intoxication is due to sodium-channel blockade and should be treated with sodium bicarbonate.

COMPLICATIONS

- Numerous, including dysrhythmias, MI, ischemic bowel, CNS bleed, rabdoymyolysis, and IDU-related complications

Amphetamines

This is a large class of structurally related drugs. Medical indications include attention deficit hyperactivity disorder, narcolepsy, and weight loss.

SPECIFIC PREPARATIONS

- Methamphetamine ("crank, ice") synthesized from ephedrine; readily absorbed from oral, parenteral, and inhalational routes
- 3,4 methylenedioxymethamphetamine (MDMA, "ectasy, E")
- Ephedrine/ma-huang found in over the counter preparations, Chinese herbal preparations, and legal stimulants; less potent than other amphetamines alone

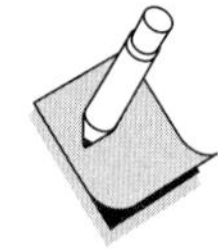

Specific anticonvulsant medications, such as phenytoin, are not indicated for toxicologic seizures.

MECHANISM/TOXICITY

- ↑ Release of neurotransmitters (primarily norepinepherine and dopamine) from presynaptic nerve terminals.
- $5\text{-}HT_2$ agonism and D_2 antagonism → hallucinations.

SYMPTOMS/EXAM

- Similar to cocaine, but duration of action is considerably longer and may last >24 hours
- Na^+ channel blockade does **not** occur.

DIAGNOSIS

- Usually clear from history and exam
- Urine screens are available in most hospitals
  - The results may be positive 2–3 days beyond period of toxicity.
  - Many drugs may cross react.

TREATMENT

- As with cocaine toxicity above

COMPLICATIONS

- Similar to cocaine
- **Hyponatremia may occur with MDMA** and is associated with
  - Increased release of vasopressin (ADH)
  - Isotonic fluid loss related to dancing and sweating, replaced with free water
- Serotonin syndrome: With MDMA

Opiates

See "Opiates," page 366.

BODY PACKERS AND STUFFERS

Body packers

- Purposefully swallow large amounts of prepared packets of drugs (cocaine, heroin most common) for the purpose of smuggling
- Packets are less likely to rupture, but contain potentially lethal amounts of drug.

Body stuffers

- Rapidly consume bags or vials of drugs, to avoid police detection
- Typically smaller amount of drug ingested, but increased chance of exposure given the poorly packaged drug load

SYMPTOMS/EXAM

- Toxidrome consistent with packaged substance

DIAGNOSIS

- Clinical diagnosis is based on history and examination.
- Abdominal radiography (X-ray or CT) may identify packets, vials.
  - May help assess body burden and location
  - Repeat CT with contrast may document passage of drug.

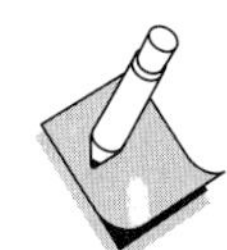

Stuffers are more likely to be symptomatic, but packers, if symptomatic, are more likely to have lethal amounts of drug.

TREATMENT

- Supportive therapy
- Treat toxidrome, if present.
- Multiple-dose activated charcoal and whole-bowel irrigation to bind any available drug and decrease transit time, respectively
- A body packer who develops symptoms should undergo emergent laporotomy to remove the packets.

PCP

MECHANISM/TOXICITY

- σ Receptor stimulation → dysphoria.
- Antagonism of glutamate activity at NMDA receptor → sedation.

Symptoms/Exam

- Altered perception of reality (including pain perception) without loss of consciousness
- CNS effects
  - AMS, hallucinations (lower doses)
  - Coma, seizures (higher doses)
- Tachycardia, hypertension, hyperthermia
- Nystagmus (vertical or rotatory)
- Increased secretions
- Muscular rigidity

Treatment

- Supportive care
- Aggressive cooling for hyperthermia
- Sedation to control agitation and hyperthermia
- Place patient in a quiet room with minimal stimulation.
- Evaluate for concomitant injuries/infections.

Ketamine

- PCP derivative with similar presentation and management
- "K-hole": Overdose/adverse reaction consisting of severe hallucinations, dysphoria, vomiting, and catatonia

Dextromethorphan

- **Opioid** with a chemical structure similar to PCP
  - Acts at the same σ receptor as PCP
  - May cross react on PCP urine toxicology screens
- Less respiratory depression compared to other opioids
- May precipitate serotonin syndrome

Gamma-Hydroxybutyrate

The only FDA-approved use is for treatment of cataplexy. It is used illicitly by body-builders, within the rave culture, and in sexual assault.

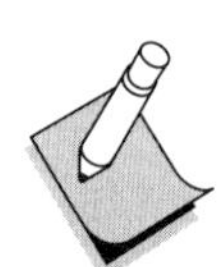

Sedation with marked agitation on stimulation? Think GHB intoxication.

Mechanism/Toxicity

- Structurally resembles gamma amino butyric acid (GABA) and readily crosses the blood-brain barrier

Symptoms/Exam

- Primarily CNS
  - Euphoria, drowsiness (low doses)
  - Sedation with amnesia (moderate doses)
  - Coma (high doses)
- Hallmark is coma with episodes of marked agitation on stimulation.
- Bradycardia, hypothermia, respiratory depression (high doses)
- Variable neuromuscular activity: Hypotonia, myoclonus, seizures
- Patients will characteristically awake spontaneously within a few hours after ingestion and rapidly return to baseline.

The duration of GHB coma is typically short (2–8 hours).

TABLE 6.19. Toxicity of Common Inhaled Drugs of Abuse

Inhalant	Toxicity
Hydrocarbons (gasolines, oils)	Sudden sniffing death Peripheral axonopathy
Methylene chloride (paint stripper)	Carbon monoxide poisoning
Toluene (glue)	Non–anion gap metabolic acidosis (hippuric acid)
Nitrites	Methemoglobinemia Syncope
Nitrous oxide	Sedation and coma Vitamin B_{12} deficiency

Treatment

- Supportive therapy
- Airway management and aspiration precautions

Complications

- Rhabdomyolysis

Inhalants

Inhaled drugs of abuse are a diverse group of substances (see Table 6.19) that are inhaled for their euphoric effects. Toxicity is unique to each substance.

Hydrocarbons

Found in readily available household products, typically in the propellant; inhaled via three common routes:

- Sniffing: Directly inhaling from the source
- Huffing: Inhaling from soaked cloth
- Bagging: Inhaling from a bag that has been sprayed

Hydrocarbons are rapidly absorbed when volatilized and rapidly distribute to the CNS because of their high lipid solubility.

Mechanism/Toxicity

- Exact mechanism is not known.

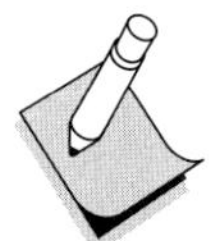

Hydrodrocarbon's effect rapidly resolves when exposed to fresh air. Prolonged AMS suggests other etiologies or hypoxic damage.

Symptoms/Exam

- Short-lived inebriation, euphoria, coma
- Chronic abuse may result in an organic brain syndrome or peripheral axonopathy.
- "**Sudden sniffing death**": Sensitization of the heart to catecholamines results in VT or Vfib when startled.

Treatment

- Supportive care

HORMONAL AGENTS

Thyroid Hormones

Thyroid hormones are used as replacement therapy in hypothyroidism. Levothyroxine (T_4, Synthroid) is the most commonly used agent, though levothyronine (T_3) is also available.

Onset of symptoms from levothyroxine (T_4) overdose may be delayed by several days as T_4 requires in vivo conversion to the active hormone, T_3. Hence, T_3 ingestions will produce symptoms more quickly.

MECHANISM/TOXICITY

- Excessive sympathetic activity

SYMPTOMS/EXAM

- Tremor, confusion, agitation, hyperreflexia
- Tachycardia, hypertension, palpitations, flushing, diaphoresis
- Mydriasis
- Diarrhea
- Patient may report fever, weight loss, and heat intolerance with chronic overdose (facticious hyperthyroidism).

DIFFERENTIAL

- Primary hyperthyroid states (Graves disease)
- Sympathomimetic toxicity (cocaine, amphetamines)
- Methylxanthine toxicity (theophylline, caffeine)

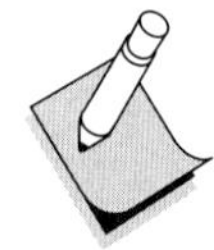

Acute ingestions of levothyroxine will not produce symptoms for several days.

DIAGNOSIS

- Clinical diagnosis based on history and physical examination.
- Elevated serum T_4 and T_3 levels
- An elevated T_4:T_3 ratio is suggestive of chronic, excess levothyroxine intake.

TREATMENT

- β-Antagonists, such as propranolol or esmolol, to control the effects of excessive sympathetic activity
- Agents that block endogenous thyroid hormone production (PTU, methimazole) have limited utility.

INDUSTRIAL TOXINS

Hydrogen Fluoride

Hydrogen fluoride (HF, hydrofluoric acid) is a water soluble gas that is most commonly encountered as a solution.

HF is encountered commonly in rust removers, oven cleaners, and automotive wheel cleaners. Commercial uses include glass etching, graffiti removal, and manufacture of semiconductors and certain fuels.

Mechanism/Toxicity

- Absorbed through skin and mucous membranes → free fluoride ion avidly binds extracellular Ca^{++} and Mg^{+} → pain
  - Systemic hypocalcemia and hypomagnesemia may occur with ingestion or heavy dermal exposure.
  - Hyperkalemia may be delayed in onset due to cellular breakdown, acidosis and direct fluoride effects on K^{+} efflux.
- HF is a weak acid and exposure to low-concentration (< 10%) solutions does not produce caustic injury.
- High-concentration solutions can produce direct tissue injury similar to other strong acids.

Symptoms/Exam

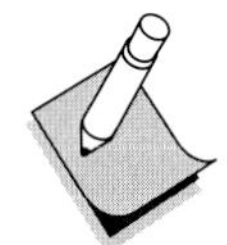

Onset of symptoms from dermal exposure to low concentrations of HF may be delayed up to 24 hours.

- There is a direct relationship between solution concentration and symptom onset.
  - Concentrated solutions produce symptoms earlier.
  - Onset can be delayed up to 24 hours after exposure to a dilute solution.
- Dermal exposure to low concentrations:
  - Local pain, erythema, swelling, and a white-blue discoloration (especially subungual)
  - Pain "out of proportion" to skin findings
- Oral ingestion or large dermal exposure to concentrated solutions:
  - Local pain of direct tissue injury
  - Systemic hypocalcemia → tetany, weakness, Chvostek's sign, dysrhythmias, and sudden death.

Diagnosis

- Usually determined from the patient's history and examination
- ECG findings with severe hypocalcemia include prolonged QT interval and peaked T waves.
- Direct measurement of total or ionized Ca^{++} confirms severe toxicity.

Treatment

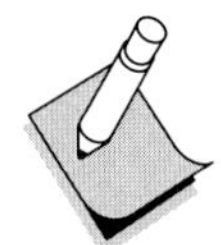

Calcium gluconate paste, injection, and arterial infusions are key to treating ongoing pain and toxicity from dermal HF exposure.

- **Copious water irrigation** for surface decontamination
- **Calcium gluconate** administration (to bind fluoride ions):
  - Topical paste
  - Subcutaneous and intradermal injections
  - Regional intraarterial infusion
  - Nebulized (for inhalation exposure)
- Systemically ill patients should be monitored carefully and aggressively treated with intravenous calcium.
- **Avoid calcium *chloride* injection,** which can cause skin necrosis.

Lead

Lead is a heavy metal used extensively in commercial products and manufacturing processes. Adult lead exposure is primarily occupational (construction, mining, welding, smelting, manufacture of batteries, plastic and rubber, "moonshine"). Pediatric exposure usually results from accidental ingestion of lead-containing material, especially paint chips.

Most lead toxicity is due to chronic, low-level exposure. Acute toxicity from single exposures is rare.

MECHANISM/TOXICITY

- Inhibits a wide variety of cellular enzymes
- Directly damages peripheral nerves

SYMPTOMS/EXAM

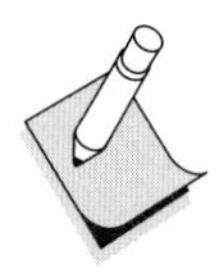

Most lead toxicity is chronic and causes subtle neurologic changes and anemia.

- **Chronic lead toxicity** produces subtle, insidious, and nonspecific symptoms, including headache, peripheral motor neuropathy, HTN, anemia, gout, and cognitive impairment.
- **Acute lead toxicity**
  - Nausea/vomiting, abdominal pain
  - Ataxia
  - **Encephalopathy** and seizures

TOXICOLOGY

DIAGNOSIS

- Diagnosis of lead toxicity requires a high index of suspicion.
- Lead can be directly measured in whole blood.
- Ingested lead-containing material is usually visible on X-ray.

TREATMENT

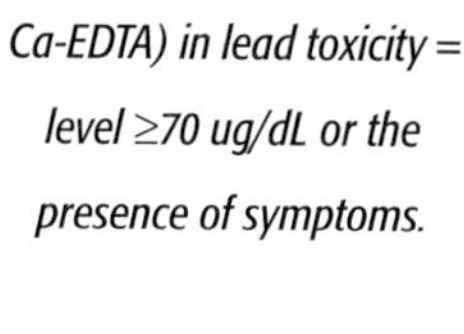

Indications for immediate IV chelation therapy (BAL and Ca-EDTA) in lead toxicity = level ≥70 ug/dL or the presence of symptoms.

- Remove the patient from the source of exposure.
- Activated charcoal does **not** bind metals.
- Whole-bowel irrigation is indicated in cases of lead ingestion with visible material on X-ray.
- **Antidote = BAL (British anti-lewisite, dimercaprol) and Ca-EDTA (calcium disodium ethylenediaminetetraacetic acid).**
  - Use for the severely poisoned patient or level > 70 μG/dL
  - Both are parenteral chelating agents.
- **DMSA** (2,3-dimercaptosuccinic acid, succimer) oral chelation therapy if no acute symptoms and level < 70 μG/dL

Arsenic

Arsenic-containing compounds are used in a wide variety of applications:

- Pesticides, wood preservatives, metal alloys, chemical synthesis, and glass manufacturing
- Arsenic trioxide is used as a chemotherapeutic agent for acute promyelocytic leukemia.

MECHANISM/TOXICITY

- Inhibits multiple key enzymes in cellular oxidative metabolism
- Arsine gas causes acute hemolysis by an unknown mechanism.

SYMPTOMS/EXAM

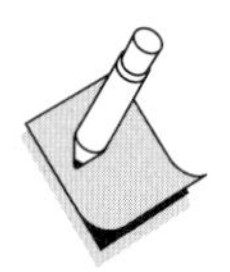

Mee's lines appear weeks to months after arsenic exposure.

- Chronic poisoning
  - Peripheral neuropathy, headache, ataxia, confusion
  - Diarrhea, constipation
  - Hyperpigmentation, **Mees' lines** (transverse white lines on nails), alopecia, various rashes
  - Malaise, anorexia, fatigue

- Acute poisoning
  - GI symptoms predominate: **Violent gastroenteritis**
  - Confusion, coma, seizures
  - Hypotension, tachycardia, prolonged QT interval, dysrhythmias
  - ARDS-like syndrome
- Arsine gas poisoning
  - Findings consistent with acute hemolysis: Hematuria, jaundice, renal failure
  - Abdominal pain, N/V
  - Hypotension, tachycardia, pulmonary edema

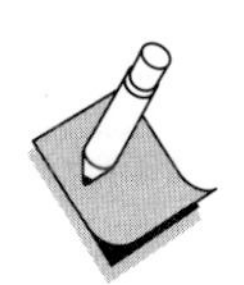

Acute arsenic exposure is characterized by violent gastroenteritis.

DIAGNOSIS

- Suspect based on clinical presentation and possible exposure.
- Blood or 24-hour urine arsenic levels
  - Levels may be elevated following consumption of seafood because of the presence of nontoxic, organic arsenic compounds.
- Ingested arsenic-containing material is usually visible on X-ray.

TREATMENT

- In chronic poisoning cases, identify and remove the source of arsenic exposure.
- Whole-bowel irrigation: If radiopaque objects visible on X-ray
- **Antidote = BAL** (British anti-lewisite, dimercaprol)
  - In cases of severe, acute toxicity
- **DMSA** (2,3-dimercaptosuccinic acid, succimer)
  - In cases of chronic poisoning
- Arsine gas toxicity does not usually require chelation.

TOXICOLOGY

Mercury

Mercury is pervasive in industrial processes and commercial products. It is encountered in three forms:

- Elemental mercury (quicksilver): Mercury-containing devices in workplace or home
- Inorganic mercury salts: Disk batteries
- Organic mercury: Occupational/agricultural exposure

Each form of mercury has differing toxicity. Elemental mercury primarily causes toxicity when inhaled, while the principal route of exposure for mercury salts and organic mercury is through GI absorption.

MECHANISM/TOXICITY

- Inhibition of multiple cellular enzyme systems
- Inhalation of elemental mercury may lead to severe pneumonitis.

SYMPTOMS/EXAM

- Elemental mercury (quicksilver) inhalation: Rapid onset of shortness of breath, cough, chills, fever, respiratory distress
- Acute ingestion of inorganic mercury: Corrosive gastroenteritis with shock (from massive fluid loss), renal failure, grayish discoloration of mucous membranes, metallic taste

- Acute ingestion of organic mercury: Characterized by delayed (and permanent) neurotoxicity—ataxia, dysarthria, constricted visual fields
  - GI symptoms and dermatitis may occur acutely.

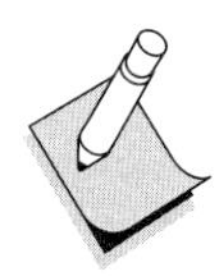

Elemental mercury (inhaled) → respiratory distress. Inorganic mercury (ingested) → severe corrosive gastroenteritis. Organic mercury (ingested) → delayed neurotoxicity.

DIAGNOSIS

- Based on presenting symptoms and history of exposure
- Mercury can be measured in whole blood or urine.
- Ingested mercury-containing material is usually visible on X-ray.

TREATMENT

- Whole-bowel irrigation: If radiopaque objects visible on X-ray
- **Antidote = BAL** (British anti-lewisite, dimercaprol) **or DMSA** (2,3-dimercaptosuccinic acid for symptomatic patients

INHALED TOXINS

Simple Asphyxiants

Simple asphyxiants include carbon dioxide, nitrogen dioxide (silo filler's disease), nitrous oxide, methane gas, and helium. Methane gas is present in high concentrations in bogs of decaying organic matter and in natural gas.

MECHANISM/TOXICITY

- Produce toxicity by displacing O_2 → hypoxia

SYMPTOMS/EXAM

- Rapid onset
- Tachycardia, tachypnea, shortness of breath
- Dizziness and confusion to coma
- If untreated may lead to cardiac arrest

DIAGNOSIS

- Clinical diagnosis is based on history of exposure

TREATMENT

- Remove patient from source of exposure.
- Supportive care
- Administration of O_2

A 40-year-old female presents to the ED with complaints of headache, nausea, and dizziness. Other family members have recently reported similar symptoms. She reports recent problems with her water heater at home. What diagnostic test can most easily aid in the diagnosis?

Carbon monoxide poisoning should always be suspected when several members of the same household have mild flulike symptoms. A venous or arterial carboxyhemoglobin level greater than 5% (10% in a smoker) confirms the diagnosis.

Carbon Monoxide

Carbon monoxide (CO) is an odorless and colorless gas produced by incomplete combustion of fuels or organic material.

Common sources of CO include vehicle exhaust, ovens, house fires, furnaces, and portable generators.

Methylene chloride, a solvent found in paint removers, degreasers, and other similar products, is metabolized in vivo to CO following absorption.

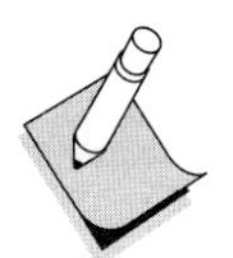

The solvent methylene chloride is metabolized to carbon monoxide after absorption.

Mechanism/Toxicity

- Binds to hemoglobin → carboxyhemoglobin (COHb), which is incapable of carrying O_2 → impaired O_2 delivery, cellular hypoxia, lactic acidosis
- Shifts the oxyhemoglobin dissociation curve to left → ↓ release of O_2 to tissues from normal hemoglobin
- Binds to heme groups in mitochondira and triggers oxidative injury
- CO has even greater affinity for fetal hemoglobin → higher fetal levels and toxicity for any given maternal exposure.

TOXICOLOGY

Symptoms/Exam

The symptoms and signs of CO toxicity are vague and nonspecific, and, if not severe, will resolve shortly after removal from CO source.

- Headache, dizziness, weakness
- Tachycardia, chest pain
- Dyspnea
- Nausea/vomiting (no diarrhea)
- Confusion, memory impairment (delayed)
- In severe cases: Myocardial ischemia, seizures, syncope, coma, cardiac arrest

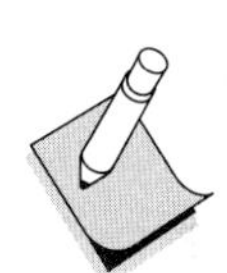

CO poisoning:
Normal pulse oximetry
ABG with metabolic acidosis and normal PaO_2

Diagnosis

- Direct measurement of COHb in either arterial or venous blood via co-oximetry
  - Normal nonsmoker = 2–3%
  - Smokers = <10%.
- Pulse oximetry **cannot** distinguish COHb from oxyhemoglobin.
- Expected ABG findings:
  - Normal PaO_2 (measuring dissolved O_2)
  - Metabolic acidosis (from **lactate** accumulation)
  - Normal **calculated** O_2 saturation (calculated from PaO_2)

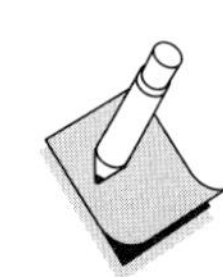

Elimination half life of CO
Room air: 4–5 hours
100% O_2: 1 hour
Hyperbaric O_2: 20–30 minutes

Treatment

- Removal of the patient from CO source
- Acute stabilization as required
- Administration of **100%** O_2:
  - Reduces the elimination half-life of CO from approximately 4–5 hours (room air) to 1 hour
  - Continue until COHb level is ≤ 5%.
- **Hyperbaric O_2 (HBO)**
  - Further reduces the elimination half-life of CO to 20–30 minutes
  - Indications are listed in Table 6.20.

TABLE 6.20. Indications for HBO Treatment of CO Poisoning

Any history of syncope
Evidence of major end-organ damage
Persistent neurologic symptoms
Pregnancy
COHb level > 20–25%

Complications

- Delayed or persistent neurocognitive deficits on neuropsychiatric testing.
  - HBO therapy may prevent the development of these effects but studies are not conclusive.

A 25-year-old male is brought to the ED after being found unresponsive inside a burning house. He was intubated by EMS en route. On arrival he is hypotensive, comatose, and markedly tachypnic. There is no evidence of trauma or skin/airway burns. ABG reveals a severe metabolic acidosis and a normal measured PaO_2. What is the most appropriate next step?

This patient should be presumed to have a combined CO and cyanide (CN) poisoning based on his hemodynamic instability and coma. Initial treatment of CO poisoning consists of O_2 therapy, which has already been initiated. The next most appropriate step, therefore, is administration of either hydroxycobolamin or sodium thiosulfate for treatment of CN poisoning. In the smoke inhalation victim, administration of nitrites is not recommended, as a nitrite-induced methemoglobinemia will further decrease tissue O_2 delivery in the CO-poisoned patient. If the COHb level is low on co-oximetry, nitrites may be initiated.

Cyanide

Cyanide (CN) is a rapid-acting, highly toxic poison found in a wide variety of chemicals. Poisoning is rare in the United States as few household products contain CN.

Sources of CN include:

- Combustion of plastics, synthetic fibers, or wool
  - House fires (smoke inhalation) represent the most likely source of exposure.
- Prolonged infusion of nitroprusside
- Industry, including mining, plastics manufacturing, welding, fumigation, chemical synthesis, and research
- The pits and seeds of certain fruits (apricots, bitter almonds) contain a compound amygdalin, which releases CN in vivo during its metabolism.

MECHANISM/TOXICITY

- Inhibits cytochrome oxidase, disrupting oxidative phosphorylation → cellular hypoxia and lactic acidosis

SYMPTOMS/EXAM

Suspect CN poisoning if patient presents with rapid onset of coma, shock, and severe metabolic acidosis.

- Effects are very rapid following CN inhalation or absorption.
- In contrast, toxicity due to amygdalin may be delayed by hours as CN is released by metabolism.
- Early symptoms of N/V, headache, and confusion are followed rapidly by seizures and coma.
- Cardiovascular findings include hypertension and tachypnea (initially), dysrhythmias, pulmonary edema, and cardiac arrest.
- Skin may appear flushed or cyanotic.

DIFFERENTIAL

Any other cause of coma, shock, or lactic acidosis

DIAGNOSIS

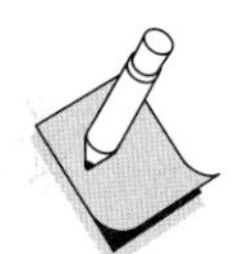

Laboratory clues to CN poisoning: Marked lactic acidosis, arterial appearance of venous blood, elevated measured venous O_2 saturation

- CN poisoning should be considered in any patient presenting with rapid onset of coma, shock, and marked lactic acidosis.
- ABG findings are similar to *severe* CO poisoning.
- Clues to the diagnosis include:
  - A history of smoke inhalation or occupational access to CN
  - Evidence of decreased tissue extraction of O_2:
    - Arterial appearance of venous blood
    - Elevated measured venous O_2 saturation (>90%)
    - Marked lactic acidosis
  - Patient has a distinct, almond-like smell. Many individuals are genetically incapable of detecting this odor.
- Blood CN levels can be directly measured, but are not available in a timely manner.

TREATMENT

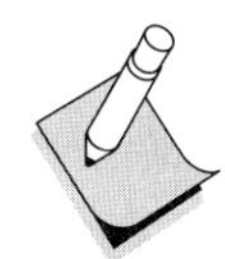

Sodium thiosulfate should be administered empirically if CN poisoning is considered.

Avoid using sodium nitrite in smoke inhalation victims with suspected CO poisoning. Use sodium thiosulfate alone.

- Acute stabilization as required
- Surface decontamination, if indicated
- **Antidote = cyanide antidote kit**; three components:
  - **Amyl nitrite pearls (for inhalation)**
    - Use until IV access is obtained.
    - Induces methemoglobinemia
    - Methemoglobin strongly binds CN, pulling it away from cellular enzymes.
    - Is used illicitly as "poppers"
  - **IV sodium nitrite**
    - Induces methemoglobinemia
  - **IV sodium thiosulfate**
    - Binds to CN to form thiocyanate, a much less toxic compound that is renally excreted
- A smoke inhalation victim with suspected CN poisoning should only receive sodium thiosulfate. There is the potential for worsening tissue oxygenation from nitrite-induced methemoglobinemia.
- **Antidote = hydroxycobalamin.**

- Recently approved as an antidote for cyanide poisoning in the United States
- It reacts with CN to form cyanocobalamin (vitamin B_{12}), a nontoxic compound which is readily excreted in urine.
- It may replace the cyanide antidote package in the future due to its ease of use and improved risk profile.

Hydrogen Sulfide

Hydrogen sulfide (H_2S) is a gas formed as a byproduct of organic decomposition. It has a very strong, distinct "rotten egg" odor.

Sources of H_2S include:

- **Sewer or manure gas**
- Chemical or industrial processes, such as tanning, rubber vulcanizing, mining, and manufacture of paper, silk, rayon, refrigerants, soap, and petroleum products
- Natural sources include hot springs and volcanic eruptions.

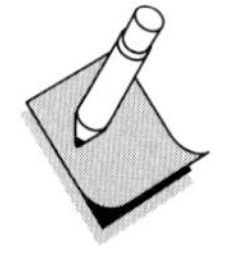

Sewer or manure gas exposure? Rotten egg odor? Think hydrogen sulfide toxicity.

Mechanism/Toxicity

- H_2S is a stronger inhibitor of cytochrome oxidase than CN → disruption of oxidative phosphorylation → cellular hypoxia and lactic acidosis.
  - **Spontaneously dissociates** from cytochrome oxidase
- Direct mucous-membrane irritant

Symptoms/Exam

- Severity of symptoms depends on the concentration and duration of exposure. Low concentration exposure may only produce mild mucous membrane irritation. Brief exposures to very high concentrations can cause immediate loss of consciousness.
- Mucous membrane irritation: Conjunctivitis, rhinitis, bronchorrhea, pulmonary edema
- Headache, seizures, loss of consciousness, coma
- Hypotension, bradycardia, dysrhythmias, cardiac arrest
- N/V

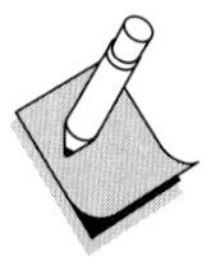

Hydrogen sulfide toxicity: Rapid coma, shock, and lactic acidosis (as with CN); spontaneous improvement after exposure is ended

Diagnosis

- H_2S poisoning should be considered in any patient presenting with rapid onset of coma, shock, and marked lactic acidosis.
- Clues to the diagnosis include:
  - Relevant occupational setting
  - Odor of rotten eggs at scene
  - Evidence of decreased tissue extraction of O_2:
    - Arterial appearance of venous blood
    - Elevated measured venous O_2 saturation (>90%)
    - Marked lactic acidosis
- Blood levels of sulfide and thiosulfate can serve as markers of H_2S exposure, but are not readily available in most clinical laboratories.

Treatment

- Acute stabilization as required
- Administer 100% O_2.

- Most patients will not require further therapy.
- **Antidote = sodium nitrite** (if prolonged symptoms).
  - Induces methemoglobinemia
  - Methemoglobin binds H_2S, producing sulfmethemglobin.

A 30-year-old male on chronic lithium therapy for bipolar disorder is brought to the ED by his mother for mental-status changes. She reports he has had a flulike illness over the past few days with vomiting and diarrhea. On examination the patient appears dehydrated, lethargic, and confused, but has normal VS. His lithium level returns at 1.5 (upper level of normal). What is the single most important therapeutic intervention for this patient with presumed lithium toxicity?

This patient likely has chronic lithium toxicity related to a decreased GFR from dehydration. In chronic toxicity, CNS effects predominate. The single most important therapy for this patient is to reestablish GFR with IV hydration.

LITHIUM

Lithium is a mood stabilizer used to treat bipolar disorder. It has a narrow therapeutic window.

Mechanism/Toxicity

- Lithium is a cation and behaves like Na^+ or K^+. It is thought to affect catecholamine and serotonergic neurotransmission.
- CNS uptake **and** elimination are slow, therefore serum lithium levels do NOT correlate with CNS effects.
- Lithium elimination is glomerular filtration rate (GFR) dependent.
- Precursors to chronic toxicity:
  - ↑ Therapeutic dose
  - ↑ Renal reabsorption in dehydration
  - ↑ GFR (renal insufficiency, use of NSAIDs, ACE–I)
  - Drug-drug interactions with SSRIs and antipsychotic agents

A decrease in GRF (↓ drug clearance) is a common precursor to chronic lithium toxicity.

Symptoms/Exam

The expected effects from lithium intoxication depend on whether the ingestion is acute or chronic.

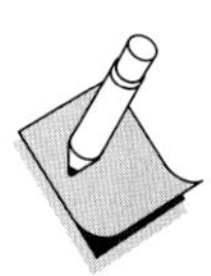

Acute lithium ingestion → high serum levels, minimal CNS effects.

Chronic lithium toxicity → lower serum levels, significant CNS effects.

Acute ingestion

- Occurs in patients who do not normally take lithium but acutely ingest a large quantity
- GI toxicity >> CNS toxicity (no time for CNS uptake).
- GI toxicity = nausea/vomiting/diarrhea.
- CNS findings are typically mild.
  - Severe ingestion: hyperreflexia, clonus, agitation, AMS, seizures
- **Chronic ingestion**
  - Patient on chronic lithium therapy with toxicity due to:
    - CNS toxicity >> GI toxicity
    - CNS effects may range from lethargy and confusion to coma and seizures.
    - ECG changes are common, including prolonged PR, QRS, qTc, nonspecific ST-T changes, bradycardia.

TABLE 6.21. **Indications for Hemodialysis in Lithium Toxicity**

Renal failure
Inability to handle aggressive hydration
Severe CNS toxicity
Level >4.0 mEq/L in acute ingestion
Level >2.5 mEq/L with moderate CNS symptoms in chronic ingestion

Diagnosis

- Clinical diagnosis based on history and examination
- Lithium levels:
  - Measure 4–6 hours postingestion, follow until clear peak and decline.
  - Peak serum level with large ingestion, especially sustained-release preparations, may occur >12 hours postingestion.
  - Falsely elevated if placed in a green-top tube (lithium heparin)

Treatment

- Supportive therapy
- **GI decontamination** for acute ingestions (**ineffective for chronic ingestions**)
  - Lithium does **not** bind to charcoal.
  - Gastric lavage—if <1 hour and large ingestion.
  - **Whole-bowel irrigation**
- **Kayexelate** administration has been shown to decrease serum lithium levels due to lithium's similarity to K^+, but its effect on outcome is uncertain.
- **Hydration** is essential to correct dehydration and increase GFR.
- **Hemodialysis**
  - Lithium is effectively removed by hemodialysis (see Table 6.21).
    - Because HD removes lithium only from the plasma, a "rebound lithium level" may occur. Levels should be checked after HD and 6 hours later.
- Benzodiazepines for seizures and agitation
- **Avoid**
  - **Phenytoin:** Decreases renal excretion of lithium
  - Forced diuresis or diuretics (not effective)

Complications

- Hypothyroidism (concentrates in the thyroid)
- Nephrogenic diabetes insipidus (via blockage of antidiuretic hormone)
- Increased risk of serotonin syndrome when taken with serotonergic agents

LOCAL ANESTHETICS

Local anesthetics are typically divided into two classes:

- **Esters**: Procaine, tetracaine, benzocaine
- **Amides**: Lidocaine, bupivacaine, mepivacaine

Effect is usually local only, but may become systemic with:

- Inadvertent injection into a blood vessel
- Use of large volumes
- Premature release of cuff with intravenous regional anesthesia (Bier block)

Severity is related to dose and route.

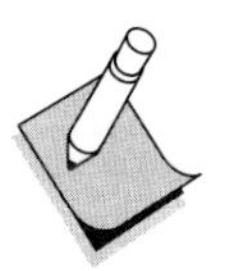

All amide local anesthetics have two "i"s in their name.

MECHANISM/TOXICITY

- Inhibition of Na^{++} channels → reversible blockade of the initiation and propagation of action potentials along affected nerve.
- Methemoglobinemia is possible with exposure to benzocaine or prilocaine.

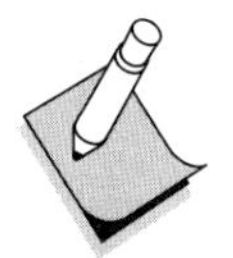

Toxicity is characterized primarily by neurologic symptoms, but may include cardiovascular symptoms in large overdoses.

SYMPTOMS/EXAM

- Mild overdose
  - Headache, drowsiness, dizziness/lightheadedness
  - Anxiety, tinnitus, numbness of mouth
  - Hypertension, tachycardia
- Severe overdose
  - Confusion, tremors, seizures and coma
  - Respiratory depression and apnea
  - Hypotension, bradycardia, asystole
  - Widening of PR interval and QRS complex, VT or Vfib
- Bupivicaine
  - More cardiotoxic than other local anesthetics
  - Not indicated for IV regional anesthesia

Pregnant women are disproportionately affected by bupivicaine, and it is no longer indicated for obstetric anesthesia.

DIAGNOSIS

- Usually clear from history and exam
- ECG, as needed
- Co-oximetry if methemoglobinemia is suspected

TREATMENT

- Supportive care
- Benzodiazepines for seizures
- Standard ACLS for cardiac dysrhythmias
- Discontinue use of agent.
- No role for decontamination or enhanced elimination

COMPLICATIONS

- Allergic reactions
  - Ester anesthetics are responsible for most, likely due to metabolite **para-aminobenzoic acid (PABA)**.
  - Preservative **methylparaben** is found in multidose vials of amide anesthetics and is chemically related to PABA.
- Inadvertent IV injection of epinephrine (in "with epi" preparations)

METHYLXANTHINES

Agents in this class include:

- **Caffeine:** Most commonly used drug in the world; marketed for increased alertness, weight loss, migraine therapy, and neonatal apnea and bradycardia

- **Theophylline:** While it was once a very popular therapy for asthma and COPD, newer, safer, and more selective medications are more common now. This agent is still used in neonatal apnea and bradycardia.
- **Theobromine**: Found in chocolate and various teas

MECHANISM/TOXICITY

- Mechanism of toxicity is not fully understood but includes:
  - Triggers release of preformed epinephrine and norepinephrine → adrenergic receptor stimulation and hypokalemia
  - Phosphodiesterase inhibition
  - Adenosine receptor antagonism

SYMPTOMS/EXAM

- **Severe N/V** in majority of patients
- CNS stimulation ranging from elevated mood to nervousness, agitation, and seizures
- Cardiovascular stimulation with tachycardia, hypertension, and dysrythmias
- At high concentrations: Peripheral vasodilation and hypotension

DIAGNOSIS

- Usually clear from history and exam
- Serum theophylline levels, repeated every 2–4 hours until peak and decline
- In chronic ingestions, severe symptoms may occur at significantly lower levels.
- Caffeine may cross react with the theophylline assay in overdose.

TREATMENT

- Supportive and symptomatic therapy
- Most patients autodecontaminate with profuse vomiting.
- **Multiple-dose activated charcoal:** To both decrease absorption and increase elimination
- **Whole-bowel irrigation:** For large ingestion of sustained release preparations
- Charcoal hemoperfusion or hemodialysis for severe toxicity
- Benzodiazepines for CNS stimulation

OPIATES

The opioid toxidrome may result from exposure to any of the following:

- Prescription medications (eg, fentanyl, methadone, oxycodone)
- Over-the-counter medications (eg, diphenoxylate, dextromethorphan)
- Illicit drugs (eg, heroin)

MECHANISM/TOXICITY

- Stimulate opiate receptors in the CNS

SYMPTOMS/EXAM

- The classic triad includes CNS depression, respiratory depression, and pinpoint pupils.
  - Pinpoint pupils may not be seen with propoxyphene (Darvon), pentazocine (Talwin), meperidine (Demerol).
- Bradycardia, hypotension
- Hypothermia
- Muscle flaccidity
- Noncardiogenic pulmonary edema
- Seizures: After exposure to propoxyphene or meperidine
- Wide complex dysrhythmias: Associated with Na^{++} channel blockade after propoxyphene overdose

Opiate toxidrome = CNS depression, respiratory depression, and pinpoint pupils.

DIAGNOSIS

- Clinical diagnosis based on exposure history and physical exam
- Reversal of symptoms by naloxone

TREATMENT

- Support ventilation, as needed
- **Antidote = naloxone (Narcan).**
  - Pure antagonist at opiate receptor
- Sodium bicarbonate for wide complex dysrhythmias (propoxyphene)
- Seizures are typically self-limited.

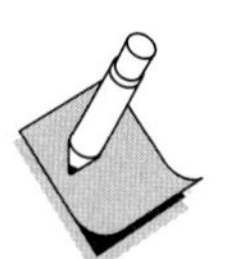

Naloxone is only indicated for reversal of hypoventilation and is not useful in the intubated patient.

COMPLICATIONS

- Aspiration
- Rhabdomyolysis: From prolonged immobilization

OVER-THE-COUNTER MEDICATIONS

Acetaminophen

Acetaminophen ingestions are typically divided into acute overdoses (**single ingestion**) and repeated supra-therapeutic ingestions (**chronic exposure**). A single ingestion of greater than 150 mg/kg (children) or 7.5 g (adults) should be considered toxic.

MECHANISM/TOXICITY

- Acetaminophen is primarily metabolized by the liver.
- In therapeutic doses, about 90% of acetaminophen is conjugated with glucuronide or sulfate to nontoxic metabolites, while about 5% is oxidized by cytochrome P-450 to a **toxic metabolite, N-acetyl-p-benzoquinoneimine (NAPQI)**.
- Hepatic stores of **glutathione** rapidly combine with NAPQI to form nontoxic metabolites.
- In APAP overdose, normal glucuronide and sulfate conjugation is overwhelmed and a large amount of NAPQI is produced.
- When NAPQI formation exceeds glutathione stores, free NAPQI binds to cellular proteins causing hepatotoxicity (centrilobular or zone III).
- High-risk patients: Patients with decreased glutathione stores (alcoholics, malnourished) and those on cytochrome P-450–inducing medications (INH, anticonvulsants) may have increased risk of hepatotoxicity.

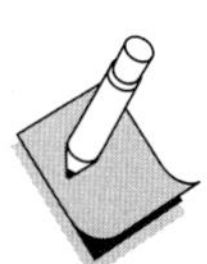

In acetaminophen toxicity, glutathione stores become depleted, allowing NAPQI (toxic metabolite) to accumulate.

Symptoms/Exam

- **Acute toxic ingestion:** Typically divided into four stages or phases (see Table 6.22).
- The most severe cases will develop fulminate liver failure with hepatic encephalopathy, severe coagulopathy, renal failure, cerebral edema, and acidosis. Liver transplantation may be indicated.
- **Repeated supra-therapeutic ingestion (chronic exposure):**
  - Ingestion of >7.5 g (adults) or 150 mg/kg (child) in a 24-hour period
    - Use a 24-hour dose of 4 g (adults) and 90 mg/kg (child) if patient is high risk for hepatotoxicity or is a febrile child <5 years.
  - Due to a subacute course, patients may present anywhere along a spectrum: Normal LFTS to asymptomatic elevation of enzymes to hepatic failure.

Diagnosis

- **Acute ingestion (time of ingestion known)** of both immediate *and* extended-release formulations:
  - Obtain a 4-hour (up to 24 hours) postingestion serum acetaminophen level and plot the level on the Rumack-Matthew nomogram (see Figure 6.2).
    - The dotted line (Rumack-Matthew line) is the original line developed from the study above which hepatotoxicity will likely occur.
    - The solid line (treatment line) is the line accepted as the standard of care in the United States and is 25% lower as a safety margin.
  - If the patient's serum APAP level falls above the treatment line (150 μg/mL), start treatment with N-acetylcysteine (NAC).
- **Acute ingestion (time of ingestion unknown) or repeated supra-therapeutic ingestion.**
  - An acetaminophen level **CANNOT** be plotted on the Rumack-Matthew nomogram.
  - Draw an APAP level and AST/ALT at time of presentation.
  - If the APAP level is >10 mcg/mL **OR** the AST/ALT are elevated, treatment with NAC is recommended.

Unknown time of acetaminophen ingestion? If the APAP level is >10 mcg/mL or the AST/ALT is elevated → treat with NAC.

TABLE 6.22. Stages of Acetaminophen Poisoning Following Acute Toxic Ingestion

Stage of Toxicity	Time From Ingestion	Clinical Findings
Stage 1 (preinjury)	1/2–24 hrs	Nonspecific symptoms–N/V, anorexia, malaise
Stage 2 (injury begins)	12–72 hrs	RUQ pain, rising AST/ALT, INR, bilirubin
Stage 3 (peak injury and sequelae)	72–96 hrs	Hepatic necrosis with resultant hepatic failure and sequelae; AST/ALT usually peak at 72 hours, regardless of clinical status
Stage 4 (Recovery)	4 days–2 wks	Regeneration of liver, AST/ALT return to baseline

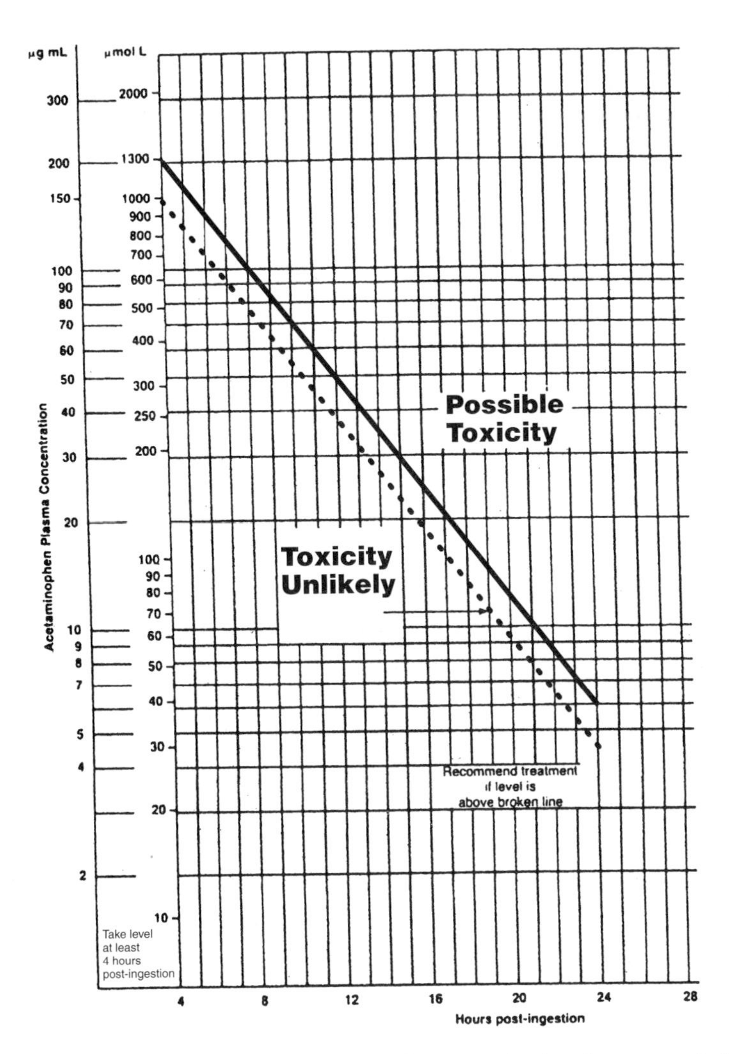

FIGURE 6.2. Rumack-Matthew nomogram. Serum acetaminophen concentration vs time after acute ingestion.

(Reproduced, with permission, from Rumack BH, Matthew H. Acetaminophen poisoning and toxicity. *Pediatrics* 55:871, 1975.)

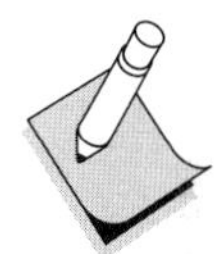

NAC is most effective if given within 8 hours of ingestion.

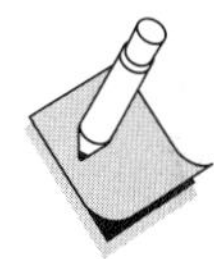

Even late administration of NAC can be beneficial.

TREATMENT

- Supportive therapy as indicated.
- Activated charcoal: If <4 hours (2 hours per recent study) from time of ingestion
- **Antidote: N-acetylcysteine (NAC)**
  - Very effective if given *within 8 hours* of ingestion, but even late administration is beneficial (**always** give NAC).
  - If no acetaminophen level available and patient approaching (or exceeding) 8 hours from ingestion → give NAC.
  - Oral dose (Mucomyst): 140 mg/kg load, then 70 mg/kg every 4 hours.
  - Intravenous (Acetadote) administration is indicated for fulminant hepatic failure, intractable vomiting, or pregnancy.
    - May cause dose-, rate-, and concentration-dependent anaphylactoid reactions

Acetaminophen toxicity:
Toxic single dose = 150 mg/kg (about 7.5 g for adults)
Toxic level at 4 hours = 150 mcg/mL
Oral NAC loading dose = 140 mg/kg

COMPLICATIONS

- Liver failure →
  - Metabolic acidosis
  - Hepatorenal syndrome
  - Coagulopathy
  - Infection
  - Cerebral edema
  - Hypoglycemia
  - **Indications for liver transplantation** include pH < 7.3 after resuscitation, INR > 7, Creatinine > 3.4, grade 3 or 4 encephalopathy.

> A 33-year-old female presents to the ED with complaint of N/V and back pain. The back pain has been ongoing since she lifted some heavy boxes 2 days earlier and was severe enough that she took a "handful" of aspirin 4 hours earlier to treat the symptoms. On examination she is tachypnic, but otherwise alert and hemodynamically stable. ABG reveals a pH of 7.51, PCO_2 of 13.9, PO_2 of 110 mmHg. Serum HCO_3^- = 12 mEq/L. What is the goal of initial therapy in this patient?
>
> Therapy with sodium bicarbonate boluses, and then drip should be initiated with a goal of urinary alkalinization to a pH of 7.5–8.0. Alkalinization keeps salicylate in the nonionized form, which increases renal clearance and decreases CNS uptake of salicylate.

Salicylates

Salicylates are found in a variety of over-the-counter preparations such as analgesics (eg, Bayer aspirin), cold medicines, antidiarrheal agents (bismuth subsalicylate in Pepto Bismol), and topical dermatological products for warts (methyl salicylate), and as combination products in decongestants, antihistamines, and narcotic medications.

Salicylic acid is a weak acid that at normal serum pH is mostly ionized, therefore will not cross the blood-brain barrier or the renal tubules (for reabsorption). As the blood becomes more acidemic, a more nonionized form develops, allowing salicylate to enter the brain and be reabsorbed by the kidneys (decreasing renal excretion). Treatment is logically geared toward keeping salicylate in the ionized form.

Chronic excessive use of salicylates (chronic ingestion) is seen primarily in the elderly and is associated with a higher clinical toxicity for a given serum salicylate level.

MECHANISM/TOXICITY

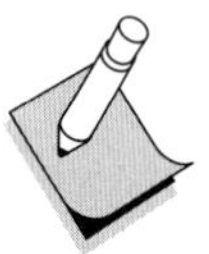

Chronic salicylate ingestion is associated with higher toxicity for a given salicylate level.

- **Direct stimulation of respiratory center** → hyperventilation and respiratory alkalosis.
- **Stimulation of chemoreceptor trigger zone** → vomiting.
- **Uncoupling of oxidative phosphorylation** → anaerobic metabolism, lactate production anion-gap acidosis and hyperthermia.
- **Increased fatty acid metabolism** → metabolic acidosis (ketones).
- Platelets permanently lose their ability to aggregate at therapeutic aspirin doses. Bleeding is rare in overdose.
- **Ototoxicity** → tinnitus and hearing loss correlate with salicylate level.

SYMPTOMS/EXAM

- **Acute ingestion**
  - Early symptoms include N/V, tinnitus, hearing loss, hyperventilation, and hyperthermia.
  - The classic presentation of mild to moderate toxicity is a mixed acid-base picture with a respiratory alkalosis, wide anion-gap metabolic acidosis, and (possibly) a metabolic alkalosis (from dehydration).
    - Blood gases early on often show a respiratory alkalosis with pH > 7.5.
    - Less respiratory alkalosis (and therefore greater overall acidosis) is seen in children.
  - Severe intoxication results in profound metabolic acidosis, marked hyperthermia, cerebral edema (coma and seizure), hypoglycemia, pulmonary edema.
- **Chronic ingestion**
  - Symptoms of toxicity overlap with those of acute ingestion, but are slower in onset and often less severe.
  - Neurologic symptoms are common, including confusion, hallucinations, agitation, coma.
  - Pulmonary edema, seizures, and renal failure occur more frequently compared to acute ingestions.

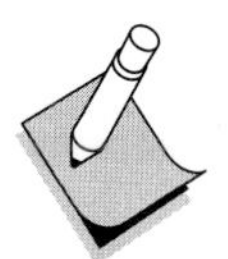

Patient with respiratory alkalosis and increased anion-gap metabolic acidosis? Think salicylate toxicity.

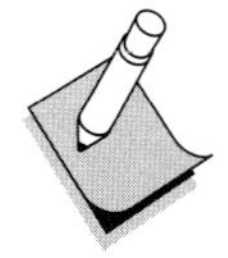

Suspect chronic salicylate intoxication in elderly patients with altered mental status or hearing complaints.

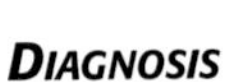

DIAGNOSIS

- Based on history, physical exam and acid-base findings
- Maintain high level of suspicion in patients with:
  - Unexplained respiratory alkalosis
  - Mixed metabolic disorders
  - Metabolic acidosis
  - Elderly with altered mental status
  - Patients with hearing complaints
- Key labs: Salicylate level, ABG, electrolytes
- **Urine ferric chloride test** will confirm exposure, but not toxicity.
- The Done nomogram should **NOT** be used!

TREATMENT

The goal of treatment is to keep salicylate in the ionized form, thereby inhibiting its movement into the brain and tissues *and* enhancing its urinary excretion.

- Supportive and symptomatic care
  - Avoid CNS/respiratory depressants, which may decrease the respiratory alkalosis and thereby worsen the acidemia.
  - If intubated, match the preintubation pCO2.
- Activated charcoal: If no significant CNS depression and <1 hour from ingestion
- IV hydration (**not** forced diuresis) to maintain renal perfusion
- **Sodium bicarbonate therapy:**
  - 1–2 mg/kg IV bolus, followed by drip
  - Goal is **urinary alkalinization** to pH 7.5–8.0.
- **Correct hypokalemia**
  - Results from intracellular shifts and body losses
  - Urinary alkalinization will not occur unless hypokalemia is corrected.
- Obtain salicylate levels every 2 hours until levels are declining.
- **Hemodialysis:** Indications listed in Table 6.23.

TABLE 6.23. Indications for Hemodialysis in Salicylate Toxicity

Level >100 mg/dL (acute ingestions)
Altered mental status
Renal failure
Severe persistent acid-base disturbance
Pulmonary edema
Failure to respond to intensive treatment

TOXICOLOGY

Nonsteroidal Anti-Inflammatory Drugs

NSAIDs inhibit the enzyme cyclooxygenase, causing decreased prostaglandin formation. Prostaglandins have a variety of functions including mediating pain and inflammation, maintaining the gastric mucosa, and regulating blood flow in the kidneys. Ibuprofen is the most common NSAID seen in overdose.

MECHANISM/TOXICITY

- Gastrointestinal irritation (nausea and vomiting) caused by disruption of the gastric mucosa
- Large overdoses result in systemic effects from unclear mechanism.
- Renal insufficiency and GI bleeding are **rare** in acute overdose.

SYMPTOMS/EXAM

- Abdominal pain, N/V
- Altered mental status, seizure, metabolic acidosis

DIAGNOSIS

- Based primarily on history and physical exam

TREATMENT

- Supportive and symptomatic therapy

Iron

- For any given iron compound, it is the amount of elemental iron that determines its toxicity.

MECHANISM/TOXICITY

- **Direct corrosive effect** on gastrointestinal tract
- **Toxicity from free circulating iron** → cellular uncoupling of oxidative phosphorylation and production of free radicals → anaerobic metabolism and multiorgan failure.

A key feature of iron toxicity is the uncoupling of oxidative phosphorylation → anaerobic metabolism.

SYMPTOMS/EXAM

Classically described as five phases of toxicity (see Table 6.24), as follows:

TABLE 6.24. The Five Phases of Iron Toxicity

Phase
Phase 1: Gastrointestinal phase
Phase 2: Latent phase
Phase 3: Systemic toxicity
Phase 4: Fulminant hepatic failure
Phase 5: Delayed sequelae

- **Phase 1: Gastrointestinal phase**
  - N/V/D, gastrointestinal bleeding from corrosive effect
  - No vomiting within 6 hours = no toxicity.
- **Phase 2: Latent phase (6–24 hours postingestion)**
  - Clinically stable after resuscitation
  - Patients with mild toxicity will not progress beyond this stage.
- **Phase 3: Systemic toxicity**
  - Recurrence of GI symptoms
  - Anaerobic metabolism → shock, lactate production, anion gap metabolic acidosis.
  - Multiorgan involvement with cardiac dysfunction, bleeding, renal failure
- **Phase 4: Fulminant hepatic failure (2–5 days postingestion)** from cellular oxidative injury
- **Phase 5: Delayed sequelae** from gastrointestinal scarring

Patients without onset of vomiting 6 hours after iron exposure will not have significant systemic toxicity.

DIFFERENTIAL

- Most ingested metals cause gastrointestinal effects with large doses such as mercuric salts, lead, arsenic.

DIAGNOSIS

- History of ingestion and presence of GI (phase 1) symptoms indicate toxicity.
- Presence of anion gap metabolic acidosis (primarily lactate) indicating cellular toxicity.
- Total serum iron level at 4–6 and 6–8 (for SR or EC preparations) hours postingestion.
  - Level >500 mcg/dL = severe toxicity.
- Measurement of TIBC has little or no value.
- Abdominal radiograph: A negative radiograph for radiopaque pills does **not** rule out ingestion.

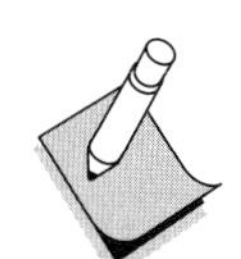

Not all iron pills are visible on abdominal X-ray.

TREATMENT

- Supportive and symptomatic care
- Remember, no GI symptoms within 6 hours = no toxicity.
- Decontamination
  - Activated charcoal does **not** bind iron.
  - Whole-bowel irrigation: If large amounts of pills visualized on X-ray and levels rising

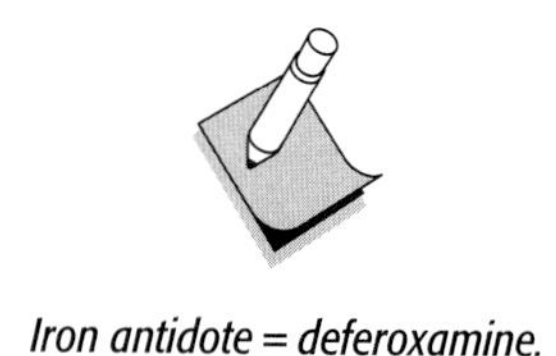

Iron antidote = deferoxamine.

- **Antidotal therapy: Deferoxamine**
  - Chelating agent
  - Indications:
    - Systemic illness (severe acidosis, shock)
    - Serum iron levels >500 mcg/dL (with clinical symptoms)
  - Urine color may change to pink-red ("vin-rose") color when deferoxamine-iron complex excreted in urine may be seen.

COMPLICATIONS

- ***Yersenia enterocolitica*** GI infection or sepsis may occur from chronic iron overload or deferoxamine therapy (both foster the growth of the organism).

Dextromethorphan

Structurally related to levorphanol, a synthetic opioid agonist.

MECHANISM/TOXICITY

- Antagonizes NMDA receptors and inhibits serotonin reuptake

SYMPTOMS/EXAM

- Mild to moderate overdose: Agitation, ataxia, nystagmus, visual and auditory hallucinations
- Severe overdose: Coma and respiratory depression
- Serotonin syndrome is rare but may occur when ingested with other serotonergic agents.

TREATMENT

- Supportive and symptomatic therapy

Diphenhydramine

- Diphenhydramine is a sedating antihistamine medication with anticholinergic, antitussive, antiemetic, and local anesthetic properties.

MECHANISM/TOXICITY

- Antagonizes histamine-induced responses at H_1 receptors → smooth muscle relaxation.
- Antagonism of H_1 receptors in the brain → sedation.
- Antagonism of cholinergic muscarinic receptors → anticholinergic effects.
- Na^{++} channel blockade (at high doses)

SYMPTOMS/EXAM

- CNS depression
- Cholinergic toxidrome
- Extremely large doses may cause seizures and dysrhythmias.

DIAGNOSIS

- Based on history and clinical presentation

TREATMENT

- Supportive and symptomatic therapy
- Benzodiazepines for agitation or seizures
- Sodium bicarbonate if wide complex dysrhythmias occur

PESTICIDES/INSECTICIDES/RODENTICIDES

> EMS presents with a 54-year-old male farm worker who called EMS after ingesting insecticide in a self-harm attempt. On ED arrival, he is confused and smells of garlic. Further examination reveals pinpoint pupils, excessive salivation, lacrimation, and muscle fasiculations. What is the most appropriate initial medication to give in the treatment of this patient?
>
> This patient is presenting with cholinergic excess consistent with organophosphate poisoning. Atropine is the initial medication and should be used to control airway secretions and symptomatic bradycardias. Large doses are often needed.

Cholinergic toxidrome—

SLUDGE
Salivation
Lacrimation
Urination
Defecation
GI symptoms
Emesis

and the
Killer Bs:
Bronchorrhea
Bronchospasm
Bradycardia

Organophosphates and Carbamates

Organophosphates and carbamates are insecticides used extensively in agricultural and commercial applications.

MECHANISM/TOXICITY

- Inhibition of cholinesterase → increased activity at all nicotinic and muscarinic receptors.
- Carbamates bind cholinesterase transiently (minutes to hours).
- Organophosphates can undergo "aging" → irreversible binding of the insecticide to cholinesterase.

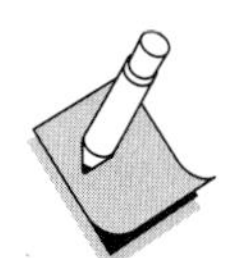

Unlike carbamates, the organophosphate bond to cholinesterase will "age" and become irreversible over time.

SYMPTOMS/EXAM

- Cholinergic toxidrome
- Altered mental status (delirium to coma), seizures

DIFFERENTIAL

- Toxicity from nerve agents (VX, Soman, Tabum) or nicotine

DIAGNOSIS

- Usually apparent from clinical symptoms and a history of exposure
- Measured RBC cholinesterase or pseudocholinesterase (plasma cholinesterase) levels
  - Reduced in toxicity, but are not available in a timely manner

TREATMENT

- Immediate surface decontamination, as indicated
- Supportive therapy
- Benzodizepines or phenobarbital for seizures
- **Antidote = atropine,** used for
  - Hemodyamically unstable bradycardia
  - Excessive secretions (endpoint is drying of airway secretions)
  - Very high doses often needed (>10 mg)
- **Antidote = pralidoxime (2-PAM)**
  - Can potentially reactivate inhibited cholinesterase
  - Indicated in organophosphate poisoning, but is ineffective in after aging has occurred

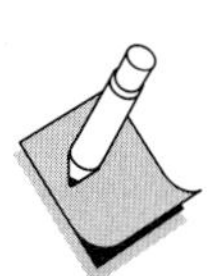

Antidotes to organophosphate poisoning: Atropine and pralidoxime

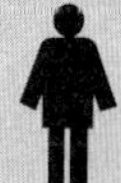

A 2-year-old girl is brought in to the ED by her parents following suspected ingestion of rat poison containing difenacoum 1 hour earlier. She has no past medical history, is acting normally, and the physical examination is unremarkable. What workup and intervention should be considered at this time?

Nothing at this time. It is very unlikely that the labs will be abnormal and very rare to have clinically significant bleeding after a one-time unintentional ingestion. A conservative approach is to have follow-up coagulation studies done daily for 2–3 days.

Superwarfarins

Most home rodenticide products contain a superwarfarin such as brodifacoum. Symptoms occur 1–2 days following ingestion.

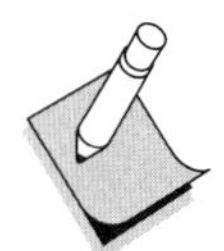

Duration of anticoagulation following superwarfarin ingestion may extend for weeks.

Mechanism/Toxicity

- Superwarfarins act similarly to warfarin by inhibiting production of vitamin K dependent clotting factors (II, VII, IX, X); however, the duration of anticoagulation may extend for weeks.

Symptoms/Exam

- Symptoms are due to bleeding (brain, GI, vaginal, etc.).
- Onset of symptoms is 1–2 days following ingestion.

Diagnosis

- PT/INR measurement can determine the extent of anticoagulation from superwarfarins.

Treatment

- Vitamin K supplementation for elevated INR. Large ingestions may require high doses for prolonged periods of time.
- Prophylactic vitamin K (prior to elevation of INR) is **not** indicated (duration of action of superwarfarin is much longer than that of vitamin K).
- Acute bleeding requires FFP or cryoprecipitate to reverse anticoagulation.

Strychnine

A rodenticide with significant human toxicity, its use in home products has largely been supplanted by the superwarfarins.

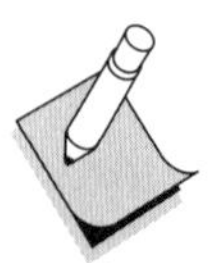

Generalized, uncontrolled muscular activity with normal mental status is suggestive of strychnine poisoning.

Mechanism/Toxicity

- Inhibits glycine receptors within the spinal cord → uncontrolled muscular contraction

Symptoms/Exam

- Strychnine poisoning produces rapid onset involuntary muscle contractions, opsithotonus, hyperreflexia, clonus, and trismus. Mental status is not affected.

DIAGNOSIS

- Specific testing for strychnine is not available.

TREATMENT

- Benzodiazepines or barbituates are administered to relieve excessive muscular activity.
- More severe cases may require intubation and neuromuscular blockade.

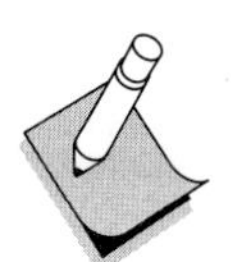

Severe barbiturate intoxication depressed/decreased:
HR
BP
RR
Temperature
CNS

SEDATIVE HYPNOTICS

Sedative-hypnotic agents are medications used to treat anxiety, panic disorders, and insomnia.

Medications in this class include barbiturates, benzodiazepines, antihistamines, antidepressants, and other agents with sedating side effects.

This section is limited to a discussion of barbiturates and benzodiazepines.

Barbiturates

Barbiturates are used as sedatives, to induce anesthesia, and to treat epilepsy, including status epilepticus.

They are categorized by their duration of action.

- Ultrashort-acting (eg, methohexital, thiopental)
- Short-acting (eg, pentobarbital)
- Intermediate-acting (eg, amobarbital)
- Long-acting (eg, phenobarbital)

The magnitude and duration of effect depends on the agent and dose. Chronic exposure often leads to tolerance.

MECHANISM/TOXICITY

- Bind to GABA-A chloride channel → depression of neuronal firing
- Depress medullary respiratory centers
- Inhibit myocardial contractility and conduction

SYMPTOMS/EXAM

- Mild to moderate intoxication: Lethargy, nystagmus, ataxia, slurred speech (similar to alcohol intoxication)
- Severe intoxication: Small/midsized pupils, hypothermia, coma, respiratory depression, hypotension, bradycardia

DIAGNOSIS

- Usually based on history of exposure and clinical examination
- Serum levels may be available for agents used to treat epilepsy (eg, phenobarbital).
  - In overdose, clinically correlate levels, and monitor for peak and decline.

TREATMENT

- Supportive therapy
- Gastric lavage if life-threatening ingestion **and** <60 minutes from ingestion

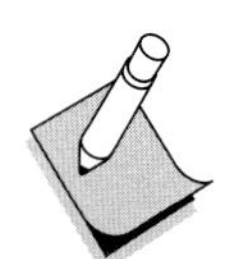

Urinary alkalinization is effective for long-acting barbiturates (phenobarbital) only.

- **Activated charcoal**
  - Multiple-dose activated charcoal: If large phenobarbital overdose
- **Whole-bowel irrigation** if long-acting agents
- **Urinary alkalinization**
  - For long-acting barbiturates (eg, phenobarbital) only
  - **Not** effective for shorter-acting agents
  - To urine pH of 8.0
- Hemodialysis for severely intoxicated patients refractory to above therapy

Benzodiazepines

Benzodiazepines are used as sedatives, to induce anesthesia, and to treat epilepsy, including status epilepticus.

They are categorized by their duration of action.

- Short-acting (eg, midazolam)
- Intermediate-acting (eg, lorazepam)
- Long-acting (eg, diazepam)

The shorter-acting agents are more lipophilic, and therefore cross the blood-brain barrier more rapidly (rapid on, rapid off). Half-life is **not** a good indicator of duration of effect.

Severe toxicity from benzodiazepine exposure is rare unless combined with other agents that have synergistic effects.

Mechanism/Toxicity

- Enhanced binding of GABA to GABA-A channels → depression of neuronal firing.
- Peripheral vasodilatation

Symptoms/Exam

- Mild to moderate intoxication: Lethargy, slurred speech, ataxia
- Severe intoxication: Coma, respiratory depression, hypotension

Diagnosis

- Usually based on history of exposure.
- Many urine toxicology tests screen for benzodiazepines.

Treatment

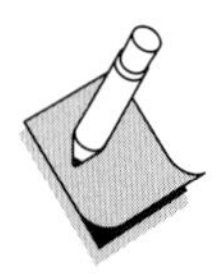

Flumazenil contraindications:
Chronic benzodiazepine use
Coingestion of seizure-inducing meds
Suspected ↑ ICP

- Supportive therapy
- Activated charcoal (if <1 hour and no significant CNS depression)
- **Antidote: Flumazenil**
  - Benzodiazepine receptor antagonist
  - Duration of effect = 1 hour (recurrent sedation possible)
  - Limited utility in the ED (mostly for reversal of procedural sedation)
  - Contraindications:
    - Chronic benzodiazepine use (may induce withdrawal)
    - Coingestion of seizure-inducing medication (eg, TCAs)
    - Suspected increased ICP

A 21-year-old male is brought in by the police after being found running naked in the park on a hot summer night. Physical examination reveals an agitated patient chewing on the restraints and fighting to get loose. His airway and breathing are intact and the nurse states that his pulse is "fast." What are the first actions to take in treating this patient?

Sedation with benzodiazepines and temperature control are essential with the undifferentiated sympathomimetic patient. Although it would be ideal to know what he took, determining the temperature and reversing the psychomotor agitation are of paramount importance.

SYMPATHOMIMETICS

The sympathomimetic toxidrome may result from exposure to any of the following:

- Prescription medications: ADD/ADHD medications (Ritalin, Adderall)
- Over-the-counter medications and herbal preparations: Ephedrine, pseudoephedrine, Ma Huang
- Illicit drugs: Cocaine, methamphetamines

MECHANISM/TOXICITY

Excessive epinephrine or norepinephrine due to:

- Increased release from α- and β-adrenergic receptors *or*
- Decreased enzymatic breakdown *or*
- Decreased reuptake
- Cocaine → Na^+ channel blockade causing wide complex dysrhythmias.

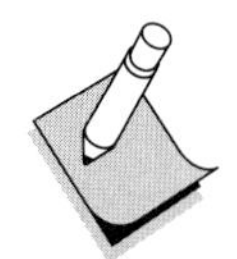

Sympathomimetic toxidrome:
Agitation
Tachycardia
Hypertension
Large pupils
Diaphoretic

SYMPTOMS/EXAM

- Agitations, hallucinations
- Tachycardia, hypertension
- Hyperthermia with diaphoretic skin
- Mydriasis
- Muscular rigidity

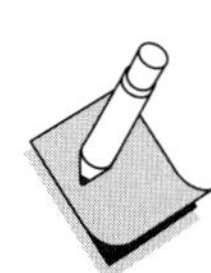

Diaphoretic, not dry, skin is the key to differentiating the sympathomimetic toxidrome from the anticholinergic toxidrome.

DIAGNOSIS

Clinical diagnosis based on exposure history and physical exam
ECG to establish rhythm and screen for ischemic changes
CT of abdomen and pelvis may be indicated if body packer or stuffer.

TREATMENT

- Supportive care
  - Passive and active cooling measures, as needed
  - Intravenous hydration
- **Benzodiazepines:** For sedation, hyperthermia, tachycardia, seizures, muscular rigidity
- **Sodium bicarbonate:** For wide complex dysrhythmias
- **Avoid**
  - β-Blockers due to concern for unopposed α-receptor stimulation

TABLE 6.25. **Antidotes for Specific Toxicologic Agents**

Antidote	Ingestion/Exposure	Indications for Treatment
Atropine	Cholinergic poisoning	Symptomatic bradycardia Excessive secretions
Black widow spider antivenom	Black widow spider (*Latrodectus*)	Persistent symptoms despite analgesia Pregnancy Very young or elderly
Calcium	Hydrofluoric (HF) acid exposure	Local symptoms or burns (dermal application) Hypocalcemia or high-concentration exposure (IV dosing)
CroFab	Family Viperidae: Rattlesnakes Copperheads Water moccasins	Progressive swelling Increased pain Coagulopathy Systemic symptoms
Cyanide antidote kit	Cyanide	Suspicion for exposure in patients with acidosis coma, seizures, and hypotension
Deferoxamine	Acute iron intoxication	Systemic symptoms Iron level >500 mcg/dL
Digoxin-specific Fab	Digoxin toxicity	Ventricular dysrhythmias Bradycardia unresponsive to therapy K > 5.0 mEq/dL in acute ingestion Potentially massive overdose
Flumazenil	Benzodiazepine overdose	Severe respiratory depression Contraindicated in: chronic use; if coingestion of seizure-inducing medication; elevated ICP
Fomepizole	Ethylene glycol Methanol	Metabolic acidosis or known ingestion of a toxic alcohol
Glucagon	Ca^{++} channel blocker toxicity β-Blocker toxicity	Symptomatic bradycardia Hypotension
Hydroxocobalamin	Cyanide	Suspicion of exposure in patients with acidosis coma, seizures, and hypotension
Insulin/glucose	Ca^{++} channel blocker toxicity β-Blocker toxicity	Symptomatic bradycardia Hypotension
Methylene blue	Methemoglobinemia	Levels >30% Mental status changes Chest pain Shortness of breath

TABLE 6.25. **Antidotes for Specific Toxicologic Agents (*Continued*)**

Antidote	Ingestion/Exposure	Indications for Treatment
N-acetylcysteine (NAC)	Acetaminophen	Acute single ingestion: Use Rumack-Matthew nomogram Unknown time or repeated supra-therapeutic ingestion: Elevated AST/ALT APAP level > 10 μcg/mL
Naloxone	Opioid toxicity	Respiratory depression
Octreotide	Sulfonlyurea overdose	Recurrent hypoglycemia
Physostigmine	Anticholinergic toxidrome (rarely indicated)	Delirium Seizures Dysrhythmias
Pralidoxime (2-PAM)	Organophosphates	Symptomatic poisonings
Vitamin K	Warfarin	Increased INR (escalating dosing) Bleeding

Complications

- Cardiac ischemia
- Aortic dissection
- Ruptured abdominal aorta
- Ischemic bowel
- Perforated viscus
- Rhabdomyolysis

CHAPTER 7

Endocrine, Metabolic, Fluid, and Electrolyte Disorders

Kenny V. Banh, MD

FLUID AND HYDRATION

Basic Definitions

- Solvent: Solution or medium, usually H_2O
- Solute: Crystalloid (cation or anion) or colloid (plasma protein)
- Osmosis: Movement of solvent (usually H_2O) across a membrane through an osmolar gradient
- Osmolality: Pressure exerted by the number of particles in the solution

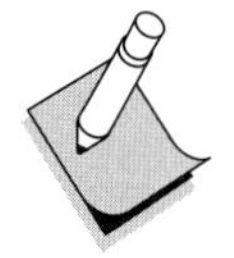

Total blood volume in adults is 70 mL/kg or about 5 L in a 70-kg person. Total blood volume is 80–90 mL/kg in children.

Total Body Water and Distribution

- Total body water = about 60% of total body weight
- Two-thirds of TBW is intracellular = 40% of total body weight (see Table 7.1).

Physiology

- Cell membranes are semipermeable and allow free passage of solvent but not solute, hence water moves freely between intracellular, interstitial, and plasma compartments to maintain equilibrium.
- Normal serum osmolality is around 285 mOsm/L.
- Osmolality can be calculated using this formula:

$$2[Na^+] + \frac{Glucose}{18} + \frac{BUN}{2.8} = \text{calculated osmolality}$$

In patients with altered mental status and an unexplained increased anion gap, use the osmolal gap as a screening test for methanol or ethylene glycol toxicity.

- Hyperosmolar states include:
  - Alcohol
  - Hypernatremia
  - Hyperosmolar hyperglycemic nonketotic coma
  - Ketoacidosis
  - Uremia
- Hypo-osmolar states are usually caused by hyponatremia.
- The osmolal gap is the difference between the calculated and measured osmolality and should be < 10 mOsm/L.
- High osmolal gaps are caused by increases in measured (but not calculated) serum osmolality.
- Account for ethanol's contribution to the osmolar gap by dividing by the blood ethanol in mg/dL by 4.6.
- Causes of high osmolal gaps include:
  - Ethanol—most common
  - Isopropyl alcohol
  - Mannitol
  - Sorbitol
  - Glycerol
  - Acetone
  - **Methanol**
  - **Ethylene glycol**

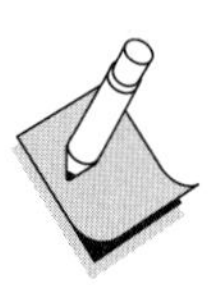

An increased osmolar gap that is explained by an elevated serum ethanol level is normal in a drunk patient.

ENDOCRINE, METABOLIC, FLUID, AND ELECTROLYTE DISORDERS

TABLE 7.1. Comparison of Intracellular and Interstitial Fluid

	% TBW	% WEIGHT	Na^+	Cl^-	HCO_3^-	K^+	Ca^{2+}	Mg^{2+}	INCLUDES
Intracellular	2/3	40%	14	4	10	150	< 1	30	Proteins
Interstitial	1/3	20%	140	113	27	5	9	3	Plasma

Fluid Balance

WATER

- Adults need 2000–3000 mL of water a day on average.
- Water loss can be categorized as sensible and insensible.
- Sensible water loss = urinary output = approximately 1500 mL/day.
- Cellular function creates approximately 300 mL of water/day.
- Minimum normal urine output of a hydrated adult without renal compromise is approximately 0.5 mL/kg/hour.
- Insensible water loss includes:
  - Respiratory losses of approximately 600 mL/day
  - Integumentary/evaporative skin losses of about 300 mL/day
  - GI/Feces losses of about 100 mL/day
- The body handles water regulation with three major mechanisms:
- Antidiuretic hormone (ADH)
  - Dehydration → decreased free water → increased serum osmolality → stimulate ADH release → retention of free water.
- Aldosterone and renal tubule water absorption
  - Hypovolemia → renin released by kidneys → aldosterone released by adrenals → sodium retention in renal tubules → water retention.
- Hypothalamic thirst center
  - Driven by increases in serum osmolality, renin-angiotensin, β-adrenergic stimulation and drugs such as lithium, as well as by drops in intracellular and extracellular volume.

An 86-year-old male with urosepsis presents dehydrated. How much intravascular fluid does 1 L of 0.9 NS provide? How about 1 L of 0.45 NS or D5W?

Following redistribution with extra vascular space, 1 L of NS provides 250 mL of intravascular fluid, while 0.45 NS provides only 125 mL of intravascular fluid. D5W initially provides 333 mL of intravascular fluid, but only a minimal amount of that remains once the sugar is metabolized.

FLUIDS AND DEHYDRATION

- Fluid tonicity
  - 0.9% NS and lactated Ringer's are approximately isotonic to plasma.
  - D5W is approximately isotonic, but sugar is then metabolized leaving hypotonic free water.
- Fluid distribution
  - 1 L of 0.9 NS will distribute 250 mL intravascularly and 750 mL in the interstitial space.
  - 1 L of 0.45 NS places only 125 mL in the intravascular space.
  - 1 L of D5W places 333 mL initially in the intravascular spaces, but after the sugar is metabolized only one-quarter (83 mL) remains.
- Dehydration
  - Dehydration can be broken up into three categories related to its osmolality: Hypotonic, isotonic, and hypertonic (see Table 7.2).
  - For more detailed information on hypo- and hypernatremic states, see "Sodium."
  - In patients with hypernatremia, the total free water deficit can be calculated with the equation

$$\text{Water deficit (L)} = 0.6 \times \text{wt (kg)} \times (Na^{+}/140 - 1)$$

TABLE 7.2. Categories of Dehydration

Type	Hypotonic Dehydration	Isotonic Dehydration	Hypertonic Dehydration
Etiology	Na^+ loss > H_2O loss	Na^+ loss = H_2O loss	Na^+ loss < H_2O loss
Common causes	Vomiting	Vomiting	Diarrhea
	Diuretics		HHNK
	Third spacing		DI
	Adrenocortical insufficiency		Inability to drink

- Rehydration should commence immediately and can usually be safely done with isotonic 0.9 NS, at least initially, with one-half of the deficit given to the patient over the first 24 hours.

ELECTROLYTE PUMP PHYSIOLOGY

- While water freely moves between cells, it follows the gradient set up by electrolyte cell pumps.
- Pumps can be active (requiring ATP) or passive. The most important ones to be familiar with are:
  - Na^+/K^+ ion pump: The major active pump in the human body exchanges 3 Na^+ for 2 K^+. This creates Na^+ and K^+ gradients across the cell membrane and also an electrical gradient that is used for many processes from neurotransmitters to myocardium.
  - H^+/K^+ ion pump
- In acidosis, H^+ is pumped intracellularly in place of K^+ to act as a buffer for the cell.
- This is why patients with diabetic ketoacidosis are initially hyperkalemic. With longstanding DKA, K^+ is lost in the urine. When the acidosis is corrected, the hypokalemia is unmasked. This only occurs with organic acids such as ketones that do not freely cross the cell membrane, not with lactate or alcohol.

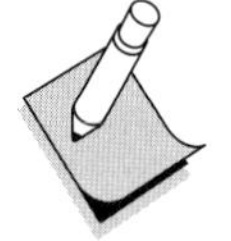

Digoxin directly inhibits the Na^+/K^+ pump. Severe hypokalemic and hypercalcemic states increase digoxin's inotropic effect on myocardium.

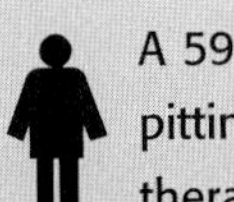

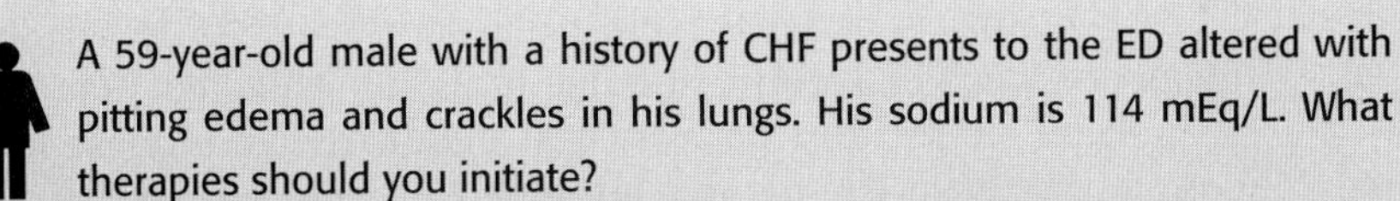

A 59-year-old male with a history of CHF presents to the ED altered with pitting edema and crackles in his lungs. His sodium is 114 mEq/L. What therapies should you initiate?

This patient needs water restriction, diuresis with furosemide, hypertonic saline and treatment of his underlying CHF. Consider dialysis if he has end-stage renal disease.

SODIUM

- Sodium is the major extracellular cation as opposed to K^+ and Mg^{2+}, which are the major intracellular cations.
- Sodium regulation is followed passively by water regulation, hence problems with sodium usually represent problems with water balance.

Hyponatremia (Na^+ < 135 mEq/L)

SYMPTOMS

- Headache
- Confusion
- Seizures
- Many patients are asymptomatic.

EXAM

- Besides often presenting with altered mental status, patients may have findings consistent with the underlying cause of their hyponatremia, including:
  - CHF
  - Cirrhosis
  - Vomiting
  - Diarrhea
  - Excessive thirst or water intake

> **Differential for altered mental status–**
>
> **AEIOU TIPS**
> **A**cidosis/Alcohol
> **E**pilepsy
> **I**nfection
> **O**verdose
> **U**remia
> **T**rauma to head
> **I**nsulin
> **P**sychosis
> **S**troke

DIFFERENTIAL

- A wide differential of altered mental status should include vital sign abnormalities (hypoxia, hypotension), head injury, toxic/metabolic abnormality, infection, or psychiatric illness.

DIAGNOSIS AND CAUSES

- Na^+ <120 mEq/L is considered severe hyponatremia. Most patients will be symptomatic.
- If etiology of hyponatremia is not clearly evident on history, checking serum and calculated osmolality will help differentiate pseudohyponatremia from true hyponatremia.
- Figure 7.1 charts the basic algorithm for evaluation of hyponatremia.
- Pseudohyponatremia (falsely elevated)
  - Normal to high measured osmolality
  - If low calculated osmolality state:
    - Low water state with high amounts of unmeasured solute found in multiple myeloma and hyperlipidemia
  - If high calculated osmolality state:
    - Water moves from intracellular into higher solute extracellular space in conditions like hyperglycemia and radio contrast or mannitol administration.
    - Hyperglycemia is by far the most common cause of hyperosmolar hyponatremia. The correction factor is an expected decrease in sodium by 1.6 mEq/L for every 100 mg/dL rise in glucose for glucose levels above 100 mg/dL. For glucose levels >400 mg/dL, some authors advocate a correction factor of 2.4 mEq/L.
- True hypo-osmolar hyponatremia (elevated TBW)
  - Measured and calculated osmolality are low and similar.
  - Checking volume status and urine sodium will help differentiate the type of disorder.
  - Hypervolemic hypo-osmolar hyponatremia
    - Signs of fluid overload
    - Etiology is usually from a perceived low intravascular volume by the kidneys and active water reabsorbtion in excess to sodium retention.
    - If urine sodium is low (<10 mEq/L) = loop diuretic, cirrhosis, CHF, or nephrotic syndrome.
    - If urine sodium is high (>20 mEq/L) = acute or chronic renal failure.

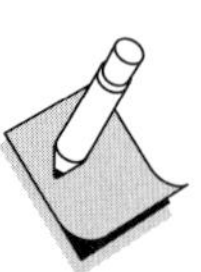

*Hypervolemic hyponatremia may be caused by **liver** failure, **heart** failure, or **renal** failure.*

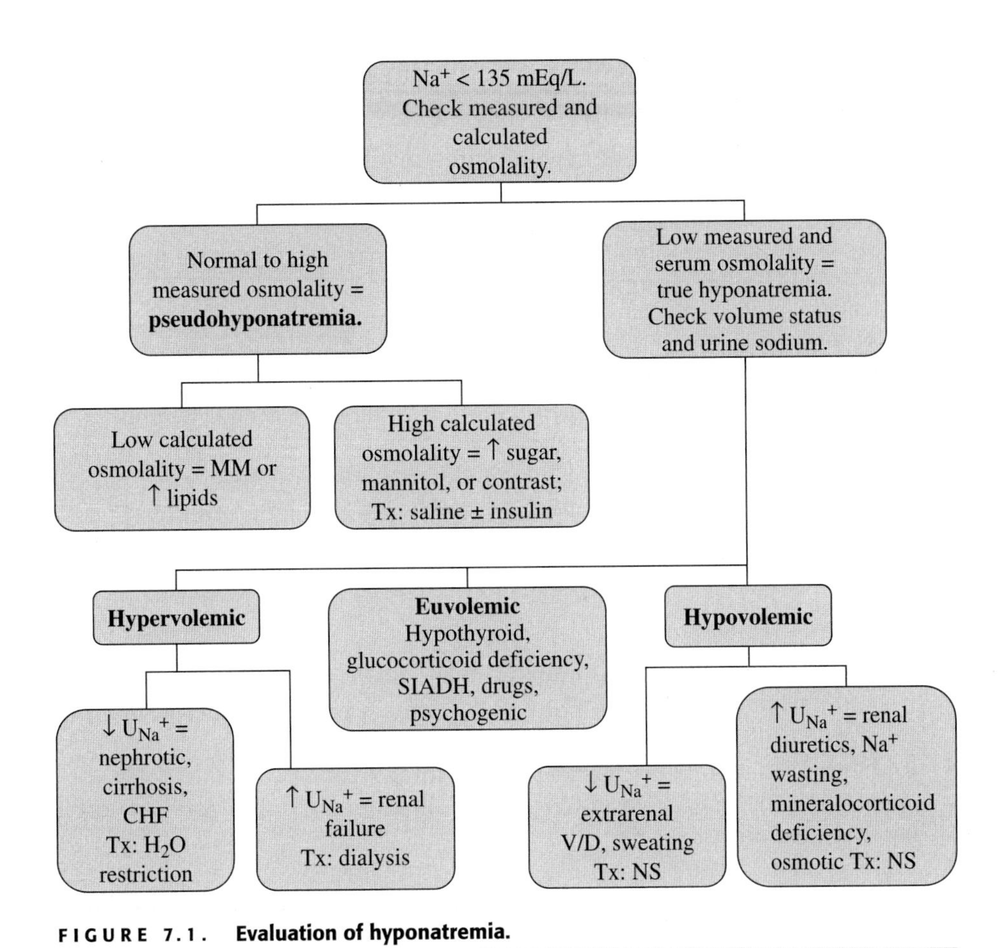

FIGURE 7.1. Evaluation of hyponatremia.

- Euvolemic hypo-osmolar hyponatremia
  - Urine sodium is usually high (>20 mEq/L)
  - Etiology is either endocrine or nonendocrine caused:
    - Endocrine: Hypothyroidism, SIADH, and glucocorticoid deficiency
    - Nonendocrine: Drugs or psychogenic polydipsia
  - SIADH is a diagnosis of exclusion but typical lab findings are:
    - High urine Na^+ (>20 mEq/L)
    - High urine osmolality (>150)
    - Low BUN
- Hypovolemic hypo-osmolar hyponatremia (dehydrated)
  - Caused by dehydrated states where the kidney is actively trying to reabsorb water
  - Signs of dehydration including poor skin turgor and tachycardia.
  - If urine sodium is low (<10 mEq/L), the etiology is likely extrarenal sodium loss such as vomiting diarrhea, fistula, sweating, or traumatized muscle.
  - If urine sodium is high (>20 mEq/L), the etiology is likely renal sodium loss such as from diuretics, hyperglycemia, nephropathy, or mineralocorticoid deficiency.

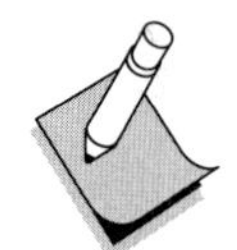

A high urine sodium (>20 mEq/L) in a patient with hyponatremia suggests a renal-related etiology (SIADH, nephropathy, diuretics, hyperglycemia, or mineralcorticoid deficiency).

TREATMENT

- Treatment focuses on identification and correction of the underlying cause.
- Emergent hyponatremia requiring hypertonic 3% saline is reserved for patients with an altered level of consciousness or seizures with Na^+ <115.
- Patients who are dehydrated and hyponatremic need to be volume resuscitated as well, hence should be resuscitated with 0.9 NS.

- Sodium deficit can be approximated with this equation:

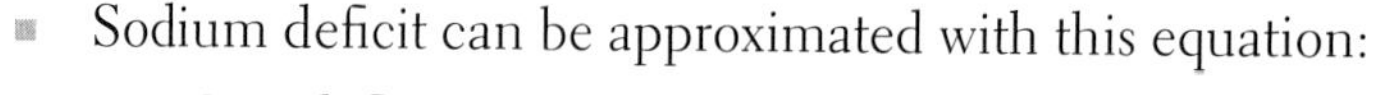

$$Na^+ \text{ deficit (in total mEq)} = 0.6 \times \text{wt(kg)} \times (140 - \text{serum } Na^+)$$

- Nonemergent treatment of hyponatremia involves treating the various underlying causes of hyponatremia.
  - Pseudohyponatremia secondary to
    - Multiple myeloma or hyperlipidemia does not require treatment
    - Mannitol or contrast agents requires saline
    - Hyperglycemia requires insulin and saline
  - Hypervolemic hypo-osmolar hyponatremia secondary to
    - Renal failure requires dialysis
    - CHF, cirrhosis, or nephritic syndrome requires fluid restriction and treating the underlying disorder
    - Euvolemic hypo-osmolar hyponatremia requires free water restriction, saline, and possibly furosemide, depending on severity
    - Hypovolemic hypo-osmolar hyponatremia requires aggressive hydration with saline

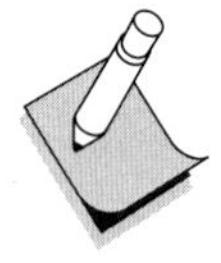

Reserve use of hypertonic saline for emergent cases of hyponatremia such as seizures or decreased mental status, typically in patients with Na <115 mEq/L.

Complications

- Rapid correction of hyponatremia has been associated with neurologic deterioration known as central pontine myelinosis or osmotic demyelinating syndrome (ODS).
- ODS presents with flaccid paralysis, dysarthria, dysphagia, and hypotension.
- Alcoholics, malnourished or chronically ill patients, women, and children are at increased risk.
- ODS has been associated with rates of correction >0.6 mEq/L/hr or >25 mEq/48 hours in patients with hyponatremia >2 days. It has also been associated with correction rates >2.5 mEq/hr with patients with hyponatremia between 1 and 2 days. No such risk has been seen in patients with acute (<24 hours) hyponatremia.

Hypernatremia (Na^+ >145 mEq/L)

Hypernatremia results from either a hypovolemic state or iatrogenic Na^+ gain.

Symptoms and Exam

- Headache, seizures, altered mental status
- Vomiting, sweating, and hyperpnea may be symptoms of the underlying disease causing the hypernatremia.
- Poor skin turgor, tachycardia, low urine output

Causes

- Three major types:
  - Dehydration
    - Inadequate water intake from physical or neurologic disability
    - Common in elderly and disabled patients
    - Osmotic diuresis secondary to hyperglycemia, DKA, or hyperosmolar nonketotic coma
  - Iatrogenic: Drugs such as lithium or fluoride
  - Salt wasting: Diabetes insipidus whether central or nephrogenic

Treatment

- Rehydration for hypovolemic patients initially with 0.9 NS as well as correction of the underlying mechanism
- Furosemide and D5W for hypervolemic patients

Complications

- Overly aggressive correction of chronic hypernatremia can lead to cerebral edema.

> A patient with a history of renal failure missed her last few dialysis sessions and presents with weakness. When attached to the cardiac monitor you notice a very wide QRS complex resembling a sine wave. What treatments should be initiated? Which of these treatments is definitive?
>
> Initiate treatment with calcium, insulin with glucose, kayexalate, and dialysis. Consider sodium bicarbonate and albuterol as adjuncts. Ultimately only kayexalate and dialysis are definitive.

POTASSIUM

- While 98% of K^+ is intracellular, serum K^+ is usually a good indicator of total body stores.
- Changes in intracellular/extracellular gradient assist propagation of electrical impulses.
- K^+ is freely filtered through the glomerulus, absorbed in the proximal and ascending tubules, and secreted in the distal tubules through a Na^+/K^+ gate.

Hypokalemia (K^+ <3.5 mEq/L)

Symptoms

- Nonspecific
- Weakness
- Abdominal distention

Exam

- Muscle weakness
- Hyporeflexia in severe cases but DTRs usually preserved
- Paralysis if severe, ie, hypokalemic periodic paralysis
- Ileus
- Cardiac findings: not sensitive, but see Figure 7.2
  - Bradycardia and AV block
  - VFib or V-Tach
  - U waves and flat T waves
  - ST depression if severe
  - QT prolongation if severe

Differential

- CVA
- Infection
- Primary neuromuscular disorders such as:
  - Amyotrophic lateral sclerosis
  - Guillain-Barré syndrome
  - Myasthenia gravis
  - Botulism

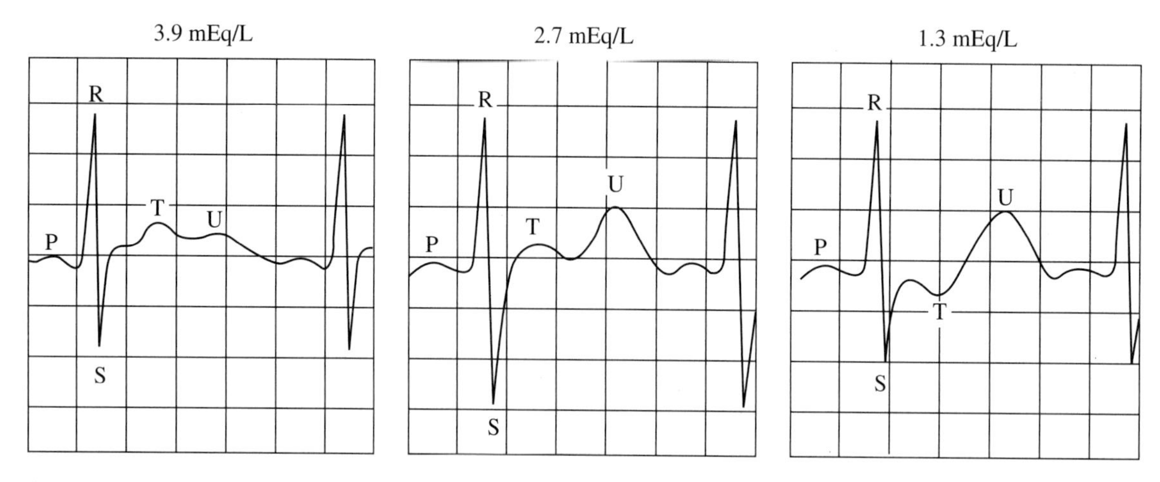

FIGURE 7.2. ECGs of hypokalemia with characteristic U waves and ST depression.

CAUSES

- History and physical are usually sufficient in diagnosing the cause of potassium loss.
  - Renal losses
    - With metabolic acidosis include renal tubular acidosis and postobstructive diuresis.
    - With metabolic alkalosis include diuretics, Cushing syndrome, and licorice ingestion (causes increased cortisol).
  - Nonrenal losses, which include
    - Vomiting, diarrhea, or suctioning
    - Colon cancer
    - Villous adenoma
    - Excessive sweating
  - Decreased intake
  - Intracellular shift
    - Familial periodic paralysis
    - Insulin or albuterol administration
  - Endocrine: Hyperthyroidism

TREATMENT

- Acute hypokalemia
  - Uncommon but considered life-threatening
  - 40 mEq of K^+ raises the serum level approximately 1 mEq/L acutely, but total body K^+ deficit may be much larger.
  - Goal is to correct K^+ to at least 3.5 mEq/L.
  - Cardiac monitoring
- Chronic hypokalemia
  - Not usually life-threatening
  - K^+ replacement should be done orally if there is no contraindication.

COMPLICATIONS

- Both inadequate and overzealous K^+ replacement can lead to cardiac dysrhythmias and death.
- Oral replacement safer than IV but 10 mEq/hour IV is safe.

- Always remember to check for and correct any associated hypomagnesemia. In patients with hypokalemia and malnutrition, it is appropriate to presumptively **give magnesium along with potassium** replacement.

Do not forget to replace K^+ in DKA patients, even if they have normal serum K^+ initially. Correction of acidosis can lead to a precipitous and dangerous drop in the K^+.

Hyperkalemia (K^+ >4.5 mEq/L)

SYMPTOMS

Similar to hypokalemia

EXAM

- Weakness and areflexia
- Hypotension
- Dysrhythmias: Peaked T waves → widened QRS → sine waves (M or W complexes) (see Figure 7.3).

CAUSES

- Common
  - Pseudohyperkalemia
    - Errors: Lab errors (hemolysis most common) and prolonged tourniquet application
    - Thrombocytosis or leukocytosis
  - Renal insufficiency or failure
  - DKA or other states of acidosis
- Uncommon
  - Increased potassium intake
  - Increased cellular breakdown or turnover from trauma, burns, tumor lysis, or rhabdomyolysis
  - GI bleed
  - Potassium salt substitutes
  - High-dose Pen-VK
  - Decreased renal excretion of K^+
  - Type IV renal tubular acidosis most commonly from diabetes
  - Drugs such as K^+ sparing diuretics and ACE inhibitors, β-blockers, digoxin, or succinylcholine
  - Adrenal and/or aldosterone insufficiency (Addison disease)

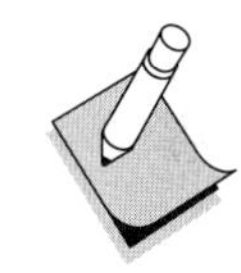

Hyperkalemia due to digoxin toxicity needs digibind, not calcium.

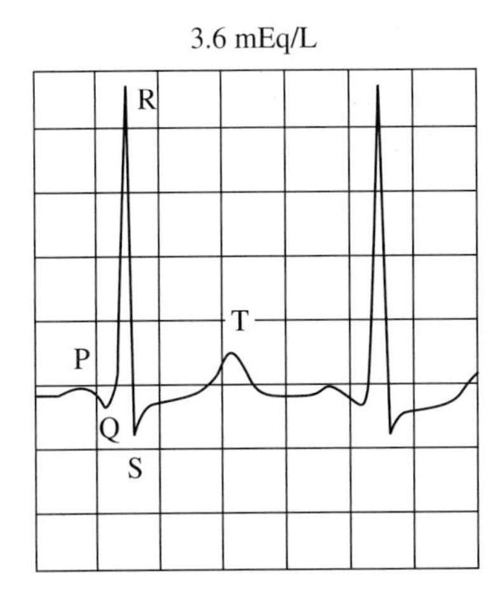

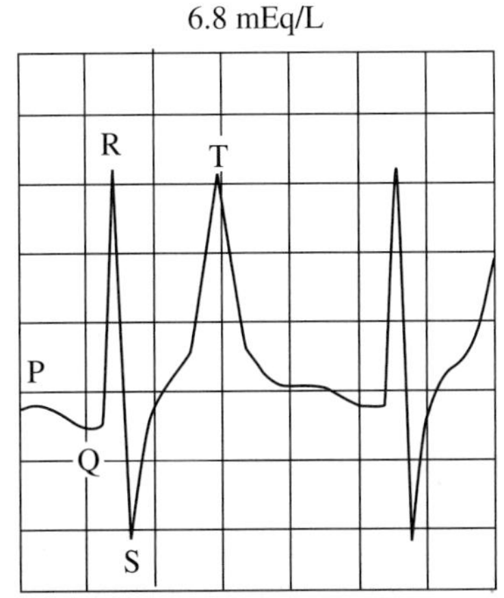

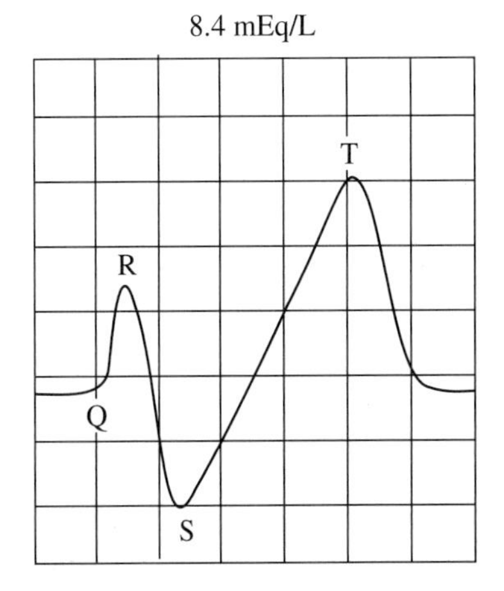

FIGURE 7.3. ECGs of hyperkalemia with peaked T waves progressing to sine waves.

TABLE 7.3. Treatments for Hyperkalemia

INTERVENTION	MECHANISM CATEGORY	USUAL DOSE	ONSET OF ACTION	DURATION OF EFFECT ON K^+
Kayexalate	Excretory	15 g PO or 30 g PR	1–2 hrs	4–6 hrs
Furosemide	Excretory	40 mg IV	<1 hr	6 hrs
Dialysis	Excretory	–	Immediate	Continuous
Insulin and glucose	Redistribution	10–15 U regular insulin and 50 g of D50	30 min	4–6 hrs
Sodium bicarbonate	Redistribution	1 mEq/kg IV	5 min	2 hrs
Albuterol	Redistribution	10–20 mg inhaled	30 min	2–4 hrs
Calcium gluconate/ chloride	Membrane stabilization	10–20 mL IV of 10%	1–3 min	30–60 min

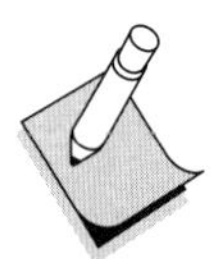

Do not use succinylcholine for RSI on patients who have known or suspected hyperkalemia or in patients with neurologic conditions (Guillaine-Barré, muscular dystrophy, old CVA, old burn, crush, or spinal cord injury) that may predispose them to a large increase in serum K^+ with succinylcholine.

TREATMENT

- Three categories of treatment (see Table 7.3)
- Without ECG findings, treatment can be limited to decreased intake and potassium excreting drugs.
- ECG findings prompt use of protective agents such as insulin and calcium until definitive excretory methods can take effect. Generally, **give calcium if there is QRS widening.**
- Sodium bicarbonate has no effect on nonacidotic patients.

COMPLICATIONS

- Inadequate treatment of hyperkalemia can lead to life-threatening cardiac arrhythmias.
- Only kayexalate, dialysis, and diuretics remove potassium. The other measures are temporizing measures that protect against high potassium levels without changing total body potassium.

A 54-year-old female undergoing treatment for breast CA presents to your ED with abdominal pain, nausea, and vomiting. Her electrolytes show a creatinine of 3.1 mg/dL and a Ca^{2+} of 13.6 mg/dL. What treatments should you initiate?

Treat this patient with fluid, furosemide, hydrocortisone, and either calcitonin, mithramycin, or a bisphosphonate.

CALCIUM

- Almost all calcium (99%) is in bone. The rest is in the plasma with half bound to proteins and half as free (ionized or active) ions.
- Normal plasma calcium levels are maintained by Vitamin D and parathyroid hormone with normal concentrations of about 8.8–10.3 mg/dL.

- Ca^{2+} has a host of critical functions, including:
  - Control of cell membrane depolarization
  - Coagulation and platelet aggregation
  - Hormone secretion
  - Contractile protein function
  - Intracellular enzyme regulation
- Drops in pH increase levels of ionized calcium because Ca^{2+} binds to protein in place of H^+. This is known as relative hypercalcemia.
- The same relative hypercalcemia occurs with hypoalbuminemia with no change in total calcium.

Hypocalcemia (Ca^{2+} <8.5 mg/dL)

Symptoms

- Parasthesias, particularly perioral and distally
- Muscle spasms, particularly carpopedal
- Seizures

Exam

- Hyperreflexia
- Chvostek sign (spasm when tapping along the facial nerve)
- Trousseau sign (arm spasm when BP inflated)
- Cardiovascular findings
  - Hypotension due to loss of vascular tone
  - CHF
  - Arrhythmias
  - QT prolongation

Causes

- Vitamin D disorder
  - Malabsorption of Vitamin D from chronic diarrhea
  - Impaired production of 1,25-dihydroxy vitamin D, usually secondary to renal or hepatic failure or anticonvulsants
- Hypoparathyroidism
- Hypomagnesemia
- Acute pancreatitis as fat binds calcium
- Alkalosis, either respiratory or metabolic
- Rapid and massive blood transfusions
- Rhabdomyolysis
- Drugs: Dilantin, cimetidine, steroids, foscarnet, and anticonvulsants

Treatment

- Emergent treatment of acutely symptomatic patients with 10% calcium chloride
- Transfusion-associated hypocalcemia is transient in most patients and will resolve without treatment. Since citrate is metabolized through the liver, patients with liver disease may require calcium during transfusions.

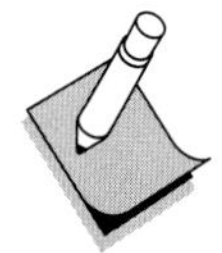

Hypocalcemia can protect against digitalis toxicity; treatment of hypocalcemia can expose digitalis toxicity.

Hypercalcemia (Ca^{2+} >10.5 mg/dL)

Hypercalcemia is generally a product of another underlying disorder and not a primary process in itself.

CAUSES

Causes are grouped into four categories:

- Malignancy: **Most common in hospitalized patients**
  - Primary hematologic or metastatic to bone
  - Parathyroid producing tumor
- Hyperparathyroidism: Most common in nonhospitalized patients
- Increased intake
  - Milk-alkali syndrome
  - Vitamin D or A toxicity
- Increased bone breakdown
  - Immobilization
  - Paget disease

> ***Symptoms of hypercalcemia–***
>
> **Stones, bones, abdominal groans, psychiatric overtones**
> **S**tones (renal)
> **B**ones (fractures/mets)
> **A**bdominal groans (vomiting, constipation)
> **P**sychiatric overtones (weakness, AMS)

SYMPTOMS

- Lethargy and weakness
- Constipation
- Anorexia

EXAM

- Neuromuscular
  - Confusion → lethargy → stupor → coma with increasing Ca^{2+}
  - Weakness, hypotonia, and hyporeflexia
  - Apathy or depression
- Cardiovascular effects
  - Hypertension
  - Arrhythmias
  - Digitalis sensitization
  - Shortened QT interval
  - ST and T-wave coving or T-wave widening
- Renal
  - Renal failure
  - Nephrolithiasis
  - Polyuria

TREATMENT

- Hydration
- Furosemide increases calcium excretion, especially useful in patients with fluid overload
- Hydrocortisone
- Drugs that decrease bone absorption: Calcitonin, bisphosphonates, and mithramycin
- Potassium replacement
- Treatment of underlying cause

MAGNESIUM

- Approximately 60% of the 24 g of magnesium are contained in bone with the remaining 40% intracellular. Because of this, magnesium regulation is related to calcium and phosphate.
- Intake is generally through leafy green vegetables.
- It plays crucial roles in the clotting cascade and neuromuscular activity.

> You respond to a code on the floor to find an elderly man seizing. After treating the seizures you review the chart to see the patient has been admitted for pneumonia and has been receiving IV fluids for the last few days. With a basic metabolic panel that shows a normal sodium and potassium, what electrolyte abnormality could cause the seizure?
>
> This patient likely has iatrogenic hypomagnesemia.

Hypomagnesemia (Mg^{2+} <1.4 mEq/L)

Causes

- Inadequate intake/absorption
  - Malnutrition
  - Inadequate supplementation in IV fluids
  - Malabsorption
- Alcoholism
- Pancreatitis
- Endocrine disorders
- Aminoglycosides

Symptoms

- Lethargy
- Muscle spasms
- Seizures

Exam

- Neuromuscular
  - Irritability
  - Hyperreflexia, tremor, tetany, or carpopedal spasms
- Cardiovascular
  - Hypotension
  - Arrhythmias: **Digoxin potentiation for toxicity**
  - QT and PR prolongation
  - Widened QRS
  - ST depression
  - T-wave flattening and inversion
- Hypokalemia
- Hypocalcemia

Treatment

- Emergent replacement of life-threatening dysrhythmias or seizures should include 1–2 g of $MgSO_4$ IV over 1–5 minutes.
- Nonemergent magnesium replacement rate is 1–2 g over 1 hour, followed by 0.5 g/hour.
- Check and correct for associated hypokalemia and hypocalcemia.

Hypermagnesemia (Mg^{2+} >2.2 mEq/L)

Causes

- Iatrogenic, most commonly from administration to preeclamptic patients
- Renal failure
- DKA
- Adrenal insufficiency

Symptoms

- Weakness
- Slurred speech
- Drowsiness → lethargy → coma and respiratory failure.

Exam

- Hyporeflexia
- Cardiovascular
- Hypotension
- Prolonged PR and QT
- ST and T-wave elevation
- Bradycardia → AV block → asystole.

Always remember to regularly check the reflexes of any preeclamptic patient getting magnesium. Decreased reflexes indicate toxicity.

Treatment

- Diuretics → calcium → dialysis for severe cases.

CHLORIDE

- Extracellular anion that follows changes of other anions
- Disorders in chloride are rarely the primary problem, but a reflection of another process.
- Chloride functions in water, osmotic, and acid-base balance.

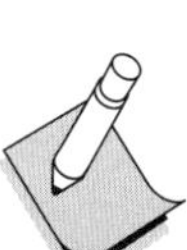

Hypochloremic hypokalemic metabolic alkalosis is the classic electrolyte disorder seen with pyloric stenosis.

Hypochloremia (Cl^- <100 mEq/L)

Causes

- Vomiting or diarrhea
- Excessive sweating or heat exhaustion
- Hyokalemic alkalosis
- Acute infections

Treatment

- Replace chloride with normal saline.
- Check and correct for other associated electrolyte abnormalities.

Hyperchloremia (Cl^- >110 mEq/L)

Causes

- Dehydration
- Cardiac decompensation
- Gastrointestinal or renal losses of bicarbonate

Treatment

- For gastrointestinal loss administer saline.
- For renal loss administer oral bicarbonate.

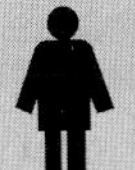

A 70-year-old female presents with fever, tachypnea, and AMS. Her ABG shows pH = 7.44, Po_2 = 90, Pco_2 = 20, HCO_3^- = 12. The chemistry panel shows an increased anion gap. What acid-base disorders are present?

Primary anion gap metabolic acidosis and primary respiratory alkalosis, consider salicylate toxicity.

ACID-BASE DISORDERS

Interpreting Blood Gases

Basic Definitions

- Acidosis/alkalosis: A process → acidemia/alkalemia
- Acidemia: pH <7.40
- Alkalemia: pH >7.40
- Metabolic disorder: Change in HCO_3^-
- Respiratory disorder: Change in Pco_2
- Respiratory or renal compensation: Other system alterations that bring the blood gas toward a normal pH of 7.40

Diagnosis

Use the history and exam for clues to the disorder.

- Respiratory status (increased RR suggests respiratory alkalosis; decreased RR or respiratory failure suggests respiratory acidosis)
- Dehydration/vomiting = metabolic alkalosis; diarrhea = metabolic acidosis.
- Past medical history, medication, and toxin exposures

Now look at the blood gas and chemistry.

- Look at the pH to determine if there is an acidemia or alkalemia.
- Check the Pco_2 to determine if there is a respiratory acidosis or alkalosis.
- Examine the HCO_3^- to determine if there is a metabolic acidosis or alkalosis.
- Calculate the anion gap [$Na^+ - (K^+ + Cl^-)$]. If ≥20, there is an underlying metabolic gap acidosis.

Classify the disturbance.

- Respiratory alkalosis (Pco_2 <40) caused by CHF, hypoxia, ↑ ICP, toxic salicylates, and sympathomimetics
- Respiratory acidosis (Pco_2 >40) caused by respiratory failure, sedatives, and opiates, common and often chronic in patients with COPD, considered a sign of respiratory failure in asthmatics
- Metabolic alkalosis (↑ HCO_3^-) caused by hypovolemia, hyperaldosteronism and Bartter syndrome.
- Metabolic acidosis (↓ HCO_3^-) causes are subdivided by the presence of an anion gap.
  - Low gap (anion gap <1) states caused by:
    - Increases in unmeasured serum cations (seen in myeloma)
    - Decreased serum albumin
    - Bromide or iodine poisoning (which are mistaken for chloride in many labs)
  - Normal anion gap acidosis (variously reported as 3–11, 8–16, or 1–20 mmol/L depending on analyzer) caused by:
    - Diarrhea
    - Renal tubular acidosis

Causes of a high anion gap—

MUDPILES
Methanol, **M**etformin
Uremia
Diabetic (or alcoholic) ketoacidosis
Paraldehyde
INH/iron/inhalant (ie, CO) poisoning
Lactic acidosis (sepsis, shock, hypoxia, seizures, cyanide)
Ethylene glycol
Salicylates, **S**olvents

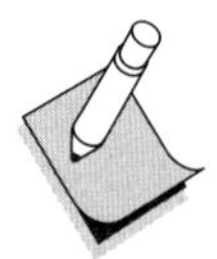

There are only three endogenous causes of an anion gap acidosis: Lactate, ketones, and uremia. All other causes are exogenous.

Compensation for an acid-base disorder never completely normalizes the pH. A pH of 7.45 in a patient with a low HCO_3^- indicates a second disorder (in this case a primary respiratory alkalosis) (see Table 7.4).

    - Ketone wasting
    - Toluene
  - High anion gap (anion gap >20) caused by increased concentrations of anions other than K^+ and Cl^-

Three rules assist in identifying a mixed disorder:

1. Neither respiratory nor renal compensation completely normalizes the pH.
2. The PCO_2 in patients with a metabolic acidosis is predicted by Winter's formula: $PCO_2 \approx 1.5\ HCO_3^- + 8$.
   - PCO_2 below predicted by Winter's formula = respiratory alkalosis.
   - PCO_2 above predicted by Winter's formula = respiratory acidosis.
3. Δ gap = measured anion gap − normal anion gap. The Δ gap should approximate the decrease in HCO_3^-; if the drop in HCO_3^- cannot be explained completely by the Δ gap a nongap acidosis is also present.

Metabolic Acidosis (↓ pH + ↓ HCO_3^-)

An extremely common presentation both in the emergency department and on the exam, patients are often ill- or septic-appearing on presentation.

Symptoms and Exam

- Tachypnea is a compensatory response in any patient with a metabolic acidosis, but may be greatest (ie, Kussmaul) in DKA or salicylate poisoning.
- Severe hypoxia or hypotension may precipitate lactic acidosis.
- Intoxicated appearance or visual complaints and a high anion gap acidosis should prompt an evaluation of serum osmolar gap to screen for toxic alcohols.
- Volume overload may be due to acute renal failure with associated acidosis.
- Adrenal insufficiency
- Diarrhea

Diagnosis and Causes

- A metabolic acidosis is present in any patient with a pH <7.35 and HCO_3^- <20 mEq/L. In patients with mixed disorders, the pH may be normal or >7.40. Use the anion gap and the serum K^+ to help narrow the differential.

- Normal anion gap $[Na^+ - (K^+ + Cl^-)] \approx 12$
  - Look for chloride losses.
    - Hypokalemic normal gap acidosis:
      - Renal losses: Renal tubular acidosis or acetazolamide
      - GI losses: Diarrhea or malabsorption

TABLE 7.4. Commonly Tested Acid-Base Disorders

pH	PCO_2	HCO_3^-	Anion Gap	Causes
↓ or ↑	↓↓	↓	↑	Salicylates
↓	↓	↓	↑	DKA, toxic alcohol, sepsis
↓	↑↑	–	–	Narcotic OD, COPD (pure respiratory acidosis)

- Hyperkalemic normal gap acidosis:
  - Adrenal insufficiency
  - Renal insufficiency
  - Posthypocapnia
- Increased anion gap $[Na^+ - (K^+ + Cl^-)] > 20$
  - Causes of a high anion gap acidosis can be remembered with the MUDPILES mnemonic.
  - For patients with a high anion gap without obvious identifiable cause, such as DKA, lactic acidosis, or known ingestion, calculating a serum osmolar gap is a screen for the presence of toxic alcohols. See "Fluids" for a more detailed explanation.

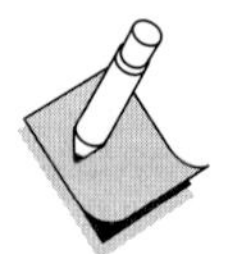

Measure the serum osmolar gap to screen for toxic alcohol ingestion in patients with AMS and an increased anion gap. Normal rate is <10 mOsm/L.

Treatment

Treating the underlying cause is the most important action.

- Sodium bicarbonate treatment is a controversial and potentially dangerous treatment because of the risk of electrolyte disturbances and paradoxical cerebral acidosis. The cerebral acidosis occurs 2° to the inability of HCO_3^- to quickly cross the blood-brain barrier. Bicarbonate for the treatment of acidosis should only be considered for extremely ill patients with severe acidosis.
- A brief reminder of some special treatments of underlying causes of metabolic acidosis includes:
  - Ethylene glycol and methanol: Ethanol or 4-methylpyrazole and dialysis
  - Salicylate toxicity: HCO_3^- to keep serum pH between 7.3 and 7.5 with resultant urine alkalinization; dialysis
  - Iron overdose: Deferoxamine
  - Isoniazid: Pyridoxine (vitamin B_6)

Metabolic Alkalosis (↑ pH + ↑ HCO_3^-)

Causes

Increased bicarbonate usually occurs in the setting of:

- Gastric acid loss from vomiting or NG suctioning
- Diuretic use
- Adrenocrotical hormone excess

Diagnosis

Diagnosis of type can be categorized as:

- Chloride (saline) sensitive (most common)
  - Diuretic or GI losses of K^+ and Cl^- → responds to replacement.
- Chloride (saline) resistant
  - Mineralocorticoid excess → renal absorption of Na^+ and HCO_3^- and excretion of K^+, H^+, and Cl^- → large K^+ replacement required.

Respiratory Acidosis (↓ pH + ↓ HCO_3^-)

Causes

Primarily caused by inadequate ventilation or increased dead space. Causes include:

- Head or chest trauma
- Oversedation, obtundation, or coma
- Neuromuscular disorders

- Pickwickian syndrome (obesity-hypoventilation syndrome)
- COPD

Renal compensation occurs after 48 hours of steady state.

Compensation, whether renal or respiratory, should never completely correct the pH by itself. Complete or overcorrection is an indicator of another process occurring.

TREATMENT

- Ventilatory support
- O_2 may be necessary to treat hypoxia, but may worsen hypercapnia in patients with COPD or in heavily sedated patients.

Respiratory Alkalosis (↓ pH + ↓ HCO_3^-)

CO_2 ventilation outpaces production. The most common cause of respiratory alkalosis in ill patients is a 2° compensatory respiratory alkalosis in response to a metabolic acidosis (seen in sepsis, DKA).

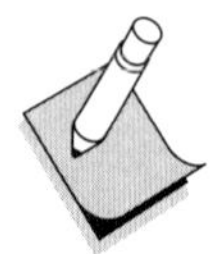

Be careful administering O_2 to COPD patients. Chronic hypercapnia in COPD patients lowers the CO_2 respiratory drive, leaving hypoxia as the only respiratory trigger.

CAUSES

Primary causes of respiratory alkalosis include:

- Hyperventilation secondary to anxiety
- CNS disorder
- Hypermetabolic states
- Hypoxia
- Hepatic insufficiency
- Aspirin toxicity

TREATMENT

Treatment focuses on identifying and addressing the underlying cause of tachypnea.

HYPO-/HYPERGLYCEMIA

Insulin Physiology

- Functions in glucose liver uptake and storage as glycogen
- Increases lipogenesis and inhibits lypolysis leading to increased triglycerides

Ketones

Production increased during states of cellular starvation. Three types are produced:

- β-Hydroxybutyrate: Not detected by serum or urine ketone tests
- Acetoacetate
- Acetone: Neutral pH

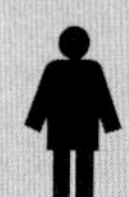

A lethargic 5-year-old boy is brought in with an empty bottle of his father's glipizide. His accucheck is 30 mg/dL, and upon administration of glucose the boy returns to baseline. When can he be discharged home?

This patient needs to be observed for a minimum of 24 hours with normal sugars before discharge, usually prompting admission.

Hypoglycemia (Blood Sugar <70 mg/dL)

One of the most common causes of altered mental status in the emergency department

Causes

- Systemic infection
- Hypoglycemia of infancy
  - Seen in 4 in 1000 births, usually with one of the following risk factors:
    - Diabetic or narcotic-abusing mothers
    - Premature or small for gestational age infants
- Postprandial hypoglycemia
  - Occurs within 6 hours of eating and caused by:
    - Alimentary hyperinsulinism or NIDDM
    - Fructose intolerance, leucine sensitivity, or galactemia
- Fasting hypoglycemia
  - Occurs about 6 hours after eating usually by:
    - Islet cell pancreatic or extrapancreatic tumor
    - Starvation
    - Adrenocortical insufficiency or hypopituitarism
    - Hepatic or renal disease
    - Autoimmune disease
    - Prolonged exercise
    - Late pregnancy
- Idiopathic/drug-induced
  - Hypoglycemic agents
    - Insulin: Treatment length depends on type of insulin
    - Metformin: Usually potentiated by alcohol abuse
    - Sulfonylureas: Summarized in Table 7.5

Symptoms

Patients usually become symptomatic below 50 mg/dL. They can present with complaints of:

- Tremors and agitation
- Sweating
- Seizures

Exam

Patient exams are usually consistent with their symptoms but you may also find:

- Altered mental status or focal neurologic signs
- Tachycardia

TABLE 7.5. Sulfonylureas

Medication	Tolbutamide	Glipizide	Glyburide	Chorpropamide
Associated medication interactions	Warfarin	TMP/SMX	TMP/SMX,	Warfarin
	Sulfa	Miconazole	Ciprofloxacin	Chloramphenicol
	Chloramphenicol	ASA	H_2-blockers	Probenecid
	Rifampin		Rifampin	Allopurinol
	Digoxin			Rifampin
Duration	6–12 hrs	12–24 hrs	12–24 hrs	4–5 days

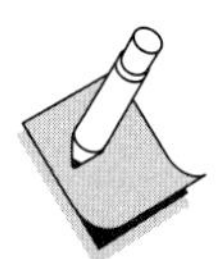

Sepsis should be considered in all patients with a low blood sugar.

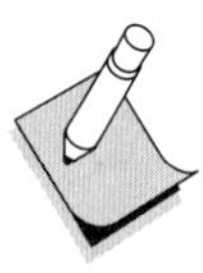

Sulfonylureas (glipizide, glyburide) increase insulin release. Octreotide inhibits insulin release.

Do not discharge patients with an overdose of a long-acting hypoglycemic agent until they have been observed beyond the duration of the drug.

DIFFERENTIAL

A patient presenting with seizures or altered mental status without a known reason deserves an immediate bedside glucose. Administering glucose to a hypoglycemic patient should quickly resolve their symptoms. If not, further investigation is required.

- Alcohol: Inhibition of gluconeogenosis and depletion of glycogen stores
- Salicylate: Primary hypoglycemia and seizures in children are common
- β-Blockers: Potentiate hypoglycemic effects of medications in diabetics
- Haloperidol
- Phenothiazines
- Disopyramide: In malnourished elderly patients without glycogen stores
- MAO inhibitors
- Cimetidine

TREATMENT

- IV glucose is the mainstay of treatment.
- IM glucagons can also be used when IV access is not available, but may not be effective on elderly or alcoholic patients who do not have adequate glycogen stores. Octreotide, which inhibits insulin release, may also be used, particularly for recurrent hypoglycemia following sulfonylurea overdose.
- IV dextrose is fast and effective but not a large or long-lasting source of carbohydrate. An amp of D50 provides only 25 g or 100 calories.
- A complex meal consisting of protein, fat, and complex carbohydrates is preferable to simple sugars such as fruit juice or candy bars.

Hyperglycemia

Hyperglycemia is a common ED complaint. DKA and hyperglycemic hyperosmolar nonketotic coma are life threatening emergencies and must be considered in all ED patients with an elevated blood sugar. Patients with isolated hyperglycemia with a blood sugar less than 400 can generally go home without ED treatment but with a consideration of changes in medications and close follow up.

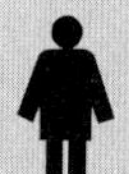

An elderly nursing home resident with a history of DM presents with altered mental status. She appears ill and dehydrated. Her bedside blood glucose is 950. What is her most likely diagnosis?

This patient has a hyperglycemic hyperosmolar nonketotic coma.

Diabetic Ketoacidosis

The diagnosis of DKA requires the presence of **hyperglycemia** (may be mild), **ketosis**, and an **anion gap metabolic acidosis**. Serum HCO_3^- may be normal due to the presence of both an anion gap acidosis and metabolic alkalosis due to vomiting and dehydration. Do not ignore an increased anion gap. Multiple factors induce diabetic patients into DKA, including:

- Relative insulin insufficiency → inability of glucose to enter cells → hyperglycemia → cellular starvation → stress hormone upregulation → increased gluconeogenesis, glycogenolysis, and lipolysis → further elevated hyperglycemia → increased free fatty acids → ketone formation (β-hydroxybutyrate and acetoacetate).
- High extracellular sugar levels create an osmotic diuresis. Patients with DKA are usually severely dehydrated, acidotic, and electrolyte depleted.

A precipitating factor usually initiates this cascade of events:

- Lack of insulin
- Infection
  - Urinary tract infection
  - Pneumonia
- Acute myocardial infarction or CVA
- Trauma or surgery
- Pregnancy
- Hyperthyroidism
- Pancreatitis
- Alcohol or illicit drug use
- Steroids
- Pulmonary embolism

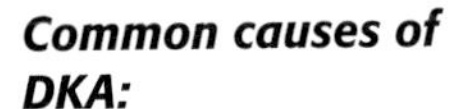

Common causes of DKA:

Insulin (lack of)
Infection
Ischemia (MI, CVA)
Illicit drug use (cocaine)

SYMPTOMS

- Patients usually present with a history of one of the precipitating factors, but may also complain of:
  - Thirst
  - Nausea/vomiting
  - Abdominal pain
  - Agitation or altered mental status

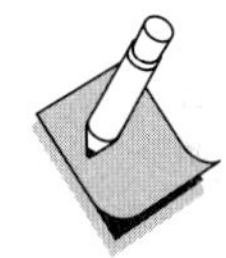

Hyperglycemia depresses serum sodium by dilution. To correctly interpret the sodium level, add 1.6 mEq/L for each 100 mg/dL of glucose above 100 mg/dL.

EXAM

- Elevated glucose
- Dehydration
- Tachycardia
- Deep and rapid breathing (Kussmaul respirations)
- Hypotension
- Acidosis
- Pan electrolytes depletion, particularly potassium

DIFFERENTIAL

- Hyperosmolar nonketotic coma
- Other acidosis (eg, alcoholic ketoacidos, lactic acidosis)

DIAGNOSIS AND CAUSES

- Patients presenting with suspected DKA need a thorough evaluation.
- Bedside glucose will indicate level of hyperglycemia.
- Urine dip or urinalysis
  - Ketones (acetoacetate, β-hydroxybutyrate, and acetone)
  - A positive nitroprusside tests is consistent with DKA but only tests for acetoacetate. **β-Hydroxybutyrate is not measured** with the nitroprusside test and ketone tests may be normal in patients with DKA.
- Glucose usually >350 mg/dL unless recently used insulin
- ABG and bicarbonate indicate level of acidosis (pH <7.30).
- CBC is a marker for infectious etiology.
- Individual serum ketones, which may be missed on urinalysis or serum ketone level
- Electrolytes including magnesium, calcium, and phosphorus
- BUN/creatinine: Indicator of renal function and dehydration
- Chest X-ray and urinalysis to look for signs of infection
- ECG and cardiac enzymes if appropriate for patient

TREATMENT

- DKA treatment encompasses a multisystem approach including hydration, electrolyte replacement, and insulin administration under careful monitoring.
- Rehydration
  - Patients are usually significantly dehydrated. Most patients will benefit from an initial 2-L saline bolus followed by additional fluids to total 4–6 L in the first 6 hours.
  - Use 0.9 NS unless the patient is severely dehydrated where 0.45 NS or combination are acceptable as well.
  - Once the patient's glucose falls <250 mg/dL switch to a glucose solution to avoid hypoglycemia and cerebral edema.
  - In pediatric patients, overly aggressive fluid resuscitation has been associated with cerebral edema. Do not exceed 40 mL/kg in the first 4 hours.
- Insulin
  - Bolusing large doses of insulin may cause hypoglycemia and hypokalemia. Instead infusing 0.1 units/kg/hr is a safe and effective way to initiate insulin. If the patient fails to respond after a few hours, infusion rates may be increased. Do not initiate insulin therapy until you know the patient's serum potassium. Giving insulin to a DKA patient with low serum potassium is a way to stop his heart. If the serum potassium is low, replace potassium before initiating insulin treatment.

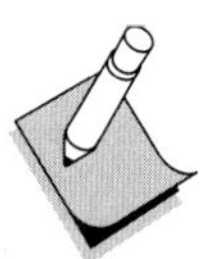

In DKA, insulin should start late and end late. Start insulin late because you need to wait for the serum potassium. End insulin late because you need to close the anion gap (not just bring down the glucose).

- Potassium replacement
  - DKA may causes significant hypokalemia that is sometimes only unmasked once the acidosis is reversed and the remaining extracellular K^+ shifts back into the cell.
  - After the initial fluid bolus patients with normal K^+ should receive at least 20–40 mEq/L in infusion fluids.
- Sodium bicarbonate should be reserved for critically ill patients with a pH <7.0 and evidence of shock, renal failure, or respiratory depression. Risks of sodium bicarbonate administration include:
  - Paradoxical CSF acidosis
  - Hypokalemia
  - Hyperosmolarity from sodium overload worsening dehydration
  - Decreased O_2 dissociation from red blood cells, ie, leftward shift of the oxyhemoglobin dissociation curve delaying O_2 deliver and recovery
- Phosphate replacement
  - Not routinely given 2° to possibly disposing patients to seizures
  - Do not give as initial management and reserve for levels below 1 mg/dL

COMPLICATIONS

- DKA has a host of life-threatening complications that result from the 1° disease as well as the treatment.
- Primary-disease related:
  - MI and cardiovascular collapse
  - DIC
  - Cerebral edema
  - Rhabdomyolysis
- Therapy-related
  - Hypoglycemia (from insulin)
  - Hypokalemia
  - Hypophosphatemia
  - Cerebral edema (insulin)
  - Alkalosis and paradoxical CSF acidosis (from bicarbonate)
  - CHF and ARDS (fluids)

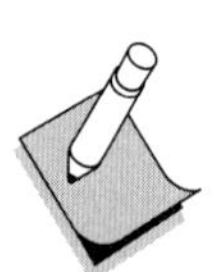

The most common cause of death in children with DKA is cerebral edema, which is associated with bicarbonate therapy and overly aggressive fluid resuscitation.

Hyperglycemic Hyperosmolar Nonketotic Coma

This is a rarer condition than DKA and a slower process, usually occurring in the elderly diabetic patient. The degree of volume contraction is generally greater in HHNK than DKA.

- Hyperglycemia and stress → insulin resistance → increased insulin → gluconeogenesis and glycogenolysis → hyperglycemia without ketosis → chronic osmolality and dehydration → dehydration without acidosis.

Symptoms

- Weakness and fatigue
- Thirst
- Anorexia

Exam

- Most patients have some altered mental status but are not comatose (despite the name).
- Focal neurologic signs
- Dehydration

Diagnosis

- Extremely elevated blood glucose (>400 mg/dL but often >800 mg/dL)
- Negative ketones
- No acidosis on ABG

Treatment

- IV fluids
  - Patients have incredibly large water deficits averaging 8–12 L. Hydration should be initiated as in DKA.
  - Approximately half of the estimated water deficit should be replaced during the first 8 hours and the rest during the next 24 hours.
- Insulin
  - Initiating 0.1 units/kg/hour is a safe and effective dose and should be continued until the patient's glucose reaches approximately 300 mg/dL.
  - Aggressively replete potassium and magnesium as in DKA.

Complications

- HNNK carries a high mortality rate of 8–25%.

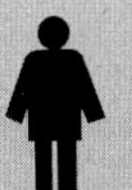

A 50-year-old homeless man is brought in altered and dehydrated with a history of chronic alcohol use. His labs are negative for alcohol or ketones, but he has an anion gap of 22 mEq/L and a glucose of 150 mg/dL. What is his diagnosis?

Likely alcoholic ketoacidosis. Check an osmolar gap to exclude the possibility of methanol or ethylene glycol poisoning.

ENDOCRINE, METABOLIC, FLUID, AND ELECTROLYTE DISORDERS

ALCOHOLIC KETOACIDOSIS

PHYSIOLOGY

- Chronic alcohol consumption and inadequate nutrition → decreased insulin and increased glucagons and ethanol inhibition of gluconeogenesis → lypolysis → increased ketone (acetoacetate and β-hydroxybutyrate) production → nausea and vomiting → severe dehydration and acidosis.

SYMPTOMS AND EXAM

- Nausea and vomiting
- Lethargy or altered mental status
- History of alcohol consumption but not usually intoxicated at time of evaluation

DIFFERENTIAL

- DKA
- Lactic and uremic acidosis
- Alcohol intoxication

DIAGNOSIS

Nondistilled alcohol (beer, wine) contains lots of carbohydrates, which is why AKA doesn't usually occur while a patient is still drunk.

- Key points in diagnosing alcoholic ketoacidosis and differentiating this from DKA are based on these facts:
  - A low bicarbonate level (<10) indicating acidosis
  - A high anion gap (>16) primarily from β-hydroxybutyrate
  - The nitroprusside test is negative or weakly positive because it does not test for this ketone. The test often becomes positive as patient becomes more hydrated and there is a shift from acetoacetate to β-hydroxybutyrate.
  - **A low or negative blood alcohol level**
  - Blood glucose is usually only minimally elevated (< 200 mg/dL).
- Concomitant hypokalemia, hyponatremia, and hypophosphatemia may be present.

TREATMENT

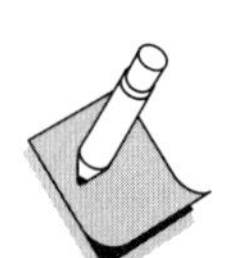

The primary treatment of alcoholic ketoacidosis is the administration of glucose and volume. Give D5NS.

- Insulin is not required.
- IV hydration with D5NS: The combination of fluid and carbohydrate corrects the ketoacidosis quicker than fluid alone
- Thiamine 50–100 mg IV to prevent Wernicke encephalopathy
- Correction of electrolyte losses
- Bicarbonate only if the patient is severely ill or acidotic

LACTIC ACIDOSIS

Lactate is a byproduct of anaerobic metabolism. Both acute and chronic conditions can cause elevated lactate levels. A normal lactate level is typically given as <2 mEq/L. Levels >4–5 mEq/L are considered significantly elevated. Typically, such patients will have an increased anion gap acidosis.

Acute conditions:

- **Inadequate tissue perfusion** due to either hypotension or hypoxia
- Toxic causes of disruption in cellular metabolism such as cyanide
- Exercise
- Hyperventilation
- Glucose, saline, or bicarbonate infusions that contain lactate
- Insulin or epinephrine injections

Chronic conditions:

- CHF
- Diabetes mellitus
- Liver disease
- Pulmonary disease

DIFFERENTIAL

- Other causes of high anion gap acidosis must be considered. See "Acid-Base Disorders" for more information.

DIAGNOSIS AND CAUSES

- History should lead to one of the four categories of lactic acidosis.
  - Type A: Inadequate tissue perfusion → hypoxia.
  - Type B1: Disorders
    - Diabetes
    - Renal or hepatic failure
    - Leukemia or cancer
    - Seizures
    - Infectious etiology
  - Type B2: Toxins
    - Ethanol or methanol
    - Fructose and sorbitol
    - Epinephrine
    - Metformin
  - Type B3: Inborn errors of metabolism and hepatic fructose-biphosphate deficiency

TREATMENT

- Hydration as indicated
- Support oxygenation and blood pressure as needed.
- Treat infection.
- Sodium bicarbonate should be reserved for extremely acidotic and deteriorating patients.
- Thiamine for alcoholic patients

THYROID DISORDERS

PHYSIOLOGY

- Hypothalamus releases thyrotropin releasing hormone (TRH) → anterior pituitary releases thyroid stimulating hormone (TSH) → thyroid gland releases T_3 and T_4.
- Disorders are either 1° disorders of T_3 and T_4 production at the thyroid gland or 2° disorders of the hypothalamus or pituitary.

Hypothyroidism and Myxedema Coma

ETIOLOGY

- 1° hypothyroidism by far most common.
  - Iatrogenic: Treatment of Graves disease with radiation or thyroidectomy most common
  - Autoimmune disorders such as Hashimoto thyroiditis

- Iodine deficiency
- Antithyroid drugs such as lithium, amiodarone, iodine and iodinated contrast, sulfonamides, or phenylbutazone
- Spontaneous hypothyroidism from Graves
- Congenital
- 2° hypothyroidism
  - Pituitary tumors
  - Postpartum hemorrhage: Sheehan syndrome
  - Sarcoidosis
  - Hypothalamic dysfunction: Tertiary hypothyroidism

SYMPTOMS

- Fatigue, lethargy, coma in extreme cases
- Weakness
- Cold intolerance
- Weight gain
- Menstrual irregularity
- Muscle cramps
- Thinning hair or hair loss
- Urinary retention

EXAM

- Hypothermia
- Respiratory failure
- Cardiovascular findings
  - Bradycardia and hypotension
  - Cardiomegaly
  - Low voltage 2° to pericardial effusion
  - Prolonged QT
- Dry skin and thinning hair
- Abdominal distention
- Nonpitting edema
- Cheyney reflexes (brisk upstroke but delayed relaxation)

DIAGNOSIS

- TSH, FT4 can confirm diagnosis and indicate type of disorder.
- Glucose: Normal to low
- Electrolytes: Hyponatremia and hypochloremia (hypocalcemia in thyroidectomy patients)
- CBC: Left shift
- Elevated serum cholesterol, CPK, LDH, and AST sometimes found
- Elevated protein >100 mg/dL in CSF

TREATMENT

- Thyroid hormone: 300–500 μg IV thyroxine
- Supportive
  - Correction of electrolytes, blood glucose, hypothermia, and respiratory support
  - Antibiotics if underlying infection

- Vasopressors for hypotension
- Hydrocortisone empirically for adrenal insufficiency

> A 75-year-old female presents to the ED with the chief complaint of lethargy, weakness, and weight loss. On exam she has sleepy-looking eyes, a palpable goiter, and atrial fibrillation on the cardiac monitor. Her TSH is markedly elevated. What is her diagnosis?
>
> Apathetic hyperthyroidism.

Hyperthyroidism and Thyroid Storm

Symptoms

- Anxiety and restlessness
- Manic behavior or frank psychosis
- Weakness
- Weight loss
- **Apathetic hyperthyroidism** is seen in elderly patients: Lethargy, weakness, weight loss, blepharoptosis (eye drooping), and atrial fibrillation with CHF

Exam

- Febrile and diaphoretic
- Tachycardia
- Exopthalmus
- Goiter
- Myopathy

Differential

- Most commonly presents in patients with Graves disease and set off by a stressful event, such as:
  - Infection
  - DKA or hypoglycemia
  - Withdrawal of antithyroid drugs
  - Contrast or radioactive iodine administration
  - CVA or MI
  - Trauma
  - Emotional stress
  - Palpation of thyroid

Levothyroxine (synthroid) is synthetic T_4. Levothyroxine overdose is usually asymptomatic because the breakdown of T_4 occurs more rapidly than the conversion to T_3. Overdose is not a cause of thyroid storm.

Diagnosis

Confirmed by an elevated free T_4

Treatment

- Supportive therapy
  - Oxygen
  - Cooling
  - Hydration and electrolyte replacement
  - Digitalis and diuretics for AFib and CHF

- Glucocorticoids dexamethasone or hydrocortisone: Dexamethasone has the additional advantage of decreasing T_4 to T_3 peripheral conversion
- β-Blockers: Propranolol is preferred because it also decreases T_4 to T_3 conversion. Consider esmolol in patients with CHF.

- Thyroid medications
  - Antithyroid drugs block the synthesis of thyroid hormone.
    - Propylthiouracil: Preferential 2° to conversion inhibition and rapid onset
    - Methimazole
  - Iodide
    - Inhibits stored thyroid release
- Treat underlying stressful event.

Thyroid Treatment–

***P**roptotic **P**olly **(W**ait**) I**s **D**ying*
Propranolol
Propylthiouracil
Wait 1 hour
Iodide
Dexamethasone

COMPLICATIONS

- Near 100% mortality if left untreated
- CNS dysfunction = confusion → obtunded → coma → death.
- Cardiovascular = tachycardia → CHF → cardiovascular collapse.
- **Avoid ASA** for hyperthermia because ASA displaces thyroid hormone from thyroglobulin, increasing the availability of active hormone.

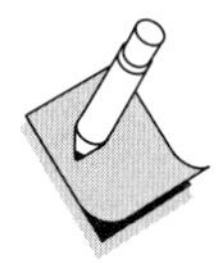

Always administer PTU at least 1 hour before iodide to prevent increased thyroid hormone synthesis.

An elderly patient presents with pneumonia and sepsis. After treatment with antibiotics and fluid the patients remains hypotensive. Labs reveal a blood glucose of 50 and a sodium of 124. What other diagnosis might this patient have and how do you treat it?

Adrenal insufficiency. Give dexamethasone (doesn't interfere with cortisol level testing) + fludrocortisone or hydrocortisone.

ADRENAL INSUFFICIENCY AND CRISIS

PHYSIOLOGY

- Adrenals produce
  - Glucocorticoids: Cortisol is the major glucocorticoid. Hypothalamus secretes corticotropin releasing factor → pituitary secretes ACTH → adrenal cortex secretes cortisol.
  - Mineralocoricoids: Aldosterone is the major mineralocorticoid and is controlled by the renin-angiotensin system and K^+ concentrations.
  - Catecholamines: Epinephrine and norepinephrine
  - Androgens: In small amounts
- Insufficient glucocorticoid and mineralocorticoid for physiologic demands leads to adrenal insufficiency; can be caused by 1° or 2° insufficiency.
  - 1° adrenal insufficiency known as Addison disease and is 2° to destruction of the adrenal cortex.
    - Idiopathic: Associated with DM, Hashimoto disease, and Graves disease
    - Infectious/infiltrative: TB, fungal, AIDS, sarcoid, CA
    - Drugs: Methadone, rifampin, and ketoconazole
    - Adrenal apoplexy (bilateral adrenal hemorrhage)
    - Anticoagulation
    - Neonatal sepsis causing:
      - Infarction known as Waterhouse-Friderichsen syndrome
      - Hemorrhage

- 2° adrenal insufficiency from pituitary dysfunction; causes include:
  - Suppression from prolonged steroid use
  - Pituitary tumor or infarction
  - Basilar skull fracture
  - Infiltrative disease like sarcoidosis
  - Infection
  - Internal carotid artery aneurysm

Addison Disease

SYMPTOMS

- Weakness and fatigue
- Abdominal pain, nausea/vomiting, and anorexia
- Syncope

SIGNS

- Dehydration and shock
- Hypoglycemia
- Postural hypotension
- Inaudible heart sounds
- **There is brownish pigmentation of the skin**, particularly on pressure points and hand creases. Increased pigmentation is seen with primary adrenal insufficiency (in which ACTH and related peptides are elevated) but not secondary adrenal insufficiency.
- Electrolyte abnormalities: ↓Na^+, ↑K^+, and ↑Ca^{2+}
- Azotemia
- ECG changes
  - Hyperkalemia: Tall T, long PR and QT, and absent P waves
  - Low voltage
  - Inverted T waves and a depressed ST segment

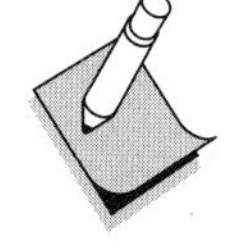

The endogenous mineralocorticoid, aldosterone, maintains volume by stimulating renal sodium reabsorption. In adrenal insufficiency, the BP is low and the sodium is low.

TREATMENT

- Glucocorticoid replacement: Hydrocortisone or prednisone
- Mineralocorticoid replacement: Fludrocortisone acetate
- Androgen replacement: Fluoxymesterone

Adrenal Crisis

DIAGNOSIS

- Adrenal crisis presents with more extreme findings than adrenal insufficiency. Patients are usually very ill and near cardiovascular collapse. Refractory hypotension and hypoglycemia are extremely common.
- Diagnosis is made with a cosyntropin stimulation test, which evaluates the ability of the adrenals to release cortisol in response to the administration of synthetic ACTH. Hydrocortisone interferes with the cortisol stimulation test, but dexamethasone does not.

TREATMENT

- IV fluids
- Glucose if hypoglycemic

- Glucocorticoid replacement: Dexamethasone 6–8 mg IV is preferred over hydrocortisone 100 mg IV initially as it does not interfere with any diagnostic tests.
- Mineralocorticoid replacement: Fludrocortisone should be administered with dexamethasone, but is unnecessary with hydrocortisone at the doses used to treat adrenal crisis.
- Search for underlying condition causing the adrenal crisis, eg, infection, acute coronary syndrome.

CHAPTER 8

Infectious Disease

Ross I. Donaldson, MD, MPH

SELECTED VIRUSES

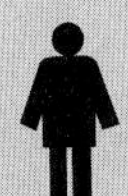

A 60-year-old male with a history of COPD presents with 12 hours of flulike symptoms in the middle of a known outbreak of influenza. What antiviral agent is contraindicated in this patient?

Zanamivir (because of COPD history).

Influenza

- A single-stranded RNA, orthomyxoviridae virus
  - Types: A (pandemic; tends to be more pathogenic), B (epidemic), and C (sporadic)
- Spread by droplets (highly contagious)
- Maximal transmission November–April (Western hemisphere)

Symptoms/Exam

- Incubation period: ~2 days
- Characterized by:
  - Sudden onset, high fever (2–4 days)
  - Headache
  - Nonproductive cough
  - Myalgias
  - Sore throat
  - Fatigue and malaise (can last weeks)
  - Children frequently note GI symptoms.

Differential

Bacteremia, parainfluenza, RSV, adenoviruses, coronaviruses, echoviruses

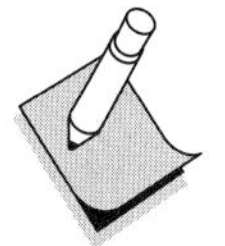

All antivirals for influenza are only efficacious if started within 48 hours of symptoms.

Diagnosis

- Clinical (during known outbreak ~85% accurate)
- Rapid antigen test

Treatment

- See Table 8.1.
- Antivirals:
  - Treatment (only if symptom duration <48 hours)
  - Prevention (if exposed during known outbreak)

Complications

- 1° (viral) and (bacterial) 2° pneumonia
  - Occur most frequently in the elderly and those with comorbidities
- Rare: Aseptic meningitis, pericarditis, Guillain-Barré

Mononucleosis

- Epstein-Barr virus (EBV)
- Transmitted by saliva (ie, the "kissing" disease)
- >90% of population has developed antibodies to EBV

TABLE 8.1. Influenza Antiviral Treatment

Drug	Indication	Side Effect	Cautions
Amantadine	Influenza A	Insomnia, anxiety, nausea, and confusion (elderly)	Caution in renal failure
Rimantadine	Influenza A	Insomnia, anxiety, nausea, and confusion (elderly)	Not approved for treatment in children
Zanamivir	Influenza A Influenza B	Wheezing	Contraindicated with asthma/COPD
Oseltamivir	Influenza A Influenza B	Nausea	Adjust dose for kidney disease Caution in children, possible increased suicide risk

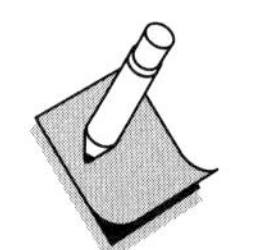

If patients with mono are falsely diagnosed with strep pharyngitis and given antibiotics, they can develop a diffuse maculopapular rash and be incorrectly told they have a drug allergy.

Symptoms/Exam

- Characterized by:
  - Fever and malaise
  - Exudative pharyngitis
  - Cervical lymphadenopathy (particularly posterior LAN)
  - Splenomegaly in half of cases
  - Rash common following antibiotics (classically amoxicillin; also levaquin and azithromycin)

Differential

Strep pharyngitis, hepatitis

Diagnosis

- Transaminitis is common.
- Atypical lymphocytes in peripheral blood smear
- Heterophil antibody tests, eg, Monospot (viral capsid IgM) = definitive
  - May have false-negatives early in disease

Treatment

- Supportive
- Steroids if significant tonsillar hypertrophy
- **Avoid contact sports** if splenomegaly.

Complications

Rare: Burkitt lymphoma, nasopharyngeal carcinoma

Hantavirus

- Single-stranded RNA virus of the Bunyaviridae family
- Vector: Rodents (eg, **deer mouse**)
  - Spread via inhalation of feces/urine or direct bite
- In North America, majority of cases occur in **southwestern United States.**

Symptoms/Exam

- Hantavirus pulmonary syndrome
  - Initial flulike prodrome (3–4 days)
  - Followed by:
    - Pulmonary edema/hypoxia
    - Thrombocytopenia
    - Metabolic acidosis
    - Hypotension
  - Sin Nombre virus (a close relative to Hanta) may also cause Hantavirus pulmonary syndrome

Differential

Influenza, bacterial pneumonia, ARDS

Diagnosis

- History of exposure and clinical diagnosis
- Confirmed by immunofluorescent or immunoblot assays

Treatment

Supportive care (mortality 50–70%)

West Nile Virus

- Vector: **mosquitoes**
- **RNA virus**
- Seasonal epidemics (summer and fall)

Symptoms/Exam

- Incubation: 3–14 days
- Most (>70%) who are infected are asymptomatic.
- Symptoms usually last for 3–6 days.
  - West Nile fever
    - Fever and flulike illness
    - URI symptoms
    - Maculopapular rash (50%)
  - Meningoencephalitis (1 in 150), which can result in acute asymmetric flaccid paralysis, and bowel or bladder dysfunction, but no sensory abnormalities

Diagnosis

- CSF = viral meningoencephalitis.
  - ↑lymphs, ↑protein, nl glucose
- Definitive: Viral isolation or serology (IgM antibody) in CSF or serum

Treatment

Supportive

Complications

- Older patients are primarily at risk for encephalitis/death. Immunocompromised and diabetics also at risk.
- Hospitalized patients with WNV have a mortality rate of 4–18%.

A 25-year-old male with known HIV/AIDS (last CD4 count <200) presents with hypoxia, a chronic cough, and a CXR showing diffuse interstitial infiltrates. In addition to normal bacterial pneumonia treatment, what other organism should be emergently covered and what test needs to be done before initiating treatment?

Pneumocystis carinii pneumonia (PCP) and an ABG to determine the need for prednisone.

HIV/AIDS

- RNA retrovirus
- Risk factors
  - Male with male sex
  - IVDA
  - Unprotected intercourse
  - Blood transfusion prior to 1985
  - Maternal transmission

DIAGNOSIS

- Sequential enzyme-linked immunoassay (EIA) and Western blot (~99% sensitive/specific)
  - Positive 3–12 weeks after exposure
  - Confirm with two tests.
  - Rapid HIV test may substitute for EIA.
- **Time course**. See Table 8.2.

TABLE 8.2. HIV Time Course

Stage	CD4 Count	Time Course	Clinical
Exposure	Normal	N/A	Via blood/blood products, semen, vaginal secretions, breast milk, or transplacentally
Acute HIV syndrome	Normal	2–4 wk after exposure	Flulike illness for 1–3 wk
Seroconversion	Normal	3–12 wk after exposure	Lab tests become positive.
Asymptomatic (incubation) period	>500	Mean: Adults = 8 yr Children = 2 yr	Asymptomatic, generalized lymphadenopathy
Early symptomatic	200–500	Variable	Thrush, pneumonia, herpes zoster, hairy leukoplakia, B-cell lymphoma, Hodgkin disease, ITP, Kaposi sarcoma (KS), tuberculosis (TB)
Late symptomatic (AIDS)	<200	Variable	Esophageal candidiasis, cytomegalovirus (CMV) retinitis, PCP, HIV encephalopathy, disseminated histoplasmosis, *Salmonella* septicemia
End-stage AIDS	<50	Variable	Disseminated CMV, *Mycoplasma avium*

Pulmonary Complications

See Table 8.3 for CXR differential diagnosis.

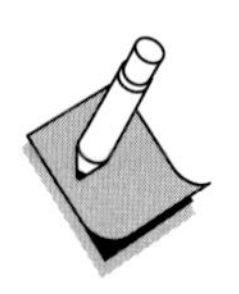

When treating for PCP, steroids should be given prior to starting antibiotics if the A-a gradient is >35 or Pa_{O_2} is <70 mm Hg.

COMMUNITY ACQUIRED PNEUMONIA (NONOPPORTUNISTIC)

- This is the #1 cause of pulmonary infection in HIV+ patients (*S. pneumoniae*, *H. influenzae*, *P. aeruginosa*).

P. carinii **pneumonia** (newly named *Pneumocystis jiroveci*) is the #1 cause of AIDS-associated mortality.

SYMPTOMS/EXAM

- Fever
- Cough (nonproductive)
- Dyspnea

TABLE 8.3. Differential Diagnosis for AIDS-Associated CXR Findings

CXR	DIFFERENTIAL DIAGNOSIS
Normal	Histoplasmosis (40%)
	PCP (20%)
	TB
	Cryptococcosis
Focal consolidation	Bacterial pneumonia
	Mycoplasma pneumoniae
	PCP
	TB
	Mycoplasma avium
Nodular lesions	Kaposi's sarcoma
	TB
	M. avium
	Fungal lesions
	Toxoplasmosis
Cavitary lesions	PCP
	TB
	Bacterial abscess
	Fungal abscess
Diffuse interstitial infiltrates	PCP
	CMV
	TB
	M. avium
	Histoplasmosis
	Coccidioidomycosis
	Lymphoid interstitial pneumonitis
	M. pneumoniae

DIAGNOSIS

- CXR
  - Classically: Diffuse interstitial infiltrates
  - Other: Focal consolidation, cavitary lesion, or normal
- LDH and A-a gradient frequently elevated

TREATMENT

- TMP-SMX (sulfa allergy = clindamycin + primaquine)
- Prednisone if A-a gradient > 35 or Pao_2 < 70 mm Hg

MYCOBACTERIUM TB

- 50–200 times higher incidence in HIV+ patients
- False-negative PPDs common due to immunosuppression

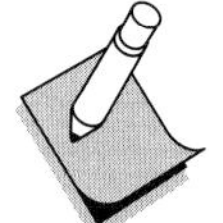

HIV+ patients with CD4 counts <200 can have active (highly contagious) TB with a normal CXR.

SYMPTOMS/EXAM

- Fever
- Cough
- Hemoptysis
- Night sweats
- Weight loss/anorexia

DIAGNOSIS

- CXR
- Classically: Upper lobe infiltrates and cavitary lesions
- CD4 <200: Negative or have almost any finding

Neurologic Complications

See Table 8.4 for head CT findings.

TABLE 8.4. Head CT and CSF Findings in HIV

DISEASE	HEAD CT	CSF	DEFINITIVE DIAGNOSIS
HIV encephalopathy	Atrophy	Normal	Diagnosis of exclusion
C. neoformans	Normal	↑Opening pressure (66%), ↑Monos, + India ink (70%)	+ Cryptococcal antigen
T. gondii	Multiple ring-enhancing lesions (subcortex or basal ganglia)	↑Opening pressure, ↑monos	Brain biopsy
CNS lymphoma	Solitary ring-enhancing lesions (periventricular)	↑Protein	Monoclonal malignant lymphocyteson CSF cytology
Progressive multifocal leukoencephalopathy	Nonenhancing white matter lesion(s)	Normal or ↑protein	PCR of JC virus
Mycobacterial meningitis (#1 *M. avium intracellulare*)	Intracranial/spinal cord abscesses	Frequently normal	Brain biopsy, normally

HIV ENCEPHALOPATHY (AIDS DEMENTIA)

- Progressive impairment of memory/cognitive processes caused directly by HIV
- Diagnosis of exclusion (work up any progressive signs of AMS).

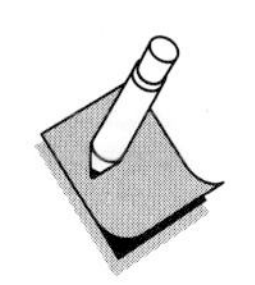

*Any **new** alteration of mental status must be fully worked up in a patient with HIV including head CT and lumbar puncture.*

CRYPTOCOCCUS NEOFORMANS

- Fungal CNS infection causing focal cerebral lesions or diffuse meningoencephalitis
- Most common with CD4 <100

SYMPTOMS/EXAM

- Fever
- **Chronic or subacute headache**
- Nausea/vomiting
- AMS
- Focal neuro deficits
- **Meningismus uncommon**

DIAGNOSIS

- **Head CT negative**
- Elevated opening pressure (~66% of cases)/lymphocytic pleocytosis
- India ink stain (~70% sensitive)
- Fungal Cx (~95% sensitive)
- **CSF cryptococcal antigen (100% sensitive/specific)**
- **Serum cryptococcal antigen (95% sensitive)**

TREATMENT

- Normal mental status: fluconazole PO
- AMS: Amphotericin B IV (± flucytosine)

COMPLICATIONS

- High intracranial pressure → sudden cerebral herniation
- Fatal if untreated
- With treatment, mortality ~6%

TOXOPLASMA GONDII (TOXOPLASMOSIS)

#1 cause of focal intracranial mass in HIV (latent resurgence)

SYMPTOMS/EXAM

- HA
- Fever
- Focal neuro deficits (80%)
- AMS
- Seizures

DIFFERENTIAL

- Lymphoma, cerebral TB, fungi, progressive multifocal leukoencephalopathy (PML), CMV, KS, hemorrhage

DIAGNOSIS

- Serologic testing not helpful (high antibody prevalence)
- CT: Multiple subcortical lesions
  - Most common in basal ganglia (often multiple)
  - Contrast shows ring enhancement.

TREATMENT

- Pyrimethamine + sulfadiazine (+ folinic acid)
- Significant edema: Add steroids + phenytoin

CNS LYMPHOMA

- Polyclonal tumor from EBV
- Most frequent with CD4 <100

SYMPTOMS/EXAM

- Subacute AMS

DIFFERENTIAL

Toxoplasmosis

DIAGNOSIS

CT: Hyperdense/isodense periventricular enhancement

TREATMENT

- Chemotherapy + radiation
- Median survival 0.5–2 years

PROGRESSIVE MULTIFOCAL LEUKOENCEPHALOPATHY

Jacob-Creutzfeldt (JC) virus reactivation

SYMPTOMS/EXAM

- Weakness
- Headache
- Speech disturbance
- Cognitive dysfunction

DIAGNOSIS

- CT: Single or multiple nonenhancing white-matter lesions
- PCR of the JC virus

TREATMENT

Highly active antiretroviral therapy (HAART)

HIV is an indication for a head CT before performing an LP.

TUBERCULOSIS MENINGITIS

Initiate treatment with isoniazide, rifampin, and pyrazinamide (all of which enter CSF in presence of meningeal irritation).

HIV Neuropathy

- Rarely emergent
- Painful sensory symptoms in feet

Gastrointestinal Complications

Thrush (Oral Candidiasis)

- *Candida albicans*
- Affects >80% of patients with AIDS
- Whitish plaques that (unlike hairy leukoplakia) easily scrape off to leave an erythematous base

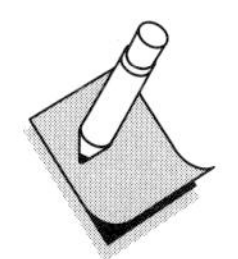

Hairy leukoplakia (unlike oral candidiasis) is normally located on the lateral portions of the tongue.

Esophagitis

Symptoms/Exam

Odynophagia and/or dysphagia

Differential

Candida, herpes simplex, CMV

Treatment

- Empiric with antifungal
- Nystatin wash or troche, fluconazole, or ketoconazole
- F/U with endoscopy if persistent

Diarrhea

Very common

Differential

Normal bacterial organisms, *Giardia, Cryptosporidium, Isospora belli*, CMV, *M. avium intracellulare*, antibiotic/HAART adverse reaction

Hepatomegaly (AIDS-Associated)

- Elevated alkaline phosphatase is disproportionately high compared to other LFTs.
- Jaundice is rare.
- Consider coinfection with Hepatitis B and/or C (HBV/HCV).

Proctitis

Symptoms/Exam

Tenesmus
Pain with defecation
Rectal discharge

Differential

Neisseria gonorrhoeae, Chlamydia trachomatis, Treponema pallidum, HSV, fissures, masses.

Cutaneous Complications

Kaposi Sarcoma

More common in men who have sex with men

Symptoms/Exam

- Pink, red, or purple
- Papules or nodules
- Painless/nonblanching
- Commonly on lower limbs, face, mouth, and genitals

Shingles in a multidermatomal pattern is suspicious for HIV coinfection or other immune compromise.

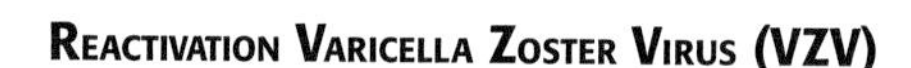

Reactivation Varicella Zoster Virus (VZV)

- 17× higher incidence in HIV
- Frequently multidermatomal

Treatment

- Oral acyclovir, famciclovir, or valacyclovir
- IV antiviral therapy if severe, systemic, or ophthalmologic

Ophthalmologic Complications

CMV Retinitis

- #1 cause of AIDS-associated blindness
- Severe necrotic vasculitis and retinitis

Symptoms/Exam

- Visual acuity changes, photophobia, floaters, scotoma, redness and/or pain
- Retina: Fluffy white perivascular lesions

Treatment

Ganciclovir

Adverse Medication Reactions

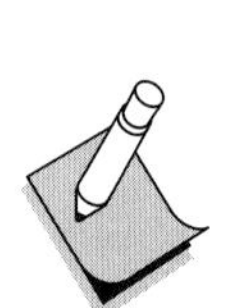

NRTIs can cause a life-threatening lactic acidosis.

- Drug fever, rash, nausea, diarrhea, headache, neuropathy, and liver disease are associated with several different medications.
- Lactic acidosis can be seen with nucleoside reverse transcriptase inhibitor (NRTI) HIV drugs.
  - Classically associated with stavudine, zidovudine, didanosine, and lamivudine
  - Typically present with nausea/vomiting, abdominal pain, muscle weakness
  - Elevated lactate level
  - Untreated mortality rate as high as 50%
- For specific HIV medication side effects, see Table 8.5.

Other HIV Complications

- Cardiovascular
  - Pericardial effusion, cardiomyopathy, myocarditis, cardiotoxic medications
- Renal
  - Prerenal azotemia (secondary to concomitant infection); renal-toxic medications; HIV-associated nephropathy

TABLE 8.5. Specific Side Effects for HIV-Associated Medications

Drug	Side Effect
Didanosine	Pancreatitis
Foscarnet	Nephrotoxicity, seizures
Indinavir	Nephrolithiasis
Lamivudine	Cough
Ritonavir	Paresthesias

- Psychiatric
  - Depression, AIDS psychosis

Treatment

- Highly active antiretroviral therapy
- Treatment of HIV+ patients frequently requires discussion with a consultant.
- Admit AIDS (CD4 <500) with:
  - New fever of unknown origin
  - Hypoxia worse than baseline (or $Pa_{O_2} < 60$)
  - Suspected PCP or TB
  - New CNS symptom
  - Intractable diarrhea
  - Suspected CMV retinitis or herpes zoster ophthalmicus
  - Inability to care for self

SYSTEMIC STDs

A 24-year-old female presents with several days of fever and tenderness over the dorsum of one wrist and one ankle, with decreased range of motion of both. She also notes hemorrhagic pustules on her distal extremities. What is the most likely diagnosis and treatment?

Disseminated GC. Admit for ceftriaxone 1 g daily and possible surgical drainage, along with empiric coverage for chlamydia.

Gonococcal (GC) Infections

- Gram-negative diplococcus *N. gonorrhoeae*
- Second most common STD (after chlamydia)

Symptoms/Exam

- Incubation period: 1–14 days
- Asymptomatic infection common

- Uncomplicated
  - Men: Urethritis, epididymitis, prostatitis
  - Women: Cervicitis, PID
  - Both: Pharyngitis, conjunctivitis
- Disseminated (~2% of patients; usually women)
  - Primary (febrile) stage
    - Fever/chills
    - Rash
      - Tender pustules on red/hemorrhagic base
      - Peripherally located
    - Tenosynovitis (~66%)
      - Most often dorsum of wrist, hand, and ankle
  - Second stage
    - Monoarticular or oligoarticular septic arthritis

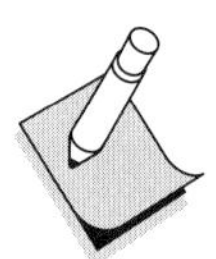

Empirically treat all patients with suspected gonorrhea for chlamydia, because of the high rates of coinfection.

DIAGNOSIS

- Uncomplicated
  - Cervical/urethral swab using nucleic acid amplification tests (NAAT; sensitivity ~95%)
  - Urine test (less sensitive)
- Disseminated
  - BCx, biopsy of skin lesions, or synovial fluid (positive in only 20–50%)
  - Cultures
    - Chocolate agar if sterile site (eg, CSF, synovial fluid)
    - Martin-Lewis agar if nonsterile site (eg, cervix, urethra, rectum, oropharynx)

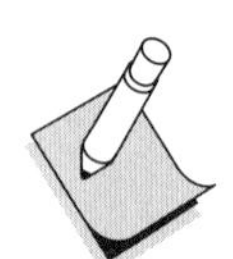

Consider 2° syphilis in any patient with a rash involving the palms and/or soles.

TREATMENT

- All cases should also be empirically covered for chlamydia
- Uncomplicated (not PID)
  - Ceftriaxone 125 mg IM × 1 or cefixime 400 mg PO
  - Avoid fluoroquinolones (increasing resistance)
- PID
  - See Gynecology section.
- Disseminated
  - Treat empirically if high suspicion as test sensitivity is low.
  - Ceftriaxone 1 g IV daily × 10 days
    - Or ceftriaxone × 3 days followed by cefixime PO for 7 days
  - Refractory tenosynovitis may require surgical washout.

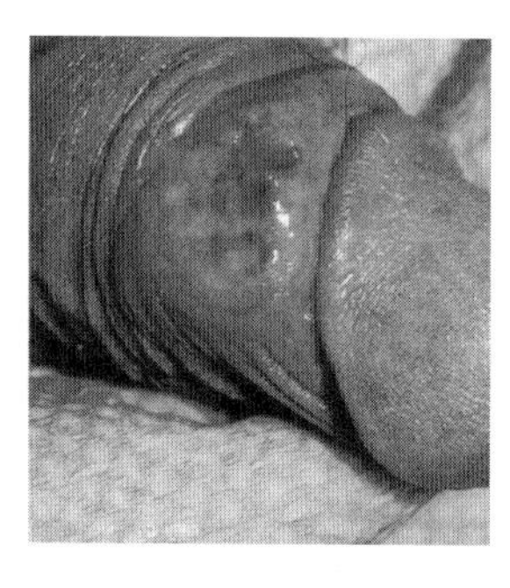

FIGURE 8.1. Primary syphilis.

(Reproduced, with permission, from Bondi EE et al. *Dermatology: Diagnosis and Therapy*. Stamford, CT: Appleton & Lange, 1991:394.)

Syphilis

- The spirochete *Treponema pallidum*

SYMPTOMS/EXAM

- Incubation period: ~3 weeks
- 1° syphilis (see Figure 8.1)
  - Painless genital ulcer with indurated border (chancre)
  - Heals spontaneously over 2–6 weeks
- 2° syphilis
  - 4–8 weeks after healing of chancre

- Rash
  - Nonpruritic
  - Dull red maculopapular
  - Spreads trunk → extremities (may involve palms and/or soles)
- Constitutional symptoms
  - Flulike
  - Sore throat, oral lesions
  - Wartlike anogenital growths (condyloma lata)
  - Generalized lymphadenopathy
- Symptoms resolve spontaneously.

- Latent
  - Asymptomatic period (serologies positive)
  - Normally lasts 3–4 years
  - Two phases
    - Early latent (<1 year from acquisition)
    - Late latent (>1 year)
- Tertiary
  - Peripheral neuropathy (tabes dorsalis)
  - Meningitis
  - Dementia
  - Gummatous lesions of mucous membranes
  - Aortitis
    - Aortic-valve insufficiency
    - Thoracic aortic aneurysm

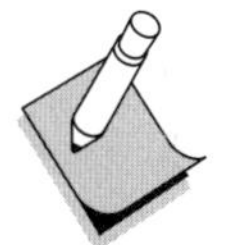

RPR and VDRL false-positives occur frequently in patients with HIV, malaria, pneumonia, and lupus.

Diagnosis

- Early stages
  - Dark-field microscopy (sensitivity ~80%)
    - From chancre or oral/genital lesions
- Later (>2 weeks after 1° chancre)
  - RPR or VDRL
    - Screening test (nonspecific antibodies)
    - False-positive rate ~2%
  - FTA-ABS
    - More specific (treponemal antibodies)
    - Used to confirm diagnosis

Treatment

- 1°, 2°, or early latent
  - Benzathine penicillin 2.4 million U IM × 1
    - Alternative: Doxycycline × 14 days
- Late latent or unknown
  - Benzathine penicillin 2.4 million U IM weekly × 3
    - Alternative: Doxycycline × 28 days
- Partners should be tested and treated empirically if sexual contact within 90 days.
- Jarisch-Herxheimer reaction
  - A transient inflammatory reaction following treatment of syphilis (1°, ~75%; 2°, ~90%)
  - Symptoms
    - Fever, chills, headache, myalgias, and exacerbation of cutaneous lesions
    - Duration = several hours
- Also seen with borreliosis, brucellosis, typhoid fever, and trichinellosis

POSTEXPOSURE PROPHYLAXIS (PEP)

A 28-year-old surgical intern presents after being stuck with a bloody 18G needle while placing a femoral line. The patient has known AIDS with a high viral load. What is the HIV transmission risk and what treatment should be initiated?

High-risk source; high-risk exposure. Although the transmission rate is probably <1% for this exposure, should recommend expanded HIV PEP regimen with first dose given as soon as possible. Confirm Hep B vaccination.

- Needlestick injuries are associated with risk for bacterial infections, hepatitis B, hepatitis C, and HIV.

Occupational Exposure

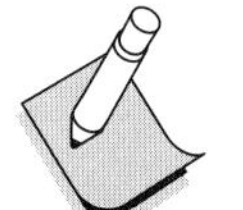

Exposure of bodily fluids onto intact skin is not a risk for HIV transmission.

HIV Transmission Risk

- Greatly reduced by universal precautions
- Majority of occupational seroconversions are percutaneous.
  - Occasionally mucocutaneous
  - No confirmed HIV seroconversions to date with a suture needle
- See Table 8.6 for HIV transmission rates.
- See Table 8.7 for risk stratification.

Treatment

- Tetanus immunization; see "Special Wound Infections"
- Hepatitis B PEP for nonvaccinated exposed individuals (see below)
- No current PEP is available for Hepatitis C, but testing of source and patient should be conducted to document if patient converts.
- HIV PEP
  - Consider source patient testing if not known.
    - Depends on patient agreement and state law
      - Rapid HIV
      - Hepatitis panel
      - Consider RPR or other tests given clinical scenario.

TABLE 8.6. Risk for HIV Transmission by Route (per Episode)

Type	Exposure	Estimated Risk (%)
Occupational	Percutaneous	0.3
	Mucocutaneous	0.09
Nonoccupational (assumes no condom use)	Needle-sharing injection drug	0.7
	Receptive anal intercourse	0.5
	Receptive penile-vaginal intercourse	0.1
	Insertive anal intercourse	0.07
	Insertive penile-vaginal intercourse	0.05
	Receptive oral (male) intercourse	0.01
	Insertive oral (male) intercourse	0.005

TABLE 8.7. **Risk Stratification for HIV Transmission**

Type	Low Risk	High Risk
Source	Asymptomatic HIV	Symptomatic HIV/AIDS
	Viral load <1500 copies/mL	Acute seroconversion
		High viral load
Exposure	Superficial	Deep injuries
	Solid needle	Visible blood on device
	Contact with intact skin = no risk.	Injuries sustained placing a catheter in a vein/artery

- Associated with 79% reduction in transmission
- Initiate ASAP (goal = 1–2 hours).
- >36 hours: Normally deferred, unless particularly high risk
- Common side effects = constitutional, gastrointestinal.
- See Table 8.8 for general guidelines.
  - CDC website lists specific regimens.

Nonoccupational Exposure

- Sexual-assault victims, sexual partners, or needle-sharing partners of sources with possible transmission
- Accounts for ~80% of all HIV PEP given

Symptoms/Exam

- For sexual assault, keep records of detailed exam.
  - Frequently performed by specialized professional
- See Table 8.6 for HIV transmission rates.

Treatment

- Tetanus immunization
- Pregnancy prophylaxis if appropriate
  - Initiate <72 hours
  - Check pregnancy test, then
    - Plan B or Ovral (several suggested regimens)
- If considering prophylaxis, CDC recommends baseline HIV, CBC, BUN/creatinine, LFTs, Hepatitis B and C serology of exposed patient.

TABLE 8.8. **Occupational HIV Postexposure Treatment Guidelines**

Regimen	Application	Treatment[a]
Basic	Exposures for which there is a recognized transmission risk	4-wk, two-drug regimen (normally zidovudine and lamivudine)
Expanded	High-risk exposures	Basic regimen + protease inhibitor (eg, indinavir or nelfinavir)

[a]If source has a known resistant HIV strain, consult specialist for specifically tailored regimen.

TABLE 8.9. Nonoccupational HIV *Post-Substantial-Risk* Exposure Treatment Guidelines

Time Course	Source = Unknown HIV Status	Source = Known HIV+
<72 hours	Case-by-case determination	28-day course of HAART (three-drug regimen), start ASAP
>72 hours	No HAART recommended	No HAART recommended

- HIV prophylaxis nonoccupational algorithm
  - Negligible exposure risk
    - Urine, nasal secretions, saliva, sweat, or tears not visibly contaminated with blood
    - HIV Postexposure Prophylaxis not recommended
  - Substantial exposure risk
    - Exposure of vagina, rectum, eye, mouth or other mucous membrane, nonintact skin, or percutaneous contact
    - Blood, semen, vaginal secretions, rectal secretions, breast milk, or any body fluid visibly contaminated with blood
    - See Table 8.9 for treatment guidelines.

Hepatitis B

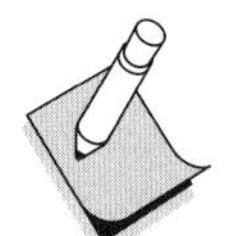

*Patients with a known response to Hep B vaccination (ie, **HBsAg positive**) are considered **protected** and do not require Hep B PEP following a possible exposure.*

Health care workers in the United States are required to receive Hepatitis B vaccination. For this reason, health care workers generally do not need to receive PEP to prevent Hep B transmission following possible exposure. Nonvaccinated individuals and those known not to have responded to vaccination with a high-risk exposure should receive:

- Hepatitis B immunoglobulin (HBIG)
- Hepatitis B vaccination: Usually given as three doses over 4–6 months with first dose given with HBIG in different site
- Individuals who have been vaccinated but who did not receive postvaccine testing to confirm the presence of the HBsAg should receive a vaccine booster.

SPECIAL WOUND INFECTIONS

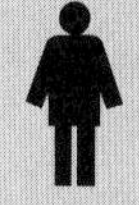

An 80-year-old male presents with pain and stiffness in his masseter muscles 1 week after stepping on a rusty nail. Muscle rigidity has progressed to his neck, torso, and upper extremities. What treatment needs to be initiated before wound debridement?

Tetanus immunoglobulin.

Tetanus

- The spore-forming, anaerobic, Gram-positive rod *Clostridium tetani*
- Ubiquitous in soil, dust, and animal feces
- Risk factors
  - IV drug users
  - Temperate climates (Texas, Florida, California)
  - Elderly (>60 years old)

- Puncture wounds
- Wounds with crushed/devitalized tissue
- Inadequate immunization
- Produces tetanospasmin
  - Neurotoxin blocks inhibitory nerves
  - Causes overstimulation of
    - Skeletal muscle motor endplates
    - Autonomic nervous system
    - CNS

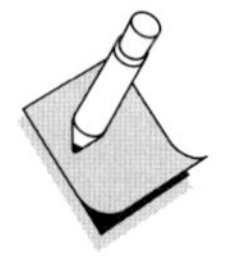

A significant portion of patients with tetanus do not report specific trauma.

SYMPTOMS/EXAM

- Traumatic injury (~30% do not report a specific event)
- Incubation period: 1 day to >1 month (shorter = more severe)
- Types:
  - Generalized (#1)
    - Trismus due to masseter spasm ("lockjaw")
    - Muscle rigidity/spasms
      - Shortest nerves affected first
      - Progresses from head to feet
    - Hydrophobia/drooling
    - Leads to
      - Respiratory failure
      - Autonomic instability
        - Starts in second week
        - Generally hypersympathetic (ie, tachycardia, HTN, diaphoresis)
  - Localized
    - Persistent muscle spasms near site of injury
    - Spontaneously resolves in weeks to months
    - Normally no permanent sequelae
  - Cephalic
    - After head wound or otitis media
    - Cranial nerve dysfunction (most common = CN VII)
  - Neonatal
    - Inadequately immunized mother
    - Unsterile handling of umbilical stump
    - Irritability and poor feeding in first week of life
    - Close to 100% case fatality rate

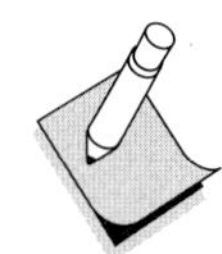

Strychnine acts by blocking an inhibitory glycine receptor, rapidly causes convulsions and death, and is treated with benzos and dantrolene.

DIFFERENTIAL

Strychnine poisoning, dystonic reaction, hypocalcemia, encephalitis, meningitis, rabies

DIAGNOSIS

Clinical

TREATMENT

Symptomatic:

- Aggressive supportive care
  - Benzodiazepines are mainstay for muscle relaxation.
  - Magnesium sulfate will improve spasm control.
  - Labetalol indicated for sympathetic hyperactivity.
    - Avoid isolated β-blockade.

- Intubation and long-term neuromuscular blockade with vecuronium if necessary
  - Succinylcholine safe for RSI
- Tetanus immune globulin (TIG)
- 3000–5000 units IM
  - Neutralizes circulating tetanospasmin
    - Does not affect toxin already absorbed by CNS
  - Significantly reduces mortality (but not acute symptoms)
- Tetanus immunization (give opposite site of TIG)
- Wound treatment
  - Delay wound debridement and irrigation until after TIG (additional toxin may be released during procedure).
  - Antibiotics
    - Metronidazole
    - Penicillin theoretically contraindicated (may potentate neurotoxin effects)

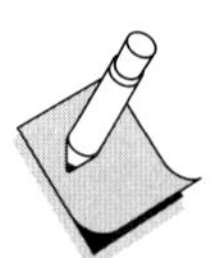

In addition to Td vaccination, give tetanus immunoglobulin (TIG) for high-risk wounds with uncertain or <3 prior immunizations.

WOUND PROPHYLAXIS

For prophylaxis in the absence of clinical tetanus, see Table 8.10.

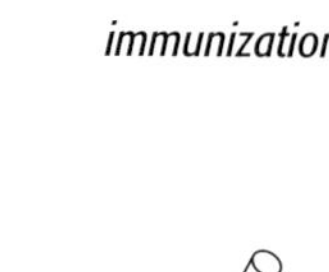

MRSA biochemistry:
mecA*—a gene that conveys methicillin resistance found in all MRSA*
Panton-Valentine leukocidin (PVL)—a virulence factor found in CA-MRSA

Methicillin-Resistant *Staphylococcus aureus*

- Began as a hospital-acquired disease (HA-MRSA), but now the community-acquired form of MRSA (CA-MRSA) is becoming more prevalent and the two forms are becoming epidemiologically blurred.
- Resistance to methicillin in both CA-MRSA and HA-MRSA is through the presence of the *mecA* gene, which is not found in MSSA.
- CA-MRSA is more likely to encode the putative virulence factor, **Panton-Valentine leukocidin**.
- CA-MRSA infections should be considered in all patients with soft-tissue infections. Populations at increased risk include: children at day care centers, athletic team members, military personnel, prisoners, IVDU patients, HIV+ patients, and Native Americans. Additional risk factors include skin trauma, contact sports, shaving, higher body mass index, and poor hygiene.
- HA-MRSA is most commonly spread from one patient to another by health care workers whose hands or gloves have become transiently contaminated with MRSA. Three major reservoirs of HA-MRSA are patients, health care workers, and the inanimate environment. The disease is commonly found in ICUs.

TABLE 8.10. Tetanus Prophylaxis

PRIOR IMMUNIZATION	LOW-RISK WOUND (CLEAN/MINOR)	HIGH-RISK WOUND[a]
≥3	dT (if >10 yr since last dose)	dT (if >5 yr since last dose)
Uncertain or <3	dT	dT and TIG (250 units IM)

[a]High risk is defined as >6 hours old; contaminated (eg, dirt, saliva, feces); puncture, crush wounds, or avulsions; foreign bodies, burns, frostbite.

SYMPTOMS/EXAM

- CA-MRSA patients frequently present with skin or soft tissue infections (especially nonhealing wound infections), but may develop necrotizing pneumonia, necrotizing fasciitis, or rapidly fatal septicemia, endocarditis, or osteomyelitis.
- HA-MRSA infection is also most frequently found in skin and soft tissue infections. It is also commonly found in the bloodstream, followed by the lower respiratory and urinary tracts.

DIAGNOSIS

- The most accurate methods are PCR to detect the *mec*A gene and latex agglutination tests to detect the protein product of *mec*A, penicillin-binding protein 2a.
- Traditional culture and sensitivity techniques are acceptable, such as oxacillin–salt agar screening plates and cefoxitin disk diffusion tests.

TREATMENT

- CA-MRSA is typically responsive to a variety of common antibiotics, eg, trimethoprim-sulfamethoxazole, rifampin, minocycline, doxycycline, levofloxacin, and clindamycin. Local sensitivities may vary.
- Suspected HA-MRSA should be treated empirically with **vancomycin**. Patients unable to tolerate vancomycin or who develop vancomycin-resistant MRSA may use linezolid or daptomycin.
- Culture sensitivities should be reviewed when available to guide therapy.
- Eradication of nasal colonization can be accomplished by using mupirocin 2% ointment 0.5 g in each nostril twice a day for 5 days.

Rabies

>80% of cases in the United States attributed to bats

SYMPTOMS/EXAM

- Incubation period: 30–90 days
- Prodrome (days 1–4): flulike symptoms + pain/paresthesia at bite site (80%)
- CNS involvement:
  - Agitation
  - Hydrophobia (violent inability to swallow)
  - Muscular spasms → paresis of mouth/periphery
  - Altered mental status/opisthotonos

Symptomatic rabies infections are almost invariably fatal, thus wound prophylaxis is the key to surviving the disease.

DIFFERENTIAL

Other CNS infection (eg, encephalitis, meningitis), tetanus, cholinergic poisoning, Guillain-Barré, polio

DIAGNOSIS

- ED = clinical (may see elevated CSF protein)
- Final = postmortem brain analysis/CSF titers

Treatment

Symptomatic treatment:

- ICU admission and supportive care
- Symptomatic disease almost invariably fatal (normally within a week of onset)

Wound Prophylaxis

- Wound care
    - Aggressive washing with soap and virucidal agent (eg, 2% benzalkonium chloride or povidone-iodine)
    - Debridement of devitalized tissue
    - Do not suture.
- Treatment guidelines (see Table 8.11)
    - Human rabies immune globulin (H-RIG)
        - 20 IU/kg dose at initial treatment
        - Can be given up to 7 days after the first vaccine in the series.
        - As much of the immunoglobulin as possible should be infiltrated around the wound site.
    - Human diploid cell vaccine (HDCV)
        - IM in deltoid (1-mL doses) on days 0, 3, 7, 14, and 28

Fewer than half of rabies cases due to bats have a documented bite so treatment is indicated even if there is no documented bite, eg, found a bat in sleeping room.

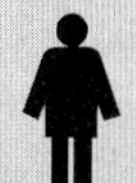

A 4-month-old boy presents with 4 days of constipation and poor feeding. He is afebrile, appears lethargic, and has decreased muscle tone with depressed deep tendon reflexes. What food product did the child likely consume?

Honey.

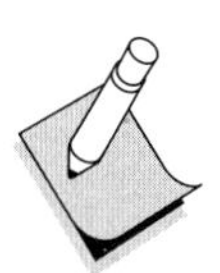

Rabies wound prophylaxis: Clean the wound, give the vaccine, give immune globulin at the wound site.

Botulism

- Gram-positive, spore-forming rod *Clostridium botulinum.*
- Produces neurotoxin that blocks the release of acetylcholine
    - Results in neuromuscular blockade
- Potential bioterrorism agent.

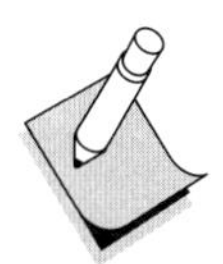

Bites from ***skunks, raccoons, foxes, and bats*** *are high risk for rabies. Treat empirically with both human rabies immune globulin and vaccine if unvaccinated.*

TABLE 8.11. Postexposure Rabies Prophylaxis

Animal	Animal Disposition	Recommendation[a]
Dog, cat, ferret	Healthy/captured	Observe animal for 10 days, no treatment unless clinical signs develop
	Escaped	Consult public health
	Sick	H-RIG + HDCV
Skunks, raccoons, foxes, bats	Captured	H-RIG + HDCV (stop series if euthanized animal tests negative)
	Escaped	H-RIG + HDCV
Squirrels, hamsters, guinea pigs, gerbils, chipmunks, rats, mice, rabbits	N/A	Almost never requires treatment (consult public health for specific recommendations)

[a]If treated with preexposure vaccine → finish vaccine course, but do not give H-RIG.

SYMPTOMS/EXAM

- Food-borne
  - Direct toxin ingestion (eg, canned foods)
  - Incubation: ~1 day (range: 6 h–10 days)
  - Descending weakness
    - Cranial nerve palsies (eg, diplopia, dysphagia, dysarthria)
    - Followed by descending paralysis and respiratory failure
- Wound
  - From open wounds and IVDA (eg, "black tar" heroin)
  - Incubation period ~1 week
  - Lower mortality than food-borne
- Infantile (usually <1 year old)
  - Ingestion of spores (typically in honey)
  - Constipation followed by
    - Poor feeding (fever absent)
    - Weak cry
    - Decreased muscle tone/loss of head control
      - Depressed deep tendon reflexes
      - Respiratory failure (50%)

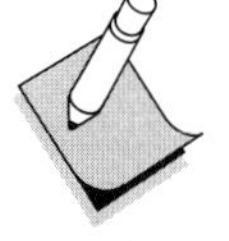

Adults don't get botulism from eating honey because the presence of normal intestinal flora prevents colonization of the GI tract.

DIFFERENTIAL

Gastroenteritis, myasthenia gravis, Guillain-Barré, Bell palsy, tick paralysis, poliomyelitis, diphtheria, Eaton-Lambert, anticholinergic or organophosphate toxicity

DIAGNOSIS

Clinical (EMG may be useful)

TREATMENT

- Supportive care
  - Respiratory (early intubation)
- Decontamination
  - Bowel irrigation in food-borne and infant types
  - Wound irrigation in wound type
- Botulinum antitoxin
  - Trivalent antibodies to toxin Types A, B, and E (derived from horse serum)
  - Neutralizes only circulating toxin
  - Not recommended in infant type due to low efficacy and risk of anaphylaxis
    - Human botulism immunoglobulin available for infants
- Avoid antibiotics!
  - May increase cell lysis and promote toxin release.
  - In wound type may use for concomitant infection after antitoxin given

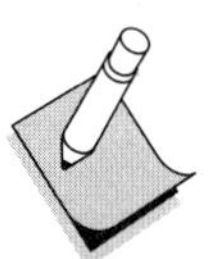

In cases of clear-cut botulism, withhold antibiotics until antitoxin administered.

COMPLICATIONS

- Respiratory failure
- Mortality 50% (without ICU) to 8% (with ICU)

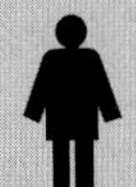

A 30-year-old otherwise healthy male gardener presents with ulcerating lesions progressing up his arm 3 weeks after planting a new rose bush. What is the diagnosis and treatment?

Sporotrichosis and itraconazole.

Sporotrichosis

- Infection caused by the traumatic inoculation of *Sporothrix shenckii* (a fungus)
- Found on plants and in the soil (classically on rose thorns)

SYMPTOMS/EXAM

- Incubation period: 1–10 weeks
- One or more suppurating subcutaneous nodules
- Normally progress proximally along lymphatic channels

DIAGNOSIS

- ED = treat based on clinical suspicion
- Definitive = biopsy/fungal culture

TREATMENT

- Itraconazole for 3–6 months
- Disseminated: Amphotericin B
- Unless disseminated, most can be treated as outpatient

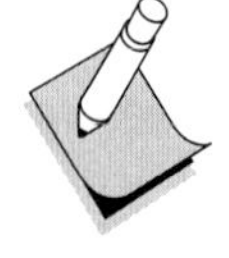

*Colorado tick fever is a tick-borne **self-limited viral infection** that requires only symptomatic treatment.*

TICK-BORNE ILLNESSES

Lyme Disease

- The spirochete *Borrelia burgdorfei*
- Ticks *Ixodes scapularis* (deer ticks) and *Ixodes pacificus*
  - Nymph stage (1–2 mm) responsible for most transmission
- Peak transmission in summer months
- Endemic foci
  - Northeast Coast (Connecticut, Rhode Island)
  - Midwest (Wisconsin, Minnesota)
  - West Coast (California, Oregon)

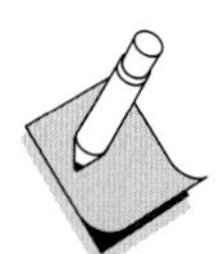

The majority of people with Lyme disease do not recall a tick bite.

SYMPTOMS/EXAM

- **>66% of people do not recall bite.**
- Early localized
  - ~1 week later
  - Flulike symptoms
  - Rash (90%)
    - Erythema migrans (migrans, because it grows)
    - Spreading redness with central clearing ("target lesion") occurs at site of bite (average 16 cm diameter). (See Figure 8.2.)
- Early disseminated
  - Weeks to months after exposure
  - Large joint arthritis
  - Neurological
    - Cranial neuropathies (may mimic Bell palsy)
    - Meningitis
    - Radiculopathy (motor or sensory)
  - Carditis (~7%)
    - Typically AV blocks
- Late
  - >1 year after exposure
  - Chronic arthritis
  - Peripheral neuropathy

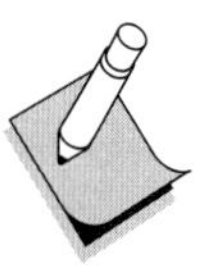

Target lesion differential:

1. *Lyme disease: Single lesion, increases in size, central clearing*
2. *Erythema multiforme (Stevens-Johnson syndrome): Multiple lesions with central blister or necrosis*

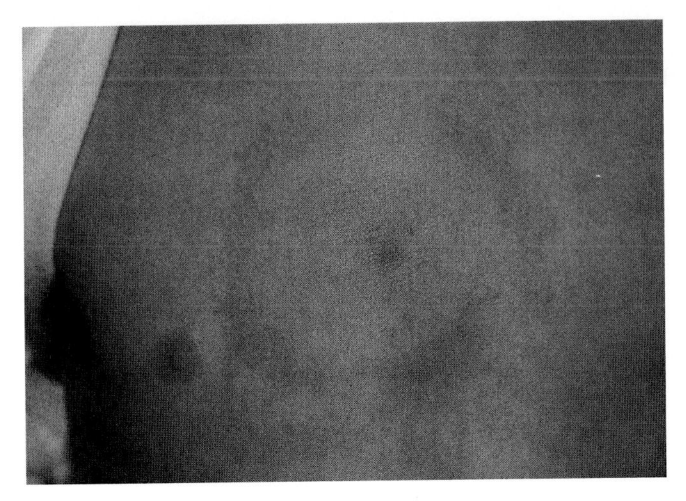

FIGURE 8.2. Erythema migrans. Spreading redness with central clearing in patient with Lyme disease.

(Reproduced, with permission, from Rudolph CD et al. *Rudolph's Pediatrics*, 21st ed. New York: McGraw-Hill, 2003: Color Plate 22.)

Differential

Enteroviral diseases, aseptic meningitis, acute rheumatic fever, encephalitis, multiple sclerosis, rheumatoid arthritis, Reiter syndrome

Diagnosis

- Summer visit to endemic area + suggestive clinical symptoms (eg, rash, meningitis)
- CSF: ↑Lymphs, ↑protein, normal glucose
- Definitive diagnosis: Serum/CSF serologies
- Frequent false-positives
- Requires two positive tests

Symptomatic Treatment

- For treatment regimens see Table 8.12.

TABLE 8.12. Lyme Disease Treatment Regimens

Staging	Treatment[a]
Early localized	Doxycycline × 21 days
Early disseminated (arthritis)	Doxycycline × 30 days
Early disseminated (neurologic)	Doxycycline × 21 days (if isolated CN palsy) or Ceftriaxone IV at meningitic doses (all others)
Early disseminated (cardiac)	Doxycycline × 21 days (if first-degree AV block) or Ceftriaxone IV at meningitic doses (all others)

[a]Substitute amoxicillin for doxycycline in children <8 years old.

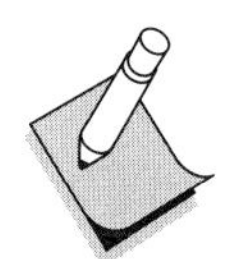

Give a single dose of doxycycline for the prophylaxis of high-risk tick bites.

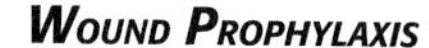

WOUND PROPHYLAXIS

- Prophylaxis
  - *Ixodes* tick bite (other ticks do not infect)
  - Only if tick attached >48 hours
  - Single 200-mg dose doxycycline <72 hours after bite

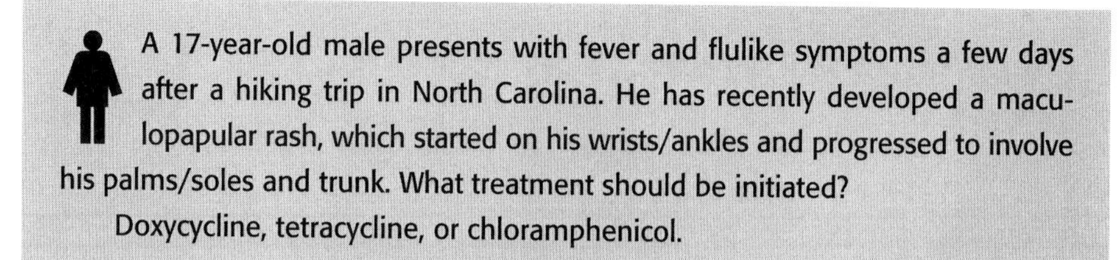

A 17-year-old male presents with fever and flulike symptoms a few days after a hiking trip in North Carolina. He has recently developed a maculopapular rash, which started on his wrists/ankles and progressed to involve his palms/soles and trunk. What treatment should be initiated?

Doxycycline, tetracycline, or chloramphenicol.

Rocky Mountain Spotted Fever

- Obligate intracellular coccobacillus *Rickettsia rickettsii*
- Carried by *Dermacentor* sp. ticks (on deer, horses, cats, dogs)
- Peak transmission between April and September (95%)
- Majority of cases in **south Atlantic states** (eg, North Carolina, South Carolina), not the Rockies!
- Two-thirds of cases in children

The classic triad of tick exposure, fever, and rash is only initially present in a minority of RSMF cases.

SYMPTOMS/EXAM

- Incubation period: 2–14 days
- Sudden onset of flulike, AGE-like, or meningitislike symptoms (headache = prominent feature).
- Classic triad (present in only ~18% initially)
  - History of tick exposure (~65%)
  - Fever (~75%)
  - Rash (~50%)
    - Maculopapular → petechial/purpuric.
    - Starts on wrists/ankles
    - Spreads centripetally (extremities → trunk)
    - Classically involves **palms** and **soles**

DIFFERENTIAL

Viral illnesses (eg, enterovirus, mononucleosis, measles, rubella), meningococcal infection, gonococcemia, leptospirosis, typhus

DIAGNOSIS

- Treat empirically if suspected on clinical grounds
- CXR abnormalities in 25% (eg, interstitial infiltrate)
- Serology (positive 6–10 days after onset) or rash biopsy

TREATMENT

- Doxycycline, tetracycline, or chloramphenicol
- Untreated = 25% mortality

COMPLICATIONS

- Interstitial pneumonitis leading to ARDS
- Myocarditis, CHF, DIC, shock
- Seizures, encephalomyelitis, coma

Ehrlichiosis

- Obligate intracellular Gram-negative coccobacillus of the *Ehrlichia* sp.
- Transmitted by *Ixodes* or *Amblyomma* ticks (reservoir = deer, mice, other mammals)
- Geographic and temporal distribution similar to Lyme disease

Symptoms/Exam

- Incubation period: 1–21 days (median = 7 days)
- Initially flulike symptoms
- 10% develop a RMSF-like rash.

Differential

Rickettsial diseases (eg, RMSF), bacterial meningitis

Diagnosis

- Leukopenia, thrombocytopenia, transaminitis (~75%)
- Mulberrylike clusters (morulae) of the tiny bacteria form inside leukocytes (seen on peripheral blood smear).
- IgG antibody titers confirm diagnosis.

Treatment

Doxycycline, tetracycline, or chloramphenicol

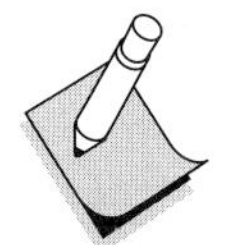

If suspected, both RMSF and ehrlichiosis must be treated immediately (based on clinical suspicion), since the illnesses can be rapidly fatal.

Complications

- ARDS, renal failure, DIC, cardiomegaly, encephalitis
- Neurologic sequelae, death (~2%)

Babesiosis

- Malarialike protozoan parasites of the genus *Babesia* infect red blood cells, leading to hemolytic anemia
- Vector: *Ixodes* ticks (same as Lyme disease)
- Reservoir: Deer, mice
- Scattered areas in the United States (especially Northeast) during summer months

Symptoms/Exam

- Incubation: 1–4 weeks
- Flulike illness with:
  - High spiking fevers
  - Dark urine (from hemolytic anemia)
  - No rash
- More severe if splenectomy

Differential

Malaria, Lyme disease

Diagnosis

- Thick and thin Giemsa-stained smears
  - Budding tetrad in "Maltese cross" formation

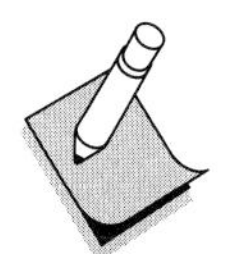

Babesiosis is of greatest concern in the splenectomized patient.

TREATMENT

- Mild disease → no treatment.
- Severe disease or splenectomy → quinine + clindamycin × 10 days.
- Exchange transfusion if fulminant

COMPLICATIONS

- Mortality ~6.5% (from acute renal failure, DIC, ARDS)
- Poorer prognosis if asplenic, elderly, or immunocompromised

Consider Q Fever in the differential diagnosis of patients who have significant exposure to animal byproducts (eg, abattoirs).

Q Fever

- *Coxiella burnetii*
- Transmitted by tick bites, blood transfusions ingestion of raw milk, and inhalation of dried byproducts of cattle, sheep, or goats
- Possible bioterrorism agent

SYMPTOMS/EXAM

- Incubation: 2–6 weeks
- Flulike symptoms, pneumonia, hepatitis

DIAGNOSIS

- Acute = clinical
- Definitive = serologies (positive 2–3 weeks after infection)

TREATMENT

- Doxycycline, tetracycline, or chloramphenicol

COMPLICATIONS

- Culture-negative endocarditis, granulomatous hepatitis

PULMONARY FUNGAL INFECTIONS

- All found in soil (see Table 8.13)
  - Commonly in people who disturb soil (eg, construction workers, dirt bike riders, farm workers)
  - Coccidiomycosis exhibits increased rates of disseminated disease in Filipinos, blacks, and Hispanics.

SYMPTOMS/EXAM

- Frequently asymptomatic
- Granulomas and hilar adenopathy on CXR

TABLE 8.13. Pulmonary Fungal Infections

DISEASE	ORGANISM	LOCATION
Coccidioidomycosis	*Coccidioides immitis*	SW desert (eg, San Joaquin valley of central California), Latin America
Histoplasmosis	*Histoplasma capsulatum*	Mississippi and Ohio river valleys; birds, bats, and construction sites
Blastomycosis	*Blastomyces dermatitides*	SE central and midwestern states bordering the Great Lakes

- Acute or chronic pneumonia
- Disseminated disease
- Reactivation possible in immunocompromised

Cocci—**C**alifornia
Histo—O**h**io
Blasto—**B**ordering Great Lakes

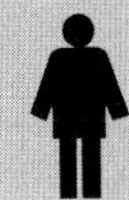

A 3-year-old boy presents with nightly perianal itching and a normal physical exam. What is the most likely diagnosis?

Pinworm (*Enterobius vermicularis*).

COMMON PARASITIC HELMINTHS

- Most cause eosinophilia.
- Most helminths are uncommon within the continental United States, with the exception of *E. vermicularis* (prevalence ~10% in some studies).
- Other less commonly identified helminths (mainly in rural southeast United States) include hookworm (1.5%), *Trichuris trichiura* (1.2%), *Ascaris lumbricoides* (0.8%), *Strongyloides stercoralis* (0.4%), *Hymenolepis nana* (0.4%), and *Taenia* species (0.1%).

Intestinal Nematodes (Round Worms)

- Worldwide distribution (see Table 8.14)
- Treat with mebendazole, albendazole, or pyrantel pamoate.
- Pulmonary symptoms (ie, Löeffler syndrome, including cough, wheezing, and pulmonary consolidations) due to worm migration through the lungs may be seen in infections with *Ascaris*, hookworm, *Strongyloides*.

TABLE 8.14. Intestinal Nematodes

Name	Nematode	Route	Symptoms/Exam	Diagnosis
Pinworm	*E. vermicularis*	Fecal-oral (most commonly among children)	Nocturnal **perianal itching**	Scotch-tape swab
Common roundworm	*A. lumbricoides*	Ingestion	Pneumonitis, abdominal cramps, worm passage (~30 cm long), obstruction	O&P
Hookworm	*Ancylostoma duodenale* *Necator americanus*	Soil contact (ie, bare feet)	Localized dermatitis (normally feet), pneumonitis, abd pain, **anemia**	O&P
Whipworm	*T. trichiura*	Ingestion, soil contact, flies on food	Dysentery, tenesmus, rectal prolapse	O&P
Strongyloides	*S. stercoralis*	Soil contact, ingestion	Eosinophilia, perianal rash, abd pain, **overwhelming infection in immunosuppressed**	Serology, O&P
Trichinella	*Trichinella sprialis*	Ingestion of **raw pork**, walrus, or bear	Fever, periorbital edema, myalgias, CNS abnormalities	Serology, muscle biopsy

TABLE 8.15. Blood and Tissue Nematodes

Name	Distribution	Vector	Symptoms/Exam	Treatment
Lymphatic filariasis	SE Asia (*Brugia malayi*) Tropics (*Wuchereria bancrofti*) Indonesia (*Brugia timori*)	Mosquito	Elephantiasis (lymphangitis and lymphedema), pneumonitis	DEC
Onchocerca vovulus	Africa, Central/South America	Blackfly (*Simulium*)	**Blindness** (sclerosing keratitis), subcutaneous nodules	Ivermectin
Loa loa	Africa	Deerfly (*Chrysops*)	Larvae migrating across eye conjunctiva	DEC
Dracunuculus medinensis	Africa	Ingestion of infected water (copepods)	Painful worm extruding from lower extremity	**Wrap worm around stick**, metronidazole

DEC = diethylcarbamazine.

In endemic areas, cysticercosis (T. solium) *is responsible for over one-third of the cases of adult-onset epilepsy.*

Blood and Tissue Nematodes (Filaria)

See Table 8.15.

Cestodes (Tapeworms)

- Treat with praziquantel (intestinal) and albendazole (extraintestinal).
- Diagnosis is made on O&P or biopsy.
- See Table 8.16.

TABLE 8.16. Cestodes

Parasite	Ingestion	Clinical Findings
Taenia saginata	Raw beef	Muscle cysts
Cysticercosis *(Taenia solium)*	Raw pork	**New onset seizures**, CNS cysts
Diphyllobothrium latum	Undercooked fish	Megaloblastic anemia due to **B_{12} deficiency**
H. nana and *H. diminuta*	Rodent feces or fleas	Abdominal cramps, diarrhea
Dipylidium caninum	Dog fleas	Abdominal cramps, diarrhea
Echinococcus *(E. granulosus, E. multilocularis,* and *E. vogeli)*	Feces of sheepdogs, cattle, wolves, foxes	Hydatid disease (liver, lung, and/or CNS abscesses)

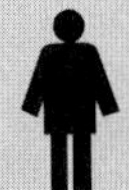

A 60-year-old ill-appearing woman presents with high fevers followed by drenching sweats a week after returning from visiting relatives in West Africa. What diagnostic test should be sent and (if positive) what treatment should be initiated?

Thick and thin smears; quinidine gluconate and doxycycline.

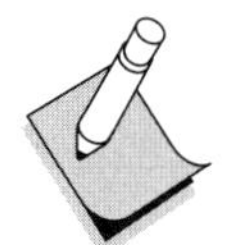

As malaria symptoms are often nonspecific, consider the diagnosis in any febrile person with a history of travel to the tropics.

Malaria

- *Plasmodium falciparum*, *P. vivax*, *P. ovale*, and *P. malariae*
- Transmitted by *Anopheles* mosquito bite
- Globally endemic

Symptoms/Exam

- Incubation period: 1–4 weeks
  - Longer with partial immunity or antimalarial use
- Begins with flulike prodrome
  - Frequently presents with misleading symptoms (eg, chest pain, abdominal pain, vomiting, diarrhea, arthralgias, etc.)
- Progresses to high fever, chills, and rigor
  - Classic febrile cycles (from RBC lysis) frequently absent
- Symptoms/exam
  - High fever
  - Tachycardia
  - Pallor/anemia
  - Splenomegaly
- ***P. falciparum*** **responsible for most mortality**
  - Most *P. falciparum* cases acquired in sub-Sahara Africa
  - Hepatomegaly, icterus, peripheral edema, seizures (cerebral malaria)

Differential

- Influenza, hepatitis, viral syndromes, multiple other infections

Diagnosis

- Basic labs: Normochromic normocytic anemia, thrombocytopenia, hypoglycemia, mild LFT abnormalities
- Definitive diagnosis: Plasmodial parasites on Giemsa-stained thick and thin smears
- Speciation important as *P. falciparum* infections should be hospitalized (mixed infections uncommon in travelers)

Treatment

- DEET and mosquito nets for prevention
- See Table 8.17 for treatment regimens.
- Admit for:
  - Suspected *P. falciparum*
  - Significant hemolysis or parasitemia >3% on smear
  - Significant comorbid conditions

TABLE 8.17. Malaria Treatment Regimens

SETTING	ADULT DRUG REGIMEN[a]	PEDIATRIC DRUG REGIMEN[a]
Uncomplicated, chloroquine-sensitive (Central America and Caribbean)	Chloroquine phosphate	Chloroquine phosphate
Uncomplicated, chloroquine-resistant (South America, South Asia, Africa)	Quinine sulfate (PO) + doxycycline or Atovaquone/proguanil or Mefloquine	Quinine sulfate (PO) + primethamine sulfadoxine[b] or Atovaquone/proguanil or Mefloquine
Complicated (possible *P. falciparum*, unable to tolerate PO)	Quinidine gluconate (IV) + doxycycline	Quinidine gluconate (IV)

[a]For *P. vivax, P. ovale*, also add primaquine phosphate to prevent relapse (test first for G6PD deficiency).

[b]Contraindicated in infants <2 months old.

- Infants, elderly, or pregnant women
- Patients with complications

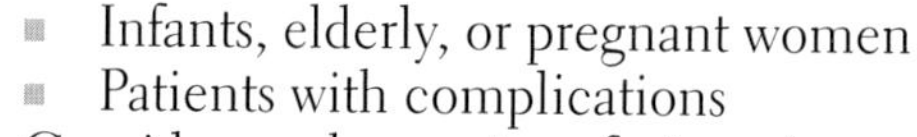

- Consider exchange transfusions (removing patient RBCs and transfusing donor RBCs) for:
  - Parasitemia >10%
  - Pulmonary edema
  - Cerebral malaria
  - Renal complications

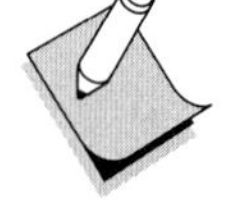

If unsure about chloroquine sensitivity in the region, treat as if resistant.

COMPLICATIONS

P. falciparum:

- General
  - Lactic acidosis
  - Severe hypoglycemia
  - Noncardiogenic pulmonary edema, DIC, death
- Cerebral malaria
  - Mortality ~20%
  - Prostration, leading to delirium, coma, and seizures
- Blackwater fever
  - Massive intravascular hemolysis leading to acute renal failure
  - Characterized by jaundice and hemoglobinuria (black urine)

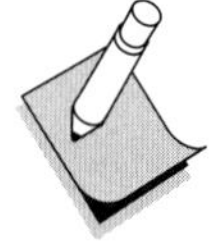

Patients must be first tested for G6PD deficiency before taking primaquine due to a potentially fatal hemolysis reaction.

Dengue

- Globally endemic
- Transmitted by the *Aedes aegypti* mosquito
- Four serotypes

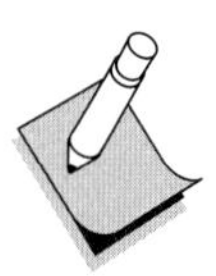

Falciparum malaria can be rapidly fatal.

SYMPTOMS/EXAM

- Incubation: 5–10 days
- High fever
  - Saddleback pattern
    - Several days of fever, a period of improvement, followed by several days of resumed symptoms
- Flulike symptoms
- Severe myalgias
  - Dramatic bone pain ("break-bone fever")
- Rash (scarlatiniform, maculopapular, or petechial)
- Dengue hemorrhagic fever (DHF)
  - Occurs when exposed to second serotype
  - Increased vascular permeability and bleeding with thrombocytopenia
    - Grade 1: Platelets <100,000
      - +tourniquet test (petechiae below cuff) = 98% PPV
    - Grade 2: Spontaneous bleeding
    - Grade 3: Circulatory failure
    - Grade 4: Profound shock

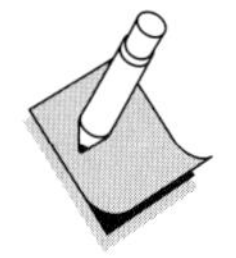

Dengue presents with fever and dramatic bone pain in the traveler.

DIAGNOSIS

- Clinical: Leukopenia and thrombocytopenia common
- Definitive: Serologies

TREATMENT

- Supportive
- DHF mortality
  - 50% without care
  - <5% with care

A 35-year-old male presents with fever and the worst headache of his life 2 weeks after returning from a white-water rafting trip to Peru. Physical exam reveals bilateral conjunctivitis. An LP shows aseptic meningitis. If untreated, what life-threatening syndrome may develop?

Weil syndrome.

Leptospirosis

- The mobile spirochete *Leptospira interrogans*
- #1 zoonosis affecting humans worldwide
- Contaminated freshwater from the urine of rodents, livestock, or domestic animals (through damaged skin or exposed mucous membranes)
- Risk factors: Walking in creeks, rodents in food storage area
- After periods of heavy rainfall/flooding

SYMPTOMS/EXAM

- Incubation: 2–30 days
- Acute (3–7 days)
  - Symptoms ranges from mild illness to abrupt high fever/chills, intense HA (worst HA), severe myalgias. Conjunctival suffusion (redness without exudates) is pathognomonic.

- Leptospiruric/immune phase (1 month)
  - Aseptic meningitis
- Weil syndrome (10%)
  - Progresses to severe, life-threatening jaundice
  - ARF, hemorrhage, ARDS
  - Mortality = ~5%

DIFFERENTIAL

Meningitis, dengue, malaria, viral hepatitis, typhus.

DIAGNOSIS

- Clinical in acute phase
  - ↑ WBC, ↑ bilirubin (relatively mild increase Alk-phos and transaminases)
  - CSF = aseptic meningitis
- Blood and urine cultures
- Serology (ELISA)

TABLE 8.18. Geographically Limited Causes of Acute Fever

NAME	VECTOR	ORGANISM/DISTRIBUTION	SYMPTOMS/EXAM	DIAGNOSIS/TREATMENT
Schistosomiasis	Penetration of skin by fresh water cercariae (eg, while swimming)	*S. mansoni* (Africa, Caribbean, S. America, Middle East) *S. japonicum* (China, SE Asia) *S. mekongi* (Cambodia, Laos) *S. hematobium* (Africa, Middle East)	*Acute*: Severe fever, HA, cough, urticaria, hypereosinophilia (Katayama fever) *Chronic*: Dermatitis, hematochezia, hepatic cirrhosis, *S. hematobium* hematuria	O&P Serologic testing Praziquantel
Chagas disease (American trypanosomiasis)	Reduviid (kissing) bug	*Trypanosoma cruzi* (South and Central America)	*Acute*: Unilateral periophthalmic cellulitis (Romaña's sign) *Chronic*: Cardiomyopathy megaesophagus, megacolon	Blood smear or xenodiagnosis Nifurtimox
West African trypanosomiasis (sleeping sickness)	*Glossina* (tsetse) fly	*Trypanosoma brucei gambiense* (West and Central Africa)	Posterior cervical LAD (Winterbottom sign), pruritis, personality changes, with slow progression to coma	Increased serum IgM Pentamidine or Melarsoprol
East African trypanosomiasis (sleeping sickness)	*Glossina* (tsetse) fly	*Trypanosoma brucei rhodesiense* (East and Southeast Africa)	High fever, rash, leading rapidly to encephalitis and coma	Increased serum IgM Suramin or Melarsoprol
Visceral leishmaniasis (Kala-Azar)	Sandflies (*Phlebotomus* sp.)	*L. donovani, infantum, chagasi* (South Asia, Middle East)	Hepatosplenomegaly, anemia, cachexia, grayish skin coloration	Sodium stibogluconate

LAD = lymphadenopathy.

Vaccine ▼ / Age ▶	Birth	1 month	2 months	4 months	6 months	12 months	15 months	18 months	24 months	4–6 years	11–12 years	13–14 years	15 years	16–18 years
Hepatitis B	HepB	HepB		*HepB[1]*		HepB					HepB Series			
Diphtheria, Tetanus, Pertussis			DTaP	DTaP	DTaP		DTaP			DTaP	Tdap		Tdap	
Haemophilus influenzae type b			Hib	Hib	*Hib[3]*	Hib								
Inactivated Poliovirus			IPV	IPV		IPV				IPV				
Measles, Mumps, Rubella						MMR				MMR			MMR	
Varicella							Varicella					Varicella		
Meningococcal								Vaccines within broken line are for selected populations	MPSV4		MCV4		MCV4 / MCV4	
Pneumococcal			PCV	PCV	PCV	PCV			PCV			PPV		
Influenza						Influenza (Yearly)						Influenza (Yearly)		
Hepatitis A										HepA Series				

This schedule indicates the recommended ages for routine administration of currently licensed childhood vaccines, as of December 1, 2005, for children through age 18 years. Any dose not administered at the recommended age should be administered at any subsequent visit when indicated and feasible. ▒ Indicates age groups that warrant special effort to administer those vaccines not previously administered. Additional vaccines may be licensed and recommended during the year. Licensed combination vaccines may be used whenever any components of the combination are indicated and other components of the vaccine are not contraindicated and if approved by the Food and Drug Administration for that dose of the series. Providers should consult the respective ACIP statement for detailed recommendations. Clinically significant adverse events that follow immunization should be reported to the Vaccine Adverse Event Reporting System (VAERS). Guidance about how to obtain and complete a VAERS form is available at **www.vaers.hhs.gov** or by telephone, **800-822-7967**.

▒ Range of recommended ages ▒ Catch-up immunization ▒ 11–12 year old assessment

FIGURE 8.3. Recommended childhood and adolescent immunization schedule (2006).

(Adapted from the Department of Health and Human Services, Centers for Disease Control and Prevention. www.Cispimmunize.org.)

TABLE 8.19. Common Vaccines and Their Contraindications

Vaccine	Contraindications
All	Previous anaphylactic reaction to specific vaccine or vaccine constituent
Live vaccines MMR Varicella OPV Influenza (live) Oral yellow fever typhoid Smallpox (vaccinia)	1° or 2° immunodeficiency Pregnancy Significant contacts of above[a]
Influenza (inactivated)	Anaphylactic reaction to eggs
HBV	Anaphylactic reaction to baker's yeast
HAV	Anaphylactic reaction to 2-phenoxyethanol or alum
DTaP	History of encephalopathy <7 days from prior DTaP

[a]For live flu and vaccinia vaccines.

OPV = oral polio vaccine; HAV = hepatitis A virus; HBV = hepatitis B virus; MMR = measles, mumps, rubella vaccine; DTaP = diphtheria, tetanus, acellular pertussis vaccine.

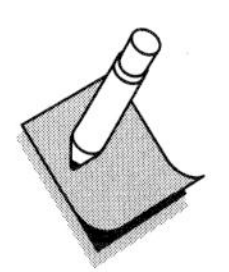

Consider empirically covering for leptospirosis in the traveler presenting with aseptic meningitis.

Treatment

- Most effective in first 4 days
- Sensitive to multiple medications
- Severe = penicillin (as with syphilis) or ceftriaxone
- Mild = doxycycline (as with Lyme disease)

Others

- For other causes of fever in the traveler, see Table 8.18.

VACCINATIONS

- See Figure 8.3 for standard immunization schedule.
- For vaccine contraindications see Table 8.19.
- Live vaccines
  - Give either together or > 30 days apart.
  - Contraindications
    - 1° immunodeficiency (eg, HIV/AIDS with low CD4 count)
    - 2° immunodeficiency
      - High-dose corticosteroids for >14 days
      - Other immune-modulating agents (eg, chemotherapy)
    - Pregnant patients
    - Significant contacts of the above

CHAPTER 9

Hematology, Oncology, Allergy, and Immunology

Alex Ho, MD

An HIV-positive African American male recently began trimethoprim-sulfamethoxazole for PCP prophylaxis. The patient presents to the ED with shortness of breath and is found to have a hemoglobin of 7 with normal MCV. His rectal exam shows no occult blood. What diagnosis should be considered, and how would you confirm the diagnosis?

G6PD deficiency with hemolysis following exposure to sulfonamide. Diagnose using hemolysis labs (elevated lactate dehydrogenase [LDH], elevated indirect bilirubin, decreased haptoglobin), G6PD enzyme level, and peripheral smear showing Heinz bodies.

ANEMIA

Hemoglobin < 12 g/dL in women and < 14 g/dL in men. The MCV is used to classify anemia (see Table 9.1).

Microcytic anemias—

FALTS
Fe deficiency
Anemia of chronic disease (may also be normocytic)
Lead poisoning
Thalassemia
Sideroblastic anemia

SYMPTOMS/EXAM

- Depends on chronicity and extent of anemia
- Palpitations, dizziness, fatigue, orthostasis
- Pale, tachycardia, hyperdynamic precordium, syncope

DIAGNOSIS

- CBC with indices, reticulocyte count, peripheral smear

TABLE 9.1. Classification of Anemia

TYPE	PATHOPHYSIOLOGY	CAUSES
Microcytic anemia (MCV <80 fL)	Decreased production of hemoglobin	Iron deficiency Thalassemia Anemia of chronic disease Lead poisoning Sideroblastic anemia
Macrocytic anemia (MCV >100 fL)	Decreased DNA synthesis	Vitamin B_{12} deficiency Folate deficiency Sulfa drugs Alcohol abuse
Normocytic anemia	Decreased marrow production of RBCs *or* increased loss or destruction of RBCs	Hemorrhage Hemolysis (G6PD deficiency, hereditary spherocytosis, microangiopathic hemolytic anemias) Aplastic anemia Sickle cell disease Anemia of chronic disease Anemia of renal disease

TREATMENT

- Treat underlying cause.
- Provide PRBC transfusion as needed. Most sources recommend maintaining hemoglobin above 10 g/dL in patients with evidence of cardiac ischemia. Young, healthy patients may tolerate lower hemoglobin levels.

HEMOLYTIC ANEMIA

Hemolytic anemia results from the destruction of RBCs due to an **inherited** or **acquired** disorder (see Table 9.2). Destruction may occur within the blood vessels (intravascular hemolysis) or as a result of sequestration elsewhere in the body (extravascular hemolysis).

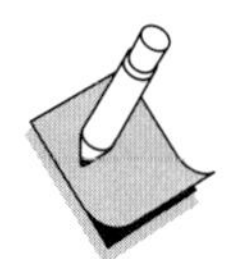

Red cell production, measured by a reticulocyte count, should be increased in patients with hemolytic anemia.

Signs and symptoms are generally attributed to the resultant anemia and include shortness of breath, fatigue, and pale or yellow skin. The spleen may be enlarged, indicating splenic sequestration and destruction of RBC. Patients with hemolysis may also present with symptomatic cholelithiasis or cholecystitis as a result of **bilirubin** gallstone formation.

A variety of tests are useful in the evaluation of the patient with suspected hemolytic anemia (see Table 9.3).

Hereditary Spherocytosis

This autosomal dominant disease with a defect in red cell membrane protein is common among persons of Northern European descent. Severity of hemolysis ranges from mild to severe.

PATHOPHYSIOLOGY

- RBCs take on a microspherocytic shape that is unable to pass through the spleen → RBC destruction.

SYMPTOMS/EXAM

- Anemia, jaundice, splenomegaly
- Symptoms/findings consistent with cholelithiasis are common.

DIAGNOSIS

- Peripheral smear with spherocytes
- Negative Coombs test (to rule out autoimmune hemolytic anemia)
- MCV may be decreased, indicating chronic hemolysis.
- Osmotic fragility test is confirmative.

TABLE 9.2. Classification of Hemolytic Anemia

HEREDITARY	ACQUIRED
Hereditary spherocytosis	Immune-mediated
Thalassemia	Microangiopathic
G6PD deficiency Sickle cell disease	Infection (eg, malaria, babesiosis)

TABLE 9.3. Tests Used in the Evaluation of Hemolytic Anemia

CBC	Anemia (normocytic if acute)
Peripheral smear	
Spherocytes	RBC membrane destruction, seen in autoimmune hemolytic anemia and hereditary spherocytosis
Schistocytes	RBC fragmentation, seen in microangiopathic hemolytic anemia
Heinz bodies	RBCs with precipitated hemoglobin, indicating G6PD deficiency
Reticulocytes	Should be elevated in hemolysis
Haptoglobin	Binds to free hemoglobin, therefore decreased in hemolysis
Lactate dehydrogenase	Elevated in hemolysis
Indirect bilirubin	Elevated indirect (unconjugated) bilirubin in hemolysis
Direct Coomb test	Positive if IgG or complement present on RBC surface
Osmotic fragility test	Positive in hereditary spherocytosis

Treatment

- Folic acid, splenectomy

Thalassemia

This genetic disorder is characterized by underproduction of either **alpha** or **beta** globin chains of the hemoglobin molecule. Thalassemia occurs in people of Mediterranean, African, Middle Eastern, Indian, and Asian descent.

Alpha Thalassemia

Occurs when one or more of the four alpha globin chain genes fails to function. Severity of disease depends on number of genes deleted or mutated.

- **Carrier state:** One deletion
  - No anemia, asymptomatic
  - CBC: No abnormalities on CBC
- **Alpha thalassemia minor:** Two deletions
  - Usually asymptomatic
  - CBC: Mild microcytic anemia
- **Hemoglobin H disease:** Three deletions
  - Splenomegaly, jaundice, chronic microcytic anemia
  - Avoid oxidative drugs (same drugs to be avoided with G6PD deficiency); see Table 9.3.
- **Hydrops fetalis:** Four deletions
  - Fetal demise, total body edema

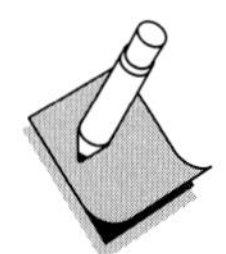

Patients with severe forms of thalassemia are at risk of heart failure due to anemia and iron toxicity resulting from numerous blood transfusions.

BETA THALASSEMIA

Occurs when one or both beta globin chain genes fails to function normally

- **Thalassemia minor**
  - Asymptomatic
  - Hypochromic, microcytic anemia (Hb > 10 g/dL)
- **Thalassemia intermedia**
  - Symptoms of anemia
  - Hypochromic, microcytic anemia (Hb 7–10 g/dL)
  - May require transfusions
- **Thalassemia major** (Cooley anemia)
  - Severe anemia, splenomegaly, frontal bossing
  - Requires transfusions to sustain life
  - Iron chelation therapy is required to prevent complications from chronic transfusions.
  - Splenectomy may reduce transfusion requirements.

G6PD Deficiency

This X-linked recessive disorder results in RBCs that are more susceptible to oxidant stress. Level of G6PD deficiency ranges from mild to severe. The disease is common in people of African, Asian, and Mediterranean descent.

PATHOPHYSIOLOGY

- Oxidant stress (see Table 9.4) → hemoglobin precipitation within the RBC → removal of cell from circulation via spleen.

SYMPTOMS/EXAM

- Asymptomatic unless exposed to precipitant
- Exposure results in hemolysis.
- Hemolytic crisis = severe hemolysis with hemoglobinuria, jaundice, splenomegaly, and possible vascular collapse.
- Symptoms/findings consistent with cholelithiasis are common.

DIAGNOSIS

- Peripheral smear showing **Heinz bodies** (RBCs with precipitated hemoglobin)
- Measurement of enzyme levels

TABLE 9.4. Common Precipitants of Hemolysis in G6PD Deficiency

Drugs (oxidizing agents)
Dapsone, methylene blue, **nitrofurantoin, phenazopyridine (pyridium)**, primaquine sulfonamides, antimalarials
Infection
Fava beans

TREATMENT

- Supportive care if hemolysis occurs
- Avoid precipitants.

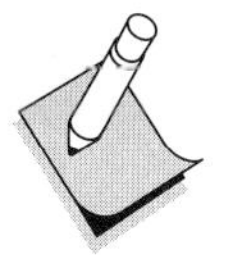

The classic story for hemolysis due to G6PD deficiency is the ***African American male*** soldier in Vietnam receiving ***treatment for malaria***.

Sickle Cell Disease

This autosomal recessive disease is caused by an abnormal structure to both beta-globin chains of hemoglobin, resulting in sickling of deoxygenated RBCs.

Patients with sickle cell trait have the defect in only one beta-globin chain and sickle only under conditions of *severe* hypoxia.

PATHOPHYSIOLOGY

- Deoxygenated RBC takes on sickle shape → obstruction of RBC in microcirculation → vaso-occlusive ischemic tissue injury.
- Sickled cells are sequestered and destroyed by liver and spleen.

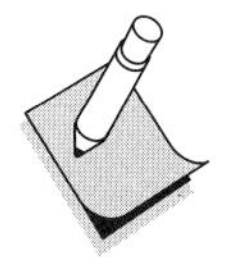

Patients should avoid hypoxia or dehydration because they may precipitate or exacerbate sickling.

VASO-OCCLUSIVE PAIN CRISIS

Most common manifestation of sickle cell crisis

SYMPTOMS/EXAM

- Pain in ribs, back, limbs
- Pattern of pain is usually consistent from crisis to crisis and may last 5–7 days.

DIAGNOSIS

- CBC: Evaluate for aplastic crisis.
- Reticulocyte count: Evaluate for aplastic crisis.
- UA, CXR, cultures: Evaluate for infection.

TREATMENT

- Fluid hydration (PO if able to tolerate, otherwise IV hydration)
- Analgesia
- Antibiotics if indicated
- Folic acid

ACUTE CHEST SYNDROME

This disease is caused by a combination of pulmonary vascular **infarction** and/or **infection**, most often by *Chlamydia*, *Mycoplasma*, RSV, *Staphylococcus aureus*, and *Streptococcus pneumoniae*.

SYMPTOMS/EXAM

- Chest pain, fever, cough
- Lung consolidation, hypoxia

DIAGNOSIS

- CXR: New pulmonary infiltrate

Treatment

- O_2 supplementation
- Antibiotics: Macrolide or cephalosporin
- Hydration
- Analgesia
- **Exchange transfusion** for multiple lobe involvement, hypoxia, worsening disease

Splenic Sequestration Crisis

Rapid sequestration of RBCs in spleen causing splenomegaly and severe anemia; occurs in **children** 6 months to 6 years old

Symptoms/Exam

- Abdominal pain, pallor, shock, splenomegaly

Diagnosis

- Very low hemoglobin with evidence for reticulocytosis

Treatment

- Hemodynamic support
- PRBC transfusion
- Splenectomy for recurrent events

Aplastic Crisis

Sudden decrease in hemoglobin production by bone marrow resulting in severe anemia; usually precipitated by infection (**parvovirus B19**)

Symptoms/Exam

- Pallor, lethargy, shock

Diagnosis

- Very low hemoglobin without reticulocytosis

Treatment

- Hemodynamic support
- PRBC transfusion

Stroke

May be thrombotic or hemorrhagic

Symptoms/Exam

- Aphasia, hemiparesis, vision changes

Diagnosis

- CT, MRI

TREATMENT

- **Exchange transfusion** to decrease HbS <30%

LEG ULCERS

Commonly found on malleoli

TREATMENT

- Rest, leg elevation
- Local wound care

INFECTIONS

- Sepsis, meningitis, pneumonia, osteomyelitis occur at an increased frequency secondary to functional asplenia. There is increased susceptibility to **encapsulated** organisms (*Haemophilus influenzae, S. pneumoniae*).

TREATMENT

- Low threshold for broad spectrum antibiotics
- Adhere to immunization schedule.

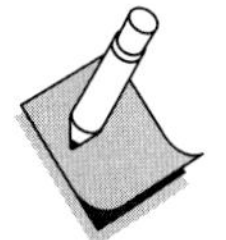

Sickle cell patients with suspected osteomyelitis should receive antibiotics to cover for S. aureus *and* Salmonella typhi.

CHOLELITHIASIS

Bilirubin stone formation from increased hemolysis

TREATMENT

- Elective cholecystectomy

OSTEONECROSIS

Typically affects femoral and humeral heads

TREATMENT

- Analgesics
- Avoid weight bearing
- Arthroplasty

PRIAPISM

- Painful erection secondary to vaso-occlusive crisis

TREATMENT

- Terbutaline sub-Q
- Hydration
- PRBC transfusion
- Analgesia
- Urology consultation

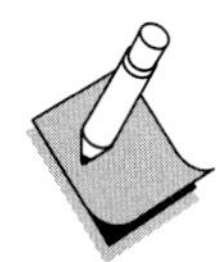

Exchange transfusions *are indicated for sickle cell patients with cardiopulmonary collapse, acute CNS event, and priapism.*

Immune-Mediated Hemolytic Anemia

Mediated by antibody formation to antigens on the RBC surface, these antibody-coated RBCs are partially digested by macrophages in the spleen (resulting in microspherocytes) and removed from circulation.

TABLE 9.5. Classification of Immune-Mediated Hemolytic Anemia

Autoimmune		
Warm antibody	IgG autoantibody Bind at body temperature	Lymphoproliferative disorders
Cold antibody	IgM autoantibody (cold agglutinins) Bind at cool temperatures	Acute: *Mycoplasma pneumonia* or Epstein-Barr infection Chronic: lymphoma or Waldenstrom macroglobulinemia
Alloimmune	Antibodies against foreign RBC antigens	Transfusion reaction Hemolytic disease of newborn
Drug-induced	Three possible mechanisms:	
	IgG autoantibody	α-Methyldopa, cephalosporins, ibuprofen
	Hapten formation	Penicillin, cephalosporin
	Immune complex formation	Amphotericin B, INH, quinidine, sulfonamides

May be further divided (see Table 9.5)

- Autoimmune (warm and cold antibody) hemolytic anemia
- Alloimmune (transfusion reaction) hemolytic anemia
- Drug-induced hemolytic anemia

ALLOIMMUNE

Mediated through antibodies against foreign RBC antigens either through transfusion of ABO incompatible blood or sensitization to maternal Rh factor in hemolytic disease of the newborn

DRUG-INDUCED HEMOLYTIC ANEMIA

Mediated through formation of drug-induced antibodies, hapten formation, or immune complex formation

Hemolysis stops with cessation of drugs.

DIAGNOSIS

- Microspherocytes on peripheral smear
- Positive Coombs test

TREATMENT

- Treat underlying cause or stop implicated medication/transfusion.
- Warm antibody hemolytic anemia may respond to high-dose corticosteroids, IV gamma globuline, cytotoxic agents, or splenectomy.
- Cold antibody hemolytic anemia is generally not responsive to medical therapy, therefore primary treatment is avoidance of cold.

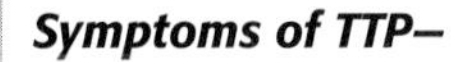

Microangiopathic Hemolytic Anemia

Mechanical disruption of RBCs in circulation, resulting in fragmentation hemolysis

Symptoms of TTP–

FAT RN
Fever
Anemia
Thrombocytopenia
Renal Failure
Neurologic problems

Causes

- Disseminated intravascular coagulation (DIC)
- Thrombotic thrombocytopenic purpura (TTP)
- Hemolytic uremic syndrome (HUS)
- Artificial heart valve
- Pregnancy
- Malignant HTN
- Malignancies

Thrombotic Thrombocytopenic Purpura

- Pregnancy, HIV, cancer, and noncancer immunosuppressive medications (eg, cyclosporine) are associated with TPP.
- Patients often present with fever and vague symptoms. Low platelets on CBC usually prompts consideration of the diagnosis.
- The classic pentad (fever, anemia, thrombocytopenia, renal failure, and neurology problems) is rarely seen on presentation.
- Neurologic symptoms may include AMS, seizures, and focal neurologic deficits.
- The cornerstone of treatment for TTP is **plasma exchange transfusion.** Other treatments to be considered include:
  - Plasma transfusion (if exchange not available)
  - High-dose steroids (unclear benefit)
  - Splenectomy (if unresponsive to plasma exchange)
  - Aspirin (controversial)
- Platelet transfusion is associated with **rapid deterioration** and should not be given to patients with TTP.

E. coli *0157:H7 is found in the GI tract of healthy cows.*

Hemolytic Uremic Syndrome

- HUS is typically **preceded by infectious diarrhea** (90%) caused by enterohemorrhagic *E. coli*, particularly *E. coli* 0157:H7, shigella, or salmonella containing the Shiga toxin. It may be preceded by URI (10%).
- Identified exposures to *E. coli* 0157:H7 include unwashed lettuce, poorly cooked hamburger, unpasteurized dairy products, and petting cows.
- Antimotility drugs and antibiotics may increase the risk of HUS.
- HUS is more common in children than adults.
- Patients typically present with diarrhea. The diarrhea may be grossly bloody. Petechiae and purpura are also common.
- Most patients will recover with only supportive therapy. Severe cases of HUS are treated with plasma exchange. **Antibiotics are generally discouraged** and may increase the likelihood of HUS and increase toxin production.

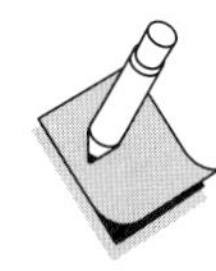

HUS: *Microangiopathic hemolytic anemia with renal failure usually precipitated by infectious bloody diarrhea*
HSP: *Vasculitis with abdominal pain, palpable purpura, and hematuria usually precipitated by a URI; bloody diarrhea may occur as a result*

POLYCYTHEMIA

Polycythemia is characterized by an increase in RBC count, hemoglobin (men >17 g/dL, women 15 g/dL), and blood volume. **Primary** polycythemia is called polycythemia vera and is regarded as a hematologic malignancy. **Secondary** causes include conditions that increase EPO levels such as lung disease, heart disease, high altitude, EPO secreting tumors.

SIGNS/SYMPTOMS

- Symptoms are generally due to sludging of blood flow leading to (ironically) poor O_2 delivery. Common complaints include weakness, headache, vision changes, and bleeding.
- Ruddy complexion, hypertension, pruritus are also common.

DIAGNOSIS

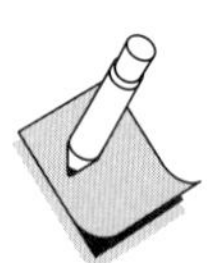

Thrombosis and hemorrhage due to ischemia secondary to thrombosis are the main causes of death in patients with polycythemia vera.

- CBC, serum EPO level, splenomegaly
- A low EPO level and elevated hemoglobin level indicate polycythemia vera; a high EPO level suggests a secondary cause.

TREATMENT

- Treat underlying cause, phlebotomy.

> A 20-year-old female presents with complaint of easy bruising. She also reports a history of heavy menstruation and prolonged bleeding after dental extraction. Exam shows multiple areas of petechiae and purpura. Her aPTT is increased with normal platelet count and PT. What is your suspected diagnosis?
>
> Von Willebrand disease.

DISORDERS OF HEMOSTASIS AND CLOTTING CASCADE

Primary Hemostasis

Immediate response to vessel injury. Platelets and von Willebrand factor (vWF) form a primary plug.

Secondary Hemostasis

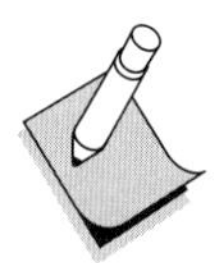

Tissue plasminogen activator (tPA) converts plasminogen to plasmin, which accelerates fibrin breakdown.

- Slower process, which activates the coagulation cascade to form a fibrin clot
- **Intrinsic** pathway
  - Measure with **PT**.
  - Tissue factor → factor VII → factor X.
- **Extrinsic** pathway
  - Measure with **aPTT**.
  - Factor XII → factor XI → factor IX → factor VIII → factor X.
- Intrinsic and extrinsic coagulation pathways share a common final pathway:
  - Factor X → factor V → thrombin formation → conversion of fibrinogen to fibrin (see Figure 9.1).

SYMPTOMS/EXAM

- Prolonged bleeding, easy bruising
- Petechiae, purpura, ecchymosis

DIAGNOSIS

- CBC, bleeding time, PT, aPTT, thrombin time, vWF activity (see Table 9.6)

Thrombocytopenia

Thrombocytopenia may result from decreased platelet production, increased platelet destruction, or splenic sequestration (see Table 9.7).

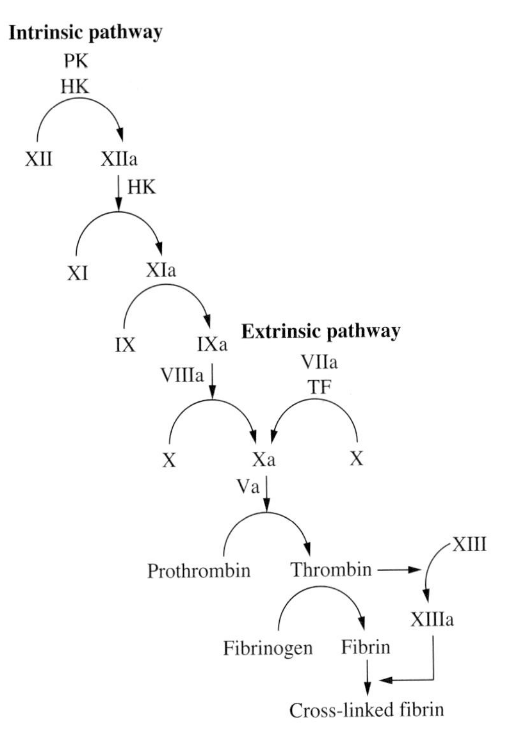

FIGURE 9.1. The coagulation cascade. The intrinsic pathway is measured by the activated partial thromboplastin time (PTT). The extrinsic pathway is measured by the prothrombin time (PT).

(Reproduced, with permission, from Lichtman MA, Beutler E, Kipps TJ, et al. *Williams Hematology*, 7th ed. New York: McGraw-Hill, 2006:1684.)

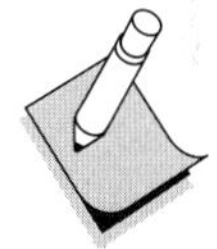

Patients with clotting-factor problems tend to suffer from prolonged bleeding after an injury or surgery and bleeding into joints; patients with platelet problems tend to suffer from petechiae, epistaxis, gum bleeding, and vaginal bleeding.

SYMPTOMS/EXAM

- Petechiae or ecchymosis of mucus membranes or skin
- Epistaxis, gum bleeding, menorrhagia, or GI bleeding

DIAGNOSIS

- Increased bleeding may occur when platelets are below 50,000/μL.
- Risk of life-threatening spontaneous hemorrhage occurs with counts <20,000/μL and substantially increases with counts <10,000/μL.

TREATMENT

- Treat underlying cause.
  - Significant hemorrhage or major procedure with platelets < 50,000/μL

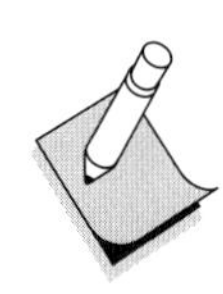

Thrombocytopenia in patients with alcoholism results from direct toxicity to the bone marrow from alcohol, folic acid deficiency, and increased sequestration from splenomegaly.

TABLE 9.6. Use of Laboratory Values to Identify Cause of Increased Bleeding

LABORATORY FINDING	CAUSES
Low platelets	See Table 9.9.
Prolonged PT	Liver disease, vitamin K deficiency, warfarin
Prolonged PTT	Hemophilia A and B, von Willebrand disease, heparin
Low fibrinogen level	Disseminated intravascular coagulation, large volume transfusion, liver disease, severe malnutrition

TABLE 9.7. Common Causes of Thrombocytopenia

Decreased bone marrow production	Marrow infiltration Drugs Toxins Infection
Increased platelet destruction	Immunologic Idiopathic thrombocytopenic purpura (ITP) Collagen vascular disease (eg, systemic lupus erythematosus [SLE]) Leukemia, lymphoma Drug-induced (eg, heparin) Infection (typically viral) Mechanical Thrombotic thrombocytopenic purpura Hemolytic uremic syndrome Disseminated intravascular coagulation HELLP syndrome Vasculitis
Splenic sequestration	Hypersplenism

- Platelet transfusion if
  - Life-threatening hemorrhage and abnormal platelet level or function
  - Platelets < 10,000/μL for bleeding prophylaxis, except in ITP, TTP, HIT

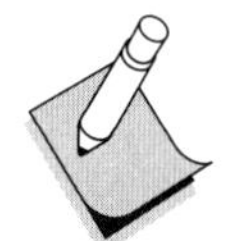

ITP is the most common hemorrhagic disease in children. It is usually self-limited, resolving in weeks to months.

IDIOPATHIC THROMBOCYTOPENIC PURPURA

Idiopathic thrombocytopenic purpura is thrombocytopenia without an underlying causative disease or offending medication. Platelets are removed prematurely by reticuloendolethial system. Peak incidence occurs in children (2–6 years old) and adults (20–50 years old). Acute ITP is more common in children and chronic ITP is more common in adults. Platelet counts of <20,000/mm^3 may cause life-threatening hemorrhage.

SYMPTOMS/EXAM

- In children, often follows a **viral** infection
- Petechiae, gingival bleeding, epistaxis, menorrhagia, GI bleeding, intracranial hemorrhage

DIAGNOSIS

- Isolated thrombocytopenia on CBC
- Peripheral smear with a small number of well-granulated platelets
- Bone marrow biopsy shows no primary bone marrow disorder.

TREATMENT

- Treatment is reserved for severe bleeding with platelets <50,000/mm^3 or platelet count <10,000/mm^3 without bleeding.
- For children, treatment is usually conservative since the majority have a favorable outcome. Children should avoid physical activity or NSAIDs.

- Prednisone 1–1.5 mg/kg/day
- IVIG or anti-D immunoglobulin
- Platelet transfusion is not normally indicated and should be limited to patients with life-threatening hemorrhage.
- Those unresponsive to steroids and IVIG may need splenectomy or immune modulation therapy.

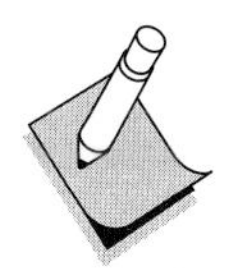

ITP—IVIG, steroids

TTP—exchange transfusions

Disseminated Intravascular Coagulation

Disseminated intravascular coagulation is widespread activation of the **coagulation** and **fibrinolytic** cascade leading to a life-threatening bleeding disorder. Common causes are listed in Table 9.8.

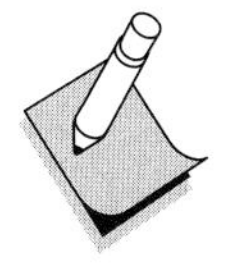

Infection is the most common cause of DIC. Specific causes include Gram-positive and Gram-negative sepsis, meningococcemia, typhoid fever, and Rocky Mountain spotted fever.

Symptoms/Exam

- Purpura, petechiae
- **Bleeding,** involving skin, mucus membranes, venipuncture sites, surgical wounds, GI tract, GU tract, CNS
- **Thrombosis,** causing focal ischemia in areas of end circulation (extremities, nose, genitalia), mental status changes

Diagnosis

- Prolonged PT and aPTT, low platelet count, low fibrinogen level, elevated fibrin degradation products, elevated D-dimer, increased thrombin time, decreased antithrombin III levels
- Schistocytes (from fibrin deposition in small vessels and resultant RBC destruction) on peripheral smear

Treatment

- Supportive care
- Treat underlying cause.

TABLE 9.8. Common Causes of DIC

Common Causes of DIC
Infection (bacterial, viral, fungal)
Carcinoma (adenocarcinoma, lymphoma, acute leukemia)
Trauma (burns, crush, head injuries)
Shock
Liver disease
Pregnancy (placental abruption, amniotic fluid emboli, fetal death in utero)
Envenomation
ARDS
Transfusion and drug reactions
Surgical procedures
Heat stroke

- FFP if bleeding predominates
- Cryoprecipitate to replace fibrinogen
- Platelet transfusion if <50,000/μL with active bleeding or if <10,000/μL
- Vitamin K 10 mg parentally
- Heparin if thrombosis fibrin deposition predominates or if purpura fulminans is present

Von Willebrand Disease

This is the most common hereditary bleeding disorder. The von Willebrand factor facilitates adherence of platelets to injured blood vessels and also stabilizes factor VIII in plasma.

There are three forms of vWF characterized by their quantitative or qualitative defects:

- Type I, the most common form, has a partial decrease in vWF.
- Type II has dysfunctional vWF.
- Type III has almost no vWF.

SYMPTOMS/EXAM

- Epistaxis, gingival bleeding, menorrhagia, GI bleeding

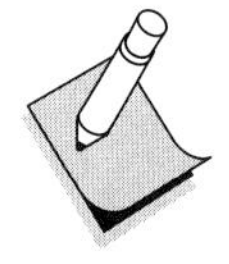

*Bleeding disorder with normal platelet count, PT, and PTT suggests **von Willebrand disease**.*

DIAGNOSIS

- aPTT may be **normal or prolonged**, normal platelet count, normal PT, increased bleeding time
- Abnormal assay of vWF activity, vWF antigen, or factor VIII coagulant (C) activity

TREATMENT

- **Desmopression (DDAVP)**
  - Stimulates release of vWF (and factor VIII) stored in vascular endothelial cells
  - Indicted for type I disease
- Factor VIII concentrates with vWF (Humate-P, Koate HS)
  - Primary therapy for types II and III disease
  - Should be used in all cases of serious bleeding
- Cryoprecipitate
  - Contains vWF, but carries risk of infectious disease transmission, therefore is only recommended when factor VIII concentrate with vWF are not available

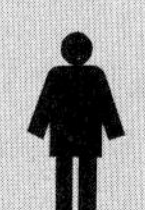

A 25-year-old hemophiliac weighing 70 kg presents with a head injury and decreased mental status after a high speed MVC. What is the level of factor (in %) that is desired in this patient?

This patient must be presumed to have intracranial hemorrhage and requires 100% factor replacement. Based on a starting factor level of 0% and with each unit/kg of factor VIII raising the plasma level by 2%, the number of units of factor required is 3500 (0.5 U/kg × 70 kg × 100% increase needed).

Hemophilia

Hemophilia A (classic hemophilia) and **Hemophilia B** (Christmas disease) are X-linked coagulation disorders characterized by a deficiency in factor **VIII** and factor **IX**, respectively. Patients may have mild, moderate, or severe disease depending on their factor activity.

Treatment is guided by the type of hemophilia, bleeding site, bleeding severity, and presence or absence of an inhibitor. Patients may develop **inhibitor** antibodies against replacement factors, limiting their effectiveness and leading to risk of anaphylaxis during factor replacement in patients with hemophilia B. Patients with low levels of inhibitors may be treated with factor VIII or IX replacement by overwhelming the inhibitor. Hemophiliacs with serious bleeding and high inhibitor levels should be treated with factor VII, which serves as a factor VIII inhibitor bypassing agent.

SYMPTOMS/EXAM

- Easy bruising, hemarthrosis, hematuria
- Muscle hematoma, intracranial hemorrhage, retroperitoneal hematoma

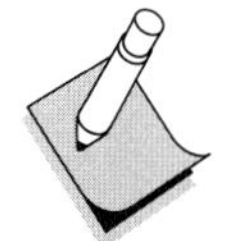

Inhibitors are present in all patients with acquired hemophilia and also develop in about 20% of patients with inherited hemophilia.

DIAGNOSIS

- Prolonged PTT, normal PT, abnormal factor assay
- The clotting factor mixing test mixes normal plasma with a patient's serum. Under normal circumstances the PTT should normalize. If the PTT remains prolonged, then the patient's serum contains an inhibitor.

TREATMENT

- Factor replacement is required prior to any invasive procedure, including central line, lumbar puncture, arterial puncture.
- Tranexamic acid and aminocaproic acid (Amicar) are used to help prevent clot dissolution in patients with hemophilia.

Hemophilia A

- Desmopressin (DDAVP)
  - Indicated for mild to moderate hemophilia with minor bleeding
  - Increases plasma factor VIII levels by three- to five-fold in 30 minutes
  - 0.3 mcg/kg IV
- Factor VIII replacement
  - See Table 9.9 for factor replacement guidelines.
  - Each U/kg of factor VIII raises factor VIII levels by 2%.
  - **Units of factor VIII required = weight (kg) × 0.5 × (% activity desired– % intrinsic activity).**
  - For those with low concentrations of inhibitors, an increased factor dose can be given in attempt to overwhelm existing antibodies.
- Factor VIIa
  - Indicated for patient with high titer inhibitor levels

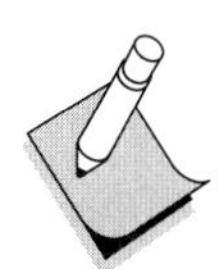

Assume the present level of factor VIII is zero unless it is previously known.

Hemophilia B

- See Table 9.9 for factor replacement guidelines.
- Factor IX replacement
  - Each U/kg of factor IX raises factor IX levels by 1%.
  - **Units of factor IX required = weight (kg) × 1 × (% activity desired – % intrinsic activity).**
- Factor VIIa
  - Indicated for patient with high titer inhibitor levels

TABLE 9.9. Factor Replacement Guidelines

Bleeding Site	Desired Factor Level (%)
Deep muscle	40–50
Joint	30–50
Epistaxis	80–100
Oral mucosa	50
GI tract	100
CNS	100

ANTICOAGULATION AND ANTIPLATELET AGENTS

Anticoagulant and antiplatelet therapy are used to treat and prevent thrombosis.

Warfarin

Oral anticoagulant that prevents reduction of **vitamin K** to its active form

CONTRAINDICATIONS

- Hypersensitivity, active bleeding, pregnancy, liver failure

DOSING

- Start warfarin 5 mg PO daily.

MONITORING

- For most indications, therapeutic INR is 2.0–3.0.
- For mechanical valves, therapeutic INR is 2.5–3.5.
- Table 9.5 shows a list of medications that can interfere with **INR**.

The vitamin K–dependent cofactors are factors II, VII, IX, X, protein C, and protein S. Upon starting warfarin, the patient may initially be hypercoagulable because of the rapid loss of the anticoagulants protein C and protein S.

COMPLICATIONS

- Major bleeding occurs in about 3% of patients.
- Many medications can alter the effect of warfarin on clotting factor production (see Table 9.10). The most common mechanism is by induction of hepatic enzymes leading to increased drug clearance.
- Thrombosis and warfarin-induced skin necrosis can occur between the third and 10th day after initiating therapy. Risk is greatly reduced by concurrent use of heparin or low-molecular-weight heparin

REVERSAL

See Table 9.11.

Unfractionated Heparin

Inhibits thrombin and other factors in the intrinsic cascade; prevents clot propagation

TABLE 9.10. Medications Affecting INR

Increase INR	Decrease INR
Allopurinol, amiodarone, azithromycin, cimetidine, clotrimazole, fluroquinolones, INH, metronidazole, omeprazole, penicillin, phenytoin, prednisone, propoxyphene, quinidine, statins, sulfonyureas, tetracycline, tamoxifen, zafirlukast	Carbamazepine, cholestyramine, dicloxacillin, griseofulvin, haloperidol, nafcillin, ranitidine, rifampin

Contraindications

- Hypersensitivity, active GI bleeding, intracranial hemorrhage, current bacterial endocarditis, heparin-induced thrombocytopenia (HIT)

Dosing

- Bolus 70–80 units/kg IV followed by infusion 15–18 units/kg/hour

Monitoring

- Follow aPTT and titrate based on therapeutic range (usually 1.5–2.5 × the normal value).

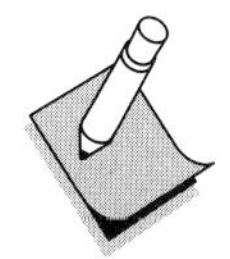

HIT syndrome is less common with low-molecular-weight heparin (LMWH) than with heparin. In patients with HIT, stop the heparin or LMWH and start a direct thrombin inhibitor.

Complications

- Major bleeding
- HIT syndrome (autoimmune response to heparin → low platelets, **thrombosis**)

Reversal

- Stop heparin—short half-life
- Protamine sulfate, 1 mg IV for every 100 units of heparin, over the previous four hours to a maximum of 50 mg

Low-Molecular-Weight Heparin

Inhibits activity of factor Xa; includes enoxaparin, dalteparin, ardeparin

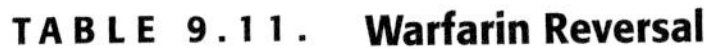

TABLE 9.11. Warfarin Reversal

INR	Bleeding	Treatment
< 5	No	Hold dose, recheck INR in 24 hours
5–9	No	Hold dose, consider oral vitamin K 1–2 mg PO, recheck INR in 24 hours
> 9	No	Hold dose, vitamin K 2–4 mg PO, recheck INR in 24 hours
Any elevation	Major bleeding	Hold dose, FFP transfusion or factor concentrates, vitamin K 5–10 mg slow IV or sub Q
Any elevation	Minor bleeding	Hold dose, vitamin K 2–4 mg PO

CONTRAINDICATIONS

- Hypersensitivity, active bleeding

MONITORING

- Factor Xa levels (monitor in patients with CrCl <30)

COMPLICATIONS

- Major bleeding

REVERSAL

- Protamine 1 mg IV for every 1 mg of enoxaparin

The dosing of low-molecular-weight heparin must be reduced in patients with severe renal impairment.

Direct Thrombin Inhibitors

Inhibit circulating and clot bound thrombin; include lepirudin, argatroban; indicated in patients with HIT

Aspirin

Aspirin irreversibly inhibits cyclooxygenase, which prevents synthesis of thromboxane needed for platelet aggregation.

CONTRAINDICATION

- Hypersensitivity reaction, severe hepatic disease, bleeding disorder, major GI bleed

DOSE

- ASA 81–162 mg PO daily

COMPLICATIONS

- Bleeding, allergic reactions

TREATMENT OF BLEEDING

- Transfuse platelets to keep platelets >50,000/μL.

Thienopyridines

Irreversibly inhibit platelet aggregation via adenosine diphosphate receptor antagonism; includes clopidogrel, ticlopidine

CONTRAINDICATION

- Active severe bleeding, hypersensitivity

COMPLICATIONS

- GI bleeding, hypersensitivity, TTP (more common with ticlopidine), neutropenia (more common with ticlopidine)

TREATMENT

- Bleeding
  - Transfuse platelets to keep platelets >50,000/μL.

Glycoprotein IIb/IIIa Inhibitors

GP IIb/IIIa inhibitors prevent binding of fibrinogen on the IIb/IIIa receptor which inhibits platelet activation. Most sources recommend addition of GP IIb/IIIa inhibitors to conventional anticoagulation for patient receiving percutaneous coronary intervention. GP IIb/IIIa inhibitors include abciximab, tirofiban, eptifibatide.

CONTRAINDICATION

- Hypersensitivity, bleeding disorder, severe hypertension (SBP >200 mmHg), severe renal insufficiency, major surgery in the preceding 6 weeks, history of hemorrhagic stroke, ischemic stroke within past 30 days

COMPLICATION

- Bleeding, hypersensitivity

DYSHEMOGLOBINEMIAS

A 60-year-old patient is undergoing placement of a nasogastric tube. Benzocaine is used to anesthetize the posterior pharynx. The patient's O_2 saturation drops to 83% without improvement with supplemental treatment. What is your suspected diagnosis?

Methemoglobinemia.

Metheomoglobinemia

In the presence of non-O_2 oxidizing agents, Fe^{2+} changes to Fe^{3+}. Hemoglobin-containing Fe^{3+} does not bind O_2 and is referred to as methemoglobin.

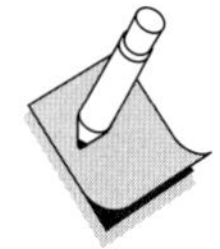

Treat methemoglobinemia with methylene blue.

CAUSES

- Nitrates (in well water or vegetables)
- Medications: Lidocaine, benzocaine, nitrates, nitroglycerin, nitroprusside, sulfonamides, dapsone, phenazopyridine (pyridium)

SYMPTOMS/EXAM

- Bluish skin discoloration, anxiety, headache, lightheadedness
- Symptoms include tachypnea, tachycardia, myocardial ischemia, seizures, coma. Classically see pulse oximetry of 80–85% without response to supplemental O_2. However, pulse oximetry is an unreliable test in the presence of methemoglobinemia. Actual tissue O_2 availability may be much lower than suggested by pulse oximetry.
- **Chocolate brown blood** on venipuncture
- May become more symptomatic at lower levels with underlying anemia or pulmonary disease

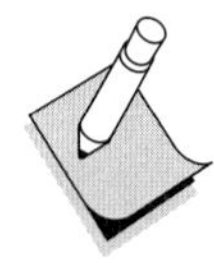

The amyl nitrite and sodium nitrite in the Cyanide Antidote Kit or "Lilly Kit" work by inducing a methemoglobinemia, which scavenges cyanide. Use the "Lilly Kit" to treat cyanide toxicity, not methemoglobinemia.

DIFFERENTIAL

- Hypoxemia
  - Decreased FiO_2 (altitude)
  - Hypoventilation
  - Ventilation-perfusion mismatch
  - Right-to-left shunt
- Dyshemoglobinemia (methemoglobinemia or sulfhemoglobinemia)

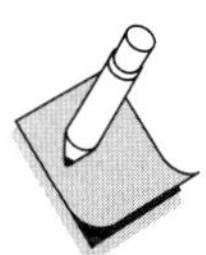

Paradoxical methemoglobinemia—excess methylene blue can cause methemoglobinemia.

DIAGNOSIS

- **Co-oximetry** can differentiate between oxy-, deoxy-, carboxy-, and methemoglobinemias and allows confirmation of the diagnosis.
- In patients with methemoglobinemia the partial pressure of O_2 in the blood is usually normal, and an ABG typically yields a normal PaO_2 and O_2 saturation.

TREATMENT

- **Methylene blue** (1–2 mg/kg IV) facilitates the reduction of Fe^{3+} changes to Fe^{2+}.

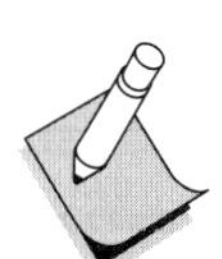

*Inhaled **hydrogen sulfide** (H_2S) acts as a mitochondrial toxin similar to cyanide and is treated with **nitrates** in order to induce a methemoglobinemia. The primary described mechanism of toxicity is not via sulfhemoglobinemia.*

Sulfhemoglobinemia

Pathophysiology and causes are similar to methemoglobinemia, though usually less severe because sulfhemoglobinemia causes a rightward shift of the O_2 dissociation curve, favoring the release of O_2 (whereas methemoglobinemia causes a leftward shift).

CAUSES

- Nitrates, sulfonamides, trinitrotoluene

DIAGNOSIS

- **Co-oximetry** will identify the presence of an abnormal hemoglobin but cannot differentiate between met- and sulfhemoglobin. Adding cyanide to the blood sample changes the absorption pattern of methemoglobin and allows for the identification of sulfhemoglobinemia.

TREATMENT

- Supportive care
- Transfusions may be necessary for severe toxicity.
- Methylene blue does not reduce sulfhemoglobin. Because of the potential side effects of methylene blue (including paradoxical methemoglobinemia), an effort should be made to differentiate between sulf- and methemoglobinemia.

Causes of Hypercalcemia—

MISHAP
Malignancy
Ingestion vitamin D, calcium
Sarcoidosis
Hyperparathyroidism
Alkali-milk syndrome
Paget disease, **p**araneoplastic syndrome

ONCOLOGIC EMERGENCIES

Hypercalcemia of Malignancy

In the setting of cancer, hypercalcemia results from bone destruction (metastasis, multiple myeloma), paraneoplastic syndrome (parathyroid hormonelike substance), or osteoclast activation (lymphoma, leukemia).

SIGNS/SYMPTOMS

- Generally present when levels exceed 12 mg/dL
- Polyuria, nephrolithiasis, anorexia, nausea, vomiting, constipation, weakness, confusion, pathologic fracture

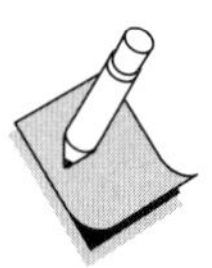

Symptoms of hypercalcemia: Stones, bones, abdominal groans, and psychiatric overtones

DIAGNOSIS

- Chemistries, serum PTH level
- ECG with shortened QT interval

TREATMENT

- IV fluids—maintain a positive fluid balance
- Saline diuresis—causes calcium excretion after fluid volume is restored; may add furosemide to assist in diuresis
- Bisphosphonates (pamidronate, zoledronate) inhibit bone resportion.
- Calcitonin inhibits bone resorption and increases calcium excretion.
- Glucocorticoids have direct cytolytic effect on some tumor cells, inhibit calcium absorption from intestines, increase calcium excretion.
- Phosphate binds calcium, but not part of routine ED treatment due to the possibility of causing calcium-phosphate deposition.
- Mithramycin decreases bone resorption
- Dialysis is indicated for patients with renal failure.

Hyperviscosity Syndrome

This syndrome is characterized by sludging and the term is used to describe decreased perfusion secondary to increased products (paraproteins, RBC, WBC) in the bloodstream.

CAUSES

- Waldenstrom macroglobulinemia (increased IgM)
- Multiple myeloma (increased IgG or IgA)
- Leukemias with blast transformation
- Polycythemia vera

SIGNS/SYMPTOMS

- Blurred vision, headache, fatigue, somnolence, stroke, mesenteric ischemia

DIAGNOSIS

- Peripheral smear may show rouleaux formation, which describes stacks of RBCs that form in the presence of increased serum proteins, particularly fibrinogen and globulins.
- Increased WBC, Hb, serum proteins

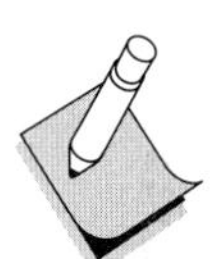

The tendency of RBCs to stack in the presence of fibrinogen causes them to settle faster and provides the basis for the erythrocyte sedimentation rate test.

TREATMENT

- Two unit phlebotomy with replacement with IV fluids
- Plasmaphoresis: Dysproteinemias
- Leukaphoresis: Blast transformations
- Chemotherapy

A 60-year-old male presents with complaints of fever. His temperatures at home have been running 38.5°C. He has an indwelling catheter in place that is red and tender. Otherwise, he denies other symptoms and does not appear toxic. His CBC shows an absolute neutrophil count (ANC) of 400/μL. What are your next steps in management?

Obtain cultures and start ceftazidime and vancomycin. Remove indwelling catheter. Also do a careful skin exam and check CXR and urine for alternative source of infection.

Neutropenic Fever

Neutropenic fever is defined as sustained temperatures <38°C or single temperature <38.3°C in the presence of neutropenia (ANC **<500 cells/µL**). Fever may be the only presenting sign. Risk of death increases as the ANC decreases.

CAUSES

Sources of infection:

- Most likely sources include respiratory, urinary, GI, and line infection.
- Bacterial infection
  - Gram-negative (*Pseudomonas, E. coli, Proteus, Klebsiella*)
  - Gram-positive (*Staphylococcus, Streptococcus*)
- Viral infection
  - CMV, herpes
- Opportunistic infections

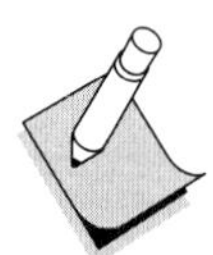

Typhlitis is inflammation or necrosis of the ileum and cecum in neutropenic patients. The mortality rate is 40–50%.

SIGNS/SYMPTOMS

- Range from minimal symptoms to septic shock

DIAGNOSIS

- CBC, chemistries, LFTs, coagulation panel
- Cultures from indwelling catheter, blood, urine, sputum, stool
- CXR

TREATMENT

- Hemodynamic support
- Initiate broad spectrum antibiotic
  - Antipseudomonal aminoglycoside plus antipseudomonal PCN or
  - Antipseudomonal third generation cephalosporin (**Ceftazidime**) plus vancomycin
- Control source of infection with debridement if appropriate or surgical consultation for intra-abdominal infections.

A 70-year-old male with a history of prostate cancer presents with low back pain. The pain is worse in the recumbent position and worse with palpation. He describes retaining urine and problems with ambulation. Exam shows decreased rectal tone, postvoid residual of 500 mL, and motor/sensory changes. What is your suspected diagnosis and next step in management?

Acute spinal cord compression; administer dexamethasone and call neurosurgery and/or radiation oncologist.

Spinal Cord Compression

Presents with back pain at the level of compression with motor, sensory, autonomic dysfunction below the level of compression. Etiologies include multiple myeloma, lymphoma, metastatic cancer (lung, breast, prostate). The most common site is the thoracic spine followed by lumbar and cervical spine.

SIGNS/SYMPTOMS

- Back pain, bilateral motor weakness, sensory changes, bladder/bowel dysfunction
- Vertebral tenderness, motor weakness, abnormal rectal tone, loss of anal wink, areflexia, saddle anesthesia

DIAGNOSIS

- Plain films: Identify fracture
- MRI spine: Gold standard
- Myelography: If MRI is unavailable

TREATMENT

- Pain control
- Dexamethasone
- Radiation therapy
- Neurosurgery: Decompression laminectomy

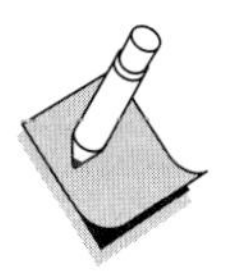

Cauda equina syndrome is a form of spinal cord compression involving the terminal portion of the cord. Patients present with some combination of low back pain, saddle anesthesia, bowel and bladder dysfunction, and lower extremity motor and sensory loss.

Superior Vena Cava (SVC) Syndrome

SVC syndrome is obstruction of the SVC from underlying malignancy. Obstruction may be due to external pressure on the SVC or invasion of the SVC by tumor and resultant thrombosis.

CAUSES

Common causes include bronchogenic carcinoma, small cell lung CA, squamous cell lung CA, and lymphoma.

SIGNS/SYMPTOMS

- Facial/upper extremity edema, shortness of breath, headache, chest pain
- Facial plethora, distended neck/chest veins

DIAGNOSIS

- CXR: Evaluate for widened mediastinum
- CT chest with IV contrast
- MRI: If neck pain is also present, to rule out spinal cord compression

TREATMENT

- Supplemental O_2
- Raise head and upper body
- Steroids
- Diuretics
- Vascular stents, thrombolytics, and radiation may be used to improve SVC flow depending on the type of tumor and its location.

An 18-year-old patient with Burkitt's lymphoma presents 3 days after his last chemotherapy with fatigue, muscle spasms, and palpitations. Labs obtained show elevated potassium, uric acid, and phosphate levels, and decreased calcium level. The patient's monitor shows a widened QRS complex. What is your suspected diagnosis and next step in management?

Tumor lysis syndrome and hyperkalemia. Administer calcium gluconate, insulin IV, one ampule D50, one ampule bicarbonate, albuterol nebulizer, and kayexylate.

Tumor Lysis Syndrome

Death of numerous neoplastic cells causes release of large quantities of **intracellular** content and uric acid in the bloodstream. This typically follows **1–3 days** after the last chemotherapy of hematologic malignancies (most commonly Burkitt's lymphoma). Tumor lysis syndrome is also more likely to develop in patients with underlying renal insufficiency.

SIGNS/SYMPTOMS

- Fatigue, lethargy, nausea, vomiting, cloudy urine, muscle spasm, altered mental status
- Acute renal failure, ventricular dysrrhythmias

DIAGNOSIS

- Hyperuricemia
- Hyperkalemia
- Hyperphosphatemia
- Hypocalcemia

TREATMENT

- Hyperkalemia: Treat in standard fashion.
- Hyperuricemia: Treat with alkalinization of the urine to maintain urine pH 7.1–7.5.
- Hemodialysis with refractory hyperkalemia >6 mEq/L or hyperuricemia >10 mg/dL, phosphate levels >10 mg/dL, creatinine >10 mg/dL, symptomatic hypocalcemia or volume overload.

DERMATOLOGIC MANIFESTATIONS OF MALIGNANCY

The skin may show signs of internal disease. The following are skin disorders associated with internal malignancy:

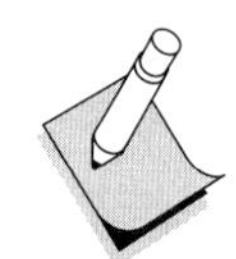

To make a bicarbonate drip, add three ampules of bicarbonate to D5W.

Ancanthosis Nigricans

- Hyperpigmentation and hyperkeratosis of skin folds (axilla, antecubital fossa, neck, and groin)
- Associated with GI malignancies (adenocarcinoma), lung and breast CA; also seen in patients with DM

Dermatomyositis

- Systemic disease characterized by
  - Violaceous rash of eyelids and periorbital region
  - Erythema of face, neck, and upper trunk
  - Progressive proximal muscle weakness
- Associated with breast, ovarian, uterine, stomach, colon, and lung CAs.

Erythema Multiforme

- Erythematous plaques with pale centers and bright red borders distributed in a symmetric fashion on extremities and oral mucosa
- Associated with leukemias and Hodgkin disease, although herpes simplex and *M. pneumoniae* infections are more common causes

Erythema Nodosum

- Painful, erythematous nodules on extensor surfaces of lower extremities
- Associated with leukemia, Hodgkin disease, and metastatic carcinoma, though streptococcal infections and sarcoidosis are more common causes

Erythroderma

- Diffuse erythema of the skin
- Associated with Hodgkin disease, leukemia, and mycosis fungoides

Ichthyosis

- Diffuse, dry scaling lesions
- Associated with lymphoma, breast, cervical, lung, and colon CAs

Pruritus

- Itching and burning sensation of the skin
- Associated with Hodgkin disease, leukemia, multiple myeloma, polycythemia vera, adenocarcinoma, carcinoid syndrome

Sister Mary Joseph Node

- Periumbilical nodule
- Associated with advanced adenocarcinoma (gastric, ovarian)

Urticaria

- Transient areas of raised, red wheals
- Associated with Hodgkin disease, leukemia, internal carcinoma, multiple myeloma

Purpura

- Red or purple discoloration of the skin
- Associated with Hodgkin disease, acute leukemias, lymphoma, multiple myeloma, polycythemia vera

MULTIPLE MYELOMA

Malignant plasma cell disorder accompanied by urine/serum paraprotein

SYMPTOMS/EXAM

- Hypercalcemia, anemia, lytic bone lesions, acute renal failure

DIAGNOSIS

- Bone survey, serum/urine protein electrophoresis

TREATMENT

- Oral alkylating agent, steroids, local radiation for bony lesions

HYPERSENSITIVITY REACTIONS

There are four classes of immune-mediated (hypersensitivity) reactions (see Table 9.12).

A 40-year-old male with an allergy to peanuts presents with hives and hypotension after a peanut exposure. The patient has a history of hypertension for which he takes atenolol. The patient's BP remains low after two doses of IM epinephrine and a 2-L NS bolus. What is the most appropriate next therapy?

Glucagon (1 mg every 5 minutes) is indicated in the treatment of anaphylaxis with refractory hypotension in patients on β-blockers.

TABLE 9.12. Hypersensitivity Reaction

TYPE OF REACTION	MECHANISM	EXAMPLE
Type I: Anaphylactic	IgE-mediated degranulation of mast cells with release of mediators	Anaphylaxis Urticaria Angioedema
Type II: Cytotoxic	IgG or IgM antibodies react with cell antigens with resultant complement activation	Autoimmune hemolytic anemia Goodpasture syndrome
Type III: Immune complex	Immune complex deposition and subsequent complement activation	Serum sickness SLE RA
Type IV: Cell-mediated	Activated T cells against cell surface bound antigens	Contact dermatitis

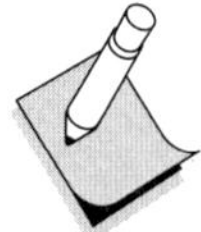

Most serious reactions may usually occur within minutes of exposure. Some patients, however, may experience a recurrence of symptoms in 4–8 hours.

Anaphylaxis and Anaphylactoid Reactions

Anaphylaxis is an **IgE**-mediated systemic, immediate hypersensitivity reaction to a specific antigen. IgE causes release of histamine, serotonin, leukotrienes, and prostaglandins from basophils and mast cells. Common causes are listed in Table 9.13.

Anaphylactoid reactions result from **direct release** (no IgE) of mediators listed above. Common causes are listed in Table 9.13.

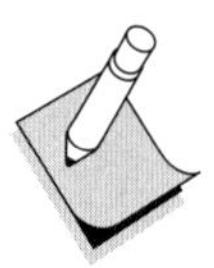

Penicillins and cephalosporins cause >100 anaphylaxis deaths each year in the United States and are among the most common causes of fatal anaphylaxis.

SYMPTOMS/EXAM

- Urticaria, pruritis, angioedema, wheezing, stridor, hypotension, abdominal cramps, nausea/vomiting, diarrhea
- Hypotension during anaphylaxis is a form of distributive shock (like sepsis) in which systemic vascular resistance is decreased. The skin should be warm.

DIAGNOSIS

- Clinical diagnosis: Angioedema, cutaneous manifestations, history of inciting antigen, respiratory, or cardiovascular collapse

TABLE 9.13. Common Causes of Anaphylaxis and Anaphylactoid Reactions

ANAPHYLAXIS	ANAPHYLACTOID REACTION
Medications (any prescription or OTC medications)	Radiographic IV dye
Food (shellfish, nuts, milk, eggs)	Blood products
Insect stings (hymenoptera)	Opioids (morphine)
Latex	Scombroid

TREATMENT

- Stop offending agent.
- Ensure adequate airway, supplemental O_2, IV fluids.
- **Epinephrine,** 0.3–0.5 mg (1:1000) IM (pediatric, 0.01 mL/kg)
- Generally, reserve epinephrine for patients with hypotension or airway complaints (swelling, voice change, difficulty breathing). Patients with cardiovascular collapse should receive intravenous epinephrine (0.1 mg IV over 5 minutes).
- **H_1 blocker** (diphenhydramine) and H_2 blocker (ranitidine, famotidine)
- **Steroids** (prednisone, methylprednisolone)
- Albuterol for bronchospasm
- **Glucagon:** For patients on β-blockers who are refractory to fluids and epinephrine
- Observe patients who receive epinephrine for at least 4 hours prior to discharge. Admit patients with recurrent symptoms.

A 40-year-old male with hypertension presents with angioedema involving his tongue. He was prescribed an ACE inhibitor last month. After treatment with steroids, H_1/H_2 blockers, and epinephrine, he reports feeling better but continues to have swelling on exam. Nasopharyngoscopy shows laryngeal edema. What is the patient's disposition?

Admit to ICU to closely monitor his airway.

Angioedema

Edema of the deeper dermal and subcutaneous layers of the skin

CAUSES

- Hereditary angioedema, an autosomal dominant hereditary disorder associated with C1 inhibitor deficiency
- ACE inhibitor (ACE-I) or angiotensin II receptor blockers use, mediated through bradykinin and substance P
- IgE-mediated hypersensitivity
- Direct mast cell stimulation

Sixty percent of cases of ACE-I-induced angioedema occurs within 1 week of starting the medication. It may, however, occur years after starting the medication.

SYMPTOMS/EXAM

- Edema may occur anywhere in the body but most concerning is its involvement with tongue, face, and neck.
- Other common locations involve hands, feet, eyelids, and scrotum.
- Upper airway involvement may lead to dyspnea, cough, hoarseness, stridor.

DIAGNOSIS

- Clinical diagnosis but may obtain a C4 level to screen for hereditary angioedema (HAE); the C4 level is usually low in affected individuals
- Nasopharyngoscopy can be used to evaluate for laryngeal edema.

TREATMENT

- Stop offending medication.
- First-line agent = antihistamines (H_1/H_2 blockers).
- Epinephrine can be used for severe cases.
- Corticosteroids may help limit response.

TABLE 9.14. Common Causes of Urticaria

Drugs	PCN, sulfa, ASA, local anesthetics, diuretics, NSAIDs, morphine, codeine, progesterone
Infection	EBV, HBV, coxsackie, parasitic infections
Environmental	Heat, cold, exercise, metals, animal saliva
Food	Fish, eggs, nuts, shellfish, fruits
Other	Latex, pregnancy, malignancy

- C1-inhibitor replacement or fresh frozen plasma (contains C1 inhibitor) may shorten duration, if hereditary angioedema.
- Epinephrine, antihistamines, and steroids are of limited benefit in hereditary angioedema and uncertain benefit in ACE-I and ARB angioedema.

Urticaria (Hives)

Pruritic, raised, erythematous, well-demarcated skin lesions; causes listed in Table 9.14

Treatment

- Avoid causative agent.
- Antihistamines: first or second generation
- Steroids and/or epinephrine for severe cases

Serum Sickness

A **type III (immune complex) hypersensitivity reaction,** serum sickness results when injection of an offending agent (see Table 9.15) results in antigen-antibody complex formation. These complexes deposit in vessel walls and result in activation of the complement cascade.

Symptoms/Exam

- Onset of symptoms is typically 7–10 days after exposure to causative agent.
- Fever, arthralgias, and malaise (flulike symptoms)
- Rash (most commonly angioedema/urticaraia)

TABLE 9.15. Common Causes of Serum Sickness

Medications	Envenomation
Antibiotics (eg, PCN, sulfonamides)	Hymenoptera
Phenytoin	
Thiazide diuretics	
Barbiturates	
Horse serum antivenin	

DIAGNOSIS

- Clinical diagnosis with history of inciting agent
- Serum complement (C3,C4) levels will be decreased.

TREATMENT

- Stop offending agent.
- Antihistamines, NSAIDs, steroids
- Plasmaphoresis for severe symptoms is not responsive to other treatments.

*Serum sickness occurs 6–21 days after exposure to foreign antigen or 1–4 days after a reexposure. Symptoms that occur during the initial treatment of a crotalidae envenomation are **not** due to serum sickness.*

INFLAMMATORY DISORDERS

Reiter's Syndrome

Seronegative spondyloarthropathy that is predominantly seen in young males. The triad of symptoms is usually preceded by an infection caused by *Chlamydia*, *Shigella*, or *Salmonella*. The syndrome lasts from one to several months and may recur.

Reiter's syndrome symptoms:

Can't see (conjunctivitis)
Can't pee (urethritis)
Can't climb a tree (arthritis).

SYMPTOMS/EXAM

- Asymmetric oligoarthritis: Especially of lower extremities
- Urethritis
- Conjunctivitis

TREATMENT

- Treat urethritis for *Chlamydia* and *Gonorrhea* because of frequency of coexisting infection.
- Patients with recurrent ocular inflammation may require immunosuppresants.
- NSAIDs for arthritis

SLE is associated with accelerated ischemic coronary artery disease, and has earned, along with diabetes, the status of "CAD-risk equivalent."

Systemic Lupus Erythematosus

This multisystem inflammatory disorder is mediated by **autoantibodies**. SLE is usually first diagnosed in women of childbearing age. Disease course is highly variable and patients may have acute flares. Drug-induced SLE is often reversible.

SYMPTOMS/EXAM

- Constitution symptoms, including fatigue, malaise, weight loss, fever
- Malar or discoid rash, photosensitivity
- Oral ulcerations
- Arthralgias, arthritis, myalgias
- Serositis: Pleuritis, pericarditis
- Seizure, stroke, psychosis

DIAGNOSIS

- Hematologic findings include hemolytic anemia, thrombocytopenia, leukopenia.
- Persistent proteinuria (nephritis) is common.
- The presence of four of 11 criteria outlined in mnemonic DOPAMINE RASH is diagnostic.
- During acute flares, there is a decrease in C3, C4 levels but an increase in ESR and CRP levels.

SLE criteria—

DOPAMINE RASH
Discoid rash
Oral ulcers
Photosensitive rash
Arthritis
Malar rash
Immunologic criteria (+anti-dsDNA test or +anti-Sm test)
NEeurologic or psychiatric symptoms
Renal disease
ANA+
Serositis (pleural, pericardial, peritoneal)
Hematologic disorders

> ***Drugs That induce SLE–***
>
> **HIPPS**
> **H**ydralazine
> **I**NH
> **P**henytoin
> **P**rocainamide
> **S**ulfonamides

TREATMENT

- NSAIDs for arthritis, arthralgias, serositis
- Hydroxychloroquine for rash, malaise, arthralgias
- Steroids for life-threatening manifestations, acute flares, symptoms refractory to conservative therapy
- Immunosuppressive therapy

COMPLICATIONS

- Nephrotic syndrome or renal failure
- Purulent pericarditis (*S. aureus*)
- Pleural effusion/tamponade
- Interstitial lung disease, pulmonary hypertension
- Coronary artery vasculitis with acute myocardial infarction
- Libman-Sacks endocarditis: A noninfectious endocarditis
- Mesenteric vasculitis

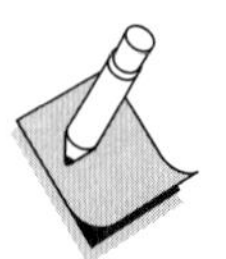

The ESR is elevated above 50 mm/hr in most patients with giant cell arteritis. Start prednisone 1–2 mg/kg/day immediately to prevent irreversible blindness.

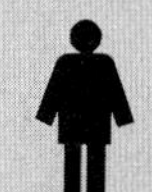

A 70-year-old woman presents with new-onset severe, throbbing, unilateral headache. She has also noted proximal muscle weakness and blurry vision. Physical exam shows tender, pulseless temporal artery and vision loss. What's the suspected diagnosis and next step?

Temporal arteritis (giant cell arteritis). The patient will require immediate high-dose oral steroids and temporal artery biopsy within 1–2 days.

Vasculitis

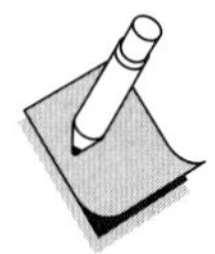

The classic case of Henoch-Schönlein purpura is a boy between 2 and 11 years old who presents with palpable purpura on his legs, edema, and abdominal pain with a history of recent URI.

Vasculitis is inflammation and necrosis of blood vessels leading to tissue damage. This may affect different types and sizes of blood vessels. See Tables 9.16, 9.17, and 9.18.

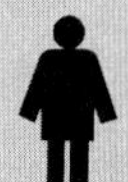

An infant is status post–cardiac transplant for myocarditis. How might acute cardiac rejection present?

Feeding intolerance, fever, or fussiness.

TABLE 9.16. Large Vessel Vasculitis

SYNDROME	SIGNS/SYMPTOMS	DIAGNOSIS	TREATMENT
Giant cell arteritis	Involvement of branches of carotid artery → headache, jaw claudication, scalp tenderness, vision changes.	Temporal artery biopsy ESR >50 mm/hr	Prednisone
Takayasu's arteritis	Involvement of aorta and major branches → finger ischemia, arm claudication.	Aortic arch arteriogram	Prednisone

TABLE 9.17. Medium Vessel Vasculitis

SYNDROME	SIGNS/SYMPTOMS	DIAGNOSIS	TREATMENT
Polyartertis nodosa	Skin ulcers Nephritis Mesenteric ischemia	Biopsy (skin, kidney) Mesenteric angiogram HBV/HCV testing	Prednisone Cyclophosphamide
Wegener granulomatosis	Sinusitis Pulmonary infiltrates Nephritis	c-ANCA Lung biopsy	Prednisone Cyclophosphamide
Behçet disease	Recurrent painful oral and genital ulcers Uveitis, iritis, or optic neuritis	Biopsy of affected tissue	Prednisone Immunosuppressants
Microscopic polyangitis	Pulmonary infiltrates Nephritis	p-ANCA Renal biopsy	Cyclophosphamide

TRANSPLANT REJECTION

Immunosuppressants for transplant recipients:

- **Cyclosporine** (Sandimmune, Neoral): Acute toxicity causes reversible vasoconstriction and renal ischemia. Ca channel blockers and antibiotics (doxycylcine, erythromycin) can increase cyclosporine levels.
- **Mycophenolate** (Cellcept): Side effects include diarrhea, N/V, leukopenia.
- Tacrolimus (Prograf): Side effects include nephrotoxicity, seizures, neuropathy.
- Corticosteroids

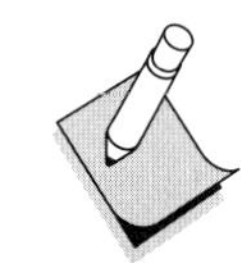

A transplant patient's failure to take immunosuppressant medications should be considered an emergency.

TABLE 9.18. Small Vessel Vasculitis

SYNDROME	SIGNS/SYMPTOMS	DIAGNOSIS	TREATMENT
Hypersensitivity vasculitis	Palpable purpura	Skin biopsy	Prednisone
Henoch-Schonlein purpura	Palpable purpura (buttocks, lower extremities) Abdominal pain, N/V/D Hematuria	Skin biopsy Rectal biopsy	Supportive Prednisone
Goodpasture's syndrome	Cough and dyspnea Hemoptysis Glomerulonephritis	Renal or lung biopsy showing basement membrane antibodies	Supportive Prednisone Cyclophosphamide Plasmapheresis

There are three categories of transplant rejection: Hyperacute, acute, and chronic.

- **Hyperacute**: Occurs from a few minutes to hours after surgery and results in irreversible graft destruction
- **Acute**: Generally occurs 1–12 weeks after transplant and may be reversed
- **Chronic**: Progressive, insidious decline results in tissue fibrosis, ischemia, and death; no effective therapy

Renal Transplant

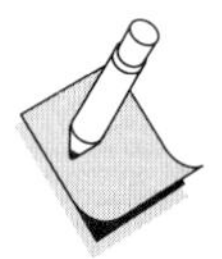

Complications in transplant patients:
Rejection
Infection
Immunosuppressant drug ***toxicity***

Symptoms/Exam

- Tenderness over allograft (in the left or right iliac fossa)
- Decreased urine output, increased edema, and weight gain
- Elevated serum creatinine
- Worsening hypertension

Differential

- Volume contraction, cyclosporine nephrotoxicity

Diagnosis

- UA, chemistries, renal ultrasound, cyclosporine level

Treatment

- Methylprednisolone, 500 mg IV

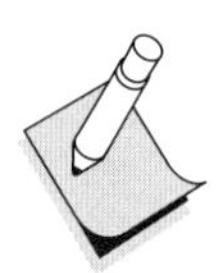

A subtle rise in creatinine may be the only indication of acute rejection of a transplanted kidney.

Lung Transplant

Symptoms/Exam

- Cough, dyspnea
- Chest tightness
- Fever (>0.5 degrees C above baseline)

Differential

- Infection

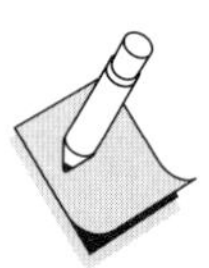

Findings on CXR for acute lung rejection are usually nonspecific and may include perihilar infiltrates, interstitial edema, pleural effusions.

Diagnosis

- CXR, ABG, spirometry, drug levels

Treatment

- Methylpredisolone, 500 mg–1 g IV

Heart Transplant

Symptoms/Exam

- Patient may be asymptomatic or complain of generalized fatigue.
- Heart failure: Orthopnea, JVD, PND
- Dysrhythmias

Diagnosis

- ECG, cardiac enzymes

Treatment

- Methylprednisolone, 1 g IV
- Isoproterenol for bradydysrhythmias
- Dopamine or dobutamine for hypotension

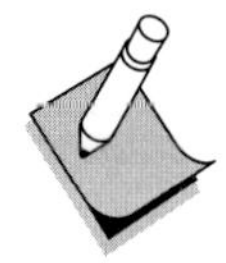

***Atropine does not increase HR** in patients with a heart transplant. Use isoproterenol, dopamine, or dobutamine.*

Transplanted hearts are denervated. Myocardial ischemia will not present with angina but will present as heart failure or with sudden death.

Liver Transplant

Symptoms/Exam

- Fever
- Anorexia
- Abdominal pain, ascites
- Decreased bile output or change in color
- Abnormal liver function tests

Differential

- Vascular thrombosis, biliary anastomotic leak/obstruction, infection, drug toxicity

Diagnosis

- CBC, chemistries, coagulation panel, cultures, hepatic ultrasound

Treatment

- Methylprednisolone, 500 mg 1 g IV
- Broad spectrum antibiotics if biliary leak is present

INFECTION IN TRANSPLANT RECIPIENTS

Infection is the primary cause of death after transplantation and must be considered in all transplant recipients who appear to be suffering from rejection. Transplant recipients are at risk of infections transmitted from donor to recipient at the time of transplantation, or reactivation of latent infections that become symptomatic following the initiation of immunosuppressive treatment.

Infections in the First Month

- Bacteria—most often related to the surgery itself (eg, IV lines, intubation, nosocomial pathogens).
- Candida
- HSV

Infections From First to Sixth Month

- Viruses
  - **CMV:** Presents with pneumonitis, gastrointestinal, renal, skin, or CNS infection and can trigger or exacerbate organ rejection; treat with IV ganciclovir
  - EBV—clinical effects similar to CMV, also causes a mononucleosis-like syndrome.
  - Hepatitis

*Symptomatic infection with **CMV** begins a median of 40 days after transplantation.*

- Listeria
- Pneumocystic
- Aspergillosis

Infections After 6 Months

- Chronic viral infections
  - CMV, EBV, hepatitis B or C, HSV
  - **Varicella-zoster virus:** Primacy varicella infection can result in disseminated diseases. Seronegative patients should receive varicella-zoster immune globulin after exposure to chickenpox or zoster. Hospitalization with IV acyclovir should be considered in transplant patients with cutaneous herpes zoster.
- Increased risk of community-acquired infections (pneumonia, UTIs)
- Also consider *Strongyloides* hyperinfection syndrome, *Tuberculosis*, *Toxoplasmosis*, fungal infections.

IMMUNODEFICIENCY/IMMUNOSUPPRESSION

Immunodeficiency results in increased susceptibility to infection. Patients with defects in **antibody-mediated** immunity (also known as humoral or B-cell–mediated immunity) are at particularly increased risk of infection by encapsulated bacteria. By contrast, **cellular** immunity (also known as T-cell–mediated immunity) is more important in protecting patients against viral, intracellular, bacterial, and fungal infections as well as malignancies.

Evaluation for suspected immunodeficiency:

- CBC with differential, quantitative immunoglobulin levels, complement levels, HIV test

Antibody-Mediated Immune Dysfunction

- IgA deficiency (a selective immunoglobulin deficiency)
  - Recurrent sinus and pulmonary infections
  - At risk for developing severe transfusion reactions
- Common variable immunodeficiency (CVID)
  - Low or dysfunctional IgG, IgA, IgM antibodies
  - Recurrent sinus and pulmonary infections
- Hyper-IgE syndrome (Job syndrome)
  - Recurrent pyogenic infections of the skin and lower respiratory tract
- Multiple myeloma
  - Defect in production of opsonizing antibodies
- Splenectomy patients
  - Increased susceptibility to encapsulated bacteria
  - Administer pneumococcal, meningococcal, *H. influenzae* type B vaccines.

Cellular Immune Dysfunction

- Congenital causes:
  - Bruton agammaglobulinemia
    - Recurrent bacterial infections
    - DiGeorge syndrome
    - Recurrent viral, fungal, and protozoan infections

- Chronic mucocutaneous candiasis
  - Recurrent candida infections
- Severe combined immunodeficiency syndrome
  - Recurrent viral, bacterial, fungal, and protozoan infections
- Wiskott-Aldrich syndrome
  - Recurrent pyogenic infections, eczema, thrombocytopenia.

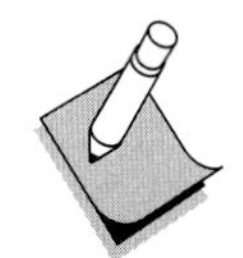

Patients with cellular immune dysfunction are susceptible to intracellular infections including listeria, mycobacterium, cryptococcus, fungi, HSV, CMV, and Pneumocystis carinii.

- Hodgkin disease
  - Impaired delayed type hypersensitivity recall to antigens
- AIDS
  - Lymphopenia and depleted CD4 T cell
  - Opportunistic infections with PCP, *Cryptococcus meningitis*, CNS toxoplasmosis, *Mycobacterium avium* complex, tuberculosis, candiasis, CMV
  - Please see section on AIDS for further discussion.
- Treatment of transplant rejection
  - Immunosuppressive therapies

Neutropenia

- Absolute neutrophil count <500 cells/μL
- Susceptible to pseudomonas and staphylococci infection
- May have bacteremia, pneumonia, perirectal/perineal infections

Medical Therapies

- Various medications may cause reduced resistance to infections.
  - Glucocorticoids, methotrexate, azathioprine, mycophenolate mofetil, cyclophosphamide, tumor necrosis factors inhibitors, chemotherapeutic agents
- Plasmaphoresis
  - Removal of plasma from the body also removes antibodies, which leaves the body susceptible to bacterial infection.
- Radiation
  - May impair production of leukocytes

Diabetes Mellitus

- Diabetics have a higher incidence of infections.
  - Cystitis, pyelonephritis, candida vulvovaginitis, pneumonia, bronchitis, bacteremia, lower-extremity infections, surgical wound infections, tuberculosis, otitis externa, mucormycosis, Fournier gangrene
- Mechanisms of increased susceptibility to infection:
  - Impaired neutrophil function
  - Circulatory insufficiency, leading to delayed response to infection
  - Sensory deficits, causing decreased awareness of skin trauma
  - Autonomic dysfunction, causing urinary retention

CHAPTER 10

Thoracic and Respiratory Disorders

Christian Merlo, MD, MPH and Lauren Grossman, MD, MS

SIGNS AND SYMPTOMS

Cough

CAUSES

Cough results from stimulation of irritant receptors in the larynx, trachea, and major bronchi. Triggers include mucus, allergens, gastric acid (and more). Likely etiologies differ depending on whether the cough is acute or chronic (>3-week duration).

Acute Cough

- Acute upper respiratory infection (most common)
- Lower respiratory infection
- Postnasal drip (rhinitis, sinusitis)
- Asthma/COPD exacerbation
- Airway foreign body
- CHF
- Aspiration (disordered swallow)

Chronic Cough

- Chronic bronchitis/smoking
- Postnasal drip (rhinitis, sinusitis)
- GERD
- Asthma
- ACE inhibitor
- Think about *Bordetella pertussis.*
- Other causes include bronchiectasis, CHF, environmental irritants, and aspiration.

SYMPTOMS/EXAM

- Inquire about postnasal drip symptoms, asthma, GERD, treatment with ACEIs, and smoking.
- Determine if cough is productive (infection, bronchiectasis) or bloody (malignancy, infection, Goodpasture syndrome, Wegener granulomatosis).
- The physical exam should focus on the nasal mucosa, lungs, heart, and extremities (for clubbing).

DIAGNOSIS/TREATMENT

- Evaluation should be guided by history and exam findings (eg, CXR if abnormal lung sounds).
- Treatment should be geared to underlying cause.

Dyspnea

Dyspnea is the uncomfortable awareness of difficult, labored, or unpleasant breathing. Normal resting patients are unaware of the act of breathing. For most patients presenting with dyspnea, there is either a cardiac or pulmonary cause of their symptoms (see Table 10.1). Other, less common, causes include psychogenic factors, GERD, and deconditioning.

SYMPTOMS/EXAM

Look for signs of impending respiratory failure (severe tachypnea/tachycardia, stridor, agitation) and evidence for underlying etiology (eg, rash and hypotension with anaphylaxis).

THORACIC AND RESPIRATORY DISORDERS

TABLE 10.1. Differential Diagnosis of Dyspnea

	ACUTE DYSPNEA (MINUTES TO HOURS)	CHRONIC DYSPNEA (DAYS TO YEARS)
Pulmonary disorders	Pneumonia/bronchitis Pulmonary embolism Pneumothorax Bronchospasm (asthma, COPD) Obstruction (anaphylaxis, aspiration)	COPD Asthma Intertstitial lung disease Pulmonary hypertension
Cardiovascular disorders	Ischemia CHF Cardiac tamponade	Cardiomyopathy

DIAGNOSIS/TREATMENT

- Conduct a systematic diagnostic and therapeutic evaluation for the cause of dyspnea.
- Obtain a CXR at minimum. Obtain other studies (CT-PE, echocardiogram) based on clinical suspicion.

TREATMENT

Treat underlying condition.

Wheezing

A wheeze is a continuous musical sound lasting >100 msec. Wheezes can be high or low pitched, consist of a single or multiple tones, and occur during inspiration or expiration.

Wheezing is most likely to occur in obstructed airways (see Table 10.2) but may occasionally be heard in a normal airway.

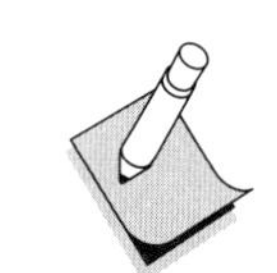

All that wheezes is not asthma.

SYMPTOMS/EXAM

Look for symptoms/findings that suggest an underlying cause (eg, unilateral wheezing in toddler suggesting foreign body aspiration).

DIFFERENTIAL

- **Rhonchi**: Lower in pitch and longer in duration; a "snoring" quality
- **Crackles**: Intermittent, explosive sounds of very brief duration; fine crackles are higher pitched than coarse crackles

DIAGNOSIS

- Conduct a systematic diagnostic and therapeutic evaluation for the cause of wheezing.
- If no prior history of wheezing, obtain a CXR at minimum. Obtain other studies based on clinical suspicion.

TREATMENT

Treat underlying disorder.

TABLE 10.2. **Causes of Wheezing**

Upper airway (more likely to be stridor, may have element of wheezing)
Angioedema: allergic, ACE inhibitor, idiopathic
Foreign body
Infection: croup, epiglottis, tracheitis
Lower airway
Asthma
Transient airway hyperreactivity (usually caused by infection or irritation)
Bronchiolitis
COPD
Foreign body
Cardiovascular
Cardiogenic pulmonary edema ("cardiac asthma")
Noncardiogenic pulmonary edema (ARDS)
Pulmonary embolus (rare)
Psychogenic

(Reproduced, with permission, from Tintinalli JE Kelen GD, Stapczynski JS. *Emergency Medicine: A Comprehensive Study Guide,* 6th ed. New York: McGraw-Hill, 2004:440.)

Cyanosis

Cyanosis is a bluish discoloration of the skin due to the presence of deoxygenated hemoglobin (deoxyhemoglobin or abnormal hemoglobin) in skin capillaries. It is generally detected when there is 5 g/dL (**absolute level**) of deoxygenated hemoglobin in the circulating capillary blood, although it can sometimes be detected at lower levels. The presence of cyanosis suggests (but does not diagnose) tissue hypoxia.

Central Cyanosis

- When abnormal or deoxygenated hemoglobin is circulated
- **Causes** include:
  - R to L cardiac shunt
  - V/Q mismatch (eg, PE, polycythemia)
  - Impaired diffusion (eg, interstitial fibrosis)
  - Hemoglobinopathy (eg, methemoglobinemia)
  - Toxins (eg, cyanide)
  - Polycythemia
  - High altitude

Peripheral Cyanosis

- This is due to slowing of flow of normally oxygenated hemoglobin to the extremity or extremities resulting in ↑ O_2 extraction.
- Causes include shock and arterial/venous obstruction (eg, thrombus, vasoconstriction).

Symptoms/Exam

- Central cyanosis is best seen on perioral skin, oral mucosa, or conjunctivae.
- Look for symptoms/findings that suggest an underlying cause (eg, LE cyanosis, hypotension, and abdominal pain in ruptured AAA, murmur and central cyanosis in cardiac shunt).

DIFFERENTIAL

Pseudocyanosis from heavy metals or drugs (amiodarone, phenothiazine); skin does not blanch with pressure

DIAGNOSIS

- Conduct a systematic diagnostic and therapeutic evaluation for the cause of cyanosis.
- The presence of clubbing suggests a chronic hypoxemic state.
- If central cyanosis is present, the presence of an abnormal form of hemoglobin must first be ruled out by co-oximetry.
- Other tests that may be helpful include a CBC and CXR.

TREATMENT

- Administer supplemental O_2, although this will not improve cyanosis in hemoglobinopathy, cyanide poisoning, and anatomic shunt.
- Treat underlying cause.

Hemoptysis

Defined as the coughing up of blood from the lower (below larynx) respiratory tract. Hemoptysis can range from blood-streaked sputum to life-threatening bleeding. **Massive hemoptysis** carries a high mortality and is defined as the coughing up of >100–600 mL of blood in a 24-hour period.

Bronchitis, bronchogenic carcinoma, and bronchiectasis are the most common causes of hemoptysis (see Table 10.3), but up to 30% of patients have no identifiable cause even after extensive evaluation.

TABLE 10.3. Causes of Hemoptysis

MOST COMMON CAUSES	OTHER CAUSES
Bronchitis	Infection
Lung neoplasm	Pneumonia
Bronchiectasis	Aspergilloma
	Lung abscess
	TB
	Autoimmune disorder
	Goodpasture syndrome
	Wegener granulomatosis
	Cardiovascular
	Pulmonary embolism
	Arteriovenous malformation
	Mitral stenosis
	CHF
	Arterial-tracheal/bronchial fistula
	Bleeding disorder
	Trauma
	Cystic fibrosis

Symptoms/Exam

Historical clues that suggest a cause:

- A history of TB or sarcoidosis → aspergilloma.
- Frequent, multiple episodes of pneumonia as a child → bronchiectasis.
- A diastolic heart murmur → mitral stenosis.
- A history of epistaxis, telangiectasias, and a bruit in the posterior aspect of the lungs → hereditary hemorrhagic telangiectasia with a ruptured pulmonary AVM.
- Renal insufficiency and hemoptysis → Wegener granulomatosis or Goodpasture syndrome.
- Weight loss, tobacco abuse, and cachexia → malignancy.

Differential

Blood expectorated from the upper respiratory tract and the upper GI tract can mimic blood coming from the trachea and below.

Diagnosis

- Obtain a CXR in all patients with hemoptysis.
- Laboratory studies include CBC with differential, coagulation studies, UA, BUN, creatinine.
- Further diagnostic options include high-resolution CT scan with contrast (stable patients) and bronchoscopy.

Treatment

Nonmassive Hemoptysis

- Treatment is directed at the specific cause (eg, antibiotics for superinfected aspergilloma).

Massive hemoptysis:

- Treatment is directed toward bringing about abrupt cessation of bleeding.
- Place the patient with bleeding-side down to maximize V/Q ratio.
- Intubate with a large bore single-lumen endotracheal tube; selectively intubate the nonbleeding mainstem bronchus, when possible. Double-lumen endotracheal tubes are **not** preferred (difficult to place, small lumens).
- Urgent bronchoscopy may help localize the site of bleeding.
- Angiography of the bronchial arteries (a more common site of bleeding than the pulmonary arteries) has been shown to identify the bleeding site in >90% of patients.
- When angiography is combined with embolization, bleeding can successfully be stopped in >90% of cases.
- Emergency surgery for massive hemoptysis is controversial and usually reserved for those with failed embolization.

ACUTE UPPER AIRWAY OBSTRUCTION

The upper airway extends from the lips and nares to the first tracheal ring. When upper airway obstruction is present, patients typically develop dyspnea when the obstruction is <8 mm in diameter and stridor when the diameter is <5 mm.

Causes

- **Infection:** Epiglottitis, croup, retropharyngeal abscess, peritonsillar abscess, Ludwig angina
- **Medical conditions:** Anaphylaxis, angioedema, laryngospasm, neoplasm
- **Trauma:** Blunt or penetrating trauma; tongue in presence of altered mental status
- **Physical and chemical agents:** Foreign body, burn, caustic ingestion

Symptoms/Exam

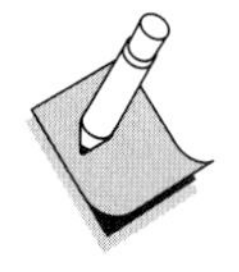

__Inspiratory__ stridor is associated with obstruction above the glottis. __Expiratory__ stridor is more likely to result from intrathoracic obstruction.

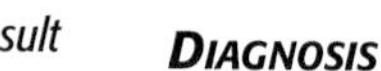

- The patient will typically appear anxious or agitated and will often prefer to sit upright.
- Dyspnea, stridor
- Drooling or spitting secretions
- Other symptoms depend on underlying cause (eg, fever and sore throat with epiglottitis).

Diagnosis

- Often based on clinical presentation alone
- **Soft-tissue neck XR:** May reveal foreign body or inflammation (**steeple sign,** which is supraglottic swelling on the AP view typically found in croup; **thumbprint sign** in epiglottitis; or an **irregular tracheal margin** in bacterial tracheitis)
- **Direct laryngoscopy:** Can define degree of obstruction

Treatment

- Treatment depends on the underlying cause of the obstruction.
- Allow the patient to maintain a position of comfort (typically a sniffing position) and provide supplemental O_2.
- Immediate procedures to control the airway are needed if the obstruction is severe or progressing.
- If foreign body is present or suspected:
  - Heimlich maneuver (see Chapter 1) if patient is awake
  - Direct laryngoscopy and removal with Magill forceps if patient is unconscious

HYPOXEMIA

Defined as a ↓ in blood O_2 (in general, a PaO_2 of <60 mmHg). Hypoxemia may (or may not) result in inadequate delivery of O_2 to tissues (tissue hypoxia). Five distinct causes or a combination thereof may → hypoxemia (see Table 10.4).

Symptoms/Exam

Hypoxemia can → **tissue hypoxia** and cause impaired judgment, motor dysfunction, fatigue, drowsiness, respiratory distress, and respiratory failure.

Diagnosis

- Formal diagnosis of hypoxemia requires arterial blood gas analysis.
- Perform history, examination, and obtain studies (eg, CXR, CT-PE), as indicated, to search for underlying cause.
- Calculate the alveolar-arterial (A-a) O_2 gradient (to narrow the etiology):

TABLE 10.4. Etiologies of Hypoxemia

CAUSE	MECHANISM	DISEASE STATES	COMMENTS
Reduced inspired O_2	O_2 is replaced by other gases *or* low total O_2	Enclosed spaces, fire High altitude, air travel	Normal alveolar-arterial (A-a) gradient
Diffusion abnormality	Reduction in diffusion capacity → low PaO_2	Interstitial lung disease	An uncommon cause of hypoxemic respiratory failure
Hypoventilation	↓ Minute ventilation results in ↑ $PaCO_2$ and ↓ PaO_2	See Table 10.5.	Normal A-a gradient
Ventilation-perfusion (V/Q) mismatch	Altered ratio of perfusion to ventilation	Pulmonary embolus, pulmonary hypertension, COPD, asthma	↑ A-a gradient. PaO_2 corrects with supplemental O_2
Shunt	Physiologic shunt: Perfusion to nonventilated lung. Anatomic shunt: Communication between the arterial and venous systems.	ARDS, pneumonia Pulmonary AVM, congenital heart disease, patent foramen ovale with right-to-left flow	↑ A-a gradient. PaO_2 does not correct with supplemental O_2

THORACIC AND RESPIRATORY DISORDERS

- A-a gradient = $PiO_2 - (PaO_2 - PaCO_2/8)$.
- Assuming sea level, an FiO_2 of 0.21 and 37°C, PiO_2 becomes 150 mmHg.
- A conservative estimate of a normal A-a gradient is 4 + age (years) / 4.

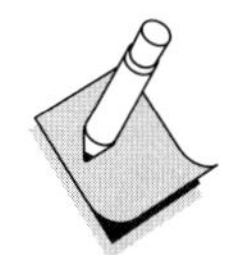

Hypoxemia due to shunt does not correct with 100% O_2 therapy.

TREATMENT

- All patients with hypoxemia should be treated with supplemental O_2. However, be careful with chronic COPD patients whose respiratory drive is O_2 dependent. No improvement with supplemental O_2? Suspect anatomic shunt.
- Treat underlying cause.

HYPERCARBIA

Hypercarbia is elevated CO_2 in the blood ($PaCO_2$ > 45 mmHg). It is nearly always a result of alveolar hypoventilation from a variety of disease processes. In rare cases, this can be the result of exogenous CO_2 poisoning (dry ice, volcanic eruption).

ETIOLOGIES

See Table 10.5.

TREATMENT

- Treatment depends on underlying cause (eg, narcan in opiate-induced hypoventilation).
- In all cases, provide supplemental O_2 and support ventilation via bag-valve mask ventilation, noninvasive positive-pressure ventilation, or intubation (depending on cause).

TABLE 10.5. Etiologies of Hypercarbia

CAUSE	MECHANISM	DISEASE STATES
Depressed central respiratory drive	↓ Minute ventilation	Drug overdose CNS lesion/infarction Central sleep apnea Hypothyroidism
Peripheral nerve disorders	Same as above	Guillain-Barré syndrome ALS Poliomyelitis West Nile virus
Neuromuscular junction disorders	Same as above	Myasthenia gravis, botulism
Muscle disorders	Same as above	Muscular dystrophy Glycogen storage disease
Lung disorders	↓ Alveolar ventilation due to obstructive lung disease	COPD Asthma Cystic fibrosis
Chest wall disorders	Chest wall mechanics are altered, leading to ↓ alveolar ventilation.	Kyphoscoliosis Massive obesity

ASTHMA

Reactive airway disease consists of three classical components: **Airway inflammation, bronchial hyperresponsiveness, and reversible airflow obstruction.** Asthma is more prevalent in blacks than whites, and, in childhood, asthma is more prevalent in boys than girls.

CAUSES

Common triggers include respiratory infections, environmental allergens/irritants, weather changes, and exercise. Rarer causes include aspirin or NSAID hypersensitivity, β-blocker use, and emotional stressors.

Risk factors for death include:

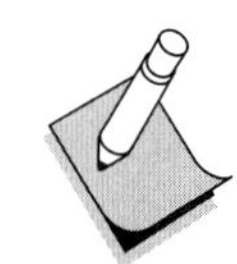

Death due to asthma is rising.

- Previous ICU admission/intubation
- More than two hospitalizations or three ED visits in the past year
- Use of corticosteroids or >2 canisters of β_2 agonist MDIs per month
- Difficulty perceiving presence or severity of airflow obstruction
- Low socioeconomic status
- Illicit drug use
- Serious comorbidities

SYMPTOMS/EXAM

- Dyspnea, wheezing, coughing, chest tightness
- Fever and purulent sputum usually represent a complicating process such as pneumonia.

- Wheezes are usually present, but may be absent in either mild or severe cases (minimal airflow). Presence of inspiratory wheezing or stridor should prompt evaluation for upper airway obstruction.
- Prolonged expiratory phase
- Findings suggestive of **severe airway obstruction** include:
  - Poor air movement that can manifest itself as **absence of wheezing**
  - Tachypnea (>30 bpm)
  - Tachycardia (>130 bpm)
  - Pulsus paradoxus (>15 mmHg)
  - Accessory respiratory muscle use
  - Altered mental status
  - Hypoxemia
  - Peak expiratory flow rate (PEF) < 100 L/min before treatment or PEF < 300 L/min after aggressive treatment.

DIFFERENTIAL

- "**All that wheezes is not asthma.**" Consider CHF, upper airway obstruction, foreign-body aspiration, vocal cord dysfunction.
- Other causes include COPD, bronchiectasis, CF.

DIAGNOSIS

- **PEF** is most predictive of the severity of exacerbation and should guide therapy. PEF <100 is considered severe exacerbation.
- **Pulse oximetry** is helpful to establish adequate oxygenation, but it is not a good indicator of ventilation. **Capnography** is the noninvasive method of choice for monitoring ventilation.
- **ABG analysis** does not predict clinical outcome and should not supersede clinical findings in determining need for intubation. However, stages of asthma have been described based on ABG findings (see Table 10.6).
- **CXR** is usually normal or show hyperinflation and is necessary only when a secondary process is suspected such as pneumonia, CHF, pneumothorax, or foreign body. Obtain CXR for all first episodes of wheezing.

TREATMENT

Treatment should proceed as follows (see Table 10.7):

- **O_2 therapy** to keep the O_2 saturation >90%.
- **Inhaled β_2-agonist**
  - Amount and frequency depends on the degree of airflow obstruction.
  - **Drug delivery is equivalent** with handheld MDIs and nebulizer therapy in multiple studies; however, the latter is clinically more effective in patients who are in acute distress.
  - **Combination therapy** with ipratropium bromide should be used for the first three treatments in all patients with severe exacerbations.

TABLE 10.6. ABG Findings in Asthma

SEVERITY	PH	P_{CO_2}	P_{O_2}
Mild	↑	↓	Normal
Moderate	Normal	Normal	↓
Severe	↓	↑	↓

THORACIC AND RESPIRATORY DISORDERS

TABLE 10.7. Treatment of Acute Asthma Exacerbations

ALL PATIENTS	SELECTED PATIENTS	NOT USEFUL/HARMFUL
Inhaled bronchodilators	Antibiotics	Theophylline
Corticosteroids	O_2-assisted ventilation	Injected bronchodilators
	Magnesium sulfate	Mucolytic agents

- **Systemic corticosteroids**
  - Oral and intravenous delivery equally effective
  - Decreases the need for hospitalization and subsequent relapse rate
  - Requires about 4 hours to take effect; so, **administer early**!
  - Discharged patients should continue oral therapy for 3–10 days.
- **Inhaled steroid therapy**
  - **Mainstay of outpatient treatment** for controlling exacerbations
  - Beware the expense of treatment.
- **Antibiotics** are generally unnecessary. Reserve for patients if an underlying bacterial pneumonia is suspected.
- **Magnesium sulfate** is somewhat controversial but has been shown to improve airflow obstruction in patients with severe exacerbations.
- **Heliox** may be helpful. Usually delivered in an 80% (helium)/20% (O_2) mixture. As the proportion of O_2 rises, this modality becomes less effective.
- **Assisted ventilation** in severe cases of ventilatory failure
  - **Noninvasive mechanical ventilation (BiPAP)** may be helpful but not as well established as in CHF and COPD.
  - **Mechanical ventilation:** Use low tidal volumes (<6 mL/kg) and low RRs (6–8 bpm) that allow maximum time for expiration.
  - Beware of auto-PEEP and breath stacking leading to barotrauma as asthma is primarily a **disease of prolonged expiratory phase**!

CHRONIC OBSTRUCTIVE PULMONARY DISEASE

This disease state is characterized by chronic airflow limitation that is no longer fully reversible. COPD is usually progressive and results from chronic bronchitis and emphysema.

- **Chronic bronchitis** is defined clinically as chronic productive cough for 3 consecutive months in 2 consecutive years.
- **Emphysema** is defined pathologically as abnormal enlargement of the airspaces distal to the terminal bronchioles, with wall destruction.
- The most important risk factor for developing COPD is cigarette smoking. α_1-Antitrypsin (AAT) deficiency is also a well-characterized genetic abnormality that predisposes individuals to the development of early onset COPD.

SYMPTOMS/EXAM

- Symptoms are usually not present until the individual has smoked >1 pack of cigarettes per day for 20 years.
- The patient typically presents with chronic cough in the fourth or fifth decade of life. Dyspnea usually occurs only with moderate exercise and not until the sixth or seventh decade of life.

- Chest wall hyperinflation, prolonged expiration, wheezing, and distant breath and heart sounds may be present.
- The patient may use accessory muscles and pursed-lip breathing **(pink puffer)**, and cyanosis may be present as well **(blue bloater)**. Neck vein distention, a tender liver, and lower-extremity edema suggest cor pulmonale.

DIFFERENTIAL

Acute bronchitis, asthma, bronchiectasis, CF, CHF

DIAGNOSIS

Along with a history and physical exam, testing modalities that are useful in diagnosing COPD and evaluating the disease progression include CXR, PFTs, and ABG analysis.

- **CXR:** Typically demonstrates ↓ lung markings, ↑ retrosternal airspace, and flattened diaphragms
- **PFTs:** Essential for diagnosis as well as for the evaluation of treatment and disease progression
- **ABG analysis:** Acute exacerbations show hypoxemia and hypercarbia, with acute respiratory acidosis
- **BODE index:** This is more effective than FEV_1 at predicting the risk of death from any cause in patients with COPD. The **BODE** index consists of:
  - BMI
  - Obstruction of airflow (FEV_1)
  - Dyspnea (as measured by the modified Medical Research Council dyspnea scale)
  - Exercise capacity (6-minute walk)

THORACIC AND RESPIRATORY DISORDERS

TREATMENT

- **Acute exacerbations:** Where possible, the cause of the exacerbation should be treated.
- **β_2-adrenergic** and **anticholinergic agents** are first-line therapy.
- Treatment includes **O_2 therapy** titrated to maintain an O_2 saturation of around 90%. *Excessive* O_2 administration may → hypercarbia from a ↓ respiratory drive or from ↑ V/Q mismatch, but O_2 therapy must not be withheld because of fears of hypercarbia.
- **Systemic corticosteroids** in oral or IV form help ↓ the length of exacerbations and improve FEV_1 in hospitalized patients.
- **Antibiotics** are recommended by the American Thoracic Society for patients with acute exacerbation who have a **change in sputum amount, consistency, or color.**
- **Noninvasive positive pressure ventilation** is of benefit for patients with **severe** acute exacerbations of COPD as it reduces in-hospital mortality, ↓ the need for intubation, and diminishes hospital length of stay.

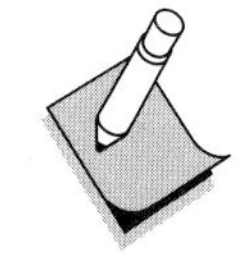

O_2 therapy is the only intervention known to ↑ life expectancy in hypoxemia COPD patients.

BRONCHIECTASIS

Defined as the irreversible dilatation and destruction of bronchi with inadequate clearance of mucus in the airways. Cycles of infection and inflammation → dilated airways and focal constrictive areas.

CAUSES

Causes of bronchiectasis include:

- Inability to clear secretions (cilliary abnormalities, CF)
- Severe or repeated episodes of pneumonia

- Recurrent aspiration (eg, severe GERD, disordered swallow)
- Lower airway obstruction with tumor

SYMPTOMS

Patients often have cough productive of yellow or green sputum together with dyspnea and hemoptysis.

EXAM

- Lung exam reveals crackles and wheezes.
- Acute exacerbations typically include changes in sputum production, ↑ dyspnea, ↑ cough and wheezing, fatigue, low-grade fever, ↓ pulmonary function, changes in chest sounds, and radiographic changes.

DIFFERENTIAL

COPD, interstitial fibrosis, pneumonia, asthma

DIAGNOSIS

- Suspect based on history and patient risk factors
- Evaluation primarily consists of PFTS and chest CT.

TREATMENT

- **Inhaled bronchodilators:** Helpful when used routinely as many patients have hyperresponsiveness that likely results from airway inflammation
- **Inhaled corticosteroids:** Can reduce inflammation and improve dyspnea, cough, and pulmonary function in severe cases
- **Antibiotics:** The standard of care for acute exacerbations, a reasonable first-line choice would include a fluoroquinolone.
- Other treatment aimed toward specific underlying cause (eg, percussive vests to aid in clearance of secretions in patients with CF)
- **Surgical resection** remains an option for patients with localized focal bronchiectasis.
- **Double-lung transplantation** has been performed in patients with severe bronchiectasis.

COMMUNITY-ACQUIRED PNEUMONIA

An infection of the lower respiratory tract in an individual who has not been recently hospitalized

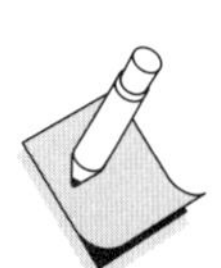

S. pneumoniae and S. aureus are common causes of postinfluenza pneumonia.

CAUSES

The single leading cause of community-acquired pneumonia is *Streptococcus pneumoniae*. Common organisms are listed in Table 10.8. Less common pathogens will be discussed further.

PATHOPHYSIOLOGY

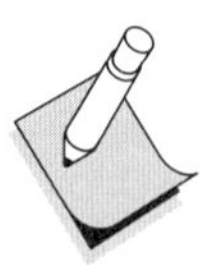

Pneumonia in alcoholics is most likely due to S. pneumoniae, anaerobes, or coliforms.

- Decreased mucociliary clearance of airway (eg, cystic fibrosis, smoking, COPD, elderly) → ↓ host defenses.
- Relative/absolute immunosuppression (eg, chronic disease, HIV) → ↓ susceptibility to bacterial infection.
- Hematogenous spread of organism to lung (eg, IDU, *Pneumococcus*)

Patients at risk for the above pathophysiologic process are most likely to get pneumonia.

TABLE 10.8. Common Community-Acquired Pneumonia Pathogens

ORGANISM	CLASSIC PATIENT	CLASSIC CLINICAL PRESENTATION
Typical aerobic organisms		
S. pneumoniae	Extremes of age and chronically ill immunocompromise (eg, HIV, splenectomy)	Peak incidence in winter and early spring Abrupt onset of **single**-shaking chill **Rusty-colored sputum** Sepsis or multisystem illness
Haemophilus influenzae	Elderly Underlying lung disease (eg, **COPD**)	Peak incidence in winter and early spring Less abrupt in onset
Klebsiella sp.	Alcoholic or chronically debilitated patient	Abrupt onset rigors (multiple) and chills **Currant-jelly sputum** Right upper lobe infiltrate with **bulging fissure**
Staphylococcus aureus (MSSA, MRSA)	Elderly Hematogenous (**IVDA**) Postinfluenza pneumonia	Insidious onset Low-grade fever Necrotizing pneumonia (empyema, lung abscess)
Anaerobes		
Peptostretococcus *Fusobacterium* *Bacteroides* *Prevotella*	Aspiration Poor dental hygiene	Subacute or chronic presentations Necrotizing pneumonia (empyema or lung abscess)
Atypical organisms		
Mycoplasma sp.	Younger, healthy patient	Year round Subacute illness May see extrapulmonary manifestions (eg, rash, bullous myringitis, pericarditis)
Legionella sp.	Immunosuppressed Smokers Outbreaks associated with aerosolized water (eg, showers)	Year round Mild to multisystem illness **GI symptoms** **Hyponatremia** Pleuritic CP and pleural effusions common
Chlamydophila (formerly *Chlamydia*) *pneumoniae*	Younger, healthy patient	Mild, subacute illness
Viral pathogens		
RSV Parainfluenza Influenza	Infants and young children	Autumn and winter months

THORACIC AND RESPIRATORY DISORDERS

SYMPTOMS/EXAM

- Fever, dyspnea, or cough productive of purulent or bloody sputum are most common.
- Pleuritic chest pain, tachypnea, and abnormal breath sounds
- In the elderly, the presenting complaint may be vague and nonspecific, eg, altered mental status, poor appetite, or a fall.

DIFFERENTIAL

- **Hospital-acquired pneumonia:** Occurs after at least 5 days of inpatient care and frequently caused by *Pseudomonas*, *Enterobacter*, *Legionella*, or *S. aureus*.
- Also consider pulmonary embolism, bronchiectasis, bronchitis, CHF.

DIAGNOSIS

- Suspect based on clinical presentation
- It is not possible to differentiate atypical from typical infections based on clinical criteria.
- **CXR**
  - Radiographic findings cannot accurately predict the microbial cause, but lobar infiltrates are more likely due to typical bacterial pathogens and interstitial infiltrates due to atypical pathogens.
  - The initial CXR may be negative in patients with significant dehydration.
- Microbiological diagnosis is reserved for more seriously ill admitted patients:
  - Blood cultures: Low yield overall but accurately identifies organism when positive
  - Sputum Gram stain and culture. Diagnostic sample must have **<10 epithelial cells and >25 WBC/hpf**. See Table 10.9 for Gram stains of common organisms that cause pneumonia.
  - Specific culture and antigen testing if *Legionella* suspected
  - Pleural fluid evaluation, if present.
- **Findings associated with poor outcome:**
  - Pleural effusion
  - Multilobar involvement
  - Pleural effusion

TABLE 10.9. Gram Stains of Common Organisms That Cause Pneumonia

ORGANISM	GRAM STAIN FINDINGS
S. pneumoniae	Gram+ lancet-shaped cocci, usually in pairs, PMNs
H. influenzae	Gram– coccobacillus, PMNs
S. aureus	Gram+ cocci in clusters, PMNs
Klebsiella sp.	Gram– rod, PMNs
Legionella sp.	Weakly Gram– rod, PMNs
Oral flora (aspiration)	Mixed Gram+ and – cocci and rods, PMNs
Atypicals Viral *Legionella*	Few bacteria, many PMNs or monos

- Cavitation
- WBC count >30,000 or <4000 cells/mm^3

TREATMENT

- The **Pneumonia Patient Outcomes Research Team (PORT)** score can help guide decisions regarding the need for hospitalization in **immunocompetent adults** (see Tables 10.10 and 10.11).

TABLE 10.10. PORT Prediction Rule for CAP

PATIENT CHARACTERISTIC	POINTS ASSIGNED[a]
Demographic factor	
Age: men	Number of years
Age: women	Number of years minus 10
Nursing home resident	10
Comorbid illnesses	
Neoplastic disease[b]	30
Liver disease[c]	20
CHF[d]	10
Cerebrovascular disease[e]	10
Renal disease[f]	10
Physical examination finding	
Altered mental status[g]	20
Respiratory rate ≥30 breaths/min	20
Systolic BP <90 mmHg	20
Temperature ≤35°C or ≥40°C	15
Pulse ≥125 bpm	10
Laboratory or radiographic finding	
Arterial pH <7.35	30
BUN ≥30 mg/dL	20
Sodium <130 meq/L	20
Glucose >250 mg/dL	10
Hematocrit <30%	10
Arterial Po_2 <60 mmHg	10
Pleural effusion	10

(Adapted, with permission, from Fine MJ et al. "A prediction rule to identify low-risk patients with community-acquired pneumonia." *NEJM*. 1997(336):243.)

[a]A total point score for a given patient is obtained by summing the patient's age in years (age minus 10 for women) and the points for each applicable characteristic.

[b]Any cancer except basal or squamous cell carcinoma of the skin that was active at the time of presentation or diagnosed within 1 year before presentation.

[c]Clinical or histologic diagnosis of cirrhosis or another form of chronic liver disease.

[d]Systolic or diastolic dysfunction documented by history, physical examination and CXR, echocardiogram, multiple uptake gated acquisition (MUGA) scan, or left ventriculogram.

[e]Clinical diagnosis of stroke or TIA or stroke documented by MRI or CT scan.

[f]History of chronic renal disease or abnormal BUN and creatinine concentration documented in the medical record.

[g]Disorientation (to person, place, or time, not known to be chronic), stupor, or coma.

THORACIC AND RESPIRATORY DISORDERS

TABLE 10.11. **Risk Stratification Based on PORT Score**

NUMBER OF POINTS	RISK CLASS	MORTALITY AT 30 DAYS (%)	RECOMMENDED SITE OF CARE
Absence of predictors	I	0.1–0.4	Outpatient
≤ 70	II	0.6–0.7	Outpatient
71–90	III	0.9–2.8	Outpatient or brief inpatient
91–130	IV	8.2–9.3	Inpatient
≥ 130	V	27.0–31.1	Inpatient

(Data from Fine MJ et al. "A prediction rule to identify low-risk patients with community-acquired pneumonia." *NEJM*. 1997(336):243.)

- **Outpatient empiric therapy**
  - Healthy adults: Macrolide (azithromycin or clarithromycin) or doxycycline.
  - Adults with comorbidity (or recent antibiotic use): Antipneumococcal fluoroquinolone **or** combination of macrolide (azithromycin or clarithromycin) + a β-lactam against *S. pneumoniae* (high-dose amoxicillin or amoxicillin-clavulanate or cefpodoxime or cefuroxime).
- Inpatient empiric therapy not admitted to the ICU
  - Ceftriaxone or cefotaxime IV + azithromycin or antipneumococcal fluoroquinolone
- Inpatient empiric therapy admitted to the ICU
  - Patients are more likely to have risk factors for resistant pathogens, including community-associated MRSA and *Legionella* spp, therefore intravenous combination therapy with a potent antipneumococcal β-lactam (ceftriaxone or cefotaxime) + either azithromycin or a respiratory fluoroquinolone (levofloxacin or moxifloxacin).
- Special considerations
  - Suspected *Pseudomonas:* Add combination therapy with both an antipseudomonal β-lactam antibiotic **and** fluoroquinolone such as piperacillin-tazobactam, imipenem, meropenem, cefepime, ceftazidime + ciprofloxacin, or levofloxacin. For β-lactam allergic patients, options include: aztreonam + levofloxacin or moxifloxacin **plus** an aminoglycoside.
  - Suspected *Legionella* spp: Add fluoroquinolone or azithromycin.
  - Suspected MRSA: Add vancomycin or linezolid.
  - Suspected aspiration pneumonia: Add piperacillin-tazobactam or clindamycin.

Fungal Pneumonia

Fungal pneumonia occurs when disruption of contaminated soil results in inhalation of fungal spores.

HISTOLASMOSIS

The fungus *Histoplasma capsulatum* is endemic in the moist soil of the **Mississippi** and **Ohio River valleys**. It can be found in bat and bird droppings. Severe or disseminated infection is more common in immunocompromised patients.

SYMPTOMS/EXAM

- Infection can be clinically silent.
- Primary infection is characterized by cough and flulike symptoms.
- Chronic illness typically manifests as TB-like symptoms (weight loss, fevers, malaise, hemoptysis).

DIAGNOSIS

- **CXR:** Often normal or showing isolated hilar adenopathy in primary infection; scattered nodules (histoplasmomas) or upper lobe cavitary lesions may develop in chronic illness
- Positive fungal stains, cultures, antigen detection, or serologic testing is confirmative.

TREATMENT

Antifungals are reserved for patients with moderately severe acute disease or those with chronic illness.

COMPLICATIONS

- Disseminated disease with multiorgan involvement
- Mediastinal fibrosis (SVC syndrome, airway obstruction, dysphagia)

COCCIDIOMYCOSIS (VALLEY FEVER)

The fungus *Coccidioides immitis* is endemic to the arid soils of the **southwestern United States**. Infection results from inhalation of dust from disturbed soil. Severe or disseminated infection is more common in immunocompromised patients.

SYMPTOMS/EXAM

- Primary infection is clinically silent in most individuals.
- Classic presentation is triad of pneumonitis, rash (erythema nodosum), and arthritis.
- Cough, fevers/chills, and flulike symptoms are common.

DIAGNOSIS

- **CXR:** In acute infection it may be normal or show hilar adenopathy, thin-walled cavities, or unilateral infiltrates.
- Positive fungal stains, cultures, or serologic testing is confirmative.

TREATMENT

Ketoconazole, fluconazole, itraconazole; amphotericin B only in severe cases

COMPLICATIONS

Disseminated disease with multiorgan involvement

BLASTOMYCOSIS

The fungus *Blastomyces dermatides* is found in the **Midwest** and **the southeastern United States.**

SYMPTOMS/EXAM

- Many cases are subclinical.
- Fever, cough, headache, dyspnea

DIAGNOSIS

- CXR: Fibronodular, interstitial, or alveolar infiltrates
- Positive fungal stains, cultures, or serologic testing are confirmative.

TREATMENT

- Pulmonary blastomycosis
  - Life-threatening: Amphotericin B
  - Mild to moderate: Itraconazole, ketaconazole, fluconazole
  - Many cases resolve spontaneously. Observation is a valid option in the immunocompetent patient.
- Disseminated blastomycosis
  - CNS or life threatening: Amphotericin B
  - Mild to moderate: Itraconazole
- Immunocompromised and pregnant patients: Amphotericin B

COMPLICATIONS

Dissemination to skin, bones, joints, prostate

Psittacosis (Parrot Fever)

CAUSES

Caused by organism *Chlamydia psittaci*, which is transmitted from **birds** to humans

SYMPTOMS/EXAM

- History of occupational or recreational exposure to birds
- Subacute illness with protracted symptoms
- Headache and relative bradycardia

TREATMENT

- Tetracyclines, eg, doxycycline and tetracycline
- Erythromycin as second-line agent
- Chloramphenicol and rifampin have also been used effectively.

COMPLICATIONS

Renal failure, encephalitis, endocarditis, DIC

Q Fever

CAUSES

Caused by the organism *Coxiella burnetii*, which is transmitted to humans from **sheep, goats, and cattle**

SYMPTOMS/EXAM

- History of occupational or recreational exposure to sheeps, goats, or cattle
- Flulike illness along with dry cough and pleuritic chest pain
- Confusion and GI symptoms are common.

DIAGNOSIS

- Diagnosed by serologic testing

TREATMENT

Doxycycline

COMPLICATIONS

Endocarditis or hepatitis

Pneumocystis Pneumonia

CAUSES

PCP results from reactivation of a previously acquired *Pneumocystis jiroveci* (formerly *carinii*) infection in an immunocompromised host (eg, HIV, transplant). It is the most common AIDS-defining illness in HIV+ patients with a **CD4 count <200**.

SYMPTOMS/EXAM

- Symptom progression over a 2- to 3-week period
- Dyspnea, dry cough
- Low-grade fever
- Hypoxic, tachypneic, tachycardic
- The patient may have normal lung sounds or rales.

DIAGNOSIS

- **CXR:** May be normal if early in the disease process or may have a classical bilateral interstitial infiltrate that projects out from the perihilar region
- **Chest CT:** More sensitive than CXR in early disease.
- **Ambulatory pulse oximetry:** If CXR is normal but diagnosis is suspected.
- O_2 desaturation to <90% with ambulation is enough to initiate treatment.
- An LDH >450 is common, and the degree of elevation is prognostic.
- **Immunofluorescent staining** of sputum or BAL sample (gold standard) is confirmative.

TREATMENT

- **TMP-SMX** is the preferred agent.
  - High-dose oral therapy (two DS tabs TID) may be used for patients with mild or early disease.
  - IV therapy should be given to all admitted patients.
- Second-line agents include pentamidine or dapsone.
- **Steroids** are also considered first-line adjuvant therapy in patients with PO_2 <70 mmHg and/or an A–a gradient >35.

Tuberculosis

Approximately one-third of the world's population is infected with TB; however, only about 10% of infected hosts develop active disease.

CAUSES

- *Mycobacterium tuberculosis*, a slow-growing aerobic rod
- Transmitted human-to-human via respiratory droplets
- Humans are the only natural reservoir and usually must be in confined environments over extended periods of time to transmit the disease.
- See Table 10.12 for TB risk factors.

PATHOPHYSIOLOGY

- **Primary infection** in immunocompetent host → small number of organisms contained in gramulomas or spread through the body → **latent (dormant) infection** and +PPD.

TABLE 10.12. TB Risk Factors

Immunocompromise
Older age
Substance abuse
Malnutrition
Silicosis
Close contact with infected person
Crowded living conditions
Travel to endemic areas
Health- or residential-care work
Recent immigration

- Host becomes immunocompromised (eg, HIV, malignancy, immunosuppressant medications) → **reactivation** of latent disease and symptoms.
- Hematogenous spread during primary or reactivation → **miliary TB**.

SYMPTOMS/EXAM

- **Primary TB**
  - Usually asymptomatic, but a small number of cases may develop progressive primary infection, resembling CAP
- **Latent TB**
  - No symptoms of active disease, PPD+
- **Active TB/reactivation disease**
  - **Pulmonary TB**: Persistent cough, malaise, night sweats, fever, weight loss, and hemoptysis
  - **Extrapulmonary TB:** Sites include lymph node (most common), pleura, genitourinary tract, bones and joints, pericardium, and meninges. See Table 10.13 for clinical clues.

TABLE 10.13. Clinical Clues with Extrapulmonary TB

EXTRAPULMONARY LOCATION	CLINICAL CLUE
Meninges	Lumbar puncture: High opening pressure and protein Lymphocyte predominance ↓Glucose
Pleura	Exudative pleural effusion with predominance of lymphocytes
Genitourinary tract	Urinary tract complaints WBCs without bacteria on UA
Miliary	Abnormal CBC Hepatosplenomegaly Lymphadenopathy Hyponatremia CXR with millet seed-like densities

DIAGNOSIS

- CXR
  - **Primary TB:** May be completely normal or reveal nonspecific infiltrate in any region of the lung. This infiltrate in association with regional lymphadenopathy is termed the **Ghon complex**. PPD will be positive.
  - **Reactivation TB: Upper lobe infiltrates** with or without cavitation
- **Sputum smears** are stained for **acid-fast bacilli**.
- Cultures of sputum, blood, or tissue are the gold standard for diagnosing active infection but may take weeks to grow.
- **PPD test** is the gold standard for diagnosing latent infection. Positive test is based on the degree of induration (not redness) in a given patient risk group.
  - Low-risk individuals (eg, >aged 4 years, without any risk factors): >15 mm
  - Average risk individuals: >10 mm
  - High risk patients (see Table 10.12): >5 mm
  - Many foreign-born patients may have been immunized with BCG, the therapeutic effectiveness of which is unclear. Therefore, the CDC recommends that history of such is ignored when interpreting the PPD response.

TREATMENT

- **Latent TB (newly +PPD)**: 6–9 months of INH
- **Active TB: Initial therapy with four drugs is now recommended until a multi–drug-resistant strain can be ruled out by culture**. There are six first-line drugs now commonly employed: INH, rifampin, pyrazinamide, ethambutol, rifabutin, and rifapentine. The drugs are selected for treatment based on local practice, patterns of resistance, and patient tolerance. Baseline labs, particularly liver function tests, are indicated before use of these drugs.
- **Corticosteroids:** For TB meningitis and pericarditis

COMPLICATIONS

- Hyponatremia, anemia, elevated LFTs, thrombocytosis
- Pneumothorax empyema
- Adverse drug reactions, eg, hepatitis, secondary to INH
- Inadequate therapeutic effect of warfarin, steroids, OCPs, oral hypoglycemics, digoxin, anticonvulsants, and methadone secondary to treatment with INH

Bioterrorism Agents

Pulmonary infections related to biological weapons of mass destruction include anthrax, plague, and tularemia. These are discussed further in Chapter 20, "EMS and Disaster Medicine."

ASPIRATION PNEUMONITIS AND PNEUMONIA

This disease occurs when normal protective mechanisms of the airway are compromised and foreign material enters the tracheobronchial tree. The aspiration can occur either in community or hospital settings. The airway becomes inflamed and the parenchyma collapses.

CAUSES

Common pathogens include:

- **Anaerobes: *Peptostretococcus, Fusobacterium, Bacteroides, Prevotella***
- *Klebsiella pneumoniae*
- *Staphylococcus aureus*
- *Streptococcus*

Risk factors include any process that alters the gag/cough reflex.

- Drug or alcohol intoxication
- General anesthesia/sedation
- Use of the esophageal obturator airway
- Seizures
- Brain injury and dementia

PATHOPHYSIOLOGY

- Aspiration of gastric contents → immediate inflammatory response and chemical pneumonitis.
- Aspiration of bacterial pathogens → delayed polymicrobial pneumonia.
- Severity of the insult depends on the volume of the aspirate, presence of particulate matter, and the pH of the material. High-risk aspirates include those with **volumes >25 mL, particulate food matter, a low pH, and bacterial contamination**.

SYMPTOMS/EXAM

- Aspiration event may be immediately followed by coughing or choking in the awake patient.
- Tachypnea, shortness of breath
- Cough productive of bloody or purulent sputum
- Wheezing, rhonchi, or rales over involved lung fields

DIAGNOSIS

- Suspect based on clinical history and presentation.
- **CXR:** May be completely normal immediately after event; infiltrate will appear, most frequently in the **RLL**, within the first 12 hours

TREATMENT

- Supportive care
- Indications for antibiotic therapy (piperacillin-tazobactam or clindamycin) include:
  - Unexplained deterioration
  - Expanding infiltrate
  - New fever >36 hours after aspiration event
- **Avoid**: Systemic corticosteroids, which are of no benefit and may be harmful

COMPLICATIONS

- Respiratory failure and shock
- Empyema/abscess development
- Pulmonary fibrosis
- If the pH of the aspirated material is <2.5, the lungs have suffered a chemical burn in addition to the ensuing 2° bacterial infection, and the mortality rate may be as high as 70%.

Lung Abscess

A lung abscess is defined as necrosis of the lung parenchyma by a microbial infection, most commonly associated with aspiration.

CAUSES

Common organisms include

- Anaerobes (most common)
- *S. aureus*

- *K. pneumoniae*
- Gram-negative bacilli
- *Streptococcus pyogenes*
- *Nocardia asteroids*
- *Actinomyces* sp.

SYMPTOMS/EXAM

Indolent course of fever, chest pain, weight loss, and night sweats

DIFFERENTIAL

The differential diagnosis of the cavitary lung lesion includes fungal infections, neoplasm, Wegener granulomatosis, sarcoidosis.

DIAGNOSIS

- CXR: Usually confirms the presence of cavitary lesion with air-fluid levels
- Chest CT: May occasionally be needed to confirm cavitation

TREATMENT

Piperacillin/tazobactam or clindamycin

THORACIC AND RESPIRATORY DISORDERS

Empyema

Defined as pus in the pleural space or pleura fluid with presence of organisms on Gram stain

Risk factors for empyema include:

- Pneumonia with parapneumonic effusion (most common)
- Penetrating trauma
- Esophageal perforation/rupture
- Presence of hemothorax, hydrothorax, or chylothorax

PATHOPHYSIOLOGY

The infection generally progresses through three stages:

- **Exudative stage:** Free-flowing fluid present
- **Fibrinopurulent stage:** Fibrin strands develop → loculations
- **Organizational stage:** Thick pleural peel present
- Identification and treatment in the exudative stage is essential to ensure good patient outcome.

SYMPTOMS/EXAM

- Presence of risk factor, eg, recent pneumonia
- Persistent fevers, dyspnea, pleuritic chest pain, and cough
- Dullness to percussion and ↓ breath sounds over the effusion

DIAGNOSIS

- **CXR:** Can confirm the presence of pleural effusion
- **Decubitus CXR:** To determine if fluid is free-flowing or loculated
- **Pleural fluid evaluation**. Findings consistent with empyema include:
  - Aspiration of frank pus
  - Pleural fluid pH <7.2
  - Positive Gram stain or culture
- **Chest CT:** To further delineate underlying pathology and evaluate extent of loculations and/or pleural peel, as needed

TREATMENT

- **Drainage of pleural space:** Required in all cases
- If exudative stage: Tube thoracostomy and IV antibiotics
- Fibrinopurulent and organizational stage empyemas often require more aggressive surgical management (eg, intrapleural fibrinolytics).

Acute Respiratory Distress Syndrome

The root problem underlying the development of ARDS is acute lung injury (ALI), which arises for many different reasons. Not all ALI progresses to ARDS, but all cases of ARDS begin as ALI.

CAUSES

See Table 10.14.

PATHOPHYSIOLOGY

- Triggering event → complex inflammatory response → both alveolar epithelial cell and vascular endothelial cell injury.
- Cell injury → capillary leak, cell death, and loss of surfactant resulting in diseased alveoli that do not participate in oxygenation (shunt).
- Diseased segments of the lung are interspersed with healthy segments.

SYMPTOMS/EXAM

Presents with rapid onset of dyspnea, tachypnea, and diffuse crackles

DIFFERENTIAL

Includes cardiogenic pulmonary edema, pneumonia, diffuse alveolar hemorrhage

TABLE 10.14. Causes of Acute Lung Injury and ARDS

Direct pulmonary injury
Pneumonia
Aspiration
Toxic inhalation
Ventilator associated
Indirect pulmonary injury
Infection (systemic)
Pancreatitis
Drugs (heroin, ASA)
Trauma

TABLE 10.15. Diagnosis of Acute Lung Injury and ARDS

	Onset of Symptoms	Oxygenation	Hemodynamics	CXR
ALI	Acute	$Pao_2/Fio_2 \leq 300$	Low or normal left atrial pressure	Bilateral infiltrates
ARDS	Acute	$Pao_2/Fio_2 \leq 200$	Low or normal left atrial pressure	Bilateral infiltrates

Diagnosis

Both ALI and ARDS are clinically defined by rapidity of symptom onset, oxygenation, hemodynamic criteria, and CXR findings (see Table 10.15). Additional findings are as follows:

- **CT chest:** May demonstrate alveolar filling and consolidation in dependent lung zones with sparing of other areas
- **Bronchoalveolar lavage (BAL):** May help differentiate the etiology (eg, *Pneumocystis* in the immunocompromised patient)

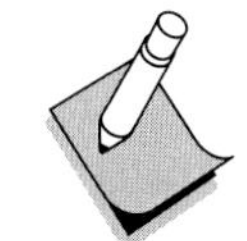

To improve mortality in patients with ARDS, target a tidal volume of 6 mL/kg ***predicted*** *body weight.*

Treatment

- Search for and treat the underlying cause of acute respiratory failure (ARF).
- Most patients with ARDS require mechanical ventilation during the course of the disease.
  - **Use of tidal volumes ≤6 mL/kg of predicted body weight has been shown to ↓ mortality.**
  - Add positive end-expiratory pressure (PEEP) as needed to maintain Fio_2 <60%.
  - Inverse ratio ventilation with permissive hypercarbia allows for more inspiratory time and may improve oxygenation.
  - Plateau pressure must be kept at <30 cm H_2O to prevent barotrauma (see the discussion of ventilator management).
- A conservative fluid management strategy (ie, one involving less volume) is preferred over a liberal fluid strategy. In a recent randomized trial comparing such strategies, both techniques yielded similar 60-day mortality rates, but conservative management was found to be associated with shorter mechanical ventilation and ICU times.
- Corticosteroids have been given in the proliferative phase of ARDS, but their use in this context is still considered experimental.
- The use of inhaled vasodilators, exogenous surfactant, high-frequency ventilation, liquid ventilation, and antioxidant therapy has been studied with no proven benefit.
- Approximately 25% of survivors have no pulmonary impairment at 1 year, 50% have mild impairment, 25% moderate impairment, and a small fraction severe impairment.

PLEURAL EFFUSION

Defined as the abnormal accumulation of fluid in the pleural space, in the United States, the most common causes are CHF, pneumonia, and cancer. It is classified as **transudative** or **exudative.**

Transudative Effusion

- Occurs because of an imbalance between hydrostatic and oncotic pressures in the pleural space
- The main causes are CHF, cirrhosis, nephrotic syndrome, and PE.

Exudative Effusion

- Occurs when inflammation → altered vascular permeability and protein-rich pleural fluid
- Common causes include malignancy, bacterial, and viral pneumonia, TB, PE, pancreatitis, esophageal rupture, collagen vascular disease, chylothorax, and hemothorax.

SYMPTOMS/EXAM

- Dyspnea
- Pleuritic chest pain
- Dullness to percussion, ↓ or absent fremitus, and ↓ breath sounds on the affected side
- Findings of underlying disease process (eg, productive cough, fever, and consolidation in parapneumonic effusion)

DIAGNOSIS

- **CXR:** Upright CXR confirms diagnosis in most cases. Decubitus films help determine if fluid is free-flowing or loculated. The presence of >1 cm of fluid on decubitus CXR suggests the presence of a significant amount of fluid.
- **Diagnostic thoracentesis:** Perform on clinically significant effusions; analyze fluid to distinguish transudate from exudate using Light's criteria (see Table 10.16).
- If exudative effusion is suspected or confirmed, additional pleural fluid analysis should occur (see Table 10.17), guided by clinical suspicion for underlying disease process.
- **Chest CT**: Can confirm diagnosis and aid in differentiating underlying disease process (eg, PE, malignancy)

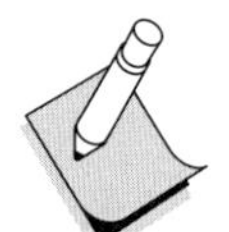

Drain a pleural effusion if pH is <7.2, glucose is <60 mg/dL, or Gram stain is ⊕.

TREATMENT

- **Transudative pleural effusion:** Treatment is aimed at the underlying cause with therapeutic thoracentesis if the patient is symptomatic.
- **Parapneumonic effusion:** Chest tube placement for drainage of the pleural space is indicated if there is evidence of empyema (pH <7.2, pus, glucose <40 mg/dL, Gram stain ⊕).
- **Hemothorax:** Drainage is required or fibrothorax will likely develop.

TABLE 10.16. Light's Criteria for Distinguishing Transudative From Exudative Effusion

Pleural fluid/serum protein ratio >0.5
Pleural fluid LDH >2/3 upper limit of serum reference range
Pleural fluid/serum LDH ratio >0.6
The fluid is an exudate if at least one of the above criteria is present. The fluid is a transudate if none of the above criteria is present.

TABLE 10.17. Exudative Pleural Fluid Analysis and Interpretation

PLEURAL FLUID TEST	INTERPRETATION
RBC count	Grossly bloody or >100,000 cells/mm^3 suggests trauma, malignancy, PE, pneumonia
Neutrophils	>50% suggests acute pleural process (infection, PE).
Lymphocytes	>50% suggests chronic pleural process (TB, malignancy)
Eosinophils	Presence suggests air or blood in pleural space.
Glucose	<60 mg/dL suggests a complicated parapneumonic effusion, malignancy, ruptured esophagus, TB, or rheumatoid arthritis.
Triglycerides	>110 mg/dL suggests chylothorax.
pH	Pleural pH < 7.2 with parapneumonic effusion indicates the need for drainage.

SPONTANEOUS AND IATROGENIC PNEUMOTHORAX

Pneumothorax is defined as the presence of air in the pleural space.

- **Spontaneous pneumothorax:** Not caused by any obvious external factor (eg, trauma)
  - **1° spontaneous pneumothorax:** No clinically apparent lung disease; usually tall, thin males
  - **2° spontaneous pneumothorax:** Occurring in patients with underlying pulmonary disease process (see Table 10.18)
- **Iatrogenic pneumothorax**: The result of diagnostic (thoracentesis) or therapeutic intervention (central venous catheter placement)

Symptoms/Exam

- Most patients present with unilateral chest pain (either sharp or steady pressure) and acute shortness of breath.
- Patients with significant underlying lung disease may present with significant distress, even with a small pneumothorax.

TABLE 10.18. Common Causes of Secondary Spontaneous Pneumothorax

COPD (most common)
Asthma
Pneumonia (eg, PCP)
TB
Interstitial lung disease
Cystic fibrosis
Malignancy
Endometriosis

- The physical exam may be normal if the pneumothorax is small.
- If the pneumothorax is large, exam may reveal ↓ chest movement, hyperresonance, ↓ fremitus, and ↓ breath sounds.
- Tachycardia, hypotension, and tracheal deviation should raise suspicion of tension pneumothorax.

DIFFERENTIAL

Acute PE, MI, pleural effusion, pneumonia, pericardial tamponade

DIAGNOSIS

- **CXR** is usually confirmative. An expiratory film may identify small apical pneumothoraces. A **deep sulcus sign** (deep lateral costophrenic angle) suggests pneumothorax on the supine radiograph.
- CT can be used to assess the stable patient with underlying lung disease when the diagnosis is in question (eg, differentiating bleb from pneumothorax).

TREATMENT

- **Small 1° pneumothoraces:** This usually can be resolved with simple observation and O_2 therapy. Supplemental O_2 accelerates the reabsorption of gas from the pleural space to about 8–9% per day.
- **Larger, more symptomatic primary spontaneous pneumothoraces:** May be drained either with simple aspiration or with placement of a small-bore chest tube
- **2° spontaneous pneumothorax:** Treat with a larger-bore chest tube attached to a water-seal device.
- Persistent air leaks and recurrences are more common with 2° than with 1° spontaneous pneumothorax.
- For those with 2° spontaneous pneumothorax, recurrence is often prevented with instillation of sclerosing agents (eg, talc) through the chest tube, video-assisted thoracoscopic surgery, or limited thoracotomy.
- Interventions to prevent recurrence in patients with 1° spontaneous pneumothorax are usually recommended only after the second ipsilateral pneumothorax. Pilots and divers with 1° spontaneous pneumothorax should be cautioned against such activity in the future because of the risk of contralateral pneumothorax.

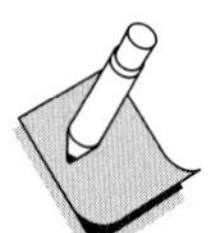

Tension pneumothorax is a medical emergency requiring immediate decompression of the pleural space with a 14-gauge needle in the second intercostal space at the midclavicular line.

PNEUMOMEDIASTINUM

Results from ↑ intra-alveolar pressures → rupture of peribronchial vascular sheaths and dissection along the hilum into the mediastinum. Usually occurs spontaneously in young, healthy patients in their second to fourth decades but has been associated with heavy physical exertion, eg, coughing, weight lifting, vomiting, inhaling recreational vapors ("huffing"), Valsalva maneuvers, iatrogenic procedures, mechanical ventilation, and trauma. Generally, this is a benign, self-limiting condition unless associated with esophageal perforation or mediastinitis.

SYMPTOMS

- Chest pain worsened by inspiration, often radiating to back, neck, or shoulders
- Dyspnea
- Dysphagia and dysphonia

EXAM

- Crepitus suggestive of subcutaneous air is the most common finding.
- **Hamman sign** is a crunching sound that is synchronous with the heart beat. It is uncommonly seen, but when present, it is highly suggestive of pneumomediastinum.
- Often there is no physical abnormality.

DIAGNOSIS

- CXR: Most easily seen on lateral view; a thin line of radiolucency that outlines the heart and mediastinal structures
- CT: More sensitive than CXR; may also provide the etiology of the air, eg, esophageal perforation
- Esophagoscopy if esophageal perforation is suspected
- Bronchoscopy if tracheobronchial perforation is suspected

TREATMENT

- Most cases resolve spontaneously.
- Admission or observation is indicated if symptoms are severe or if there is suspicion for pneumothorax, tension pneumothorax, or mediastinitis.
- Surgery is rarely needed.
- Antibiotics are indicated if esophageal perforation is suspected.

COMPLICATIONS

Pneumothorax, tension pneumothorax, mediastinitis

MEDIASTINITIS

- A very serious, life-threatening condition that usually occurs after a medical procedure, eg, cardiac surgery, endoscopy, or bronchoscopy
- Can also result from esophageal perforation, trauma, upper respiratory infection, or an odontogenic infection (resulting in descending necrotizing mediastinitis)
- Risk factors include malignancy, immunocompromise, autoimmune disease, diabetes, and illicit drug use.
- *S. aureus* and *S. epidermidis* account for the majority of cases (70–80%) after cardiac surgery. Anaerobic organisms are common in non-iatrogenic infections. Mixed infections, including *Pseudomonas*, are common. Rarely, *Histoplasmosis* infection may cause a fibrosing mediastinitis.

SYMPTOMS

- Chest pain often worsened by inspiration radiating to the neck or upper back
- Dyspnea
- Confusion
- Sore throat or dental pain if odontogenic
- Drainage from surgical site

EXAM

- Fever and tachycardia
- Audible click of an unstable sternum
- Subcutaneous emphysema

- Redness and swelling around surgical site
- Hamman sign (systolic crunching sound)

DIFFERENTIAL

Cellulitis, necrotizing fasciitis, pharyngitis, pneumonia, Ludwig angina

DIAGNOSIS

- Mainly a clinical diagnosis
- CXR and CT may reveal findings of pneumomediastinum, air fluid levels or precervical, retropharyngeal, and paratracheal soft tissue swelling.
- MRI is not useful if recent surgery with metallic hardware

TREATMENT

- Ensure adequate airway protection.
- Broad-spectrum antibiotics including coverage for MRSA, pseudomonas, and oral and GI flora
- Treat sepsis if present.
- Surgical consult if debridement is necessary.

COMPLICATIONS

Sepsis, pneumoperitoneum, pneumothorax

PULMONARY IRRITANTS

Pneumoconiosis

Pneumoconiosis is a lung disease caused by inhalation of organic or inorganic dusts. It usually develops over long periods of time and is often occupation related. The chronic inflammation caused by these dust particles eventually → pulmonary fibrosis.

CAUSES

Common dusts include: asbestos, silica minerals, talc, and carbon materials (see Table 10.19), and rarely, beryllium and hard metals (cobalt, tungsten carbide, aluminum).

SYMPTOMS/EXAM

- Often asymptomatic for 20–30 years from time of initial exposure
- Depends on severity and length of exposure
- Insidious onset of shortness of breath or dyspnea on exertion
- Made worse with cigarette smoking
- Cough, sputum production, and wheezing are **unusual**
- Fine bibasilar and end-inspiratory crackles

DIFFERENTIAL

COPD, TB, fungal infection, interstitial lung disease, cancer, rheumatoid nodules, sarcoidosis

DIAGNOSIS

- Reliable exposure history
- Evidence of interstitial fibrosis by:

TABLE 10.19. Common Pneumoconiosis

SUBSTANCE	SOURCE	OCCUPATIONS
Asbestos	Home insulation, fireproof materials, tiles for floors	Construction workers, miners, demolition workers, ship builders, and auto mechanics
Silicon dioxide	Sand, sandstone, slate, clay, granite	Sandblasters, miners, tunnel builders, quarry workers
Carbon	Coal, graphite	Coal miners
Talc	Talc mining and milling	Miners and millers, IVDU
Kaolin (china clay)	Ceramics, papers, medicines, costmetics, toothpaste	Miners and millers
Siderosis	Iron	Welders or silver polishers

- CXR: Generally signs of interstitial fibrosis
  - Asbestosis: Coarse honeycombing in advanced disease; **pleural plaques**
  - Silicosis: **Basilar alveolar filling pattern** in acute silicosis; **nodular opacities** in simple silicosis; **large upper- or midzone opacities** in progressive massive fibrosis
  - Carbon (coal miners lung): Small, rounded opacities first seen in the upper lobes
- PFTs reveal **reduced lung volumes**, particularly vital capacity and total lung capacity, diminished single breath DLCO, ↓ compliance, usually **absence of obstruction**.
- Absence of other causes of interstitial fibrosis

TREATMENT

- Mainly prevention and supportive
- Smoking cessation
- Supplemental O_2 as needed
- Pneumococcal and influenza vaccination
- Corticosteroids may be helpful

COMPLICATIONS

- Respiratory failure, especially with concomitant pulmonary infection
- Cancer
- TB in cases of silicosis

Toxic Gases, Fumes, Vapors

Chemical irritants in the form of gases, fumes, and vapors are readily absorbed by the lung lining and can cause inflammation and edema that can → chronic bronchitis. Toxicity depends on concentration and duration of exposure.

TABLE 10.20. **Common Toxic Gases, Fumes, and Vapors**

Substance	Source	Toxicity
Phosgene	Plastics, textiles, pharmaceuticals	Hydrolyzes to CO_2 and HCl
Chlorine	Water purification, paper manufacturing	Forms acids and oxidants causing inflammation
Nitrogen oxide	Combustion	Converts to nitric acid; causes delayed alveolar injury and pulmonary edema
Ammonia	Fertilizers	Forms ammonium hydroxide
Hydrocarbons	Fuels, lubricants, cleaning solvents	Depends on physical characteristics (volatility, viscocity, and surface tension), chemical characteristics (aliphatic, aromatic, or halogenated) and presence of toxic additives
Hydrogen sulfide	Organic decomposition	Disrupts oxidative phosphorylation causing cellular asphyxia and anaerobic metabolism **similar to cyanide**

Causes

Common substances and their sources are found in Table 10.20.

Symptoms/Exam

- **Phosgene:** Odor of freshly mowed hay, respiratory irritation, skin irritation
- **Chlorine:** Distinctive odor of "swimming pool"; ocular and respiratory; nausea and vomiting are common
- **Nitrogen oxides: Triphasic illness** of flulike symptoms followed by transient improvement, then pulmonary edema
- **Ammonia:** Distinctive odor of cleaning product, severe mucous membrane irritation
- **Hydrocarbons:** Odor may be noted; respiratory irritation; stimulation followed by ↓ alertness
- **Hydrogen sulfide:** Odor of rotten eggs, ocular and respiratory irritation; high concentrations cause rapid LOC and seizures

Diagnosis

- Clinical diagnosis primarily from history of exposure
- Helpful studies may include ABG with COHb and MetHb levels, lactate, RBC cyanide levels, ECG, and CXR.

Treatment

- Removal from source
- 100% O_2
- Irrigation of exposed areas, especially eyes and skin

- Early intubation if signs of airway edema and obstruction
- Bronchodilators may be helpful.
- Antibiotics are not helpful.
- Steroids may be helpful in nitrogen oxide poisoning to prevent bronchiolitis obliterans.
- Cyanide antidote kit in hydrogen sulfide poisoning

COMPLICATIONS

Pulmonary edema (often delayed) from a chemical pneumonitis is a common complication among most toxic gases, fumes, and vapors. Other possible complications include:

- **Nitrogen oxides:** Methemoglobinemia bronchiolitis obliterans
- **Ammonia:** Corneal burns
- **Hydrocarbons:** Persistent airway irritation, CNS depression, peripheral neuropathy, dysrhythmias, hepatic toxicity, eg, CCl_4, renal failure, blood dyscrasias
- **Hydrogen sulfide:** Severe metabolic acidosis

CYSTIC FIBROSIS

This is the most common lethal autosomal-recessive disorder in Caucasians, affecting 1 in 3500 births. It is classically characterized by multisystem involvement of the sinuses, lungs, pancreas, liver, gallbladder, intestines, bones, and, in males, the vas deferens.

CAUSES

CF is caused by mutations in the CF transmembrane conductance regulator (CFTR) → chloride channel dysfunction.

SYMPTOMS/EXAM

- Most CF patients are diagnosed during childhood. A history of failure to thrive as a child, persistent respiratory infections *(Pseudomonas)*, nasal polyposis, sinusitis, intestinal obstruction, malabsorption, recurrent pancreatitis, hepatobiliary disease, and male infertility are suggestive of CF.
- Seven percent of CF patients are diagnosed as adults, and these patients tend to present with upper lobe bronchiectasis.
- **Exam** may reveal ↑ chest AP diameter, upper lung field crackles, nasal polyps, hepatomegaly, and clubbing.
- Acute exacerbations are typically characterized by ↑ sputum production, dyspnea, fatigue, weight loss, and a decline in FEV_1.

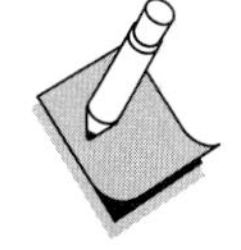

Although most CF patients are diagnosed in childhood, 7% are diagnosed as adults and tend to have upper-lobe bronchiectasis.

DIFFERENTIAL

Immunodeficiency, asthma, ABPA

DIAGNOSIS

Diagnosis requires both clinical and laboratory evidence of CFTR dysfunction.

- **Sweat chloride concentration:** The best screening test for CF for a patient with a suggestive clinical picture; normal sweat chloride is <40 mmol/L
- **Genotyping:** Screening for the presence of two CFTR mutations known to cause CF; newer tests screen for >1000 different known mutations

- **Nasal potential difference:** Directly evaluates CFTR function by measuring ion transport in the epithelial cells lining the interior of the nose
- **CXR:** Shows hyperinflation, bronchiectasis, and upper lobe infiltrates; nodules often represent mucoid impaction in the airways

TREATMENT

- **Acute pulmonary exacerbations:** Treat with chest physical therapy, bronchodilators, DNase, and usually two antipseudomonal antibiotics.
- **Chronic stable CF**
  - **Inhaled tobramycin:** Slows the decline in FEV_1 and is used for long-term therapy
  - **Nebulized DNase:** Improves FEV_1 and should be offered to patients with daily cough, sputum production, and airflow obstruction
  - **Azithromycin:** Improves FEV_1 and reduces pulmonary exacerbations in those infected with *Pseudomonas*
  - **Aerobic exercise, flutter devices, external percussive vests:** Help with regular airway clearance
  - **Pancreatic enzymes** and the **fat-soluble vitamins A, D, E, and K:** Given for malabsorption
  - **Nutritional counseling:** Essential for proper health maintenance and to help prevent diabetic complications, osteoporosis, and weight loss
  - **Double-lung transplantation:** Remains an option for severe progressive pulmonary disease

SARCOIDOSIS

This is a systemic autoimmune disorder that primarily affects the lungs and lymphatics and is characterized by noncaseating granulomas. It is primarily a self-limited disease of young and middle-aged adult black Americans or those of Scandinavian descent.

SYMPTOMS/EXAM

- Nonspecific constitutional symptoms such as fever, fatigue, anorexia, weight loss, and arthralgias
- Physical examination may reveal dry crackles, lymphadenopathy, **parotid enlargement**, splenomegaly, uveitis, or skin changes (erythema nodosum).

DIFFERENTIAL

Tuberculosis, fungal infections, rheumatoid arthritis, lymphoma, Wegener granulomatosis

DIAGNOSIS

- Suspect based on findings of bilateral hilar adenopathy, pulmonary infiltrates, and skin lesions
- Diagnosis is made by a combination of clinical, radiographic, and histologic findings along with exclusion of other diseases that have a similar clinical picture.

TREATMENT

Systemic corticosteroids

SOLITARY PULMONARY NODULE

This is defined as an isolated round lesion <3 cm in diameter that is surrounded by pulmonary parenchyma. Abnormalities >3 cm are termed masses and are usually malignant. Cancer affects 10–70% of those with solitary pulmonary nodules. Most benign lesions are infectious granulomas.

SYMPTOMS/EXAM

- Patients are often asymptomatic but may present with cough, hemoptysis, and dyspnea.
- Older age and a history of cigarette smoking raise the suspicion of cancer.
- Patients should be questioned about prior TB and histoplasmosis.
- Physical examination of the lungs is frequently normal. However, examination of the lymphatic system may demonstrate lymphadenopathy.

DIFFERENTIAL

Granuloma (old TB, histoplasmosis, foreign body reaction), bronchogenic carcinoma, metastatic disease (usually >1), bronchial adenoma, round pneumonia

DIAGNOSIS

- Solitary pulmonary nodules are usually discovered incidentally.
- **Comparison of serial CXRs:** The **initial** step in determining the progression and extent of the nodule, stability of findings on CXR for 2 years is considered a sign that the lesion is benign.
- **Chest CT:** This offers improved estimation of nodule size, characteristics (eg, pattern of calcification), and interval growth. Contrast enhancement allows for the simultaneous evaluation of the mediastinum for lymphadenopathy.
- **PET scan:** This may help provide staging information in the case of lung cancer. The diagnostic accuracy of detecting mediastinal involvement among patients with lung cancer is 65% by CT, 90% by PET, and >95% using a combination of CT and PET.

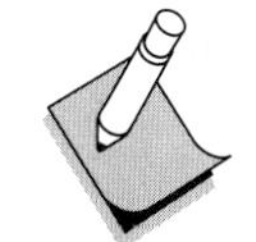

Lesions that ↑ in size or change in character are likely malignant and should be resected, assuming low surgical risk and no evidence of metastatic disease.

TREATMENT

- When the probability of cancer is low (age <35 years, nonsmokers, smooth nodules with a diameter <1.5 cm), the lesion should be monitored with serial high-resolution CT at 3-month intervals.
- When the probability of cancer is high (age >35, smokers, spiculated nodules with a diameter >2 cm), the lesion should be resected if preoperative risk is acceptable and there are no other contraindications to surgery.
- When the probability of cancer is intermediate, additional testing (PET, transthoracic needle biopsy) may be warranted.

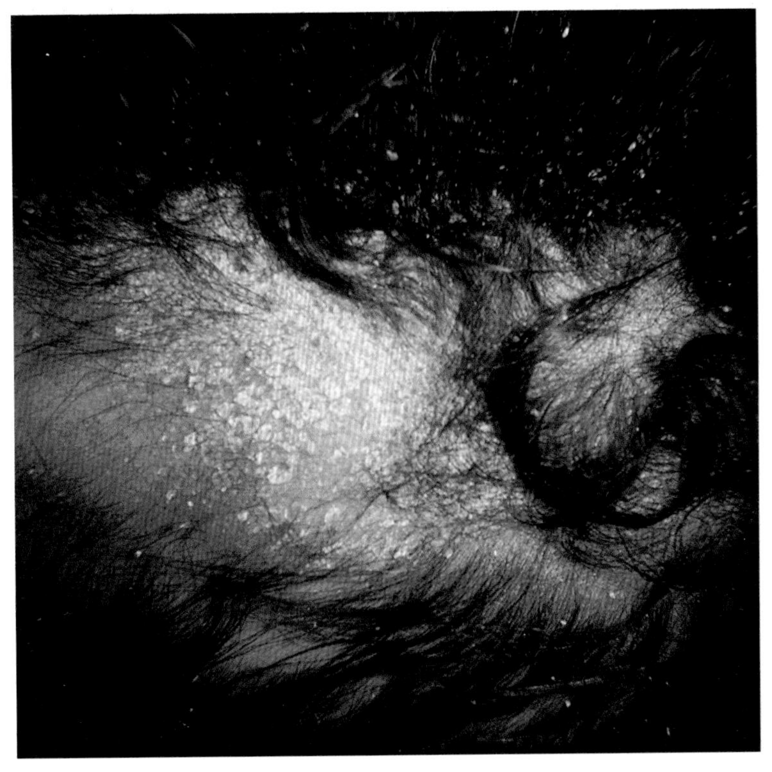

FIGURE 5.3. Seborrhea.

(Reproduced, with permission, from Shah BR, Lucchesi M. *Atlas of Pediatric Emergency Medicine*. McGraw-Hill, 2006:295.)

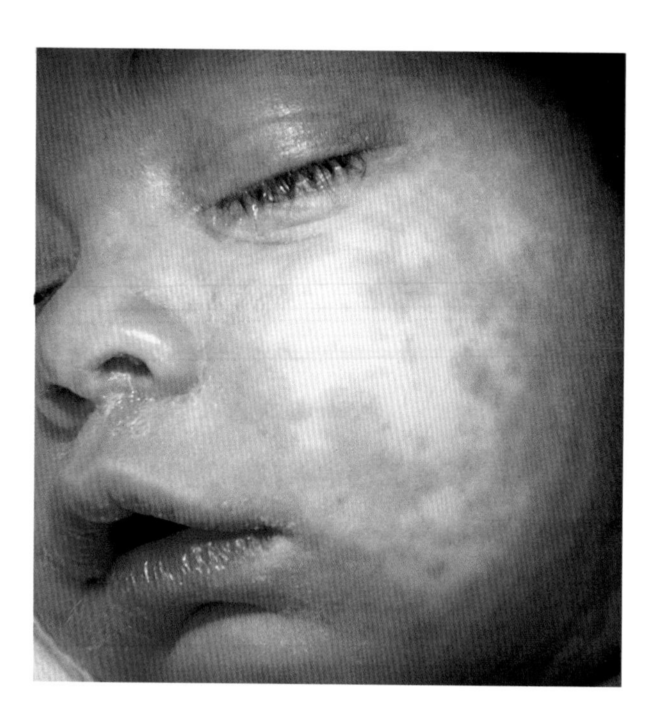

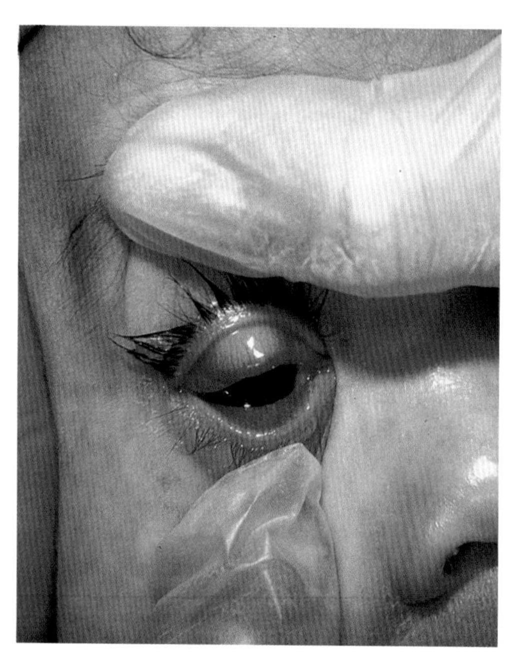

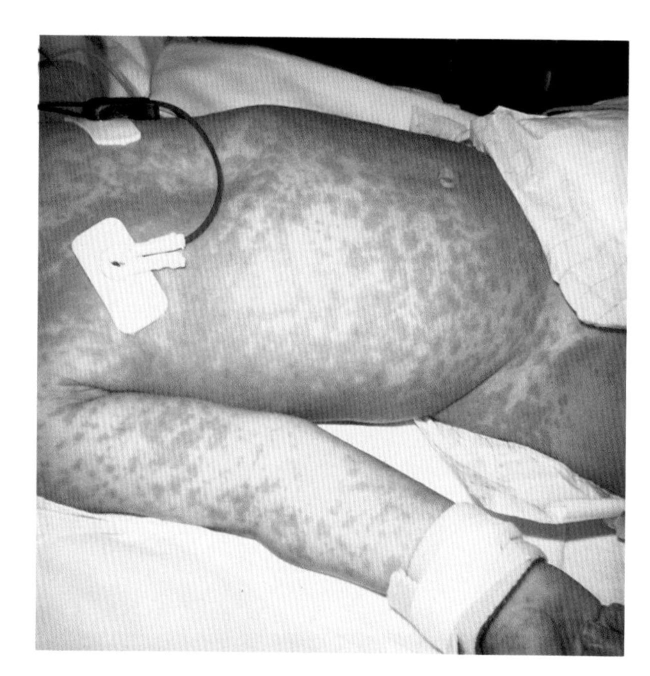

FIGURE 5.7. Measles (rubeolla).

(Reproduced, with permission, from Shah BR, Lucchesi M. *Atlas of Pediatric Emergency Medicine*. New York: McGraw-Hill, 2006:135.)

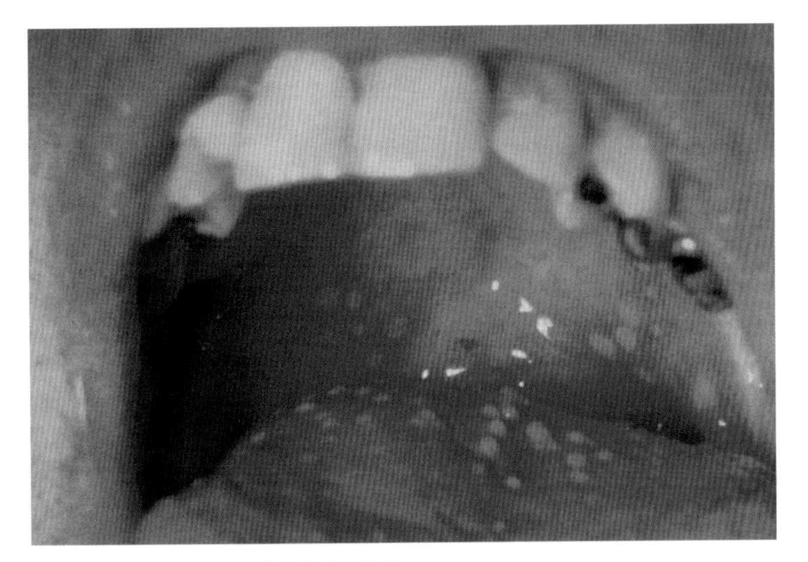

FIGURE 5.8. Measles (rubeolla).

(Reproduced, with permission, Mei Kane KS, Ryder JB, Jonson RA, et al. *Color Atlas & Synopsis of Pediatric Dermatology*. New York: McGraw-Hill, 2002:585.)

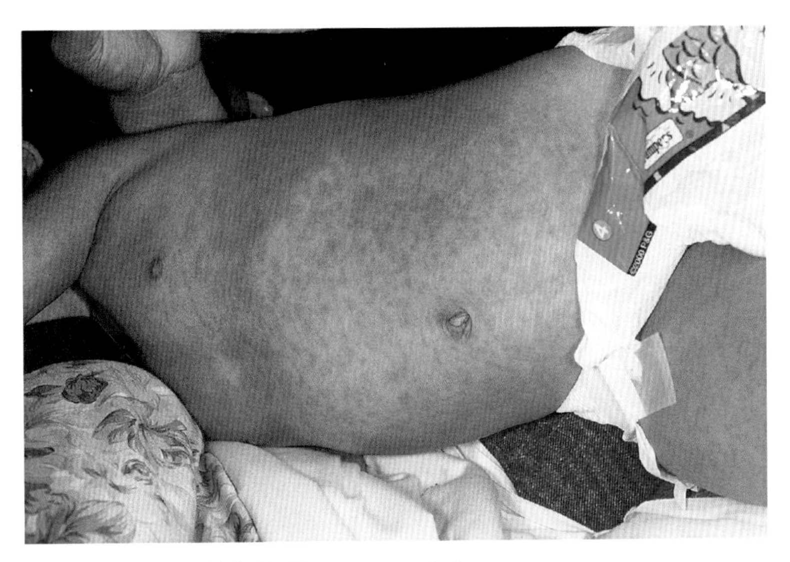

FIGURE 5.9. Rubella (German measles).

(Reproduced, with permission, from Shah BR, Lucchesi M. *Atlas of Pediatric Emergency Medicine*. New York: McGraw-Hill, 2006:137.)

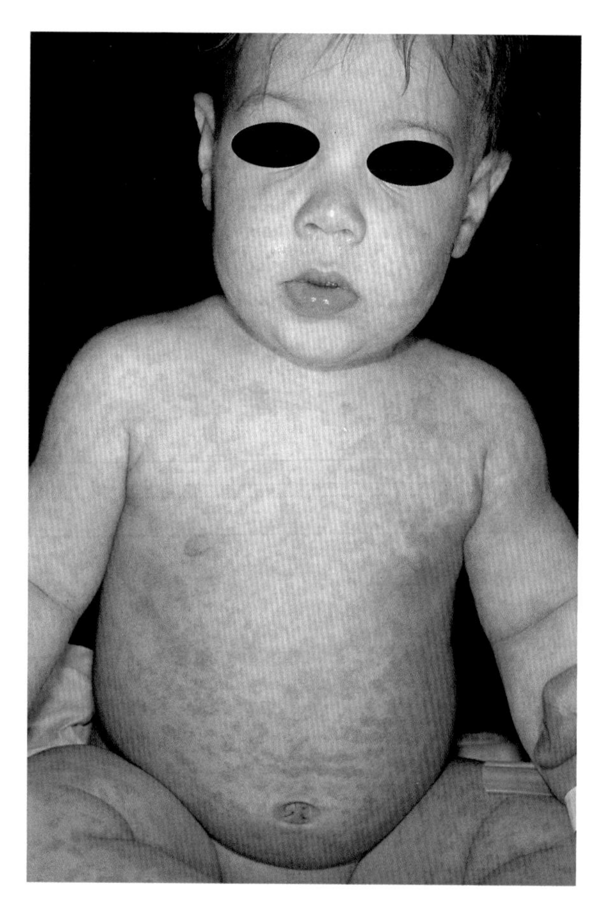

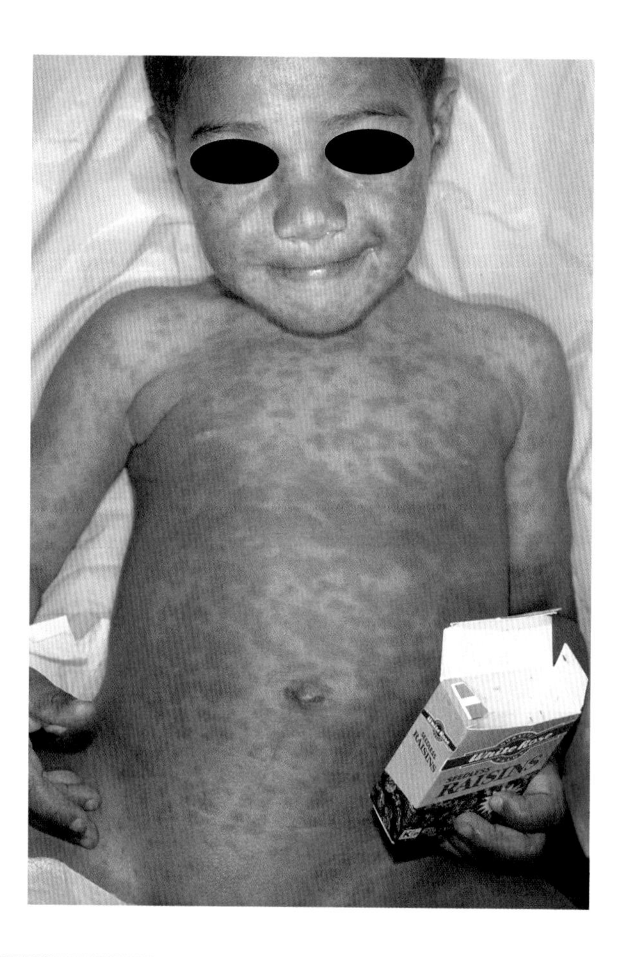

FIGURE 5.10. Roseola.

(Reproduced, with permission, from Shah BR, Lucchesi M. *Atlas of Pediatric Emergency Medicine*. New York: McGraw-Hill, 2006:137.)

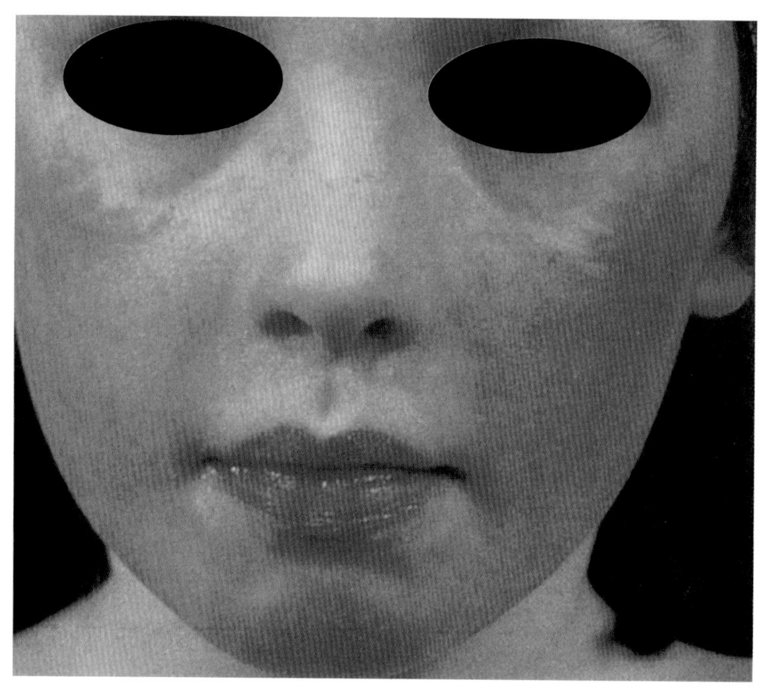

FIGURE 5.11. Erythema infectiosum.

(Reproduced, with permission, from Mei Kane KS, Ryder JB, Jonson RA, et al. *Color Atlas & Synopsis of Pediatric Dermatology*. New York: McGraw-Hill, 2002:579.)

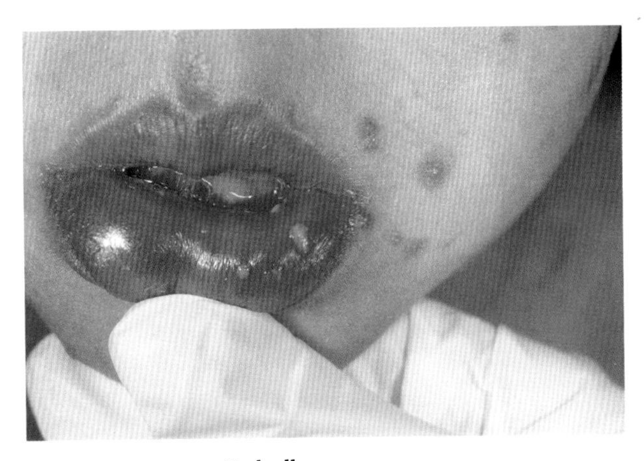

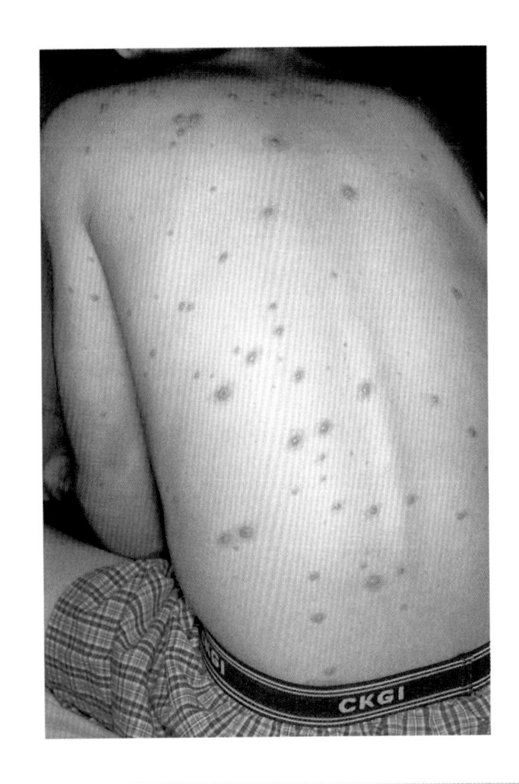

FIGURE 5.12. Varicella.

(Reproduced, with permission, from Shah BR, Lucchesi M. *Atlas of Pediatric Emergency Medicine*. New York: McGraw-Hill, 2006:119.)

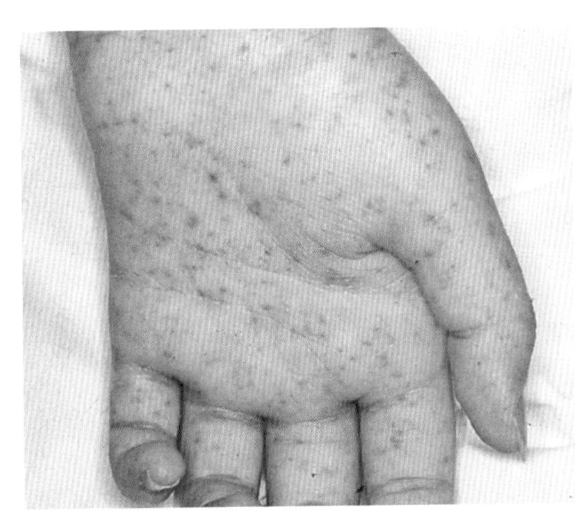

FIGURE 5.14. Rocky Mountain spotted fever.

(Reproduced, with permission, from Weinberg S, Prose NS, Kristal L., *Color Atlas of Pediatric Dermatology*, 4th ed. New York: McGraw-Hill, 2008:56.)

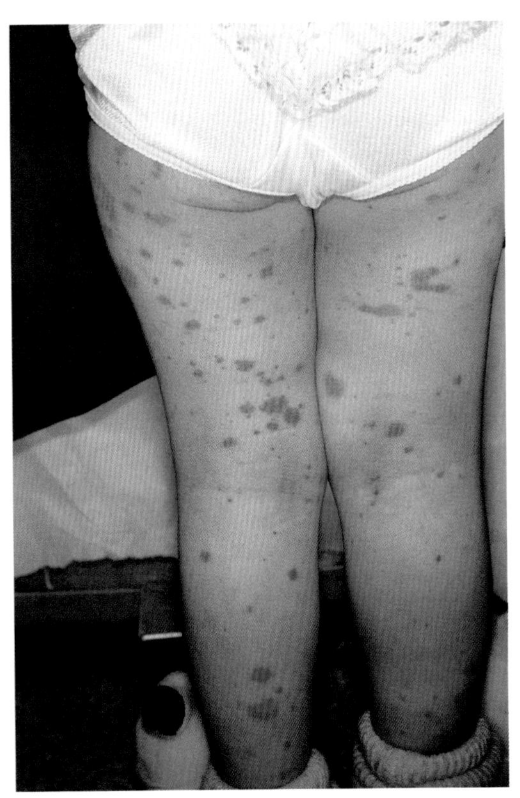

FIGURE 5.19. Henoch-Schonlein purpura.

(Reproduced, with permission, from Shah BR, Lucchesi M. *Atlas of Pediatric Emergency Medicine*. New York: McGraw-Hill, 2006:109.)

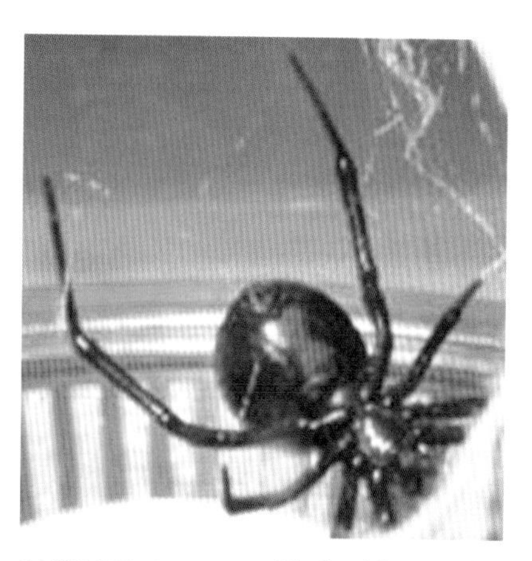

FIGURE 13.1. Black widow spider.

(Courtesy of Fred Severyn, MD.)

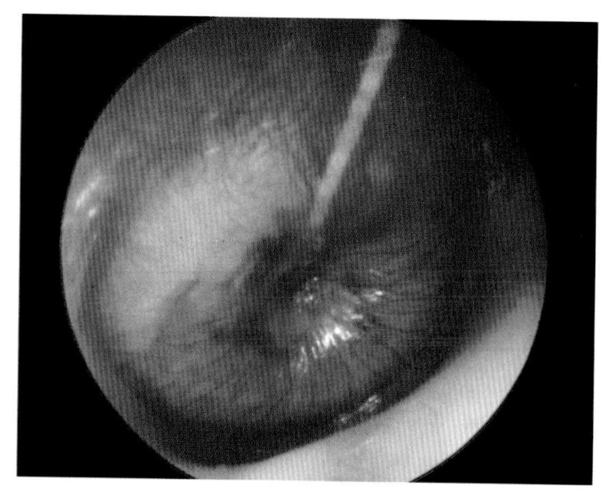

FIGURE 14.2. Otitis media with red, bulging tympanic membrane.

(Courtesy of Richard A. Chole, MD, PhD as published in Knoop KJ, Stack LB, Storrow AB. *Atlas of Emergency Medicine*, 2nd ed. New York: McGraw-Hill, 2002:118.)

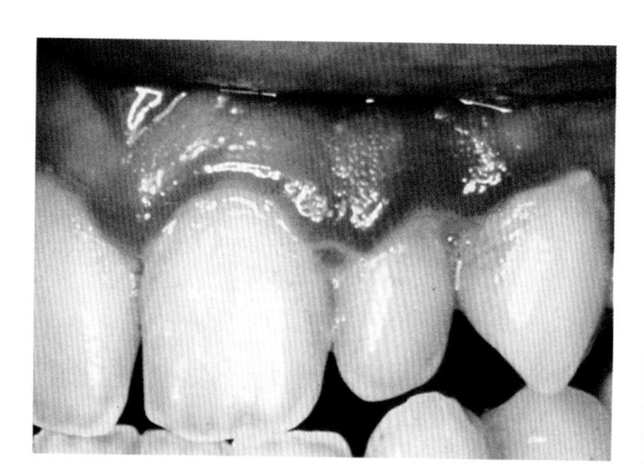

FIGURE 14.25. Acute necrotizing ulcerative gingivitis.

(Courtesy of David P. Kretzschmar, DDS, MS as reproduced, with permission, from Knoop KJ, Stack LB, Storrow AB. *Atlas of Emergency Medicine*, 2nd ed. New York: McGraw-Hill, 2002:174.)

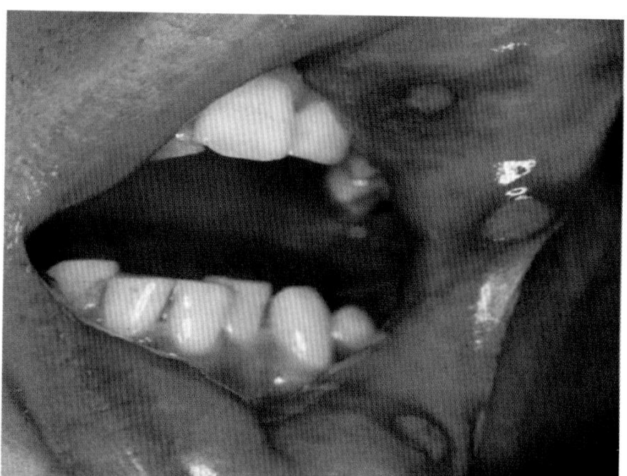

FIGURE 14.26. Aphthous stomatitis.

(Reproduced, with permission, from Wolff K, Johnson RA, Suurmond D. *Fitzpatrick's Color Atlas & Synopsis of Clinical Dermatology*, 5th ed. New York: McGraw-Hill, 2005:1017.)

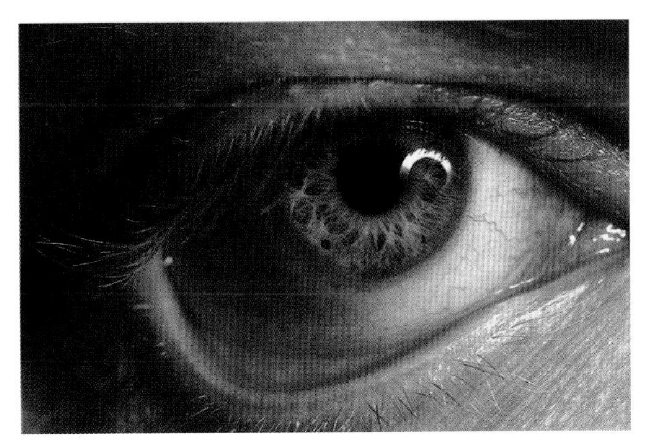

FIGURE 14.34. Metallic foreign body with rust ring at 8 o'clock. position

(Reproduced, with permission, from Knoop KJ, Stack LB, Storrow AB. *Atlas of Emergency Medicine*, 2nd ed. New York: McGraw-Hill, 2002:100.)

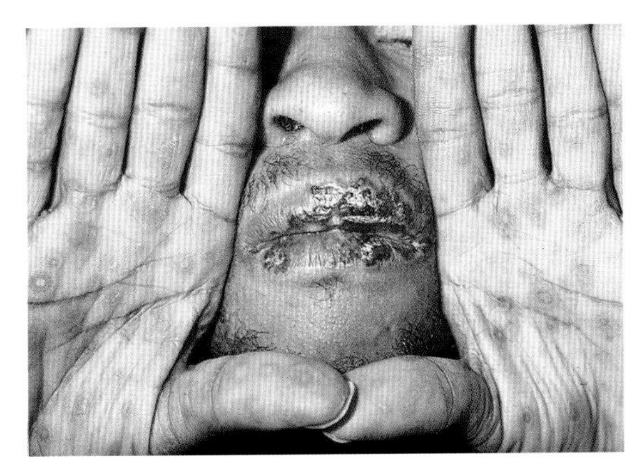

FIGURE 17.1. Stevens-Johnson syndrome. Note the target lesions on the hands of this patient.

(Reproduced, with permission, from Knoop KJ, Stack LB, Storrow AB. *Atlas of Emergency Medicine*, 2nd ed. New York: McGraw-Hill, 2002:379.)

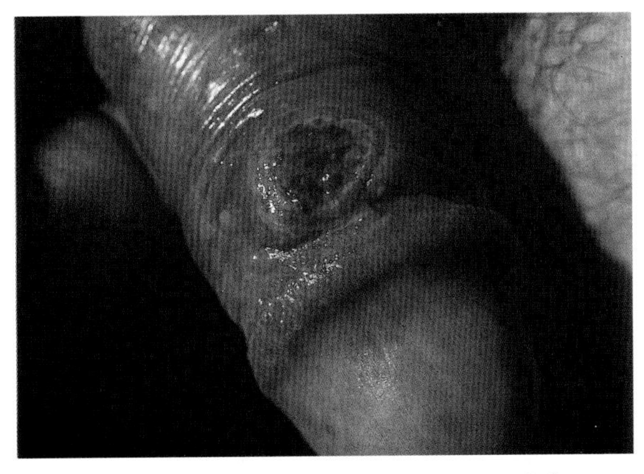

FIGURE 18.2. Syphilis. Painless, indurated chancre.

(Reproduced, with permission, from Wolff K, Johnson RA, Suurmond D. *Fitzpatrick's Color Atlas & Synopsis of Clinical Dermatology*, 5th ed. New York: McGraw-Hill, 2005:915.)

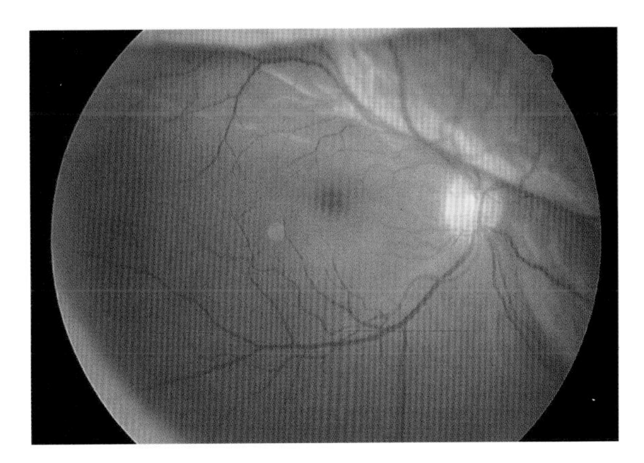

FIGURE 14.42. Retinal detachment from 11 o'clock to 4 o'clock. Note the dunes on a beach appearance.

(Reproduced, with permission, from Kasper DL, Braunwald E, Fauci AS, et al. *Harrison's Principles of Internal Medicine*, 16th ed. New York: McGraw-Hill, 2005:170.)

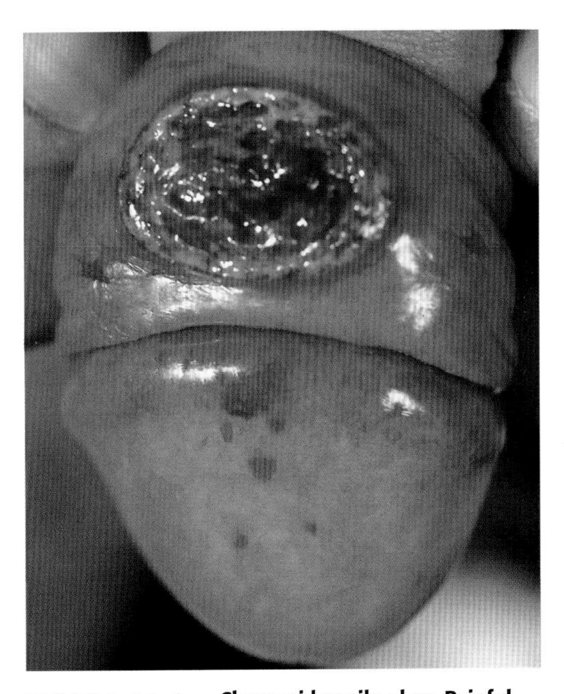

FIGURE 18.1. Chancroid penile ulcer. Painful sharply demarcated ulcer with undermined edges.

(Courtesy of Professor Alfred Eichman, MD as reproduced, with permission, from Wolff K, Johnson RA, Suurmond D. *Fitzpatrick's Color Atlas and Synopsis of Clinical Dermatology*, 5th ed. New York: McGraw-Hill, 2005:926.)

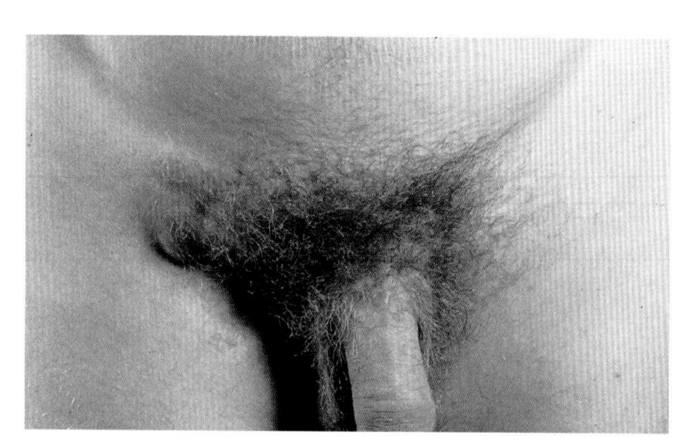

FIGURE 18.3. Lymphogranuloma venerum. Unilateral tender lymphadenopathy.

(Reproduced, with permission, from Wolff K, Johnson RA, Suurmond D. *Fitzpatrick's Color Atlas & Synopsis of Clinical Dermatology*, 5th ed. New York: McGraw-Hill, 2005:935.)

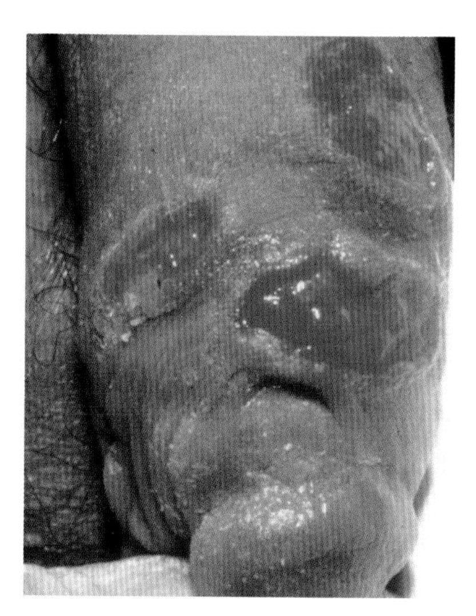

FIGURE 18.4. Granuloma inguinale. Beefy red, highly vascular, painless ulcers.

(Reproduced, with permission, from Kasper DL, Braunwald E, Fauci AS, Hauser SL, Longo DL, Jameson JL. *Harrison's Principles of Internal Medicine*, 16th ed. New York: McGraw-Hill, 2005:933.)

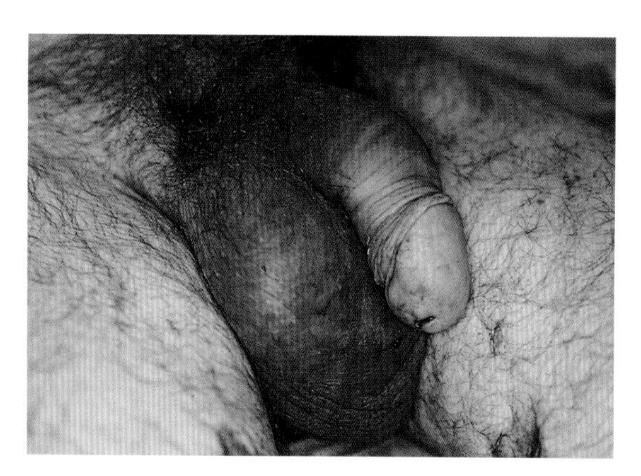

FIGURE 18.7. Penile fracture. Swollen, deformed, and discolored penis.

(Reproduced, with permission, from Knoop KJ, Stack LB, Storrow AB. *Atlas of Emergency Medicine*, 2nd ed. New York: McGraw-Hill, 2002:228.)

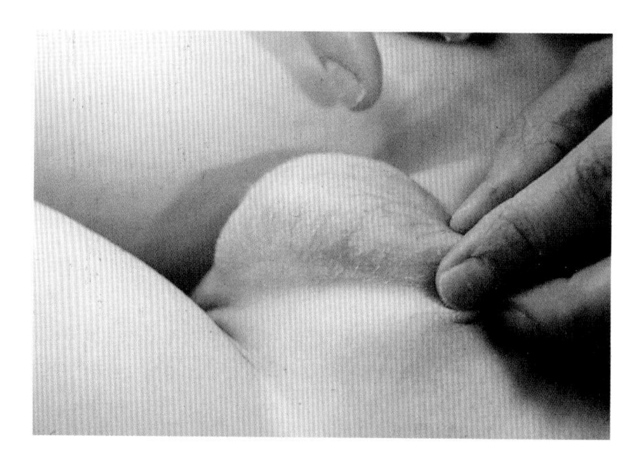

FIGURE 18.8. Blue-dot sign indicating appendageal torsion of the testicular appendix.

(Courtesy of Javier A. Gonzalez del Rey, MD as published in Knoop KJ, Stack LB, Storrow AB. *Atlas of Emergency Medicine*, 2nd ed. New York: McGraw-Hill, 2002:220.)

CHAPTER 11

Abdominal and Gastrointestinal Emergencies

Allison L. Hobelmann, MD, Ann C. Czarnik, MD,
Emilie J. B. Cavello, MD, MPH, and Charles H. Brown IV, MD

ESOPHAGEAL DISORDERS

Infectious Esophagitis

Infectious esophagitis is usually seen in patients who are immunosuppressed, ie, AIDS patients.

SYMPTOMS

Chest pain, odynophagia, dysphagia, symptoms of dehydration

EXAM

- Oral lesions are not reliable diagnostic indicators.
- Shoddy cervical lymphadenopathy

DIFFERENTIAL

- **Noninfectious esophagitis:** Reflux, pill, caustic ingestion, radiation, eosinophilic, autoimmune (eg, Crohn's, Behçet's)
- Functional dyspepsia, esophageal stricture, mass lesion, motility disorders, graft-versus-host disease
- Cardiac disease

DIAGNOSIS

- Endoscopy and biopsy
- Viral infections (eg, CMV, HSV, EBV) and fungal infections are less common but may be seen in patients with severe immunosuppression.

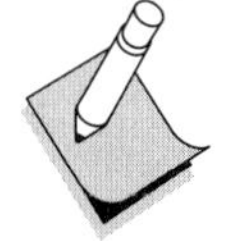

Advanced AIDS (CD4 count <200) should make you more aware of the potential for esophageal candidiasis.

TREATMENT

- Treat or adjust underlying immunosuppression.
- ***Candida albicans:*** Treatment depends on host immune status.
  - **Immunocompetent patients:** Topical therapy; nystatin swish and swallow five times a day × 7–14 days; test for HIV
  - **Immunocompromised patients:** Oral therapy, initially with fluconazole 100–200 mg/day; if the patient is unresponsive, consider increasing fluconazole or giving itraconazole, other azoles, caspofungin, or amphotericin
- **CMV:** Ganciclovir 5 mg/kg IV BID × 3–6 weeks
- **HSV:** Acyclovir 200 mg PO five times a day or valacyclovir 1000 g PO BID
- **Idiopathic ulcers:** Trial of prednisone

COMPLICATIONS

- Dehydration, requiring admission for IV resuscitation
- Stricture, malnutrition, hemorrhage

Inflammatory Esophagitis

This inflammatory response in the esophagus may be caused by medications and pills, eg, bisphosphonates, tetracyclines (especially doxycycline), and NSAIDs.

SYMPTOMS

Chest pain and odonyphagia

EXAM

Cardiac and abdominal exam to rule out perforation and other causes of pain

DIFFERENTIAL

Infectious and other noninfectious esophagitis, gastroesophageal reflux disease (GERD), functional dyspepsia, esophageal stricture or mass lesion, esophageal motility disorders

- Cardiac disease
- Pulmonary disease

DIAGNOSIS

Endoscopy and empiric treatment with resolution of symptoms

TREATMENT

- Discontinue the suspected drug. Expect symptom relief within 1–6 weeks.
- Patients should drink 8 ounces of water with each pill and remain upright at least 30 minutes afterward.
- Proton pump inhibitors (PPIs) may facilitate healing in the setting of concurrent GERD.

COMPLICATIONS

Perforation and strictures

Gastroesophageal Reflux Disease

Affects approximately 20% of adults; often related to incompetence of the lower esophageal sphincter, hiatal hernia, or incomplete emptying of stomach

SYMPTOMS

- **Typical presentation:** A retrosternal burning sensation (heartburn) is accompanied by regurgitation that begins in the epigastrium and radiates upward (typically occurring within 1 hour of a meal, during exercise, or when lying recumbent) and is at least partially relieved by antacids. **Water brash** (excess salivation), **bitter taste,** globus sensation (throat fullness), odynophagia, dysphagia, halitosis, and otalgia are also commonly seen.
- **Atypical symptoms (up to 50%):** Nocturnal cough, asthma, hoarseness, noncardiac chest pain

EXAM

Exam is often normal, or patients may present with **poor dentition** and wheezing.

DIFFERENTIAL

Infectious esophagitis (CMV, HSV, *Candida*), pill esophagitis (alendronate [Fosamax], tetracycline), PUD, dyspepsia, biliary colic, angina, esophageal dysmotility

DIAGNOSIS

- For **typical symptoms,** treat with an empiric trial of PPIs for 4–6 weeks. Response to PPIs is diagnostic.

- If the patient is **unresponsive** to therapy or has **alarm symptoms** (dysphagia, odynophagia, weight loss, anemia, long-standing symptoms, blood in stool, age >50), proceed as follows:
  - **Barium esophagography:** Has a limited role but can identify strictures
  - **Upper endoscopy with biopsy:** Standard workup in the presence of **alarm symptoms;** normal in >50% of patients with GERD (most have nonerosive reflux disease) or may reveal endoscopic esophagitis grades 1 (mild) to 4 (severe erosions, strictures, Barrett esophagus); strictures can be dilated
  - **Ambulatory esophageal pH monitoring:** The gold standard, but often unnecessary; indicated for correlating symptoms with pH parameters when endoscopy is normal and (1) symptoms are unresponsive to medical therapy, (2) antireflux surgery is being considered, or (3) there are atypical symptoms (eg, chest pain, cough, wheezing)

TREATMENT

See Table 11.1.

- **Behavioral modification:** Elevate the head of the bed 6 inches; stop tobacco and alcohol use. Advise patients to eat smaller meals, reduce fat intake, lose weight, avoid recumbency after eating, and avoid certain foods (eg, mint, chocolate, coffee, tea, carbonated drinks, citrus, and tomato juice). This is effective in 25% of cases.

TABLE 11.1. Treatment of GERD/Peptic Ulcer Disease

AGENT	MECHANISM	EXAMPLE
Antacid	Neutralizes gastric acid	Calcium carbonate, aluminum hydroxide, magnesium hydroxide
Histamine antagonist (H-2 blocker)	Inhibits gastric acid secretions	Cimetidine, ranitidine, famotidine, nizatidine
Proton pump inhibitor	Inhibits H^+/K^+ ATPase enzyme in parietal cells, prevents acid release	Omeprazole, lansoprazole, pantoprazole
Misoprostol	Prostaglandin E analog, prevents NSAID-induced ulcers only	Misprostol
Sucralfate	Binds to ulcer site	Sucralfate
Bismuth	Diminishes pepsin activity, used with triple therapy for *Helicobacter pylori* eradication	Bismuth subsalicylate
H. pylori eradication	95% of duodenal ulcers and 70% of gastric ulcers are due to *H. pylori,* Gram-negative, spiral-shaped organism; eradication with triple therapy treatment for 10–14 days	Amoxicillin, clarithromycin, omeprazole or bismuth, tetracycline, metronizadole, omeprazole; other PPIs acceptable to substitute for omeprazole

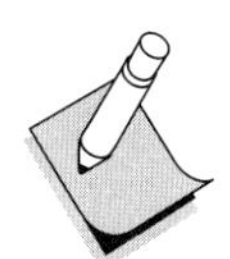

Both ACS and GERD or esophageal spasm may be relieved by nitroglycerin.

- **Antacids (calcium carbonate, aluminum hydroxide):** For mild GERD; fast but afford only short-term relief
- **H_2-receptor antagonists (cimetidine, ranitidine, famotidine, nizatidine):** For mild GERD or as an adjunct for nocturnal GERD while the patient is on PPIs; effective in 50–60% of the cases
- **PPIs (omeprazole, lansoprazole, rabeprazole, pantoprazole, esomeprazole):** The mainstay of therapy for mild to severe GERD; generally safe and effective but now associated with pneumonia, atrophic gastritis (hypergastrinemia), enteric infections (*Clostridium difficile*), and hip fractures; daily dosage effective in 80–90% of patients; **fewer than 5%** of patients are **refractory** to twice-daily dosage

Caustic Ingestions

May be a suicide attempt in adults, whereas most ingestions in children are accidental

Symptoms

Presents with chest pain, dysphagia, and drooling

Exam

Local burns to the oropharynx, edema, and sloughing of GI tract that may → obstruction

Diagnosis

- History and physical
- CXR to identify perforation
- Endoscopy or bronchoscopy to identify extent of burns

Treatment

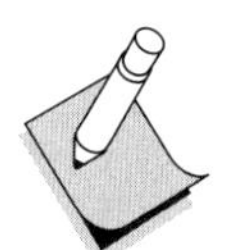

Alkali burns cause liquefaction necrosis (much more serious), whereas acidic burns cause coagulation necrosis.

- IV fluids and antibiotics
- Do not induce vomiting.
- Severe burns may require emergent esophagectomy.
- Serial exams to rule out esophageal stenosis and need for stenting should be performed.

Complications

Perforation, stenosis, strictures

Dysmotility

Dysmotility can be broken down into two classifications (see Table 11.2). **Oropharyngeal dysphagia** describes abnormality in transferring food from the pharynx to the esophagus. **Esophageal dysphagia** describes difficulty in transfer to the stomach from the upper esophagus.

Foreign Bodies

Eighty percent of ingestions are by children. Others at risk include psychiatric patients, prisoners, and those with altered mental status. More than 50% of ingestions are coins. Objects remained lodged in places of physiological narrowing. In children, this is the level of the cricopharyngeus muscle (C6). In adults, the most common place is just above the lower esophageal sphincter.

TABLE 11.2 Dysmotility Syndromes

	Oropharyngeal Dysphagia	Esophageal Dysphagia
Etiology	Neurological lesions	Motility or obstruction
Differential	CVA, multiple sclerosis, Parkinson disease, myasthenia gravis, neuropathy	Achalasia, esophageal spasm, obstructions (tumors), strictures
Presentation	Gagging and drooling, liquids more difficult than solids	Chest pain, food sticking, painful swallowing, solids worse than liquids
Treatment	Swallow evaluation	Spasm may be treated with Ca channel blockers or nitrates to relax smooth muscle. Achalasia may need esophageal dilatation as do strictures.

Foreign bodies that pass the pylorus are rarely problematic and can be managed expectantly. **Button batteries** are problematic due to the alkali contents and may cause liquefaction necrosis or rupture of the esophagus within 4–6 hours.

Symptoms

- Children may present with signs of acute airway obstruction.
- Other symptoms include retching or vomiting, coughing or gagging.
- Retrosternal pain may be a sign of esophageal perforation.

Exam

- Examine the neck for crepitus or subcutaneous air, suggesting esophageal perforation.
- Examine the abdomen for peritonitis indicative of GI perforation.

Imaging

- CXR and soft-tissue lateral neck to identify radio-opaque objects.
  - AP view: Coins in the esophagus will be seen in the coronal plane (see Figure 11.1).
  - Lateral view: Coins in the trachea will be seen in the sagittal plane.
- CT scan is better than plain films for locating the foreign body.

Treatment

- Direct laryngoscopy if airway compromise and retrieval of foreign body
- Endoscopy for diagnosis and treatment
- Button batteries in the esophagus require emergent removal secondary to alkali contents. Once in the stomach, they can be allowed to pass but close follow-up is warranted because if they do not pass in 48 hours, endoscopic removal is indicated.
- Smooth objects <5 cm (length) and <2 cm (width) will usually pass spontaneously.
- Food boluses may be removed via endoscopy or pharmacologically with nitroglycerin or nifedipine to relax the sphincter; IV glucagon may also be used to expel food boluses. Proteolytic enzymes such as papain are no longer recommended.
- Sharp objects, eg, razor blades, need to be removed via endoscopy to prevent perforation.

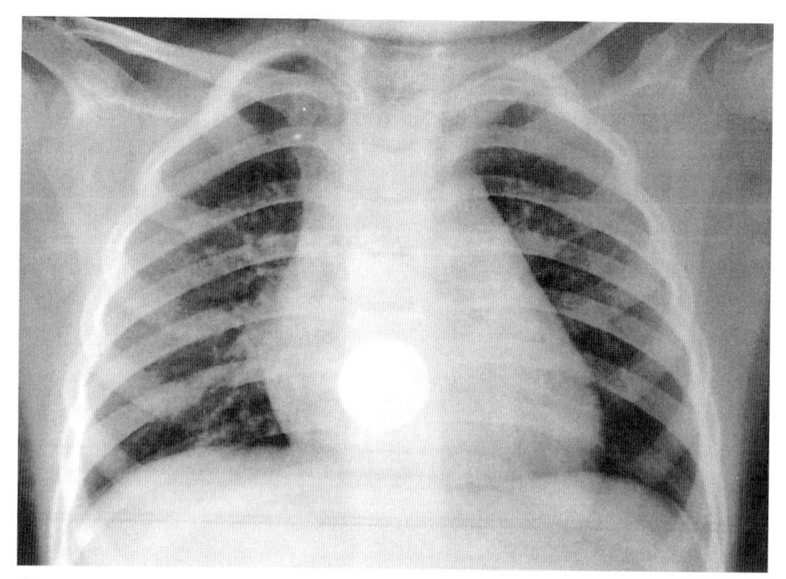

A

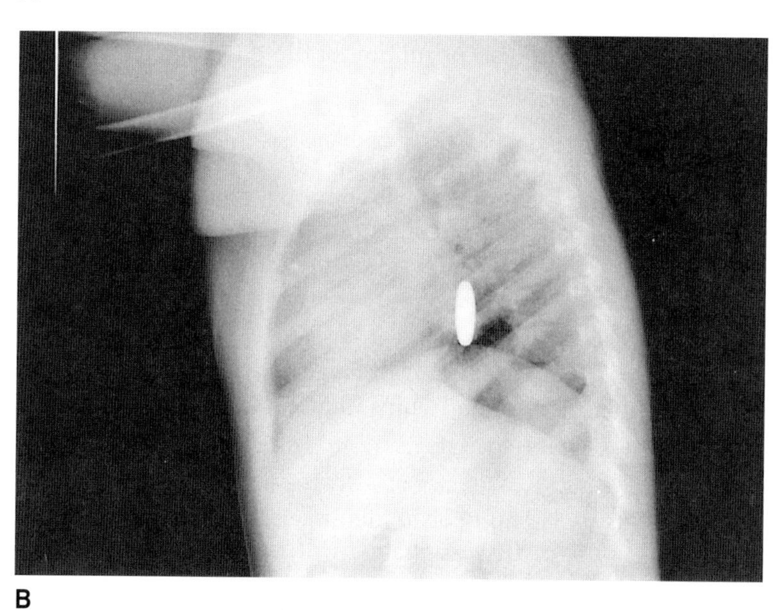

B

FIGURE 11.1. Posteroanterior (A) and lateral (B) chest X-rays, showing esophageal foreign body.

(Reproduced, with permission, from Stone CK, Humphries, RL. *Current Emergency Diagnosis and Treatment*, 5th ed. New York: McGraw-Hill, 2004:1092.)

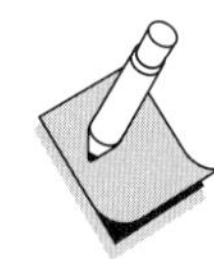

Ninety percent of esophageal foreign bodies pass spontaneously.

DISPOSITION

- **Eighty to ninety percent** of objects pass spontaneously; ten percent require further intervention.
- Esophageal foreign bodies may be managed in the ED or admitted.
- Patients with small smooth objects that have passed the esophagus may be discharged and followed with serial imaging and stool monitoring.
- Esophageal perforation requires emergent surgery.

Structural Abnormalities

MALLORY-WEISS TEAR

Partial esophageal tear, usually due to retching or vomiting; longitudinal mucosal tears seen at the gastroesophageal junction

SYMPTOMS

Hematemesis after forceful retching

EXAM

Rule out crepitus of the neck or peritonitis, which would suggest complete esophageal perforation.

DIFFERENTIAL

Esophagitis, Boerhaaeve syndrome, peptic ulcer disease

DIAGNOSIS

History or endoscopy

TREATMENT

- May cause upper GI Bleed (see "GI Bleeding" for treatment)
- Usually no treatment required

BOERHAAVE SYNDROME

This is a postemetic perforation. **Ten percent** of cases involve patients with underlying pathology that causes leakage of nonsterile substances into the mediastinum. Boerhaave's is a cause of rapid overwhelming sepsis. Iatrogenic perforations account for 80% of cases of esophageal perforation. Rupture of all layers of the esophageal wall is possible, most commonly on the left posterolateral aspect.

SYMPTOMS

- Most common presentation is chest or midepigastric pain that radiates to the neck and occasionally the back.
- Most reliable presentation is pleuritic pain in the esophageal region that is **worsened by neck flexion and swallowing**.
- Often associated with pneumothorax or hydrothorax
- Mediastinal crunch (**Hamman sign**) may be heard on auscultation of the heart.
- Fever or shock may be present as well.

DIAGNOSIS

- Plain CXR and/or soft-tissue lateral neck XR reveals mediastinal air. Other findings include subcutaneous emphysema, left-sided pleural effusion, pneumothorax, and widened mediastinum.
- An esophagram using water soluble contrast and EGD are the definitive studies to diagnose and locate a perforation.
- CT scan may show mediastinal air.
- Thoracentesis will show high amylase level secondary to esophageal contents in the pleural space.

TREATMENT

- In the ED, immediate broad spectrum antibiotics should be started.
- Antibiotics should cover *Staphylococcus, Streptococcus, Pseudomonas,* and *Bacteroides.*
- The majority of perforations are treated surgically; therefore, a surgical consult should be immediately requested.
- Keep the patient NPO and treat shock with IV fluids and vasopressors if necessary.
- H2 blockers have no role in treatment of Boerhaave syndrome.

DISPOSITION

- There is a 10% mortality rate when the disease is immediately recognized; this ↑ to 50% survival when perforation has occurred >24 hours before ED presentation.
- Most patients will require ICU level of care.

ESOPHAGEAL VARICES

Varices are dilated submucosal veins that become distended when portal pressure is elevated. They are found in half of patients with ascites. One-third of cases cause upper GI bleeding. (See also "Upper GI Bleeding.")

SYMPTOMS

Usually presents as an upper GI bleed

TREATMENT

- Bleeding may be life threatening; adequate fluid resuscitation with IV fluids and blood products if needed
- Over-resuscitation can increase portal pressure and increase rate of bleeding (hematocrit >30% is associated with elevated portal pressures).
- Coagulopathic patients may require FFP or platelets.
- **IV octreotide**
- IV antibiotics (third-generation cephalosporin or floroquinolone)
  - Balloon tamponade (Sengstaken-Blakemore and Minnesota tubes) may be used to stop hemorrhage. Strongly advise prior airway protection.
- Emergent endoscopy is needed for banding or sclerotherapy of bleeding varices.

DISPOSITION

- In-house mortality rates are 15%.
- Patients require ICU care.

ACHALASIA

SYMPTOMS

Dysphagia, odynophagia, regurgitation of undigested food

DIFFERENTIAL

Spasm, stricture, tumor

DIAGNOSIS

Bird's beak on barium swallow, dilation of upper esophagus with narrowing at cardioesophageal junction (see Figure 11.2).

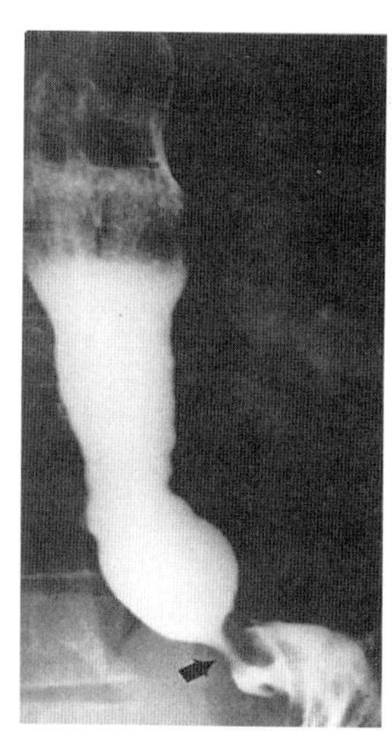

FIGURE 11.2. Achalasia seen on barium swallow.

(Reproduced, with permission, from Chen MYM, Pope TL, Ott DJ. *Basic Radiology*. New York: McGraw-Hill, 2004:258.)

Treatment

- Nifedipine 10–20 mg before meals
- Botulinum toxin injection endoscopically
- Esophageal dilation
- Surgery

Complications

Dehydration

Esophageal Web

Symptoms

Dysphagia

Differential

Spasm, stricture, tumor, achalasia

Diagnosis

Barium swallow or EGD

Treatment

Disruption of webs by endoscopy, treat iron deficiency

Complications

Dehydration, iron-deficiency anemia.

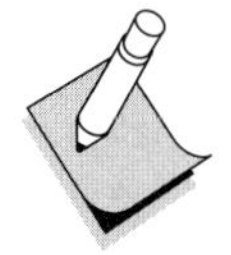

IV antibiotics can reduce the absolute mortality associated with an upper GI bleed in cirrhotic patients by up to 9%.

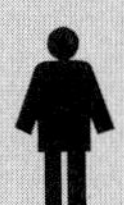

A 47-year-old male presents with massive hematemesis, hypotension, and altered mental status. On exam, he has scleral icterus, a distended abdomen, and spider telangectasias on his chest. What is the likely diagnosis?
Esophageal varices.

GI BLEEDING

Potentially life-threatening disease; incidence 100 in 100,000 for upper GI bleeds and 20 in 100,000 for lower GI bleeds with an overall mortality rate of about 10%; classified as upper or lower GI bleed defined by its relationship to the ligament of Treitz

Upper GI bleeds—

GUM BLEED
Gastritis
Ulcers
Mallory-Weiss tears
Biliary
Large esophageal varices
Esophagitis
Enteric-aortic fistula (seen in patients with aortic grafts)
Dieulafoy lesions (gastric vessel aneurysm)

Upper GI Bleeding

Etiology

Peptic ulcer disease (most common), esophagitis, Mallory-Weiss tears, gastritis, esophageal varices, stress ulcers, AVM, and malignancy

Symptoms

- Hematemesis or "coffee-ground" emesis
- Hypovolemia, syncope, abdominal pain, chest pain, and dyspnea

- Mallory-Weiss tears present with bright red hematemesis after an episode of forceful retching or vomiting.
- Gastric ulcers typically present with pain immediately after eating. Duodenal ulcers typically present with night time pain or pain 2–3 hours after eating.

EXAM

- Skin for signs of shock, as well as for signs of liver dysfunction such as jaundice or hemangiomas
- Abdominal exam to assess for organomegaly or ascites, as well as abdominal tenderness
- Heme occult

DIAGNOSIS

- History, rectal exam, nasogastric lavage
- Inquire about medications, alcohol consumption, risk factors for viral hepatitis, and previous history of GI bleeds.
- NGT to evaluate ongoing bleeding
- Hematocrit, platelets, coagulation profile, type, and crossmatch
- Note that the initial HCT may not reflect blood loss due to hemoconcentration.
- Serial HCT to follow trend
- Early endoscopy for both diagnostic and therapeutic purposes

TREATMENT

See Figure 11.3.

- Treatment begins with securing an airway if necessary. Most common cause of early death in upper GI bleeding is aspiration.
- Insert a nasogastric tube to see if the patient is actively bleeding or if bleeding has stopped.
- Lavage with water until aspirate clears.
- Volume replacement should be initiated with crystalloid.
- Failure to achieve adequate resuscitation after 2 L of crystalloid is generally an indication for blood replacement.
- Patients who are on Warfarin or have liver dysfunction may require coagulation replacement with FFP and Vitamin K.
- Proton pump inhibitors: Omeprazole IV bolus at 80 mg and a drip at 8 mg/hr for presumed ulcer or variceal hemorrhage
- IV octreotide (25–50 μg bolus followed by drip at 25–50 μg/hour) and IV antibiotics (third-generation cephalosporin/fluoroquinolone) if cirrhosis is suspected
- **Early endoscopy** for direct interventions for hemostasis (focal cautery, epinephrine injection, banding, and sclerotherapy)
- Balloon tamponade (Sengstaken-Blakemore and Minnesota tubes) may be used to stop hemorrhage; strongly advise prior airway protection
- Transjugular intrahepatic portosystemic shunt (TIPS) may be required for refractory variceal bleeding.
- Treat concomitant *H. pylori* infection if suspected peptic ulcer disease (see Table 11.1).

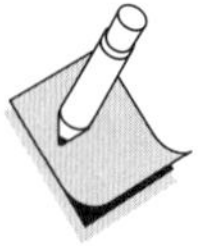

Predictors of high mortality include initial HCT < 30, advanced age, hypotension or presence of shock, and a physical exam consistent with advanced liver disease.

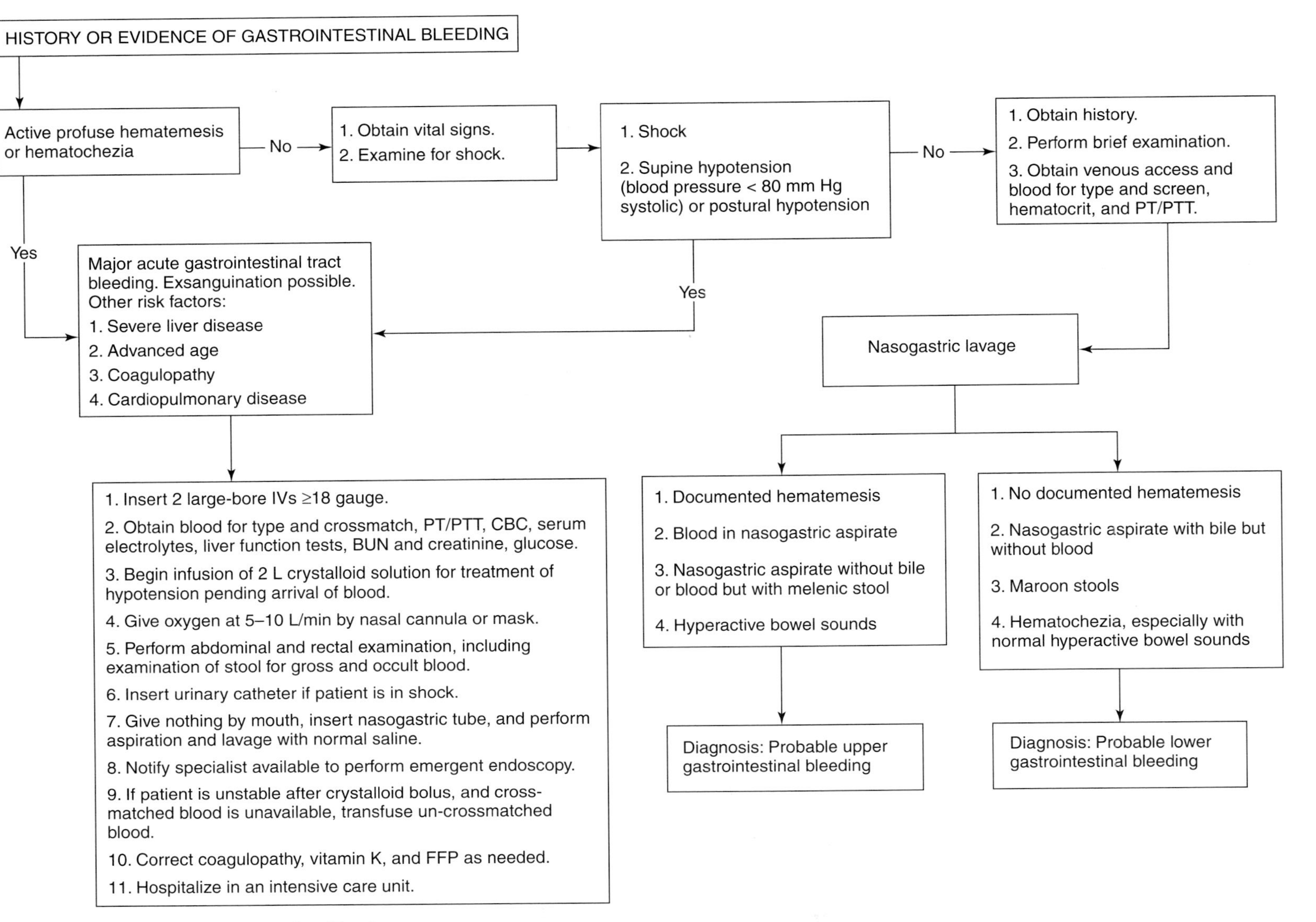

FIGURE 11.3. Management of GI bleeds.

(Reproduced, with permission, from Stone CK, Humphries, RL. *Current Emergency Diagnosis and Treatment*, 5th ed. New York: McGraw-Hill, 2004:284.)

DISPOSITION

- Disease associated with high rate of mortality
- Admit for intervention and continual resuscitation.
- Early consultation with gastroenterologist or surgical specialist is highly advised.
- Consider ICU admission.

Lower GI Bleeds–

DRAIN
Diverticulosis
Radiation or Ischemic Colitis
AVMs, angiodysplasia
Inflammatory bowel disease (IBD)
Neoplasms (Cancer)

Lower GI Bleeding

ETIOLOGIES

Diverticulosis (most common), tumors, angiodysplasia, polyps, hemorrhoids or brisk upper GI bleeds, and aortoenteric fistula in patients with history of aortic stent

SYMPTOMS

- Hematochezia
- Abdominal pain
- Weight loss
- Change in bowel pattern
- Hypovolemia or signs of shock

DIAGNOSIS

- Rectal exam for presence of blood and anoscopy as indicated.
- Angiography can localize site of bleeding if rate >0.5 mL/min.
- Tagged red blood scan can localize the site of bleeding if rate >0.1 mL/min; not as good at localizing site of bleeding as angiography.
- Colonoscopy (after bowel prep if patient is stable)
- CBC, coagulation profile, type, and crossmatch

TREATMENT

- Fluid resuscitation
- Packed red blood cells if patient has ongoing bleeding or is symptomatic after 2 liters of IVF
- Replace coagulation factors as needed.
- Vitamin K if INR is high
- Vasopressin after angiography may be beneficial.
- Definitive treatment includes selective embolization, endoscopic coagulation, and surgical resection.

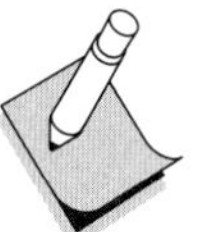

Ten percent of apparent lower GI bleeds are actually caused by upper GI bleeds.

DISPOSITION

- Most GI bleeds should be admitted.
- Low-risk patients (hemorrhoids, fissures, and proctitis) may be safely discharged if they have adequate follow-up care.

STOMACH

Gastritis

May be due to stress, burns, sepsis, drugs (ASA and NSAIDs), alcohol, autoimmune conditions, or *H. pylori* bacterial infection

Symptoms

Abdominal pain, nausea and vomiting, anorexia

Differential

Cardiac disease, ulcers, hernia, GERD, gastroparesis, functional dyspepsia, pancreatitis, hepatitis, AAA, cholelithiasis

Exam

Epigastric pain on palpation

Diagnosis

- Endoscopy with gastric biopsy
- Nonbleeding gastritis is managed medically.

Treatment

- Discontinue ASA, NSAID, or alcohol use.
- Suspected gastritis without steroid evidence of bleeding may be treated with a trial of viscous lidocaine and an antacid.
- Consider prescribing a PPI or an over-the-counter H2 blocker.
- Test for the presence of *H. pylori* and treat with triple therapy if present (see Table 11.1).

H. pylori serologic tests are useful for past exposure but cannot be used for test of cure. Urea breath test, endoscopic biopsy, and stool antigen may be used for diagnosis and to confirm adequate treatment.

Complications

- Ulcers or GI bleeding
- Chronic atrophic gastritis may → lead to loss of gastric parietal cells (and intrinsic factor production) → vitamin B_{12} deficiency and pernicious anemia.

Gastric and Duodenal Ulcers

Symptoms

- Abdominal pain, nausea and vomiting, anorexia
- Burning epigastric pain is the most common symptom. It may be relieved by milk, antacids, and food. Food typically worsens gastric ulcers and relieves duodenal ulcers. Duodenal ulcers get worse 2–3 hours after eating.

Differential

Cardiac disease, hernia, gastritis, GERD, irritable bowel disease

If a patient has received H. pylori treatment but has persistent symptoms, test for eradication. If not eradicated, treat again with a different regimen. If eradicated, refer for endoscopy.

Exam

- Epigastric pain on palpation
- Abdominal distention due to obstruction, GI bleeding on rectal exam or NGT tube placement, and abdominal rigidity from perforation indicate acute complications.

Diagnosis

Endoscopy with biopsy to rule out *H. pylori* infection and carcinoma

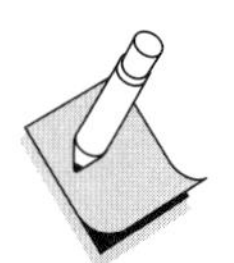

Gastric ulcers get worse shortly after eating, and duodenal ulcers get better.

TREATMENT

- Discontinue ASA, NSAID, or alcohol use.
- Test for presence of *H. pylori* and treat with triple therapy if present (see Table 11.1).

COMPLICATIONS

Ulcers or GI bleeding

Pyloric Stenosis

Pyloric stenosis is caused by an increase in the musculature of the pylorus. Seen in about 1 in 1000 live births. More common in firstborn males. Seen between 2 and 8 weeks of life (median, 5 weeks).

SYMPTOMS

Projectile vomiting of nonbilious emesis, dehydration, hypochloremic, metabolic alkalosis

DIFFERENTIAL

GERD or bowel obstruction

EXAM

Olive-sized mass in the subhepatic region

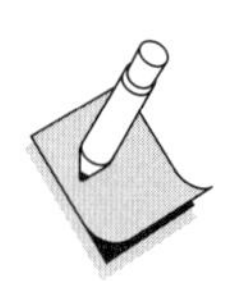

Pyloric stenosis causes nonbilious emesis, whereas intestinal obstruction causes biliary emesis.

DIAGNOSIS

Ultrasound or via visualization of "**string sign**" on upper GI series

TREATMENT

Surgery for pylorotomy and IV-fluid resuscitation

Gastrinoma (Zollinger-Ellison Syndrome)

Gastrin-secreting neuroendocrine tumor; two-thirds are malignant

SYMPTOMS

- Recurrent and intractable peptic ulcer disease
- Diarrhea is common with ZES.

DIFFERENTIAL

PUD, GERD, gastritis

EXAM

Epigastric tenderness on palpation

DIAGNOSIS

- Elevated serum gastrin level
- Multiple ulcers in abnormal locations on endoscopy

TREATMENT

- Proton pump inhibitors
- Resect local disease if found before it has metastasized to the liver.

Eighty percent of ZES is sporadic, whereas 20% is associated with multiple endocrine neoplasia type 1 (MEN 1).

Gastric Cancer

Adenocarcinoma is the most common worldwide. This is a highly aggressive cancer with a poor prognosis.

SYMPTOMS

- Usually asymptomatic until the disease is advanced
- Abdominal pain, weight loss, anemia, GI bleeding

DIFFERENTIAL

PUD, GERD, gastritis

EXAM

- Lymphadenopathy
- Sister Mary Joseph nodule, which is a firm, red, nontender nodule from metastatic spread within the falciform ligament

DIAGNOSIS

- Abdominal CT scan
- Endoscopy

TREATMENT

Surgery, chemotherapy, palliative care

COMPLICATIONS

Gastric-outlet obstruction, anemia, dehydration, blood loss, bowel obstruction, death

SMALL INTESTINE

Crohn Disease

Crohn disease is a chronic, recurrent, inflammatory disease of the GI tract that may affect any segment from mouth to anus. Crohn disease has a propensity for the ileum and proximal colon (see Table 11.3). Incidence is higher among Ashkenazi Jews, smokers, and those with a family history. All layers of the bowel wall are involved, and the disease may extend to mesenteric lymph nodes. The disease is discontinuous, with skip areas that are free of ulceration. Deep ulcerations of the bowel wall → fistulas and abscesses.

SYMPTOMS

Abdominal pain, anorexia, diarrhea, fever, weight loss, malaise, extra-intestinal complications

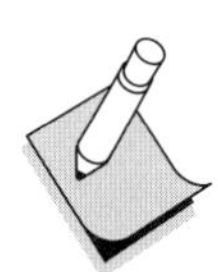

Twenty-five to thirty percent of patients with Crohn disease will manifest extraintestinal complications.

EXAM

Abdominal tenderness, abdominal mass, anal fissures, fistulas

TABLE 11.3. **Distinguishing Features of IBD**

Feature	Crohn Disease	Ulcerative Colitis
Age at onset	Bimodal: 15–25, 55–65 yr	Bimodal: 20–40, 60–70 yr
Abdominal pain	Sharp, focal	Crampy, associated with bowel movement
Bowel obstruction	Common	Rare
Gross hematochezia	Occasionally	Common
GI involvement	Mouth to anus; typically terminal ileum/proximal colon; perianal involvement common	Colon only; rectum always involved with continuous progression proximally Perianal involvement uncommon
Abscesses	Common	Uncommon
Pattern	Segmental, transmural, Eccentric	
Ulceration	Superficial to deep, linear, serpiginous	Superficial
Histology	Noncaseating granulomas	Crypt abscesses
Fistula/stricture	Common	Uncommon
Toxic megacolon	Uncommon	Common
Extraintestinal manifestations	Uncommon	Common
Infliximab response	Often	Occasionally
Surgery curative	Never	Often

Differential

IBS, ulcerative colitis, infectious enterocolitis (*Yersinia* sp., TB, *Entamoeba histolytica*, etc), celiac sprue, lymphoma, mesenteric ischemia, carcinoma of the colon

Diagnosis

- Anemia, leukocytosis, elevated ESR and CRP, B12 deficiency
- Colonoscopy reveals skip lesions, linear ulcerations, and granulomas, particularly, at the terminal ileum.
- Biopsy demonstrates chronic and acute inflammation and evaluates for the presence of colorectal cancer.
- Small bowel follow-through (SBFT)
- CT scan evaluation for abscess, mesenteric inflammation, obstruction, and fistulas

TREATMENT

- Initial treatment in the ED includes fluid resuscitation and electrolyte replacement, NGT placement if obstruction or toxic megacolon are suspected, and broad spectrum antibiotics for patients with peritonitis, abscess, or fulminant colitis.
- Patients with severe disease should receive intravenous steroids.
- Admission is required for severely ill patients.
- Medical therapy
  - Anti-inflammatories: Sulfasalazine and mesalmine, administered orally or rectally
  - Antibiotics, eg, metronidazole and ciprofloxacin, with uncertain benefit
  - Corticosteroids: Prednisone, budesonide
  - Immune modifiers: Azathioprine, methotrexate, infliximab
- Surgery: May be required for obstruction, abscesses; avoid if possible because of future strictures, adhesions, fistulas

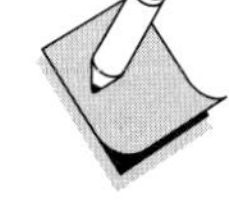

Closed-loop obstruction occurs at two points and often results in strangulation.

COMPLICATIONS

Obstruction, abscess, toxic megacolon, colorectal cancer, fistulas, strictures

Small-Bowel Obstruction/Ileus

Mechanical obstruction is the most common surgical emergency of the small intestine. Mechanical small-bowel obstruction results from a physical barrier that prevents passage of intestinal contents. It may be partial or complete and occur at one or two points. Simple obstruction blocks the lumen only, while strangulation impairs the blood supply to the intestine as well. Adynamic or paralytic ileus implies failure of peristalsis to propel intestinal contents through the bowel in the absence of a mechanical barrier.

ETIOLOGY

See Tables 11.4 and 11.5.

TABLE 11.4. Causes of Mechanical Small-Bowel Obstruction

Adhesions (most common)
Hernias: Inguinal, femoral, internal
Crohn disease
Volvulus
Intusussception
Neoplasms
Strictures
Gallstone ileus
Foreign body

TABLE 11.5. Causes of Adynamic Ileus

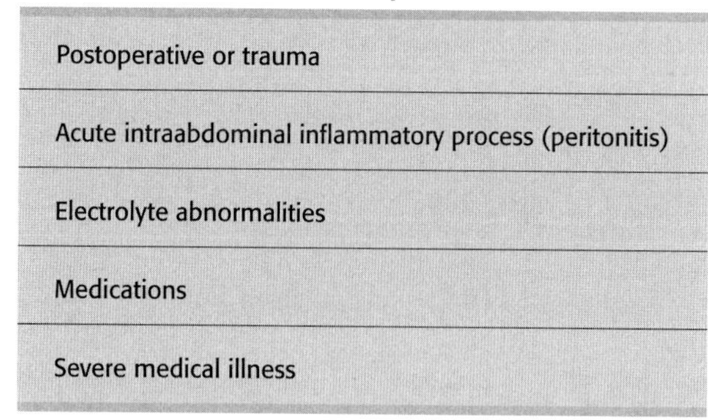

Causes of Adynamic Ileus
Postoperative or trauma
Acute intraabdominal inflammatory process (peritonitis)
Electrolyte abnormalities
Medications
Severe medical illness

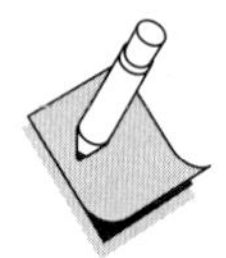

Pain from adynamic ileus is usually more constant and less intense than mechanical small-bowel obstruction.

SYMPTOMS

- The site and cause of the obstruction will determine presentation.
- Crampy and intermittent abdominal pain, bilious emesis with proximal obstruction and feculent emesis with distal obstruction, and inability to pass stool or flatus
- Ileus is associated with nausea, vomiting, obstipation, abdominal pain, and distention.

EXAM

- **Early:** Mild abdominal distention, abdominal tenderness may be mild and diffuse, tympanic to percussion, increased high-pitched bowel sounds
- **Late:** Distention, decreased peristaltic waves and bowel sounds, acute abdomen with strangulation and perforation
- **Ileus:** Mild abdominal tenderness, minimal distention, and decreased bowel sounds

DIFFERENTIAL

Acute appendicitis, pancreatitis, gastroenteritis, large-bowel obstruction, pseudo-obstruction

DIAGNOSIS

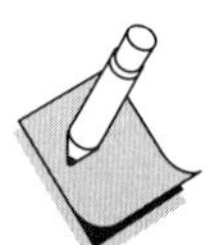

Plain abdominal radiographs are 70–80% sensitive for detection of SBO as ileus may mimic AXR findings. CT is 80–90% sensitive.

- Labs: Leukocytosis, hemoconcentration, electrolyte abnormalities, elevated serum amylase
- AXR: Dilated small-bowel loops with air fluid levels (findings may be absent in early, closed-loop, or high SBO); **"string of pearls"** sign, which are small air pockets, may be present; absence of air in colon if late obstruction (see Figure 11.4); free air with perforation
- CT: Contrast-enhanced CT is highly accurate for making the diagnosis. It delineates partial vs complete obstruction, level, and type of obstruction, and may demonstrate the cause. It is also helpful in differentiating between ileus and obstruction.

TREATMENT

- Partial SBO: It may be managed expectantly. NGT suction, bowel rest, and fluid and electrolyte replacement are required. Surgery may be required if obstruction does not resolve with conservative management.
- Complete SBO: Surgical intervention is often required. NGT suction, NPO status, and fluid and electrolyte resuscitation should be initiated preoperatively.

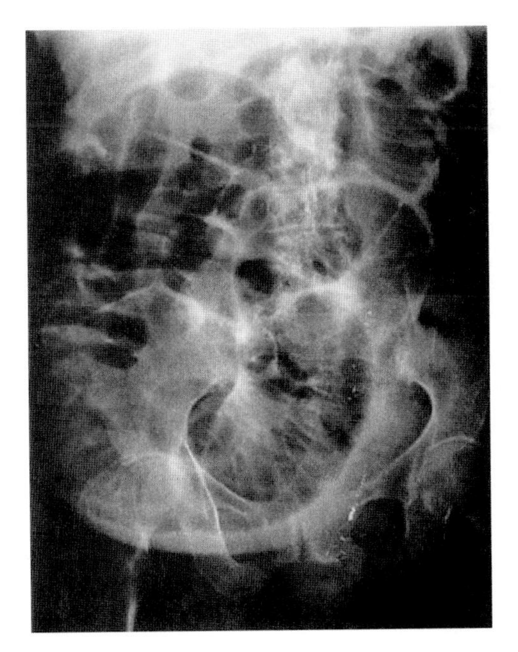

FIGURE 11.4. Small-bowel obstruction. Plain AXR demonstrates dilated small-bowel loops and paucity of air in the colon.

(Reproduced, with permission, from Brunicardi FC, Andersen DK, Billiar TR, Dunn DL, Hunter JG, Pollack RE. *Schwartz's Principles of Surgery*, 8th ed. New York: McGraw-Hill, 2004:1027.)

- Ileus: NGT suction, bowel rest, and removal or correction of precipitating factors

COMPLICATIONS

Strangulation of blood supply, perforation of small bowel, peritonitis, septic shock

Aorto-Enteric Fistula

Fistula between the aorta and the bowel should be considered in all patients with unexplained GI bleeding. The duodenum is most commonly involved. Patients with recent aortic graft placement remain at highest risk for this complication, but it may be secondary to erosion of an AAA into the bowel.

SYMPTOMS/EXAM

- Symptoms include massive GI bleeding including hematemesis, melena, hematochezia. A mild GI bleed may signify impending rupture with massive bleeding.
- Rectal bleeding, decreased distal blood flow, high-output heart failure, and hemodynamic instability may be found on exam.

DIAGNOSIS

- Diagnosis may be difficult and may be largely based on a high level of clinical suspicion. It may be difficult to differentiate from graft infection.
- Upper GI endoscopy if the patient is stable
- CT angiography may aid in identifying an associated infection.

TREATMENT

Treatment consists of large-bore IV placement, vigorous fluid resuscitation with crystalloid and blood products, cardiac monitoring with institution of vasopressors as needed, and emergent surgical consultation. If the patient is unstable, do not wait for further diagnostic studies. Emergent laparotomy is the only life-saving treatment for massive bleeding.

Meckel Diverticulum

This is the most prevalent congenital anomaly of the GI tract. Approximately 2% of the population is affected. Males are more commonly affected. Most are found in the ileum within 2 feet of the ileocecal valve. Many contain heterotopic tissues, the most common of which are gastric mucosa and pancreatic acini.

Rule of 2s for Meckel diverticulum: 2% prevalence, 2:1 male-to-female ratio, 2 feet proximal to ileocecal valve, and half of those symptomatic are <2 years of age

SYMPTOMS/EXAM

Symptoms may include rectal bleeding and abdominal pain, distention, nausea and vomiting with obstruction, strictures, or intussusception.

DIAGNOSIS

Diagnosis is most often made incidentally during radiographic imaging, endoscopy, or surgery. Radionuclide scanning and angiography can be used to locate the source of bleeding during acute hemorrhage from the diverticulum.

TREATMENT

- Surgical resection of the diverticulum is indicated in patients with complications.
- Expectant management in patients with asymptomatic diverticulae found incidentally is acceptable.

COMPLICATIONS

Intussusception, SBO, bleeding from heterotopic gastric mucosa, strictures from diverticulitis

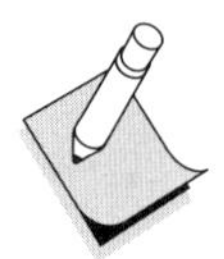

The small bowel is most commonly infiltrated by metastases from distant sites or by direct invasion of a malignancy of an adjacent organ. Melanoma has a predilection for metastases to the small intestine.

Small-Bowel Neoplasms

Primary small-bowel cancers are rare. Adenocarcinomas, carcinoid tumors, and lymphomas make up the majority of these malignancies. Other benign neoplasms of the small bowel include adenomas, fibromas, lipomas, and neurofibromas, which are generally found incidentally in the duodenum during EGD. Most patients with small-bowel cancer are in their fifth and sixth decades. Risk factors include ingestion of red meat and smoked or cured foods, Crohn disease, hereditary nonpolyposis, colorectal cancer (HNPCC), familial adenomatous polyposis (FAP), and Peutz-Jeghers syndrome.

SYMPTOMS/PHYSICAL EXAM

- Most small-bowel neoplasms remain asymptomatic until they are large.
- Abdominal distention, nausea, and vomiting associated with small-bowel obstruction.
- Exam may be benign as only 25% of small intestinal tumors are associated with abdominal mass. Findings of small-bowel obstruction, cachexia, jaundice, hepatomegaly, and ascites are late findings.

DIFFERENTIAL

- Metastasis from distant site
- Invasion of malignancy from adjacent organ
- Benign polyp
- Endometrioma

DIAGNOSIS

- Rarely diagnosed preoperatively
- Laboratory tests are generally nonspecific.
- Upper GI series with small-bowel follow-through, CT scanning, and angiography

TREATMENT

- Surgical resection and pathologic diagnosis are the mainstays of therapy.
- Adjuvant therapy depends on tissue diagnosis.

LARGE BOWEL

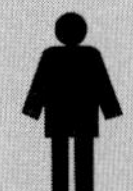

A 25-year-old female presents with copious foul-smelling diarrhea, crampy abdominal pain, and flatus. She recently returned from a camping trip in the mountains where she drank from a stream. What is the likely diagnosis?
Giardia lamblia.

Gastroenteritis

Gastroenteritis is characterized by the acute onset of vomiting and diarrhea. It is often difficult to identify the causative agent or pathogen in the acute setting; however, up to 70% of cases are caused by viruses (see Table 11.6). The remaining cases are largely caused by bacteria, with a small subset due to parasites. Infectious gastroenteritis may be invasive (dysenteric), causing systemic illness, or noninvasive, causing secretory diarrhea and few systemic symptoms (see Table 11.7).

SYMPTOMS/EXAM

See Tables 11.6 and 11.7.

- **Noninvasive**
  - Mild systemic symptoms, including nausea, vomiting, and diarrhea, generally not associated with fever or abdominal pain
  - Patients may have diffuse abdominal tenderness to palpation and signs of dehydration.
- **Invasive**
  - Fever, bloody diarrhea, abdominal cramps, myalgias, headache, anorexia, and weight loss
  - Diffuse abdominal tenderness to palpation, dehydration, evidence of systemic infection.

DIFFERENTIAL

- Food poisoning
- Antibiotic-induced gastroenteritis
- *C. difficile* infection
- Viral, parasitic, bacterial gastroenteritis

TABLE 11.6. **Common Causes of Noninvasive Gastroenteritis**

CAUSATIVE AGENT	INCUBATION AND TRANSMISSION	DESCRIPTION	THERAPY
Viral gastroenteritis	11–72 hr; person-to-person, fecal-oral, contaminated food or water	Norwalk and Rotavirus most common agents; nausea, vomiting, and watery diarrhea; usually afebrile; may have mild abdominal cramps and myalgias	Self-limiting; supportive care with PO or IV hydration and antiemetics
G. lamblia	1–4 wk; contaminated food or water, person-to-person, fecal-oral	Backpackers, campers, the elderly; also homosexual males, persons in institutions; most common intestinal parasite in the U.S.; abdominal cramping, bloating, flatus, malabsorptive chronic diarrhea	Metronidazole
Staphylococcus aureus	1–6 hr; previously cooked food (ham, egg salad, potato salad)	Nausea, severe vomiting, diarrhea, mild abdominal cramps; symptoms caused by preformed entertoxins	Supportive care with IV fluids and symptomatic treatment; antibiotics ineffective
Bacillus cereus	1–6 hr; previously cooked meats, fried rice, vegetables and dried fruits	Abrupt onset of nausea, vomiting, and mild diarrhea; caused by preformed enterotoxins	Supportive care with IV fluids and symptomatic treatment; antibiotics ineffective
Clostridium perfringens	8–24 hr; previously cooked or reheated meats and poultry	Abdominal cramps, nausea, minimal vomiting, and watery diarrhea; caused by enterotoxins	Supportive care with IV fluids and symptomatic treatment
Vibrio cholerae	11–72 hr; raw or undercooked seafood, fecal-oral, contaminated water	Explosive rice-water diarrhea; vomiting, fever, abdominal cramps, dehydration, lactic acidosis; enterotoxins are formed before and after bacterial colonization	Fluid resuscitation is critical; ciprofloxacin, bactrim, or tetracycline may shorten the course of disease
Enterotoxigenic *Escherichia coli*	11–72 hr; contaminated water	Traveler's diarrhea; profuse watery diarrhea; caused by enterotoxins	Self-limiting; supportive care; if severe, ciprofloxacin
Antibiotic-associated enteritis	Temporally associated with antibiotic use	Mild severity without cramps, fever, or fecal leukocytes	Withdrawal of antibiotic

TABLE 11.7. Common Causes of Invasive Gastroenteritis

Causative Agent	Incubation and Transmission	Description	Treatment
Salmonella sp.	8–72 hr; contaminated food (eggs or poultry) or water, pet turtles, chicks, or lizards	Fever, abdominal pain, myalgia, headache; risk of sepsis in very young, elderly, immunocompromised; many fecal WBCs and few RBCs	Ciprofloxacin if severe illness, sepsis, or immunocompromise; alternatives: Ceftriaxone or Azithromycin
Shigella sp.	1–3 days; fecal-oral, person-to-person, contaminated food	Fever, headache, myalgia, diarrhea, little vomiting; common in kids 1–5 yr; many fecal WBCs and RBCs	Ciprofloxacin if severe illness, sepsis, or immunocompromise; alternatives: Ceftriaxone or Azithromycin
Campylobacter sp.	1–7 days; contaminated water, food (poultry, eggs), animals or pets	Common in children and young adults; low-grade fever, abdominal pain, and vomiting may precede diarrhea; fecal RBCs and WBCs common	Ciprofloxacin if severely ill or septic; alternative: Azithromycin
Yersinia enterolitica	1–5 days; contaminated food or water (milk, pork), fecal-oral, person-to-person, pets or wild animals	Children and young adults; may mimic appendicitis; anorexia, fever, RLQ abdominal pain, and vomiting precede diarrhea; many fecal WBCs and RBCs	Usually self-limiting; treat with Ciprofloxacin; Alternative: Bactrim
C. difficile	1–11 wk; recent antibiotic use; PCN, clindamycin, cephalosporins most commonly implicated	Fever, abdominal pain, copious foul-smelling diarrhea, rarely vomiting; fecal WBCs and RBCs; stool *C. difficile* toxin confirms diagnosis	Metronidazole orally preferred; vancomycin orally; IV vancomycin ineffective; IV metronizadole may be beneficial
Entamoeba histolytica	1–11 wk; contaminated food or water, poor sanitation, travel to developing countries	Acute amebic dysentery: abrupt onset of fever, abdominal pain, tenesmus, and bloody diarrhea; chronic dysentery: malaise, weight loss, bloating, and bloody diarrhea; may develop hepatic abscess; fecal RBCs, WBCs common	Metronidazole then Iodoquinol; chloroquine may be added; antibiotics will usually sufficiently treat abscess as well

(Continued)

ABDOMINAL AND GASTROINTESTINAL EMERGENCIES

TABLE 11.7. Common Causes of Invasive Gastroenteritis (*Continued*)

Causative Agent	Incubation and Transmission	Description	Treatment
Enterohemorrhagic *Escherichia coli* O157:H7	3–8 days; contaminated food or water; undercooked meats, person-to-person, fecal-oral	Fever, abdominal pain, vomiting, grossly bloody diarrhea; hemolytic uremic syndrome (HUS) in 5% of patients fecal WBCs also common	Supportive care; antibiotics not recommended as they may increase the incidence of HUS especially in children
Entamoeba histolytica	8–72 hours; contaminated food or water, raw or undercooked shellfish	Common in summer months in adults fever, abdominal cramps, diarrhea, nausea with little vomiting; fecal WBCs and RBCs common	Self-limiting; supportive care, antibiotics are not recommended

Diagnosis

- Diagnosis is based on history and physical.
- If the causative agent is invasive, stool testing will reveal fecal leukocytes and erythrocytes.
- Stool culture is expensive and labor intensive, and plays a small role in ED diagnosis. Reserve for severely ill patients, outbreaks, and patients recently on antibiotics.
- Parasitic enteritis may be difficult to distinguish from other invasive causes. Consider in patients who travel to developing countries, the immunocompromised, the institutionalized, and patients with a prolonged course not responsive to traditional therapy. Send stool for ova and parasite analysis.

Treatment

- Oral rehydration may be acceptable in patients with mild to moderate dehydration if they are able to tolerate oral intake. These patients may be discharged with instructions to return if symptoms persist or worsen.
- Give IV-fluid resuscitation with LR or NS and antiemetics for patients unable to tolerate PO and those with severe dehydration.
- Consider hospitalization for the severely dehydrated patient. Other treatment considerations depend on suspected etiology. (See Tables 11.6 and 11.7.)

Complications

Dehydration, electrolyte imbalances, bacteremia, sepsis, shock

Appendicitis

Acute appendicitis begins with obstruction of the lumen due to food, adhesions, fecalith, or enlarged lymphoid tissue. Mucosal secretion continues with increasing intraluminal pressure and eventual compromise of venous and lymphatic drainage. As a result, epithelial breakdown with bacterial invasion of the bowel wall may result, causing inflammation. Finally, arterial stasis and tissue infarction occur with perforation of the appendix and leakage of bowel contents into the peritoneum.

SYMPTOMS/EXAM

- The classic symptom is diffuse periumbilical abdominal pain with migration to the right lower quadrant.
- Fever may be present in only 20% of cases.
- Pain is followed by anorexia, nausea, and vomiting.
- Diffuse tenderness to palpation early with tenderness to deep palpation over **McBurney point** as the illness progresses
- **Rovsing sign** is pain in the RLQ with palpation of the LLQ.
- The **obturator sign** is induced by passively flexing the right hip and knee and internally rotating the hip. A positive sign is indicative of an irritated obturator internus muscle from a presumed inflamed appendix.
- The **psoas sign** is elicited by placing the patient in the left lateral decubitis position and extending the right leg at the hip. It may also be performed by providing resistance against the leg as the patient attempts to lift his thigh off the table. These maneuvers will cause pain by stretching the psoas muscle, which may be irritated by adjacent inflamed appendix or mass.
- Involuntary guarding, rebound tenderness, voluntary guarding, and tenderness on rectal exam may also be present.

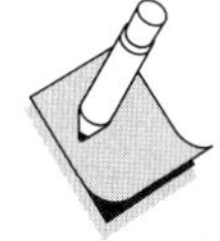

The obturator sign is induced by passively flexing the right hip and knee and internally rotating the hip. An inflamed appendix may irritate the obturator internus muscle.

DIFFERENTIAL

- Appendicitis may be confused with any condition that causes abdominal pain.
- Appendicitis is particularly difficult to diagnosis in the elderly, the pregnant patient, and the pediatric patient.
- Most common findings during laparotomy when appendicitis is diagnosis in error are mesenteric lymphadenitis, no disease, PID, acute gastroenteritis.
- Cholecystitis, perforated ulcer, diverticulitis, pancreatitis, small-bowel obstruction, renal calculus, pylonephritis
- Ovarian pathologies like abscess, torsion, cyst, or ectopic pregnancy

DIAGNOSIS

- WBC, urinalysis, and temperature are of limited value but may be abnormal.
- Plain radiographs are abnormal in 24–95% of cases but are of limited value. Findings may include appendiceal fecalith, appendiceal gas, and free air.
- CT scan is considered the best choice for initial evaluation. It has excellent sensitivity (87–100%) and specificity (89–90%). Thin-slice CT with rectal contrast has the highest specificity (98%) and avoids oral contrast. However, rectal contrast can be difficult and inconvenient to administer.
- CT is positive if it shows an inflammed appendix that does not fill with contrast, pericecal inflammation, abscess, phlegmon, or fluid collection.
- Graded compression ultrasound has a 94.7% sensitivity and 88.9% specificity if the appendix is noncompressible, >6 mm in diameter, or demonstrates appendicolith or abscess. This is the test of choice in children and pregnant patients.
- Barium enemas, nuclear medicine scans, and MRI have also been used.

The psoas sign is elicited by placing the patient in the left lateral decubitis position and extending the right leg at the hip. The maneuver will cause pain by stretching the psoas muscle, which may be inflamed by an adjacent mass.

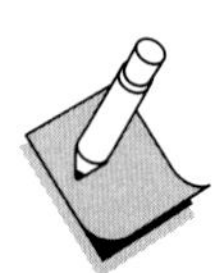

Ultrasound is the initial study of choice in children and pregnant women to rule out appendicitis.

TREATMENT

- Appendectomy is the standard of care.
- Clinical observation with serial abdominal exams may be warranted if diagnosis is not clear.
- The patient should be NPO and should receive IV fluids and antibiotics that cover anaerobes, enterococci, and Gram-negative GI flora.

COMPLICATIONS

- Perforation—seen in almost 20% of cases
- Periappendical abscess
- Peritonitis

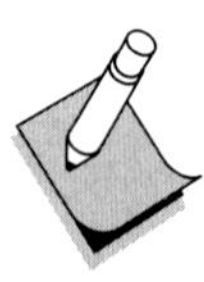

Appendicitis remains the most common extrauterine surgical emergency in pregnancy. The diagnosis should be considered in pregnant women with abdominal pain and gastrointestinal symptoms.

Necrotizing Enterocolitis

The most serious and frequent GI disorder of predominantly premature infants, it presents around 10 days after birth. It is characterized by necrosis, ulceration, and sloughing of intestinal mucosa; and may progress to full-thickness bowel necrosis. Clustering of cases in nurseries suggests an infectious etiology, but other risk factors include intestinal ischemia and immunologic immaturity of the gut. More than 80% of cases are found in premature infants weighing <2500 g, but it is seen in a small proportion of term infants as well.

SYMPTOMS/EXAM

- Bilious vomiting, abdominal distention, bloody stools, lethargy
- Exam may reveal abdominal distention, abdominal wall erythema, crepitus, and edema.
- Bradycardia, hypotension, apnea, and temperature instability are also possible findings.

Beware of atypical presentations of appendicitis in the very young and the very old and in pregnant patients. These groups of patients have much higher rates of delayed diagnosis and postoperative complications.

DIAGNOSIS

- Labs: Leukocytosis or leukopenia, thrombocytopenia, and acidosis
- AXR: May demonstrate dilated bowel loops, pneumatosis, and free air with perforation; contrast-enhanced studies contraindicated due to risk of perforation

TREATMENT

- Stop feedings, begin fluid resuscitation, correct electrolyte abnormalities, and initiate broad spectrum antibiotic coverage.
- Emergent surgical consultation is required.
- Bowel resection is indicated for perforation or severe extensive disease.

COMPLICATIONS

- Bacteremia, sepsis, shock, ascites with SBP, extensive bowel resection → short gut syndrome, intestinal strictures.

Ulcerative Colitis

This chronic, recurrent disease is characterized by mucosal and submucosal inflammation of the colon. Less than 20% involve the entire colon with most cases isolated to the rectum and sigmoid colon. Bimodal distribution: onset is typically from 15–35 years old, but another spike occurs at 50–70 years of age.

Course involves repeated flares and remissions. More common among nonsmokers, Ashkenazi Jews, and those with a family history. See Table 11.3 for a comparison with Crohn disease.

Symptoms/Exam

- Bloody diarrhea, crampy abdominal pain, fecal urgency, tenesmus
- Abdominal tenderness to palpation grossly bloody stool on digital rectal exam
- Extraintestinal manifestations common (see Table 11.8)

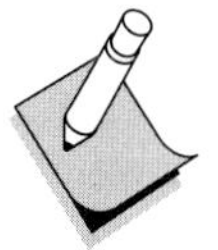

Avoid sigmoidoscopy and colonoscopy in patients with ulcerative colitis if there is a severe flare because they increase the risk of perforation.

Differential

Infectious etiology, Crohn disease, ischemic, toxic, pseudomembranous, radiation colitis

Diagnosis

- Sigmoidoscopy or colonoscopy demonstrates continuous circumferential ulceration.
- Biopsy shows acute and chronic inflammation, crypt abscesses, no granulomas.

Treatment

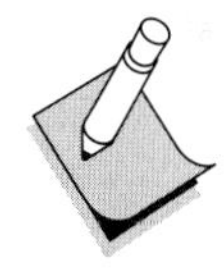

Surgery can be curative and can eliminate the risk of colorectal cancer in patients with ulcerative colitis.

- Treatment depends on location and severity of disease. Mild disease can be managed outpatient with follow-up.
- Fluid resuscitation, electrolyte replacement, broad spectrum antibiotics and admission are indicated for patients with fulminant colitis.
- Distal disease: Mesalamine or hydrocortisone enema or suppository
- Diffuse disease: Oral or IV medications
- Mild to moderate:
  - Sulfasalazine
  - Mesalamine
  - Prednisone
- Severe disease: Methylprednisolone, occasionally infliximab
- Colectomy may be indicated if no response in 7–10 days.

Complications

Lower GI bleeding, toxic megacolon, colorectal cancer, extraintestinal manifestations (see Table 11.8)

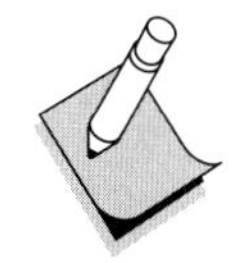

There is a 10- to 30-fold increase in the risk of developing colorectal cancer with ulcerative colitis. Risk increases with duration and extensiveness of disease.

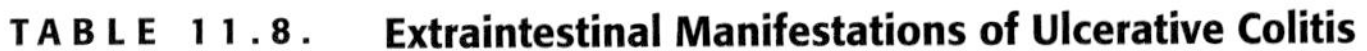

TABLE 11.8. Extraintestinal Manifestations of Ulcerative Colitis

Arthritic	Peripheral arthritis, ankylosing spondylitis
Opthalmologic	Uveitis, episcleritis
Dermatologic	Pyoderma gangrenosum, erythema nodosum, oral apthous ulcers
Hepatobiliary	Pericholangitis, chronic active hepatitis, cirrhosis, cholelithiasis, bile duct carcinoma

Hirshprung Disease

Disease characterized by functional obstruction of the colon due to failure of cephalocaudal migration of parasympathetic myenteric nerve cells into the distal bowel. The bowel fails to relax in response to distention → constipation. The aganglionic segment begins at the anus and extends varying distances proximally. There is a greater incidence in males, those with a family history, and Down syndrome.

Symptoms

Severity is variable but almost always presents shortly after birth. Infants pass little or no meconium in the first 24 hours after birth. Constipation is subsequently chronic or intermittent. Other symptoms include abdominal distention, bilious emesis, diarrhea, listlessness, reluctance to feed, and developmental delay.

Exam

- Normal or contracted rectum on digital rectal exam with absence of feces
- Distended abdomen, abdominal mass on palpation due to impacted stool in the sigmoid colon

Differential

Rectal or colonic atresia, meconium ileus, meconium plug syndrome, hypothyroidism, electrolyte imbalances

Diagnosis

- Contrast enema demonstrates narrowed (aganglionic) colon, and proximal bowel dilatation.
- Biopsy showing lack of ganglion cells is definitive.

Treatment

Surgical resection of aganglionic bowel segment

Complications

Enterocolitis, postoperative fecal incontinence, postoperative episodic abdominal distention, constipation.

Irritable Bowel Disease (IBD)

A chronic functional bowel disorder of unknown etiology that is characterized by abdominal pain or discomfort and alterations in stool frequency and form. There is also a lack of structural GI abnormality and underlying medical disease. The disorder is more common in women and the average age of onset is 20 years. Onset can follow a bout of gastroenteritis.

Symptoms

- Chronic or intermittent diffuse colicky or crampy abdominal pain
- Abdominal distention and bloating
- Temporary relief with passage of flatus or bowel movement
- Association with emotional upset or stress

Exam

Abdominal exam is generally benign but may reveal a cordlike mass in the LLQ.

DIFFERENTIAL

Crohn disease, ulcerative colitis, infectious enterocolitis, colorectal cancer, celiac sprue, endometriosis

DIAGNOSIS

- Exclude organic causes
- Labs: CBC, LFTs, albumin, ESR, celiac sprue serologies
- Stool: O&P, *C. difficile* toxin
- Consider referral for endoscopy and colonoscopy if symptoms are severe.

TREATMENT

- Provide reassurance.
- Tactfully explain visceral hypersensitivity and validate symptoms.
- **Dietary trials:** Lactose-free, high-fiber diet
- **Antispasmodics:** Dicyclomine, hyoscyamine, peppermint oil
- **Antidepressants:** Desipramine, amitriptyline, fluoxetine, paroxetine
- **Constipation-predominant type:**
  - ↑ Fluid intake.
  - Provide bowel habit training.
  - Tegaserod 6 mg BID
  - Osmotic laxatives
- **Diarrhea-predominant type:** Loperamide, cholestyramine

Large-Bowel Obstruction

Mechanical colonic obstruction is due to a physical barrier that prevents the passage of bowel contents through the GI tract. Unlike SBO, the cause is rarely adhesions or hernias. The common causes are listed in Table 11.9.

SYMPTOMS/EXAM

- Symptoms include abdominal pain, distention, nausea, vomiting, and inability to pass flatus or stool.
- Exam is notable for abdominal distention, hypogastric abdominal tenderness to palpation, vomiting that is feculent if the obstruction is low, tympanitic abdomen, high-pitched increased bowel sounds early, and decreased or absent bowel sounds late in the course.

DIFFERENTIAL

Small-bowel obstruction, pseudo-obstruction, paralytic ileus, constipation, fecal impaction

DIAGNOSIS

- AXR: May demonstrate air fluid levels, free air, masses, and may localize the obstruction to the large bowel
- Labs: Leukocytosis, hemoconcentration, and electrolyte abnormalities
- CT: Contrast-enhanced exam may delineate location of obstruction, etiology, and partial vs complete obstruction.
- Contrast enema/sigmoidoscopy: May reveal location and cause of obstruction

TREATMENT

- Insertion of NGT, NPO status, fluid resuscitation, electrolyte replacement, and broad spectrum preoperative antibiotics are required.

TABLE 11.9. **Common Causes of Large Bowel Obstruction**

Etiology	Pathophysiology	Diagnosis/Treatment
Colorectal cancer	Most common cause of LBO; history may reveal change in bowel habits, rectal bleeding, weight loss	Diagnosis can be made with contrast enema or colonoscopy. CT may be helpful in evaluating extension and metastases. Treatment in cases of LBO is resection of involved segment.
Diverticulitis	Second most common cause of LBO; infection of the walls of diverticuli leads to bowel edema and secondary obstruction; second most frequent cause of large-bowel obstruction Occurs in 10–25% of pts with diverticuli; incidence increases with age. Right-sided diverticular disease is more common in pts of Asian and African descent.	CT is diagnostic. Treatment is conservative and includes broad spectrum antibiotics, NPO, NGT decompression, and fluid, electrolyte repletion.
Sigmoid volvulus	Rotation of a segment of bowel on an axis formed by its mesentery; older pts, bedridden pts, and those w/ psychiatric illness taking anticholinergic medications are at risk for sigmoid volvulus; history of constipation	AXR: A single distended loop of bowel is seen rising out of the pelvis. Contrast enema: A dilated bowel loop with bird's beak shape. CT is also diagnostic. Treatment: Decompression with a scope or rectal tube may be successful. Resection and fixation are indicated for unsuccessful attempts and strangulation.
Cecal volvulus	Congenital defect in the peritoneum resulting in the twisting of the mobile segment of the cecum; most common in younger men and gravid females	AXR or contrast enema is diagnostic: Distended ovoid cecum that takes a "coffee bean" shape. Treatment is surgical.
Intussusception	Proximal segment of bowel invaginates into more distal segment; primarily a disease of children	Contrast enema is diagnostic and therapeutic in 60–80% of cases Diagnosis may also be made with abdominal ultrasound or CT; unsuccessful reduction with enema or evidence of perforation treated with operative resection
Acute colonic pseudo-obstruction (Ogilvie syndrome)	Seen in elderly patients hospitalized with severe illness; massive dilatation (>10 cm in diameter) usually of the cecum and right colon in the absence of a mechanical obstruction; often an underlying surgical disorder or precipitated by a medical disorder	CT is diagnostic; correct underlying precipitating disorder. Initial conservative management with bowel rest, hydration and correction of electrolyte abnormalities; avoid medications that slow colonic motility; pharmacologic treatment with neostigmine or colonoscopic decompression may be effective in cases that do not resolve with conservative management Surgical intervention is reserved for refractory cases or cases complicated by perforation.

- Emergent surgical consultation is imperative as operative management is often necessary. Management may vary depending on etiology. (See Table 11.9.)
- Antibiotic regimens include tazobactam-piperacillin, cefotetan, ertapenam, or combination of a fluoroquinolone and metronizadole.

COMPLICATIONS

- Bowel perforation carries up to 40% risk of mortality.
- Acute colitis may occur due to bowel ischemia.

ANORECTAL

Perianal/Anal Abscess

Common in middle-aged males

SYMPTOMS/EXAM

- Easily palpable tender mass, close to the anal verge, usually posterior midline
- Pain may be worse before defecation and with valsalva maneuvers.

DIFFERENTIAL/DIAGNOSIS

- Crohn's disease, fissures, cancer, pilonidal disease, hidradenitis suppurativa, cancer, STDs.
- CT or ultrasound to assess rectal involvement.

TREATMENT

- Isolated and fluctuant abscesses may be drained in the ED. Use a cruciate incision (+/– packing) so that wound edges do not close. Simple linear incisions may be used but require packing and 24-hour follow-up.
- Antibiotics as a rule are not necessary but should be used with fever, leukocytosis, overlying cellulitis, or in immunocompromised patients.
- Warm sitz baths

COMPLICATIONS

Recurrence, fistulas, sphincter injury, sepsis

Perirectal Abscess

SYMPTOMS/EXAM

- See Figure 11.5 for common locations of perirectal abscesses.
- Ischiorectal abscess: Dull pain with few outward signs; signs may be more lateral to anal verge than perianal abscess
- Intersphincteric abscess: Pain with defecation, rectal discharge, fever, mass on rectal exam
- Supralevator abscess: Buttock or perirectal pain; few outward signs

DIAGNOSIS

CT/US/MRI to determine the extent of tissue involvement

TREATMENT

- Surgical consult: All perirectal abscesses should be drained in the operating room because of the high incidence of recurrence.
- Daily warm sitz baths; antibiotics

COMPLICATIONS

Recurrence, fistulas, sphincter injury, sepsis

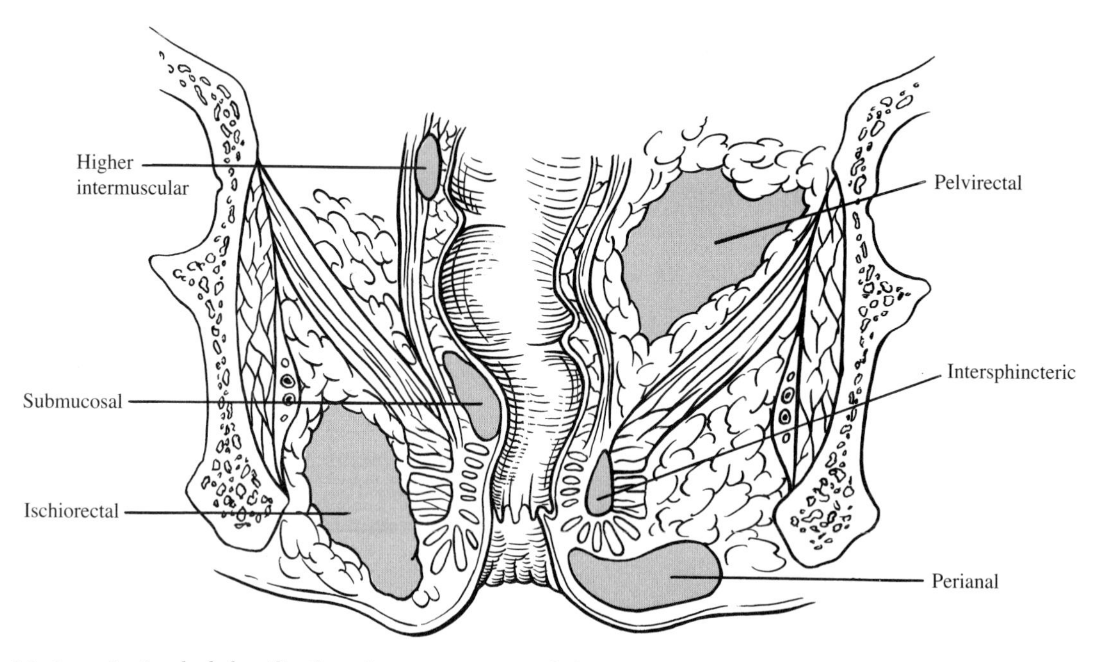

FIGURE 11.5. Anatomical classification of common anorectal abscesses.

(Reproduced, with permission, from Tintinalli JE, Kelen GD, Stapczynski JS. *Emergency Medicine: A Comprehensive Study Guide*, 6th ed. New York: McGraw-Hill, 2004:544.)

Pilonidal Cyst

Pilonidal abscesses are acquired, chronic infections of gluteal cleft hair follicles over the sacral/perianal region. Pilonidal cysts are not related to the anorectum in any way; however, because of their proximity, **they are often usually not for perirectal abscesses and vice-versa**.

SYMPTOMS/EXAM

- Tender, swollen, purulent nodule along superior gluteal fold
- Abscessed pilonidal sinus is always located in posterior midline over sacrum/coccyx. On the other hand, fistulas from perirectal abscesses are usually not midline.

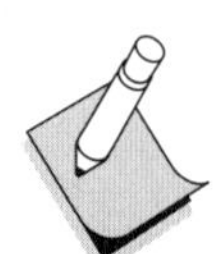

Pilonidal cysts are always midline and usually a couple of centimeters above the anus.

TREATMENT

- Incision, drainage, packing +/– surgical follow-up for wide excision
- No antibiotics necessary unless accompanying cellulitis present

COMPLICATIONS

Carcinoma is a rare complication of recurrent pilonidal sinus disease, usually in men.

Proctitis

Sexually transmitted diseases of the anus may be caused by anal sex or occasionally by spread from the vagina or scrotum (see Figure 11.6). If a patient has one of these STDs, assume that others are present as well. Table 11.10 lists STDs that commonly cause proctitis.

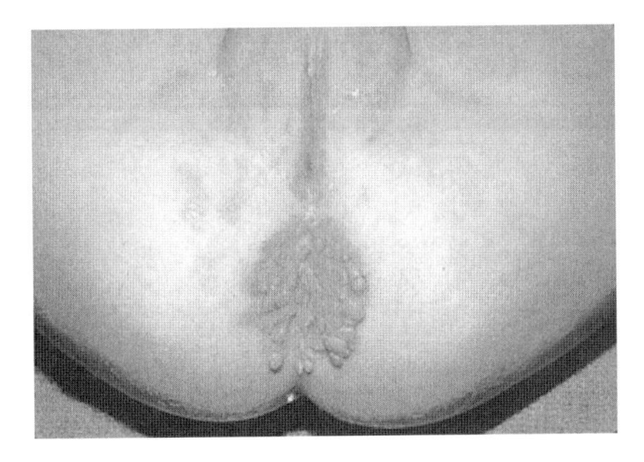

FIGURE 11.6. Perianal condylomata acuminata.

(Reproduced, with permission, from Gonzales R, Zeiger R (online eds.) *Current Medical Diagnosis & Treatment* 2008. Online edition. New York. McGraw-Hill, 2008. www.accessmedicine.com. April 2008.)

TABLE 11.10. STDs That Cause Proctitis

	SYMPTOMS/DIAGNOSIS	TREATMENT	COMPLICATIONS
Condyloma acuminata (HPV)	Perianal soft fleshy growths See Figure 11.6; may spread from vagina/scrotum Anoscopy to check for intranal disease	Chemotherapy or definitive therapy (ablation, cryotherapy, etc.)	40% recurrence associated with squamous cell carcinoma
Gonorrhea	Asymptomatic to rectal pain and discharge. Gram stain/ cultures for diagnosis.	Ceftriaxone	Dissemination to heart, liver, CNS, joints
Chlamydia	Asymptomatic to rectal pain and discharge; ulcerations Gram stain/cultures, ELISA, direct immunofluorescence, PCR assays for diagnosis	Azithromycin, doxycycline: 21-day course for LGV chlamydia	Rectal scarring, abscesses, fistulas
Syphilis	Primary: Chancre in the anus may be painful Secondary: Perianal condyloma lata	Penicillin	Good prognosis if treated
Chancroid	Multiple painful bleeding lesions with indurated, draining lymph nodes	Azithromycin Ceftriaxone Fluoroquinolones	
Herpes	Pruritus, pain Discrete vesicles on erythematous base progressing to ulcers	Analgesic Stool softener Acyclovir	Recurrent bouts Constipation common

Anal Fissure

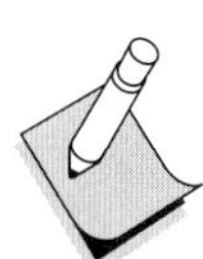

Anal fissures are the most frequent cause of rectal bleeding in infants due to hard stools.

Superficial linear tear in the anal canal; common in children and young adults; most common cause of rectal bleeding in infants due to passage of large hard stool

SYMPTOMS

- Sharp, cutting pain, especially during and immediately after bowel movements; pain subsides between bowel movements
- Small amounts of bright red bleeding, especially on toilet paper

EXAM

- Anal fissures occur in the posterior midline (90%) or in the anterior midline (10–40% women, only 1% of men)
- May see characteristic "sentinel pile": swollen papilla just distal to fissure

DIFFERENTIAL

- Consider Crohn disease, ulcerative colitis, squamous cell carcinoma, adenocarcinoma, localized anal cancer, leukemia, lymphoma, syphilis, gonorrhea, chlamydia, tuberculous ulcer
- Definitive diagnosis requires biopsy of the ulcer edge.

TREATMENT

- Meticulous anal hygiene
- Stool softener stool-bulking agent
- Local therapy: Analgesic ointment, hydrocortisone cream, nitroglycerin ointment
- Hot sitz baths to relieve sphincter spasm and bran to diet to prevent stricture formation
- May need surgery

Anal Fistula

Anal fistulas most commonly result from perianal/perirectal abscesses.

SYMPTOMS/EXAM

- Persistent, blood-stained, malodorous discharge
- Intermittent obstruction with inflammation and abscess formation

DIFFERENTIAL DIAGNOSIS

- Consider Crohn disease, cancers, STDs, anal fissures, TB, foreign bodies
- Ultrasound, CT, or MRI for definitive diagnosis

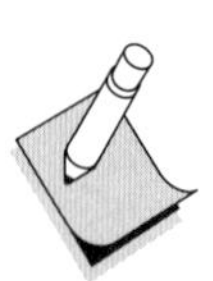

Goodsall's rule: Fistulas with anterior openings follow a direct line to the anal canal, whereas fistulas with posterior openings tend to deviate and curve.

Rectal Foreign Bodies

DIAGNOSIS

- Digital rectal exam or proctoscopic exam will localize most foreign bodies.
- X-rays are mandatory, not only to delineate the size, location, and number of foreign bodies, but also to check for the most serious complication, eg, visceral perforation.

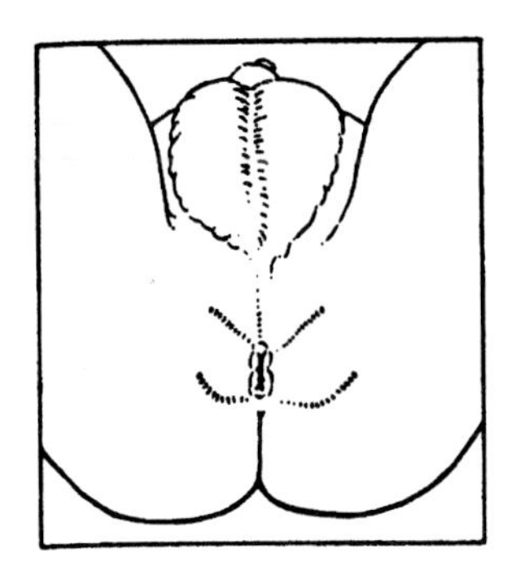

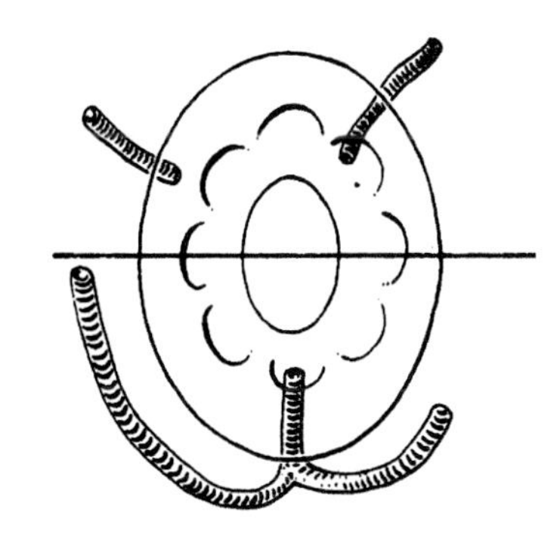

FIGURE 11.7. Goodsall's rule.

(Reproduced, with permission, from Tintinalli JE, Kelen GD, Stapczynski JS. *Emergency Medicine: A Comprehensive Study Guide*, 6th ed. New York: McGraw-Hill, 2004.)

- Clinical symptoms of perforation: Fever, leukocytosis, abdominal pain, peritoneal signs, rectal bleeding
- Radiographic signs of perforation: Free air under the diaphragm (intraperitoneal perforation) or free air tracking along the psoas muscle (retroperitoneal perforation)

TREATMENT

- Simple foreign bodies may be removed in ED. Foreign bodies that are large or with sharp edges may require surgical removal.
- Technique of ED removal
- Anesthetic: IV sedation should be considered. With patient in the lithotomy position, inject an intradermal wheal at the 6- and 11-o'clock positions of the anal canal. Insert one finger into the anal canal to guide the injection of a further 5 mL of anesthetic into each quadrant of the internal sphincter.
- Removal: Place a catheter beyond the object and inject air to overcome the vacuum created by traction on the object and pull. Alternatively, a Foley catheter may be used; after air is injected behind the object, then inflate the balloon to aid in delivery of the foreign body.

COMPLICATIONS

- Perforation may require emergency surgery.
- If perforation is suspected, serial X-rays and proctoscopic exams are indicated. If in doubt, the patient should be observed for 11 hours.
- Administer antibiotics for perforation or excessive manipulation.

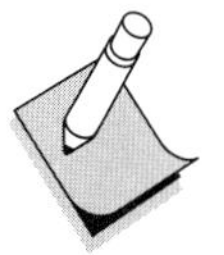

Visceral perforation is the most serious complication of rectal foreign bodies.

Hemorrhoids

Hemorrhoids are vascular complexes that line and protect the anal canal; they become symptomatic with activities that increase venous pressure, causing engorgement. Engorged, prolapsed, or thrombosed hemorrhoidal veins/arterioles cause symptoms.

Internal: Located proximal to dentate line drain; insensate area
External: Located distal to dentate line; richly innervated

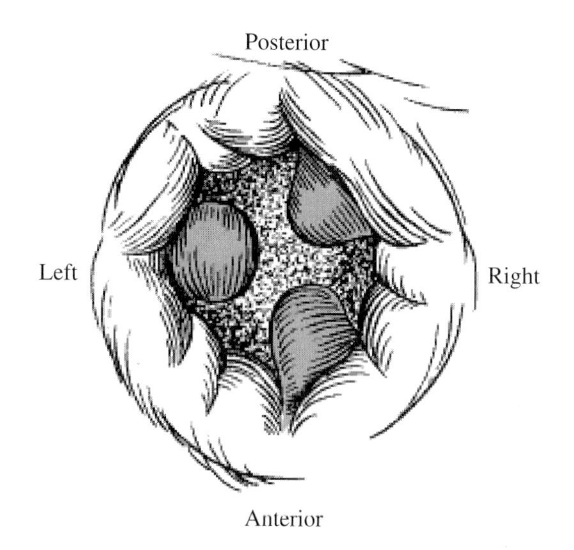

FIGURE 11.8. Common locations of internal hemmorhoids.

(Reproduced, with permission, from Tintinalli JE, Kelen GD, Stapczynski JS. *Emergency Medicine: A Comprehensive Study Guide*, 6th ed. New York: McGraw-Hill, 2004:540.)

SYMPTOMS/ EXAM

- Internal
  - Painless, bright-red rectal bleeding, mucous discharge, rectal discomfort
  - Characteristically seen at the 2-, 5-, and 12-o'clock positions on prone patients on anoscopy; see Figure 11.8
- External
  - Rectal pain if thrombosed or strangulated
  - Can be seen with visual inspection

DIFFERENTIAL

- Consider inflammatory bowel disease, diverticular disease, anal fissures/ fistulas, rectal prolapse, ulcerative colitis, Crohn disease.
- Tumors must be ruled out by sigmoidoscopy in all cases of rectal bleeding in patients >40 years old.

TREATMENT

- Conservative therapy initially: Manual reduction if uncomplicated; warm sitz baths, local hygiene, topical analgesics/steroids, bulk laxatives/bran after the acute phase is treated
- Surgical referral if needed: Options include rubber band ligation, sclerotherapy, and excision.
- External hemorrhoids that have been thrombosed for <48 hours may be excised in the ED.

COMPLICATIONS

Recurrence, infection, fistula formation, abscess formation, sepsis

Rectal Prolapse

Three types: (1) Rectal mucosa only (usually <2 years old); (2) all layers of rectum; (3) intussusception through rectum

TABLE 11.11. Classification of Anorectal Tumors by Location

Type	Location	Cell Type	Cancers	Outcome
Anal canal	Proximal to dentate line	Transition zone between squamous cell and columnar epithelium of rectum	Adenocarcinoma, melanoma, transitional cell carcinoma, Kaposi sarcoma, villous adenoma	**High-grade malignant potential;** metastasize early; poor prognosis
Anal margin	Distal to dentate line	Squamous cell	Bowen's, squamous cell carcinoma, basal cell carcinoma, Paget disease	**Lower grade malignant potential**, slow to metastasize

Symptoms/Exam

- A mass is noted in the rectum following defecation or straining, or even upon standing.
- Other symptoms include bloody mucous discharge, fecal incontinence, dull pain.

Diagnosis

- All adult patients should be referred for endoscopy to rule out tumor, polyps, IBD, or rectal ulcer.

Treatment

- Manual reduction in infants
- Surgical intervention in adults unless prolapse is minimal; if there is vascular compromise, emergent surgery

Anorectal Tumors

See Table 11.11.

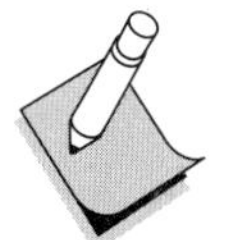

The anus is the third most common site for melanoma metastasis, after the eye and the skin.

Symptoms/Exam

- Nonspecific symptoms: Pruritus, pain, bleeding with stool, sensation of a lump
- Progressive anorexia, weight loss, diarrhea, constipation, tenesmus
- Detectable by careful visual and digital examination

Diagnosis/Treatment

- Any ulcer that fails to heal in 30 days or any discrete skin lesion that does not improve should be biopsied.
- Surgical consult

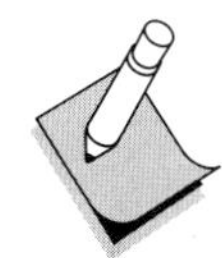

Hepatitis C is the number one reason patients require liver transplantation in the United States.

LIVER DISORDERS

Hepatitis

Viral hepatitis affects 200,000–700,000 Americans each year. Hepatitis B and C can progress to chronic hepatitis, and hepatitis C is the number one reason patients require liver transplantation in the United States.

HEPATITIS A

RNA picornavirus; endemic worldwide; in the United States, over one-third of all urban-dwelling adults seropositive for the anti-HAV antibody; common in children <15 years old; most common cause of conjugated hyperbilirubinemia in children; rare in persons >40 years old; highest rates seen in American Indians and Alaska natives

TRANSMISSION

Fecal-oral, contaminated food and water worldwide

SYMPTOMS

- Presents with flulike illness, malaise, anorexia, weakness, fever, RUQ pain, jaundice, and pruritus; children are typically asymptomatic
- Atypical presentations include acute liver failure, cholestasis (prolonged, deep jaundice), and relapsing disease (2–18 weeks after initial presentation).

DIAGNOSIS

- **History:** Inquire about ill contacts, substandard water supply, travel, and contaminated food **(shellfish and green onions).**
- **Labs:** Anti-HAV IgM (acute infection); anti-HAV IgG (prior exposure, vaccination); anti-HAV total measures IgM and IgG (acute infection, prior exposure, vaccination)

TREATMENT

- Supportive, rarely progresses into fulminant infection
- Avoid alcohol and acetaminophent (Tylenol) during acute infection.

ABDOMINAL AND GASTROINTESTINAL EMERGENCIES

HEPATITIS B

Some 400 million people worldwide have chronic HBV, including >1 million in the United States. Transmission can be perinatal (the most common cause worldwide), sexual, or percutaneous. Age at infection is **inversely related** to the risk of chronic infection. Of all patients with chronic HBV, 15–20% develop cirrhosis and 10–15% develop hepatocellular carcinoma.

TRANSMISSION

Maternal → fetal, body fluids through sexual contact, IVDA.

SYMPTOMS

Similar to acute hepatitis A

DIAGNOSIS (SEE TABLE 11.12)

- **HBsAg:** Surface antigen indicates **active** infection.
- **Anti-HBs:** Antibody to HBsAg indicates past viral infection or immunization.
- **Anti-HBc:** IgM is an early marker of infection; IgG is the best marker for prior HBV exposure. IgM may also become detectable in reactivation of HBV.
- **HBeAg:** Proportional to the quantity of intact virus and, therefore, infectivity; some HBV variants (called **precore mutants**) cannot make HBeAg.

TABLE 11.12. Serologic Patterns for Hepatitis B Infection

HBsAg	Anti-HBs	Anti-HBc	HBeAg	Anti-HBe	Interpretation
+	–	IgM	+	–	Acute hepatitis B
+	–	IgG	+	–	Chronic hepatitis B with active viral replication
+	–	IgG	–	+	Chronic hepatitis B with low viral replication
+	+	IgG	+ or –	+ or –	Chronic hepatitis B with heterotypic anti-HBs (about 10% of cases)
–	–	IgM	+ or –	–	Acute hepatitis B
–	+	IgG	–	+ or –	Recovery from hepatitis B (immunity)
–	+	–	–	–	Vaccination (immunity)
–	–	IgG	–	–	False-positive; less commonly, infection in remote past

Treatment

- **Acute exposure/needlestick prophylaxis:** The CDC recommends that hepatitis B immune globulin (HBIG) be given **within 24 hours along with vaccine** if the patient was not previously immunized.
- **Pegylated interferon-α_{2a}:** Given SQ; associated with many side effects (eg, constitutional, psychiatric, bone marrow toxicity, flare of autoimmune disease, hepatic decompensation); contraindicated in cirrhosis; the best responses to treatment obtained with active hepatic inflammation (high ALT) and low-HBV DNA levels
- **Lamivudine:** Given PO; well tolerated but resistance may develop
- **Adefovir:** Given PO; well tolerated and may be used to treat lamivudine-resistant virus; has lower rates of resistance than lamivudine; associated with renal insufficiency
- **Newer antivirals:** Entecavir, telbivudine, and emtricitabine/tenofovir (used for HIV coinfection)

Hepatitis C

Transmission

IVDA, intranasal drug use, hemodialysis, blood transfusions before 1992

Symptoms/Exam

- **Acute HCV:** Presents with flulike illness, malaise, weakness, low-grade fever, myalgias, and RUQ pain followed by jaundice; only 30% of patients symptomatic in acute disease
- **Chronic HCV:** Often asymptomatic or may present with cryoglobulinemia associated with a vasculitis skin rash **(leukocytoclastic vasculitis)**, **arthralgias**, sicca syndrome, and **glomerulonephritis;** in the setting of cirrhosis, presents with fatigue, muscle wasting, dependent edema, and easy bruising

DIAGNOSIS

- **Screening:** HCV antibody ⊕ 4–6 weeks after infection) and qualitative PCR (in acute infection; can be ⊕ 1–2 weeks after infection); screen patients with risk factors or persistently elevated transaminases
- **Confirmatory:** Qualitative PCR or recombinant immunoblot assay (RIBA)

TREATMENT

- No vaccine available
- **Acute infection/needlestick prophylaxis:** Currently not recommended
- **Chronic HCV:** Interferon alfa and ribavirin for selected patients with chronic disease can be curative.

HEPATITIS D

Defective RNA virus; **cotransmitted with hepatitis B or superinfection in chronic hepatitis B carriers (associated with high mortality)**; diagnosed by positive anti-HDV; treat HDV by treating HBV

HEPATITIS E

Rarely seen in the USA, but consider in your differential for patients returning from endemic areas, high mortality rate in pregnant patients (10–20%); illness is self-limited; no vaccine available; diagnosed by positive anti-HEV IgM (acute infection) and anti-HEV (prior exposure)

DRUG-INDUCED HEPATITIS

Ranges from subclinical disease with abnormal LFTs to fulminant hepatic failure; accounts for 40% of acute hepatitis cases in U.S. adults >50 years of age; for 25% of cases of fulminant hepatic failure; and for 5% of jaundice cases in hospitalized patients; can be characterized as intrinsic (direct toxic effect) or idiosyncratic (immunologically mediated injury) and as necroinflammatory (hepatocellular), cholestatic, or mixed; see Table 11.13 for a list of common toxins that cause liver injury; risk factors include advanced age, female gender, use of an increasing number of prescription drugs, underlying liver disease, renal insufficiency, and poor nutrition

AUTOIMMUNE HEPATITIS

Insidious onset, more common in young females

SYMPTOMS/EXAM

- Fatigue, anorexia, arthralgias
- Pruritus suggests an alternate diagnosis: Jaundice, hepatomegaly; spider angiomas
- 40% follow hepatitis A or other viral infections
- Extrahepatic features common: Coombs+ hemolytic anemia, arthritis, Sjögren syndrome, thyroiditis

TABLE 11.13. Toxins Causing Liver Injury

Toxic	Toxic and Idiosyncratic
Alcohol	Methyldopa
Acetaminophen	Isoniazid
Salicylates	Sodium valproate
Tetracyclines	Amiodarone
Trichloroethylene	**Primarily cholestatic**
Vinyl chloride	Chlorpromazine
Carbon tetrachloride	Cyclosporine
Yellow phosphorus	Oral contraceptives
Poisonous mushrooms (Amanita, Galerina)	Anabolic steroids
Idiosyncratic	Erythromycin estolate
Volatile anesthetics (halothane)	Methimazole
Phenytoin	
Sulfonamides	
Rifampin	
Indomethacin	

DIAGNOSIS

- Elevated LFTS, bilirubin, and serum gamma-globulins
- ANA and anti–smooth muscle antibody+

DIFFERENTIAL

- Viral hepatitis
- Primary biliary cirrhosis

TREATMENT

- Supportive care acutely
- Prednisone ± azathioprine

Cirrhosis

Cirrhosis is the final common pathway of many liver diseases that cause hepatocellular injury, and → fibrosis and nodular regeneration. Reversal may occur with treatment of some chronic liver diseases (eg, HBV, HCV).

SYMPTOMS

- Fatigue, anorexia, muscle wasting, loss of libido, impotence, dysmenorrhea
- Decompensation associated with GI bleeding, encephalopathy (sleep-wake reversal, ↓ concentration), ascites
- **Platypnea** (dyspnea induced by sitting upright and relieved by recumbency) and **orthodeoxia** (low PaO_2 when sitting upright that is relieved by recumbency)

EXAM

- Stigmata of chronic liver disease: Palmar erythema spider telangiectasia
- Dupuytren contractures, gynecomastia, testicular atrophy, bilateral parotid enlargement, Terry nails (white, obscure nails)

- Portal hypertension: Caput medusae, splenomegaly, ascites
- Hepatic encephalopathy: Fetor hepaticus, asterixis, confusion

DIFFERENTIAL

CHF, nephrotic syndrome

DIAGNOSIS

- Liver biopsy: The gold standard; also useful in assessing etiology
- Physical exam
- Labs: Thrombocytopenia (splenic sequestration); elevated INR and low albumin (↓ hepatic synthetic function); elevated alkaline phosphatase

COMPLICATIONS

Hepatic encephalopathy, varices, ascites/SBP, hepatorenal syndrome, hepatopulmonary syndrome, hepatocellular carcinoma; portopulmonary syndrome

Ascites and Spontaneous Bacterial Peritonitis (SBP)

In the United States > 80% of ascites cases are due to chronic liver disease (cirrhosis or alcoholic hepatitis). SBP is a spontaneous bacterial infection of ascites. The most common organism implicated is *E. coli*. Other organisms include *Streptococcus* sp. and *Klebsiella*.

SYMPTOMS/EXAM

- Abdominal pain and tenderness, ranging from mild to severe
- Other findings may include fever and altered mental status.
- Characterized by shifting dullness, fluid wave, and bulging flanks (low sensitivity, moderate specificity); imaging (ultrasound, CT) superior to examination. SBP is often asymptomatic, but patients may have fever, abdominal pain, and symptoms/signs of sepsis

DIAGNOSIS

- Diagnostic paracentesis: Indicated in any patient with ascites and abdominal pain, encephalopathy, or fever
  - Findings consistent with SBP include PMNs >250 cells/mm^3 and a +Gram stain or culture
  - The presence of multiple organisms suggests secondary peritonitis from bowel perforation.

TREATMENT

- Third-generation cephalosporin (eg, cefotaxime or ceftriaxone)
- Do not wait for culture results to begin treatment.
- SBP prophylaxis: Fluoroquinolones or TMP-SMX
  - Indicated for cirrhotics hospitalized with GI bleed (3 days); ascites with total protein <1.5 g/dL (while hospitalized); or prior SBP (if the patient has ascites)

Hepatic Encephalopathy

Hepatic encephalopathy is caused by accumulation of nitrogenous waste products in liver failure. Neuropsychiatric changes in the setting of liver disease constitute hepatic encephalopathy until proven otherwise. Look for precipitating factors, including infection, GI bleeding, dehydration, hypokalemia, constipation/ileus, hepatocellular carcinoma, dietary protein overload, CNS active drugs (narcotics, benzodiazepines, anticholinergics), uremia, hypoxia, hypoglycemia, and noncompliance with hepatic encephalopathy treatment.

SYMPTOMS/EXAM

- Insomnia, sleep-wake reversal, personality change, confusion
- Asterixis

DIFFERENTIAL

Hypoglycemia, hyponatremia, Wernicke-Korsakoff syndrome, trauma, infection

DIAGNOSIS

Diagnosis is clinical. **Blood ammonia levels are not always helpful.**

TREATMENT

- Correct precipitating factors and anticipate treatment-related adverse effects.
- Oral/NG tube or rectally administered lactulose (adverse effects include dehydration and hypokalemia); oral neomycin (adverse effects include ototoxicity and renal toxicity) or rifaxamin; oral metronidazole (adverse effects include neuropathy)
- Zinc, short-term protein restriction, branched-chain amino acid–enriched diet
- Beware of medications that are hepatically metabolized, eg, benzodiazepines such as lorazepam.

Hepatorenal Syndrome

The prognosis is grave. **Median survival is 10–14 days.** Two-month mortality is 90%.

DIFFERENTIAL

Prerenal azotemia, acute tubular necrosis, drug-induced disorders (NSAIDs, antibiotics, radiographic contrast, diuretics), glomerulonephritis, vasculitis.

DIAGNOSIS

Exclude other causes of renal failure. Discontinue diuretics and then perform a plasma volume expansion trial with 1.5 L IV normal saline or 5% IV albumin. If serum creatinine ↓, suspect another diagnosis.

TREATMENT

Identify and treat precipitants. Restrict sodium to <2 g/day if serum Na <125 mEq/L, then restrict fluids to <1.5 L/day. Treat infection; liver transplant is often required. **Renal failure from hepatorenal syndrome reverses with liver transplant.**

Hepatic Abscess

Hepatic abscesses may be pyogenic or amebic. In the United States, most cases are due to Gram-negative infections as a result of biliary obstruction, although nearly half have no identifiable cause. Primary amebic liver abscesses are due to the organism *Entamoeba histolytica*.

SYMPTOMS/EXAM

- Ill-appearing with fever; jaundice (if underlying biliary obstruction); abdominal pain
- Tender, enlarged liver

DIFFERENTIAL

Hepatocellular carcinoma, ascending cholangitis

DIAGNOSIS

- Abdominal CT scan or RUQ US
- Abscess culture is definitive.

TREATMENT

- Abscesses >5 cm may require percutaneous or surgical drainage.
- Antibiotics: Third-generation cephalosporins + metronidazole.
- Fungal abscesses usually respond to amphoterecin B.
- Metronidazole alone will treat 95% of cases of *Entamoeba histolytica*.

COMPLICATIONS

Sepsis

Tumors

Malignant tumors are called hepatocellular carcinoma (HCC). They are usually asymptomatic until disease is advanced. There are several benign liver tumors, including hemangiomas, adenomas, and focal nodular hyperplasia.

HEPATOCELLULAR CARCINOMA

SYMPTOMS/EXAM

- Abdominal distention, abdominal pain, jaundice, fatigue, weight loss
- Enlarged palpable liver and an occasional palpable mass
- Bruit over the tumor

DIFFERENTIAL

- Benign liver tumors
- Metastatic cancer
- Liver abscess or cyst

DIAGNOSIS

- Elevation in α-fetoprotein (AFP)
- Ultrasound is suggestive.
- Quad phase CT or MR in the appropriate clinical setting (cirrhosis and/or chronic HBV) can establish the diagnosis.
- Tissue biopsy may be required for confirmation or atypical cases.

TREATMENT

- Local regional therapy (radiofrequency ablation, chemoebolization) is not curative but often is performed as a bridge to liver transplantation.

- Liver transplant or surgical resection can be curative for limited stages without extrahepatic metastasis.
- Systemic chemotherapy is used for palliation only.
- Without liver transplantation or surgical resection the prognosis is poor, with 1- and 5-year survival rates of 25% and 5%, respectively.

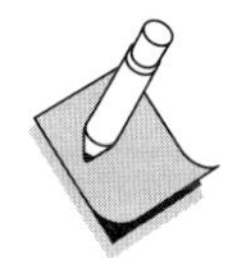

Eighty percent of hepatocellular carcinoma is associated with cirrhosis.

Benign Liver Neoplasms

Hemangioma

- Most common benign neoplasm
- More common in females
- Increases in size with use of exogenous hormones
- Biopsy may be needed to rule out malignancy.

Focal Nodular Hyperplasia

- Asymptomatic
- Hypervascular mass
- Only symptomatic patients undergo resection.

Hepatic Adenoma

- Common in women in their 30s and 40s
- Increased size with hormone use
- May cause pain if necrosis develops
- Resection advised to prevent necrosis.

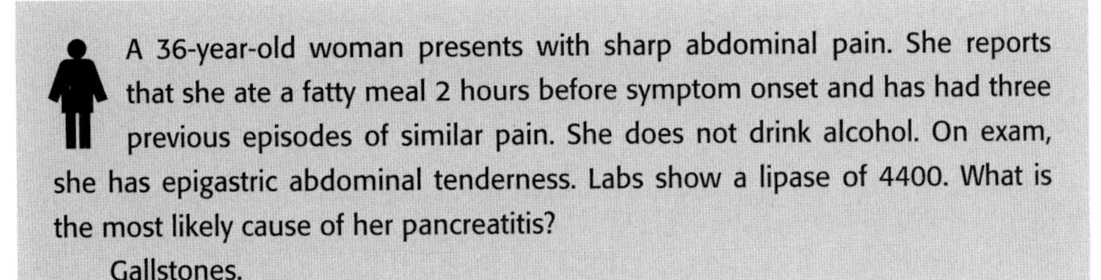

A 36-year-old woman presents with sharp abdominal pain. She reports that she ate a fatty meal 2 hours before symptom onset and has had three previous episodes of similar pain. She does not drink alcohol. On exam, she has epigastric abdominal tenderness. Labs show a lipase of 4400. What is the most likely cause of her pancreatitis?

Gallstones.

GALLBLADDER AND BILIARY TRACT DISEASES

Cholelithiasis

Colic results from transient cystic duct blockage from impacted stones. Risk factors include the 4 Fs: **female, fat, fertile, and forty**, but the disorder is common and can occur in any patient. Other risk factors include OCP use, rapid weight loss, a +family history, chronic hemolysis (pigment stones), small bowel resection, and TPN.

Risk factors for gallstones–

The **4 Fs**
Fat
Female
Fertile
Forty years old

Symptoms/Exam

- Patients present with postprandial abdominal pain (usually in the RUQ) that radiates to the right subscapular area or the epigastrum.
- Pain is abrupt, lasting minutes to hours, followed by gradual relief, often associated with nausea and vomiting, fatty-food intolerance, dyspepsia, and flatulence.
- Gallstones may be asymptomatic in up to 80% of patients.
- Exam may reveal RUQ tenderness and a palpable gallbladder.

Diagnosis

- Liver function tests are **normal** in isolated cholelithiasis.
- Plain X-rays are rarely diagnostic; only 10–15% of stones are radiopaque.
- RUQ ultrasound may show gallstones (85–90% sensitive).
- Consider upper GI series to rule out hiatal hernia or ulcer.

Treatment

- Pain relief, hydration, and electrolyte replacement if severe vomiting
- Cholecystecomy is curative and can be performed electively.
- Patients may require preoperative ERCP for common bile duct (CBD) stones.
- Treat nonsurgical candidates with dietary modification (avoid triggers such as fatty foods).

Complications

Recurrent biliary colic, acute colecystitis, choledocholithiasis, acute cholangitis, gallstone ileus, gallstone pancreatitis

Choledocholithiasis

Gallstones in the common bile duct

Symptoms/Exam

- Symptoms vary according to degree of obstruction, duration of obstruction, and extent of bacterial infection.
- Often presents with RUQ abdominal pain, jaundice, episodic colic, fever, and pancreatitis

Diagnosis

- Hallmark is increased alkaline phosphatase and total bilirubin, which may be the only abnormal lab values.
- Ultrasound may reveal a dilated common bile duct or intrahepatic ducts.
- Magnetic resonance cholangiopancreatography (MRCP) also very helpful for visualizing extra hepatic, intrahepatic, and pancreatic ducts

Treatment

- ERCP with sphincterotomy followed by semielective cholecystectomy

Cholecystitis

Prolonged blockage of the cystic duct, usually by an impacted stone → obstructive distention, inflammation, superinfections, and possible gangrene of the gallbladder (acute gangrenous cholecystitis). Acalculous cholecystitis occurs in the absence of cholelithiasis in chronically debilitated patients, classically those on TPN and trauma or burn victims.

Symptoms

- Patients present with RUQ abdominal pain, nausea, fever, and vomiting. Symptoms are typically more severe and of longer duration than those of biliary colic.

EXAM

- RUQ tenderness, inspiratory arrest during deep palpation to the RUQ (**Murphy's sign**), fever, leukocytosis, mild icterus, and possibly guarding or rebound tenderness may be present on examination.

DIAGNOSIS

- CBC, amylase, lipase, and LFT panel should be obtained.
- Ultrasound may demonstrate stones, biliary sludge, pericholecystic fluid, a thickened gallbladder wall (≥3 mm), gas in the gallbladder, and an ultrasonic Murphy sign (see Figure 11.9).
- Obtain HIDA scan when ultrasound is equivocal (see Figure 11.10).
- Nonvisualization of the gallbladder on HIDA scan suggests acute cholecystitis.
- AXR or CT may demonstrate a fluid-filled gallbladder with gas in the gallbladder wall indicative of **emphysematous cholecystitis**, a rare but life-threatening complication found in older men classically with associated diabetes.

TREATMENT

- Early surgical consultation is indicated especially if the patient is febrile, septic, or has an emphysematous or gangrenous gallbladder.
- Hospitalize patients, administer IV pain medications, antibiotics, and fluids, and replete electrolytes.
- Perform early cholecystectomy (within 72 hours of symptom onset) along with either a preoperative ERCP or an intraoperative cholangiogram to rule out common bile duct stones.
- Since 50% of cases resolve spontaneously, hemodynamically stable patients with significant medical problems, eg, diabetes, can initially be managed medically with a 4- to 6-week delay in surgical treatment.

COMPLICATIONS

- Gangrene, empyema, perforation, gallstone ileus, fistulization, sepsis, abscess formation

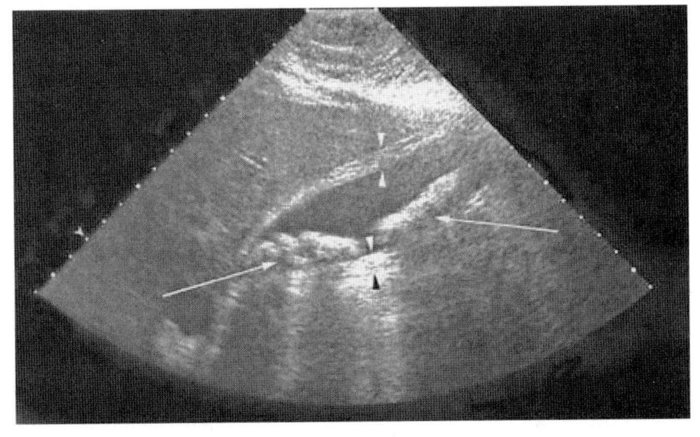

FIGURE 11.9. Acute cholecystitis. The arrowheads indicate the thickened gallbladder wall. There are several stones in the gallbladder (arrows) throwing acoustic shadows. Also seen is pericholecystic fluid.

(Reproduced, with permission, from Brunicardi FC, Andersen DK, Billiar TR, Dunn DL, Hunter JG, Pollock RE. *Schwartz's Principles of Surgery*, 8th ed. New York: McGraw-Hill, 2004:1200.)

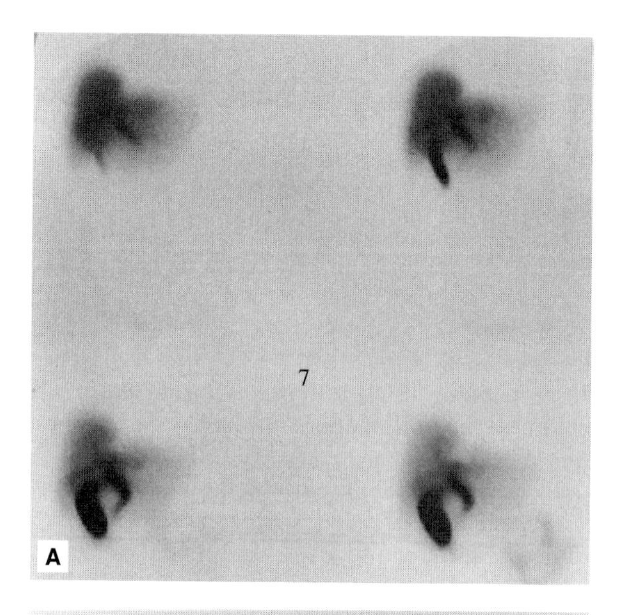

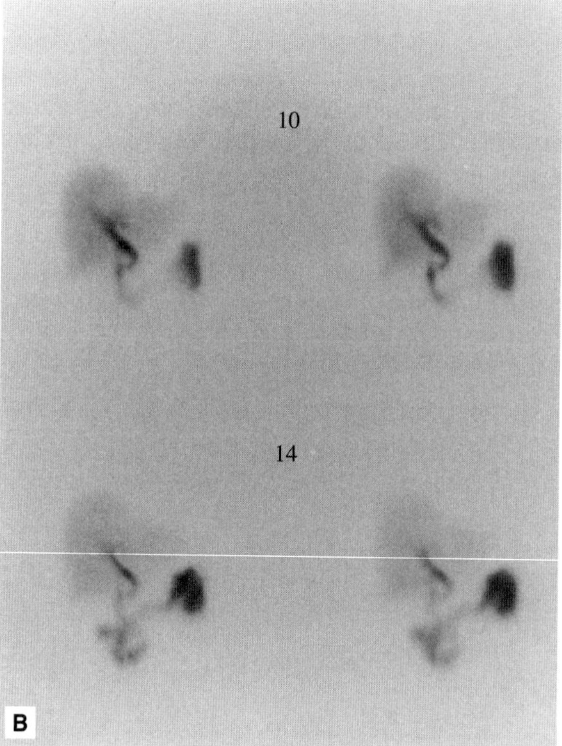

FIGURE 11.10. (A) Normal HIDA scan. IV dye is taken up by hepatocytes, conjugated, and excreted into the common bile duct. (B) Positive HIDA scan. Tracer appears in the duodenum, liver, and common duct but not the gallbladder, suggesting cystic duct obstruction due to acute cholecystitis.

(Reproduced, with permission, from Hall J, et al. *Principles of Critical Care*, 3rd ed. New York: McGraw-Hill, 2005:1258.)

Cholangitis

Cholangitis is an acute bacterial infection of the biliary tree that commonly occurs secondary to obstruction, usually from gallstones (choledocholithiasis) or primary sclerosis cholangitis (progressive inflammation of the biliary tree associated with ulcerative colitis). Gram-negative enterics (eg, *E. coli*, *Enterobacter*,

Pseudomonas) are commonly identified pathogens. Risk factors include bile duct stricture, ampullary carcinoma, and pancreatic pseudocyst.

SYMPTOMS/EXAM

- **Charcot's triad**—RUQ pain, jaundice, and fevers/chills – is classic.
- **Reynold's pentad,** Charcot's triad plus shock and altered mental status, may be present in acute suppurative cholangitis and suggests sepsis.

DIAGNOSIS

- Leukocystosis, increased bilirubin, and increased alkaline phosphatase
- Obtain blood cultures to rule out early sepsis.
- Ultrasound or CT may be a useful adjunct, but diagnosis is often clinical.
- ERCP is both diagnostic and therapeutic (biliary drainage).

Charcot's triad is fever, jaundice, and RUQ pain. Raynaud's pentad also includes decreased mental status and sepsis.

TREATMENT

- Broad spectrum IV antibiotic treatment: Penicillin/antipenicillinase, ceftriaxone + metronidazole, imipenum, or ampicillin + gentamycin + metronidazole.
- Patients often require ICU admission for monitoring, hydration, and BP support.
- Acute suppurative cholangitis requires emergent bile duct decompression via ERCP sphincterotomy, percutaneous transhepatic drainage, or open decompression.

PANCREAS

Pancreatitis

In the United States, >80% of acute pancreatitis cases result from binge drinking or biliary stones; only 5% of heavy drinkers develop pancreatitis. Twenty percent of cases are complicated by necrotizing pancreatitis. Pancreatitis can be classified as either acute or chronic (see Table 11.14).

ETIOLOGY

- **EtOH** and **gallstones** and, to a much lesser extent, trauma, account for about 90% cases of pancreatitis.
- **Drugs:** Azathioprine, pentamidine, sulfonamides, thiazide diuretics, 6MP, valproic acid, dideoxyinosine
- **Metabolic:** Hyperlipidemia or hypercalcemia
- **Mechanical:** Pancreas divisum, sphincter of Oddi dysfunction, mass
- **Infectious:** Viruses (eg, mumps, coxsackievirus B) and, to a lesser extent, bacteria and parasites (eg, *Ascaris lumbricoides*)
- **Other:** Scorpion bites, hereditary pancreatitis (an autosomal-dominant mutation of the trypsinogen gene), cystic fibrosis, pregnancy

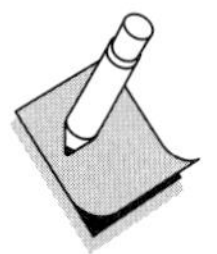

Gallstones and alcohol are the main causes of pancreatitis in the United States.

SYMPTOMS

- Sudden onset, persistent, deep epigastric pain, often radiating to the back, that **worsens when patients are supine and improves when they sit or lean forward**
- Severe nausea, vomiting, and fever are also seen.

TABLE 11.14. Acute Versus Chronic Pancreatitis

Variable	Acute Pancreatitis	Chronic Pancreatitis
Pathophysiology	Leakage of pancreatic enzymes into pancreatic and peripancreatic tissue, often secondary to gallstone disease or alcoholism	Irreversible parenchymal destruction → pancreatic dysfunction.
Time course	Abrupt onset of severe pain	Persistent, recurrent episodes of severe pain
Risk factors	**Gallstones, alcoholism**, hypercalcemia, hypertriglyceridemia, trauma, drug side effects (thiazide diuretics, steroids), viral infections, post-ERCP, scorpion bites	**Alcoholism** (90%), gallstones, hyperparathyroidism, congenital malformation (pancreas divisum); may also be idiopathic
History/PE	**Severe epigastric pain (radiating to the back)**, nausea, vomiting, weakness, fever, shock; flank discoloration **(Grey Turner sign)** and periumbilical discoloration **(Cullen sign)** may be evident on exam due to retroperitoneal hemorrhage	Recurrent episodes of **persistent epigastric pain**, anorexia, nausea, constipation, flatulence, **steatorrhea**, DM
Diagnosis	**Increased amylase, increased lipase, decreased calcium** if severe; **"sentinel loop" or "colon cutoff" sign** on AXR; ultrasound or CT may show enlarged pancreas with stranding, abscess, hemorrhage, necrosis, or pseudocyst	Increased or normal amylase and lipase, **glycosuria**, **pancreatic calcifications** and mild ileus on AXR and CT (**chain of lakes**)
Treatment	Removal of offending agent if possible; standard supportive measures: IV fluids/ electrolyte replacement, analgesia, bowel rest, NG suction, nutritional support, O_2. IV antibiotics, respiratory support and surgical debridement if necrotizing pancreatitis is present	Analgesia, exogenous lipase/trypsin and medium chain fatty-acid diet, avoidance of causative agents (EtOH), celiac nerve block, surgery for intractable pain or structural causes
Prognosis	85–90% mild, self-limited; 10–15% severe, requiring ICU admission; mortality may approach 50% in severe cases	Can have chronic pain and pancreatic exocrine and endocrine dysfunction
Complications	**Pancreatic pseudocyst, fistula formation,** hypocalcemia, renal failure, pleural effusion, chronic pancreatitis, sepsis; mortality secondary to acute pancreatitis predicted with Ranson criteria	**Chronic pain**, malnutrition/weight loss, pancreatic cancer

EXAM

- Exam reveals upper abdominal tenderness with guarding and rebound.
- Other findings include the following:
  - **Severe cases:** Distention, ileus, hypotension, tachycardia
  - **Rare:** Umbilical (**Cullen sign**) or flank (**Grey Turner sign**) ecchymosis
  - Other: Mild jaundice with stones or xanthomata with hyperlipidemia

DIFFERENTIAL

Biliary colic, cholecystitis, mesenteric ischemia, intestinal obstruction/ileus, perforated hollow viscus, inferior MI, dissecting aortic aneurysm, ectopic pregnancy

DIAGNOSIS

- Elevated amylase (more sensitive) and lipase (more specific)
- High serum glucose
- An ALT >3 × normal suggests biliary stones over EtOH; an AST/ALT ratio >2 favors EtOH. CRP declines with improvement.
- Differential for elevated amylase: Pancreatitis, pancreatic tumors, cholecystitis, perforation (esophagus, bowel), intestinal ischemia or infarction, appendicitis, ruptured ectopic pregnancy, mumps, ovarian cysts, lung cancer, macroamylasemia, renal insufficiency, HIV, DKA, head trauma; lipase usually normal in nonpancreatic amylase elevations **and therefore more specific for pancreatitis**
- AXR: May show gallstones, "sentinel loop" (an air-filled small bowel in the LUQ), and "colon cutoff sign" (abrupt ending of the transverse colon)
- RUQ ultrasound: Reveals cholelithiasis without cholecystitis; choledocholithiasis (common duct stones) often missed or have passed
- CT: Performed initially to exclude abdominal catastrophes; at 48–72 hours, exclude necrotizing pancreatitis; an ↑ risk of renal failure from contrast dye

TREATMENT

- NPO with nasojejunal tube feeds or total parenteral nutrition with severe disease and anticipated NPO status for >3–5 days
- Aggressive IV hydration
- Pain control with narcotics; avoid morphine, as it ↑ sphincter of Oddi tone
- Broad spectrum IV antibiotics (imipenem) for severe necrotizing pancreatitis
- For **gallstone pancreatitis** (elevated serum bilirubin, signs of biliary sepsis), perform ERCP for stone removal and cholecystectomy following recovery **but prior to discharge.**

COMPLICATIONS

- **Necrotizing pancreatitis**
  - Suspected in the setting of a persistently elevated WBC count (7–10 days), high fever, and shock (organ failure)
  - Has a poor prognosis (up to 30% mortality and 70% risk of complications)
  - If infected necrosis is suspected, perform percutaneous aspiration. If organisms are present on smear, surgical debridement is indicated.
- **Pancreatic pseudocyst:** A collection of pancreatic fluid walled off by granulation tissue; occurs in approximately 30% of cases but resolves spontaneously in about 50%; drainage not required unless the pseudocyst is present >6–8 weeks and is enlarging and symptomatic
- **Other:** Pseudoaneurysm, renal failure, ARDS, splenic vein thrombosis (which can → isolated gastric varices)
- **Hypocalcemia**

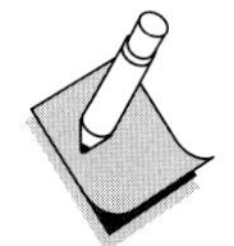

CT is prognostic in severe pancreatitis and is used to evaluate for necrotizing pancreatitis. Necrotizing pancreatitis warrants empiric antibiotics (eg, imipenem).

TABLE 11.15 Ranson Criteria for Acute Pancreatitis

On Admission	After 48 Hours
GA LAW:	C HOBBS:
Glucose >200 mg/dL	Ca^{2+} <8.0 mg/dL
Age >55	Hematocrit decrease by >10%
LDH >350 IU/L	O_2 Pao_2 <60
AST >250 IU/dL	Base deficit >4 mEq/L
WBC >16,000/mL	BUN increase >5 mg/dL
	Sequestered fluid >6 L

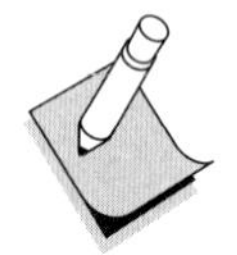

The risk of mortality in pancreatitis is <1% if 1–2 of Ranson criteria; 20% with 3–4; 40% with 4–5; near 100% with >6.

- ARDS
- Death predicted by Ranson criteria (see Table 11.15)

Pancreatic Cancer

Roughly 90% are pancreatic head adenocarcinomas. Risk factors include smoking, chronic pancreatitis, a first-degree relative with pancreatic cancer, and a high-fat diet. Pancreatic cancer is most commonly seen in men in their 60s.

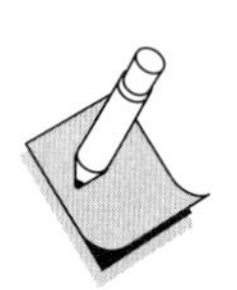

The classic presentation of pancreatic cancer is painless, progressive jaundice.

Symptoms

- Presents with abdominal pain radiating toward the back as well as jaundice, loss of appetite, nausea, vomiting, weight loss, weakness, fatigue, and indigestion

Exam

- Exam may reveal a palpable, nontender gallbladder (**Courvoisier sign**) or migratory thrombophlebitis (**Trousseau sign**).

Diagnosis

- Use CT to detect a pancreatic mass, dilated pancreatic and bile ducts, the extent of vascular involvement, and metastases. If a mass is not visualized, use ERCP or endoscopic ultrasound for better visualization and consider fine-needle aspiration.

Treatment

- Most patients present with metastatic disease, and treatment is palliative.
- Some 10–20% of pancreatic head tumors have no evidence of metastasis and may be resected using the Whipple procedure (pancreaticoduodenectomy).
- Chemotherapy with 5-FU and gemcitabine may improve short-term survival, but long-term prognosis is poor (<5% survive >5 years from diagnosis).

MESENTERIC ISCHEMIA

Mesenteric ischemia can be divided into arterial and venous disease as well as occlusive versus nonocclusive (see Table 11.16). Full-gut necrosis can occur as fast as in 6 hours. This is a disease with a high rate of morbidity and mortality (30–100%), so early identification and treatment are prudent. Acute mesenteric ischemia is most commonly (>50%) due to occlusive embolism and involves the superior mesenteric artery (SMA). Ischemic colitis is a nonocclusive process involving the inferior mesenteric artery (IMA) secondary to low-flow states.

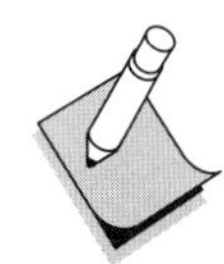

Consider acute mesenteric ischemia in patients with abdominal pain out of proportion to exam or with a persistently elevated lactate without other underlying causes.

SYMPTOMS

- Acute disease presents with abdominal pain **out of proportion** to clinical exam. Pain is severe, colicky, and poorly localized.
- History of "intestinal angina"
- Chronic disease can present as pain after eating, weight loss, or change in bowel pattern.

EXAM

- Initially soft abdomen
- Peritoneal signs once complete transmural infarct develops
- Blood on rectal exam
- Chronic mesenteric ischemia may present with an abdominal bruit.

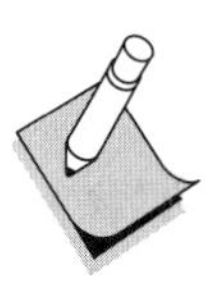

Elderly patients often present atypically with presentations that mimic other diseases.

DIFFERENTIAL

- Diverticulitis, appendicitis, MI, IBD, perforated viscous, aortic dissection, abdominal aortic aneurysm

TABLE 11.16. Causes of Mesenteric Ischemia

Occlusive Disease	
Embolism	**Atrial fibrillation**, myxoma, valvular disease
Arterial thrombosis	Atherosclerosis, low-flow state
Venous thrombosis	Hypercoaguable state
Arterial disease	AAA, AD, fibromuscular dysplasia, atherolsclerosis
Iatrogenic	Drug-induced, eg, epinephrine, post-procedure (dissection or embolism)
Trauma	Penetrating or blunt
Nonocclusive disease	
Shock	Sepsis, cardiogenic, hypovolemic
Low-flow	Myocardial infarction, arrhythmia, CHF
Drug-induced	Vasoactive drugs, cocaine, digitalis

Diagnosis

- AXR may show "**thumb-printing**" or **pneumonitis intesinalis,** which are late findings. Early findings include paucity of intestinal gas.
- CT of the abdomen may reveal indirect signs such as ascites or bowel wall edema and intraluminal gas in an arterial distribution.
- CT angiography or conventional angiography remains the diagnostic test of choice.
- Serum lactate may aid in diagnosis but is relatively nonspecific for any anaerobic metabolism.
- Diagnostic laparotomy if the patient is unstable

Treatment

- Resuscitation via IV fluids
- Immediate surgery for necrotic bowel
- IV antibiotics to cover gut flora
- Nonocclusive ischemia may be treated with intra-arterial papaverin.
- Chronic ischemia may be treated with revascularization.

Complications

- Bowel ischemia, necrosis, perforation, shock, sepsis

CHAPTER 12

Obstetrics and Gynecology

Danielle D. Campagne, MD

A 33-year-old female presents to the ED with left lower-quadrant pain. Her LMP was 2 months ago. Vital signs are BP 90/60, HR 130, RR 18. Urine pregnancy test is positive. An ultrasound is done (see Figure 12.1). What is the next appropriate step?

Emergent consultation of OB/GYN for surgical treatment of ectopic pregnancy.

ECTOPIC PREGNANCY

Ectopic pregnancy occurs when the conceptus is implanted outside of the uterine cavity.

- 95% are in the fallopian tube; other sites include ovary, abdominal cavity, and cervix.
- Ectopic pregnancy is common, occurring in 1–2% of all pregnancies.
- Heterotopic pregnancy (simultaneous IUP and ectopic pregnancy) occurs in only 1 in 4000 pregnancies but may occur in up to 3% of patients taking **fertility treatment**.
- Risk factors include pelvic inflammatory disease (PID), tubal ligation, previous pelvic surgery, current use of an IUD, history of previous ectopic, elective abortion, and fertility treatments.

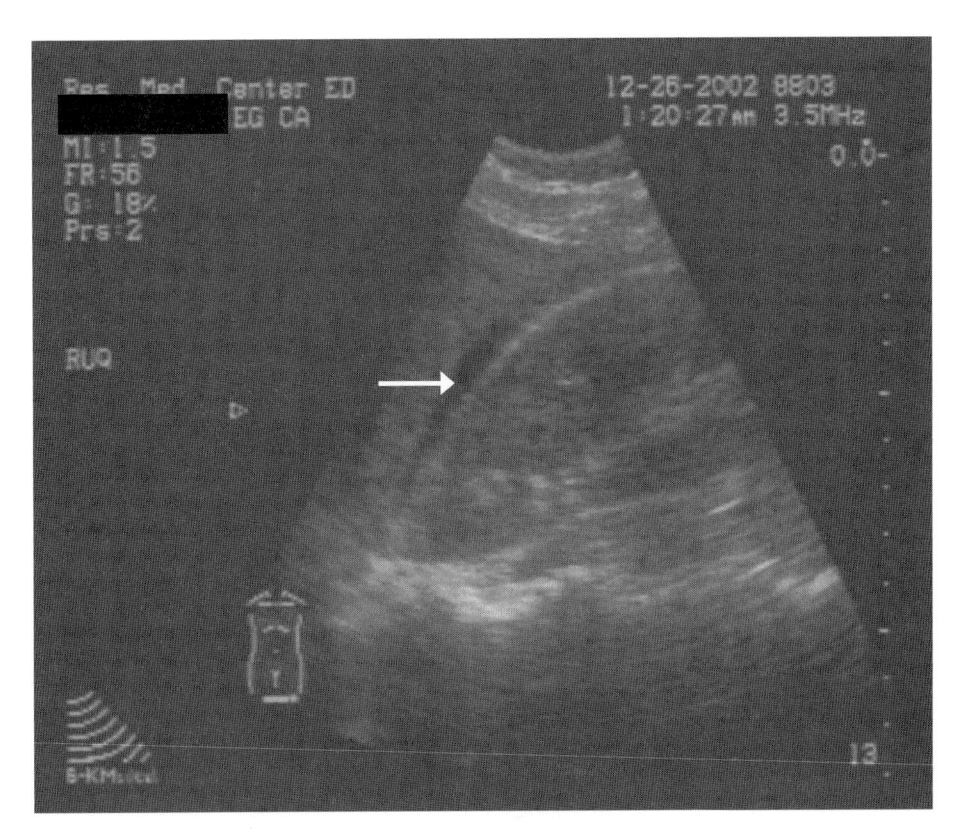

FIGURE 12.1. Ultrasound of positive FAST with free fluid.

(Reproduced, with permission, from Plantz SH, Collman D, Gossman WG, et al. *Emergency Medicine Written Board Review*, 6th ed. New York: McGraw-Hill, 2006:439.)

- A modern copper IUD does not increase the risk of ectopic compared to no contraception, but if a women becomes pregnant with an IUD, then the risk of ectopic is high (approximately 3%).

SYMPTOMS

- Abdominal pain
- Vaginal bleeding—common, but not always present
- Dizziness or syncope (less common)

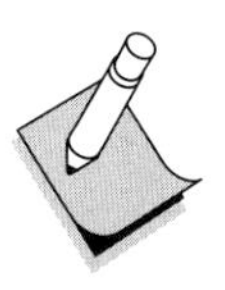

All females of childbearing age with abdominal pain should be presumed pregnant until proven otherwise.

EXAM

- Vital signs may be normal or hypotension may be present due to hemorrhagic shock.
- A relative bradycardia may be present secondary to vagal stimulation.
- The pelvic/abdominal exam may be **normal** or can have localized tenderness including CMT.
- Adnexal tenderness or adnexal mass may not always be present on exam.

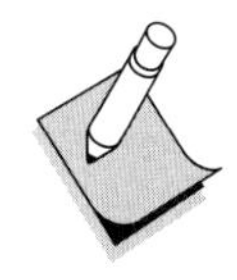

Classic triad for ectopic pregnancy:
Abdominal pain
Vaginal bleeding
Positive pregnancy test

DIFFERENTIAL

The differential for a woman of childbearing age with abdominal/pelvic pain or abnormal vaginal bleeding includes:

- Ectopic pregnancy
- Appendicitis/cholecystitis
- Ovarian cyst/torsion
- PID
- Endometriosis
- UTI/renal colic
- Inflammatory bowel disease (IBD)
- Mittelschmerz
- Intrauterine pregnancy
- Threatened abortion
- Inevitable abortion
- Molar pregnancy
- Heterotopic pregnancy
- Corpus luteum cyst

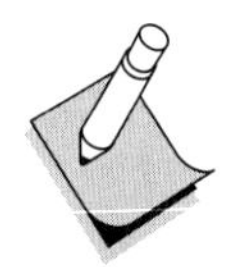

Mittelschmerz: Midcycle (half-way between periods) pain associated with ovulation, usually sharp, usually on one side

DIAGNOSIS

- Ectopic pregnancy should be considered in all women of childbearing age who present with abdominal or pelvic pain, especially those with unexplained signs/symptoms of hypovolemia.
- Positive pregnancy test is an almost universal finding in the diagnosis of ectopic (very dilute urine or switched urine samples may lead to a false negative!).
- Ultrasound is the test of choice in evaluating pregnant patients with complaints consistent with ectopic pregnancy (see Figure 12.2).
- The finding of a yolk sac, a double decidual sac, or fetal cardiac activity inside the uterus is considered diagnostic for IUP. A **gestational sac alone is not diagnostic** for IUP because it may be confused with a pseudosac, which is often present in patients with extrauterine pregnancy.
- A β-hCG facilitates ultrasound interpretation. The "**discriminatory zone**" (the β-hCG level above which an IUP should be visualized by ultrasound) for transvaginal ultrasound is 1000–1500 IU/mL; for transabdominal ultrasound it is about 4000–6500 IU/mL.
- Above the discriminatory zone, it should be possible to identify an IUP. Failure to do so mandates OB/GYN consultation for presumed ectopic.
- A β-hCG level below the discriminatory zone and an ultrasound that fails to show an intrauterine pregnancy is consistent with either an early IUP or an ectopic pregnancy.
- Heterotopic pregnancy must be considered in unstable patients with findings diagnostic for IUP. Look at the adnexa and look for signs of simultaneous ectopic pregnancy or free fluid.

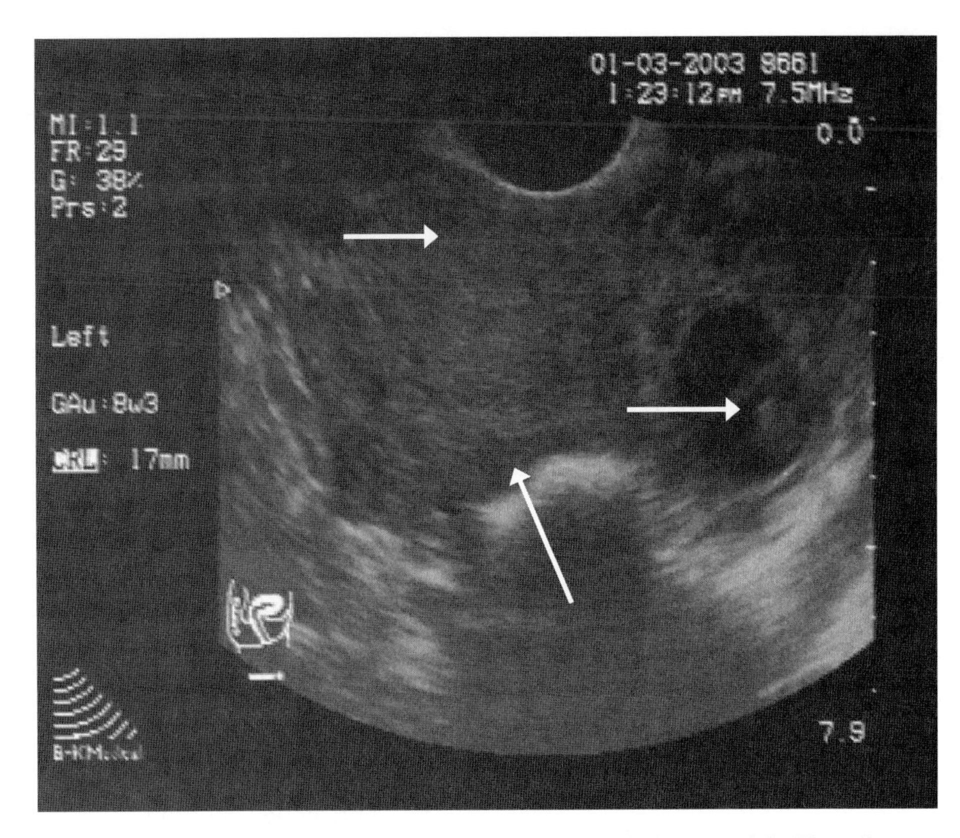

FIGURE 12.2. Endovaginal ultrasound with the uterus in the upper left side and an ectopic pregnancy on the right with a fetal pole.

(Reproduced, with permission, from Plantz SH, Collman D, Gossman WG, et al. *Emergency Medicine Written Board Review*, 6th ed. McGraw-Hill, 2006:446.)

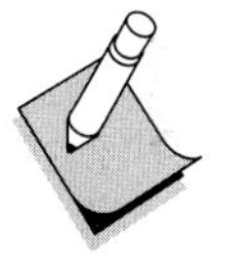

Expect to visualize an IUP using
(1) Transvaginal ultrasound and >38 days after LMP or β-hCG >1500
(2) Abdominal ultrasound and >45 days after LMP or β-hCG >4000

- Culdocentesis (placement of a needle through the posterior wall of the vagina to aspirate blood in the cul-de-sac) is rarely performed. It is indicated only in settings where sonography is not available, and ruptured ectopic is suspected. Aspiration of nonclotting blood is considered positive and indicative of an ectopic pregnancy (see Table 12.1).

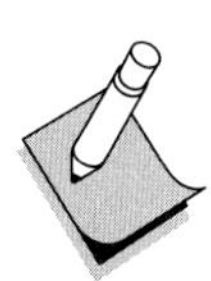

β-hCG levels in ectopic pregnancy are often below the discriminatory zone!

TABLE 12.1. Ultrasound Findings in Suspected Ectopic Pregnancy

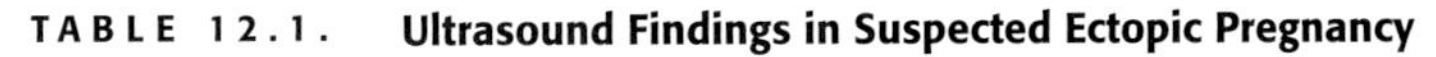

IUP	Ectopic	Suggest Ectopic	Indeterminate
Yolk sac within a gestational sac	Ectopic fetal pole	Fluid in the cul-de-sac with no IUP	Empty uterus
Intrauterine fetal pole	FHT outside uterus	Complex adnexal mass with no IUP	Echogenic material in uterus
Fetal heart tones		β-hCG above discriminatory zone with no IUP	Abnormal or single gestational sac

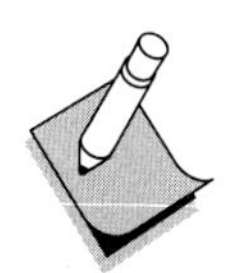

The first definitive sign of an IUP is the presence of a yolk sac within the gestational sac.

TREATMENT

Treatment is guided by the patient's hemodynamic status, quantitative β-hCG, and ultrasound findings.

- **Unstable patients:** Two large-bore IV lines with rapid infusion of crystalloid and/or packed red blood cells should be given to maintain blood pressure. OB/GYN should be consulted immediately (even before the ultrasound) for emergent laparotomy in an unstable patient with a positive pregnancy test. Lab tests including blood count and type and cross should be sent.
- **Stable patients with ectopic pregnancy**: Definitive treatment is determined by the OB/GYN consultant but may consist of laparoscopy or medical management with methotrexate.
- **Stable patients with indeterminate ultrasound**: Patients with a low β-hCG and indeterminate ultrasound may be discharged with return precautions and follow-up in 2 days for repeat β-hCG level. Women with viable pregnancies should double their serum β-hCG in 48 hours. Patients with persistent symptoms or whose β-hCG rises by $<66\%$ over 48 hours require further evaluation.

FIRST TRIMESTER BLEEDING

CAUSES

The causes of first trimester bleeding include

- Ectopic pregnancy: The most life-threatening cause of first trimester bleeding (see "Ectopic Pregnancy")
- Spontaneous abortion
- Gestational trophoblastic disease (GTD)
- Physiologic bleeding (implantation bleeding)
- Cervical pathology (eg, cervicitis)

Spontaneous Abortion

Thirty percent of all pregnancies are complicated by first trimester bleeding. About 50% of these will end in a spontaneous abortion.

Miscarriage occurs when a pregnancy ends spontaneously before the fetus has reached 20 weeks or 500 g.

TERMINOLOGY

- Threatened abortion: Abdominal pain or vaginal bleeding in the first 20 weeks gestation, **closed cervix** on exam, no passage of fetal tissue by history or exam. Fetal cardiac activity may be detected.
- Inevitable abortion: Vaginal bleeding with **open cervix** but no passage of fetal products
- Incomplete abortion: Incomplete passage of fetal parts, **open cervix**, pain, and vaginal bleeding
- Complete abortion: Complete passage of fetal parts and placenta, **closed cervix**, uterus contracted
- Septic abortion: Infection of the uterus during a miscarriage, usually due to *Staphylococcus aureus*; fever, chills, purulent cervical discharge, and uterine tenderness

- Missed abortion: In utero death of the fetus prior to 20 weeks gestation with retention of the products for a prolonged period of time

SYMPTOMS

Women usually present with a history of amenorrhea followed by vaginal bleeding and pelvic pain.

EXAM

- Cervix may be open or closed.
- Visualization of products of conception confirms a miscarriage and excludes ectopic pregnancy except in unstable patients or patients on fertility treatment.

Complications of a missed abortion include infection and coagulopathy.

DIAGNOSIS

- Vaginal exam to assess if the cervix is open
- Ultrasound with quantitative β-hCG to exclude ectopic pregnancy
- Blood type and Rh factor determination to determine need for Rhogam
- Urinalysis to exclude infection as a cause of miscarriage

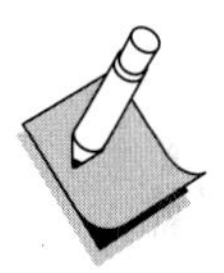

Septic abortion is a leading cause of maternal mortality in the developing world, mostly as a result of illegal and unsterile abortions.

TREATMENT

- Rh-negative women should receive Rh(D)immune globulin 300 μg, or 50 μg if $<$13 weeks gestation.
- Most patients with threatened abortion may be discharged with return precautions and OB follow-up.
- Patients with either incomplete or complete abortion with persistent bleeding should be offered dilation and curettage.
- Septic abortion mandates dilation and curettage and broad spectrum antibiotics (cefoxitin and doxycycline, ampicillin and sulbactam, or imipenem and cilastatin).

Rh INCOMPATABILITY

PATHOPHYSIOLOGY

- Approximately 15% of individuals are Rh negative.
- In Rh-negative women with an Rh-positive fetus, maternal exposure to even small amounts of fetal blood can result in the production of maternal antibodies to the foreign Rh antigen.
- The formation of maternal Rh antibodies exposes the current and subsequent pregnancies to antibody-induced hemolytic disease of the newborn.

CAUSES

- Trauma
- Vaginal bleeding
- Spontaneous or induced abortion
- Obstetric procedures
- Transfusions of Rh-positive blood may sensitize an Rh negative woman, even if she is not pregnant.

DIAGNOSIS/TREATMENT

- Rh(D) immune globulin 300 μg for Rh-negative pregnant patients with possible exposure to fetal blood.

- "Mini-RhoGAM" (50 μg) can be used for patients <13 weeks gestation.
- Give within 72 hours of exposure.
- If the volume of fetal blood to which the mother has been exposed may be large, the **Kliehauer-Betke test** can be used to quantify fetomaternal transmission.

THIRD TRIMESTER BLEEDING

Placental Abruption

Placental abruption is premature separation of the implanted placenta from the uterine wall. It occurs in 1–2% of all pregnancies. Bleeding between the placenta and uterine wall can result in significant blood loss with maternal and fetal compromise. Separations >50% result in fetal death.

Risk factors for abruption include:

- HTN
- Advanced maternal age
- Multiparity
- Smoking
- Cocaine use
- Previous abruption and abdominal trauma

SYMPTOMS

- Vaginal bleeding
- Abdominal pain

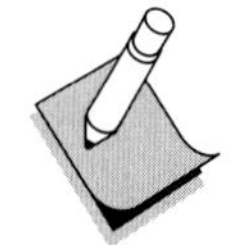

***Painful** third trimester vaginal bleeding = abruption.*

EXAM

- Uterine tenderness
- Uterine irritability with hypertonic/hyperactive contractions.
- Fetal distress and maternal DIC may occur.
- An obstetrician should be consulted prior to pelvic examination in the setting of third trimester bleeding because if placenta previa is present severe hemorrhage may result.

DIFFERENTIAL

Placental previa versus preterm labor

DIAGNOSIS

- The diagnosis is made clinically: Third trimester vaginal bleeding with abdominal pain/tenderness.
- Ultrasound is essential to rule out placenta previa; abruption is often **difficult to visualize on ultrasound**.

TREATMENT

- Assess hemodynamics and fluid resuscitate if needed. Send CBC, PT, PTT, fibrinogen levels and type, and Rh. Fibrinogen levels tend to be low in patients with placental abruption.
- **Monitoring of maternal contractions and fetal HR** provides an indication of fetal health and is the preferred method of evaluating patients with possible abruption.

- Fetus distress is suggested by: HR <120, or >160, decelerations after uterine irritability, or loss of beat-to-beat variability during continuous fetal monitoring.
- Emergent OB consultation should be obtained for assistance with monitoring and possible delivery in patients with suspected abruption.
- Rh isoimmunization prophylaxis as needed.

Placenta Previa

Placenta previa occurs when the placenta overlaps and implants on the cervix, covering the internal os to varying degrees.

Risk factors include previous placenta previa as well as any pathology that changes the inner surface of the uterus:

- Prior C-section
- Multiple gestations
- Multiple induced abortions
- Advanced maternal age

SYMPTOMS

Painless, bright red vaginal bleeding

EXAM

- Abdominal exam reveals a soft, nontender uterus.
- Do not perform a pelvic exam.
- An obstetrician should be consulted prior to pelvic examination in the setting of third trimester bleeding because if placenta previa is present, severe hemorrhage may result.

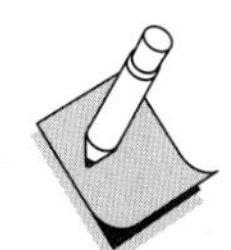

Painless, bright red, third trimester vaginal bleeding = placenta previa.

DIFFERENTIAL

Placental abruption vs rupture of membranes

DIAGNOSIS

- **Transabdominal ultrasound** is the key to the diagnosis!
- The ultrasound will show the placental location.
- This is in contrast to abruption, which cannot always be seen on ultrasound.

TREATMENT

- Emergent OB consult for maternal/fetal monitoring.
- Do not encourage vaginal delivery in a patient with placenta previa; most cases require C-section.
- Rh-isoimmunization prophylaxis as needed.

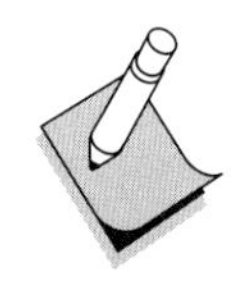

Do not perform pelvic exam on patients with third trimester vaginal bleeding.

Premature Rupture of Membranes

Defined as rupture of membranes prior to the onset of labor. Preterm premature rupture of membranes (PPROM) refers to rupture of membranes occurring prior to labor in a patient <37 weeks gestation.

SYMPTOMS

Rush of fluid or a continuous leak of fluid from the vagina

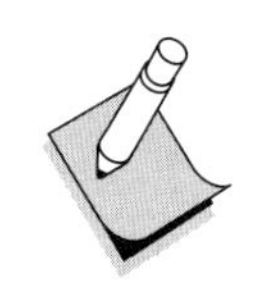

Blue nitrazine paper + ferning = amniotic fluid.

DIAGNOSIS

Confirm PROM with a sterile speculum exam showing:

- A pool of fluid in the posterior fornix
- A pH >6.5 (nitrazine paper turns **blue**!)
- Ferning of fluid as it dries on a slide; this results from the presence of proteins and electrolytes in the amniotic fluid and is also diagnostic

TREATMENT

- Immediate OB consultation and admission
- Test patients for chlamydia, gonorrhea, and group B streptococcus.
- Prophylactic antibiotics to prevent anminonitis in patients with PROM is controversial.

PREGNANCY-INDUCED HYPERTENSION

Pregnancy-induced hypertension is defined as BP >140/90 or an increase in systolic BP >20 (or diastolic >10) above baseline.

Preeclampsia/Eclampsia

Preeclampsia is defined as the presence of new onset hypertension and proteinuria with or without edema in women who are **>20 weeks gestation**. Eclampsia = preeclampsia plus seizures.

Risk factors for preeclampsia include:

- Primigravida
- Very young or advanced maternal age
- Diabetes mellitus
- Multiple gestations
- Hydatidiform mole

SYMPTOMS

- Weight gain (>5 pounds/week)
- Headache/visual disturbances
- Extremity or facial swelling
- Shortness of breath
- Decreased urine output

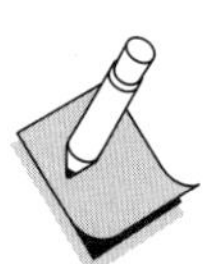

Never ignore an elevated BP in a pregnant patient. Eclampsia can kill both the mother and fetus.

EXAM

Usually a normal physical exam except for high blood pressure. Edema (peripheral or facial) can be present.

DIFFERENTIAL

- Gestational hypertension: Mild hypertension after 20 weeks gestation with no proteinuria present; may progress to preeclampsia, but usually resolves by 12 weeks postpartum
- Chronic hypertension (aka preexisting hypertension): Defined as systolic pressure ≥140 mmHg, diastolic pressure ≥90 mmHg, or both, that antedates pregnancy; present prior to the 20th week, or persists >12 weeks postpartum. Usually treated with **methyldopa (Aldomet), labetalol, or nifedipine**; avoid diuretics and ace inhibitors

- Preeclampsia superimposed upon chronic hypertension: Defined by new onset proteinuria after 20 weeks gestation in a patient with preexisting hypertension **or** development of severe hypertension (SBP ≥160 or DBP ≥110 mmHg) in a pregnant patient with a history of both hypertension and proteinuria

DIAGNOSIS

- **Preeclampsia** is new onset hypertension (systolic BP >140 and diastolic BP >90) combined with proteinuria of 30 mg/dL or 300 mg/24 hours) in patients >20 weeks gestation.
- The elevation in blood pressure should be sustained, which is generally regarded as two measurements at least 6 hours apart.

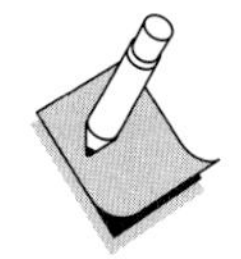

Eclampsia can occur up to 2 weeks postpartum.

TREATMENT

- The cornerstone of treatment for preeclampsia/eclampsia is delivery of the fetus.
- Expectant management can be attempted in a monitored setting for preeclamptic patients <34 weeks gestation with only mild proteinuria.
- Medical management includes **magnesium sulfate** and antihypertensive drugs (hydralazine or labetalol).
- Magnesium sulfate 4–6 g IV is given over 15 minutes followed by 1–2 g/hour.
- Watch for signs of magnesium toxicity: Hyporeflexia, loss of deep tendon reflexes, respiratory depression, and bradydysrhythmias.
- These patients are ill. Call your consultant early.

HELLP Syndrome

HELLP syndrome (hemolysis, elevated liver enzymes, low platelet count) is an uncommon but severe variant of preeclampsia. Unlike preeclampsia, which occurs in primigravida patients, HELLP syndrome is more common in the multigravid patient.

SYMPTOMS/EXAM

- Epigastric/RUQ abdominal pain and tenderness
- Patients may (or may not) have symptoms of preeclampsia.

DIFFERENTIAL

- Other causes of upper abdominal pain in pregnancy: Cholecystitis, gastritis, pancreatitis, appendicitis
- Idiopathic thrombocytopenic purpura, hemolytic uremic syndrome

DIAGNOSIS

- Primarily a laboratory diagnosis
- LDH (marker for hemolysis) >600 U/L
- Thrombocytopenia (<100,000/mm^3, but suspect if <150,000/mm^3); may predict severity
- Elevated liver enzymes with AST >70 U/L
- Peripheral smear may show evidence of microangiopathic hemolytic anemia (schiztocytes).

TREATMENT

- The cornerstone of treatment is delivery of the fetus.
- Mild cases may be treated with corticosteroids and expectant management.

- Treat preeclampsia, as above.
- Correct coagulopathy, as needed (FFP, platelets, blood transfusion).

> ***HELLP syndrome:***
>
> **H**emolysis
> **E**levated **L**iver enzymes
> **L**ow **P**latelets

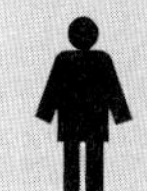

A 20-year-old, 10-week pregnant woman presents with severe nausea and vomiting. Her BP is 160/100 and her fundus is palpable at her umbilicus. What test do you perform to confirm your diagnosis?

Ultrasound to look for the "snowstorm" pattern of a molar pregnancy, and β-hCG.

HYDATIDIFORM MOLE

Gestational trophoblastic disease occurs when a nonviable embryo implants and trophoblastic cells proliferate in the uterus. The noninvasive form (no invasion of uterine wall) of GTD is the hydatidiform mole.

Hydatidiform moles are defined as either complete or partial.

- Partial mole: Triploid (two sets of paternal chromosomes/one set of maternal); has fetal parts and a higher tendency to progress to choriocarcinoma
- Complete mole: Diploid (two sets of paternal chromosomes) with the absence of fetal parts

> *Higher β-hCG and larger uterine size than expected by dates should raise suspicion of molar pregnancy.*

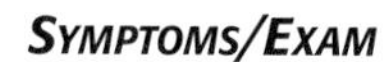

SYMPTOMS/EXAM

- Severe nausea/vomiting
- Uterus larger than expected for dates
- Vaginal passage of "grapelike" clusters of vesicles
- Intermittent vaginal bleeding during early pregnancy
- Preelampsia prior to 20 weeks gestation

DIAGNOSIS

- β-hCG is higher than expected for dates and a characteristic snowstorm appearance is seen on older ultrasound models (see Figure 12.3).
- Once a hydatidiform mole is diagnosed, a CXR should be obtained. Trophoblastic tumors metastasize to lung, liver, and brain.

TREATMENT

- Dilation and curettage in the hospital and monitoring of β-hCG levels are indicated. Failure of β-hCG to decrease to zero suggests choriocarcinoma or invasive disease.

HYPEREMESIS GRAVIDARUM

A severe form of morning sickness, with excessive pregnancy-related nausea and/or vomiting that prevents adequate intake of food and fluids.

SYMPTOMS/EXAM

- Intractable nausea/vomiting
- Weight loss (from prepregnancy weight; >5% = severe)
- Hypokalemia

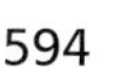

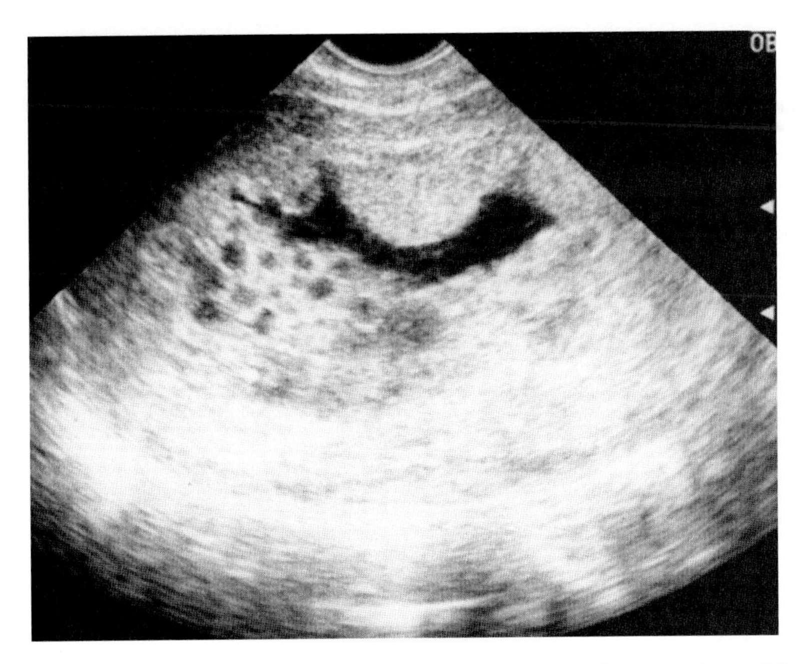

FIGURE 12.3. Molar pregnancy with intrauterine "snowstorm" pattern. Serum β-hCG in this case was >180,000 mIU/mL.

(Courtesy of Robin Marshall, MD as reproduced, with permission, from Knoop KJ, Stack LB, Storrow AB. *Atlas of Emergency Medicine*, 2nd ed. New York: McGraw-Hill, 2002:272.)

- Ketonemia
- No abdominal tenderness on exam

DIFFERENTIAL

Includes obstetric and nonobstetric causes of nausea/vomiting such as pyelonephritis, appendicitis, cholelithiasis, pancreatitis gastroenteritis, and bowel obstruction

DIAGNOSIS

- Because nausea and vomiting during pregnancy exist on a continuum, there is no clear boundary between common morning sickness and hyperemesis.

TREATMENT

- Fluid resuscitation with 5% glucose containing fluids
- Antiemetics (phenergan, compazine, reglan)
- Admit patients with persistent vomiting, electrolyte abnormalities, ketosis despite resuscitation, or weight loss >10% of prepregnancy weight.
- Consider thiamine (vitamin B1) 100 mg IV for patients with prolonged symptoms to prevent **Wernicke encephalopathy**.

NORMAL LABOR AND DELIVERY

Normal labor proceeds through three basic stages (see Table 12.2).

TABLE 12.2. **Stages of Labor**

Stage 1: Cervical stage	Onset of regular contractions to complete cervical dilation/effacement
Stage 2: Expulsion stage	Complete dilation/effacement to delivery of fetus
Stage 3: Placental stage	Delivery of fetus to delivery of placenta

Normal Vertex Delivery

Emergency delivery often proceeds rapidly and requires minimal help from the ED provider.

- Delivery of the fetal head should be controlled by applying moderate upward pressure on the fetal chin through the perineum while holding the fetal head against the pubic symphysis.
- Nose and airway suctioning, followed by palpation for a nuchal cord, should occur immediately after delivery of the fetal head.
- The anterior shoulder should be delivered first by placing hands on either side of fetal head and applying gentle downward traction. The posterior shoulder typically follows spontaneously.

DELIVERY COMPLICATIONS

Nuchal Cord

Occurs in a quarter of all cephalad presenting deliveries; can result in fetal asphyxia if not identified and treated promptly

Treatment

- Loose nuchal cord: Slip over head of fetus in between contractions
- Tight nuchal cord: Cut and clamp on perineum; prompt delivery must follow

Cord Prolapse

Occurs when the umbilical cord presents ahead of the fetal presenting part; most likely to occur with abnormal fetal presentations and with fetal prematurity

Diagnosis

- Visualization or palpation of pulsating umbilical cord at or through the cervical os

Treatment

- Elevate the presenting fetal part to reduce compression of the cord.
- This is an obstetrical emergency and a C-section is indicated. The examiner's hand should stay in the vagina elevating the presenting part until the patient undergoes surgery.
- Other adjunctive maneuvers include knee chest position and manually filling bladder with fluid (via Foley catheter).

Shoulder Dystocia

A failure of the fetal shoulders to deliver after delivery of the fetal head; occurs when the anterior shoulder impacts behind or above the pubic symphysis; most likely to occur with large fetal size or in the presence of abnormal pelvic anatomy

Symptoms/Exam

- Turtle sign: Fetal head pulled tight against perineum

Treatment

- Obtain immediate OB backup.
- Empty the bladder and make a generous episiotomy.
- Apply firm suprapubic (**not** fundal) pressure to dislodge the impacted fetal shoulder.
- McRobert maneuver: Sharply flexing hips and legs (successful alone about half the time)
- Twisting/corkscrew manipulation of fetal shoulders
- Fracture of fetal clavicle or symphysiotomy is last resort.

Breech Presentation

The major risk of breech delivery is entrapment of the fetal head and resultant fetal hypoxia.

Treatment

- The delivery should be allowed to progress as spontaneously as possible until the fetal umbilicus appears.
- At this point provider assistance and fetal rotation will be needed for delivery of fetal legs and arms.
- If the fetal head becomes entrapped apply suprapubic pressure and insert fingers to draw the fetal chin to the fetal chest.

Amniotic Fluid Embolus

Results from release of amniotic fluid into maternal circulation, typically during labor but may be also seen following uterine trauma

Symptoms/Exam

- Sudden hypoxia and hypotension
- DIC may develop.

Diagnosis/Treatment

- A clinical diagnosis after consideration and evaluation for pulmonary embolism, sepsis, and anaphylaxis
- Treatment is supportive.

POSTPARTUM HEMORRHAGE

Postpartum hemorrhage is divided into early (<24 hours) and late (>24 hours) hemorrhage. Early postpartum hemorrhage can have brisk bleeding, and shock can develop rapidly. Maternal vital signs may remain normal while large volumes of blood accumulate in the uterus.

CAUSES

The causes of postpartum hemorrhage include:

- Uterine atony (most common)
- Uterine rupture
- Laceration of the lower genital tract
- Retained placenta
- Uterine inversion and coagulopathy
- Late hemorrhage can be due to infection, retained placenta (most common), uterine inversion, coagulopathy, or sloughing of the placental site eschar.

EXAM/DIAGNOSIS

- Physical exam is the cornerstone to the diagnosis.
- An enlarged and "boggy" uterus is seen with uterine atony.
- A vaginal mass is seen with uterine inversion.
- Vaginal bleeding despite good uterine tone and size is likely due to retained products.

TREATMENT

- Depends on suspected underlying cause.
- Treat uterine atony with oxytocin and vigorous bimanual massage.
- Stabilize with crystalloid fluids or packed RBCs if needed.
- Repair lacerations.

INFECTIONS IN PREGNANCY

Urinary Tract Infections

Asymptomatic bacteriuria can be seen in up to 10% of patients. *E. coli* is responsible for most infections.

TREATMENT

- Cystitis along with asymptomatic bacteriuria should be treated with antibiotics to prevent preterm labor/delivery.
- Cephalosporins and nitrofurantoin are recommended antibiotics.
- Floroquinolones and trimethoprim/sulfamethoxazole are contraindicated secondary to teratogenic effects.

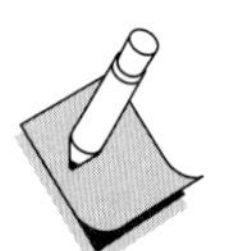

Appendicitis is the most common nonobstetrical surgical emergency in pregnancy.

Appendicitis

SYMPTOMS/EXAM

- The presentation of appendicitis during early pregnancy may be similar to that in the nonpregnant patient.
- Later in pregnancy, the enlarging uterus may shift the appendix into the right upper quadrant so the presenting complaint may be RUQ pain, although the most common presentation is still RLQ pain.

DIAGNOSIS

- Ultrasound is the imaging test of choice.

Postpartum Infections

ENDOMETRITIS

Polymicrobial postpartum infection of the endometrium

Risk factors include:

- Cesarean delivery (most important)
- Chorioamnionitis
- Duration of time since rupture of membranes
- Many vaginal exams during labor
- Presence of high-virulence organisms
- Use of an internal monitoring device

SYMPTOMS/EXAM

Fever, uterine tenderness, and foul-smelling lochia

TREATMENT

Hospitalization and IV antibiotics (ampicillin and gentimicin or cefotaxime, or zosyn).

SEPTIC PELVIC THROMBOPHLEBITIS

Develops from an infection of the placental site along with thrombosed myometrial veins. Incidence is increased after C-section. Treatment includes anticoagulation and antibiotics.

MEDICATIONS DURING PREGNANCY

See Tables 12.3 and 12.4.

EMERGENCY CONTRACEPTION

Emergency contraception refers to contraceptive measures taken after sex to prevent a pregnancy. In the United States, two medical options are available for patients who want to prevent implantation or terminate an early pregnancy.

- **Plan B** (ie, the morning-after pill): A progestin-only treatment usually consisting of levonorgesterol 1.5 mg PO × 1, or divide into 750 μg taken 12 hours apart
  - Most effective when taken in the first 72 hours after sex
  - Reduces likelihood of pregnancy from about 8% to 1%
  - Causes nausea and vaginal bleeding

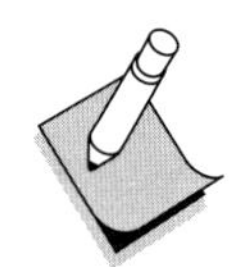

Avoid live vaccines during pregnancy.

TABLE 12.3. Vaccines and Medications Contraindicated During Pregnancy

Vaccines (any live vaccines)	MMR Live, attenuated influenza vaccine Varicella TDaP
Antibiotics	Tetracyclines Floroquinolones Sulfonamides Chloramphenicol
Antiepileptic drugs	Phenytoin Valproic acid Phenobarbital
Other	Oral hypoglycemics Warfarin

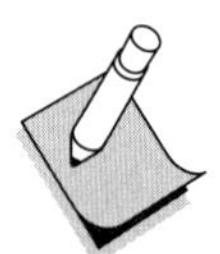

Adenosine is the drug of choice in pregnant patients with SVT. Avoid electricity if possible because of potential harm to the fetus.

TABLE 12.4. Vaccines and Medications Considered Safe During Pregnancy

Vaccines	TD (okay after first trimester) Influenza (inactivated) Pneumococcal
Antimicrobials	Penicillin Cephalosporins Azithromycin Nitrofurantoin INH Rifampin Nystatin Clotrimazole
Analgesics	Acetaminophen
Antidysrhythmics	Digoxin Adenosine
β-Adrenergics	Albuterol
GI agents	Promethazine Prochlorperazine Metoclopramide Ondansetron Cimetidine Ranitidine Tums
Antihistamines	Benadryl

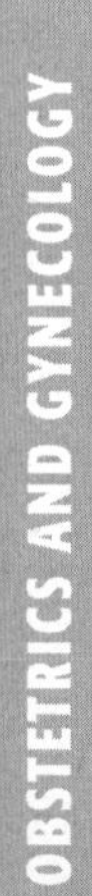

- **RU-486 (mifepristone):** A steroid that blocks progesterone receptors
  - A 10-mg dose is as effective as 1.5 mg of levonorgesterol in preventing implantation (first 72 hours).
  - A dose of 600 mg may be used as an abortifacient (approved for up to 49 days gestation in the United States).
  - Side effects include cramping and vaginal bleeding.
  - When used as an abortifacient, approximately 5% of patients will require surgical intervention for retained products.

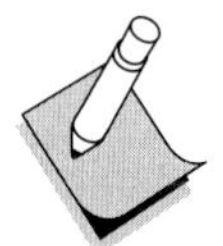

Clue cells = epithelial cells coated by bacteria = bacterial vaginosis = metronidazole or clindamycin if pregnant.

BACTERIAL VAGINOSIS

The most common cause of abnormal vaginal discharge. BV is secondary to high concentrations of anaerobic bacteria and *Gardnerella vaginalis* replacing the normal lactobacilli flora. It is seen in sexually active women.

Symptoms/Exam

- "Fishy smelling" vaginal discharge
- Itching
- Increased discharge

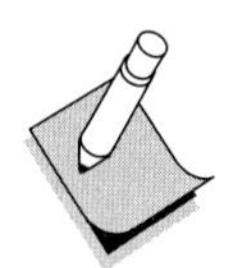

When prescribing metronidazole, warn patients about the disulfiram-like reaction when coingested with alcohol.

Differential

- Candida vaginitis
- Trichomoniasis
- Pelvic inflammatory disease

Diagnosis

- Physical exam shows a malodorous gray/white discharge.
- Wet mount shows clue cells (see Figure 12.4).
- Addition of KOH to a smear of the discharge reveals same fish smell, referred to as a "positive whiff test."

Treatment

- Metronidazole 500 mg PO BID × 7 days or a single 2-g dose
- Clindamycin is a reasonable alternative.

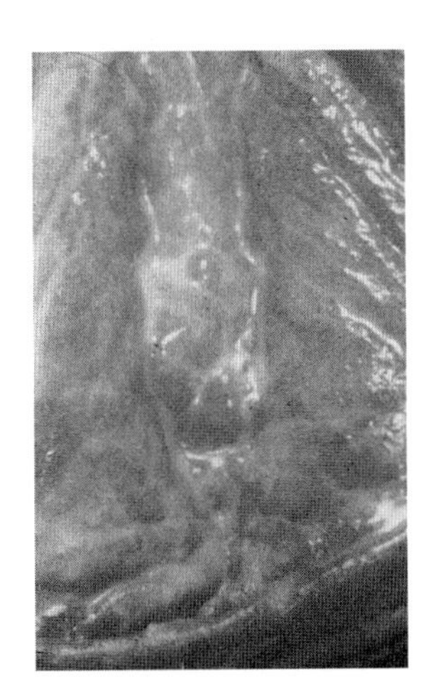

FIGURE 12.4. Clue cells in patient with bacterial vaginosis.

(Reproduced, with permission, from Kasper DL et al (eds). *Harrison's Principles of Internal Medicine*, 16th ed. New York: McGraw-Hill, 2005:767.)

CANDIDA VULVOVAGINITIS

Causes

This is caused by *Candida albicans*, which have filamentous forms that penetrate the mucosal surface, causing inflammation and lysis of tissue. Risk factors include DM, HIV, recent antibiotic use, and pregnancy (see Table 12.5).

Symptoms/Exam

- White "cottage cheese" vaginal discharge
- Red/swollen vaginal mucosa and labia
- Itching is a significant complaint along with dysuria and dyspareunia.

Differential

Bacterial vaginosis, trichomoniasis, pelvic inflammatory disease

TABLE 12.5. Vaginal Discharge

DISCHARGE	NORMAL	CANDIDIASIS	TRICHOMONIASIS	BACTERIAL VAGINOSIS
Color	Clear/white	White	Green/yellow	Gray/white
pH	<4.5	<4.5	>5.0	>4.5
Amine odor with KOH	Negative	Negative	Positive	Positive
Wet mount	Epithelial cells, lactobacilli	WBC, spores, pseudohyphae	WBC, motile trichomonads	Few WBC, clue cells

DIAGNOSIS

- Usually, visualization of the vagina allows a clinical diagnosis.
- Confirm diagnosis based on the presence of pseudohyphae and spores ("spaghetti and meatballs") on wet mount exam with a 10% KOH prep.

TREATMENT

Oral or intavaginal antifungals:

- Clotrimazole 1% cream or miconazole 2% cream topically for 3–7 days
- Fluconazole 150 mg PO × one dose

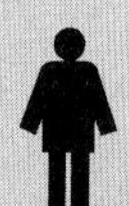

A 50-year-old female presents to the ED with the third visit in 2 months for candida vulvovaginitis that seems resistant to treatment. What do you want to check?

Accucheck to rule out underlying diabetes.

TRICHOMONIASIS

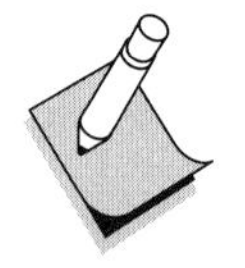

Trichomoniasis is almost always an STD!

Caused by *Trichonomas vaginalis*, a flagellated protozoan.

SYMPTOMS/EXAM

- Vaginal discharge, perineal itching, dysuria, spotting, and pelvic pain
- Physical exam shows vaginal erythema and a frothy malodorous discharge.
- Trichomoniasis is associated with premature rupture of membranes, preterm delivery, and postpartum endometritis.

DIFFERENTIAL

Bacterial vaginosis, candida vaginitis, pelvic inflammatory disease

DIAGNOSIS

The presence of motile, pear-shaped, flagellated trichomonads on wet mount (see Figure 12.5).

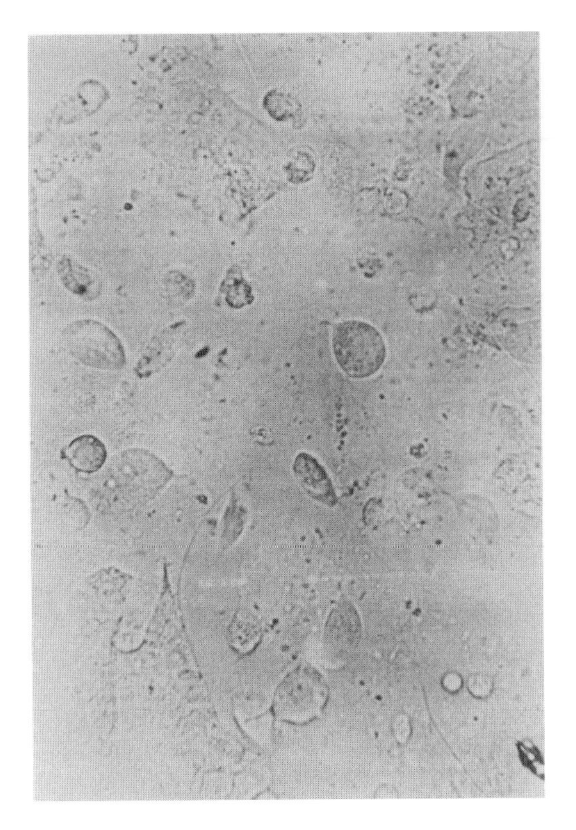

FIGURE 12.5. Trichomonads under high-power view.

(Reproduced, with permission, from Tintinalli JE, Kelen GD, Stapczynski JS. *Emergency Medicine: A Comprehensive Study Guide*, 6th ed. New York: McGraw-Hill, 2004:694.)

TREATMENT

- Metronidazole 2 g PO × one dose or 500 mg PO BID × 7 days
- Partners should also be treated.

HERPES SIMPLEX VIRUS (HSV)

SYMPTOMS/EXAM

- Painful, fluid-filled vesicles that progress to shallow-based ulcers
- Dysuria and pelvic pain may occur.
- May also see systemic symptoms of fever, malaise, headache, and myalgias

DIAGNOSIS

Genital herpes is diagnosed based on clinical examination. If necessary, confirm with culture or PCR of fluid obtained from vesicle.

TREATMENT

- Treat with antiviral agents, usually acyclovir or famcyclovir, within one day of symptom onset.
- Treatment shortens duration of symptoms but is not curative and does not affect the frequency or severity of recurrences.

CERVICITIS

- Inflammation/infection of the cervix
- Most common infectious causes are chlamydia and gonorrhea; however, herpes simplex and trichomoniasis can also cause cervicitis.
- Infectious cervicitis is usually associated with vaginitis.

SYMPTOMS/EXAM

- Vaginal discharge is the primary symptom.
- A red, inflamed, and congested cervix may be seen on exam.
- In trichomonal infection, a "strawberry" cervix can be seen.

DIFFERENTIAL

- Noninfectious cervicitis due to increased mucous discharge at ovulation
- Infectious cervicitis
- Early neoplastic process

DIAGNOSIS

Physical exam and wet mount can help identify the cause of acute cervicitis.

TREATMENT

Unless a specific etiology is identified, outpatient treatment of **both** chlamydia and gonorrhea is recommended.

- Ceftriaxone (125–250 mg IM) **and**
- Doxycycline (100 mg PO bid × 7 days) or azithromycin (1 g single PO dose)

PELVIC INFLAMMATORY DISEASE

CAUSES

PID is an ascending infection from the lower genital tract that makes up a spectrum of disease that ranges from endometritis to salpingitis and tuboovarian abscess (TOA). *Neisseria gonorrhoeae* and *Chlamydia trachomatis* are the most common causes. Simultaneous infection occurs.

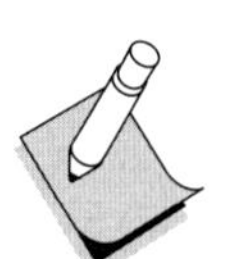

Chandelier sign = severe cervical motion tenderness seen with PID.

Risks factors for PID include multiple sexual partners, history of sexually transmitted diseases, young age, and use of an IUD.

SYMPTOMS

- Most common presenting complaint is lower abdominal pain.
- Often associated with abnormal vaginal discharge, vaginal bleeding, postcoital bleeding, dyspareunia, fever, malaise, and nausea and vomiting.
- Symptom onset is usually 2–5 days after menstruation.

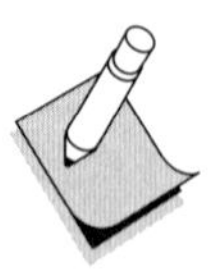

Use transvaginal ultrasound to rule out TOA in patients with PID and unilateral pelvic tenderness.

EXAM

- Lower abdominal tenderness
- Mucopurulent cervicitis
- Cervical motion tenderness
- Bilateral adnexal tenderness
- Unilateral adnexal tenderness or unilateral mass suggest TOA.

TABLE 12.6. Criteria for the Diagnosis of PID

Major criteria needed for PID diagnosis
Lower abdominal pain
Lower abdominal tenderness
CMT
Adnexal tenderness
Additional criteria that increase the specificity of the diagnosis
Fever > 38°C
Abnormal vaginal discharge
+culture for gonorrhea or chlamydia
WBC > 10,000
Elevated CRP or ESR

DIAGNOSIS

See Table 12.6.

Transvaginal ultrasound can be used to evaluate for TOA.

TREATMENT

- Treatment of PID focuses on prompt antibiotic treatment of both N. *gonorrhoeae* and C. *trachomatis*.
- Hospitalization is indicated in pregnant women, immunosuppression, documented or suspected pelvic abscess, IUD, severe vomiting, or failed outpatient management.
- All patients should be referred for HIV and syphilis testing.
- Treatment of sexual partners is needed.

Outpatient treatment:

1. Ceftriaxone 250 mg IM **plus** doxycycline 100 mg PO BID × 14 days

Inpatient treatment:

1. Cefotetan **or** cefoxitin **plus** doxycycline
2. Clindamycin **plus** gentamycin

COMPLICATIONS

- **Fitz-Hugh-Curtis syndrome**.
- Long-term consequences include infertility, ectopic pregnancy, and chronic pain.

FITZ-HUGH-CURTIS SYNDROME

An ascending pelvic infection with chlamydia (most common) or gonorrhea which results in inflammation of the liver capsule or diaphragm.

SYMPTOMS/EXAM

- Presents with RUQ pain that **may mimic cholecystitis**
- May present with referred pain to the right shoulder
- May or may not be associated with symptoms of PID

DIAGNOSIS

- Definitive diagnosis requires direct visualization of the liver capsule via laparoscopy.
- RUQ ultrasound, CT abdomen, and CXR may be used to exclude other causes of RUQ pain. CT abdomen may show a perihepatic fluid collection.
- The combination of RUQ pain, fever and/or elevated markers of infection (WBC, ESR), positive cervical cultures for chlamydia or gonorrhea, and the absence of other cause of RUQ pain (pneumonia, cholecystitis, pyelonephritis, hepatitis) allows a presumptive diagnosis of FHC syndrome.

TREATMENT

- Treatment is the same as for PID.
- Outpatient treatment is acceptable for well-appearing patients who can tolerate PO and are not pregnant.
- Discharge instructions should recommend use of condoms, treatment of partners, and further testing for HIV and syphilis.

LYMPHOGRANULOMA VENEREUM

A sexually transmitted infection caused by an aggressive L serotype of *C. trachomatis*. It is rare in the United States, but endemic in parts of Africa, Southeast Asia, South America, and the Caribbean.

SYMPTOMS/EXAM

- Inguinal, vulvar, and rectal ulceration
- Inguinal lymphadenopathy and lymphedema
- Anorectal lymphedema occurs early and leads to anal stricture.

DIFFERENTIAL

Disseminated TB, early syphilis, chancroid

DIAGNOSIS

Isolation of *C. trachomatis* from specimens confirms the diagnosis. A positive complement fixation test also aids the diagnosis.

TREATMENT

- Doxycycline 100 mg BID for 21 days **or**
- Erythromycin 500 mg QID for 21 days
- Anal strictures may need dilation or surgical management.

CHANCROID

This is a sexually transmitted disease characterized by a painful genital ulcer. The causative organism is *Haemophilus ducreyi*. It occurs more frequently in Asia and Africa but is also endemic to certain parts of the United States.

SYMPTOMS/EXAM

- Suppurative inguinal adenopathy with painful ulcers is pathognomonic.
- The early chancroid lesion is a vesicopustule on the perineum, vagina, or cervix that ulcerates and produces a heavy foul discharge that is contagious.

DIFFERENTIAL

Syphilis must be ruled out.

DIAGNOSIS

Clinical diagnosis is necessary because smears and cultures are not reliable in isolating the organism.

TREATMENT

- Azithromycin 1 g PO × 1 dose **or**
- Ceftriaxone 250 mg IM × 1 dose **or**
- Ciprofloxicin 500 mg PO BID × 3 days

SYPHILIS

Syphilis is caused by *Treponema pallidum* and is transmitted by direct contact with an infectious moist lesion.

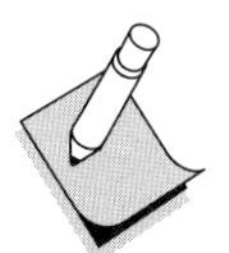

The three human diseases caused by spirochetes are treated similarly:
Syphilis → penicillin or doxycycline.
Lyme disease → doxycycline or amoxicillin.
Leptospirosis → doxycycline or amoxicillin.

SYMPTOMS/EXAM

- *Primary syphilis:* This painless genital sore (chancre) is a firm, papule or ulcer with a raised border. It occurs on the labia, vulva, vagina, cervix, or anus. Painless, rubbery regional, and then general lymphadenopathy follows. Serologic tests are positive 70% of the time.
- *Secondary syphilis:* This systemic infection becomes evident with diffuse lymphadenopathy, a "viral syndrome," and a bilateral, symmetric rash appears that is papulosquamous and involves the palms and soles. Moist papules (condyloma lata) are seen in the perineum. Serologic tests are almost always positive.
- *Tertiary syphilis:* This stage is characterized by "gummas," soft, tumorlike growths seen in the skin and mucous membranes. Other characteristics of untreated syphilis include Charcot joints (a degeneration of joint surfaces resulting from loss of proprioception), and Clutton joints (bilateral knee effusions). The more severe manifestations include neurosyphilis and cardiovascular syphilis.

DIAGNOSIS

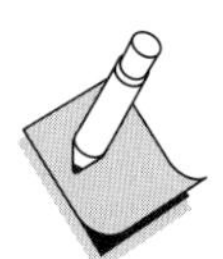

VDRL false-positives may occur with HIV, malaria, Lyme disease, and lupus.

- Diagnosis depends on a series of tests with definitive diagnosis being made only by direct visualization of spirochetes from cutaneous lesions using darkfield microscopy.
- VDRL is a nontreponemal test that will become positive 3–6 weeks after infection. The VDRL test is only about 80% sensitive in primary syphilis but 100% sensitive in secondary syphilis.
- VDRL may be used to exclude the disease in patients with a rash possibly consistent with secondary syphilis.
- The florescent treponemal antibody absorption (FTA-ABS) test and microhemagglutination assay for *T. pallidum* (MHA-TP) detect antibodies to *Treponema spirochetes.*

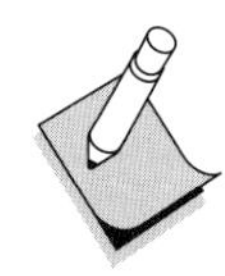

Because of its high sensitivity in patients with 2° syphilis, VDRL is the test of choice to exclude syphilis in patients presenting with a rash.

TREATMENT

- Treat primary, secondary, and early latent syphilis with Benzathine penicillin G, 2.4 million units IM × one dose.
- Late syphilis should be treated with Benzathine penicillin G 2.4 million units IM weekly × 3 consecutive weeks.
- The initial treatment of neurosyphilis requires intravenous penicillin every 4 hours.

OVARIAN TORSION

Most cases result from a mass or large cyst on an ovary or fallopian tube that stretches the pedicle and causes a rotation on its axis leading to decreased blood flow. This can occur at any age.

SYMPTOMS/EXAM

- Recurrent intermittent attacks of colicky pain with nausea, vomiting, and low-grade fever
- The abdominal pain can also be sharp and have peritoneal signs.
- Pelvic exam usually reveals adnexal fullness and tenderness.

DIFFERENTIAL

- Appendicitis
- Ruptured ovarian cyst
- Ovarian tumor
- Renal stone
- Ectopic pregnancy

DIAGNOSIS

Transvaginal ultrasound to look for ovarian cyst/mass and color flow Doppler to assess ovarian blood flow; test for pregnancy

TREATMENT

Laparoscopy or laparotomy is indicated. Failure to surgically correct the torsion can result in ischemia and necrosis of the involved ovary.

AMENORRHEA

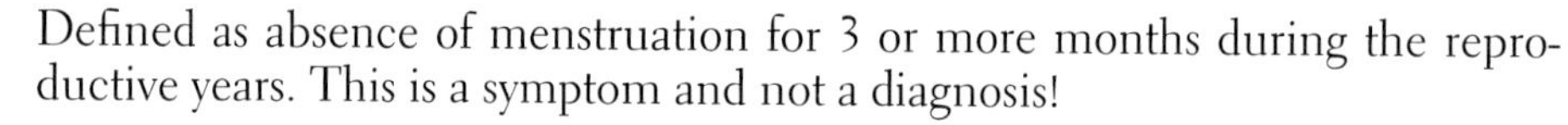

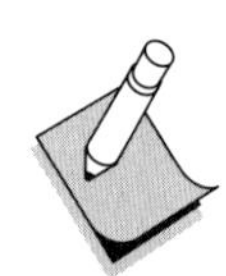

Rule out pregnancy as a cause of amenorrhea.

Defined as absence of menstruation for 3 or more months during the reproductive years. This is a symptom and not a diagnosis!

- 1° amenorrhea: Failure of menses by age 16 or within 2 years of full secondary sexual characteristic development; see Table 12.7
- 2° amenorrhea: Lack of menses for >3 months in a woman who previously had normal menstruation; mostly caused by ovarian dysfunction or ovarian failure; ovarian dysfunction (polycystic ovaries [PCOS]) due to increased androgen from the ovaries or adrenal glands that converts to excess estrogen in adipose tissue

SYMPTOMS/EXAM

- Symptoms of decreased estrogen include hot flashes, night sweats, and dyspareunia.
- Increased androgens can manifest with acne, decreased breast size, hirsutism, voice deepening, balding, and increased muscle mass.

DIAGNOSIS

Careful history and physical will help determine which organ is primarily responsible for amenorrhea. Check levels of TSH, LH, FSH, prolactin, and estradiol.

TABLE 12.7. **Causes of Primary Amenorrhea with Normal Genital Exam**

	Uterus Present	Uterus Absent
Breast development present	Hypothalamic Pituitary Ovarian Uterine	Congenital (uterovaginal agenesis) Androgen insensitivity (testicular feminization)
Breast development absent	Gonadal failure CNS (hypothalamic, pituitary disorders)	17,20-Desmolase deficiency Agonadism 17-Hydroxylase deficiency (46,XY)

Treatment

Management of the amenorrheic patient depends on the individual's desire to ovulate and the etiology of the amenorrhea.

BARTHOLIN ABSCESS

- Bartholin glands are located bilaterally at the posterior introitus and drain through ducts into the vestibule at approximately the 4 o'clock and 8 o'clock positions.
- Normally pea-sized glands are palpable if the duct becomes cystic or a gland abscess develops.
- Obstruction of the duct results in retention of the secretions and cystic dilation.

Symptoms/Exam

- Pain, tenderness, and dyspareunia are acute symptoms.
- Surrounding tissue becomes edematous and inflamed.
- A tender, fluctuant mass is usually palpable.

Treatment

- Primary treatment consists of drainage of the infected cyst/abscess followed by insertion of a word catheter or marsupialization.
- The word catheter is a small inflatable bulb-tipped catheter that allows for drainage.
- Incision and drainage alone without use of the word catheter to keep the wound open is associated with recurrent disease.
- Broad-spectrum antibiotic therapy is warranted only when cellulitis is present.

VAGINAL BLEEDING

Gynecologic causes of abnormal vaginal bleeding in nonpregnant, reproductive age females include: (1) ovulatory bleeding, (2) anovulatory bleeding, or (3) nonuterine bleeding. (See Table 12.8.)

SYMPTOMS/EXAM

- Ovulatory bleeding is associated with menses and preceded by breast tenderness, abdominal bloating, and dysmenorrhea.
- Anovulatory bleeding is seen mostly in perimenarchal or perimenopausal women. In adolescents physical exam is usually normal. If blood loss is considerable or lasting >9 days check coagulation studies. In perimenopausal women, atrophic vaginitis is a common cause.
- Nonuterine bleeding is vaginal bleeding. Bleeding from nose or gums suggests systemic etiology. **Vaginal laccrations** occur following penile or foreign body penetration and typically require suturing.

DIFFERENTIAL

- Ovulatory bleeding is due to pelvic diseases (PID, endometriosis, ovarian neoplasm) or uterine causes (leiomyomas, polyps, endometrial malignancy, or hyperplasia).
- Anovulatory bleeding in adolescents is mostly due to immature hypothalamic-pituitary-ovarian axis; in reproductive age, is usually due to fluctuating levels or estrogen that go below a critical level needed to maintain the endometrium. In menopausal patients, malignancy needs to be ruled out with an endometrial biopsy.
- Nonuterine bleeding can be from cervix or vagina. Consider also lower urinary tract or GI bleeding.

TABLE 12.8. Definitions of Vaginal Bleeding

Abnormal vaginal bleeding	Occurs outside menstrual cycle
Menorrhagia	Menses > 7 days, *or* > 60-mL blood loss *or* occurring < every 21 days
Metrorrhagia	Bleeding at irregular times
Menometrorrhagia	Heavy irregular vaginal bleeding
Dysfunctional uterine bleeding	Abnormal vaginal bleeding due to anovulation
Postcoital bleeding	Vaginal bleeding after intercourse suggesting cervical pathology
Postmenopausal bleeding	Any bleeding that occurs > 6 months after cessation of menses

Diagnosis

- Pregnancy test and CBC are needed in most cases of vaginal bleeding.
- Vaginal ultrasound can be useful to characterize the uterus and endometrium and determine the presence of leiomyomas (fibroids), tumors, and endometriosis. In stable patients, ultrasound may be deferred to the outpatient setting.
- Gynecology referral for endometrial biopsy should be obtained for women over the age of 35 with abnormal uterine bleeding and for women <35 with risk factors for endometrial cancer (obesity, chronic anovulation).

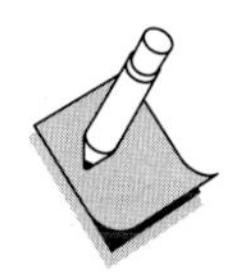

All patients of childbearing age with vaginal bleeding need a pregnancy test.

Treatment

- Treatment depends upon hemodynamic stability.
- If unstable, fluid resuscitation and blood are indicated along with emergent D&C. Intravenous conjugated estrogen 25 mg IV q 2–4 hours may be used in nonpregnant patients with bleeding not amenable to surgical intervention.
- If stable, hormonal treatment can help stabilize the endometrium.
  - Oral conjugated estrogen (Premarin) 2.5 mg PO qid for 1 day, then add medroxyprogesterone and continue both meds for 7–10 days.
  - A 7-day course of ethinyl estradiol and norethindrone may also be used.

ENDOMETRIOSIS

Disease is defined by the presence of endometrial glands/stroma outside of the uterus and seen exclusively in women of reproductive age. The size of the lesions vary from microscopic to large invasive masses that erode into underlying organs and cause extensive adhesions.

Symptoms

- Infertility
- Dysmenorrhea
- Dyspareunia
- Pelvic pain or low sacral pain that occurs premenstrually and resolves after the onset of menses is common.

Exam

Pelvic exam will show tender nodules in the posterior vaginal fornix and pain with movements of the uterus.

Diagnosis

- The diagnosis should be suspected in any woman of reproductive age complaining of pain or infertility.
- Confirmation requires direct visualization of the implants with laparoscopy or laparotomy.

Treatment

- Treatment is directed based on the woman's desire for future fertility.
- NSAIDs are the analgesic therapy of choice.
- Hormonal therapy is used to interrupt the cycles of stimulation and bleeding of endometrial tissue.

- Oral contraceptive pills and progestational agents like oral medroxyprogesterone acetate and danazol are used if fertility is not wanted.
- Surgical treatment is indicated in women with infertility or with severe disease or adhesions.

MASTITIS

Mastitis is cellulitis of breast tissue. It is most commonly due to S. *aureus*, coag-negative *Staphylococcus*, or viridans streptococci. The source of the bacteria is usually the feeding infant's nose or throat. Typically the colonized infant is asymptomatic, but localized skin and systemic infections occur.

SYMPTOMS/EXAM

Presents with erythema, edema, tenderness, malaise, and often fever

DIFFERENTIAL

- Breast abscess: Can be confirmed by ultrasound, requires incision and drainage
- Inflammatory breast cancer: Skin often has classic orange-peel appearance in addition to warmth, tenderness, and redness; confirmed by biopsy.

DIAGNOSIS

The physical exam is key for the diagnosis. If concern for an abscess exists, a breast ultrasound or needle aspiration can be helpful.

TREATMENT

- Warm compresses or frequent hot baths
- Antistaphylococcal antibiotics (dicloxacillin 250 mg or cephalexin 500 mg PO QID × 7 days)
- With puerperal mastitis, breast feeding should be continued and treatment is the same as listed above except for recommending frequent breast emptying.
- Needle aspiration of a breast abscess is thought to have little risk of spreading cancer (if present) and may be performed by an emergency physician.
- **Surgical consultation** or referral is appropriate for patients requiring **open drainage** of a breast abscess.

CHAPTER 13

Environmental Emergencies

Mashal Ahmadi, MD

BITES AND STINGS

A 31-year-old male presents to the ED for evaluation of hand pain after an altercation outside a bar. On examination there is pain, swelling, and a laceration present at the fifth metacarpal joint. The extensor tendon sheath is visible through the wound. What is the risk if this injury is left untreated?

This patient has sustained a "fight bite" or closed-fist injury from striking a person's tooth with a closed fist. If left untreated, tenosynovitis, osteomyelitis, and septic arthritis can occur, requiring surgical intervention.

Mammalian Bites

The vast majority of mammalian bite wounds seen in the ED are due to domesticated animals. Infecting organisms vary with species (see Table 13.1).

Wounds With Increased Risk of Infection (High-Risk Wounds):

- Puncture wounds
- Intraoral, hand, below knee, or joint area bites
- Cat bites > human bites > dog bites
- Immunocompromised (eg, asplenic, alcoholic) or elderly patient
- Presence of peripheral vascular disease or prosthetic valve
- Delayed presentations

TABLE 13.1. Common Infecting Organisms in Mammalian Bites

Cat	*Pasteurella multocida* *Staphylococcus aureus*
Dog	*S. aureus* *P. multocida* *Bacteroides* sp. *Fusobacterium* sp. *Capnocytophaga canimorsus*
Human	Polymicrobial Viridans streptococcus *Staphylococcus* *Bacteroides* sp. *Corynebacterium* sp. *Eikenella corrodens*
Rodent	*Streptobacillus moniliformis* *Spirillum minus* Other transmitted diseases: Leptospirosis Tularemia Sporotrichosis Plague

DIAGNOSIS

- X-ray to rule out foreign body or fracture
- Check blood sugar to see if diabetic.

GENERAL TREATMENT

- Anesthetize, clean and irrigate, debride devitalized tissue.
- Explore in full flexion and extension for ligamentous or tendon injury.
  - If present, surgical consultation and admission is warranted.
- Tetanus prophylaxis
- Consider rabies prophylaxis (animal bites).
- No evidence for infection:
  - Okay to close wound **unless** high-risk wound
  - Give antibiotic prophylaxis if high-risk wound (see Table 13.2).
- Evidence for infection:
  - Admit for IV antibiotics if high-risk wound or patient, otherwise treat with oral antibiotics.
- Arrange follow-up in 48 hours for discharged patients.

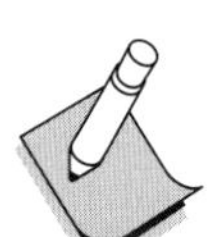

All wounds at high risk for infection should be left open and treated with antibiotic prophylaxis.

HUMAN BITES

Infections are commonly **polymicrobial**:

- Viridans streptococcus
- *Staphylococcus*
- *Bacteroides* sp.
- *Corynebacterium* sp.
- ***E. corrodens*** (a Gram-negative rod found in dental plaque)
- Other transmitted infections include syphilis, herpes
- HIV and hepatitis transmission should be considered if exposure to blood occurred.

A special concern is the closed-fist injury which is associated with joint infection, osteomyelitis, and tenosynovitis.

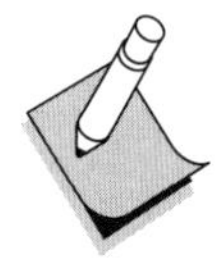

Most human bite wound infections are polymicrobial, including Gram-positive, Gram-negative, and anaerobic organisms.

TREATMENT

- General treatment, as above
- Antibiotic of choice for prophylaxis = amoxicillin/clavulanate.

TABLE 13.2. Indication for Prophylactic Antibiotics in Mammalian Bites

Cat bites
Immunocompromised or elderly patients
Presence of peripheral vascular disease
Presence of prosthetic valve
Deep puncture wounds
Intraoral, hand, below knee, or joint wounds
Delayed presentation

- Closed-fist injury requires aggressive irrigation and wound exploration. If there is evidence for deeper structure involvement, surgical consult and admission are indicated.
- Consider HIV, hepatitis B prophylaxis.

CAT BITES

The majority of untreated cat bites become infected.

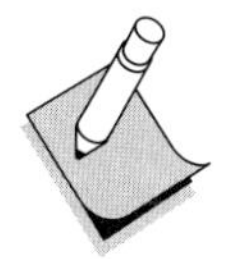

Rapid onset of infection <24 hours after a cat bite = P. multocida.

Common organisms:

- ***P. multocida***
  - A highly virulent Gram-negative anaerobic rod → infection develops within 24 hours.
- The other common organism is *S. aureus*.

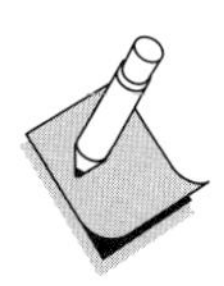

All cat bite wounds should receive antibiotic prophylaxis.

TREATMENT

- General treatment, as above
- Most wounds are puncture wounds and should be left open.
- Antibiotic prophylaxis is recommended for *all* cat bite wounds: amoxicillin/clavulanate, cefuroxime.
- *P. multocida* is highly sensitive to penicillin.

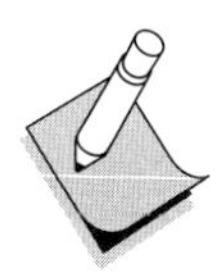

Gangrenous wound or overwhelming sepsis following dog bite = C. canimorsus.

DOG BITES

Approximately 5% of dog bites become infected.

Common organisms:

- *S. aureus*
- *P. multocida*
- *Bacteroides* sp.
- *Fusobacterium* sp.
- ***C. canimorsus***
  - Gram-negative rod → overwhelming sepsis, DIC, and cutaneous gangrene at bite site.

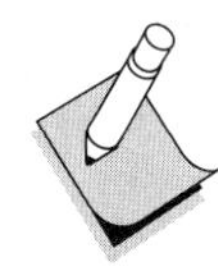

Antibiotic prophylaxis of choice for bite wounds = amoxicillin/clavulanate.

TREATMENT

- General treatment, as above
- Antibiotic prophylaxis of choice: amoxicillin/clavulanate

RODENT BITES

Rat-bite fever

- Results from infection with *S. moniliformis* and *S. minus*

SYMPTOMS/EXAM

- Abrupt onset of fevers/chills, headache, and subsequent rash
- Associated with brain, myocardial, and soft-tissue abscesses

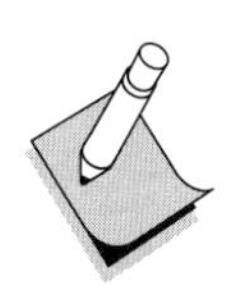

Rat-bite fever is associated with brain, myocardial, and soft-tissue abscesses.

Multiple other diseases can be transmitted via rodent bites including leptospirosis, tularemia, sporotrichosis, plague.

A 10-year-old boy is brought to the ED by his parents with c/o severe abdominal back and leg muscle cramping after being "bit by a spider" two hours earlier while playing outdoors. On examination, he appears anxious, sweaty, and is mildly hypertensive. What is the most definitive treatment for this patient?

This patient has likely been bitten by a black widow spider. Black widow spider venom is a neurotoxin that causes release of acetylcholine and norepinephrine at nerve terminals. All cases should be treated with opioid analgesia and benzodiazepines to control symptoms. Definitive treatment in this case, given the patient's age < 16 years (which increases the likelihood of severe toxicity) is the administration of black widow spider antivenom.

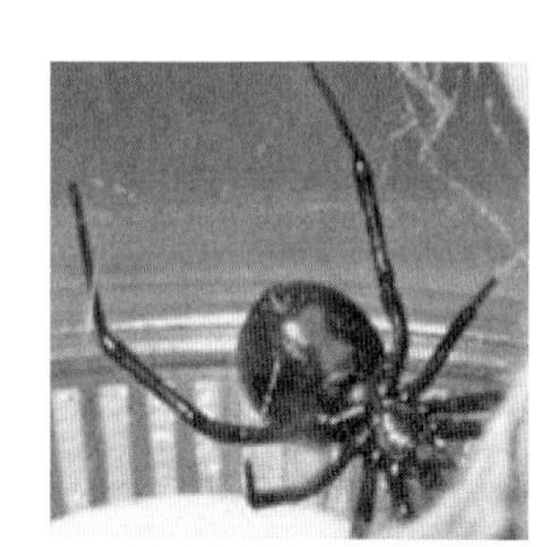

FIGURE 13.1. Black widow spider. (See also color insert.)

(Courtesy of Fred Severyn, MD.)

Spider Bites

BLACK WIDOW SPIDER (*LATRODECTUS* SP.)

The black widow spider can be found throughout the United States (except Alaska) in woodpiles, sheds, barns, and outhouses. It is classically identified by a yellow-red hourglass shape on its belly (see Figure 13.1). The venom is a neurotoxin.

MECHANISM OF TOXICITY

- Envenomation → release of acetylcholine and norepinephrine at nerve terminals → muscle cramping and systemic effects.

SYMPTOMS/EXAM

- Bite site: Target lesion with local redness and pain. Sometimes bite site cannot be seen.
- Prominent muscle cramping and pain most notably of abdominal, back, and leg muscles, starting locally and then progressing diffusely
- Tachycardia, hypertension
- Diaphoresis
- Nausea/vomiting
- Symptoms may wax and wane, but generally disappear over 2–3 days.

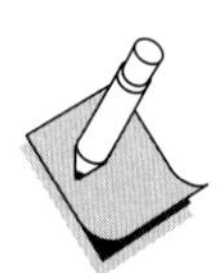

Black widow spider envenomation → severe cramping of abdominal, back, and leg muscles.

TREATMENT

- Local wound care
- Tetanus prophylaxis
- **Symptomatic treatment** is the mainstay of therapy.
  - **Opioid analgesia**
  - **Benzodiazepines** to reduce muscle spasm
  - Calcium gluconate intravenous (controversial—no proven benefit)
  - Antihypertensives as needed
- **Black widow antivenom**
  - If severe symptoms or high-risk patient (see Table 13.3)
  - A horse serum antivenom, therefore administer a test dose first

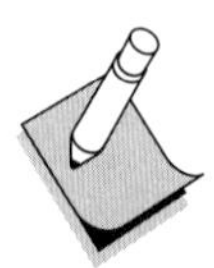

Symptomatic treatment with opioids and benzodiazepines is the mainstay of therapy.

TABLE 13.3. Indications for Antivenom in Black Widow Spider Bite

Indications
Age: <16 yr or >65 yr
Severe pain despite symptomatic treatment
Severe envenomation (seizures, uncontrolled HTN, respiratory failure)
Severe comorbidities (HTN, atherosclerotic disease)
Pregnancy

BROWN RECLUSE SPIDER (*LOXOSCELES RECLUSA*)

The brown recluse spider is identified by the brown violin shape on its cephalothorax ("**fiddleback**")(see Figure 13.2). It is found primarily in the southern midwestern United States under rocks, woodpiles, and in attics.

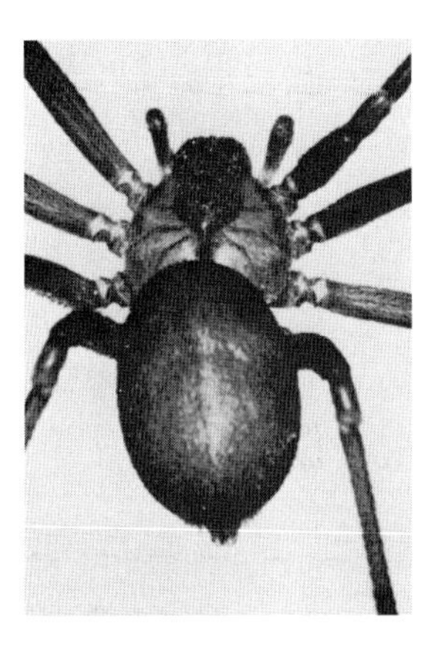

FIGURE 13.2. Brown recluse spider.

(Reproduced, with permission, from Dillaha CJ, Jansen GT, et al: North American loxocelism. *JAMA* 188:33, 1964. Copyright © 1964 American Medical Association. All rights reserved.)

MECHANISM OF TOXICITY

- Venom contains a variety of cytotoxic enzymes → local **necrotic wound** and (rarely) systemic toxicity.

SYMPTOMS/EXAM

- The initial bite is **painless** and causes a localized red lesion that usually heals.
- If severe:
  - A target lesion or pustule forms.
  - Bulla and necrotic tissue develop over 3–4 days → eschar formation.
  - Systemic effects (in 24–72 hours) with fevers, chills, nausea/vomiting
  - Hemolysis, seizures, renal failure, DIC are possible.

TREATMENT

- Supportive therapy as needed
- Local wound care and tetanus prophylaxis
- An antivenom is **not** available in the United States.
- Nitroglycerin, phentolamine, heparin, hyperbaric O_2, cyproheptadine, and steroids have all been used but show no clear evidence for efficacy.
- **Dapsone** is still recommended in some texts, but has limited benefit and is associated with hemolysis (in G6PD) and methemoglobinemia.
- **Delayed** (**not early**) excision, debridement, and possible skin grafting

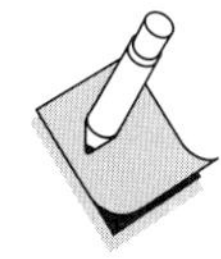

Brown recluse spider bite wounds should undergo delayed excision and debridement.

Hymenoptera Stings

The class hymenoptera include the following stinging insects:

- Bees
- Wasps
- Fire ants

Bees

- Barbed stingers → stinger remains in victim (one sting/bee).
- The process kills the bee.
- Killer bees have similar toxin potency but attack in large numbers → greater overall venom load.
- Venom contains proteins and enzymes (histamine, bradykinin, etc.).

Wasps

- Nonbarbed stinger → can sting multiple times.
- Similar venom to bees

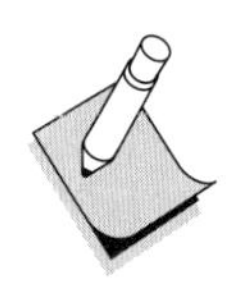

Three possible reactions to hymenoptera envenomation:

- *Local toxic reaction*
- *Allergic reaction*
- *Serum sickness*

Fire ants

- Small and light reddish-brown to brown
- Contain unique alkaloid venom

In general, three types of reactions are possible:

- **Local toxic reaction**
- **Allergic reaction**
- **Serum sickness**

MECHANISM OF TOXICITY

- Local reaction to venom
- Exposure to venom in sensitized individual → mast cell degranulation → allergic reaction.
  - Each species has unique antigens.
- Development of delayed (type III) immune response → systemic symptoms and rash (serum sickness).

SYMPTOMS/EXAM

- Local reaction
  - Bees and wasps: Irritation, itching, and redness at sting site that may last for 2–3 days
  - Fire ants: Intense burning, papules that may turn to sterile pustules in 24 hours
- Allergic reaction
  - Ranging from diffuse pruritus and urticaria to anaphylaxis
  - Vast majority occur within 30 minutes
- Serum sickness
  - Onset of symptoms 7–10 days after the sting
  - Fever, arthralgias, and malaise (flulike symptoms)
  - Rash (most commonly angioedema/urticaria)

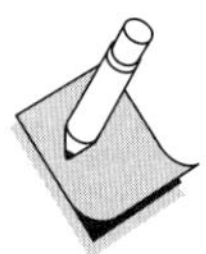

Serum sickness is a delayed immune response occurring 7–10 days after antigen exposure.

TREATMENT

- Local wound care and tetanus prophylaxis
- Remove stingers by fastest means possible to reduce venom exposure.
- Oral antihistamine
- Treat anaphylaxis
- Provide Rx for EpiPen if severe allergic reaction (up to 60% recurrence with future exposure).

Bark Scorpion Sting

Most U.S. scorpion species are not highly toxic and stings result in local pain only. Pancreatitis is associated with one species (*Tityus trinitatus*).

The bark scorpion (*Centruroides sculpturatus*, in Arizona), however, can cause systemic toxicity. Children <5 years old have a higher mortality rate than adults.

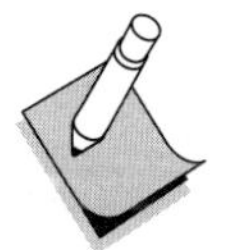

Serious bark scorpion envenomations are more common in children.

MECHANISM OF TOXICITY

- Envenomation → ↑ Na^+ channel permeability → ↑ depolarization → sympathetic, parasympathetic, and neuromuscular activation.

SYMPTOMS/EXAM

- Sensitivity to touch at site
- Numbness, tingling
- Blurred vision or **roving eye movements**
- Muscle spasms or weakness
- Hyperthermia
- Anxiety, nausea/vomiting
- Respiratory distress with **excessive secretions**
- May cause cardiopulmonary arrest

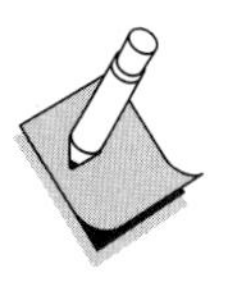

Bark scorpion envenomation → roving eye movements, muscle spasms, and excessive secretions.

TREATMENT

- Local wound care and tetanus prophylaxis
- Symptomatic treatment with
  - **Opioids** for muscle pain
  - **Benzodiazepines** for neuromuscular symptoms
  - **Atropine** for excessive secretions
- Scorpion antivenom
  - Available only in Arizona
  - Indicated in severe bark scorpion envenomation.

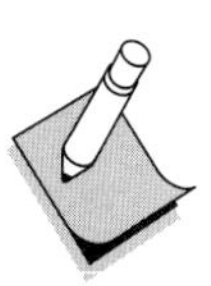

Atropine may be needed to treat excessive secretions.

> A 26-year-old man presents to the ED complaining of severe pain to his right forearm 10 minutes after being stung by a lionfish while cleaning his saltwater aquarium. His VS are normal. Physical exam shows a small puncture wounds to the forearm with mild surrounding swelling. What can you do to inactivate the venom?
>
> Lionfish are venomous fish that cause envenomation through a specialized sting apparatus. Symptoms will primarily consist of intense local pain. The venom can be inactivated by immersing the wound in hot (45°C) water for 90 minutes or until the pain subsides.

MARINE ANIMAL ENVENOMATIONS

Can be divided into three groups based on mechanism of venom delivery:

- **Stingers**
- **Nematocysts**
- **Bites**

Stingers

Marine animals with specialized sting apparatus include (see Table 13.4):

- Stingrays
- Venomous fish (catfish, zebra fish, scorpion fish, stonefish)
- Sea urchins
- Cone shells

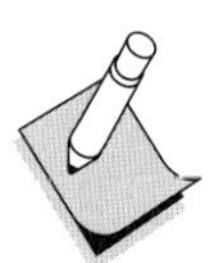

Marine animals with a stinger apparatus include stingrays, sea urchins, cone shells, and venomous fish.

TABLE 13.4. **Marine Animals That Sting**

Marine Animal	Venom Delivery Apparatus
Stingrays	Barbed stinger at end of whiplike tail
Bony fish: Catfish, zebra fish (eg, lionfish), scorpion fish, stonefish	Spines located on their fins
Sea urchins	Toxin-coated spines
Cone shells	Venom gland and teeth at end of proboscis

Mechanism of Toxicity

- Special stinger apparatus punctures skin and introduces venom → severe local symptoms and (rarely) systemic effects.

Symptoms/Exam

- Vary with species
- Most commonly, intense local pain
- Systemic symptoms may include nausea/vomiting, hypotension, muscle cramps, paralysis, cardiac arrest.

Treatment

- Supportive therapy
- Remove spines and stinger (use X-ray to verify).
- **Immediately immerse wound in hot water** (45°C for 90 minutes or until pain is relieved as this breaks down venom).
- Aggressive cleaning
- Tetanus prophylaxis
- Consider antibiotics if deep puncture wound or high-risk patient.
- Antivenom exists for stonefish toxicity.

Nematocysts

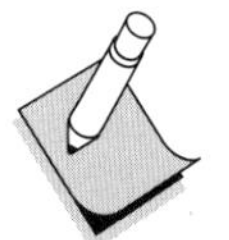

Marine animals with nematocysts include jellyfish, the Portuguese man-of-war, fire corals, sea anemones.

Marine animals with nematocysts include

- Jellyfish (Cnidaria)
- Portuguese man-of-war
- Corals
- Fire corals
- Sea anemones
- Sea wasps

Mechanism of Toxicity

- Physical contact or osmotic gradient → discharge of nematocysts ("spring loaded with venom") → local and (rarely) systemic symptoms.

Symptom/Exam

- Vary with species
- Most commonly, intense local pain
- Systemic symptoms may include nausea and vomiting, tachycardia, hypertension, respiratory paralysis, cardiac arrest.

TREATMENT

- **Immerse in 5% acetic acid (vinegar)** to inactivate nematocysts. Alternatives include:
  - Immersion in rubbing alcohol (isopropyl 40%)
  - Baking soda
- **No** fresh or tap water rinsing as this causes nematocytes to discharge via osmotic gradient
- If the nematocyte is still embedded in the skin, apply flour, or shaving cream and **shave**.
- Provide adequate analgesia.
- Treat any allergic reaction.
- Tetanus prophylaxis
- **Antivenom is available for severe box-jellyfish sting.**

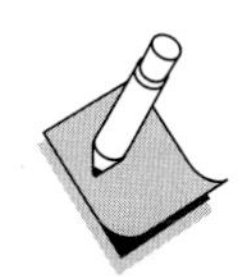

Stinger injury → Immerse in hot water. Nematocyte injury → Immerse in acetic acid.

Octopus Bites

MECHANISM OF TOXICITY

- Venom contains tetrodotoxin (TTX) → inhibition of voltage-gated Na^+ channels → paralysis.

SYMPTOMS/EXAM

- Local erythema
- Paresthesias, flaccid paralysis
- Respiratory failure

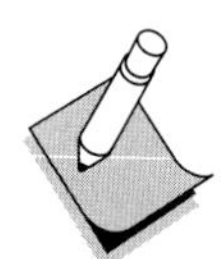

Octopus bites can → flaccid paralysis and respiratory failure via tetrodotoxin.

TREATMENT

- Supportive therapy
- Local wound care
- No known antivenom exists.

Lizard Bites

The Mexican beaded lizard and the Gila monster are venomous lizards. Approximately 70% of their bites are complicated by envenomation.

MECHANISMS OF TOXICITY

- Venom is delivered by glands in the lower jaw into the laceration created by the teeth → local and (rarely) systemic effects.
- The lizard's teeth may break and be left in the wound as a foreign body and a cause for infection.

SYMPTOMS/EXAM

- Crush and puncture wounds
- Local erythema and pain
- Systemic effects: Weakness, hypotension, and diaphoresis

TREATMENT

- Supportive therapy
- Remove animal if still attached.
- X-ray to identify any foreign body

- Irrigate copiously.
- Consider antibiotics.
- Tetanus prophylaxis

A 50-year-old male presents to the ED after sustaining a snake bite while hiking in southern North Carolina. A digital picture he took of the snake shows red/yellow/black bands with red bands touching yellow bands. The patient complains of some localized paresthesias around a small puncture wound to his L leg, but review of systems and examination is otherwise normal. Does this patient need antivenom?

Yes. The coral snake venom irreversibly binds acetylcholine receptors leading to diffuse neuromuscular symptoms, including respiratory paralysis. Early treatment of eastern coral snake bites, even if **asymptomatic**, is the key to a good outcome.

SNAKE ENVENOMATIONS

There are five families of venomous snakes worldwide. Two of these families, Viperidae (subfamily Crotalinae) and Elapidae, cause the majority of envenomations in the United States. Envenomations may be characterized by either local toxicity ± coagulopathy or neurotoxicity.

Viperidae Family

Envenomation is characterized by local tissue toxicity and, less commonly, systemic effects. Approximately 25% of bites with fang marks are "dry" bites.

The viperidae are characterized by:

- **Pit or depression midway between the eyes** (heat-sensitive thermoreceptor)
- Vertical or elliptical eyes
- Triangular shaped head
- Retractable fangs

Viperidae family includes:

- Rattlesnakes (eg, majave, diamondback)
- Copperheads
- Water moccasin (cottonmouth)

Mechanism of Toxicity

- The venom has digestive enzymes and proteins → local tissue edema and toxicity and (less commonly) systemic toxicity and coagulopathy.

Symptoms/Exam

- Local tissue toxicity (see Figure 13.3)
  - **Pain** (within 15–30 minutes)
  - Swelling (may be marked, but compartment is syndrome rare)

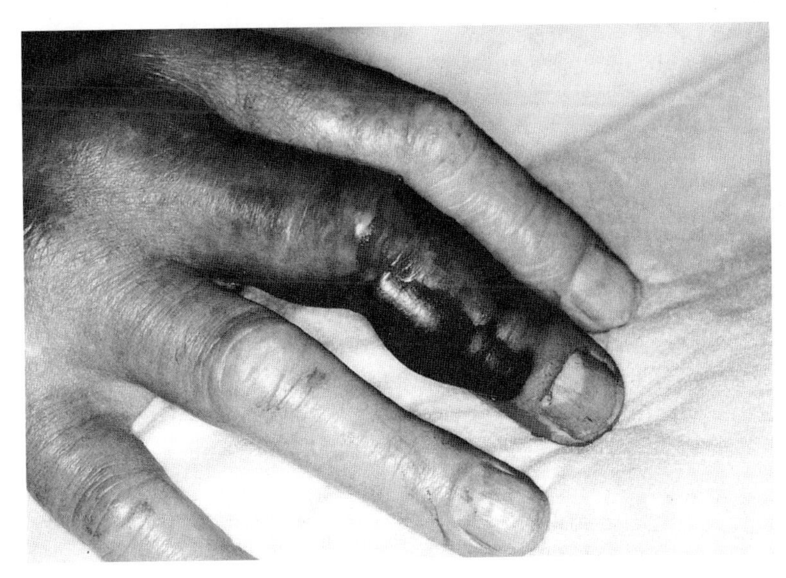

FIGURE 13.3. Local toxicity from rattlesnake envenomation.

(Courtesy of Sean P. Bush, MD as reproduced, with permission, from Knoop KJ, Stack LB, Storrow AB. *Atlas of Emergency Medicine*, 2nd ed. New York: McGraw-Hill, 2002:528.)

- Local petechiae or ecchymosis
- Bullae (may be hemorrhagic)
- Systemic toxicity
  - Oral paresthesias
  - Metallic taste
  - Fasciculations
  - Tachycardia and hypotension
  - Anaphylaxis
- Coagulopathy
  - **Thrombocytopenia**, elevated PT, decreased fibrinogen

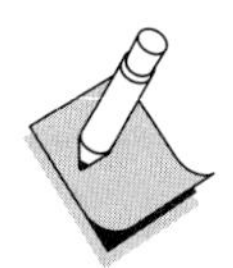

Compartment syndrome is rare as venom is in SQ tissue not fascial compartments.

TREATMENT

- Prehospital:
  - Immobilize extremity in neutral position.
  - No incision and suction
  - No tourniquet
  - Minimize physical activity, if possible, but seek medical care immediately even if it means hiking out of deep wilderness.
  - Mark leading edge of tenderness/swelling to follow progression.
- Aggressive supportive care, wound care, tetanus prophylaxis
  - Prophylactic antibiotics are **not** indicated.
  - Correct coagulopathy as needed.
- Elevate extremity and immobilize.
- Treat anaphylaxis aggressively.
- **Antivenom**
  - A newer sheep-derived antivenom (CroFab) is available (less antigenic than the polyvalent horse serum antivenom).
  - Watch closely for **allergic reaction**.
  - Indications include severe local effects or systemic illness (see Table 13.5).
  - Serum sickness can sometimes occur following administration.

TABLE 13.5. Indications for Antivenom in Snake Envenomations

Severe localized pain or throbbing
Moderate local edema and/or erythema
Progressive spreading of erythema proximally
Any coagulapathy
Any systemic symptoms
Concern for compartment syndrome
All eastern coral snake bites

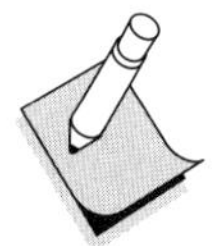

Viperidae envenomation → local tissue toxicity >> systemic effects. Elapidae envenomation → marked systemic neurotoxicity, minimal local reaction.

Elapidae Family

Envenomation is characterized by minimal local reaction with marked systemic neurotoxicity.

Poisonous coral snakes versus nonpoisonous milk and king snakes (applies to the United States only): "Red on yellow, kill a fellow" "Red on black, venom lack"

Coral snakes are primarily found in the southeastern and southwestern United States.

In the United States, Elapidae are characterized by red/yellow/black bands with red bands touching yellow bands. This does not hold true for other parts of the world.

Elapidae family includes:

- Corals (U.S.)
- Cobras
- Kraits
- Mambas

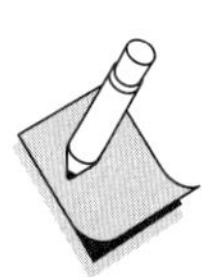

Respiratory-muscle paralysis is the immediate cause of death in most coral snake envenomations.

MECHANISM OF TOXICITY

- Coral snake venom → irreversibly binds acetylcholine receptors → systemic toxicity.

SYMPTOMS/EXAM

- Minimal local reaction
- Weakness, numbness
- Fasciculations, tremor
- Diplopia
- Bulbar palsies: slurred speech, dysphagia
- **Respiratory paralysis** (immediate cause of death)

TREATMENT

- Prehospital treatment similar to Viperidae envenomation, above
- Aggressive supportive care, wound care, tetanus prophylaxis
- **No** prophylactic antibiotics

- **Antivenom** (see Table 13.5)
  - For all eastern coral snake bites (even if asymptomatic!)
  - Otherwise, if any systemic symptoms
  - No antivenom available for Arizona coral snake (less toxic)
  - A horse-serum antivenom—administer test dose and watch for allergic reactions
- All coral snake bites require admission for observation.

A 2-year-old boy is brought to your ED after being found unconscious in his car seat. His mother left him in the locked car while shopping. His field dextrose stick is 96. His rectal temperature on arrival is 105°F. What is the preferred mechanism to rapidly lower this child's core temperature while still allowing for monitoring of vital signs?

This child has sustained heat stroke. Rapid lower of his core body temperature is essential for a good neurologic outcome. Many cooling techniques are available, but using evaporative technique where a mist of 40°C water is sprayed on the patient's skin, while air is fanned over the body (using standing fans), allows for access to the patient and limits shivering (which generates heat).

HEAT-RELATED ILLNESS

Heat-related illness is a continuum of disease extending from minor heat illness to heat exhaustion and heat stroke.

MECHANISMS OF HEAT LOSS/GAIN

- **Conduction:** Direct physical contact with another surface → heat loss or gain (eg, ice packs, heating pad).
- **Convection:** Heat transfer via circulating air or water molecules (eg, wind chill)
- **Radiation:** Heat transfer by electromagnetic waves. (eg, heat from the sun, poor insulation in cold environment)
- **Evaporation:** Heat transfer as water is vaporized (eg, sweating)

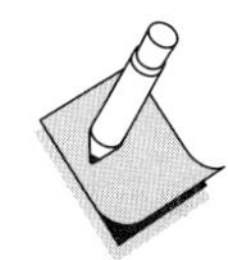

What is the difference between hyperthermia and fever?

Hyperthermia = hypothalamus overwhelmed by heat production.

Fever = ↑ hypothalamic set point from circulating cytokines.

PATHOPHYSIOLOGY

- The **anterior hypothalamus** is the body's thermostat and regulates body temperature.
- ↑ Core body temperature → peripheral vasodilation (to dissipate heat via convection), → perspiration and respiration (for evaporative heat loss).
- Acclimatization to hot environment = earlier and greater sweating, dilute sweat.

Risk factors for heat illness can be divided into three groups (see Table 13.6):

- Increased heat production
- Decreased heat loss
- Impaired ability to move to a cool environment

Malignant hyperthermia deserves special mention. It is due to a genetic instability of skeletal muscle that allows for excessive calcium release in the muscle cell when exposed to certain anesthetic agents (including succinylcholine) → muscle rigidity and profound hyperthermia.

TABLE 13.6. Risk Factors for Heat Illness

INCREASED HEAT PRODUCTION	DECREASED HEAT LOSS	IMPAIRED MOBILITY
Thyroid storm	Infants	Infants and young children
Seizures	Advanced age	Physical or mental impairment
Severe agitation	Volume depletion	Acute CNS process
Exercise	Impaired cardiac function	Alcoholism
Acute toxicologic process	Skin conditions (eg, scleroderma, prickly heat)	Tranquilizer or sedative use
Neuroleptic malignant syndrome	Medications Anticholinergics Psychiatric medications β-Blockers Diuretics	
Malignant hyperthermia		

PREVENTION OF HEAT ILLNESS

- Keep hydrated (drink solutions which help replete electrolytes)
- Wear loose, light-colored clothing.
- Stay indoors with air conditioning on hot and humid days.

Minor Heat Illness

- **Heat rash:** "Prickly heat" due to blocked sweat pores
- **Heat cramps:** These are painful contractions of large muscles that occur AFTER exertion 2° to relative hyponatremia. Individuals replace evaporative losses by drinking hypotonic fluids such as free water without replacing salt. Measured electrolytes are normal. It is usually self-limited; treatment is supportive.
- **Heat edema:** Secondary to peripheral vasodilation and orthostatic pooling of blood
- **Heat tetany:** Carpopedal spasm due to hyperventilation and ↓ P_{CO_2}
- **Heat syncope:** Syncope during heat stress 2° to peripheral vasodilation in the setting of dehydration

Heat Exhaustion

This is the most common form of heat-related illness. It is characterized by volume and/or salt depletion under conditions of heat stress. **Mental status is normal.**

SYMPTOMS/EXAM

- Dizziness, weakness, irritability
- Headache
- Perspiration

- Nausea and vomiting
- Core temperature is typically normal, but may be elevated (<40°C).

DIAGNOSIS

- Based on clinical presentation
- Electrolytes **may** be abnormal: Hyponatremia, hypochloremia, elevated BUN
- LFTs are normal.

TREATMENT

- Remove patient from heat source.
- Replete fluids with electrolyte solutions (oral or intravenous, depending on severity).

Heat Stroke

Heat stroke is severe form of heat injury with a high mortality rate in which homeostatic thermoregulatory mechanisms fail, leading to hyperthermia and multisystem organ dysfunction.

It is historically classified as **classic** or **exertional**.

- Classic heatstroke: Elderly or debilitated patients without access to air conditioning; sweating is often absent
- Exertional heatstroke: Younger individuals exercising in a hot environment

This classification has no clinical bearing as the treatment is the same.

Heat stroke = Hyperthermia with CNS dysfunction.

SYMPTOMS/EXAM

- **Altered mental status and CNS dysfunction**
- Possible seizure
- Anhydrosis: Hot/dry skin (not reliable)
- Core body temperature usually >40.5°C rectal (may be lower)
- Jaundice 24–72 hours later
- Cardiovascular dysfunction: Hypotension, pulmonary edema

Hepatic damage is nearly always present in heat stroke.

DIAGNOSIS

- Based on clinical presentation
- Marked elevation of AST/ALT is expected with peak in 24–72 hours. Complete recovery is expected.
- Renal injury is common and may be due to volume depletion, direct thermal injury, or rhabdomyolysis.
- Fluid, electrolyte, and hematologic disorders vary.

TREATMENT

- Supportive therapy
  - Continuous temperature monitoring
  - Correct electrolyte imbalances.
- **Rapid cooling** (within 1 hour) to core temperature of 39–40°C
  - Removing clothing.
  - **Evaporative cooling** (moisten skin with tepid water and fan skin with warm air) **or**
  - **Cold water immersion** (downside = less access to patient)

- Adjuncts:
  - Place ice packs to groin, axillae, and neck.
  - Cooling blanket
- If refractory, consider invasive methods.
  - Cardiopulmonary bypass
  - Gastric, pleural, or bladder lavage
- IV benzodiazepines (or paralysis) to prevent shivering (which generates heat); treat seizures
- Intravenous fluids to CVP of 12 mL H_2O or urine output = 0.5 mL/kg/hr
  - Fluid requirements vary with underlying cause.
- Dopamine for persistent hypotension despite adequate fluid resuscitation
- Dantrolene: If suspected malignant hyperthermia.
- **Avoid**
  - Antipyretics—**not** effective and may be harmful!
  - Prophylactic steroids—**not** effective.
  - Norepinephrine—causes vasoconstriction and decreases cutaneous heat exchange.
- Poor prognostic indicators:
  - Coma
  - AST > 1000 IU/L.
  - Delay in rapid cooling (morbidity and mortality are directly related to the duration of hyperpyrexia)
  - DIC
  - Hypotension
  - Renal failure in <48 hours
  - Lactic acidosis

*Antipyretics are **not** effective (and may be harmful) in treatment of heat stroke!*

COMPLICATIONS

- ARDS, electrolyte abnormalities, renal failure, rhabdomyolysis, hepatic injury, DIC
- If left untreated cerebral edema and multisystem organ failure will develop.

A homeless man presents to your ED after walking over 3 miles in freezing snow. He is complaining of numbness and swelling to his lower extremities. On exam you see diffuse erythema, edema, and both clear and hemorrhagic blisters. How will you treat this man's blisters?

With frostbite, damaged tissue releases arachidonic acid breakdown products (prostaglandins and thromboxane). These released products promote platelet aggregation, leading to thrombosis and ischemia. Blisters should be left intact or sterilely aspirated. Debride blisters only if broken.

COLD-RELATED INJURIES

There are four physiologic mechanisms of heat loss/gain (see Table 13.7). Radiation is responsible for the majority of *normal* heat loss.

TABLE 13.7. **Mechanisms of Heat Loss/Gain**

Conduction	Direct physical contact with another surface → heat loss or gain (eg, ice packs, heating pad)
Convection	Heat transfer via circulating air or water molecules (eg, wind chill)
Radiation	Heat transfer by electromagnetic waves (eg, poor insulation in cold environment)
Evaporation	Heat transfer as water is vaporized (eg, sweating, breathing)

Pathophysiology

- ↓ Core body temperature → peripheral vasoconstriction (to decrease convection) and ↓ HR (to decrease blood flow to periphery) → peripheral ischemia and cold injury.

Chillblains

Chilblains is mild tissue injury from repetitive exposure to dry cold at nonfreezing temperatures. It characteristically involves the dorsum of hands and feet, but may also involve face, ears, and thighs.

Symptoms/Exam

- Painful/inflamed skin lesions that are pruritic and erythematous.
- May evolve to plaques, blue nodules, and ulcerations.

Treatment

- Rewarming and symptomatic treatment

Trenchfoot

Trenchfoot occurs with exposure to wet cold at freezing temperatures (0–10°C) over several hours to days.

Symptoms/Exam

- Before rewarming (**prehyperemic stage**): Feet appear cold, mottled, pale
- After rewarming (**hyperemic stage**): Feet are red, painful, and swollen

Treatment

- Carefully wash and dry feet, then wrap with warm clothing.
- Elevate feet.
- Nonweight-bearing, until improved

Complications

- Wet gangrene, if untreated
- Late sequelae (**posthyperemic stage**): Cold sensitivity, pain and numbness, atrophy, weakness

Frostnip

Frostnip is a superficial freezing injury without tissue loss or tissue destruction. It typically involves exposed surfaces (face, hands).

Symptoms/Exam

- Transient numbness and tingling, resolves with rewarming
- Affected skin appears firm, cold, and white.
- Superficial blistering and peeling may occur.

Treatment

- Rewarm.
- Prevent further cold exposure.

Frostbite

The most common freezing injury of tissue that occurs when tissue temperatures drop below 0°C (32°F). Ice crystal formation damages cellular architecture leading to microvascular thrombosis, ischemia, and eventual tissue necrosis.

Only after rewarming of tissue can depth of injury can be assessed.

Traditional classification of frostbite:

- **First-degree:** Central white plaque with surrounding hyperemia
- **Second-degree:** Clear blisters
- **Third-degree:** Hemorrhagic blisters → eschar and tissue loss
- **Fourth-degree:** Focal necrosis → tissue loss

However, the above classification has no impact on treatment, so a simpler classification is often used.

- **Superficial frostbite:** No evidence for tissue loss
- **Deep frostbite:** Evidence for tissue loss

Pathophysiology

- Tissue freezing → release of arachidonic acid breakdown products (prostaglandins and thromboxane) → thrombosis and ischemia.

Symptoms/Exam

- Before rewarming:
  - Affected area appears mottled, pale, firm, and waxy.
  - Extremity may feel numb or "wooden."
- After rewarming: Blisters and focal necrosis develop.
- Dead tissue demarcates in 22–45 days.

Treatment

- Treat any associated hypothermia **first**.
- **Rapid rewarming:**
  - Immerse in **40–42°C** circulating water until tissue feels pliable.
  - Opioid analgesia is often needed.
- **Avoid:**
  - Friction or rubbing of skin
  - Dry heat
  - Refreezing (disastrous!)
- IV hydration
- Tetanus prophylaxis
- Blisters
  - Debride ONLY if broken
  - Otherwise, **aspirate or leave intact**

Rewarm by immersion in 40°–42°C circulating water.

- Debridement of skin overlying hemorrhagic blister may result in marked desiccation of the underlying tissues.
- Prevent further tissue loss:
  - Splint and elevated limb to minimized edema formation
  - Smoking cessation
  - NSAIDs (inhibit arachidonic acid cascade)
  - Topical aloe vera (inhibits thromboxane)
- **Many** other therapies have been proposed: Nifedipine, topical corticosteroids, prednisone, hyperbarics, etc., but none has been proven beneficial.
- Delayed surgical debridement and escarotomy
  - Unless severe gangrene or sepsis present

Core afterdrop: Cold peripheral blood returns core → further decrease in core temperature.

COMPLICATIONS

- **Core afterdrop**
  - Occurs when skin or extremities are warmed before the core → cold peripheral blood returns to core → core temperature drops further.
  - Rewarm core **before** periphery in all cases of hypothermia.
- Secondary bacterial/fungal infections

ACCIDENTAL HYPOTHERMIA

Hypothermia is defined as a core body temperature <35°C (95°F).

Risks for hypothermia can be divided into three groups (see Table 13.8):

- Decreased heat production
- Increased heat loss
- Impaired ability to move to warm environment

TABLE 13.8. Factors Predisposing to Accidental Hypothermia

DECREASED HEAT PRODUCTION	INCREASED HEAT LOSS	IMPAIRED MOBILITY
Hypothyroidism	Inadequate clothing	Infants and young children
Hypoadrenalism	Vasodilation	Physical or mental impairment
Malnutrition	Alcohol	Acute CNS process
Hypoglycemia	Medications	Alcoholism
Dehydration	Spinal cord injury	Tranquilizer or sedative use
Physical exhaustion	Neuropathies	
Extremes of age	Skin disorders	
Inactivity	Burns	
Impaired shivering	Exfoliative dermatitis	
	Infants	

Hypothermia is clinically defined as mild, moderate, or severe.

- **Mild hypothermia (32°–35°C):**
  - **Excitation stage:** Characterized by physiologic responses to generate heat
- **Moderate hypothermia (30°–32°C):**
  - As temperature drops below 32°C, shivering ceases and victim enters a stage of general slowing of body functions = **adynamic stage.**
- **Severe hypothermia (<30°C)**
  - Patient appears dead. Ventricular fibrillation risk increases.

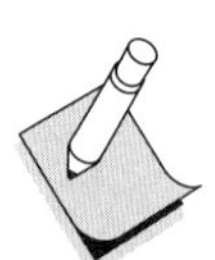

With temperatures <30°C (severe hypothermia), the patient appears dead and the VFib risk increases.

PATHOPHYSIOLOGY

- As core temperature ↓ → peripheral vasoconstriction (to limit further radiant heat loss) and shivering (to increase heat production).
- Further decrease in temperature → generalized slowing of body functions.
- **Leftward shift of oxyhemoglobin dissociation curve** → decreased release of O_2 to tissues.
- Renal dysfunction and peripheral vasoconstriction (central *hyper*volemia) → **cold diuresis** → dehydration.

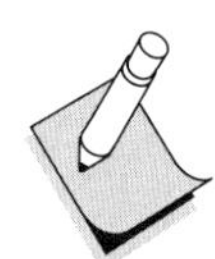

Patients with exposure to cold develop a "cold diuresis," resulting in dehydration.

SYMPTOMS/EXAM

- Mild hypothermia:
  - Tachycardia and tachypnea
  - Hyperactive reflexes
  - Shivering
- Moderate to severe hypothermia:
  - Mental status change ranging from poor judgment to lethargy to coma
  - Pupils may become fixed and dilated.
  - Poor coordination, dysarthria
  - Bradycardia or ANY atrial/ventricular dysrhythmia
  - Hypoactive reflexes, muscular rigidity

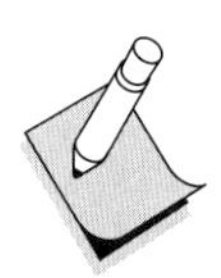

Osborne "J" waves are classic for moderate to severe hypothermia, but may be seen in other conditions.

DIAGNOSIS

- Based on history of exposure and core body temperature
- **ECG:**
  - Classic ECG = Osborne ("J") waves appear at junction of QRS complex (see Figure 13.4).
  - ST segment and QT interval are often prolonged.
  - *Any* dysrhythmia may occur.
- ABG:
  - Must be corrected for core body temperature
- Laboratory studies:
  - Hemoconcentration is common.
  - Clotting factor dysfunction
  - Thrombocytopenia
  - Hyperglycemia or hypoglycemia may be present.
  - Others, as indicated

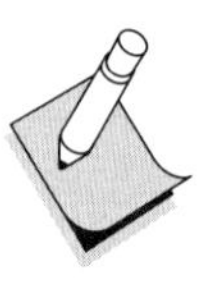

Three general methods of rewarming:
Passive (noninvasive) rewarming
Active external rewarming
Active core rewarming

TREATMENT

- Start with ABCs:
  - Continuous core temperature measurement
- **Passive rewarming:**
  - For mild hypothermia
  - Blankets

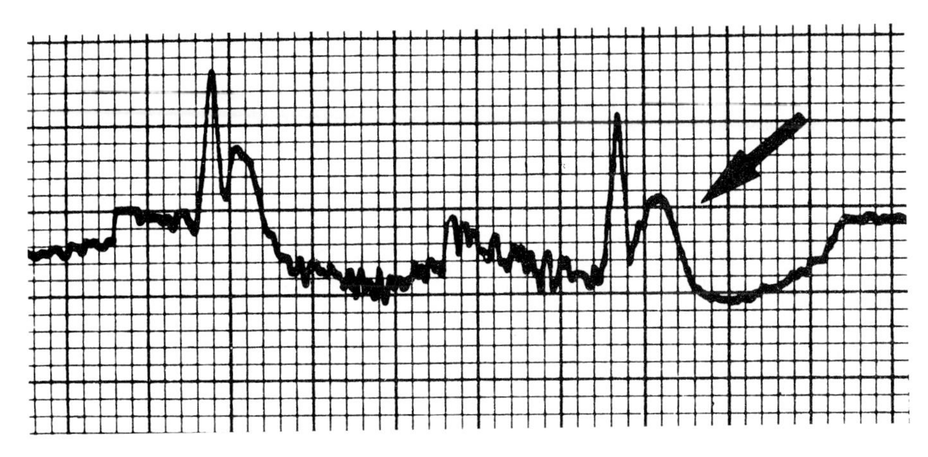

FIGURE 13.4. Osborne ("J") waves.

(Reproduced, with permission, from Tintinalli JE, Kelen GD, Stapczynski JS. *Emergency Medicine: A Comprehensive Study Guide*, 6th ed. New York: McGraw-Hill, 2004:1180.)

- Dry clothes
- Move from cold environment

- **Active external rewarming:**
  - For **severe hypothermia without cardiovascular instability**
  - Heating lamps (radiation)
  - Bair huggers (convection)
  - Warm blankets (conduction)
  - Warm intravenous fluids at 40–42°C
  - Warm humidified O_2 by mask (↓ evaporative loss)
- **Active core rewarming**
  - For severe **hypothermia with cardiovascular instability**
  - Warmed gastric, bladder, peritoneal, and pleural lavage
- The best treatment for dysrhythmias, coagulopathy, and hyperglycemia = rewarming.
- Rehydrate with warmed IV fluids (most patients are dehydrated from "cold diuresis").
- Many medications, including insulin, are ineffective until core temperature is >30°C.
- If patient is in cardiac arrest:
  - Administer CPR.
  - Consider surgical approaches to rewarming:
    - Cardiopulmonary bypass
    - Continuous arteriovenous and venovenous rewarming
    - Extracorporeal membrane oxygenation (ECMO)
    - Hemodialysis
  - Defibrillation and medications may not be effective at or below 30°C, therefore continue CPR while the patient is warmed.
  - If in VFib, only one defibrillation attempt (2 J/kg) is indicated until the core temperature exceeds 32°C.
  - Patient may be pronounced dead if core temperature is **32–35°C** and no vital signs are present.
- **Avoid**
  - Suppressing shivering response.
  - Rough handling (may induce VF).
  - Transvenous pacing (may induce VF): Use transcutaneous pacing instead.

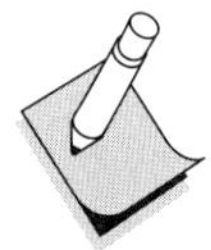

Failure to rewarm? → consider underlying endocrine failure.

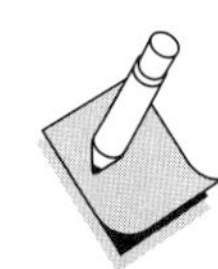

"The patient is not dead until he is warm and dead."

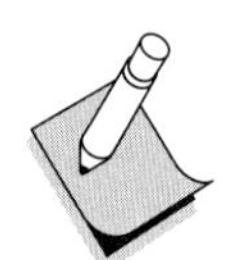

If VF develops: Defibrillate once, then hold until core temperature >32°C.

COMPLICATIONS

- Coagulopathy
- Acidosis
- Cardiac arrhythmias
- Rhabdomyolysis

> An 18-month-old female presents after sustaining an electrical injury while chewing on a power cord. On examination, there is a burn present to the corner of her mouth without marked tissue loss or evidence of other intra-oral burns. What is the most feared complication in this patient?
>
> This child has sustained a local arc burn to the commissure of the mouth. There is a risk for delayed bleeding in 3–14 days as a result of injury to the labial artery.

ELECTRICAL INJURY

Ohm's Law: Current = Voltage/Resistance.

- **Voltage** = Difference in electrical potential between two points in an electrical circuit. High voltage = ≥1000 V.
- **Current** = No. of electrons moving at any time, measured by amperage (A).
- **Resistance** = Property of the medium through which electrons pass, measured in ohms
  - Current flows through "path of least resistance"
  - Decreases with ↑ fluid content (eg, nerves, blood vessels, wet skin)
  - Increases with calloused skin

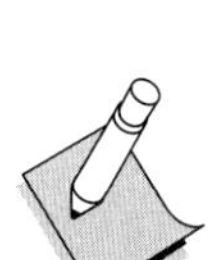

AC is more dangerous than DC at any given voltage.

There are two basic types of electrical circuits:

Alternating current (AC)

- Typical household current
- Changes its direction of current flow at a given frequency
- More dangerous than DC at any given voltage
- 1–4 mA → tingling sensation.
- 8–22 mA (the **"let go" threshold**) → tetanic muscle contraction → one cannot release the electrical source.
- >70 mA → cardiac depolarization and possible VF.

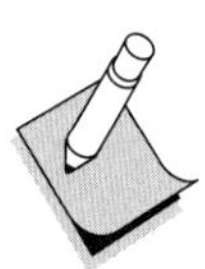

Decreasing order of electrical resistance: Bone, fat, tendon, skin, muscle, mucous membranes, blood vessels, nerves

Direct current (DC)

- Batteries and electronics
- Tends to throw the victim from the source → secondary traumatic injuries

Overall, high-voltage electrical injury is characterized by minimal external findings hiding extensive internal tissue damage.

SYMPTOMS/EXAM

- Immediate cardiac arrest may occur from asystole or ventricular fibrillation (primary cause of death).
- Patients who survive the initial electrical shock present with a variety of injuries depending on path of current flow and associated trauma.
- Loss of consciousness, confusion, amnesia

- Paresthesias
- Seizure
- Thermal source contact burns
  - Size does not correlate with underlying tissue injury.
  - Most commonly on hand
- **Arc burns** (kissing burns) = arc of extremely high voltage current across flexor creases → extensive damage.
- Visual changes from corneal burns, retinal detachment, uveitis
- Tinnitus, hearing loss, ruptured tympanic membranes
- Muscular pain
- Traumatic injuries (blunt or blast)
  - **Posterior shoulder dislocations** from being "thrown from source"

Primary cardiac arrest in electrical injuries = asystole or ventricular fibrillation.

DIAGNOSIS

- Diagnosis of electrical injury is typically obvious on presentation.
- Virtually any organ can be injured, therefore detailed evaluation is warranted.
- ECG and monitoring:
  - Dysrhythmias, heart block, QT prolongation, nonspecific ST-T changes are all possible.
- Labs include: CBC, electrolytes, UA, CK.
- Standard trauma evaluation, as necessary

TREATMENT

- ABCs
- Intravenous fluids
  - Monitor urine output (goal 1–2 mL/kg/hour).
- Treat rhabdomyolysis, if present.
  - IV fluids
  - Alkalinization of urine (three ampoules of $NaHCO_3$ in 1 L D_5W)
- Trauma management, as necessary
- Wound (burn) care and tetanus prophylaxis
- Low voltage injuries can be safely sent home.

COMPLICATIONS

- Renal failure from rhabdomyolysis
- DIC (uncommon)
- Arterial and venous thrombosis
- Labial artery burns can present with delayed severe bleeding.
- Cataracts

> A 32-year-old male is brought to the ED for evaluation after being found down in a field after a thunderstorm. He has no recollection of events. He is complaining of ringing in his ears and states that he is unable to move his extremities. What physical exam findings would help you determine if he was struck by lightning?
>
> Fernlike markings (also known as Lichtenberg figures) are pathognomonic for lightning injuries and usually fade in a few hours. Other findings consistent with lightning injury include tympanic membranes rupture (seen in 50%), tinnitus, hearing loss, and paralyzed, cold, and pulseless extremities (keraunoparalysis, a temporary condition due to sympathetic nervous system activation).

LIGHTNING INJURY

Lightning is a **unidirectional current** of **extremely high voltage**. Fortunately the duration of exposure is **very brief** and the majority of the current is transmitted via external "**flashover.**"

Lightning strike victims who reach the hospital often have many external findings, but minimal (excluding associated trauma) internal injury.

A comparison between lightning and high-voltage electrical injuries can be found in Table 13.9.

Pathophysiology of Lightning Injury

- **Direct contact**
  - Current travels directly to victim.
- **Side flash**
  - Current traverses through air from first object to victim.
- **Step or Ground current**
  - Lightning hits ground → current travels via ground to nearby victims.
- **Blunt trauma**
  - 2° to fall or falling objects
- **Blast trauma**
  - Victims suffer from pulmonary contusions, tympanic membrane rupture (up to 50%) and conductive hearing loss.
- **Thermal burns**
  - 2° to fires

Pathophysiology of Lightning Death

- Intense electrical stimulus → **asystole** (**"primary death"**) and apnea from inhibition of brainstem respiratory centers.

TABLE 13.9. Key Differences in Lightning and High-Voltage Electrical Injuries

	Lightning	High-Voltage
Duration	Short	Prolonged contact
Volts	10 million–2 billion	1000–10,000
Current	DC	AC
Side Flash	Present	Absent
Cardiac	Asystole	Ventricular fibrillation
Burns	Minor and superficial	More extensive
Myoglobinuria	Infrequent	Common
Fasciotomy	Rarely indicated	Common

- Asystole often resolves spontaneously **but** if apnea persists → "**secondary death" from hypoxia and (commonly) ventricular fibrillation.**

SYMPTOMS/EXAM

- Cardiac arrest
- The patient who survives the immediate strike may present with a variety of findings.
- Seizures, confusion, amnesia
- Dysrhythmias: May be delayed
- Anisocoria or dilated pupils
- TM rupture, tinnitus, and hearing loss
- **Keraunoparalysis:**
  - From sympathetic activation and resultant vasospasm
  - Transient paralysis and blue, mottled, pulseless lower and/or upper extremities
- Skin:
  - **Lichtenberg figures** (see Figure 13.5): Superficial fern or feather pattern from "electron shower"
  - **Linear burns:** From sweat converting to steam
  - **Punctuate burns:** Multiple small, round burns
  - **Thermal burns**
- Associated traumatic injuries

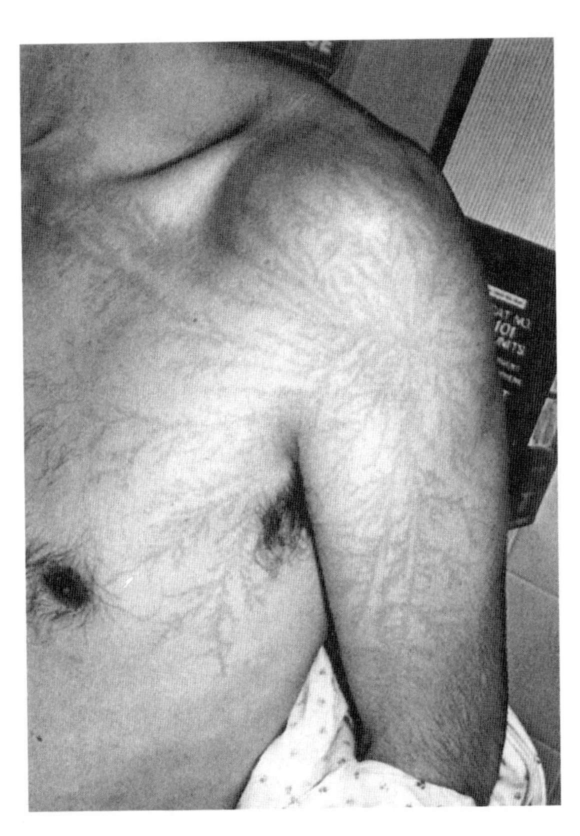

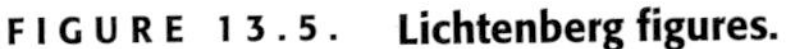

FIGURE 13.5. Lichtenberg figures.

(Reproduced, with permission, from Tintinalli JE, Kelen GD, Stapczynski JS. *Emergency Medicine: A Comprehensive Study Guide*, 6th ed. New York: McGraw-Hill, 2004:1238.)

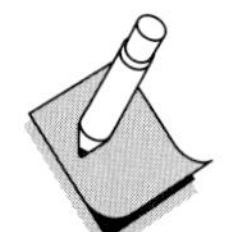

Lichtenberg figures are pathognomonic for lightning injury.

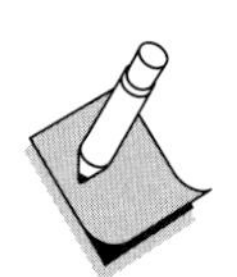

Reverse triage applies in lightning injuries → treat those that appear dead first.

DIAGNOSIS

- Typically obvious based on clinical presentation
- ECG and cardiac monitor
- Useful labs include: CBC, electrolytes, BUN, Cr, UA.

TREATMENT

- ABCs
- If on scene treat those in cardiac arrest (appear dead) FIRST. This is unlike other mass-casualty incidents.
- Trauma precautions and evaluation as indicated
- Tetanus prophylaxis
- Intravenous fluids
- Admit all patients with cardiac findings (exam or ECG), neurologic abnormalities, or significant trauma/burns.

Duration of lightning is extremely brief: Asystole is common but internal burns and rhabdomyolysis aren't typically seen.

COMPLICATIONS

- If pregnant: Fetal mortality (rate can be as high as 50%)
- Neurologic sequelae are common but lower extremity paralysis is usually only temporary.
- Cataracts (delayed)

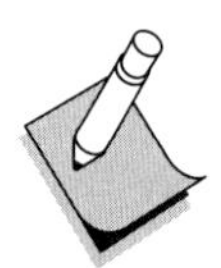

Cataracts can occur acutely or up to 3 years after lightning injury.

HIGH-ALTITUDE ILLNESS

High-altitude illness consists of three unique clinical presentations: Acute mountain sickness (AMS), high-altitude pulmonary edema (HAPE), and high-altitude cerebral edema (HACE). AMS occurs after several **hours** of exposure to altitude, while HAPE and HACE typically take days to develop.

Risk factors for developing high-altitude illness:

- Children more than adults (age >50 years decreases risk).
- Rapid ascent
- Elevation attained
- Heavy exertion
- Cold exposure (exacerbates pulmonary HTN)
- Obesity and COPD (hypoventilation)
- Sickle cell disease

PATHOPHYSIOLOGY (SEE TABLE 13.10)

- As altitude increases, partial pressure of O_2 decreases
  - Periodic breathing (exacerbates hypoxemia)
  - Pulmonary artery hypertension
  - Fluid retention
  - Cerebral hypoxia → cerebrovascular changes and damage.

High-altitude acclimatization is the body's ability to *gradually* adjust to lower O_2 concentrations by the following methods:

- Carotid body hypoxemia → hypoxic ventilatory response that stimulates ventilation to ↓ Pa_{CO_2} and ↑ Pa_{O_2}.
- In response to the acute respiratory alkalosis the kidneys excrete bicarbonate (to normalize pH).

TABLE 13.10. Altitude Classification and Pathophysiology

CLASSIFICATION	ELEVATION ATTAINED (ft)	PATHOPHYSIOLOGY
Moderate altitude	8000–10,000	↓ exercise performance ↑ ventilation to ↑ Po_2
High altitude	10,000–18,000	Maximal $Sao_2 < 90\%$ Maximal $Pao_2 < 60$ mmHg Hypoxemia
Extreme altitude	> 18,000	Severe hypoxemia Severe hypocapnia Physiologic deterioration with time

- Erythropoietin production is ↑ within 2 hours of ascent → ↑ red cell mass and ↑ O_2 carrying capacity.
- ↑ 2,3-DPG → rightward shift of oxyhemoglobin dissociation curve → improved O_2 release to tissues.

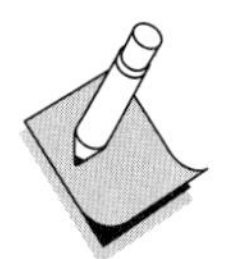

Best prevention for all types of high-altitude illness:

- *Ascend slowly and spend time at each altitude for acclimatization.*
- *Avoid alcohol and other sedatives.*
- *Avoid overexertion.*
- *Keep warm.*

Acute Mountain Sickness

Develops several hours after arrival to altitude >8000 ft in nonacclimatized individuals

SYMPTOMS/EXAM

- Symptoms are similar to viral syndrome or hangover: Anorexia, headache, nausea/vomiting, fatigue, weakness, insomnia.

TREATMENT

- Usually self-limited and resolves with acclimatization in 24–48 hours.
- No further ascent until symptoms abate
- Descend if severe symptoms
- Acetazolamide: To speed acclimatization (may start prior to ascent).
- For symptomatic relief:
  - Supplemental O_2
  - Dexamethasone
  - Tylenol, aspirin
- **Avoid:** All CNS and respiratory depressants (narcotics, alcohol, benzodiazepines).

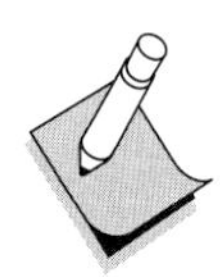

The best definitive treatment for all high-altitude syndromes is immediate descent.

High-Altitude Pulmonary Edema

HAPE is a form of noncardiogenic pulmonary edema. It typically occurs 2–4 days after arrival to high altitude.

PATHOPHYSIOLOGY

Pulmonary vasoconstriction → ↑ pulmonary hypertension → endothelial damage and capillary leak.

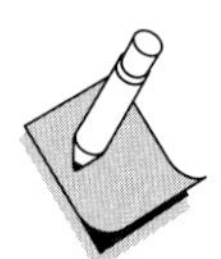

Dexamethasone can help treat HACE or AMS but has no effect for the treatment of HAPE.

SYMPTOMS/EXAM

- AMS symptoms (common)
- Cough (dry or productive)
- **Dyspnea at rest**
- Tachypnea and tachycardia
- Rales
- Fever

DIAGNOSIS

- Primarily clinical, but can be confirmed with CXR showing bilateral patchy infiltrates and *normal* heart size (see Figure 13.6)

TREATMENT

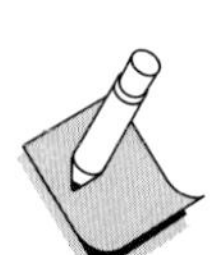

HAPE is the most life threatening of high-altitude syndromes.

- **Bed rest**
  - Mild to moderate cases may recover with bed rest ± O_2 at altitude.
- **Supplemental O_2**
- **Descent** (1500–3000 ft)
- Hyperbaric O_2 therapy
- If no descent or O_2 available: Nifedepine SL
- Morphine and furosemide are controversial regarding benefit vs harm.

High-Altitude Cerebral Edema

HACE is the most severe form of high-altitude illness. As with HAPE, onset is typically 2–4 days after arrival to altitude >12,000 ft.

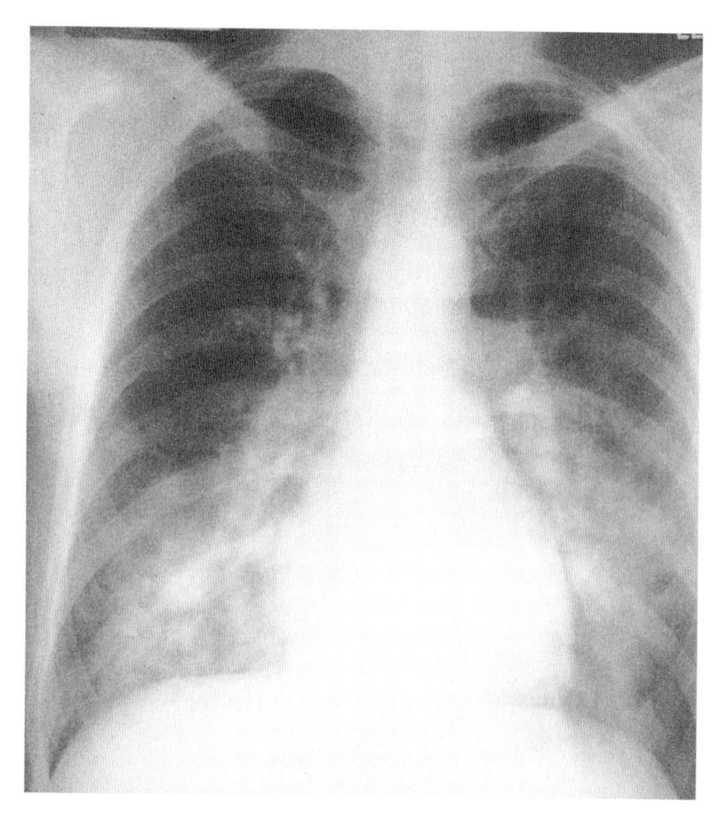

FIGURE 13.6. CXR of patient with high-altitude pulmonary edema.

(Courtesy of Peter Hackett, MD as reproduced, with permission, from Knoop KJ, Stack LB, Storrow AB. *Atlas of Emergency Medicine*, 2nd ed. New York: McGraw-Hill, 2002:515.)

SYMPTOMS/EXAM

- AMS symptoms (severe headache, nausea/vomiting)
- HAPE symptoms may also be present.
- Cerebellar ataxia: **Most sensitive sign**
- MS changes: Stupor to coma
- Seizures
- Retinal hemorrhages are common, but may occur without HACE.
- 3rd/6th cranial nerve palsies (rare)

Acetazolamide is contraindicated in sulfa allergic patients.

DIAGNOSIS

- Clinical diagnosis
- MRI, if diagnosis in question

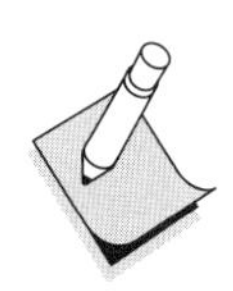

Monge disease (chronic mountain polycythemia) is a late effect of high altitude characterized by headache, trouble sleeping, and mental sluggishness.

TREATMENT

- Supplemental O_2
- Dexamethasone
- Immediate descent or evacuation
- Hyperbaric therapy
- Furosemide or mannitol may be used with caution (downside = volume depletion) [see Table 13.11].

TABLE 13.11. Medications Used For Treatment of High-Altitude Illness

MEDICATION	MECHANISM OF ACTION	INDICATION
Acetazolamide	Carbonic anhydrase inhibitor → bicarbonate diuresis and metabolic acidosis → compensatory hyperventilation	AMS prophylaxis AMS treatment Disturbing periodic breathing
Dexamethasone	↓ vasogenic edema ↓ intracranial pressure Antiemetic	Moderate to severe AMS HACE
Tylenol Aspirin Antiemetics	Symptomatic treatment	AMS
O_2 (to $Sao_2 > 90\%$)	Improves hypoxemia	Moderate to severe AMS. HAPE HACE
Hyperbaric O_2	Improves hypoxemia	Severe AMS HAPE HACE
Nifedipine	Decreases pulmonary artery pressure	HAPE (when O_2 and descent is not possible)

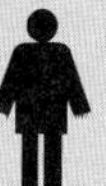

A 50-year-old male complains of a headache, and then abruptly loses consciousness 3 minutes after surfacing from a dive. What is the most likely diagnosis?

This patient has likely experienced an arterial air embolism. Any diver who develops CNS symptoms within 10 minutes of surfacing should be assumed to have an arterial air embolism. Treatment includes administering 100% O_2 by mask, placing victim supine, administering intravenous fluids, and rapid transport for hyperbaric therapy.

DYSBARISM

Dysbarism refers to diving injuries from underwater pressure changes. It is easiest to think of dysbarism in regard to timing of symptom onset (see Table 13.12):

- **Descent dysbarism** ("the squeeze")
- **Dysbarism at depth**:
  - Nitrogen narcosis
  - O_2 toxicity
  - Alternobaric vertigo
- **Ascent dysbarism**:
  - Ascent barotrauma
  - Decompression sickness (DCS)
  - Arterial air embolism

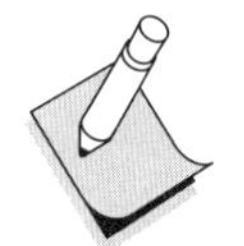

Boyle's law (for any given air space):

PV = k

where P = pressure, V = volume, k = constant; if P increases, V must ↓).

Physiology of Gases

- **Boyle's law** states that as the pressure (P) on a given air space increases, the volume of gas (V) decreases (PV = constant).
- **Henry's law** states that the amount of a gas dissolved in a liquid is directly proportional to the partial pressure of that gas.
- Atmospheric pressure at sea level = 760 mmHg or 1 atm. As one descends to 33 ft (in seawater), the atmospheric pressure ↑ to 2 atm and the volume of air-filled spaces decreases by 50%. For each gas within the space, both the partial pressure and the amount dissolved in solution (eg, blood) will ↑ accordingly.

TABLE 13.12. Types of Dysbarism

Types of Dysbarism
Descent Dysbarism ("the squeeze")
Dysbarism at depth
Nitrogen narcosis
O_2 toxicity
Alternobaric vertigo
Ascent dysbarism
Ascent barotrauma
Decompression sickness
Arterial air embolism

Descent Dysbarism

Descent dysbarism can occur in any air-filled space in the body (see Table 13.13). Overall, middle ear squeeze is the most common manifestation.

Pathophysiology

- ↑ dive depth → increased ambient pressure and "squeeze" (barotrauma) of air-filled spaces in body → symptoms if body unable to equalize pressures.

Treatment

- Depends on location and severity of injuries
  - Most injuries respond to conservative therapy (rest) alone.
- Prophylactic antibiotics if ruptured TM
- Oral steroids if 7th nerve palsy
- Topical nasal decongestants for ear and sinus squeeze
- Recompression therapy is **not** indicated.
- No further diving (until injuries have healed)

Dysbarism at Depth

Nitrogen Narcosis

Nitrogen narcosis occurs when scuba tank air (containing nitrogen and O_2) is breathed at depth. Symptoms of nitrogen narcosis typically occur after the diver has descended to ≥100 ft.

TABLE 13.13. **Descent Dysbarism**

Location of "Squeeze"	Underlying Cause	Symptoms
External ear	Obstruction of external ear canal (**no** ear plugs!)	Ear pain
Middle ear	External pressure on TM not equalized by eustacian tube	Ear pain Hearing loss TM rupture → nystagmus and vertigo Seventh nerve palsy
Inner ear	Transmission of middle ear pressure → rupture of round window	Ear pain Hearing loss Severe nystagmus and vertigo → ataxia and vomiting
Sinus	Obstruction of sinus ostia	Facial pain Epistaxis
Lung	Holding breath during descent	Shortness of breath Hemoptysis Pulmonary edema
Equipment	Tight-fitting mask or wet suit	Petechiae

Pathophysiology

- Increasing dive depth → increased ambient pressure → ↓ volume of tank air (Boyle's law) and ↑ partial pressure of nitrogen in inspired tank air → increased nitrogen dissolved in blood (Henry's law) → symptoms.

Symptoms/Exam

- Altered behavior
- Poor judgment
- Hallucinations and loss of consciousness

Treatment

- Ascend slowly with assistance.
  - Slow ascent is essential to prevent ascent dysbarism (see below).
- Use mixtures with less nitrogen in the inspired tank for dives >100 ft.

Oxygen Toxicity

Results from breathing elevated partial pressures of O_2 for extended periods of time; primarily affects the CNS and lungs

Symptoms/Exam

- Tunnel or blurred vision
- Nausea/vomiting
- Dizziness and paresthesias
- Twitching, seizures

Treatment

- Ascend slowly with assistance.
  - Slow ascent is essential to prevent ascent dysbarism (see below).

Ascent Dysbarism

Ascent Barotrauma

Ascent barotrauma is caused by expansion of gas on ascent from diving.

Pathophysiology

- ↓ In ambient pressure → ↑ in size of air-filled spaces.
- Failure of air to passively exit middle ear due to blocked eustacian tube → **alternobaric vertigo.**
- Breath-holding during ascent → air dissects into pulmonary tissue (subcutaneous emphysema to pneumomediastinum to pneumothorax).

Symptoms/Exam

- **Alternobaric vertigo**
  - Ear pain and possible TM rupture
  - Severe but transient nystagmus and vertigo
    - Nausea/vomiting may occur.
  - Transient hearing loss
- **Pulmonary barotrauma**
  - Shortness of breath
  - Hemoptysis
  - Chest pain

TREATMENT

- Typically resolves with rest
- Supplemental O_2 as needed
- Chest tube for large pneumothorax

ARTERIAL GAS EMBOLISM (AGE)

Arterial gas embolism is a form of pulmonary barotrauma that occurs during or **within 10 minutes** of ascent.

PATHOPHYSIOLOGY

- Overexpanding gas ruptures alveoli → air enters pulmonary venous circulation and travels to L heart and systemic circulation → obstruction to flow and symptoms.

SYMPTOMS/EXAM

- **Cerebral embolization (most common)**
  - Sudden stroke-like symptoms, seizure, loss of consciousness, confusion
- **Coronary artery embolization**
  - Symptoms and findings consistent with acute coronary syndrome

TREATMENT

- 100% O_2 by mask
- Recumbent/supine position
- Intravenous fluids to increase perfusion
- Rapid recompression in hyperbaric O_2 chamber

DECOMPRESSION SICKNESS

Symptoms result from formation of nitrogen bubbles in tissue or vessels. Nitrogen is highly fat soluble leading to CNS symptoms (see Table 13.14 for risk factors).

PATHOPHYSIOLOGY

- As diver ascends → ambient pressure decreases and nitrogen bubbles come out of solution → precipitate and coalesce in blood and tissues.

TABLE 13.14. Risk Factors for Decompression Sickness

Risk factors
Older age
Fatigue or heavy exertion
Dehydration
Obesity
Increased total length and depths of dive(s).
Diving at altitude
Rapid ascent
Flying after diving

SYMPTOMS/EXAM

- Symptoms depend on tissues involved. Typically symptoms begin >10 minutes after surfacing.
- **Type I decompression sickness = "the bends"** (skin, joint, and extremities).
  - Pruritis, erythema, and skin marbling
  - Limb and joint pain
  - Lymphedema
- **Type II decompression sickness** = other organ involvement (CNS, inner ear, lungs).
  - More serious manifestations
  - Mental status changes, headache, visual changes
  - Upper lumbar spine particularly susceptible → weakness, paralysis
  - **"The Staggers"**—inner ear involvement with vertigo, nystagmus, and N/V
  - **"The Chokes"**—dyspnea, cough, chest pain

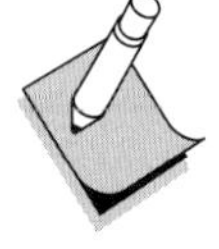

Arterial gas embolism and decompression sickness require hyperbaric therapy.

TREATMENT

- 100% O_2 by mask
- Recumbent/supine position
- Intravenous fluids
- Rapid recompression in hyperbaric chamber

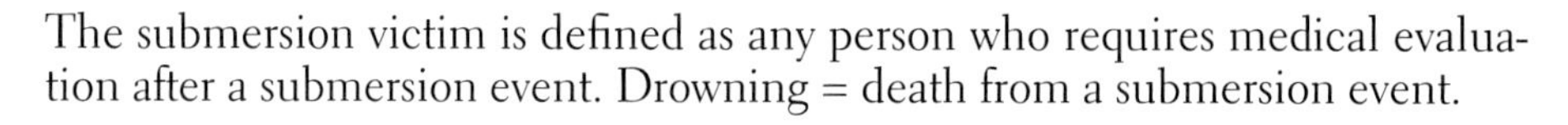

SUBMERSION INJURY

The submersion victim is defined as any person who requires medical evaluation after a submersion event. Drowning = death from a submersion event.

The effect on electrolyte status is the same regardless of seawater (oceans and some lakes) or freshwater (lakes, rivers, pools) drowning.

To contradict earlier beliefs, there appears to be no difference between freshwater and saltwater submersion unless VERY large volume of freshwater is aspirated, where hemodilution and hemolysis is possible.

Precipitating injuries include spinal cord injury, hypothermia, seizure, syncope.

PATHOPHYSIOLOGY

- In the majority of submersion events:
  - Aspiration of water into the lungs → loss of surfactant and alveolar collapse → hypoxia → brain cell death after 3 minutes.
- In 10–15% submersions are "**dry**" → hypothesized due to laryngospasm and bronchospasm (controversial).
- **Diving reflex**: (in young infants) → transiently protective bradycardia, apnea, and peripheral vasoconstriction.
- **Immersion syndrome**: immersion in very cold water → vagally mediated asystolic cardiac arrest.

Respiratory deterioration can be delayed for up to 6 hours.

SYMPTOMS/EXAM

- Respiratory distress with wheezes, rales, or rhonchi on exam
  - May be delayed up to 6 hours ("secondary drowning")
- AMS ranging from confusion to coma
- Hypothermia if cold water submersion
- Cardiac dysrhythmias

DIAGNOSIS

- Focuses on identifying associated injuries or abnormalities
- CXR—if patient symptomatic
- Cardiac monitoring
- Electrolyte studies are rarely helpful.
- Trauma evaluation (as indicated)

TREATMENT

- ABCs and supportive care
- Warm to 32–35°C.
- Treat associated injuries or trauma.
- **Not** shown to improve outcome: hyperventilation, steroids, induced coma, prophylactic antibiotics
- Asymptomatic patients can be discharged home after 4–6 hours of observation.

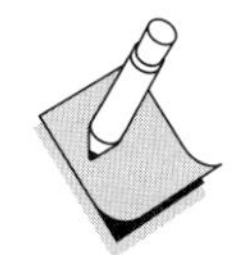

Poor prognostic factors:

Age <3 years

Delay in initiation of CPR

>5 minutes submersion time

Acidosis

GCS 3

Need for ongoing CPR

COMPLICATIONS

- Numerous pulmonary complications—pneumonia, pulmonary edema, pneumonitis, ARDS
- Hemolysis and DIC
- Hypoxia-associated complications—CNS injury, multiorgan injury
- Complete recovery in 48 hours is typical for patients not requiring CPR.

POISONOUS PLANTS

Hundreds of poisonous plants exist. This section will focus on those more commonly encountered (see Table 13.15).

Castor Bean and Jequirity Bean

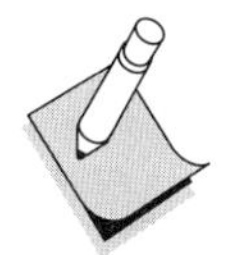

Castor beans contain ricin.

Jequirity beans contain abrin.

The castor bean and jequirity bean (rosary pea) are from the same family and contain potent toxalbumins (**ricin and abrin**, respectively). They are used for ornamental purposes, such as in prayer or rosary beads.

MECHANISM OF TOXICITY

- Chewing of bean → toxin absorption → inhibition of protein synthesis → cytotoxic cellular effects.

SYMPTOMS/EXAM

- **Fever** is the major presenting feature.
- **Delayed GI symptoms** (6 hours to days).
  - Nausea/vomiting, abdominal pain, bloody diarrhea
- Followed by delirium, seizures, liver and renal failure, coma, and death
- Castor beans are antigenic and may cause severe cutaneous hypersensitivity or systemic allergic reactions.

DIAGNOSIS

- Based on history of ingestion/exposure and clinical presentation

TABLE 13.15. Common Poisonous Plants

Plant	Toxin Mechanism of Toxicity	Major Toxic Effects
Castor bean/jequirity bean	Ricin/abrin: Cytotoxic cellular effects	Fever Delayed severe GI symptoms
Water hemlock	Antagonism of GABA	Severe status epilepticus
Azalea	Andromedotoxins: Increased permeability of Na^+ channels	Bradycardia Progressive paralysis
Cardiac glycosides Foxglove Common oleander Yellow oleander Lily of the valley	Inhibition of Na^+-K^+ ATPase pump	Symptoms of digoxin toxicity
Cyanogenic fruit seeds	Amygdalin: Metabolized to hydrocyanic acid	Cyanide poisoning
Nicotine-Containing		
Tobacco plant	Nicotine: Stimulation of nicotinic receptors	Early stimulation Later weakness, paralysis, brachycardia
Poison hemlock	Coniine alkaloids: Stimulation of nicotinic receptors	As above
Anticholinergic		
Jimsonweed	Atropine-like alkaloids: Competitive inhibition of cholinergic receptors	Anticholinergic toxidrome
Deadly nightshade	Atropine-like substance: Inhibition of cholinergic receptors	Anticholinergic toxidrome
Hallucinogenic		
Marijuana	Δ-9-Tetrahydrocannabinol (THC)	Low level: Euphoria High level: Lethargy
Mexican peyote cactus	Mescaline: Similar to LSD	Euphoria, altered perception High doses: sympathomimetic toxicity
Morning glory	D-Lysergic acid amide: Similar to LSD	Hallucinations, dilated pupils

TREATMENT

- Supportive therapy
- Gastric decontamination (consider whole bowel irrigation)
- Replace GI fluid losses with intravenous fluids.
- Electrolyte replacement

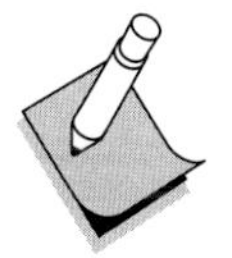

In water hemlock toxicity, seizures are often refractory to standard treatment.

Water Hemlock

Water hemlock grows throughout North America in wetlands or near streams. It is tall with small white flowers.

Toxin = **cicutoxin.**

MECHANISM OF TOXICITY

- Ingestion of plant → antagonism of GABA receptors and symptoms.

SYMPTOMS/EXAM

- Rapid onset of symptoms after ingestion
- Nausea/vomiting, abdominal pain
- Mental status changes and **severe status epilepticus**
- Death

TREATMENT

- Supportive and aggressive gastric decontamination
- Standard treatment for status epitepticus

Azalea

Exposure from ingestion of plant or contaminated honey

Toxin = andromedotoxins.

MECHANISM OF TOXICITY

- Ingestion → increased permeability of Na^+ channels.

SYMPTOMS/EXAM

- Nausea/vomiting
- Bradycardia, hypotension
- Progressive paralysis
- Death (rare)

TREATMENT

- GI decontamination
- Supportive care
- Atropine as needed for bradycardia

Cardiac Glycosides

Cardiac glycosides include:

- Foxglove (*Digitalis purpurea*)
- Common oleander (*Nerium oleander*)
- Yellow oleander (*Thevetia peruviana*)
- Lily of the valley (*Convallaria majalis*)

Foxglove contains digoxin; the others are structurally similar to digoxin.

Mechanism of Toxicity

- Inhibit the Na^+-K^+ ATPase pump.

Digoxin toxicity is covered in detail in Toxicology (see Chapter 6).

Cyanogenic Plants

Cyanide poisoning may result after ingesting large numbers of pits/seeds of a variety of fruits, including:

- Peach pits
- Apricot pits
- Pear seeds
- Crab apple seeds

Mechanism of Toxicity

- Amygdalin, a cyanogenic glycoside, is metabolized by the enzyme emulsin to **hydrocyanic** acid.
- Hydrocyanic acid may lead to acute cyanide toxicity.

Symptoms/Exam

- Acute toxicity = cyanide poisoning (see Chapter 6, Toxicology)
  - Delayed symptom onset because cyanide is released by metabolism
  - Nausea/vomiting
  - Shortness of breath
  - Headache
  - Cardiovascular collapse
- Chronic ingestion → polyneuropathies.

Treatment

- GI decontamination
- Cyanide antidote kit for acute toxicity

Nicotine-Containing Plants

Tobacco Plant

Tobacco plants contain the toxin **nicotine**. Common methods of use include cigarette smoking, cigar smoking, pipe smoking, and smokeless tobacco (snuff).

MECHANISM OF TOXICITY

- Ingestion or large skin exposure → stimulation of nicotinic receptors and symptoms.

SYMPTOMS/EXAM

- Characterized by early stimulation, followed by inhibition
- **Early stimulation**
  - Abdominal pain, nausea/vomiting
  - Salivation, bronchorrhea
  - Hypertension, tachycardia
  - Fasciculations, seizures
- **Inhibition**
  - Weakness
  - Respiratory muscle paralysis
  - Bradycardia and death

TREATMENT

- GI decontamination with activated charcoal
- **Atropine** as needed to control secretions
- **Benzodiazepines** to control agitation and seizures
- Supportive care

POISON HEMLOCK (CONIUM MACULATUM)

Poison hemlock grows along roads, ditches, and pasture areas throughout the United States. At first glance, its appearance is similar to water hemlock.

Toxin = **coniine alkaloids,** which are structurally similar to nicotine.

MECHANISM OF TOXICITY

- Ingestion of plant → stimulation of nicotinic receptors and symptoms.

Presentation and treatment as with tobacco plant exposure, above

Anticholinergic Plants

JIMSONWEED (*DATURA STRAMONIUM*)

Also known as Jamestown weed and locoweed, jimsomweed is commonly found along roadsides and in cornfields and pastures. It has broad green leaves, light purple trumpetlike flowers, and large spiny seeds. It is used intentionally for its hallucinogenic properties.

Toxin = **atropinelike** (**belladonna**) **alkaloids**.

MECHANISM OF TOXICITY

- Ingestion → competitive inhibition of cholinergic receptors.

SYMPTOMS/EXAM

- **Anticholinergic toxidrome**
  - Hallucinations
  - Hyperthermia
  - Flushed skin, dry skin, and mucous membranes
  - Mydriasis
  - Tachycardia
  - Urinary retention

TREATMENT

- Supportive (intravenous fluids, external cooling)
- Gastric decontamination (charcoal or whole bowel irrigation)
- Sedation with **benzodiazepines**
- **Physostigimine**
  - Cholinesterase inhibitor
  - Use in severe cases (failure of benzodiazepines).
  - Complications include AV block, asystole.

DEADLY NIGHTSHADE (*ATROPA BELLADONNA*)

Deadly nightshade is a black-cherry-like fruit that contains an atropine-like substance. Its Latin name means "pretty woman."

MECHANISM OF TOXICITY

Ingestion → inhibition of cholinergic receptors.

Presentation and treatment are similar to jimsonweed.

Hallucinogenic Plants

MARIJUANA: HEMP PLANT (*CANNABIS SATIVA*)

The active ingredient of marijuana is Δ-9-tetrahydrocannabinol. It can be either smoked or eaten.

SYMPTOMS/EXAM

- **Low level exposure**
  - Somnolence, euphoria, heightened sensory awareness, feeling of well-being, alteration of time perception, and paranoia
- **High level exposure**
  - Lethargy, decreased coordination, and ataxia
- Abstinence syndrome
  - Agitation, apprehension, and insomnia

DIAGNOSIS

- May be detected on urine toxicology screen

TREATMENT

- GI decontamination, if large ingestion
- Supportive care
- Benzodiazepines for agitation

COMPLICATIONS

- Severe hypertension, hyperthermia, seizures, or rhabdomyolysis

MESCALINE

Mescaline is a hallucinogenic alkaloid found in the **Mexican peyote cactus** *Lophophora williamsii.*

SYMPTOMS/EXAM

- Similar to LSD
- Euphoria, alerted perception, nystagmus, and ataxia
- Nausea/vomiting, abdominal pain
- In high doses—sympathomimetic toxicity (see Chapter 6, Toxicology)
  - Diaphoresis
  - Hypertension, tachycardia
  - Mydriasis
  - Hyperthermia

TREATMENT/COMPLICATIONS

As with marijuana, above

MORNING GLORY (*IPOMOEA VIOLACEA*)

Seeds of this plant contain D-lysergic acid amide, a compound related to LSD.

SYMPTOMS/EXAM

- Hallucinations
- Dilated pupils
- Nausea/vomiting, diarrhea
- Numbness of extremities and muscle tightness

TREATMENT/COMPLICATIONS

As with marijuana, above

GASTROINTESTINAL IRRITANTS

- **Holly (*Iiex galabra*)**—toxic berries
- **Pokeweed (*Phytolacca americana*)**—entire plant is toxic

SYMPTOMS/EXAM

- Abdominal pain, nausea/vomiting, diarrhea
- Death (rare)

TREATMENT

- GI decontamination and supportive care

A 54-year-old male presents to the ED with nausea/vomiting and abdominal pain. He reports eating some "unusual" mushrooms while out in the woods earlier in the day, but felt fine until about 7 hours later when the GI symptoms started. What can you tell this patient about his likelihood of having a serious mushroom poisoning?

Assuming his symptoms are due to ingestion of mushrooms, the onset of symptoms are > 6 hours since the time of ingestion, indicating a potential for serious toxicity. Depending on the species, hepatotoxicity, renal toxicity or seizures could develop. Consultation with a local mycologist may help determine the likely species.

MUSHROOMS

Mushroom toxicity may occur during experimental ingestions by patients looking for a "high" or in foragers who misidentify the species. The toxic dose is unknown and the amount of toxin varies widely among mushrooms.

Amanita sp. *causes most deaths.*

Mushroom toxicity can be divided into two groups based on the onset of symptoms: Early onset toxicity and delayed onset toxicity.

Early Onset Toxicity

Symptom onset 0–4 hours after mushroom ingestion typically indicates a benign course. The presentation varies with the type of mushroom ingested (see Table 13.16).

Gastrointestinal Symptoms

- Seen with many mushroom species
- Sx/Exam: Nausea/vomiting, diarrhea, abdominal pain

Muscarinic Symptoms

- Seen with *Clitocybe* sp., *Inocybe* sp.
- Sx/Exam: Symptoms of cholinergic (SLUDGE) syndrome: Excessive secretions, urination, ↑ GI motility, bradycardia

CNS Excitation

- Seen with *Amanita muscaria*
- Sx/Exam: Intoxication, dizziness, and anticholinergic effects (dry mouth/skin, mydriasis, tachycardia)

Hallucinations

- Seen with *Psilicybe* and other psilocybin-containing mushrooms
- Caused by toxin psilocybin, an LSD-like serotonin stimulator
- Sx/Exam: Visual hallucinations

Disulfiram-Like Reaction (with Coingestion of ETOH)

- Seen with *Coprinus* sp.
- Caused by toxin coprine, which inhibits ADH
- Sx/Exam: Headache, flushing, tachycardia, hyperventilation

TABLE 13.16. Mushroom Toxicity

CLINICAL SYMPTOMS	REPRESENTATIVE MUSHROOM	TOXIN	TREATMENT
Early Onset (0–4 hours)			
Gastrointestinal	Many species		Supportive and symptomatic
Muscarinic (SLUDGE)	*Cytocybe* sp. *Inocybe* sp.	Muscarine	Atropine for bradycardia and bronchorrhea
CNS excitation	*Amanita mucarinia*	Muscimol, ibotenic acid	Supportive and symptomatic
Hallucinations	*Psilocybe* sp.	Psilocybin	Supportive Benzodiazepines
Disulfarim-like reaction	*Coprinus* sp.	Coprine (with ETOH)	Supportive Benzodiazepines
Delayed Onset (6–24 hours)			
Gastroenteritis followed by hepatotoxicity	*Amanita phalloides* *Gyrometra* sp.	Amatoxins, phallotoxins Gyromitrin	Supportive and symptomtic May require transplant Supportive
Gastroenteritis followed by seizures			Benzodiazepines **Pyridoxine**
Gastroenteritis followed by renal failure	*Cortinarius orellanus*	Orellanine	Supportive May require hemodialysis

Delayed Onset Toxicity

Delayed onset toxicity is a marker for ingestion of mushrooms with potential for serious toxicity. In these cases GI symptoms (nausea/vomiting, diarrhea) do not begin until 6–24 hours after ingestion and are followed by liver, CNS, or renal toxicity:

GI Effects Followed by Hepatotoxicity

- Seen with *Amanita phalloides*
- Caused by amatoxins and phallotoxins
- Sx/Exam: Delayed nausea/vomiting and diarrhea followed by hepatic failure in 72 hours

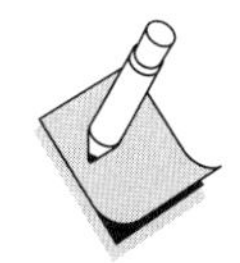

Mushroom toxicity: Early onset GI symptoms → benign course. Delayed onset GI symptoms → potential for serious toxicity.

GI Effects Followed by Seizures

- Seen with *Gyromitra* sp.
- Caused by gyromitrin toxin which **inhibits pyridoxine-dependent pathways and depletes GABA (similar to INH overdose)**
- Sx/Exam: Delayed nausea/vomiting and diarrhea followed by seizures

GI Effects Followed by Renal Failure

- *Cortinarius orellanus*
- Caused by orellanine toxin, a nephrotoxin
- Sx/Exam: Delayed nausea/vomiting and diarrhea followed by renal failure

Treatment

- Observe for development of early onset symptoms (4–6 hours).
- If no early onset symptoms, have patient return if delayed symptoms develop.
- Mainstay of therapy is supportive care.
- **Monitor *glucose*** (hypoglycemia is common).
- Atropine if symptomatic bradycardia or bronchorrhea from muscarinic syndrome
- Benzodiazepines to control agitation
- Pyridoxine: For delayed onset seizures (inhibition of pyridoxine-dependent pathways)

CHAPTER 14

Head, Eye, Ear, Nose, and Throat Emergencies

Manon Kwon, MD

EAR

Otitis Externa (Swimmer's Ear)

ETIOLOGY

- Bacterial agents—*Pseudomonas aeruginosa, Staphylococcus aureus*, Gram-negative rods
- Fungal agents—*Aspergillus, Candida*
- Increased in divers, swimmers, and regions with high humidity

SYMPTOMS/EXAM

- External ear pain
- Pain when tragus/auricle is pulled
- Localized lymphadenopathy
- Itching or burning inside the ear canal (especially if fungal)
- Exudative discharge from the ear canal
- Conductive hearing loss if severe

TREATMENT

- Suction and gentle warm irrigation of the canal are indicated.
- Administer 2% acetic acid solution or alternative drying medication (do not use if TM is ruptured).
- Topical antibiotic drops with steroid is first-line therapy (use neomycin/polymyxin/hydrocortisone otic suspension **not** solution if TM ruptured).
- If TM rupture, consider oral antibiotics (quinolones, cephalosporins, or penicillinase-resistant penicillins).
- Consider a wick to facilitate drainage and delivery of antibiotics.

COMPLICATIONS

- Mastoiditis or other cartilage/bone involvement
- Meningitis
- **Malignant otitis externa**—progression of otitis externa to cause infection of ear cartilage or osteomyelitis of the skull base (see Figure 14.1):
  - Not a malignancy
  - May see cranial nerve palsies
  - Usually occurs in immunocompromised patients or diabetics
  - ***P. aeuruginosa*** is the most common cause.
  - *Aspergillus* is the most common fungal cause.
  - IV antibiotics and admission

Acute Otitis Media

ETIOLOGY

- Viral is most common.
- Bacterial agents: *Haemophilus influenzae, Streptococcus pneumoniae, Mycoplasma pneumoniae* (bullous myringitis), *Moraxella catarrhalis*, group A strep
- Usually in children <7 years old

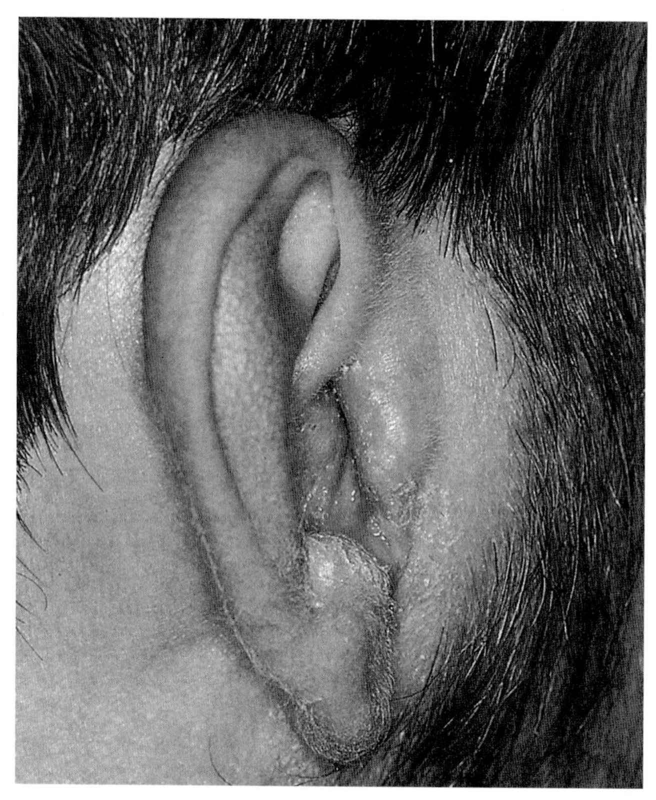

FIGURE 14.1. Malignant otitis externa.

(Courtesy of Frank Birinyi, MD as published in Knoop KJ, Stack LB, Storrow AB. *Atlas of Emergency Medicine,* 2nd ed. New York: McGraw-Hill, 2002:125.)

Symptoms/Exam

- Onset within 48 hours
- Fever, ear pain (otalgia), and otorrhea
- Conductive hearing loss
- Peripheral vertigo
- Red or cloudy tympanic membrane, possible effusion
- Bulging or retracted TM
- **Loss of TM mobility on insufflation (pneumatic otoscopy)**
- Loss of light reflex (see Figure 14.2)

Treatment

- Antipyretics, analgesics, ± antibiotics
- Some guidelines recommend delaying administration of antibiotics for 24–72 hours until patient is reassessed or reserving antibiotics for patients with fever or vomiting.
- Follow-up in 3–5 days
- Recurrent OM may require ENT referral for myringotomy.

Complications

- Hearing loss may affect speech and cause developmental delay.
- Mastoiditis
- TM perforation (most common complication)

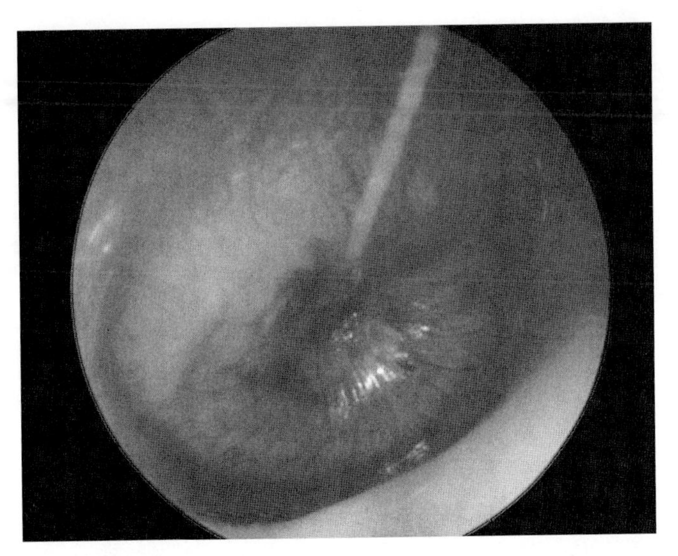

FIGURE 14.2. **Otitis media with red, bulging tympanic membrane. (See also color insert.)**

(Courtesy of Richard A. Chole, MD, PhD as published in Knoop KJ, Stack LB, Storrow AB. *Atlas of Emergency Medicine*, 2nd ed. New York: McGraw-Hill, 2002:118.)

- Meningitis (most common intracranial complication)
- Brain abscess, encephalitis, subdural emphysema
- Venous sinus thrombosis

Auricular Hematoma

Etiology

Accumulation of blood after blunt trauma

Symptoms/Exam

Hematoma and swelling of ear (see Figure 14.3)

Treatment

- Aspirate blood or I+D.
- Apply conforming pressure dressing and recheck in 24 hours.

Complications

- Reaccumulation of blood → cauliflower ear deformity.
- Infection

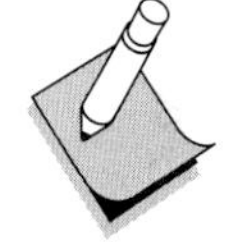

Exposed cartilage is dead cartilage. The primary goals in managing an ear laceration are (1) approximate the cartilage with absorbable suture and (2) cover the cartilage with skin.

Ear Foreign Bodies

Etiology

Insects, cleaning materials (Q tips), anything a child can put in an ear

Symptoms/Exam

- Pain
- Decrease or change in hearing
- Malodorous or purulent discharge
- Direct visualization of object

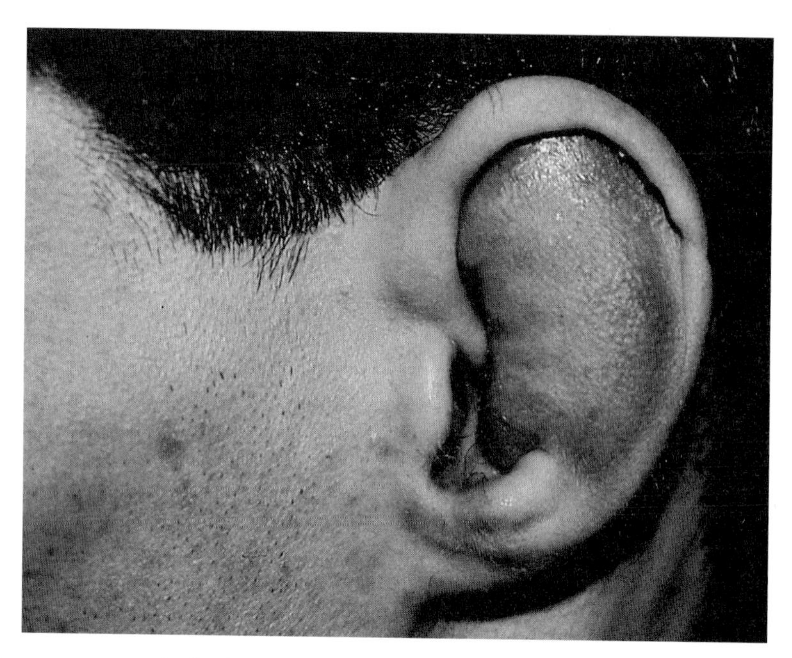

FIGURE 14.3. Auricular hematoma.

(Courtesy of C. Bruce Macdonald, MD as published in Knoop KJ, Stack LB, Storrow AB. *Atlas of Emergency Medicine*, 2nd ed. New York: McGraw-Hill, 2002:20.)

Treatment

- If alive, consider lidocaine or alcohol to sedate the insect before attempting extraction.
- Do not irrigate absorbent material (vegetables) or batteries.
- Remove FB with probe, forceps, or irrigation (use of cyanoacrylate glue on the tip of a paper clip has also been described).
- Postextraction, always reexamine to rule out TM perforation, canal damage, ossicle bone damage.
- Topical antibiotics are recommended postextraction if canal damaged.
- If unable to remove an ear foreign body, immediate consultation should be obtained for patients with severe pain, suspected TM rupture, embedded button battery or evidence of infection. Otherwise, 24-hour follow-up is acceptable.

Tympanic Membrane Perforation

Etiology

- Penetrating object
- Complication of infection (acute otitis media, myringitis)
- Blast injury (explosion, slap, or lightening)
- Barometric pressure changes (flying or scuba diving)

Symptoms/Exam

- Pars tensa most common area of the TM to perforate (thinnest part, anterior and inferior)
- Pain and decreased hearing (conductive hearing loss)
- Bleeding may be present (see Figure 14.4).

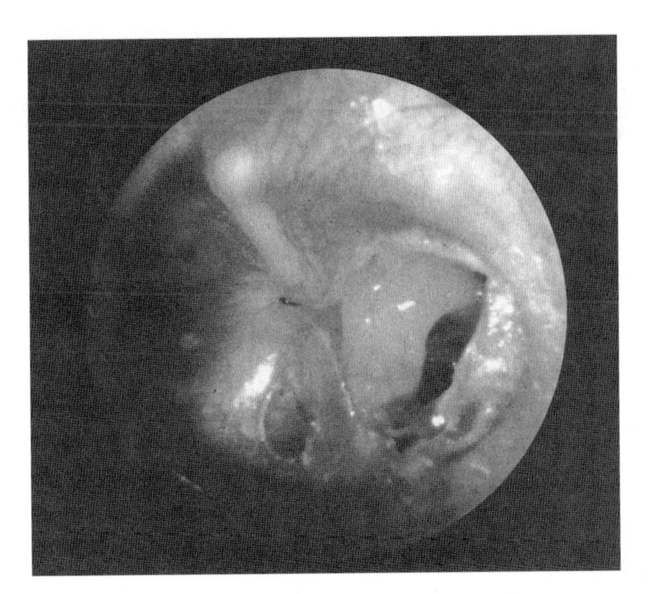

FIGURE 14.4. Tympanic membrane perforation.

(Courtesy of Richard A. Chole, MD, PhD as published in Knoop KJ, Stack LB, Storrow AB. *Atlas of Emergency Medicine*, 2nd ed. New York: McGraw-Hill, 2002:124.)

TREATMENT

- Keep ear dry.
- Analgesics
- Follow-up ENT
- Antibiotics if contaminated or infected (diving and rupture in seawater)
- Most heal in a few months (90%).

COMPLICATIONS

- Facial nerve palsy
- Vertigo
- Hearing loss

Hearing Loss

There are two types of hearing loss: sensorineural or conductive.

SYMPTOMS/EXAM

- **Rinne test:** A 512-Hz tuning fork is placed on the mastoid then placed next to external auditory canal. Normally, air conduction is better than bone. If the patient hears the sound better when the fork is placed on the mastoid, this indicates a **conductive hearing** loss in this ear.
- **Weber test:** The tuning fork is placed on the **center of the forehead**. The sound should be equal in both ears. If unequal, the side where the sound is heard better is the source of a conductive hearing problem. The side where the sound is heard less is the source of a sensorineural hearing problem (see Figure 14.5).

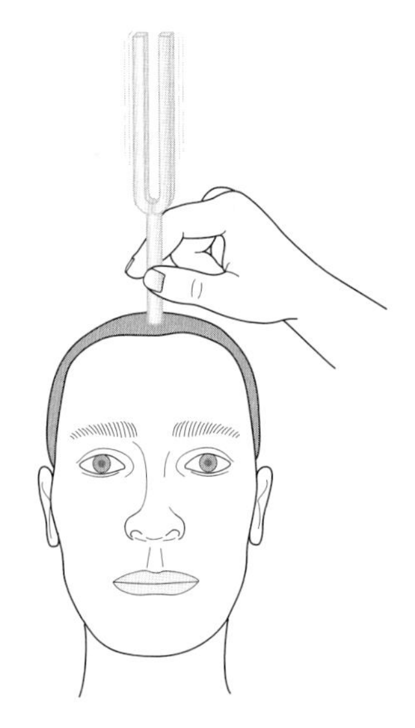

FIGURE 14.5. Weber test.

(Reproduced, with permission, from Stone CK, Humphries, RL. *Current Emergency Diagnosis and Treatment*, 5th ed. New York: McGraw-Hill, 2004:629.)

MENIERE DISEASE

Increased volume of endolymph causing unilateral sensorineural hearing loss, vertigo, tinnitus

> ***The two tests for hearing loss:***
>
> Rinne **Rings** next to the ear.
> Weber begins with **W**, which has a center point: Put the tuning fork in the center of the forehead.

LABYRINTHITIS

Infection or inflammation of labyrinth (viral mumps, measles, zoster, trauma, allergic); see peripheral vertigo, hearing loss, tinnitus, nystagmus

ACOUSTIC NEUROMA

Unilateral hearing loss, unilateral tinnitus, vertigo

OTOTOXIC AGENTS

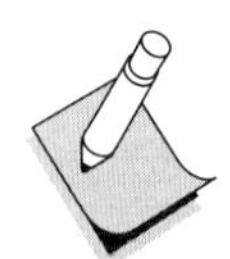

The most common cause of unilateral hearing loss is cerumen impaction.

Tinnitus and hearing loss:

- Loop diuretics
- Salicylates (usually chronic toxicity)
- NSAIDs
- Quinine
- Antibiotics (aminoglycosides, erythromycin, vancomycin)
- Chemotherapeutics

NOSE

Epistaxis

Epistaxis is a common ED complaint. Most anterior bleeds can be treated with packing and recheck in 48 hours. Posterior-bleed epistaxis and hypertension is debated, but it is reasonable to treat the BP of patients with very high BP and persistent bleeding (see Figure 14.6).

CAUSES

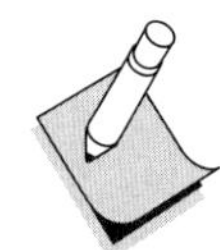

Digital trauma is the most common cause of epistaxis.

- Trauma (digital trauma, fractures)
- Infection, inflammation (sinusitis, rhinitis)
- Foreign body
- Desiccation (cold, dry winter air)
- Postsurgical bleeding.
- Hypertension
- Ischemia due to atherosclerois, insufflation (cocaine, meth)
- Systemic disease (vasculitis, Osler-Weber-Rendu syndrome)
- Bleeding disorders (hemophilia, von Willebrand, drug-induced coagulopathy)
- Polyps

ANTERIOR EPISTAXIS

SYMPTOMS/EXAM

- **Ninety** percent of all nosebleeds are anterior. **Eighty** percent are from Kiesselbach plexus (also known as Little area), an anastomotic zone on the anterior-inferior septal wall.
- Site can be directly visualized.
- Typically stops with pressure
- Is more common in children

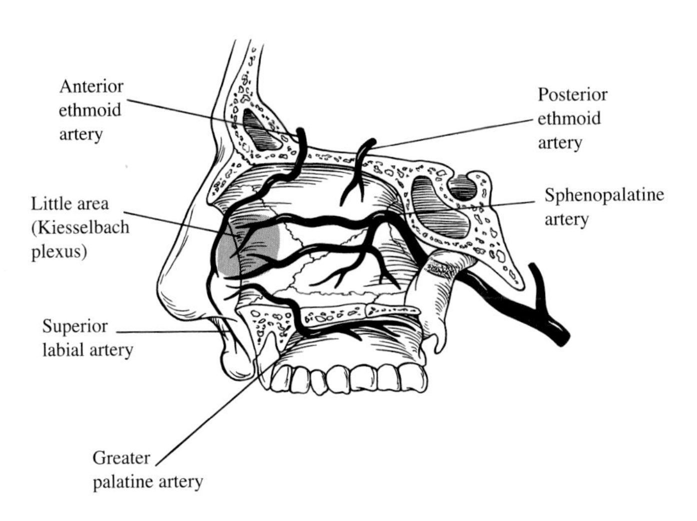

FIGURE 14.6. Arteries that contribute to anterior and posterior epistaxis.

(Reproduced, with permission, from Tintinalli JE, Kelen GD, Stapczynski SJ. *Emergency Medicine: A Comprehensive Study Guide*, 6th ed. New York: McGraw-Hill, 2004:1477.)

TREATMENT

- Direct pressure
- Expel clots (spit and blow).
- Soaked pledgets (lidocaine plus oxymetolazine, neosynephrine, or cocaine)
- Cauterize with silver nitrate 5–7 seconds max, then apply surgicel or bacitracin ointment. Avoid cauterizing both sides of the nasal septum.
- Oral antibiotics if packing placed
- Anterior packing with <10-cm tampon; remove in 2 days

> ***Four arteries of Kiesselbach***
>
> **PLE**xu**S:**
> Greater **P**alatine
> Superior **L**abial
> Anterior **E**thmoid
> **S**phenopalatine

COMPLICATIONS

Sinusitis, toxic shock syndrome, septal necrosis, rebleed

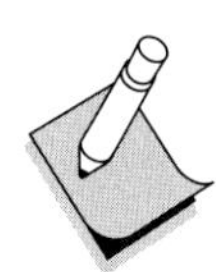

For traumatic nasal bleeding that is continuous, consider basilar skull fracture.

Posterior Epistaxis

SYMPTOMS/EXAM

- **Five** to **ten** percent of all nosebleeds
- More common in **older patients**
- Common causes: Atherosclerosis, coagulopathy, HTN
- Source is from Woodruff plexus: Anastomosis of posterior nasal, posterior ethmoid, **sphenopalatine**, and ascending pharyngeal arteries over the posterior middle turbinate
- Bilateral nasal bleeding, blood in the back of the throat, inability to visualize source or stop bleeding with anterior pack suggests posterior source

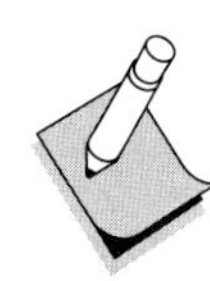

*Most common site of bleeding from the **posterior** region is the posterior lateral branch of the **sphenopalatine artery.***

TREATMENT

- First try anterior epistaxis techniques.
- Pack with posterior nasal gauze pack or 10-cm balloon tampon.

- May require 16f Foley with clamp to hold in place or two chamber intranasal balloons
- With few exceptions, patients with posterior nasal packing should receive broad-spectrum antibiotics and be admitted.
- Posterior nasal packing should be left in place for 72–96 hours.

COMPLICATIONS

- Sinusitis
- Necrosis of septum and soft palate
- Respiratory suppression with hypoxia, hypercarbia due to nasopulmonary reflex
- Bradycardia, dysrhythmias, and aspiration have been reported with posterior packing.

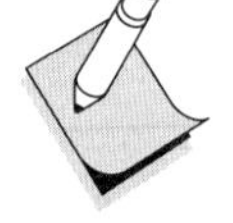

Admit patients with posterior nasal packing.

Foreign Body

A foreign body presents with unilateral foul-smelling discharge. There are various methods to extract, but if you cannot do it safely, discharge with ENT referral within 24 hours.

FACIAL TRAUMA

Fifty percent of facial trauma is caused by MVCs. This contribution has decreased with the use of seatbelts and airbags. After assessing the ABCs, the goals are to identify fractures (10% incidence of associated C-spine fractures), assess neurologic injuries, and identify/treat threats to vision.

Nasal Fracture

Nasal fracture is the most common maxillofacial fracture (#2 is mandible fracture). It is usually secondary to blunt trauma (see Figure 14.7A).

SYMPTOMS/EXAM

- Evaluate the nasal bones and facial area for swelling, tenderness, mobility, crepitus, deformity, and step-offs.
- Evaluate septum for hematoma, checking for a "dark clot" (see Figure 14.7B).

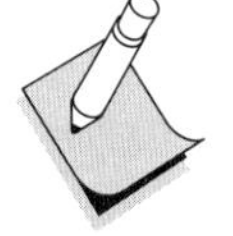

Evaluate all patients with nasal trauma for septal hematoma. Drain septal hematomas to prevent abscess formation and cartilage necrosis.

DIAGNOSIS

- A clinical diagnosis
- X-rays are insensitive and unnecessary for simple nasal fractures.

TREATMENT

- Ice to reduce swelling
- Follow up with plastics or ENT in a few weeks for cosmetic issues.
- Discharge home with pain medications, intermittent ice application, and nasal decongestants.
- Septal hematoma: I+D/pack, Doyle splint, or a bilateral pressure pack

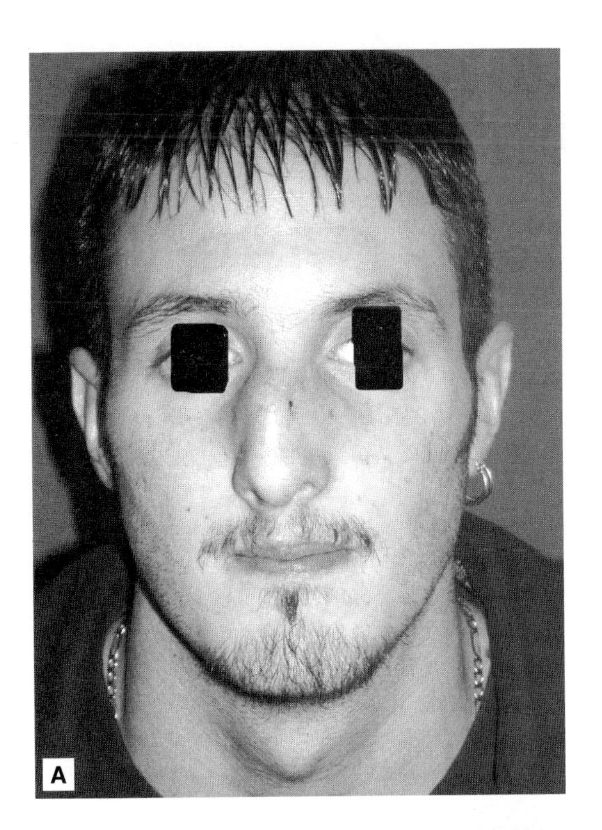

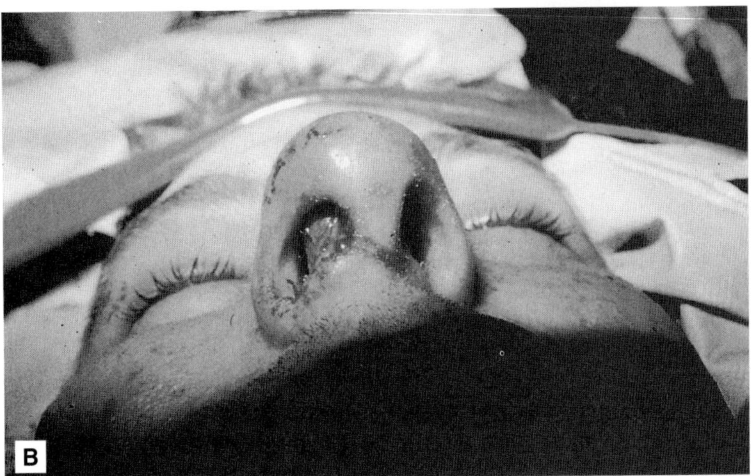

FIGURE 14.7. (A) Nasal fracture. (B) Nasal hematoma.

(A) (Reproduced, with permission, from Lalwani AK. *Current Diagnosis & Treatment in Otolaryngology: Head and Neck Surgery*, 2nd ed. New York: McGraw-Hill, 2008:251.)
(B) (Reproduced, with permission, from Knoop KJ, Stack LB, Storrow AB. *Atlas of Emergency Medicine*, 2nd ed. New York: McGraw-Hill, 2002:9.)

COMPLICATIONS

Nasal fractures may be associated with:

- CSF rhinorrhea (fracture of cribiform plate of ethmoid bone)
- Basilar skull fracture
- Untreated septal hematomas that can lead to abscess formation, necrosis, or septal perforation
- Septal damage that can lead to a saddle nose deformity

Basilar Skull Fracture

Symptoms/Exam

- A linear fracture at the base of the skull (longitudinal are the most common)
- Clinical findings include: Battle sign, raccoon eyes, hemotypanum (80%), and CSF rhinorrhea or otorrhea (15%) (see Figure 14.8).
- CSF rhinorrhea may be increased with jugular compression or leaning forward. The ring or halo sign seen on filter paper or bed sheet refers to an area of fluid beyond an area of blood and indicates the presence of CSF (not just snot).
- Additional testing for CSF includes fluid glucose (elevated compared to tears or nasal secretions) or B2 transferrin (most specific).

Diagnostics

- Skull X-ray positive in <50% (no longer used)
- CT scan with 1- to 3-mm cuts

Treatment

- ENT/neurosurgery consult
- Prophylactic antibiotics may be given, although there is not conclusive evidence that prophylaxis decreases rates of meningitis.
- Most fractures are nondisplaced and heal without surgical intervention.

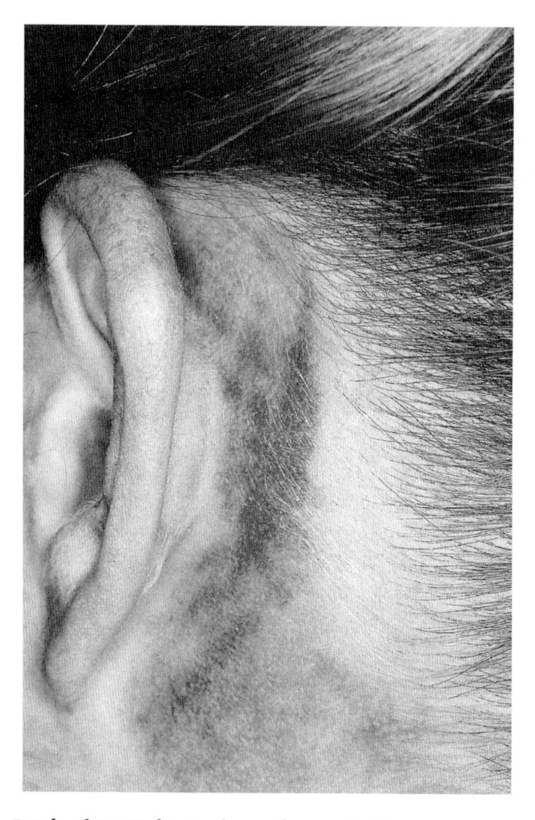

FIGURE 14.8. Battle sign: Ecchymosis on the mastoid area.

(Courtesy of Frank Birinyi, MD as published in Knoop KJ, Stack LB, Storrow AB. *Atlas of Emergency Medicine*, 2nd ed. New York: McGraw-Hill, 2002:4.)

COMPLICATIONS

Meningitis is estimated to occur in 5–10% of patients. Rates are higher in patients with CSF otorrhea or rhinorrhea.

Orbital Blowout Fracture

MECHANISM OF INJURY

- Ball or fist pushes globe, and pressure from the globe fractures the **orbital floor** down into maxillary sinus or through the lamina papyracea into the ethmoid sinus.
- Blunt trauma to orbital rim → buckle fracture of orbital floor—less likely globe injury.

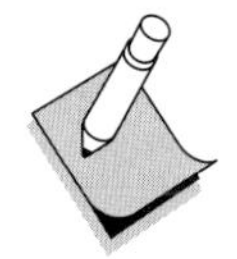

Blowout fracture with entrapment syndrome usually involves the orbital floor with entrapment of the ***inferior rectus muscle****.*

SYMPTOMS/EXAM

- Swelling, ecchymosis, and tenderness of the periorbital region or infraorbital rim (see Figure 14.9)
- Pain and diplopia may be present.
- Numb cheek or upper lip (infraorbital nerve involvement)
- Approximately 30% have associated ocular injury.
- Assess for bleeding in ipsilateral nare.

DIAGNOSIS

- Water's view shows opacity in the roof of the maxillary sinus and air-fluid level indicating fluid/blood in the affected sinus.
- Facial CT (1–3 mm axial and coronal cuts) is more sensitive than Water's view (outdated).

TREATMENT

- Ice to reduce swelling (may resolve entrapment)
- ENT consult if entrapment present
- Antibiotics
- Tetanus
- Ophthalmology consult to rule out ocular injury or if entrapment is suspected

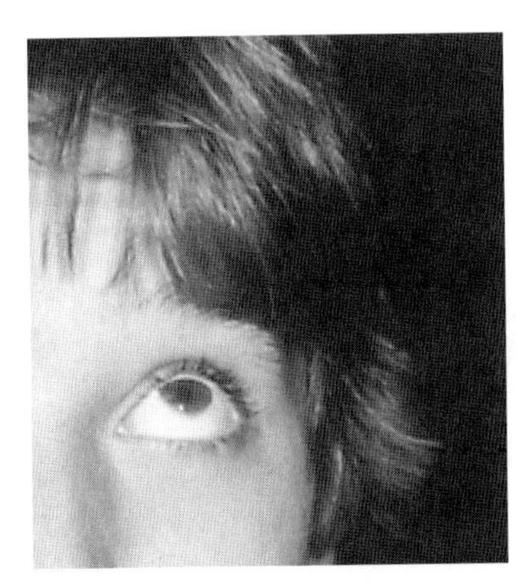

FIGURE 14.9. Entrapment of the inferior rectus after an orbital blowout fracture of the patient's left eye.

(Reproduced, with permission, from Riordan-Eva P, Whitcher JP. *Vaughan & Asbury's General Ophthalmology*, 16th ed. New York: McGraw-Hill, 2004:378.)

Mandible Fracture

- Second most common maxillofacial fracture (after nasal fractures) (see Figure 14.10)
- More common in males than females
- Most common fracture site: Condyle > body > symphysis
- Often two or more sites are fractured.
- Significant force is required to fracture the symphysis.

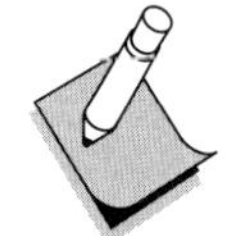

In victims of MVCs, the presence of a mandible fracture should prompt evaluation for an upper cervical spine injury.

Symptoms/Exam

- Blunt trauma is most common mechanism (fall, MVC, assault).
- Pain and swelling of jaw, asymmetry, step-off
- Trismus, malocclusion, deformity, bleeding
- Check mental nerve (lower incisors, lower lip, or chin anesthesia).
- Sublingual or buccal ecchymosis (pathognomonic)
- Blood in the auditory meatus may be seen with a condylar fracture.

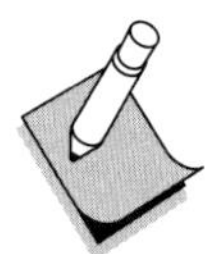

If mandible deviates toward the side with pain → fracture. If mandible deviates away from side with pain → dislocation.

Diagnosis

- When a patient bites down on a tongue blade, you should be able to twist the blade until it breaks. Inability to break the tongue blade because the patient can't hold it tight enough suggests fracture.
- Plain X-rays or mandible series usually confirm diagnosis.
- Panorex X-ray may be preferred by consultant (see Figure 14.11A).
- Consider CXR to rule out aspiration of teeth.
- Consider facial CT for evaluation of possible associated injuries.

Treatment

- Remember ABCs first!
- Maintain C-spine precautions until assessed.

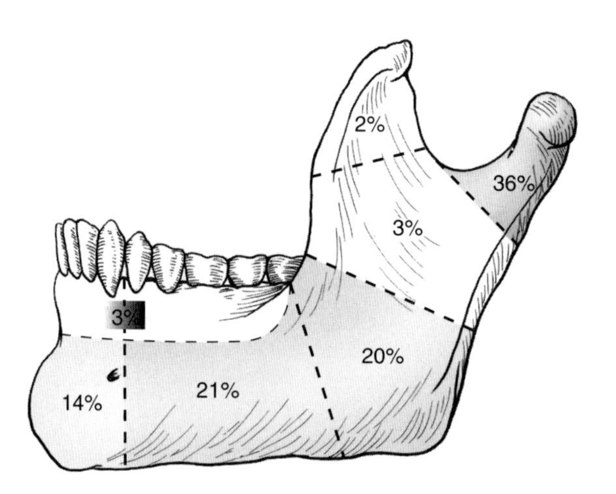

FIGURE 14.10. Distribution of fractures to the mandible.

(Reproduced, with permission, from Brunicardi FC, Andersen DK, Billiar TR, et al. *Schwartz's Principles of Surgery*, 8th ed. McGraw-Hill, 2005:513.)

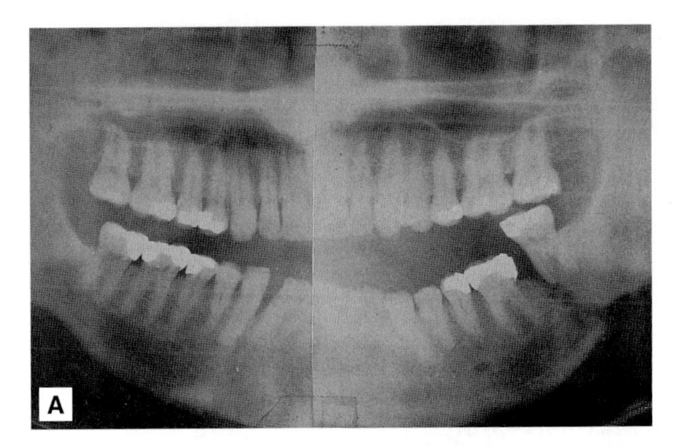

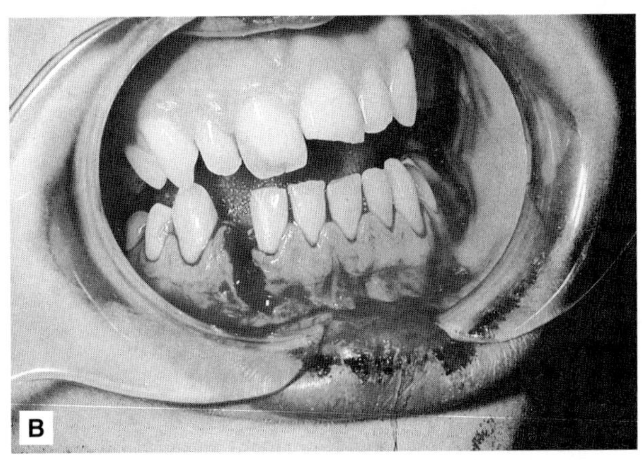

FIGURE 14.11. (A) Panorex X-ray of mandible body fracture. (B) Open mandible fracture.

(Courtesy of Edward S. Amrhein, DDS as printed in Knoop KJ, Stack LB, Storrow AB. *Atlas of Emergency Medicine*, 2nd ed. New York: McGraw-Hill, 2002:17 and 18.)

- Airway compromise may result from soft-tissue swelling and lack of tongue support from a flail mandible (bilateral mandibular body fractures).
- OMFS or ENT consult for disposition
- All open fractures (blood in mouth) require a consult and antibiotics.
- If discharged, remember to give pain meds, soft diet, and appropriate follow-up with OMFS/ENT.
- Tetanus if needed

COMPLICATIONS

- Airway compromise
- Malocclusion
- Mental nerve damage (anesthesia of the lower lip)
- Infection/osteomyelitis secondary to an open fracture

Mandibular Dislocation

- Patients usually give a history of wide mouth opening (such as with yawning or laughing) as the cause of their dislocation.
- The mandible is displaced forward and superiorly with the condyle anterior to the articular eminence, resulting in a protruding chin.
- Dislocation may be unilateral or bilateral.

SYMPTOMS/EXAM

- Malocclusion with an anterior open bite
- Pain, inability to close jaw, difficulty speaking

TREATMENT

- Reduce dislocation in a C-shaped maneuver (downward pressure on the back of the third molars and slight upward pressure on the symphysis of the mandible) (see Figure 14.12).
- Postreduction X-ray is used to rule out fracture and verify reduction.

Zygomatico-Maxillary-Orbital Complex Fracture

Tripod fractures are fractures of the zygoma (also known as cheek bone or malar bone). The fracture results from a direct blow to the zygoma (MVC or assault). The term tripod refers to the three fracture sites: (1) the zygomatic-frontal suture, (2) connection to the inferior orbit floor and rim, and (3) the zygomatic-temporal suture (zygomatic arch). See Figure 14.13.

SYMPTOMS/EXAM

- Facial flattening and asymmetry
- Paresthesia of cheek due to injury to the maxillary branch of the trigeminal nerve (CN V)
- Periorbital emphysema
- Trismus or difficulty opening and closing jaw may occur due to entrapment of the coronoid process of the mandible under a depressed zygomatic arch.
- Diplopia in setting of concurrent orbital blowout fracture

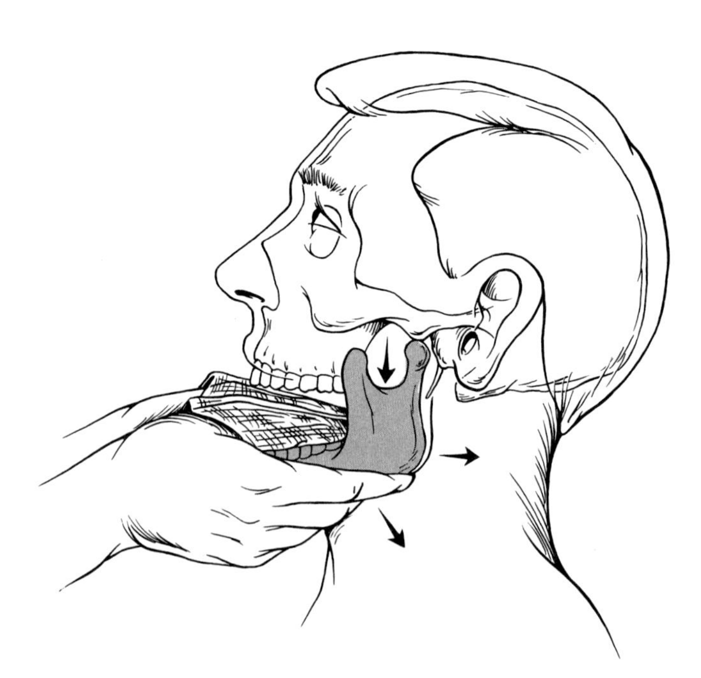

FIGURE 14.12. Reduce a dislocated mandible by pushing inferiorly and posteriorly.

(Reproduced, with permission, from Tintinalli JE, Kelen GD, Stapczynski SJ. *Emergency Medicine: A Comprehensive Study Guide*, 6th ed. New York: McGraw-Hill, 2004:1476.)

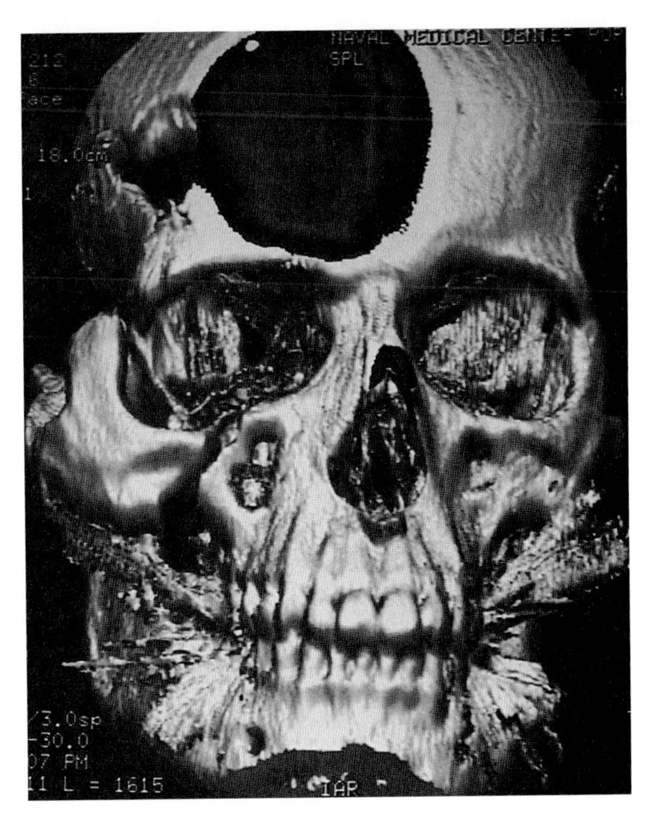

FIGURE 14.13. CT reconstruction of a right tripod fracture.

(Courtesy of Patrick W. Lappert, MD as published in Knoop KJ, Stack LB, Storrow AB. *Atlas of Emergency Medicine*, 2nd ed. New York: McGraw-Hill, 2002:11.)

- Pushing on the zygoma from inside the mouth allows you to examine the bone without pushing on soft tissue directly over the bone, which may be tender in the absence of a fracture.

Diagnostics

- Facial films: Waters and submental vertex view (outdated)
- Facial CT (1–3 mm coronal and axial cuts)

Treatment

- Sinus precautions
- Antibiotics (because of sinus involvement)
- OMFS/ENT consult for fractures with neurologic abnormalities, problems with mastication, or cosmetics

MIDFACE FRACTURES

Le Fort Fractures

See Figure 14.14.

Le Fort I

- Involves the maxilla at the level of the nasal fossa
- Upper dental arch is mobile.

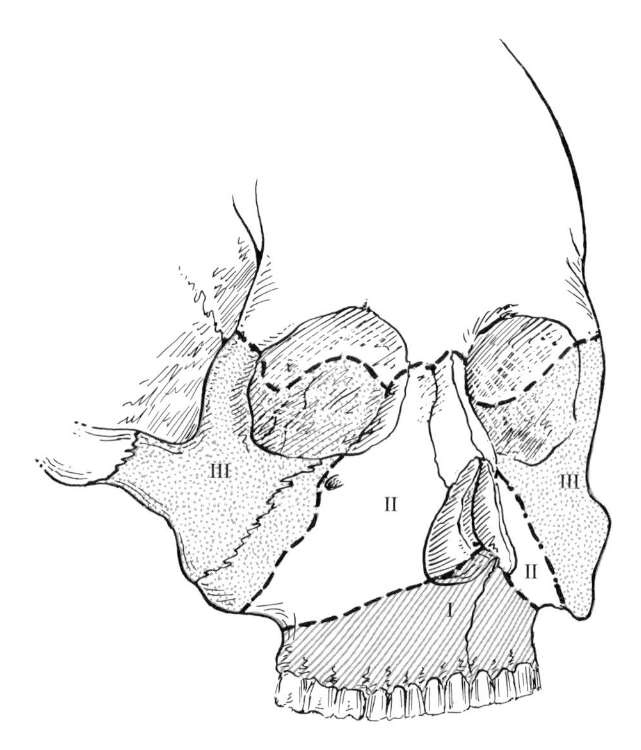

FIGURE 14.14. Le Fort fractures.

(Reproduced, with permission, from Tintinalli JE, Kelen GD, Stapczynski SJ. *Emergency Medicine: A Comprehensive Study Guide*, 6th ed. New York: McGraw-Hill, 2004:13.)

Le Fort II

- Involves the maxilla, nasal bones, and medial aspects of the orbits (pyramidal fracture)
- Upper dental arch and the nose are mobile.

Le Fort III

- Involves the maxilla, zygoma, nasal bones, ethmoids, vomer, and lesser bones of the cranial base
- The entire face is mobile: Craniofacial dysjunction.

Symptoms/Exam

- Soft-tissue swelling of the face
- Midface mobility is assessed by moving the upper teeth.
- Malocclusion
- CSF rhinorrhea is seen with Le Fort II and III.
- Usually these fractures occur in combination: Uni- or bilateral.

Diagnosis

- Mobility of the maxilla relative to the rest of the head can be assessed by moving the upper incisors.
- Facial CT is used to confirm the diagnosis and define the extent of injury.

TREATMENT

- Airway protection must be addressed or closely monitored. Blood loss may be heavy.
- All patients should receive antibiotics.
- Plastics or craniofacial consult is indicated.
- Most Le Fort fractures require surgical repair and stabilization (often with small plates).
- Early repair is considered preferable in stable patients.

COMPLICATIONS

- Airway compromise
- Malocclusion if missed diagnosis
- Infection

CAVERNOUS SINUS THROMBOSIS

This is a life-threatening infection and associated thrombosis of the cavernous sinus (see Figure 14.15). Infections usually originate in the sinuses or mid-face. Other sources of infection include facial veins, oral cavity, middle ear, and mastoid region. The most common organism is S. *aureus*.

SYMPTOMS/EXAM

- High fever
- Toxic appearance
- Periorbital edema and chemosis (conjunctival edema)
- Cranial nerve palsies (CN VI is most commonly affected, presenting as a lateral gaze palsy)
- Decreased visual acuity and sluggish pupils may be seen due to increased intraocular pressure.

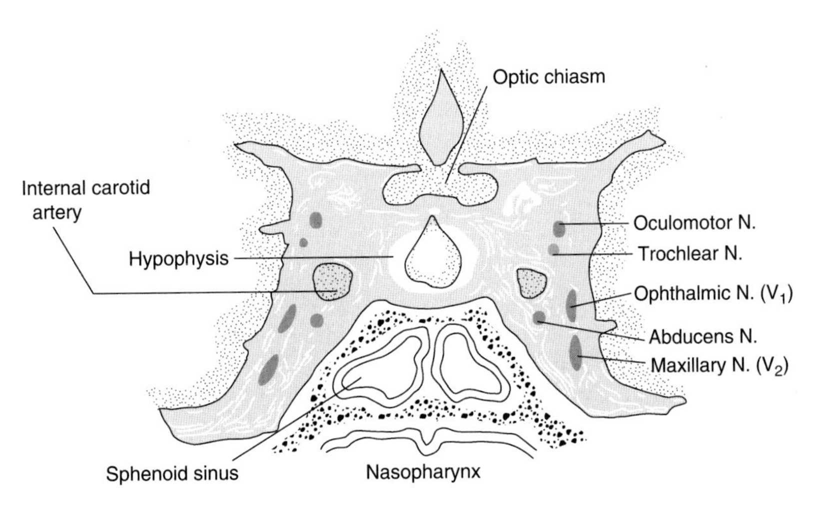

FIGURE 14.15. Diagram of the cavernous sinus.

(Reproduced, with permission, from Ropper AH, Brown RH. *Adams and Victor's Principles of Neurology*, 8th ed. New York: McGraw-Hill, 2005:229.)

Diagnostics

- MRI or CT
- Blood cultures and Gram stain to evaluate for infection and bacteremia

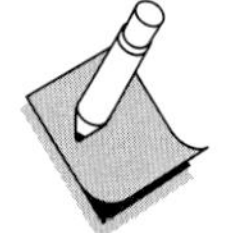

Not all infections in the head are meningitis. Cavernous sinus thrombosis must be considered in patients with cranial nerve or visual deficits.

Treatment

- Early and aggressive intravenous antibiotics
- Although evidence is limited, heparin is generally used to prevent septic emboli.
- Admit to ICU
- Surgical consultation for drainage of the sphenoid sinus if sphenoid sinusitis is present

SALIVARY GLAND PROBLEMS

Sialoadenitis

Etiology

- Inflammation/infection of the parotid (Stenson) duct or the salivary gland.
- Viral infection of the parotid gland (mumps)
- Bacterial (suppurative) infection usually due to staph or strep but often concomitant anaerobic pathogens are found
- Predisposing factors include: Recent anesthesia, dehydration, elderly, sialolithiasis, oral cancers, ductal foreign body.

Wharton duct = submandibular duct. Stensen duct = parotid duct.

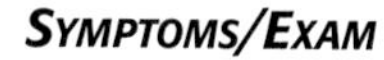

Symptoms/Exam

- Painful swelling of the parotid or salivary gland area
- Worse at mealtime
- On oral exam note drainage from the salivary ducts
- Viral
  - 90% bilateral
  - Increase in amylase
- Bacterial
  - Seen in elderly, diabetic, dehydrated patients.
  - Pus from Stensen duct
  - 30% postoperative
  - 20% bilateral

Treatment

- IV fluids for hydration
- Antibiotics to cover Gram-positive and anaerobic organisms
- Sour lozenges or sialologues to stimulate salivaries

Sialolithiasis

Etiology

- Calculi/stone in the duct
- 80% are submandibular.

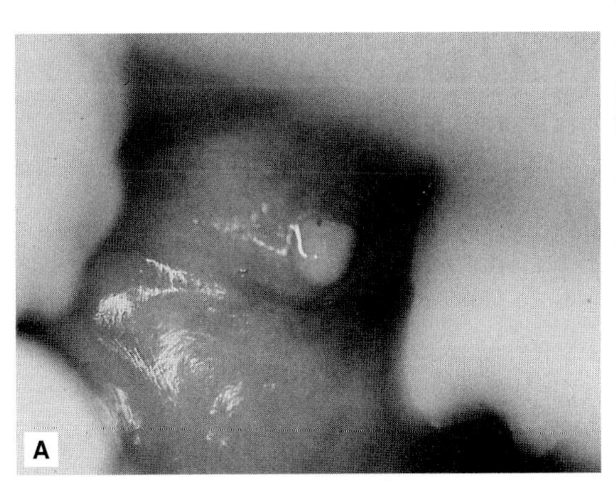
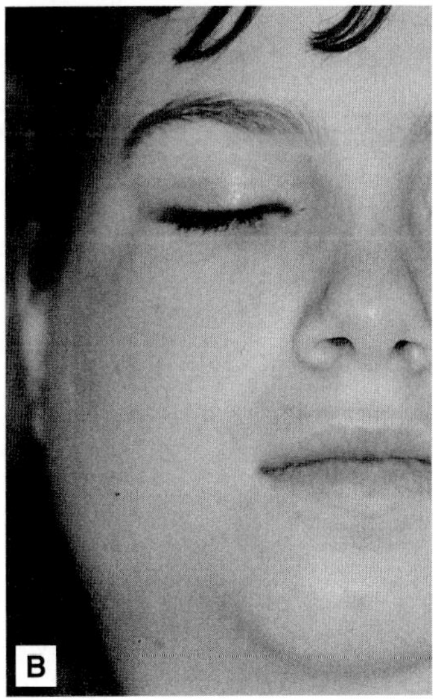

FIGURE 14.16. (A) Sialoadenitis with drainage from the parotid duct. (B) Sialoadenitis with associated inflammation of the parotid gland.

(Reproduced, with permission, from Knoop KJ, Stack LB, Storrow AB. *Atlas of Emergency Medicine*, 2nd ed. New York: McGraw-Hill, 2002:146.)

Symptoms/Exam

- Swelling of the duct area
- Tenderness and pain along the salivary duct, worse with meals
- Palpable thickened mass felt along the path of the duct when attempting to milk salivary gland (see Figures 14.16A and 14.16B)

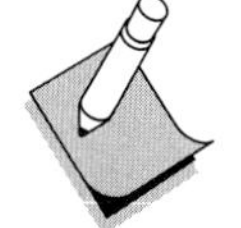

The parotid gland and facial nerve are in close proximity to each other. Assess both in infection or trauma.

Diagnosis

- Plain X-ray is used to confirm the presence of a stone (70% are radiopaque).
- CT imaging and/or sialogram may be used to characterize the duct or the presence of an obstructive lesion such as a neoplasm not seen on X-ray.

Treatment

- IV fluids
- Sour lozenges or sialologues to stimulate salivaries (most pass with this treatment)
- Possible surgical excision of the stone by ENT
- Antibiotics if secondary infection

Complications

- Infection
- Facial nerve (CN VII) palsy

OROPHARYNGEAL EMERGENCIES

Upper Airway Foreign Body

Etiology

- Children (<3 years old), eg, food, coins, toys
- Adults: Increased risk associated with elderly, alcohol, dentures, CNS disease

Symptoms/Exam

- Depends on the nature and location of the obstruction
- Stridor
  - Inspiratory = supraglottic/glottic/larynx
  - Expiratory = subglottic
- Wheezing or poor air exchange
- Voice change
- Dysphagia
- Coughing episodes
- Respiratory accessory muscle use
- Respiratory compromise and cardiopulmonary arrest

The classic PA X-ray shows a round coin in the neck. This coin is in the esophagus, which is far more common and far less scary than a coin in the trachea.

Diagnosis

- Visualization may be possible using direct laryngoscopy or indirect laryngoscopy (placing a mirror into the posterior oropharynx).
- CXR inspiratory/expiratory views might show hyperinflation distal to obstruction (air trapping and asymmetry) in acute episodes.
- X-ray or CT of soft tissues of the neck will usually identify radiopaque foreign bodies.

Treatment

- For complete obstruction
  - Adults: Heimlich, finger sweep, Magill forceps/laryngoscopy, cricothyrotomy, or tracheostomy
  - Children: Back blows, then chest thrusts; avoid blind finger sweep, transtracheal jet ventilation until definitive airway is obtained
  - If unable to remove, consider pushing FB into one bronchus and ventilating the other lung until consultant arrives.
- For incomplete obstruction
  - Do not do anything that could turn it into a complete obstruction.
  - Preferably remove under direct visualization; consultation for endoscopy may be necessary

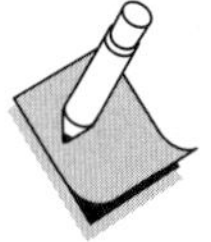

Always have the difficult airway cart (including cricothyrotomy equipment) at bedside for a potentially difficult airway.

INFECTIONS/INFLAMMATION

Epiglottitis

Etiology

- *H. influenza* type B: Classic since HIB vaccine more common in adults than children
- May also see *S. pneumonia*, *B. catarrhalis*
- Noninfectious causes include fumes, gasoline ingestion, angioedema, and super-heated steam.

Symptoms/Exam

- Dysphagia
- Rarely hoarse
- Varied presentations, but more severe in children
- Classic case is rapid onset, fever, **drooling**, tripod position.
- Pain with tracheal rock (moving the thyroid cartilage)

DIAGNOSIS

- If clinical suspicion is high, do not delay with diagnostic tests.
- Lateral neck films: "Thumb printing sign" or CT (see Figure 14.17)
- If direct laryngoscopy done (preferably in the OR) can see a cherry red epiglottis

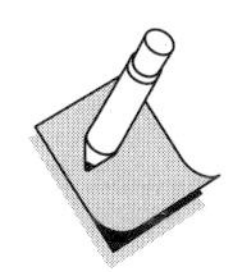

Bacterial tracheitis *looks like epiglottis–fever, stridor,* ***toxic appearance****; most common cause is* S. aureus.

TREATMENT

- Airway assessment is a priority.
- Selective intubation, preferably in a setting with personnel and equipment for difficult intubations, including fiberoptic laryngoscopy
- Antibiotics are indicated: Cefuroxime, ceftriaxone, amp/sulb, or ampicillin plus chloramphenicol. Steroids and humidified O_2 may be used (but no evidence).
- Generally, these patients are admitted to the ICU.

Croup (Laryngotracheitis)

ETIOLOGY

- Viral etiology (parainfluenza being the most common) causing subglottic edema/inflammation
- Most commonly affects children age 3 months to 3 years

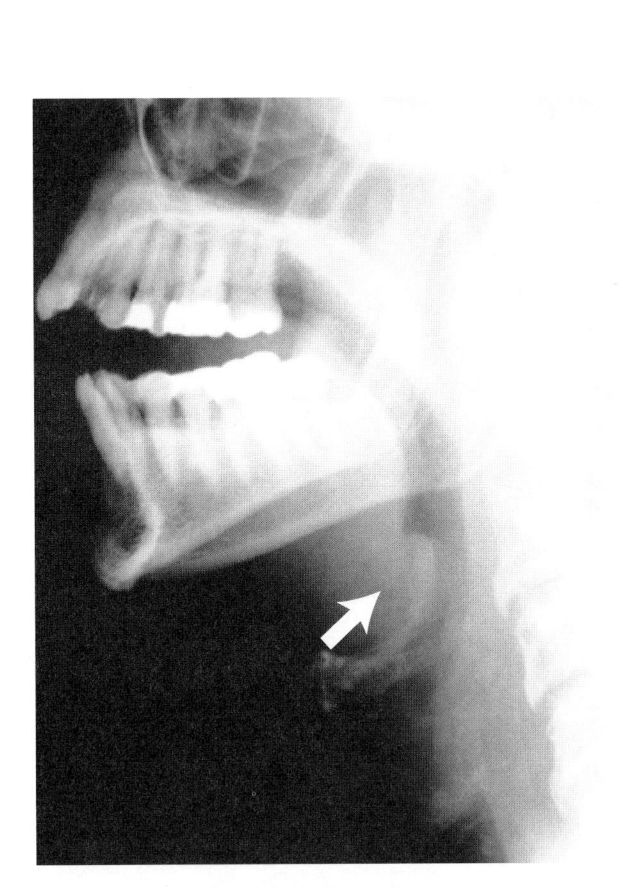

FIGURE 14.17. Lateral neck film showing thumb print sign of epiglottitis.

(Reproduced, with permission, from Tintinalli JE, Kelen GD, Stapczynski SJ. *Emergency Medicine: A Comprehensive Study Guide*, 6th ed. New York: McGraw-Hill, 2004:1497.)

SYMPTOMS/EXAM

- Respiratory distress
- Barking seal–like cough
- Severe cases may have stridor.
- Hoarseness
- URI signs and symptoms
- Low-grade fever may be present.

DIAGNOSIS

- Clinical exam
- X-ray (usually not necessary) may show "**steeple sign**" on AP view (narrowing of larynx 5–10 mm below vocal cords) (see Figure 14.18).

TREATMENT

- Steroids are indicated. Dexamethasone 0.6 mg/kg IM is a standard dose, inhaled, or oral steroids also work.
- Nebulized epinephrine
- No antibiotics needed
- Self-limiting, rarely fatal
- Consider admission if: Significant respiratory distress, persistent signs and symptoms despite ED treatment, dehydration or unable to tolerate PO, multiple doses of racemic epinephrine, or social issues.

Ludwig Angina

ETIOLOGY

- Deep space neck infection involving the submandibular, submental, and sublingual spaces (see Figure 14.9).
- Often odontogenic in origin (molars most commonly) and immunocompromised (diabetics)
- Mixed aerobic and anaerobic etiology

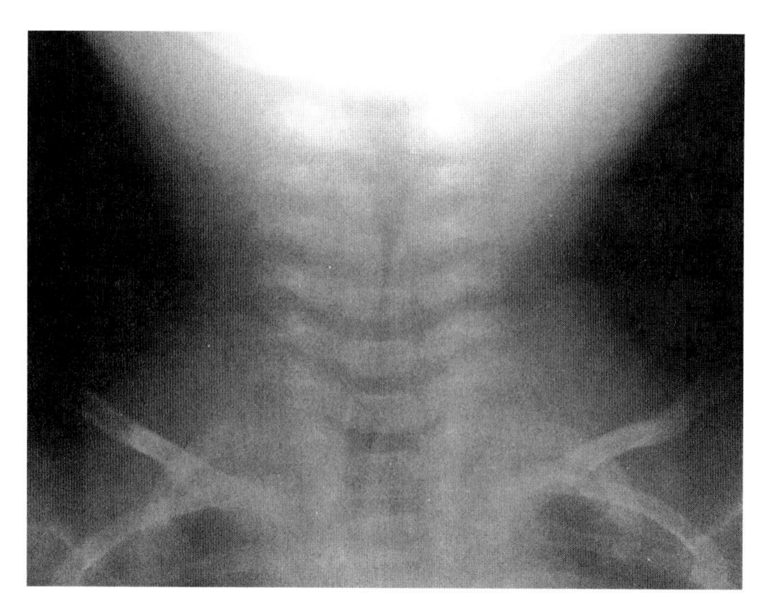

FIGURE 14.18. Subglottic narrowing, referred to as the steeple sign, in patient with croup.

(Reproduced, with permission, from Stone CK, Humphries, RL. *Current Emergency Diagnosis and Treatment*, 5th ed. New York: McGraw-Hill, 2004:648.)

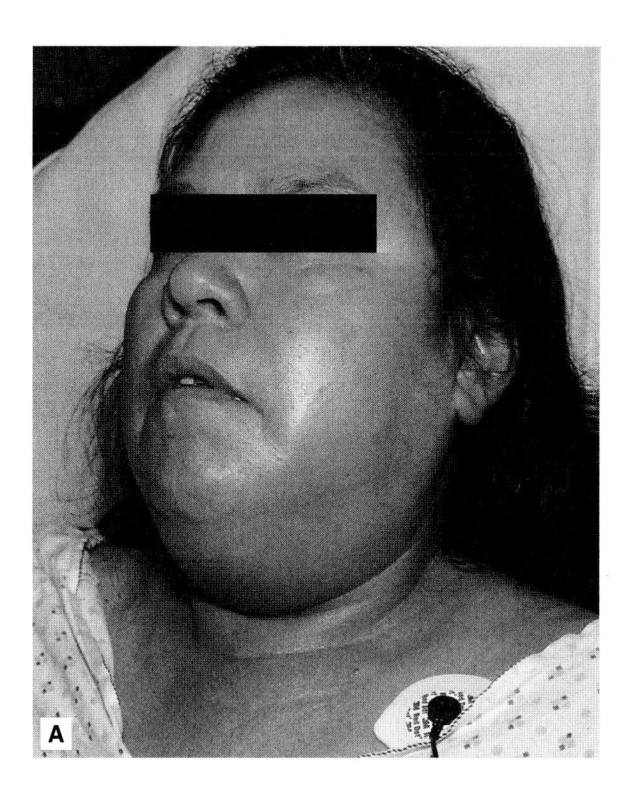

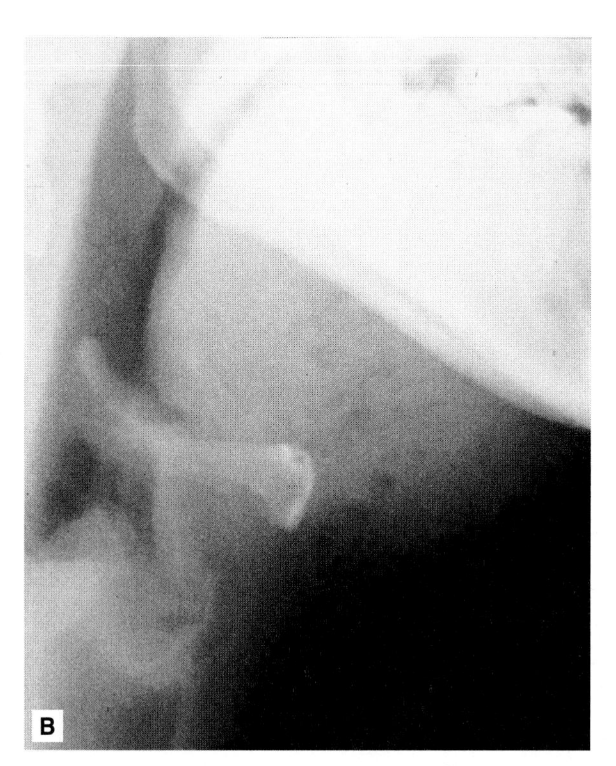

FIGURE 14.19. (A) Ludwig angina. (B) Soft-tissue swelling, air, seen on lateral neck X-ray in patient with Ludwig angina.

(A) Courtesy of Jeffrey Finkelstein, MD as published in Knoop KJ, Stack LB, Storrow AB. *Atlas of Emergency Medicine,* 2nd ed. New York: McGraw-Hill, 2002:171. (B) Courtesy of Edward C. Jauch, MD, MS as published in Knoop KJ, Stack LB, Storrow AB. *Atlas of Emergency Medicine,* 2nd ed. New York: McGraw-Hill, 2002:171.

SYMPTOMS/EXAM

- Brawny induration of the floor of the mouth (classic)
- Bilateral swelling
- Pain, edema, trismus, and drooling
- Dysphonia and dysphagia
- Tongue displaces posteriorly and superiorly, which may cause airway compromise.
- Fever, toxic appearance

DIAGNOSIS

- Clinical
- Consider later neck X-ray or CT with IV contrast, if uncertain.

TREATMENT

- ABCs, as always!
- ICU admission
- IV antibiotics (PCN or cephalosporin plus clindamycin)
- ENT consult: Incision and drainage for patients with abscess and impending complication or failure to respond to antibiotics

COMPLICATIONS

- Airway obstruction
- Extension of infection may occur, resulting in mediastinitis, intracranial infection, or IJ thrombophlebitis.

Pharyngitis

ETIOLOGY

Most commonly viral, group A strep (*Streptococcus pyogenes*) is the most common bacterial cause.

SYMPTOMS/EXAM

- Strep score (also known as Centor criteria) is a clinical rule to predict the probability of group A strep as cause of pharyngitis.
  - Tonsillar exudates
  - Anterior cervical adenopathy
  - Fever
  - Absence of cough

TREATMENT

- Various approaches have been described to decide on the use of antibiotics, including treating all patients with Centor scores of 3 or 4, or the combination of the Centor score and results of rapid strep testing.
- If thought to be bacterial, treat with PCN, cefuroxime, or erythromycin in PCN allergic patients.
- If viral only supportive care, which may include salt warm water gargles and NSAIDs
- A single dose of dexamethasone, 10 mg IM or PO, has been shown to reduce symptoms in patients receiving simultaneous treatment for strep throat.

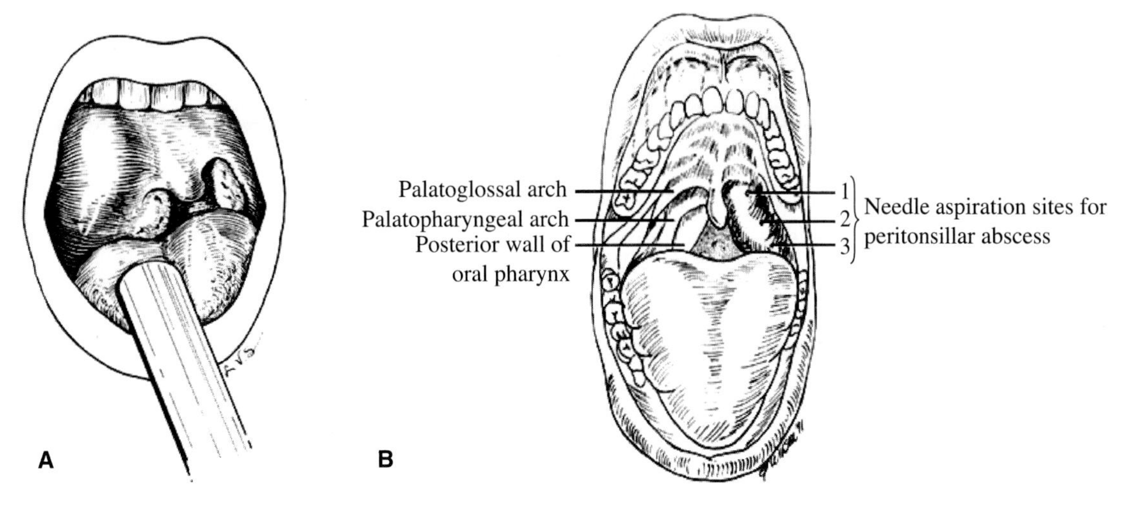

FIGURE 14.20. Peritonsillar abscess.

(Reproduced, with permission, from Stone CK, Humphries RL. *Current Diagnosis & Treatment : Emergency Medicine*, 6th ed. New York: McGraw-Hill, 2008:523 and 532.)

COMPLICATIONS

- Scarlet fever: **Sand paper rash**
- Rheumatic fever: A combination of carditis, arthritis, and dermatologic findings seen 2–6 weeks after strep pharyngitis
- Seen rarely today because of the use of antibiotics
- Abscess formation or mastoiditis (see Figure 14.20)
- Poststrep glomerulonephritis (**not prevented with antibiotics**)

Peritonsillar Abscess

ETIOLOGY

- Classically a complication of group A streptococcal pharyngitis
- Adolescents or young adults (rare in children <12 years old)
- Most common deep HEENT infection

SYMPTOMS/EXAM

- Severe sore throat and odynophagia
- Fever, trismus, and drooling
- Hot potato voice (dysarthria)
- Tender peritonsillar mass that displaces the uvula and soft palate medially
- Peritonsillar cellulitis will have minimal or no trismus and no fluctuance.

DIAGNOSIS

- Clinical
- CT with contrast (1- to 3-mm cuts) if unsure or to assess for presence of lateral or retropharyngeal abscess

TREATMENT

- Needle aspiration and/or I+D
- Outpatient antibiotics if nontoxic and tolerating PO

- Consider admission with IV antibiotics and ENT consult.
- Consider steroids and NSAIDs for inflammation.

COMPLICATIONS

- Lemierre syndrome: Throat infection leading to septicemia caused by *Fusobacterium* sp.
- Mediastinitis, intracranial extension, retropharyngeal abscess formation
- Airway compromise

Retropharyngeal Abscess

ETIOLOGY

- Mixed flora affecting the retropharyngeal space
- Commonly after trauma (popsicle stick) or upper respiratory infection
- Most common in children 3–5 years old

SYMPTOMS/EXAM

Be able to identify retropharyngeal abscess (wide retropharyngeal space), croup (steeple sign), and epiglottitis (thumb print sign) on X-rays of the soft tissues of the neck.

- Fever, neck pain, sore throat
- Dysphagia, trismus, stridor
- **Nuchal rigidity**
- Muffled voice "cri du canard" = duck-like voice
- Lymphadenopathy
- Intraoral exam shows anterior displacement of the posterior pharyngeal wall due to swelling or mass.

DIAGNOSIS

- Lateral soft tissue neck X-ray indicates retropharyngeal space at C2 is twice the size of the vertebral body. Patient should hold head in sniffing position—**slight neck extension**—to prevent false positive X-ray (see Figure 14.21).
- CT is appropriate in patients with high probability of illness and to define location of abscess.

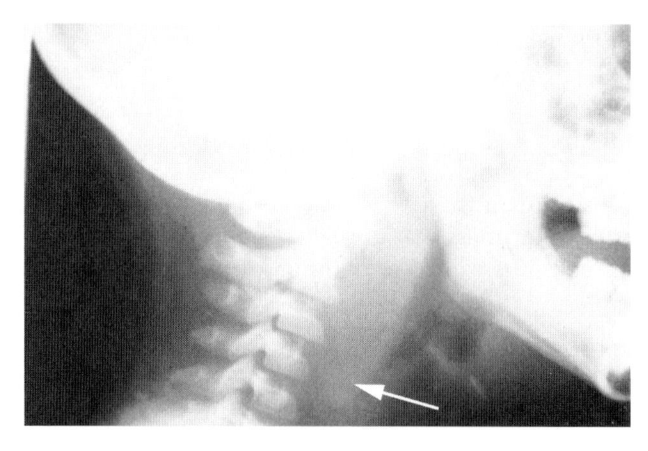

FIGURE 14.21. Lateral neck view of a child with retropharyngeal abscess and widened retropharyngeal space.

(Reproduced, with permission, from Tintinalli JE, Kelen GD, Stapczynski SJ. *Emergency Medicine: A Comprehensive Study Guide*, 6th ed. New York: McGraw-Hill, 2004:857.)

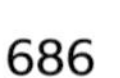

TREATMENT

- IV antibiotics (cephalosporins)
- ICU admission
- ENT/surgical consult for I + D after intubation
- Consider steroids and humidified O_2.

Diphtheria Laryngitis

ETIOLOGY

- *Corynebacterium diphtheriae* (**Gram-positive** rod)
- Local invasion with tissue necrosis
- Exotoxin production causing systemic findings
- Previously caused epidemics primarily among young children, now seen rarely in the United States
- Older adults at risk

SYMPTOMS/EXAM

- Grayish pseudomembrane (see Figure 14.22)
- Bull neck: Lymphadenopathy, edema, stridor
- Tachycardia
- Malaise
- Headache
- Immunizations not up to date

TREATMENT

- Antitoxin (horse): To neutralize the exotoxin
- Antibiotics: Penicillin or erythromycin
- Isolation

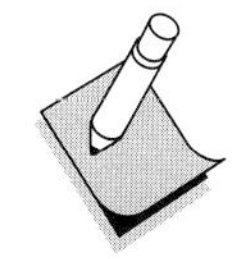

Pathogenic Gram-positive bacteria:
Staphylococcus *sp.*
Streptococcus *sp.*
Actinobacterium *sp.*
Bacillus anthracis, B. cereus
Clostridium botulinum,
C. difficile, C. perfringens,
C. tetani
Coynebacterium diphtheria
Listeria *sp.*

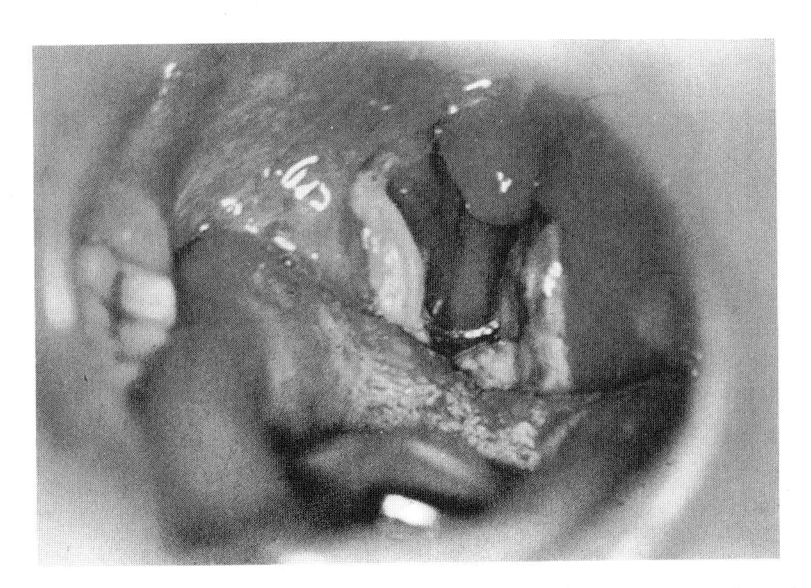

FIGURE 14.22. Pharyngeal pseudomembrane in patient with diphtheria laryngitis.

(Reproduced, with permission, from Whiting JL, Chow AW. Life-threatening infections of the mouth and throat. *J. Crit Illness* 2:36:1987.)

Complications

- Myocarditis, cardiac dysrhythmias seen after 1–2 weeks of illness
- Neurologic toxicity: Facial, pharyngeal paralysis, proximal extremity muscle weakness
- Aspiration, septicemia
- Mortality rate of 5–10%

DENTAL EMERGENCIES

Numbering Teeth

- **Primary/deciduous teeth (from about 8–12 years old)**
  - Top (going right to left) A–J
  - Bottom (going left to right) J–T
- **Secondary/permanent teeth**
  - Top (going right to left) 1–16
  - Bottom (going left to right) 17–32

Hint: If unsure, use AP X-ray to evaluate for a nonerupted developing permanent tooth.

Dental Caries/Pulpitis

Symptoms/Exam

- Dull pain worsened with stimuli
- If tenderness with percussion or fever, consider pulpitis or abscess.
- Usually associated with poor hygiene
- May have referred pain to ear, eye, temple, or neck

Treatment

- Dental blocks or other analgesics
- Antibiotics
- Dental referral

Complications

These apply for almost all dental space infections:

- Ludwig angina
- Abscess formation
- Associated facial cellulitis/abscess
- Intracranial invasion
- Descending necrotizing mediastinitis
- Airway compromise

Pericoronitis

Etiology

Gingival flap gets inflamed due to food impaction over a partially erupted or impacted tooth. Usually involves the gums over a **partially erupted third (last) molar**.

SYMPTOMS/EXAM

- Pain and swelling
- Trismus

TREATMENT

- Saline irrigation to remove food from under the gingival flap
- Antibiotics: PCN, erythromycin, or clindamycin
- I+D if abscess is present
- Referral to dentist must occur within 24 to 48 hours.
- In the case of third molar pericoronitis, tooth removal is the common, definitive treatment.

Periodontal Abscess

ETIOLOGY

- Debris and bacteria entrapped along the gingiva or between the teeth causing local swelling and infection
- Most common cause of tooth loss = gum disease.

SYMPTOMS/EXAM

- Dental and gingival pain
- Gingival swelling

TREATMENT

- Warm saline irrigation
- Antibiotics
- I+D if abscess is present

Periapical Abscess

ETIOLOGY

- Inflammation, infection, and necrosis of the apical (distal) portion of the tooth
- Usually secondary to dental caries

SYMPTOMS/EXAM

- Pain, especially when tapping on (percussing) tooth
- Facial swelling common

TREATMENT

- Analgesics
- Antibiotics
- Dental referral

COMPLICATIONS

Can erode through bone into other spaces (see Figure 14.23)

Alveolar Osteitis

ETIOLOGY

- Postextraction (usually of the molars) pain due to loss of healing clot → inflammation and local osteomyelitis.

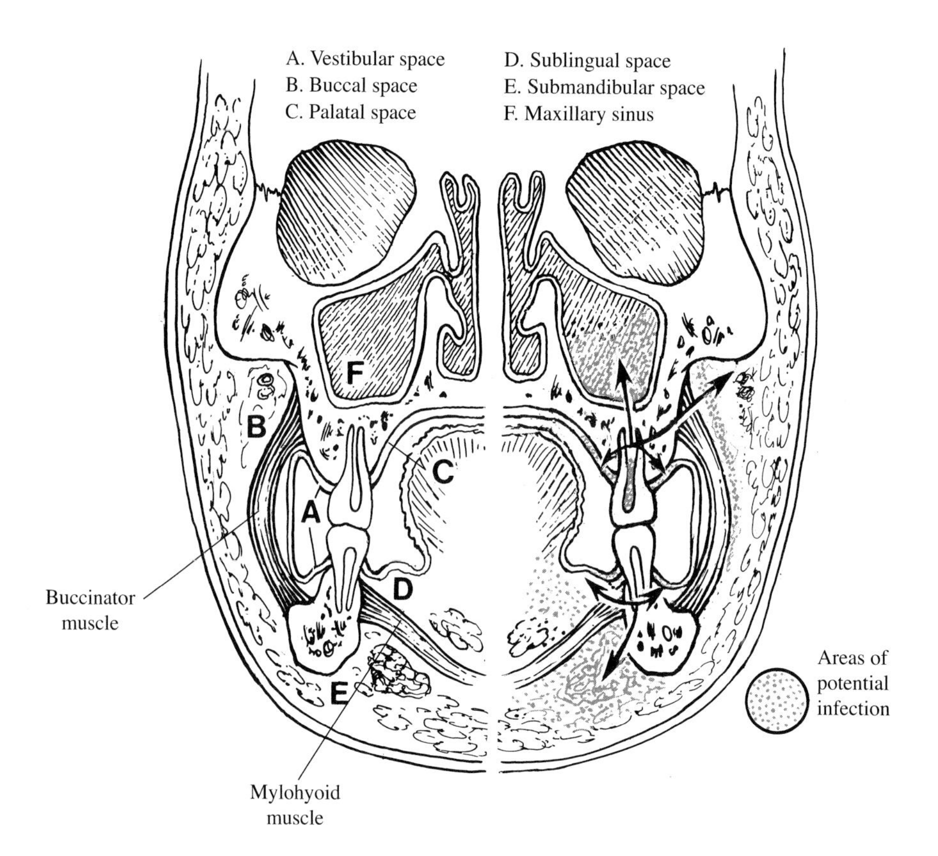

FIGURE 14.23. Periapical abscesses may erode through bone and lead to infections of the maxillary sinus, palatal space, vestibular space, buccal space, sublingual space, or submandibular space.

(Modified, with permission, from Cummings C, Schuller D. *Otolaryngology Head and Neck Surgery*. Chicago: Mosby-Year Book, 1986:1546.)

SYMPTOMS/EXAM

- Excruciating pain approximately **3–5 days post extraction** (time of onset differentiates this from post extraction pain, which occurs within the first 24 hours)
- No signs of infection or bleeding
- Fresh, clean extraction site
- Risk factors for clot loss include smoking, trauma, spitting, s/p difficult extraction of mandibular molar, females on OCPs, and local infection.

TREATMENT

- Consider a dental nerve block or other analgesia.
- Gentle irrigation of socket
- Pack socket with iodoform gauze and eugenol solution (an oil with antiseptic and analgesic properties).
- Oral antibiotics
- Dental referral in 24 hours

Avulsed Teeth

SYMPTOMS/EXAM

- Only permanent/secondary teeth need replantation.
- 1% loss of tooth survival for every minute out

TREATMENT

- Replant tooth as soon as possible, if indicated.
- Tips on transporting an avulsed tooth:
  - Touch the crown part only.
  - Gently rinse with tap water, **no scrubbing** (to avoid damaging the periodontal ligaments).
  - Transport under tongue, in saliva, saline solution, milk, or in Hank's solution (best). Avoid dry storage.
  - Temporary stabilization of tooth may be achieved with Coe Pak or other periodontal dressing or biting on a piece of gauze.
  - Immediate dental referral for splinting with adjacent teeth
  - Antibiotics
  - Tetanus
  - Soft diet postreplant

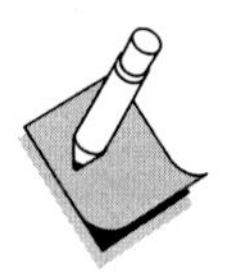

Do not reimplant baby teeth.

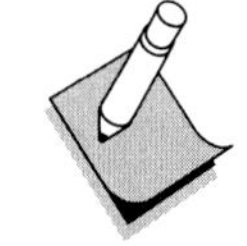

Baby teeth are naturally replaced by adult teeth between the ages of 6 and 12.

COMPLICATIONS

- Replanted baby teeth can cause bone fusion and prevent permanent teeth from erupting.

Fractured Teeth

ELLIS CLASSIFICATION

See Figure 14.24.

CLASS I

Fracture of enamel

TREATMENT

Smooth edge with file and discharge with dental follow-up.

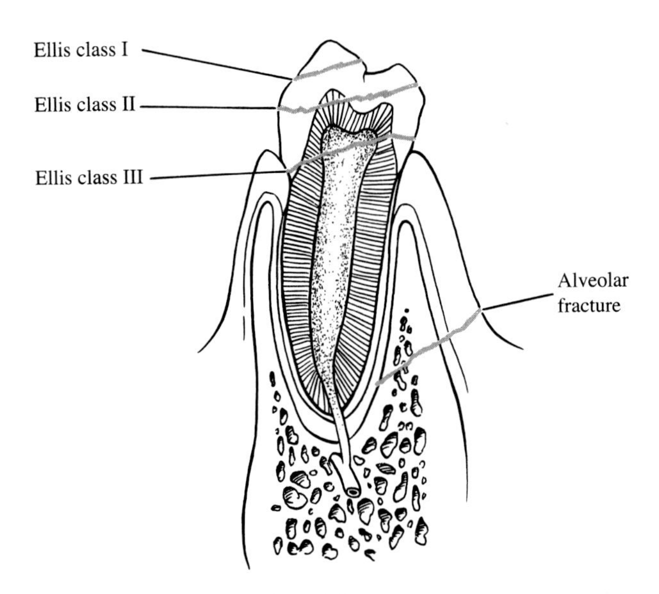

FIGURE 14.24. Ellis classification of tooth fractures.

(Reproduced, with permission, from Tintinalli JE, Kelen GD, Stapczynski SJ. *Emergency Medicine: A Comprehensive Study Guide*, 6th ed. New York: McGraw-Hill, 2004:1490.)

HEAD, EYE, EAR, NOSE, AND THROAT EMERGENCIES

CLASS II

Fracture through dentin and enamel

TREATMENT

Smooth edge with file and apply calcium hydroxide covering over exposed dentin with dental follow-up.

CLASS III

Fracture through pulp, dentin, and enamel

TREATMENT

Dental consult for pulpotomy, pulpectomy, to prevent infection

COMPLICATION

Always consider aspiration or ingestion of fractured pieces.

Acute Necrotizing Ulcerative Gingivitis

Caused by overgrowth of normal oral bacteria (usually fusobacteria or oral spirochetes) or a periodontal infection that invades nonnecrotic tissue). The name trench mouth comes from the high incidence of this disease in World War I trench-bound soldiers. It is thought to result from stress and poor hygiene and is not contagious. (See Figure 14.25.)

SYMPTOMS/EXAM

- Rapid onset
- Risk factors: Trauma, poor hygiene, smoking, immunodeficiencies, young adults

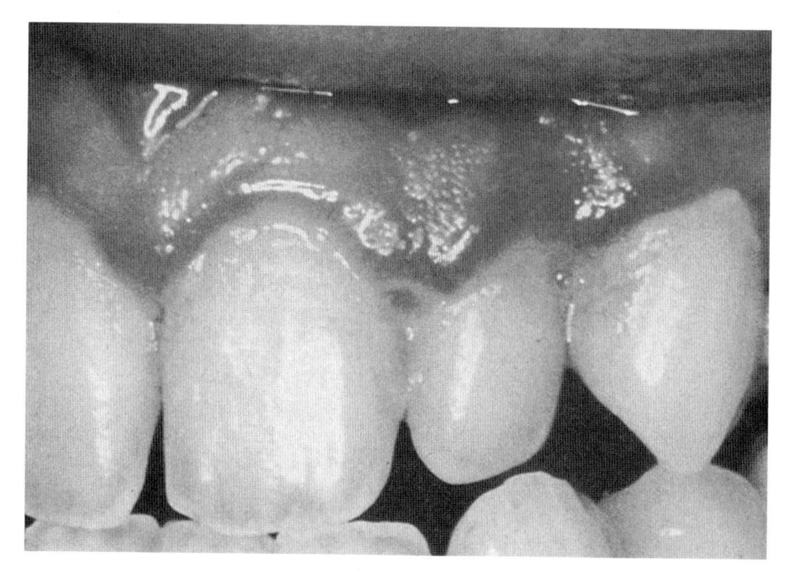

FIGURE 14.25. Acute necrotizing ulcerative gingivitis. (See also color insert.)

(Courtesy of David P. Kretzschmar, DDS, MS as reproduced, with permission, from Knoop KJ, Stack LB, Storrow AB. *Atlas of Emergency Medicine*, 2nd ed. New York: McGraw-Hill, 2002:174.)

- Diffuse red, painful, and inflamed gingiva with various degrees of erythema and ulcerations (typically peri-incisors and molars)
- Necrotic tissue in and around the gingival crest
- Metallic taste
- Foul breath/halitosis
- Grey pseudomembrane along the gingiva; may expose bleeding ulcerations when removed
- Loss of gingival tissue (especially interdental papillae)
- May be accompanied by fever, malaise, regional lymphadenopathy

TREATMENT

- Irrigate with warm saline.
- Analgesics (topical and PO)
- Antibiotics indicated include penicillin, metronidazole (Flagyl), clindamycin. Consider swish and spit rinses such as hydrogen peroxide or chlorhexidine solution.
- Dental referral for follow-up debridement
- Admit patients with extensive disease, systemic symptoms, immunocompromised, or requiring IV treatment.

COMPLICATIONS

- Vincent's angina: Spread to pharynx and tonsils
- Spontaneous bleeding gums, sloughing of the gingiva

Aphthous Stomatitis

- Chronic mucosal inflammatory/ulcerative disease of uncertain etiology (see Figure 14.26)
- Linked to cell mediated immune response, viral, genetic predisposition, stress, trauma, and malnutrition (including celiac sprue)

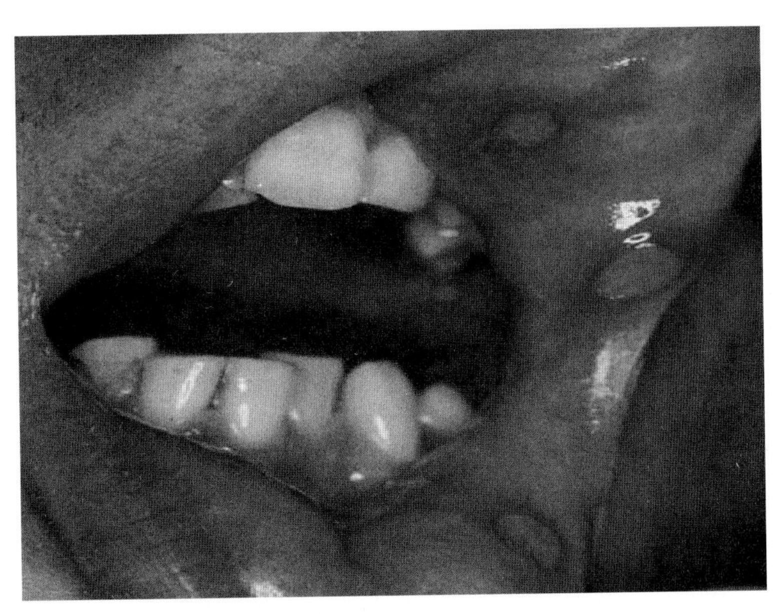

FIGURE 14.26. Aphthous stomatitis. (See also color insert.)

(Reproduced, with permission, from Wolff K, Johnson RA, Suurmond D. *Fitzpatrick's Color Atlas & Synopsis of Clinical Dermatology*, 5th ed. New York: McGraw-Hill, 2005:1017.)

- Most common oral mucosal disease in North America
- Thought to be noncontagious

SYMPTOMS/EXAM

- Painful ulcerations on the nonkeratinized mucosa of the mouth lasting weeks to months
- Varies from minor to major to herpetiform
- Typically see multiple ulcers
- Palatal or posterior oropharyngeal ulcers suggest hand-foot-and-mouth disease (coxsackievirus).
- Consider Tzanck smear (for herpes), viral culture, ESR, CBC, KOH prep.

DIFFERENTIAL

- Hand-foot-and-mouth disease
- Candidiasis
- Herpes simplex
- Behçet disease
- Reiter syndrome
- Syphilis

TREATMENT

- Supportive care
- Topical agents for analgesia and hygiene rinses (see the section Acute Necrotizing Ulcerative Gingivitus)
- Corticosteroids are first-line therapy (elixir or topical gel, PO if severe).
- Discharge with outpatient follow-up.

EYELID DISORDERS

External Hordeolum

ETIOLOGY

Acute (staphylococcal in 90–95%) infection/abscess of the oil gland associated with the follicle of a cilium (eyelash) (see Figure 14.27)

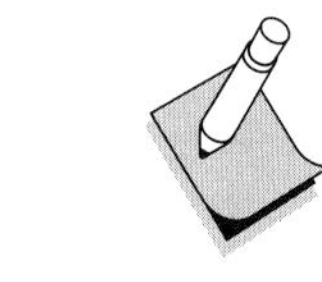

Visual acuity is the vital sign of the eye.

SYMPTOMS/EXAM

Pain, erythema, focal swelling, and tenderness of the eyelid

TREATMENT

- Warm compresses
- Antibiotic ointment
- May require incision and drainage
- Ophthalmologic referral

Internal Hordeolum: Chalazion

ETIOLOGY

- Chronic inflammation (obstruction) of the meibomian gland (see Figure 14.28)
- Clogged gland expands → lipogranulomatous foreign body reaction.

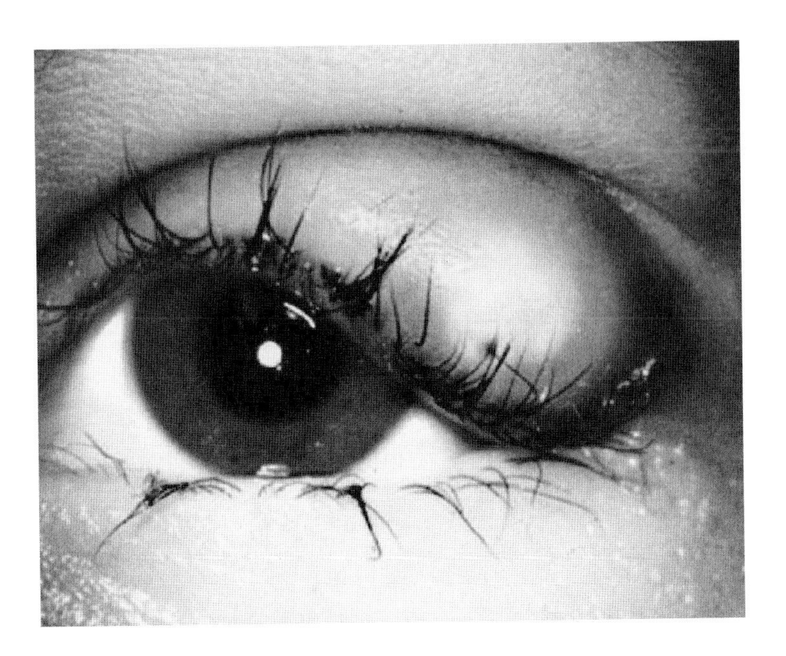

FIGURE 14.27. External hordeolum (stye).

(Reproduced, with permission, from McPhee SJ, Papadakis MA. *Current Medical Diagnosis & Treatment*, 47th ed. New York: McGraw-Hill. http://www.accessmedicine.com.)

Symptoms/Exam

- Nontender mass on eyelid
- Tender and red if secondarily infected causing a cellulitis; plugging of Meibomian gland openings (seen with slitlamp)

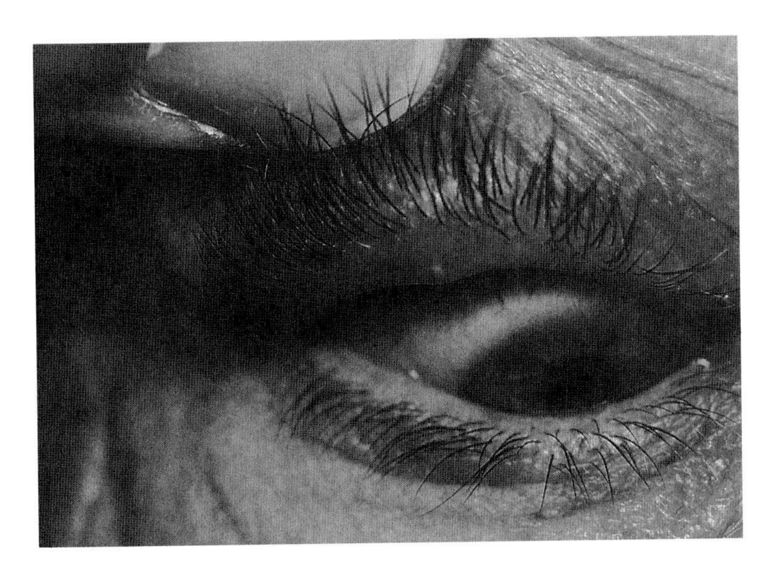

FIGURE 14.28. Internal hordeolum (chalazion).

(Reproduced, with permission, from Knoop KJ, Stack LB, Storrow AB. *Atlas of Emergency Medicine*, 2nd ed. New York: McGraw-Hill, 2002:39.)

TREATMENT

- Warm compresses
- Antibiotic ointment plus PO abx for associated cellulitis
- May require incision and drainage
- Ophthalmologic referral

Eyelid Laceration

TREATMENT

- Simple eyelid lacerations can be repaired with 6-0 or 7-0 nonabsorbable suture.
- **Involvement of the following requires ophthalmology referral:**
  - Lid margin
  - Canalicular system: Laceration medial to the punctum
  - Tarsal plate (dense connective tissue that gives form to the eyelid); may see ptosis
  - Orbital septum: Fat protruding through lid wound
  - Significant tissue loss

CONJUNCTIVITIS

ETIOLOGY

- Bacterial conjunctivitis
- Viral conjunctivitis
- Allergic conjunctivitis
- Neonatal conjunctivitis (ophthalmia neonatorum)
- When unclear, assume bacterial etiology.

SYMPTOMS/EXAM

- Discharge
  - Clear or watery discharge with allergic process, corneal abrasions, viral infections
  - Allergies can also produce a stringy white mucus
  - Yellow or purulent more common with bacterial conjunctivitis
- Preauricular andenopathy
  - Seen with most viral infections, including herpes simplex and adenovirus (pink eye)
- Membrane
  - Fibrinous membrane over palpebral conjunctiva most commonly seen with adeno or herpetic viral infections, streptococcal or gonococcal infections, and chemical burns

Opthalmia Neonatorum:

Chemical: 24–48 hours (from topical silver nitrate)

GC or HSV2: 3–5 days post delivery (from mom)

Chlamydia: 5–14 days post delivery (from mom)

Strep and staph: 5 weeks–5 years

Bacterial Conjunctivitis

ETIOLOGY

- *S. aureus*, *Streptococcus*, *H. influenza*
- *Neisseria gonorrhea*
- *Chlamydia*
- *Pseudomonas*

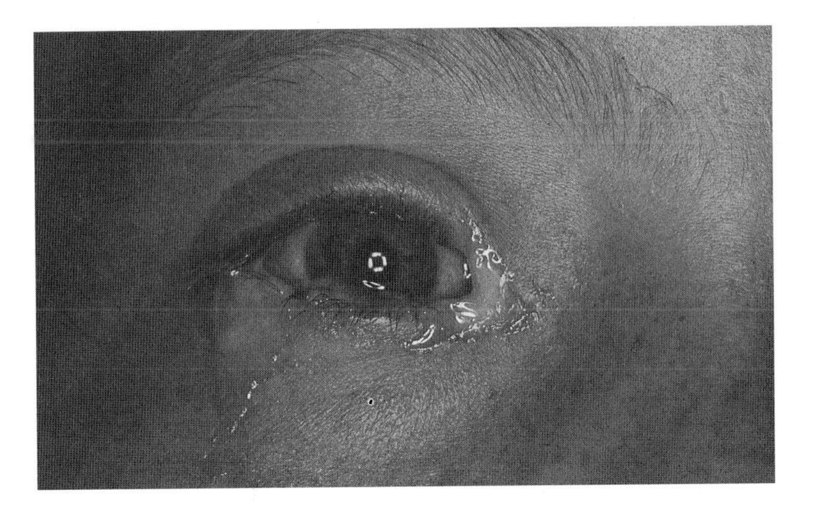

FIGURE 14.29. Bacterial conjunctivitis.

(Courtesy of Frank Birinyi, MD as published in Knoop KJ, Stack LB, Storrow AB. *Atlas of Emergency Medicine*, 2nd ed. New York: McGraw-Hill, 2002:30.)

SYMPTOMS/EXAM

- Redness or injection of the conjunctiva
- Eyelash "matting"
  - Mucopurulent discharge that reaccumulates rapidly (see Figure 14.29)
- Normal visual acuity and pupillary response
- Clear cornea and quiet anterior chamber
- Rapid response to topical antibiotics

TREATMENT

- Gram stain and culture
- Antibiotic drops or ointment
- Warm compresses

Neisseria Gonorrhea Conjunctivitis

- Rapid progression can result in corneal perforation, making this an ocular emergency (see Figure 14.30).
- Occurs in newborns and sexually active adults
- Incubation 2–5 days (neonates 3–5 days after vaginal delivery)
- Self-inoculation: Touching eye with hand after sexual contact

SYMPTOMS/EXAM

- Hyperacute onset of symptoms
- Copious purulent discharge
- Chemosis (conjunctival edema)
- Preauricular adenopathy

TREATMENT

- Gram stain and culture
- Parenteral and topical coverage:
  - Ceftriaxone 1 g IM/IV QD × 7 days
  - Topical antibiotic ointment
  - Cover for chlamydia with PO doxycycline or erythromycin

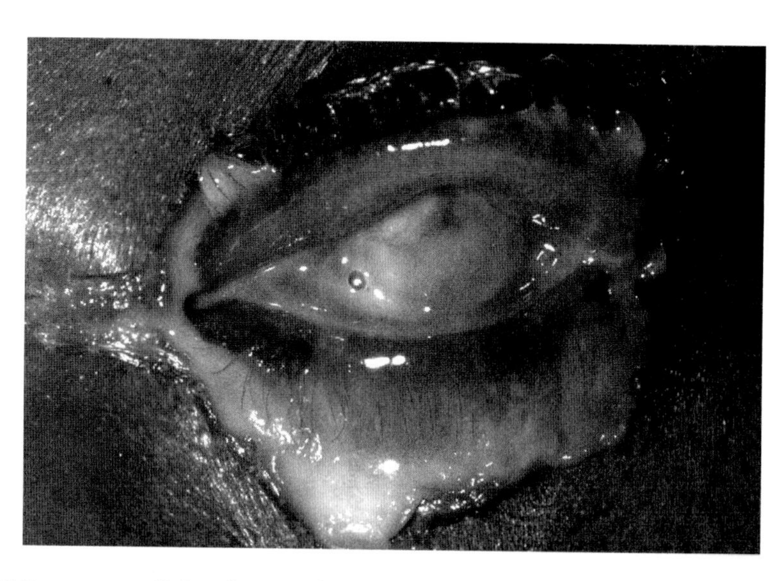

FIGURE 14.30. ***Neisseria gonorrhea*** **conjunctivitis.**

(Courtesy of L. Schwab as published in Schwab L. *Eye Care in Developing Nations*, 4th ed. London: Blackwell Publishers, 2008:128.)

- Frequent ocular irrigation with saline
- Ophthalmology consult and admission
- Evaluate and treat sexual partners.

COMPLICATIONS

Corneal ulceration and perforation

If a neonate presents with chlamydia conjunctivitis, the next appropriate test is a CXR to rule out chlamydia pneumonitis.

Chlamydia Conjunctivitis

- Leading cause of preventable blindness in young people
- Obligate intracellular parasite
- Occurs in newborns 5–7 days after delivery
- In endemic areas, transmission occurs through direct contact among young children.
- Adults with genital Chlamydia (also known as inclusion conjunctivitis)

SYMPTOMS/EXAM

- Watery discharge
- Pseudomembrane and corneal opacification may occur.

TREATMENT

- Gram stain and culture
- Topical erythromycin is given to all newborns in the United States for prophylaxis.
- Treatment includes topical erythromycin and either systemic erythromycin or tetracycline depending on age.

Complications

- Chronic untreated → trachoma/scarring → corneal abrasions/scarring.
- Risk for Chlamydia pneumonia

Viral Conjunctivitis

Etiology

- Most common cause of conjunctivitis
- Adenovirus is the most common etiology.
- 50% with constitutional URI signs and symptoms

Symptoms/Exam

- Itchy with foreign body sensation
- Tearing (watery discharge), redness/conjunctival injection (see Figure 14.31)
- Preauricular adenopathy
- Usually bilateral due to self-inoculation

Treatment

- Meticulous hygiene: Highly contagious
- Self-limiting
- Empiric topical antibiotics should be given to patients with conjunctivitis of unclear etiology.
- Ophthalmologic referral

Epidemic Keratoconjunctivitis

Etiology

Adenovirus types 8 and 19

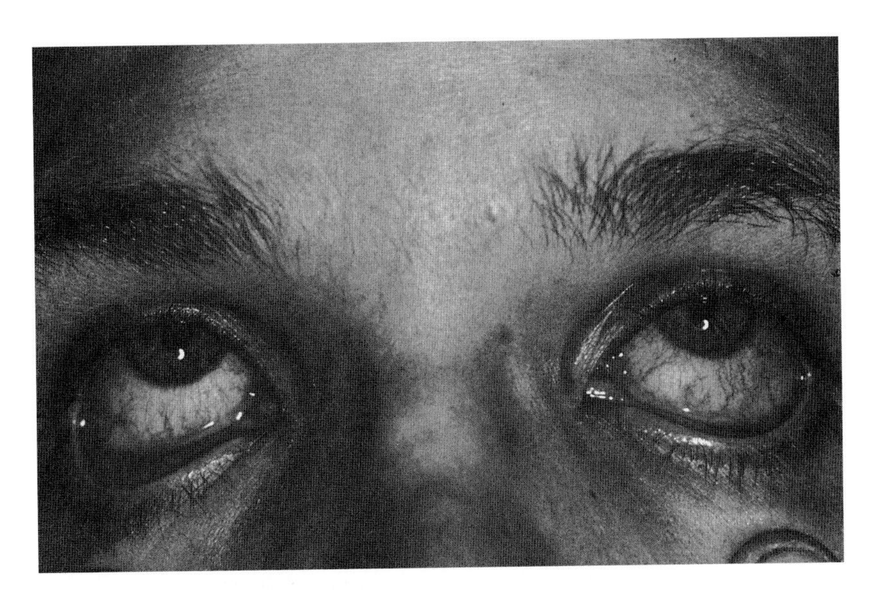

FIGURE 14.31. Viral conjunctivitis.

(Reproduced, with permission, from Knoop KJ, Stack LB, Storrow AB. *Atlas of Emergency Medicine*, 2nd ed. New York: McGraw-Hill, 2002:39.)

HEAD, EYE, EAR, NOSE, AND THROAT EMERGENCIES

Symptoms/Exam

- Pain, redness, and photophobia, subepithelial corneal infiltrates may cause decreased visual acuity.
- Tender preauricular nodes
- Superficial punctate corneal lesions
- Fibrinous membrane in some cases
- Extremely contagious
- Lasts 7–21 days

Treatment

- Diligent hand washing
- Artificial tears
- Cold compresses
- Ophthalmology may give topical steroids for membranous conjunctivitis.
- Topical antibiotics to prevent bacterial superinfection

Allergic Conjunctivitis

- Usually **recurrent**
- Results from allergen exposure, often pollen → hypersensitivity reaction in the conjunctiva.
- History of atopy, eczema, asthma

Symptoms/Exam

- Itching
- Conjunctival injection and edema (chemosis) (see Figure 14.32)
- Discharge (watery, clear, or white)

Treatment

- Topical antihistamine
- Mast cell stabilizer (cromolyn, pemirolast)
- Antibiotics if superinfection
- Oral antihistamine may be helpful if associated nasal symptoms present
- Cool compresses
- Avoid contact lenses.

Corneal Abrasion and Foreign Bodies

Symptoms/Exam

- Pain, foreign body sensation, redness
- Decreased visual acuity if central abrasion
- Fluorescein staining of epithelial defect (see Figure 14.33)

Diagnosis

- Careful slit lamp examination
- To check for foreign bodies, remember to **evert the eyelids** (see Figure 14.34).
- CT scan may be useful if suspect penetrating injury (high velocity/energy event).

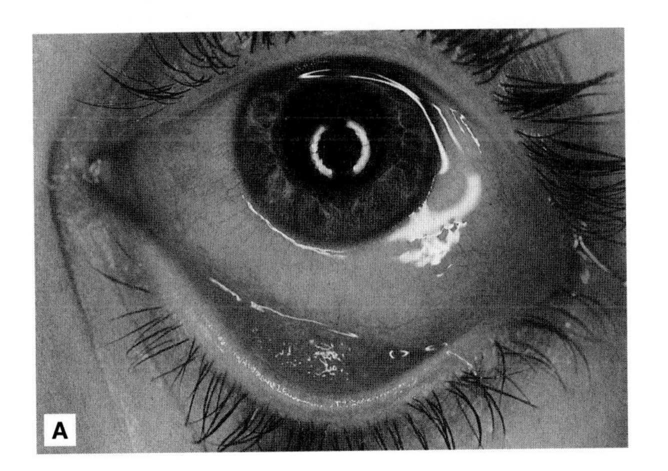

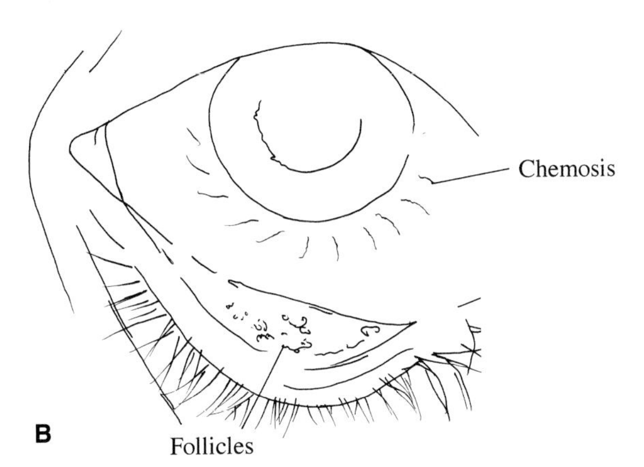

FIGURE 14.32. Chemosis seen in patient with allergic conjunctivitis.

(Courtesy of Timothy D. McGuirk, DO as reproduced, with permission, from Knoop KJ, Stack LB, Storrow AB. *Atlas of Emergency Medicine*, 2nd ed. New York: McGraw-Hill, 2002:36.)

TREATMENT

- Removal of foreign bodies and associated rust rings may be achieved with a needle, fine forceps, spud, or ophthalmic burr under magnified direct visualization using a slit lamp.
- Topical NSAIDs may be helpful. **Do not send the patient home with topical anesthetics** (eg, tetracaine, proparacaine) because they can predispose the patient to further corneal injury.
- Topical antibiotics
- Patching further impairs vision and may increase pain and incidence of infection; don't patch corneal abrasions.
- Cycloplegics are of limited benefit.
- Ophthalmology follow-up

Corneal Ulcer

A true ocular emergency; most commonly occurs following extended contact lens use

ETIOLOGY

Pseudomonas, *Staphylococcus*, and *Streptococcus*

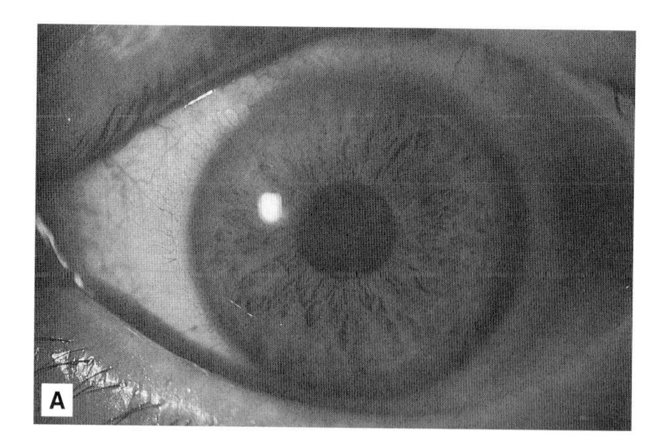

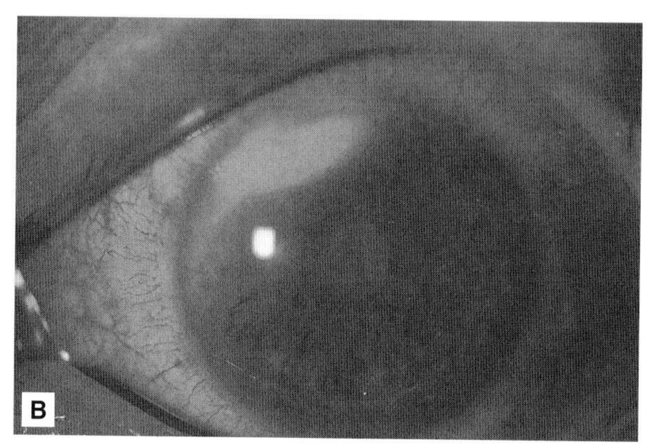

FIGURE 14.33. Corneal abrasion without (A) and with (B) fluorescein uptake.

(Courtesy of Harold Rivera as published in Knoop KJ, Stack LB, Storrow AB. *Atlas of Emergency Medicine*, 2nd ed. New York: McGraw-Hill, 2002:98.)

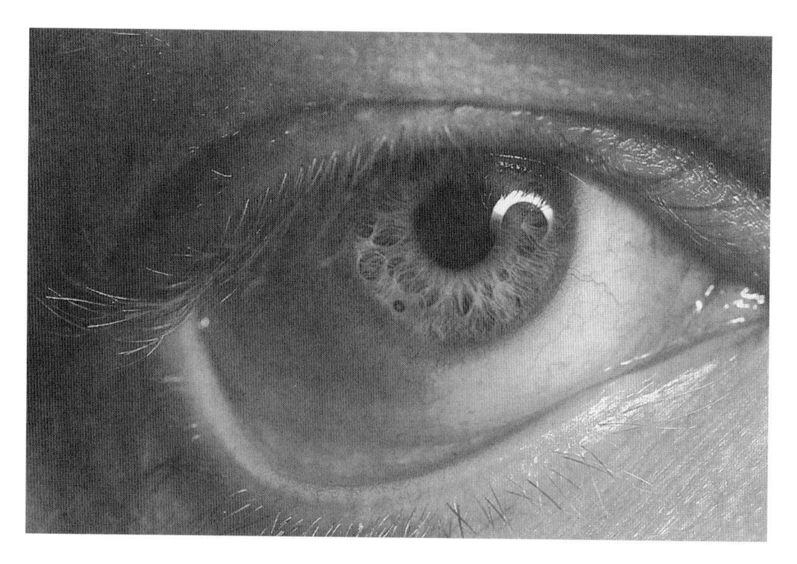

FIGURE 14.34. Metallic foreign body with rust ring at 8 o'clock. position. (See also color insert.)

(Reproduced, with permission, from Knoop KJ, Stack LB, Storrow AB. *Atlas of Emergency Medicine*, 2nd ed. New York: McGraw-Hill, 2002:100.)

Symptoms/Exam

- Severe pain, foreign body sensation
- Photophobia, blurred vision
- Conjunctival hyperemia, lid edema
- Localized whitish corneal defect with infiltrate (slit lamp)
- Anterior chamber reaction with cells and flare

Treatment

- Discontinue contact lens use.
- Eye patching is not recommended.
- Good analgesics
- Immediate ophthalmology consult is indicated. Ophthalmologist may wish to Gram stain and culture the ulcer so check if topical antibiotics should be initiated.

Hypopyon, a layered accumulation of inflammatory cells in the anterior chamber, may be seen with corneal ulcers and iritis.

Complication

Corneal perforation

Herpes Simplex Keratitis

- Occurs as a primary or recurrent infection of HSV (usually type I), the virus colonizes the trigeminal ganglion of CN V.
- Recurrences are associated with sunlight exposure and immunodeficiency (including the use of topical steroids).
- Skin and mucocutaneous lesions are typically seen in primary infection; dendritic keratitis with possible corneal scarring occurs with recurrences. (See Figure 14.35—be able to identify this pattern on pictorial.)

Symptoms/Exam

- Ocular pain, photophobia, foreign body sensation
- Visual acuity may be decreased.
- Decreased corneal sensation

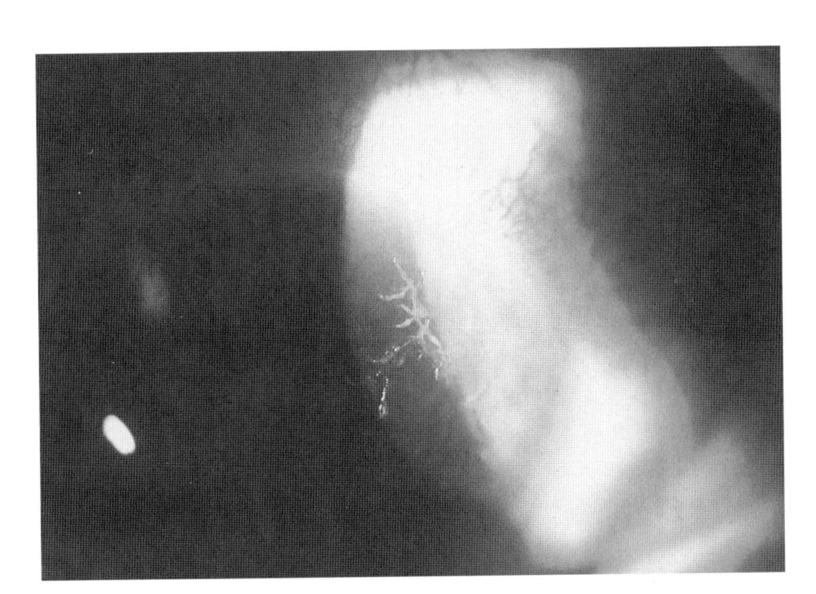

FIGURE 14.35. Dendritic pattern of herpes simplex keratitis. Be able to identify this pattern on pictorial.

(Reproduced, with permission, from Knoop KJ, Stack LB, Storrow AB. *Atlas of Emergency Medicine*, 2nd ed. New York: McGraw-Hill, 2002:57.)

- Preauricular adenopathy
- Corneal haziness
- **Classic dendritic (branching) ulcer**

TREATMENT

- Prompt ophthalmology consult
- Topical trifluridine or oral acyclovir
- Topical cycloplegic if associated iritis
- Topical steroids may be used but only in conjunction with antiviral therapy and typically only by an ophthalmologist.

Herpes Zoster Ophthalmicus

ETIOLOGY

Reactivation of latent varicella zoster virus (also known as shingles) in trigeminal ganglion

SYMPTOMS/EXAM

- Pain, paresthesia, tearing
- Unilateral vesicular eruption with dermatomal distribution (usually V1)
- Occular involvement varies (conjunctivitis, iritis, keratitis, muscle palsies, etc.).
- **Hutchinson sign:** Herpetic vesicle on the tip of the nose indicating nasocilliary nerve involvement and likelihood of ocular involvement (see Figure 14.36).
- Pseudodendritric ulcer with fluorescein staining

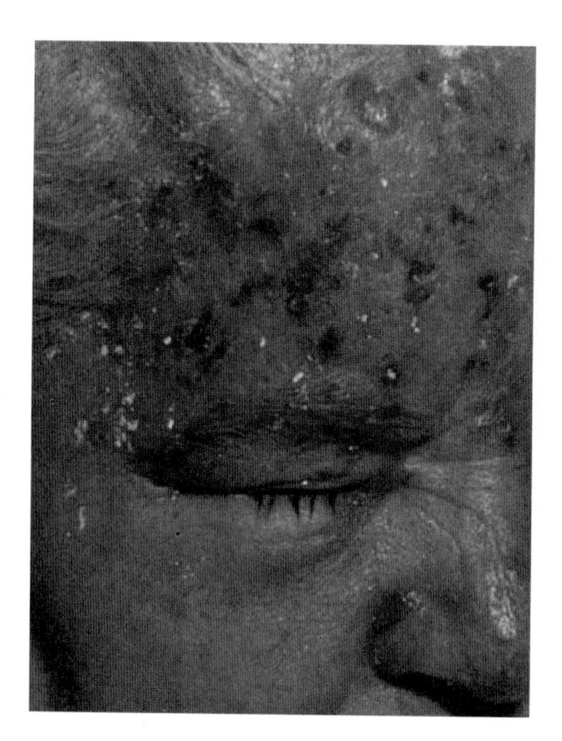

FIGURE 14.36. Herpes zoster ophthalmicus with Hutchinson sign.

(Reproduced, with permission, from Wolff K, Johnson RA, Suurmond D. *Fitzpatrick's Color Atlas & Synopsis of Clinical Dermatology*, 5th ed. New York: McGraw-Hill, 2005:825.)

TREATMENT

- Ophthalmology consult
- Oral acyclovir, famciclovir, or valacyclovir.
- Topical broad-spectrum antibiotic ointment to rash
- Steroids for iritis—leave it up to the ophthalmologist.

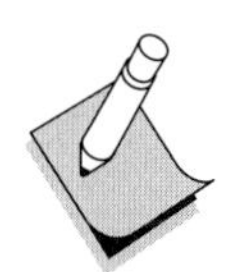

Herpes zoster is difficult to distinguish from herpes simplex on slit lamp (pseudodendritic vs dendritic keratitis). A good rule of thumb: Herpes zoster has dermatomal skin involvement and is seen in age > 60 years. Herpes simplex is typically seen in young adults.

Dacryocystitis

An acute infection/cellulitis of lacrimal sac due to nasolacrimal duct obstruction. Seen most commonly in infants and adults > 40 years. (See Figure 14.37—be able to identify on pictorial.)

ETIOLOGY

S. aureus, *S. epidermidis*, *Streptococcus* sp., and *H. influenzae*.

SYMPTOMS/EXAM

- Epiphora (excessive tearing)
- Unilateral pain, erythema, swelling over lacrimal sac
- Purulent discharge at the puncta

TREATMENT

- Broad-spectrum oral and topical antibiotics
- Warm compresses
- Good analgesics
- Gentle massage of lacrimal sac
- Ophthalmologic referral for surgical drainage

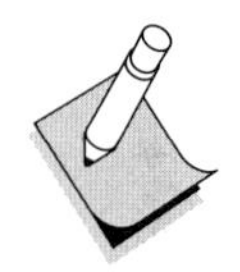

Never prescribe topical ocular steroids without an ophthamology consult.

Preseptal (Periorbital) Cellulitis

ETIOLOGY

- Infection of superficial tissues anterior to the orbital septum (fascia between eyelids and orbit)
- More common than orbital cellulitis

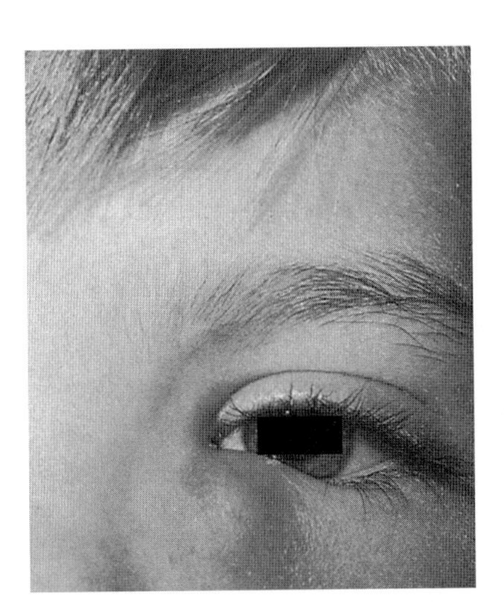

FIGURE 14.37. Dacrocystitis. Be able to identify on pictorial.

(Reproduced, with permission, from Knoop KJ, Stack LB, Storrow AB. *Atlas of Emergency Medicine*, 2nd ed. New York: McGraw-Hill, 2002:41.)

- Children <3 years old
- Culprits: *Streptococcus*, *Staphylococcus*, and *H. influenza*
- Caused by extension from ethmoid sinusitis, skin infections (bug bite), or trauma

SYMPTOMS/EXAM

- Unilateral erythema, warmth, and edema of the eyelid
- Conjunctival injection
- May see fever
- Normal visual acuity and ocular motility
- Minimal pain

TREATMENT

- Blood cultures, if febrile
- CT of orbits (3-mm fine cuts) if cannot rule out orbital cellulites
- Early/mild cases can be treated as outpatient with reliable follow-up in 24 hours.
- Broad spectrum antibiotics
- When in doubt, **admit**!

COMPLICATIONS

- Orbital cellulitis

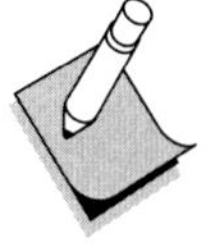

Pain with eye movements and restriction of eye movements distinguish orbital cellulitis from preorbital cellulitis.

Orbital Cellulitis

- An infection of tissues within the orbit, posterior to the orbital septum
- 90% of cases are due to spread from ethmoid sinus.
- Typical microbes are those of acute sinusitis, including *Streptococcus* sp., *S. aureus*, and *H. influenzae* type B.
- Fungal infection may occur in immunocompromised.
- Occurs in all ages, but most common in kids
- Infection may be complicated by abscess formation.

SYMPTOMS/EXAM

Eye and eyelid findings in patients with orbital cellulitis may look very similar to that of periorbital cellulitis. However, orbital cellulitis is typically distinguished by the additional findings of:

- Worse pain with eye movement
- Visual changes or diplopia
- Decreased extraocular muscle function
- Decreased papillary response
- Fever/toxic appearance
- Increased IOP

TREATMENT

- CT of orbits with 1- to 3-mm cuts
- Blood cultures
- Gram stain and culture
- Broad spectrum IV antibiotics (ceftriaxone + clindamycin or ampicillin/sulbactam)
- Urgent ophthalmology consultation and admission

COMPLICATIONS

- Vision loss
- Cavernous sinus thrombosis
- CNS involvement
- Abscess formation
- Osteomyelitis

UNILATERAL VISION LOSS

Can be divided into painless and painful types:

Painless:	Painful:
Retinal detachment	Glaucoma (acute angle closure)
CRAO	Temporal arteritis
CRVO	Optic neuritis
Vitreous hemorrhage	Corneal ulcers, abrasions, FB
Amaurosis fugax	

Open angle glaucoma presents with painless, gradual loss of peripheral vision.

PAINFUL UNILATERAL VISION LOSS

Acute Angle Closure Glaucoma

- A cause of painful, acute vision loss
- Occurs when the pupil dilates, triggered by dim light or mydriatics (tropicamide, cyclopentolate), leading to occlusion of trabecular meshwork → preventing aqueous humor from exiting → increasing intraocular pressure (IOP) (see Figure 14.38)
- Risk factors: Hyperopia, large cataract, women, Eskimo/Asian ancestry

SYMPTOMS/EXAM

- Severe, unilateral eye pain
- Blurry vision classically with "halos" around lights
- Headache
- Steamy or hazy cornea
- Injected red eye
- Mid-dilated pupil, sluggish or nonreactive to light
- Elevated IOP (40–70 mmHg) (see Figure 14.39)
- **Nausea and vomiting may mislead** the clinician.

TREATMENT

- **Block production of aqueous humor:**
  - β-Blocker topical (eg, timolol) = nonselective BB reduces aqueous humor production but is **contraindicated in patients with COPD, asthma, or congestive heart failure.**
- Alpha antagonist topical (brimonidine) = decreases aqueous humor production and increases outflow.
- Carbonic anhydrase inhibitors IV or PO (acetazolamide) = decrease aqueous humor production, thus decreasing IOP; avoid in **sulfur-allergic patients.**
- Reduce vitreous volume:
  - Osmotic agents
  - Glycerol
  - Mannitol

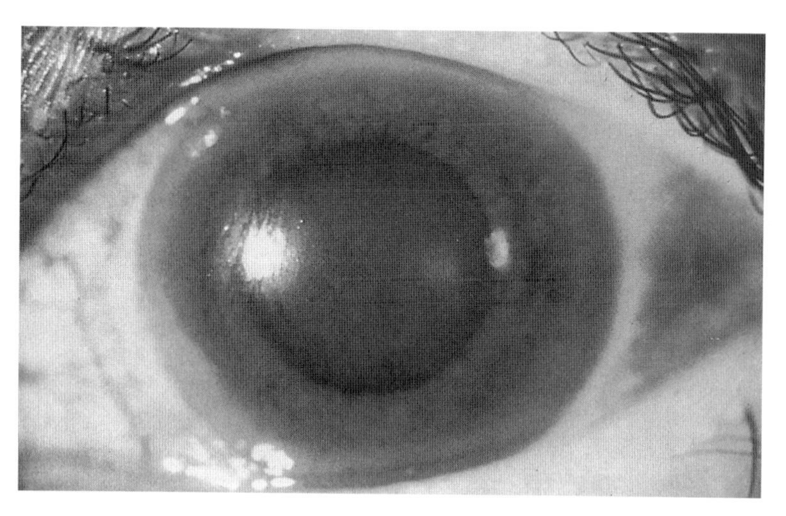

FIGURE 14.38. Acute angle closure glaucoma. Note the hazy or "steamy" cornea and mid-dilation of the pupil.

(Courtesy of Gary Tanner, MD as reproduced, with permission, from Knoop KJ, Stack LB, Storrow AB. *Atlas of Emergency Medicine,* 2nd ed. New York: McGraw-Hill, 2002:49.)

- Facilitate outflow of the aqueous humor:
  - Miotics/cholinergics (pilocarpine) = constricts the pupil thus decreasing the obstruction and allowing outflow
  - Prostaglandin agonists (latanoprost) = increases uveoscleral outflow of aqueous humor
- Emergent ophthalmology consult: The definitive treatment is laser peripheral iridotomy. This is usually performed at 24–48 hours, but may be necessary emergently if medical treatment fails to sufficiently lower IOP or break the attack.

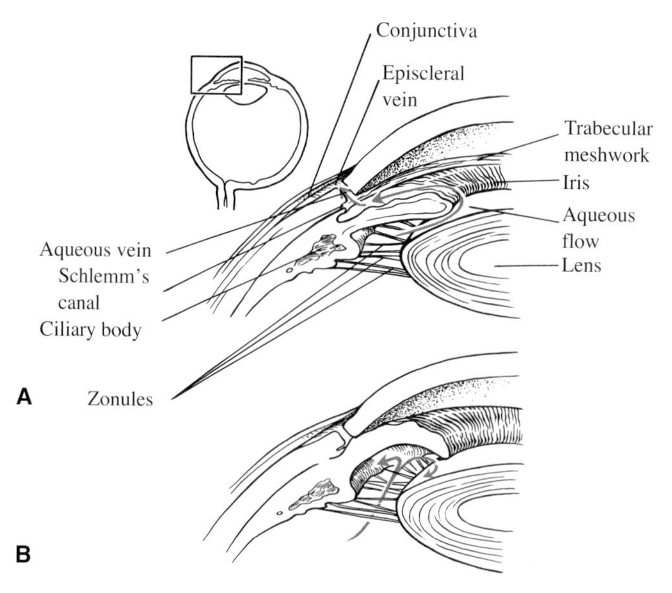

FIGURE 14.39. (A) Normal flow of aqueous from ciliary body, through the pupil and out through the trabecular meshwork and Schlemm canal, located in the anterior chamber angle. (B) Angle-closure glaucoma with pupillary block. Iris leaflet bows forward, blocking the chamber angle and prohibiting aqueous outflow. Meanwhile, aqueous production continues and IOP rises.

(Reproduced, with permission, from Tintinalli JE, Kelen GD, Stapczynski SJ. *Emergency Medicine: A Comprehensive Study Guide,* 6th ed. New York: McGraw-Hill, 2004:1459.)

Iritis/Uveitis

Etiology

- Inflammation of the iris or uveal tissue
- Iritis (also known as anterior uveitis) is most commonly caused by trauma.
- Uveitis can be caused by autoimmune disease, infection, surgery.

Symptoms/Exam

- Photophobia is a hallmark symptom.
- Decreased visual acuity, injected sclera
- Slit lamp cells and flare seen in anterior chamber (like dust particles moving through a movie projector beam).
- Can be unilateral or bilateral
- Painful

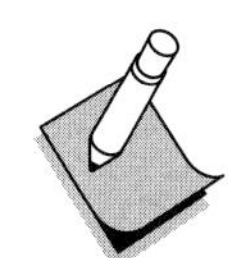

People with iritis have photophobia because light causes the iris to move.

Treatment

- Mydratics
- Analgesics
- Treat infection, if present
- Consider steroids with ophthamology consult.

HEAD, EYE, EAR, NOSE, AND THROAT EMERGENCIES

Optic Neuritis

Etiology

- Idiopathic
- Multiple sclerosis (accounts for 25% of optic neuritis)
- Sarcoidosis
- Leukemia
- TB

Optic neuritis: "The patient sees nothing and the doctor sees nothing." (Nothing abnormal on examination of the eye.)

Symptoms/Exam

- Unilateral vision loss
- Pain with EOM
- Afferent pupillary defect
- Optic-disk swelling, optic nerve pallor may be seen or exam may be normal (see Figure 14.40).

Treatment

- Ophthalmology consult
- MRI to rule out multiple sclerosis

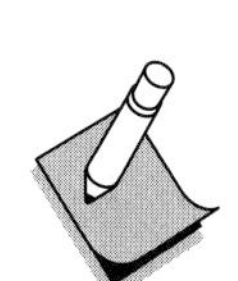

Optic neuritis = rule out multiple sclerosis.

Temporal Arteritis

Etiology

- A **segmental vasculitis** that can affect various branches of the HEENT area (eg, ophthalmic, vertebral, temporal; see Figure 14.41)
- Usually age >60 years old
- Typically women > men

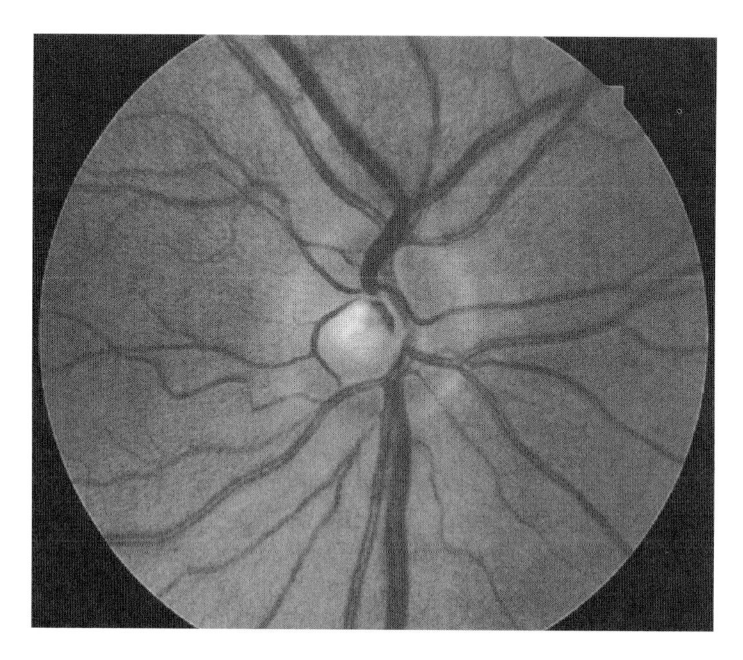

FIGURE 14.40. Optic neuritis with swollen disk. Seen in one-third of patients.

(Reproduced, with permission, from Kasper DL, Braunwald E, Fauci AS, et al. *Harrison's Principles of Internal Medicine*, 16th ed. New York: McGraw-Hill, 2005:169.)

SYMPTOMS/EXAM

- Headache over the eye or scalp
- Low-grade fever
- Eye pain
- Malaise suggests polymyalgia rheumatic.
- Jaw claudication

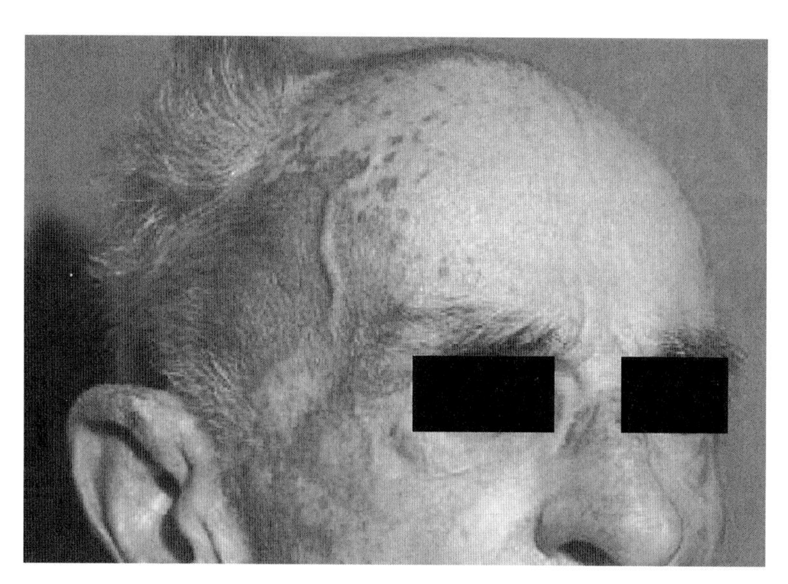

FIGURE 14.41. Patient with temporal arteritis. The superficial temporal artery is prominent, tender, and pulseless.

(Reproduced, with permission, from Wolff K, Johnson RA, Suurmond D. *Fitzpatrick's Color Atlas & Synopsis of Clinical Dermatology*, 5th ed. New York: McGraw-Hill, 2005:417.)

- Decreased vision
- Afferent pupillary defect
- Tenderness with palpation of the temporal region
- **Elevated ESR**, CRP
- Disk pallor due to decreased blood flow in the retinal artery (uncommon but significant cause of CRAO)

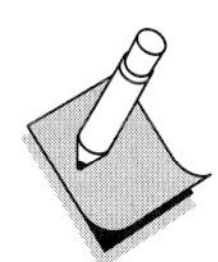

ESR is typically elevated with temporal arteritis. ESR increases with age, with the normal upper limit estimated by
Men: Age divided by 2 and
Women: (Age + 10) divided by 2.

TREATMENT

- High-dose steroids (start if clinical suspicion high)
- Admit if severe symptoms or eye involvement for IV steroids and consult ophthalmology.
- Diagnosis should be confirmed with a temporal artery biopsy (performed by ophthalmologist or vascular surgeon). As distribution is segmental or patchy, multiple biopsies may be needed.

COMPLICATIONS

If diagnosis is missed, can lead to bilateral blindness.

PAINLESS UNILATERAL VISION LOSS

Retinal Detachment

Tear in the retina allowing the vitreous fluid to separate the neurosensory retina from the pigmented epithelium underneath (see Figure 14.42)

ETIOLOGY

- Spontaneous retinal detachment associated with nearsightedness, family history, prior cataract surgery, retinopathy (diabetes, sickle cell disease)
- Also caused by trauma.

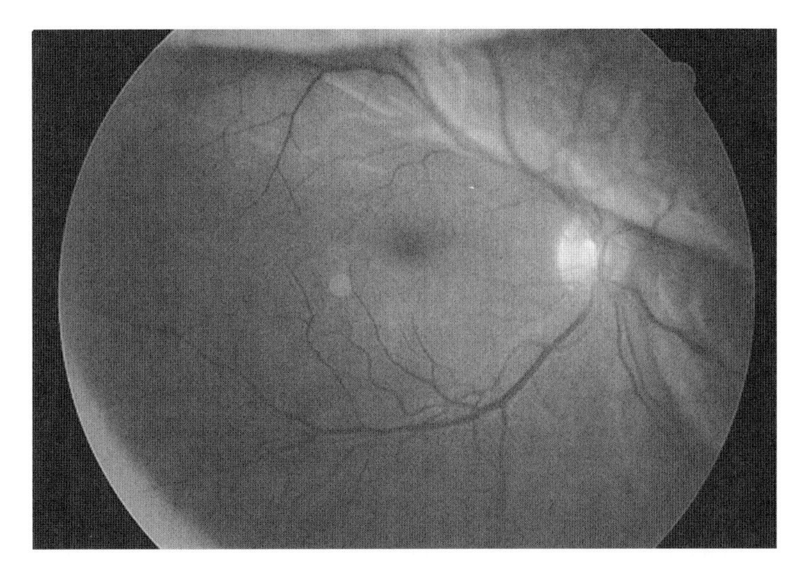

FIGURE 14.42. Retinal detachment from 11 o'clock to 4 o'clock. Note the dunes on a beach appearance. (See also color insert.)

(Reproduced, with permission, from Kasper DL, Braunwald E, Fauci AS, et al. *Harrison's Principles of Internal Medicine*, 16th ed. New York: McGraw-Hill, 2005:170.)

SYMPTOMS/EXAM

- Patients typically describe flashing lights and floaters, sometimes described as "spider webs" or "coal dust."
- Visual field defects are a late symptom.
- The retina appears like dunes on a beach or a curtain folded forward.

TREATMENT

- Ophthalmology consultation
- Urgency depends on visual acuity.
- If the macula is still attached and acuity intact, surgical repair by a retina specialist is recommended within 24–48 hours (to prevent macula from detaching also).
- If the vision is poor, the macula is likely already detached, and repair is less urgent (within 5–7 days acceptable).

Lens Dislocation

May occur anteriorly or posteriorly (more common)

ETIOLOGY

- Trauma (classically by air bag deployment)
- Idiopathic
- Marfan syndrome

SYMPTOMS/EXAM

- Iridodonesis: Trembling iris after rapid eye movements
- Monocular diplopia (two images seen with one eye)

TREATMENT

Urgent (not emergent) ophthalmology follow-up

COMPLICATIONS

Acute angle closure glaucoma

Central Retinal Artery Occlusion

ETIOLOGY

- Atherosclerotic plaque embolizes to artery (eg, from internal carotid)
- Hyperviscosity syndrome (multiple myeloma)
- Trauma with fat embolus
- Patients with sickle cell or DM
- Temporal arteritis (5% of cases)

SYMPTOMS/EXAM

- Sudden painless monocular vision loss
- Afferent pupillary defect
- Fundoscopy shows "box car" look to the retinal arterioles, a "cherry red spot" after the first few hours; a pale disk is a much later sign (seen weeks later). (See Figure 14.43.)

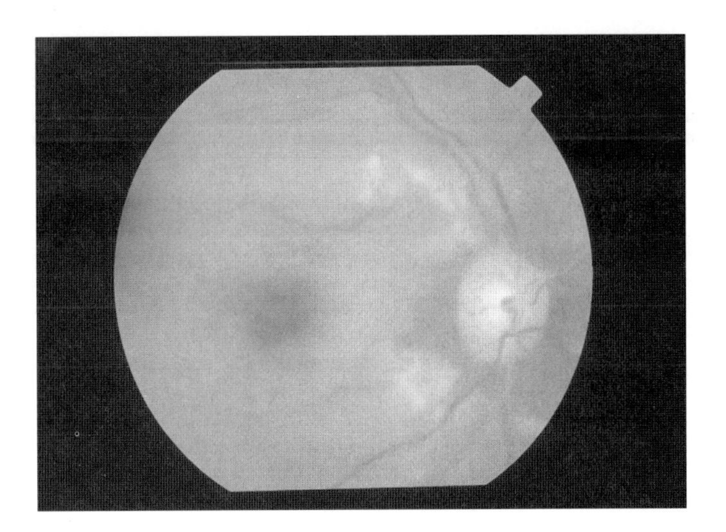

FIGURE 14.43. Central retinal artery occlusion with macular cherry red spot and pallor between macula and disk.

(Reproduced, with permission, from Tintinalli JE, Kelen GD, Stapczynski SJ. *Emergency Medicine: A Comprehensive Study Guide*, 6th ed. New York: McGraw-Hill, 2004:1461.)

TREATMENT

- Goal of therapy is to move the clot into a branch of the retinal artery and decrease infarct size. Response to treatment is rare.
- Digital massage of the globe may help dislodge the embolus.
- Increased inspired CO_2 is recommended to dilate retinal arterioles. Carbogen is recommended for this, but having the patient breathe into a paper bag can achieve similar effects.
- Consider acetezolamide or topical blockers to decrease IOP.
- Ophthalmology consult

Central Retinal Vein Occlusion

ETIOLOGY

- Atherosclerosis builds up causing occlusion and thrombosis of the central vein (see Figure 14.44).
- Risk factors include hypertension and DM.

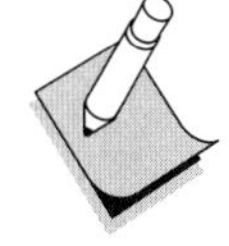

Blood and thunder = CRVO.

Cherry red spot = CRAO.

SYMPTOMS/EXAM

- Gradual painless monocular vision loss (more gradual than CRAO)
- Dilated congested veins with a "**blood and thunder**" appearance of the retina
- Numerous retinal hemorrhages = cotton wool spots and macular edema.
- Optic-disk edema

TREATMENT

- No acute treatment
- Consider same Rx for CRAO and aspirin
- Ophthamology consult

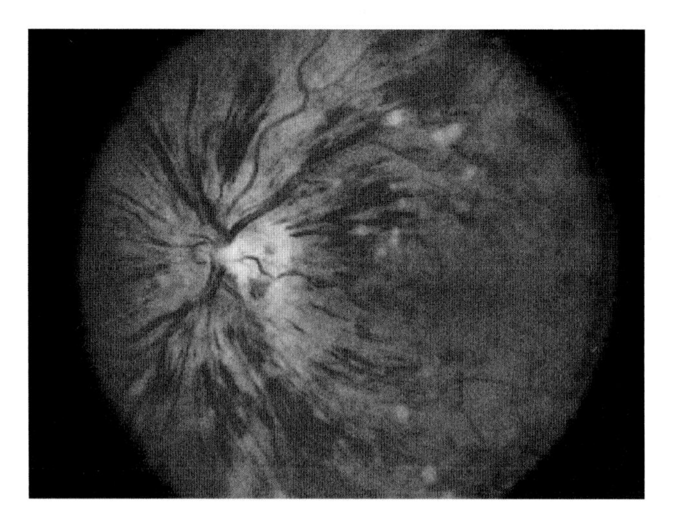

FIGURE 14.44. Central retinal vein occlusion.

(Courtesy of Department of Ophthalmology, Naval Medical Center, Portsmoutn, VA as published in Knoop KJ, Stack LB, Storrow AB. *Atlas of Emergency Medicine,* 2nd ed. New York: McGraw-Hill, 2002:83.)

OCULAR TRAUMA

Hyphema

ETIOLOGY

Blood in the anterior chamber, often secondary to trauma (see Figure 14.45)

SYMPTOMS/EXAM

- Decreased vision
- Photophobia
- Pain
- Absence of red reflex
- Layering of blood in anterior chamber when patient sitting upright
- "Eight ball hyphema" = 100% blood and requires urgent ophthalmology consult.

TREATMENT

- Rest, with elevation of HOB about 45°
- Monitor IOP.
- Avoid blood-thinning medications.
- May consider cycloplegic drops and aminocaproic acid to prevent recurrent hemorrhage.
- Avoid carbonic anhydrase inhibitor (diamox) in sicklers (increase sickling).
- Ophthalmology consult
- Patients with significant elevation in intraocular pressure typically require admission and treatment with IV mannitol.

COMPLICATIONS

- Acute glaucoma secondary to obstruction of aqueous humor
- Rebleeding 2–5 days after (most common complication)
- Corneal staining/pigmentation

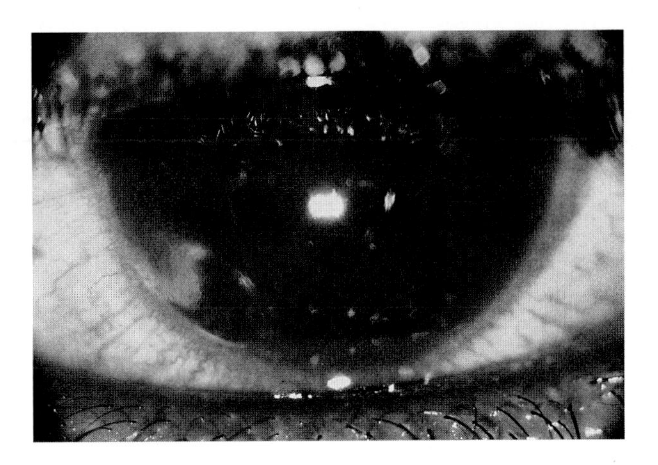

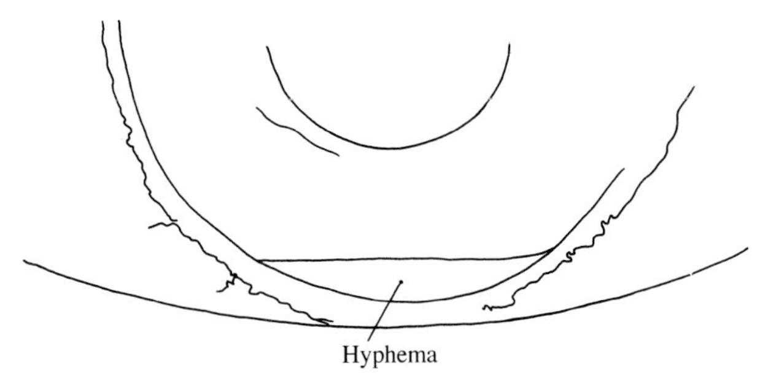

FIGURE 14.45. Hyphema present in the bottom portion of the anterior chamber seen in photo and schematic.

(Courtesy of Dallas E. Peak, MD as published in Knoop KJ, Stack LB, Storrow AB. *Atlas of Emergency Medicine,* 2nd ed. New York: McGraw-Hill, 2002:105.)

Ruptured Globe/Corneal Laceration

Symptoms/Exam

- Associated hyphema
- Prolapsed iris or other intraocular tissue
- Peaked pupil points to the rupture site (see Figure 14.46)

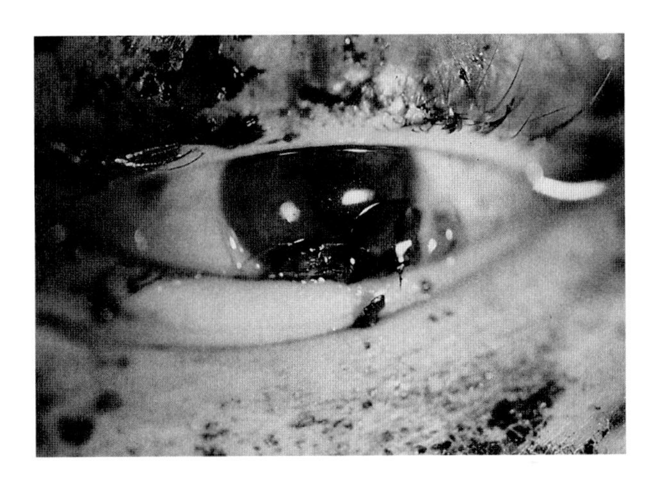

FIGURE 14.46. Ruptured globe as evidenced by herniation of Iris through the cornea and an irregular pupil shape. Do not send this patient home—surgery is needed.

(Reproduced, with permission, from Knoop KJ, Stack LB, Storrow AB. *Atlas of Emergency Medicine,* 2nd ed. New York: McGraw-Hill, 2002:109.)

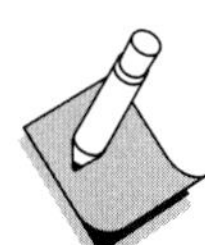

Rule out ruptured globe if you see a hyphema in the setting of trauma.

- **Seidel test** = fluorescein strip applied to wound. A positive test shows leaking aqueous humor due to corneal perforation. This is not necessary to do if iris tissue or other intraocular content is obviously prolapsed from the eye.
- Rupture globe is a cannot miss diagnosis which may have a subtle presentation. In patients with eyelid lacerations, be sure to look under the lid at the top surface of the globe.

TREATMENT

- Avoid pressure on the eye (can expel contents).
- No IOP checks
- Make sure patient is NPO!
- Shield eye.
- Antibiotics
- Pain meds
- CT scan to check for foreign bodies; no MRI as patient may retain metal foreign body
- Emergent ophthalmology consult for immediate operative repair

CHAPTER 15

Neurology

Kelly Bookman, MD

A 58-year-old female is brought to the ED as a "stroke alert." Her husband states that she woke up 1 hour prior to arrival with slurred speech and weakness in her right arm and leg. On physical exam she has aphasia, R-sided hemiparesis, and sensory deficits. Labs are drawn, and the patient is rushed to the CT scanner where a left middle cerebral artery distribution stroke (ischemic) is diagnosed. Is this patient a thrombolysis candidate?

While the patient is presenting within 3 hours of perceived onset of symptoms, we do not know the actual time the stroke occurred. The patient went to sleep 10 hours before arriving in ED, and thus stroke onset is assumed to be up to 10 hours prior to arrival, not 1 hour. This patient is not a thrombolysis candidate.

STROKE

A stroke is any process that disrupts the flow of oxygen and substrate-rich blood to the brain. Commonly an infarcted area of brain is surrounded by a region of tenuous blood flow, the **ischemic penumbra**. The focus of stroke management is to maintain the blood supply to this region, thereby limiting infarct size. Overall, 85% of strokes are ischemic and 15% are hemorrhagic.

Anatomy of Cerebral Blood Flow (CBF) (See Figure 15.1)

- **Anterior circulation (from carotid arteries, 80% of CBF)**
  - Frontoparietal lobes
  - Anterior aspect of temporal lobes

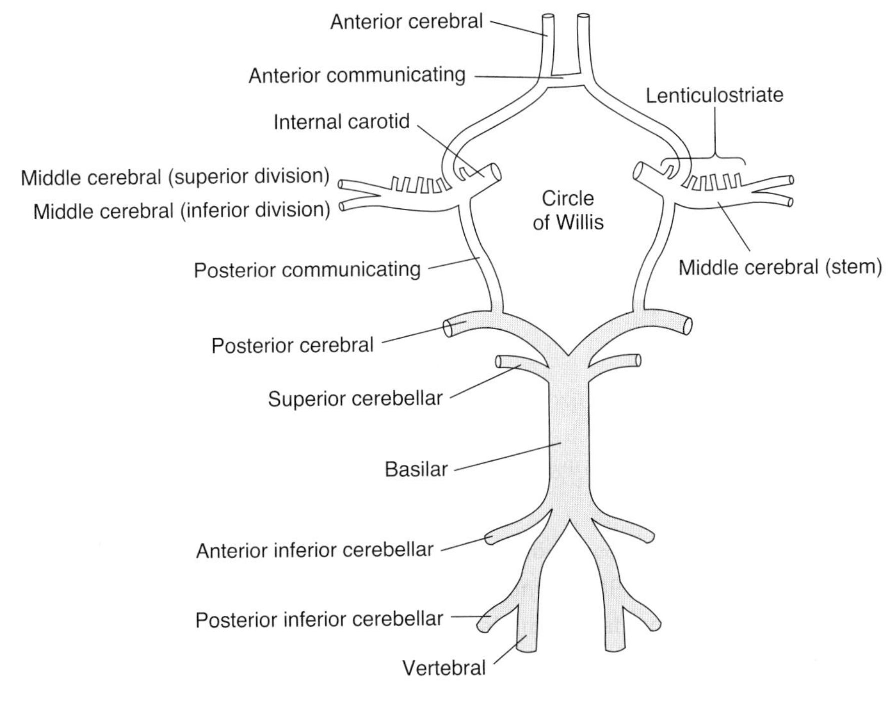

FIGURE 15.1. Anatomy of cerebral blood flow.

(Reproduced, with permission, from Aminoff MJ, Greenberg DA, Simon RP. *Clinical Neurology*, 6th ed. New York: McGraw-Hill, 2005:288.)

- Optic nerve and retina
- Deep gray matter
- **Posterior circulation (from vertebrobasilar arteries, 20% of CBF)**
  - Medial aspect of temporal lobes
  - Visual occipital cortex
  - Thalamus
  - Brainstem
  - Upper spinal cord
  - Cerebellum
  - Auditory and vestibular function
- **Circle of Willis**
  - Connection between anterior and posterior circulations

Ischemic Stroke

Ischemic stroke may be divided into three types: thrombotic, cardioembolic and hypoperfusion states.

THROMBOTIC STROKE

CAUSES

Thrombosis is the most common cause of stroke in the United States and typically results from clot formation at the site of an ulcerated atherosclerotic plaque.

Other causes include:

- Vessel narrowing from vasculitis, dissection, infectious disease, vasospasm
- Thrombophilia from hypercoagulable states
- Sickle cell disease
- Polycythemia

Symptoms generally come on gradually and may be preceded by transient ischemic attacks (TIAs) affecting the same region as the stroke.

A subset of thrombotic stroke is the **lacunar stroke**. This is a stroke of a small terminal vessel, typically deep in the subcortical cerebrum, basal ganglia, internal capsule, thalamus, corona radiate, or brainstem. There is higher incidence in African Americans, Mexican Americans, Hong Kong Chinese, and patients with hypertension and diabetes.

CARDIOEMBOLIC STROKE

The most common source of embolic stroke is mural thrombus in patients with atrial fibrillation.

CAUSES

Occurs when intravascular material (eg, clot) from a proximal source travels to the cerebral circulation, causing obstruction

Types of emboli include:

- Cardiac (mural thrombus, valvular vegetations, cardiac tumors)
- Venous thrombosis (in the presence of a ventricular or atrial septal defect)
- Proximal aortic or carotid atherosclerotic plaque
- Fat (from a broken bone)
- Air (air embolism)
- Particulate matter (eg, talc from injection drug use)

Onset is typically sudden and maximal.

Hypoperfusion States

Causes

Cerebral perfusion pressure (CPP) is dependent on mean arterial blood pressure (MAP) and intracranial pressure (ICP), and is represented by the formula: CPP = MAP – ICP. Hypoperfusion may logically result from an increased ICP or decreased MAP.

Hypoperfusion stroke is a diffuse process with regional variability depending on state of vasculature and brain in any given region. Prolonged hypoperfusion will result in permanent injury.

Stroke symptoms may wax and wane as these variables change.

Symptoms/Exam

- Symptom onset varies with stroke type.
  - Sudden and maximal at onset with embolic
  - More gradual or preceded by TIA with thrombotic
  - Waxing and waning with hypoperfusion state
- Location of symptoms varies with location of obstruction (see Table 15.1).
- **Amaurosis fugax**: Transient monocular blindness from embolization of carotid plaque to the ophthalmic artery
- **Transient ischemic attack (TIA):** Neurologic deficit that has complete clinical resolution within 24 hours.
- **Wernicke aphasia** (receptive aphasia): There is inability to comprehend language input. Speech is fluent but disorganized, due to ischemia/infarct in Wernicke's area of temporal lobe.
- **Broca's aphasia** (expressive aphasia): There is inability to communicate verbally. Speech is halting and produced with great effort, due to infarct/ischemia of Broca's area in the frontal lobe.

The hallmark of posterior circulation stroke is crossed deficits (face vs body).

Diagnosis

- Suspect based on history and examination.
- Confirmed based on CT or MRI
  - Appears as area of hypodensity on noncontrast CT (see Figure 15.2)
  - Perfusion-weighted CT angiography can identify the ischemic penumbra.
  - Ischemic stroke will not be visible on noncontrast CT until >6 hours.
- Glucose to rule out hypoglycemia
- ECG to evaluate rhythm
- Coagulation studies if coagulopathy suspected

Treatment

- ABCs (including intubation for decreased level of consciousness)
- **Hypotension:** Restore euvolemia, then use pressors (if necessary).
- **Hypertension**
  - Aggressive lowering of BP in chronically hypertensive patients (who have cerebral autoregulation curve shifted to right) may limit flow to the ischemic penumbra.
  - Treat if BP persistently elevated (systolic >220 or diastolic >140).
    - Goal = BP ≤ 185/115 mmHg.
    - Use titratable agent such as labetalol or nitroprusside.

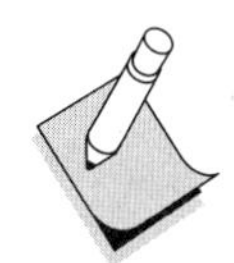

In stroke, treat BP if persistently elevated >220/140. Goal BP is ≤185/115

TABLE 15.1. Ischemic Stroke—Clinical Findings

Area of Blockage	Major Finding	Other Findings
Anterior cerebral artery	Contralateral weakness of leg > arm and face with minimal sensory findings	Altered mentation and judgment Perseveration Primitive reflexes (grasp and suck) If both arteries originate from occluded common trunk (bilateral infarct) → paraplegia and severe dysarthria
Middle cerebral artery	Contralateral weakness **and** numbness of arm and face > leg	Homonymous hemianopsia Gaze preference toward side of infarct If dominant hemisphere: Receptive/expressive aphasia Nondominant hemisphere: Inattention and neglect
Lacunar artery	Pure motor *or* pure sensory findings	Clumsy hand–dysarthria syndrome
Posterior cerebral artery	Contralateral visual field and light touch/pinprick deficit with *minimal* weakness	Memory loss
Vertebrobasilar artery	Crossed deficits: Ipsilateral cranial nerve deficits with contralateral weakness	Bilateral spasticity Syncope and drop attacks
Distal vertebral or posterior inferior cerebellar artery Lateral medullary (Wallenberg) syndrome	Crossed pain and temperature deficits: Ipsilateral loss on face, contralateral on body	Ipsilateral Horner syndrome and cranial nerve deficits may be present. Gait and limb ataxia
Basilar artery	"Locked in" syndrome (complete paralysis of voluntary muscles except eye movement; normal level of consciousness)	
Cerebellar artery	Sudden inability to walk or stand with headache, nausea/vomiting and cerebellar findings	Lateralizing dysmetria (eg, finger-nose-finger) Dysdiadokokinesis (rapid alternating movements)

- Glucose control
  - Treat hyperglycemia to keep blood glucose 100–200.
  - Avoid IV solutions with glucose.
  - Avoid steroids, if possible.
- Systemic tPA (thrombolysis)
  - Criteria
    - Symptoms <3 hours duration
    - Age >18 years
    - Blood pressure <185/110
    - Meaningful neurologic deficit that is not resolving
    - **No** finding on noncontrast CT head scan or clear ischemic penumbra on contrast perfusion images

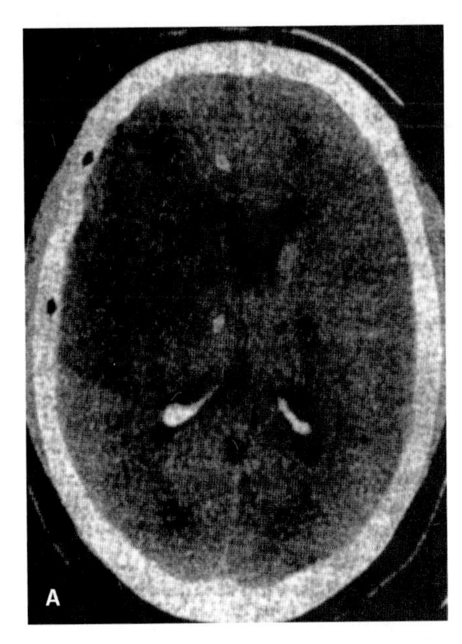

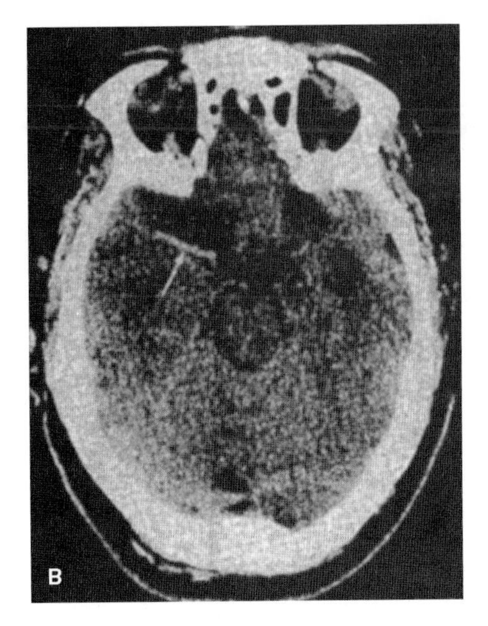

FIGURE 15.2. Noncontrast head CT demonstrating right middle cerebral artery distribution stroke. (A) Note the well-defined area of hypodensity (*arrows*) in the right middle cerebral artery (MCA) territory. (B) Acute thrombus in the right MCA (*arrow*).

(Reproduced, with permission, from Chen MYM, Pope TL, Ott DJ. *Basic Radiology*. New York: McGraw-Hill, 2004:336–337.)

- See Table 15.2 for summary of indications and contraindications to thrombolytics.
- Dose: 0.9 mg/kg with 10% given as bolus, remaining infused over 60 minutes
- **Intra-arterial tPA**
  - Used for brainstem strokes, some data supported for use in delayed time periods (>3 hours).
- **Aspirin:** 160–325mg within 48 hours (unless thrombolysis candidate) for secondary stroke prevention
  - Clopidogrel or ticlopidine if aspirin allergic
- **Aggrenox:** A combination of low-dose aspirin and dipyridamole (antiplatelet agent); greater risk reduction than aspirin alone
  - Early neurosurgical consultation for all cerebellar strokes (increased risk of herniation)
- **Avoid:**
  - Routine seizure prophylaxis
  - Heparin: No proven benefit in acute stroke (even embolic)
  - Sublingual calcium channel blockers (unpredictable drops in BP)

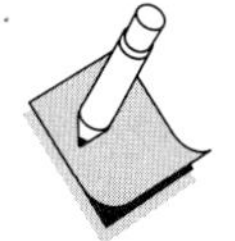

Heparin has no proven benefit in acute stroke.

NEUROLOGY

TRANSIENT ISCHEMIC ATTACK

Transient ischemic attack is a neurologic deficit that has complete clinical resolution within 24 hours. Up to 20% of patients with TIA will go on to have a stroke within 90 days, half of these within 2 days.

SYMPTOMS/EXAM

- Related to vascular distribution involved (see Table 15.1)

TABLE 15.2. Criteria for Intravenous Thrombolysis in Ischemic Stroke

INCLUSION	EXCLUSION*
Age 18 years or older	Minor stroke symptoms
Clinical diagnosis of ischemic stroke	Rapidly improving neurologic signs
Time since onset *well established* to be less than 3 hr	Prior intracranial hemorrhage
	Blood glucose <50 mg/dL or >400 mg/dL
	Seizure at onset of stroke
	GI or GU bleeding within preceding 21 days
	Recent myocardial infarction
	Major surgery within preceding 14 days
	Sustained pretreatment SBP >185 mmHg or DBP >110 mmHg
	Previous stroke within preceding 90 days
	Previous head injury within preceding 90 days
	Current use of oral anticoagulants or PT >15 s or INR >1.7
	Use of heparin within preceding 48 hr and a prolonged PTT
	Platelet count <100,000/μL

*Caution is advised before giving tPA to persons with severe stroke (NIH Stroke Scale Score greater than 22).

Abbreviations: DBP = diastolic blood pressure; GI = gastrointestinal; GU = genitourinary; INR = international normalized ratio; PT = prothombin time; PTT = partial prothrombin time; SBP = systolic blood pressure.

(Reproduced, with permission, from Tintinalli JE, Kelen GD, Stapczynski JS. *Emergency Medicine: A Comprehensive Study Guide,* 6th ed. New York: McGraw-Hill, 2004:1386 based on data from Adams HP, Brott TG, Furlan AJ, et al. Guidelines for thrombolytic therapy for acute stroke: A supplement to the guidelines for the management of patients with acute ischemic stroke. *Circulation* 94:1167, 1996.)

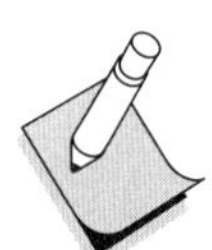

Consider intra-arterial thrombolysis in patients with brainstem strokes (even in delayed presentations).

DIAGNOSIS

- Clinical diagnosis, based on complete resolution of findings within 24 hours
- Evaluation for underlying etiology includes: ECG, carotid USN, cardiac echocardiogram (in selected patients).

TREATMENT

- Antiplatelet agent (aspirin, clopidogrel or ticlopidine) is primary therapy.
- Goal is prevention of stroke, based on suspected underlying process (eg, anticoagulation if mural thrombus).

TABLE 15.3. ABCD² Score to Predict Subsequent Stroke in Patients with TIA

Variable	Points
Age >60 years	1
BP ≥140/90 mmHg	1
Unilateral weakness	2
Speech disturbance without weakness	1
Duration ≥60 minutes	2
Duration 10–59 minutes	1
Diabetes	1
Risk for subsequent stroke: Low: 0–3 points Moderate: 3–4 points High: 6–7 points	

- The **ABCD² score** can be used to predict likelihood of subsequent stroke within 2 days (see Table 15.3).
- Patients with moderate to high risk for stroke within 2 days should be admitted for evaluation and treatment.

ABCD² Score:
Age
Blood pressure
Clinical features
Duration
Diabetes

Hemorrhagic Stroke

Can be divided into intracerebral hemorrhage and subarachnoid hemorrhage

Intracerebral Hemorrhage (ICH)

Causes

Intracerebral hemorrhage is an acute bleed into the brain parenchyma as a result of:

- Chronic hypertension (most common)
- Amyloidosis
- Cocaine or methamphetamine use
- Vascular malformation
- Anticoagulation or thrombolysis

Symptoms/Exam

- Characterized by sudden onset and rapid progression of neurologic symptoms (see Table 15.4)
- Headache
- Nausea, vomiting
- Patients usually present hypertensive.

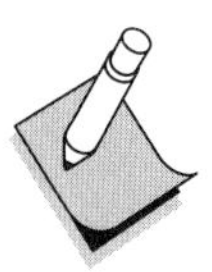

The most common location for hemorrhagic stroke is the putamen.

TABLE 15.4. **Hemorrhagic Stroke—Neurologic Findings**

LOCATION	NEUROLOGIC FINDING
Putamen (most common)	Contralateral hemiplegia Contralateral sensory deficits Contralateral conjugate gaze paresis Homonymous hemianopsia Aphasia, neglect, apraxia Usually more lethargic than middle cerebral infarcts
Cerebellar	Severe ataxia, vertigo, nystagmus Dysarthria Decreased LOC (may occur) Ipsilateral gaze palsy, facial weakness and sensory loss NO hemiparesis
Thalamic	Contralateral hemiparesis Contralateral sensory deficits Sensory loss > motor loss
Pontine	Severe headache Hyperventilation Pinpoint pupils Absence of oculovestibular reflexes Decerebrate posturing

Differential

- Hypoglycemia, Todd paralysis, complicated migraine, mass lesion, delirium

Diagnosis

- Suspect based on history and examination.
- Confirm by noncontrast CT scan (Figure 15.3).
- Lumbar puncture is necessary to rule out subarachnoid hemorrhage, when suspected.

Treatment

- Supportive therapy
- Elevated head of bed to 30°
- Hyperventilation (to P_aCO_2 of 30), mannitol and furosemide if impending herniation
- **Hypertension**
  - Treat if severe (>220/120 mmHg) with goal of gradually lowering BP to prehemorrhage levels
  - Use titratable agent—labetalol or nitroprusside.
- Seizure prophylaxis with phenytoin

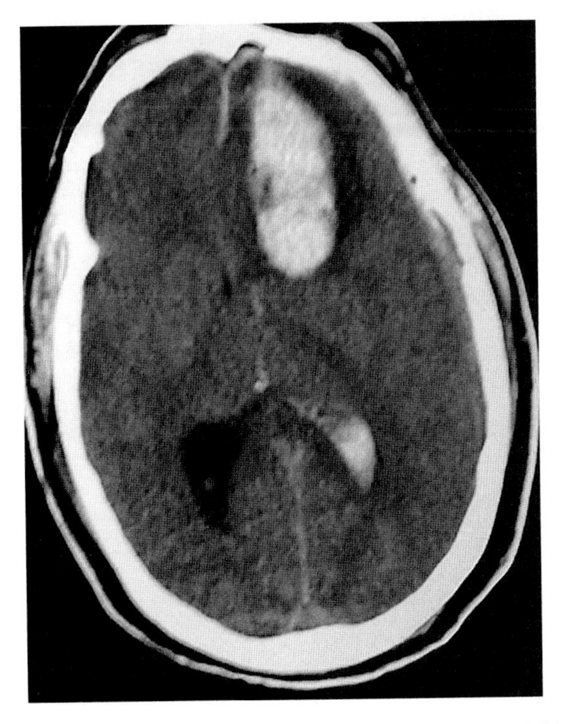

FIGURE 15.3. Noncontrast head CT demonstrating a large frontal intracerebral hemorrhage.

(Reproduced, with permission, from Stone CK, Humphries, RL. *Current Emergency Diagnosis and Treatment*, 5th ed. New York: McGraw-Hill, 2004:374.)

- Neurosurgery consult
  - Especially for cerebellar hemorrhage, which is associated with rapid deterioration and herniation

SUBARACHNOID HEMORRHAGE

See "Headache."

A 25-year-old male with a history of epilepsy presents with continous seizure activity for >30 minutes. He weighs approximately 100 kg. His glucose is normal and he has no history of alcohol use. There is no change in seizure activity after two doses of lorazepam. What is the most appropriate next agent?

Phenytoin IV is the most appropriate next agent. This patient also warrants airway control via RSI.

SEIZURES

CAUSES

Seizures result from excessive and disordered neuronal firing. They may be a primary disorder or secondary to an underlying medical condition (see Table 15.5).

TABLE 15.5. Secondary Causes of Seizures

Secondary Causes of Seizures
Metabolic derangement
Hypoglycemia
Hyponatremia
Hypocalcemia
Drugs and toxins
Anticholinergics/cholinergics
Antidepressants
Mushrooms (*Gyrometra* sp.)
Sympathomimetics
Toxic alcohols
Isoniazid
Withdrawal syndromes
CNS infection
CNS lesion or event
Neurocysticercosis
Hemorrhage
Tumors
Stroke
Vasculitis
Hydrocephalus
Febrile seizure (pediatrics)
Trauma
Eclampsia

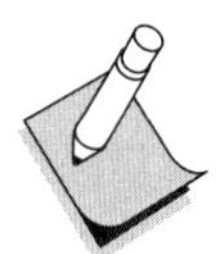

Neurocysticercosis (CNS Taenia solium *larvae infection) is the most common cause of secondary seizures in the developing world.*

Seizures are classified based on behavioral, electrophysiologic, and clinical features of the seizure rather than on anatomic or pathophysiologic features. They can generally be broken down into partial and generalized seizures.

Partial (Focal) Seizures

Partial seizures begin in localized area of the brain.

SYMPTOMS/EXAM

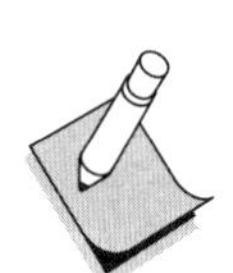

*Consciousness remains normal with simple partial seizures. Consciousness is **impaired** with complex partial seizures. Consciousness is lost with generalized seizures.*

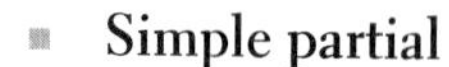

- Simple partial
  - Brief event without alteration of consciousness
  - If involving motor neurons → unilateral focal clonic movements.
  - May also manifest as isolated sensory, autonomic, or psychic symptoms
- Complex partial (temporal lobe or psychomotor)
  - Partial seizure with *impairment* of consciousness and postictal state
  - Commonly manifests as mental and psychological symptoms, including changes in affect, confusion, hallucinations, automatisms (eg, lip smacking)
- **Secondary generalized:** Partial seizure that spreads to both hemispheres (eg, generalized seizure preceded by aura)

Generalized Seizures

Primary generalized seizures begin in both hemispheres and do not have inciting focus. All except myoclonic have altered LOC.

Symptoms/Exam

- **Nonconvulsive (absence or petit mal)**
  - Alteration in mental status without motor activity
  - Most frequent in 5- to 10-year-olds
  - Rarely postictal
  - Characterized by brief 3-Hz, spike-and-wave discharges on EEG
- **Convulsive (grand mal)**
  - Abrupt loss of consciousness at onset (except with myoclonic)
  - Can be clonic, tonic, tonic-clonic, myoclonic or atonic
  - Followed by postictal state
- **Todd's paralysis:** Focal paralysis, typically following a generalized seizure; usually lasts 1–2 hours but may last 1–2 days

Nonconvulsive (absence) seizures typically develop in childhood.

Differential

- Primary considerations include syncope, dysrhythmia, psychiatric illness, decerebrate posturing, migraines.

Diagnosis

- EEG during event confirms diagnosis (if diagnosis is in question).
- ED evaluation may be limited (known seizure disorder) or extensive (seizure in febrile immunocompromised patient).
- **First-time seizure**
  - Check sodium and glucose.
  - Check urine toxicology.
  - CT scan if *any* suspicion for serious structural lesion
  - LP if *any* suspicion for meningitis or subarachnoid hemorrhage
- **Recurrent seizure**
  - Check glucose and anticonvulsant levels (if available).
    - Supratherapeutic levels of phenytoin and carbamazepine can result in seizures.
  - More extensive evaluation is necessary if change in seizure pattern, prolonged postictal state, fever, etc.
  - Status epilepticus (see "Status Epilepticus")

Serum lactate may be elevated immediately following a generalized tonic-clonic seizure, but should clear spontaneously within 1 hour.

NEUROLOGY

Treatment

- First-time seizure
  - Treat underlying cause, if identified.
  - If CNS lesion present, initiate anticonvulsant therapy.
  - Otherwise recommend outpatient follow-up for MRI and EEG if no cause found.
  - Alcohol withdrawal seizure: Treat with benzodiazepines; patients do not require chronic anticonvulsant therapy
- Ongoing seizures (see "Status Epilepticus")

Status Epilepticus

Seizure lasting >30 minutes or recurrent seizures without resolution of postictal state; may be generalized seizures (life-threatening, high mortality), absence seizures, or complex partial seizures

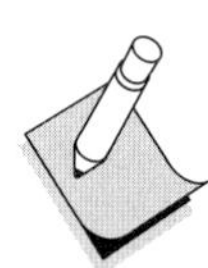

The blood prolactin level may *be elevated for 15–60 minutes following generalized seizure.*

DIAGNOSIS

- EEG is confirmative (if diagnosis is in question).
- Check glucose immediately.
- Check electrolytes, magnesium, toxicology screen, liver and renal function, pregnancy test (as indicated).
- Obtain head CT.
- Consider lumbar puncture.

TREATMENT

- Thiamine and glucose if hypoglycemic or if alcoholism suspected.
- **First-line therapy = benzodizepines**—diazepam, lorazepam, or midazolam.
  - Lorazepam has a relatively longer duration of seizure suppression.
  - Load with phenytoin if benzodiazepines are effective.
- **Second-line therapy = phenytoin and/or phenobarbital**
  - Phenytoin: Rapid administration may cause hypotension and cardiac dysrhythmias due to its propylene glycol diluent; this may be avoided with fosphenytoin (water soluble prodrug). Onset of action is 10–30 minutes.
  - Phenobarbital: Anticipate sedation, respiratory depression and hypotension. Onset of action is 15–30 minutes.
- Magnesium sulfate, if eclamptic
- Pyridoxine, if isoniazid overdose suspected
- Drug-induced coma (pentobarbital, midazolam, propofol) or general anesthesia, if resistant to above

A 23-year-old military recruit is brought in by ambulance with mental status changes. Narcan was given without effect. On arrival he is noted to be minimally responsive to painful stimuli and hypotensive. D-stick is normal. While the patient is being intubated, the skin is noted to be warm and covered with a petechial rash. What is the most appropriate next step?

This patient likely has meningococcal meningitis and needs immediate antibiotic therapy with cefotaxime or ceftriaxone IV. Until the diagnosis is confirmed, vancomycin should also be given to cover resistant strains of *Streptococcus pneumoniae*.

CNS INFECTIONS

Meningitis

Meningitis is bacterial, viral, fungal, or aseptic inflammation of the membranes covering the brain or spinal cord.

CAUSES

The causes of meningitis in adult patients include:

- Bacterial
  - *Strep. pneumoniae* (most common overall, Gram-positive diplococci)
  - *Neisseria meningitides* (younger ages, Gram-negative rod)
  - *Listeria monocytogenes* (adults >60 years, Gram-positive rod)
  - *Haemophilus influenzae* type B; disappearing with the HIB-vaccine

- *Mycobacterium tuberculosis* (uncommon)
  - Group B streptococcus, *Escherichia coli* and *Listeria monocytogenes* are the most common bacterial causes in neonates <1 month.
  - *Streptococcus pneumoniae, Staphylococcus aureus, Pseudomonas aeruginosa* and coliform bacteria are common following neurosurgical procedure or head trauma.
- Viral
  - Enteroviruses (most common, increased in summer months)
  - Herpes simplex virus should always be suspected.
  - Numerous other viruses
- Fungal (eg, *Cryptococcus*) and parasitic (eg, *Toxoplasma gondii*)—in the immunocompromised
- Noninfectious
  - SLE
  - Vasculitis
  - Drug induced
  - Carcinomatosis
  - Sarcoidosis
  - Behçet disease

A significant overlap exists between bacterial and viral meningitis presentations. Viral meningitis is a diagnosis that can be made only after other more serious pathogens have been excluded.

PATHOPHYSIOLOGY

- Bacterial infection begins with nasopharyngeal colonization → hematogenous spread (more likely with encapsulated organisms) → CNS infection.
- Viruses enter through the skin or via respiratory, GI, or GU tracts.
- Fungi primarily spread from pulmonary source.
- Meningeal inflammatory response to foreign agent resulting in:
  - Increased permeability of blood brain barrier → increased CSF proteins
  - Decreased glucose transport → decreased CSF glucose levels

SYMPTOMS

- Fever
- Headache (most common)
- Stiff neck (seen half the time)
- Photophobia
- Mental status changes or irritability (infants)
- Vomiting
- Seizures
- Symptoms may be diminished/absent in immunocompromised, very young, or elderly patients.

EXAM

- Fever
- Nuchal rigidity
- Increased deep tendon reflexes (DTRs)
- Altered mental status
- Lateral gaze ophthalmoplegia
- Petechial or purpuric rash (ominous sign)
- **Kernigs sign**: Position the patient with hips and knees flexed. Extend the knees. Flexion of neck or pain in neck is + sign.

Kernig's = Knee

- **Brudzinki sign**: Neck flexion results in flexion at hips (neck sign) *or* passive flexion of hip on one side results in contralateral hip flexion (contralateral sign).
- Look for concomitant infection, such as sinusitis, otitis, pneumonia.

DIFFERENTIAL

The differential diagnosis includes encephalitis, brain abscess, subdural, subarachnoid hemorrhage, intracranial hemorrhage, brain tumor.

DIAGNOSIS

- Meningitis should be considered in all patients presenting with a headache or stiff neck and fever.
- **Head CT**
  - Required before LP in patients >60 years old, the immunocompromised (eg, HIV), history of CNS disease (including stroke, mass lesions or recent head trauma), recent seizures within 1 week, the presence of marked CNS depression, papilledema or focal neurologic deficits.
- **Lumbar puncture (LP)**
  - Contraindications
    - Coagulopathy (relative)
    - Infection at skin puncture site (absolute)
  - CSF findings classically vary with viral, bacterial, and fungal etiologies (see Table 15.6).
    - **but**—early bacterial infections or partially treated infection may have a paucity of findings!
    - **and**—early viral infections may have significant neutrophils!
- Blood cultures may help isolate causative organism.

TABLE 15.6. Analysis of Cerebrospinal Fluid

	NORMAL LEVELS	BACTERIAL	VIRAL	FUNGAL
Opening pressure (cmH_2O)	5–20	Elevated	Normal or slightly elevated	Elevated
Leukocytes/mm^3	≤5	≥500, although may be mildly elevated early	100–500, although may be mildly elevated early	10–500
% Neutrophils	0 (≤1 PMN)	>80%	<50%	<50%
Protein (mg/dL)	20–45	>200	<200	>200
Glucose (mg/dL)	50–80% or 60–70% of serum level	≤40% or <50% of serum	Usually normal	<50
Cultures or studies		Gram stain, culture, PCR, bacterial antigen assays	HSV or enterovirus PCR	Cryptococcal antigen, yeast

TREATMENT

- Stabilization and supportive therapy, as needed
- **Immediate** empiric antibiotic therapy
  - **Vancomycin, 1 gm IV,**
    and
  - **Ceftriaxone or cefotaxime, 2 gm IV,**
    and
  - **Ampicillin** if neonate, >60 years, debilitated, alcoholic
  - Will not decrease ability to detect organism in CSF fluid if LP performed within 2 hours and antigen assays are utilized
- **Dexamethasone**
  - Appears to decrease morbidity in adults with *bacterial* meningitis (especially *S. pneumoniae*) and children with *H. influenzae* meningitis
  - Give 0.15 mg/kg IV 15 minutes before or concurrent with the first dose of antibiotics, repeat every 4–6 hours.
- Other antibiotics are indicated if fungal infection is suspected or identified.
- Viral meningitis (diagnosis of exclusion) requires no specific treatment.
- Admit all patients with high suspicion for meningitis, regardless of LP results.

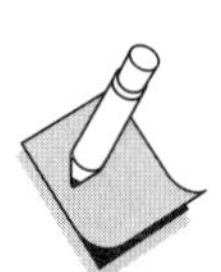

Fungal meningitis is difficult to diagnose: Low-grade fevers, variable headache, possible weight loss, lassitude; CSF with very elevated protein.

*Do **not** delay antibiotics for CT or LP.*

COMPLICATIONS

- Sepsis
- DIC
- Seizures
- Focal neurologic deficits
- Hearing loss
- Cognitive deficits
- Waterhouse-Friderichsen syndrome
- Transmission of *N. meningitidis* or *H. influenzae* type B
  - Seen in household contacts, day-care centers, schools, barracks, and mucous membrane contacts
  - Chemoprophylaxis with rifampin (four doses) is required once bacterial organism is identified.

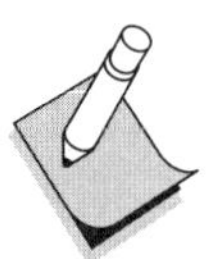

Family members and close contacts of patients with N. meningitidis *or* H. influenzae *meningitis should receive antibiotic prophylaxis.*

Encephalitis

Encephalitis is a viral infection of the brain parenchyma itself, often a progression of viral meningitis.

CAUSES

- Viruses cause the majority of cases (* = most common).
  - ***Arboviruses**
  - Mosquito and tick-borne viruses
  - Include West Nile virus, St. Louis encephalitis
  - ***Herpes simplex virus** (HSV)
  - Other herpes viruses (EBV, CMV)
  - Rabies virus
- Hypersensitivity reaction to MMR vaccination
- *Toxoplasma gondii* (immunocompromised)
- Lyme disease

Gray matter is predominantly affected in encephalitis.

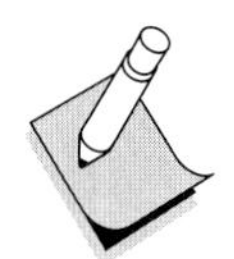

Herpes virus has a predilection for the temporal lobes. Patients often present with "psychiatric symptoms" or behavioral changes.

SYMPTOMS/EXAM

- Often begins with nonspecific acute febrile illness
- Headache and fever (common)
- Neurologic abnormalities
  - Altered mental state
  - New psychiatric symptoms
  - Emotional outbursts
  - Cognitive deficits
  - Focal neurologic deficits
  - Seizures
  - Movement disorders
- Sensorimotor deficits are uncommon.

DIAGNOSIS

- Suspect diagnosis based on presenting symptoms and exam
- **Lumbar puncture**
  - To exclude bacterial meningitis and help identify viral organism via PCR
  - Cautions and contraindications as with meningitis
- **MRI with contrast**
  - Can readily identify areas of involvement (focal edema)
  - Lesions in the temporal lobes = HSV encephalitis.
  - CT with contrast is alternative but is less sensitive.
- **EEG**
  - Suggestive EEG abnormalities may be seen.
- **Brain biopsy:** Definitive

TREATMENT

- Empiric treatment for suspected etiologic organisms
  - Acyclovir for HSV and herpes zoster virus
  - Gancyclovir for cytomegalovirus
  - Once herpes and cytomegalovirus infections have been excluded, there is no benefit from antiviral agents.

Brain Abscess

Brain abscess is an infection that becomes localized to a particular region of the brain: intraparenchymal, epidural, or subdural locations.

MECHANISMS

Infection reaches the brain via three mechanisms:

- Contiguous infection of middle ear, sinus, or teeth
- Neurosurgery or penetrating trauma
- Hematogenous spread

Common organisms include:

- Often polymicrobial
- Streptococci
- Anaerobic bacteria (esp. *Bacteroides*)
- *Staphylococcus aureus*
- Fungal and parasitic infections in the immunocompromised

Symptoms/Exam

- Often mild course that may progress slowly over weeks
- The vast majority of patients complain of headache.
- Nuchal rigidity and fever in half
- Focal neurologic deficits **may occur**.
- Papilledema is not uncommon.

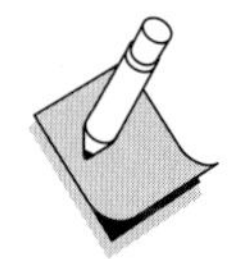

Headache is uniformly present in patients with brain abscess.

Diagnosis

- **CT or MRI with contrast**
  - Cannot exclude abscess with noncontrast studies
  - Classic finding = ring-enhancing lesion(s)

Treatment

- Supportive therapy
- Treat associated seizures.
- Empiric antibiotic therapy
  - Depends on suspected source
  - No obvious source: Cefotaxime and metronidazole
- Surgical versus medical therapy
  - Surgery for large abscesses

Neurocysticercosis

CNS infection with the larval form of the tapeworm *Taenia solium*; very common in developing countries

Mechanisms

Forms of disease:

- Invasion of brain parenchyma (most common) → formation of cysts → inflammation and fibrosis.
- Cysterci in ventricles → obstructing hydrocephalus.
- Cysterci in basilar cisterns → arachnoiditis → meningitis or communicating hydrocephalus.

Symptoms/Exam

- Seizure is the most common clinical finding.
- Headache or signs of increased intracranial pressure are seen, if hydrocephalus develops.

Diagnosis/Treatment

- Based on exposure history, CT or MRI findings and serologic testing
- Treatment depends on clinical manifestations (eg, antiseizure medications, shunting procedure).
- Antiparasitic agents

Shunt Infection

The majority of shunt infections present within 6 months of placement.

- Common infecting organisms:
  - *Staphylococcus epidermidis* (half)
  - *Staphylococcus aureus*
- Other organisms include Gram-negatives and anaerobes.

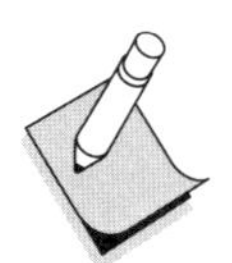

Lumbar puncture is not useful in diagnosing a shunt infection. A shunt tap is required.

SYMPTOMS/EXAM

- Shunt obstruction (most common): Headache, N/V, altered mentation
- Other findings may include fever, meningismus, and tenderness or warmth along shunt tubing.

DIAGNOSIS/TREATMENT

- Shunt tap is required to exclude diagnosis as a LP may miss the CNS infection.
- Immediate neurosurgical consultation and initiation of antibiotic therapy (vancomycin + third-generation cephalosporin and aminoglycoside).

HEADACHE

Intracranially, only the arteries at the base of the brain, their main branches, the periarterial dura mater, and the venous sinuses are pain sensitive. These pain-sensitive intracranial structures are supplied by sensory axons of the trigeminal ganglion (supratentorial structures) and by the upper cervical roots (posterior fossa structures).

Headaches are classified as **primary** (vast majority of headaches) and **secondary** (see Table 15.7). Secondary headaches are considered "secondary" to some underlying cause (eg, subarachnoid hemorrhage).

A 54-year-old female presents complaining of a severe headache. The headache was sudden in onset while she was moving boxes of books at work. The patient has neck stiffness and nausea but denies weakness or numbness in arms or legs. Her VS and neurologic examination are normal. Head CT confirms your suspicion for SAH. What is her likely prognosis? What pharmacologic agent has been shown to prevent secondary ischemic stroke in patients with SAH?

Based on the Hunt and Hess classification, this patient has a Grade I hemorrhage and should have a good neurologic outcome. Nimodipine is used to prevent vasospasm-induced ischemic stroke. Treatment is otherwise aimed toward preventing further bleeding (eg, antiemetics, seizure prophylaxis).

Subarachnoid Hemorrhage

Subarachnoid hemorrhage is an acute bleed into the subarachnoid space.

CAUSES

The majority of patients with nontraumatic SAH have a ruptured berry aneurysm. Other causes include mycotic aneurysms, arteriovenous malformations (AVMs), neoplasms, and trauma.

Conditions associated with increased incidence of berry aneurysms:

- Family history of berry aneurysm
- Coarctation of aorta

TABLE 15.7. Etiologies of Headache

Critical Secondary Causes	Reversible Secondary Causes	Primary Headache Syndromes
Vascular	Non-CNS infections	Migraine
Subarachnoid hemorrhage	Focal	Tension
Intraparenchymal hemorrhage	Systemic	Cluster
Epidural hematoma	Sinusitis	
Subdural hematoma	Odontogenic	
Stroke	Otic	
Cavernous sinus thrombosis	Drug-related	
Arteriovenous malformation	Chronic analgesic use	
Temporal arteritis	Monosodium glutamate	
Carotid or vertebral artery dissection	Miscellaneous	
CNS infection	Post–lumbar puncture	
Meningitis		
Encephalitis		
Cerebral abscess		
Tumor		
Pseudotumor cerebri		
Ophthalmic		
Glaucoma		
Iritis		
Optic neuritis		
Drug-related		
Nitrates and nitrites		
Monoamine oxidase inhibitors		
Alcohol withdrawal		
Toxic		
Carbon monoxide poisoning		
Endocrine		
Pheochromocytoma		
Metabolic		
Hypoxia		
Hypoglycemia		
Hypercapnia		
High-altitude cerebral edema		
Preeclampsia		

(Reproduced, with permission, from Tintinalli JE, Kelen GD, Stapczynski JS. *Emergency Medicine: A Comprehensive Study Guide*, 6th ed. New York: McGraw-Hill, 2004:1376.)

- Polycystic kidney disease
- Marfan syndrome
- Ehlers-Danlos syndrome
- AVMs

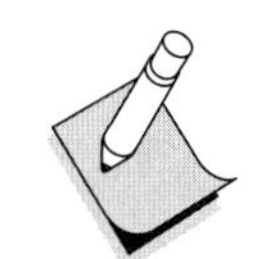

Polycystic kidney disease and headache? Think SAH!

Symptoms

- Characterized by **sudden onset** of severe headache
  - May be preceded by activities that increase ICP (intercourse, coughing, weight lifting)
  - N/V (in majority)
- Other possible symptoms include seizures, neck stiffness, preceding less severe headache ("sentinel bleed").

Exam

- Depends on degree of hemorrhage and inflammatory response
  - Fifty percent have a completely normal examination.
- **Hunt and Hess classification:**
  - **Grades I and II** have good prognosis: Headache with nuchal rigidity +/– 3rd or 6th cranial nerve palsy; normal mental status.
  - **Grade III are at risk for rapid deterioration (50% survival): Drowsiness, confusion, +/– mild focal deficit.**
  - **Grades IV, V** have poor prognosis: Stupor, hemiparesis, deep coma, decerebrate posturing.

Diagnosis

- Head CT without contrast (see Figure 15.4)
  - Symptoms <24 hours = sensitivity > 90%.
  - Symptoms for 1 week = sensitivity < 50%.
- LP if CT negative; positive CSF findings for SAH:
  - Grossly bloody
  - Persistently bloody
  - Xanthochromia (via spectrophotometry, NOT naked eye) ≥12 hours after onset of headache = gold standard.

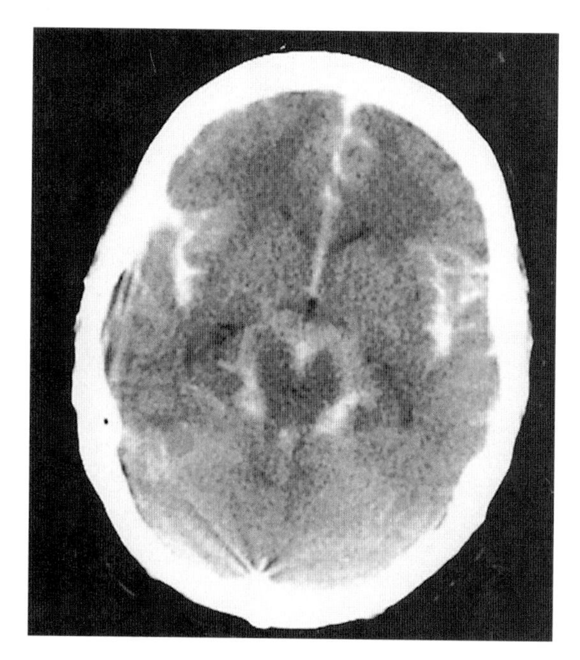

FIGURE 15.4. Noncontrast head CT demonstrating acute subarachnoid blood.

(Reproduced, with permission, from Stone CK, Humphries, RL. *Current Emergency Diagnosis and Treatment*, 5th ed. New York: McGraw-Hill, 2004:372.)

TREATMENT

- Supportive therapy
- **Nimodipine:** To prevent vasospasm and ischemic stroke
- Antiemetics to prevent N/V
- Prophylactic phenytoin to prevent seizures
- Sedation, as needed
- Definitive therapy with endovascular coil embolization or surgical clipping

Meningitis

See "CNS Infections."

Chronic Subdural Hematoma

Blood clot between the dura and the brain with symptom onset >2 weeks after trauma (some patients report minor or no injury); seen more commonly in patients with brain atrophy (elderly and alcoholics)

SYMPTOMS/EXAM

- Headache
- Unilateral weakness (up to half)
- Altered consciousness, dementia

DIFFERENTIAL

- **Subdural hygroma:** Collection of blood-tinged fluid in dural space of uncertain etiology; tends to follow trauma; on CT fluid density is same as CSF; surgical evaluation is needed, if symptomatic

DIAGNOSIS

- Noncontrast CT scan: Isodense or hypodense material in subdural space +/– mass effect (see Figure 15.5)
- MRI scan: Will appear hyperdense

TREATMENT

- Supportive therapy
- Correct any coagulopathy, if present.
- Immediate neurosurgical consultation for surgical evacuation

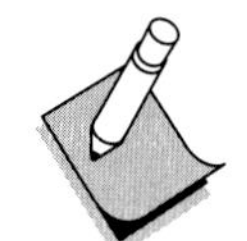

Chronic subdurals appear isodense or hypodense on noncontrast CT.

Brain Tumor

Headache is a common complaint in patients with brain tumor.

CAUSES

The most common cause is metastases from lung or breast carcinoma.

SYMPTOMS/EXAM

- Worsening headache for weeks to months
- May be worse upon awakening
- The vast majority will have focal findings on detailed neurological examination.

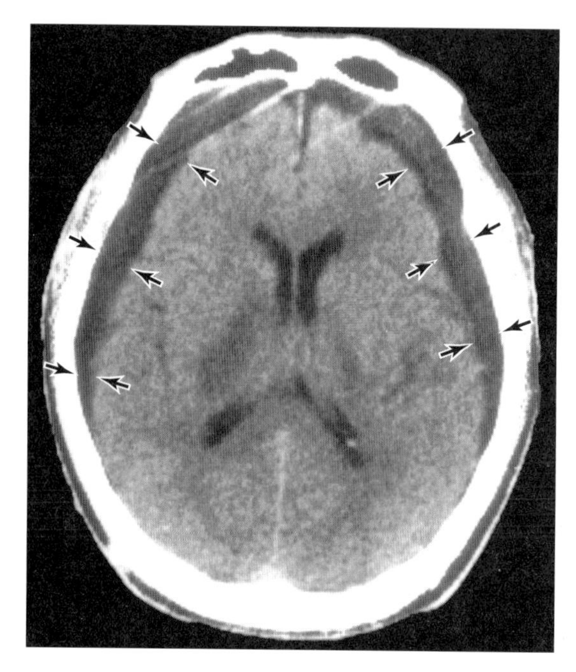

FIGURE 15.5. Noncontrast head CT demonstrating chronic subdural hematoma.

(Reproduced, with permission, from Aminoff MJ, Greenberg DA, Simon RP. *Clinical Neurology*, 6th ed. New York: McGraw-Hill, 2005:61.)

NEUROLOGY

DIAGNOSIS/TREATMENT

- CT or MRI to confirm presence of mass
- Urgent neurosurgical evaluation
- Dexamethasone if edema present on imaging or if severe symptoms

Temporal Arteritis

Temporal arteritis is an arteritis of small and medium-sized arteries that selectively involves arterial walls with significant amounts of elastin. The disease occurs predominantly in women and is rare in patients <50 years old.

SYMPTOMS/EXAM

- Severe, throbbing, frontotemporal headache
- Jaw claudication, systemic symptoms, or polymyalgia rheumatica may be present.
- Temporal artery may be nonpulsatile or tender.

DIAGNOSIS

- Three of five criteria:
  - Age >50
  - New onset localized headache
  - Temporal artery tenderness or decreased pulse
  - Erythrocyte sedimentation rate >50 mm/hour
  - Abnormal arterial biopsy findings

TREATMENT

- Start immediately if diagnosis is suspected.
- Prednisone 40–80 mg/day
- NSAIDs for pain relief

COMPLICATIONS

Severe complication → loss of vision due to ischemic optic neuritis.

Pseudotumor Cerebri

A disease primarily of young obese females

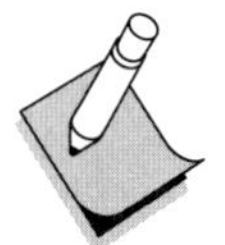

Temporal arteritis and pseudotumor cerebri may both lead to loss of vision if left untreated.

PATHOPHYSIOLOGY

Pathophysiology is uncertain, but is linked to oral contraceptives, vitamin A, chronic steroid use, tetracycline, and thyroid disorders.

SYMPTOMS/EXAM

- Longstanding headache +/– visual disturbances
- **Visual loss may occur.**
- Eye findings may include **papilledema, loss of *peripheral* vision** and **CN VI palsy.**

DIAGNOSIS

- Based on finding of increased intracranial pressure (>25 cm H_2O) with normal CSF evaluation
- Head CT may show small ventricles and an enlarged cisterna magna.

TREATMENT

- Aimed at lowering intracranial pressure
  - **Acetazolamide** or steroids to decrease the formation of CSF
  - Recurrent LP's or shunt surgery for refractory cases

Internal Carotid and Vertebral Artery Dissection

The most frequent cause of stroke in patients <45 years, internal carotid and vertebral artery dissection may be spontaneous or trauma related. Diagnosis is challenging because early symptoms are often vague and nonspecific.

SYMPTOMS/EXAM

Internal carotid dissection:

- Unilateral anterior neck pain or headache around the eye or frontal area, classically abrupt in onset
- Findings include ipsilateral Horner syndrome, contralateral stroke, or TIA symptoms.

Neck pain and neurologic symptoms? Consider internal carotid and vertebral artery dissection.

Vertebral artery dissection:

- Marked occipital or posterior neck pain with signs of brainstem TIA or stroke

DIAGNOSIS

- CT scan is **not** the imaging of choice (is often normal).
- Obtain angiography (CT angiogram has not been fully evaluated) and/or MRI/MRA to confirm diagnosis.

TREATMENT

- Surgical
- Anticoagulation

Cerebral Venous Thrombosis

CAUSES

Causes include adjacent local infection, direct injury (eg, trauma) or hypercoagulable state (eg, pregnancy).

SYMPTOMS/EXAM

- Symptoms are varied and often vague.
- Headache is the most common presenting complaint.
- Altered mental status, focal neurologic deficits, papilledema, or seizures may occur.

DIAGNOSIS

- CT and standard MRI scanning are useful only if positive (cannot exclude the diagnosis).
- **Magnetic resonance venography (MRV) combined with MRI** is imaging modality of choice and has replaced angiography.
- CT venography is being evaluated as a possible imaging method.

TREATMENT

- Heparin
- Catheter-based thrombolysis if severe symptoms

Post–Lumbar Puncture Headache

CAUSES

A post-LP headache develops within 24–48 hours of LP due to persistent CSF leak from the LP puncture site.

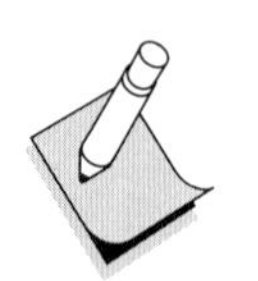

Caffeine IV can be very effective in treating post-LP headaches.

SYMPTOMS/DIAGNOSIS

Headache that is worse with upright posture and improved with lying flat

TREATMENT

- Simple analgesics
- Intravenous fluids
- **Caffeine IV**
- Blood patch, if no relief with the above measures

Migraine

PATHOPHYSIOLOGY

- Slowly spreading wave of neuronal depolorization across the brain → ion dysfunction and vasoconstriction → prodrome and aura (seen in 20%).
- Trigeminovascular activation and release of peptides → inflammation of the pain-sensitive areas and vasodilation.

Many factors can directly or indirectly trigger this neurovascular activation:

- Menstruation, contraceptive estrogens, pregnancy
- Certain foods or drinks, such as chocolate, caffeine, hard cheese, alcoholic beverages (especially red wine), monosodium glutamate (MSG), nitrites
- Alterations in circadian rhythm

SYMPTOMS

Migraine without aura ("common migraine"):

- Slow onset and lasts 4–72 hours
- Unilateral and pulsating
- Nausea, vomiting, and photo- or phonophobia

Migraine with aura ("classic migraine"):

- Headache follows aura within 60 minutes.
- Aura develops gradually over minutes, lasts <1 hour and is fully reversible.
- Types of auras
  - Visual is most common → scintillating scotomata or visual field deficit.
  - Motor → hemiparesis, ophthalmoplegia, aphasia.
  - Sensory → hemiparesthesia, dysesthesia.
  - Brainstem (basilar migraine) → vertigo, ataxia.

DIFFERENTIAL

- Includes subarachnoid hemorrhage, giant cell arteritis, cerebrovascular disease, and other secondary headaches

DIAGNOSIS

- Typically a clinical diagnosis
- Further evaluation (CT/LP) to rule out a secondary cause is needed in patients with new onset migraine or symptoms different from their typical migraine.

TREATMENT

- Goal is to abort or decrease the neurovascular effects.
- **Triptans** (eg, sumatriptan): Selective 5-HT (serotonin) agonists
  - Should not be used in patients with hypertension or other cardiovascular disease
  - Do not use within 24 hours of other ergotamine-containing medication.
- **Dihydroergotamine (DHE):** Nonselective 5-HT agonist
  - Again contraindicated in patients with cardiovascular disease or within 24 hours of triptan use
  - Nausea and vomiting are common side effects.
- **Antiemetics** (eg, prochlorpromazine, metoclopromide)
- **NSAIDs** (eg, indomethacin, ibuprofen)

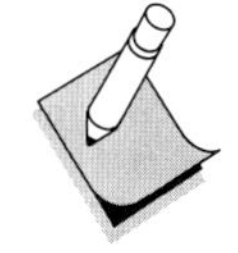

Triptans and DHE are vasoconstrictors and should not be used in patients with HTN or cardiovascular disease.

- Steroids: Controversial; may work in refractory migraines
- Opiates should be used as last resort.
- Prophylactic therapy may be indicated in patients with frequent migraines: β-blockers, Ca^{++} channel blockers, tricyclic antidepressants.

Tension-Type Headaches

PATHOPHYSIOLOGY

Thought to share a common pathophysiology with migraines

SYMPTOMS

- Bilateral, nonpulsating, not worsened by exertion
- Usually not associated with nausea and vomiting

DIFFERENTIAL

- Other primary or secondary headaches

TREATMENT

- NSAIDs
- For severe headache → treat same as migraine.

Cluster Headaches

Cluster headaches are most common in young to middle-aged men and may be precipitated by alcohol and stress. They result from dysfunction of the trigeminal nerve.

SYMPTOMS/EXAM

- Severe, unilateral orbital, supraorbital or temporal pain
- Episodes last for 15–180 minutes, but recur in clusters (eg, daily on same side for weeks).
- Associated ipsilateral findings:
  - Conjunctival injection, lacrimation, nasal congestion, rhinorrhea, facial swelling, miosis or ptosis

TREATMENT

- **High-flow O_2** is effective in 70% of patients.
- IV dihydroergotamine or sumatriptan; oral preparations take too long to be effective
- Prophylaxis with oral steroid burst, verapamil, or antiepileptic agents

A 58-year-old male is brought to the ED by his daughter for change in mental status. He was last seen 2 days earlier at work and was normal. Today he is disheveled, disoriented, and appears to be hallucinating. His daughter says the symptoms have been waxing and waning. You have trouble maintaining his attention during the examination, and you note a fine tremor. What is the most appropriate treatment for this patient?

This patient clinically has delirium. Treatment is aimed at the underlying cause.

ALTERED MENTAL STATUS

Confusional states can be broadly divided into **delirium**, **dementia**, and **psychosis** (see Table 15.8).

Delirium is a medical emergency.

Delirium

In delirium, functions of cognition and attention (arousal) are disordered due to widespread neuronal or neurotransmitter malfunction from an underlying medical (organic) cause.

CAUSES

Common causes include:

- Drug intoxication or withdrawal (most common)
- Metabolic disorders (eg, endocrine disorder, hepatic encephalopathy, uremia, hypoglycemia)
- Toxins (eg, carbon monoxide)
- Infections (eg, CNS, UTI, sepsis)
- Hypercapnia
- Trauma
- Seizures

SYMPTOMS/EXAM

- **Acute** confusional state
- Transient attention and cognition impairment

TABLE 15.8. Features of Delirium, Dementia, and Psychiatric Psychosis

CHARACTERISTIC	DELIRIUM	DEMENTIA	PSYCHIATRIC
Onset	Over days	Insidious	Sudden
Course over 24 hr	Fluctuating	Stable	Stable
Consciousness	Reduced	Alert	Alert
Attention	Disordered	Normal	May be disordered
Cognition	Disordered	Impaired	May be impaired
Orientation	Impaired	Often impaired	May be impaired
Hallucinations	Visual and/or auditory	Often absent	Usually audiotory
Delusions	Transient, poorly organized	Usually absent	Sustained
Movements	Asterixis, tremor may be present	Often absent	Absent

(Reproduced, with permission, from Tintinalli, J et al. *Emergency Medicine: A Comprehensive Study Guide*, 6th ed. New York: McGraw-Hill, 2004:229; based on data from Lipowski Z: Delirium in the Elderly Patient. *New Engl J Med* 320:578,1989.)

- **Waxing and waning** symptoms
- Hallucinations, if present, are visual and/or auditory.

DIFFERENTIAL

Dementia, psychosis

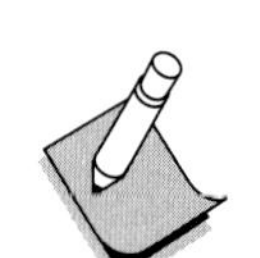

A score of <23 on the mini-mental status examination is abnormal.

DIAGNOSIS

- History of acuity of change in behavior.
- **Mini-mental status examination:** Tests orientation, memory, attention, calculation, recall, and language.
  - Score <23 is abnormal.
- General PE and ancillary tests to search for underlying cause
  - Include head CT and LP, if necessary.

TREATMENT

- Treat underlying cause.
- Sedate with haloperidol or benzodiazepines if severe agitation.

Dementia

Dementia results from a **gradual** loss of mental capacity with relatively preserved attention function.

CAUSES

Causes include

- Alzheimer disease (most common)
  - Reduction of neurons in the cerebral cortex and increased amyloid deposition → neurofibrillary tangles and plaques.
- Vascular (multi-infarct)
- Parkinson disease
- Viral infection: HIV, Creutzfeldt-Jakob disease
- Possible **treatable causes**:
  - Depression (most common treatable cause)
  - Vitamin B_{12} deficiency
  - Neurosyphilis
  - Hypothyroidism
  - Normal pressure hydrocephalus
  - Intracranial mass (eg, brain tumor)
  - Chronic drug use

Keep in mind reversible causes when evaluating the patient with dementia.

SYMPTOMS/EXAM

- **Gradual onset** confusional state
- Usually presents in the **elderly**
- Disordered cognition with normal attention
- Loss of mental capacity especially memory
  - Remote memories often preserved

DIFFERENTIAL

- Delirium, psychosis

DIAGNOSIS

- Diagnosis is primarily based on history of slow, progressive change in behavior. All patients warrant neuroimaging, TSH, and vitamin B_{12} level at minimum.
- Look for reversible cause or exacerbating comorbid condition (eg, UTI).

TREATMENT

- Treat reversible causes, if present.
- Depends on cause: For Alzheimer's, donepezil (Aricept) and tacrine (Cognex) reduce the metabolism of acetylcholine.

NORMAL PRESSURE HYDROCEPHALUS

A potentially reversible cause of dementia; results from defective CSF uptake (either a primary process or secondary to prior infection/injury/bleed) leading to increased CSF volume; most commonly occurs in older patients, but 50% are <60 years old

SYMPTOMS/EXAM

- Triad of progressive dementia, ataxia, and urinary frequency or incontinence

DIAGNOSIS

- Based on CT showing ventricular enlargement (without other pathology) and LP with normal intracranial pressure and fluid studies

NPH: Triad of dementia, ataxia, and urinary frequency/incontinence

TREATMENT

- Neurosurgical consultation for shunt placement

Psychiatric Psychosis

Functional (psychiatric) cause of confusional state

SYMPTOMS

- Loss of contact with reality
- Hallucinations, if present, are auditory
- Usually not waxing and waning
- Consciousness not clouded

DIFFERENTIAL

- Dementia, delirium ("organic" psychosis)

TREATMENT

- Environmental, psychosocial, and medical

COMA

Consciousness can be divided into arousal and content functions. Arousal functions reside in the reticular activating system (RAS) in the midbrain, pons, and medulla. Content functions reside in the cerebrum. Coma represents a failure in both arousal and content functions of the brain.

TABLE 15.9. Common Toxicologic Causes of Coma

Alcohols
Antipsychotics
Antiseizure medications
Carbon monoxide
Muscle relaxants
Opiates
Sedative/hypnotics

Causes of coma—
TIPS AEIOU
Trauma, temperature
Infection
Psychiatric, poisonings
Space occupying lesion, subarachnoid
Alcohol
Epilepsy, electrolytes, enceophalopathy
Insulin
Opioids/overdose, oxygen (hypoxia, CO_2 narcosis)
Uremia (metabolic)

Oculovestibular reflex: Direction of fast component of nystagmus, with irrigation of cold versus warm water in patient with intact brainstem—
COWS
Cold
Opposite
Warm
Same

CAUSES

Causes are myriad and include:

- Encephalopathy—metabolic, hypertensive, hypoxic, Wernicke's
- Toxins (see Table 15.9)
- Drug reaction
- Infection
- Hyper-/hypothermia
- Seizure
- Psychiatric
- CNS lesion or event (less common)
- Sepsis

SYMPTOMS/EXAM

- Eyes-closed state with inappropriate response to environmental stimuli
- Other findings vary depending on depth of coma and underlying etiology (see Table 15.10).
- Look for asymmetric findings that suggest focal or regional CNS dysfunction.

DIAGNOSIS

- Diagnosis is made based on clinical findings.
- Evaluation should focus on identifying underlying cause.
- Obtain head CT, glucose, electrolytes, renal, and liver function tests.
- Consider EEG to evaluate for nonconvulsive status epilepticus in all.

TREATMENT

- Supportive care
- Coma "protocol" (intravenous) for the undifferentiated patient
  - Thiamine
  - Glucose
  - Naloxone
- Treat underlying cause once identified.
- Empiric antibiotic coverage for meningitis if cause not readily apparent

TABLE 15.10. Pertinent Neurologic Findings in Coma

EXAM	FINDING	INTERPRETATION
Funduscopic examination	Spontaneous venous pulsations	Normal intracranial pressure
Pupillary constriction	Absent response to light Unequal pupils	Midbrain structural lesion or topical cycloplegic drug use. Structural lesion or normal variant.
Eye position	Tonic deviation	Seizure or irritant brain lesion
Corneal reflex (tests CN V and VII)	Absent	Posterior fossa or brainstem lesions
Oculocephalic reflex (doll's eye)	Conjugate deviation of eyes in direction *opposite* to passive head rotation Conjugate deviation in same direction as head rotation	Intact brainstem No brainstem function
Oculovestibular reflex (cold caloric)	Irrigate ear canal with 10 mL *cold* water: ▪ *Horizontal nystagmus* with fast component *away* from irrigated ear ▪ Tonic deviation to side of irrigation No response	 Intact cortex and brainstem Toxic/metabolic or lesion above brainstem No brainstem function
Response to painful stimuli	Decorticate posturing (elbow/wrist flexion, shoulder adduction and internal rotation, forearm supination) Decerebrate posturing (elbow/wrist extension, shoulder adduction and internal rotation, forearm pronation) Asymmetric movement	Severe damage above the midbrain Damage at the midbrain or diencephalon Structural lesions

ATAXIA

Ataxia is the failure to make smooth, intentional movements. Ataxia and gait disturbances are symptoms of particular disease processes and not diagnoses in and of themselves. In general, ataxia can be divided into two groups:

Motor (cerebellar) ataxia:

- Disorders of cerebellum (most common)
  - Sensory receptors and afferent pathways intact, but integration of proprioceptive information is poor
  - Usually ipsilateral to lesion
- Far less commonly due to infarcts in the internal capsule, thalamic nucleus, or frontal lobe

TABLE 15.11. Causes of Ataxia

GROUP	EXAMPLE
Drug intoxications	Ethanol, dilantin toxicity
Metabolic disorders	Hyponatremia
Peripheral neuropathy	Alcoholic peripheral neuropathy
Vestibulopathy	Meniere disease
Cerebellar disorder	Infarction, mass
Posterior column disorder	Vitamin B_{12} deficiency

Sensory ataxia:

- Failure of transmission of proprioception to the CNS via peripheral nerves, dorsal columns or cerebellar input tract

CAUSES

Common causes of ataxia are listed in Table 15.11.

SYMPTOMS/EXAM

- Patients may complain of difficulty ambulating, weakness, or falls.
- Ataxia that is worse with loss of visual input (eg, walking in the dark) = sensory ataxia.
- The exam should focus on differentiating motor from sensory ataxia.
- The classic **cerebellar gait** is wide based with unsteady and irregular steps.
- A **sensory ataxic gait** is characterized by abrupt movement of legs and slapping impact of feet with each step.
- Cerebellar function testing: Observe patient perform smooth, voluntary movements, and rapidly alternating movements.
- **Romberg test:** Worsened unsteadiness with eyes closed (loss of visual input) is suggestive of sensory ataxia.

DIAGNOSIS

Diagnosis is primarily made via history and physical exam.

TREATMENT

Define underlying cause. Treatment is directed toward primary disease process.

VERTIGO

Vertigo is defined as the perception of movement where no movement exists. Vertigo is typically categorized as central or peripheral.

Central Vertigo

CAUSES

Results from disorders affecting the brainstem and cerebellum

- Cerebellar hemorrhage, tumor or infarct
- Vertebrobasilar insufficiency

- Vertebral artery dissection
- Wallenberg syndrome (lateral medullary infarction of brainstem)
- Multiple sclerosis
- Migraine

*The direction of nystagmus is named by the **fast** (cortical) component.*

SYMPTOMS/EXAM

- Onset may be sudden or gradual
- Symptoms are often **ill defined and constant**
- **Vertical nystagmus**
- Associated with other CNS symptoms/findings indicating posterior fossa pathology—dipolopia, dysarthria, visual changes

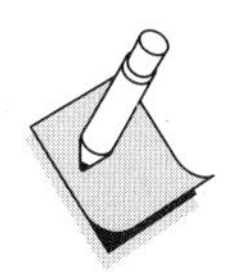

Vertigo with any CNS symptoms or findings? Assume central cause!

DIAGNOSIS/TREATMENT

MRI is imaging of choice to visualize the posterior fossa, though CT scan *may* identify cerebellar mass, hemorrhage, or infarct.

Peripheral Vertigo

CAUSES

Caused by disorders affecting VIII CN and the vestibular apparatus (see Table 15.12)

SYMPTOMS/EXAM

- Most commonly a **dramatic and sudden** onset of intense paroxysmal vertigo
- Nausea and vomiting
- Often aggravated by position
- **Rotatory-vertical or horizontal nystagmus**
- Hearing loss (not with BPPV, vestibular neuronitis)
- No central findings

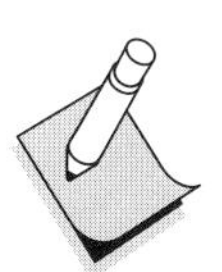

Central vertigo is classically ill defined and constant with associated vertical nystagmus. Peripheral vertigo is classically dramatic and sudden with rotatory–vertical or horizontal nystagmus.

NEUROLOGY

DIAGNOSIS

- Primarily a clinical diagnosis
- **Dix-Hallpike** test confirms posterior canal BPPV.
- MRI to visualize CN VIII lesions

TREATMENT

- Depends on underlying etiology (eg, d/c ototoxic agents in ototoxicity, Epley maneuver for posterior canal BPPV)
- Symptomatic treatment with antihistamines or antiemetics

A 50-year-old male is brought in by ambulance with a possible stroke. The patient has history of hypertension and BP 180/100 upon arrival. The findings reveal a left-sided facial droop that includes the forehead. There is no arm or leg weakness. Should this patient be worked up for a CVA?

No. This patient has isolated facial droop with forehead *included* which is consistent with a peripheral (not central) 7th nerve palsy.

TABLE 15.12. Disorders Causing Peripheral Vertigo

Disorder	Pathophysiology	Associated findings
Benign paroxysmal positional vertigo (BPPV)	Otoconia in the semicircular canals	Precipitated by sudden head movement Positive Dix-Hallpike Improvement/resolution with Epley maneuver
Meniere disease	Increased endolymph within the cochlea and labyrinth	Ear "fullness," tinnitus, *hearing loss*
Labyrinthitis	Viral or *bacterial* infection	Middle-ear findings (infection, fluid), tinnitus, *hearing loss*
Vestibular neuronitis	Viral infection	Lasts several days, no recurrence or hearing loss
Ramsay-Hunt syndrome (vestibular ganglionitis)	Viral infection of vestibular gangion	Hearing loss, vertigo, facial nerve palsy, grouped vesicles
Perilymph fistula	Trauma, sudden pressure change	Abrupt onset after inciting event +/– hearing loss Requires surgical repair
Ototoxicity	Damage to vestibular apparatus —may be irreversible	Hearing loss, vertigo, tinnitus
CN VIII lesions	Schwannomas, meningioma	Gradual onset, preceded by *hearing loss*

CRANIAL NERVE DISORDERS

Trigeminal Neuralgia

The trigeminal nerve (CN V) has three anatomic divisions, V_1-ophthalmic, V_2-maxillary, and V_3-mandibular, which innervate the cornea, the face, and the mucous membranes of the oral and nasal cavity. The motor fibers innervate the muscles of mastication.

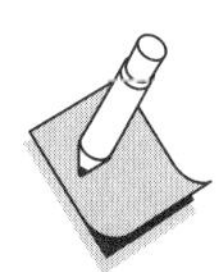

Treatment for trigeminal neuralgia = Tegretol (carbamazepine)

Symptoms/Exam

- Brief, recurrent episodes of excruciating, unilateral facial pain
- Right > left side predominance
- May be able to elicit pain by tapping the side of the face, otherwise there should be no demonstrable physical findings

Differential

- Includes vascular or space-occupying lesions (acoustic neuroma), demyelinating diseases (multiple sclerosis), herpes zoster, sinus infection, odontogenic pathology, migraine, temporomandibular joint dysfunction

Diagnosis

- Based on clinical presentation
- Imaging should be performed to rule out other etiologies if neurological findings are present.

TREATMENT

- Initiate **carbamazepine** and analgesics in ED.
- Outpatient referral to follow carbamazepine levels, CBC and liver function tests

Bell Palsy

A lower motor neuron ("peripheral") CN VII palsy

CAUSES

Bell palsy is most commonly due to herpes virus infection. Pregnant women are at greater risk. Other infections (HIV, Lyme disease) can also cause a CN VII palsy.

SYMPTOMS/EXAM

- Viral prodrome (50% of time)
- Abrupt onset of unilateral facial paralysis with forehead included (central causes will spare the forehead)
- May also have loss of taste to anterior two-thirds of tongue, hyperacusis (sound distortion or tinnitus)
- Bell's phenomenon: Eye rolls back in head when patient attempts to close the lid

DIFFERENTIAL

- **Ramsay Hunt syndrome**
  - Herpes zoster infection of geniculate ganglion
  - Characterized by facial paralysis, pain, tinnitus, hearing loss, and typical zoster lesions on the affected side, including inside external auditory canal, and/or the tympanic membrane
  - Treatment = prednisone and antivirals.
- **Lyme disease**
  - A leading cause of facial paralysis in regions where Lyme disease is endemic
  - May be unilateral or **bilateral**
  - Diagnosed via serologic titers
  - Treatment = doxycycline PO.
- **Malignant otitis externa**
  - Severe otitis externa that is typically seen in diabetes or immunocompromised patients
  - *Pseudomonas* sp. often implicated
  - Requires IV antibiotic therapy and ENT consultation
- **Acoustic neuroma**
  - Hearing loss accompanying facial weakness
  - MRI is diagnostic test of choice.
- Other causes include temporal bone trauma, mononucleosis, HIV seroconversion, other infectious organisms, mononeuropathy multiplex, Sjögren syndrome.

DIAGNOSIS

- Primarily a clinical diagnosis
- Any evidence for sparing of upper face ("central" CN VII paralysis) warrants CT or MRI to evaluate for stroke or CNS lesion.

TREATMENT

- Pharmacologic therapy should be initiated if patient presents within 1 week of symptom onset.
  - Corticosteroids
  - Antiviral therapy
- Eye protection
  - Eye patch for sleeping and artificial tears during the day

Acoustic Neuroma

Schwannoma of CN VIII that typically causes isolated CN VIII symptoms, but if large may → mass effect on adjacent structures (CN VII, CN V, 4th ventricle)

SYMPTOMS/EXAM

- Characteristic triad of sensorineural hearing loss, tinnitus, and disequilibrium

DIAGNOSIS/TREATMENT

- Audiogram to formally evaluate hearing loss
- MRI can confirm diagnosis.
- Treatment is surgical.

SPINAL CORD DISORDERS

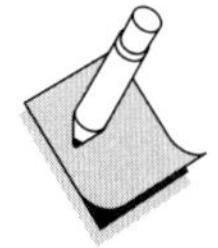

Damage to single corticospinal tract or posterior column → ipsilateral motor weakness or vibration/position loss. Damage to single spinothalamic tract → contralateral loss of pain and temperature.

Spinal cord anatomy:

- **Corticospinal tract:** Motor pathway; fibers cross in medulla then descend in cord.
- **Spinathalamic tract:** Pain and temperature pathway; fibers first cross, then ascend in cord.
- **Posterior (dorsal) columns:** Vibration and proprioceptive pathway; fibers ascend in ipsilateral posterior column to medulla, then cross.
- **Cauda equina:** Lumbar and sacral nerve roots

CAUSES

Causes of spinal cord dysfunction include:

- Trauma
- Multiple sclerosis
- Transverse myelitis
- Spinal AVM or hemorrhage
- Compression from tumor, disc, epidural abscess, or hematoma
- Syringomyelia
- Myelopathy (eg, HIV)
- Infarction

SYMPTOMS/EXAM

- Patients present with motor and sensory deficits depending on location of injury.
- **Scoring motor function**
  - **5 = Full strength**
  - **4 = Able to resist, but weak**

- 3 = Able to move against gravity
- 2 = Able to move when gravity eliminated
- 1 = Muscle fires, but no movement is generated
- 0 = No muscle firing

- Scoring reflexes
  - 0 to 4 scale with 2 being normal (0 = no reflexes, 4 = hyperactive reflexes with clonus)
- Complete injury results in complete loss of motor, sensory, and autonomic function below level of injury.
- Partial injury often presents as a spinal cord syndrome (Table 15.13).
- Table 15.14 summarizes the findings in specific disease processes.

DIAGNOSIS

- MRI is imaging of choice to evaluate for compression or mass lesion.
- Lumbar puncture is indicated to further define a suspected inflammatory or demyelinating process.

Spinal Epidural Hematoma

More likely to occur following spinal trauma or spinal procedures but may occur spontaneously in patients with coagulopathy (eg, liver disease, anticoagulation, thrombocytopenia).

SYMPTOMS/EXAM

- Abrupt severe and radicular back pain
- Weakness, loss of bowel/bladder and sensory deficits depending on degree of compression

TABLE 15.13. Spinal Cord Syndromes

SYNDROME	CHARACTERISTIC FINDINGS (BELOW LEVEL OF INJURY)	LIKELY CAUSE	COMMENTS
Central cord	Bilateral motor weakness of upper extremities > lower extremities and distal > proximal extremities	Hyperextension injury of narrowed cervical spinal canal	More common in elderly patients
Brown-Sequard (cord hemisection)	Ipsilateral motor weakness and vibration/position loss Contralateral pain and temperature loss	Penetrating trauma	Often partial syndrome Best prognosis
Anterior cord	Motor weakness, pinprick and light touch loss. Preserved vibration and position sense	Infarction of anterior spinal artery	Poorest prognosis Preservation of posterior columns
Cauda equina	Urinary retention, decreased rectal tone, saddle anesthesia, motor weakness	Ruptured L4-5 disc	Peripheral nerve (nerve root) injury

TABLE 15.14. **Clinical Features and Etiology of Spinal Cord Disorders**

SPINAL CORD DISORDER	CLINICAL FEATURES	ETIOLOGY
Diskitis	Back pain, fever, and refusal to walk in child <10 years	Inflammatory process in disc (viral or *S aureus*)
Dorsal column disorders	Loss of position sense, vibration, and light touch	Syphilis or vitamin B_{12} deficiency
HIV myelopathy	Weakness, gait problems, spasticity, sphincter dysfunction	Advanced HIV
Neoplasm	Severe pain with radiation down spine Signs of cord compression	Most common—lung cancer, breast cancer, lymphoma
Spinal epidural abscess	Severe pain with radiation down spine Signs of cord compression, fever	Expanding abscess (IDU or immunocompromise)
Spinal epidural hematoma	Severe pain with radiation down spine, signs of cord compression	Expanding hemorrhage (trauma or coagulopathy)
Syringomyelia	Disassociative anesthesia, weakness	Syrinx formation in central spinal cord
Transverse myelitis	Transverse level of sensory loss, paresis, sphincter dysfunction	Post-viral or toxic inflammation

TREATMENT

Immediate correction of coagulopathy (when present) and surgical decompression

Spinal Epidural Abscess

Typically results from hematogenous spread of infection to epidural space; **most common organism is *Staphylococcus aureus***

Major risk factors include:

- Injection drug use
- Chronic renal failure
- Dental abscess
- Bacterial endocarditis
- Alcoholism
- Diabetes
- Immunosuppression
- Recent back surgery, lumbar puncture, or epidural anesthesia

SYMPTOMS/EXAM

- Progressive pain
- Constitutional symptoms: Fevers, sweats
- Weakness, loss of bowel/bladder and sensory deficits depending on degree of compression

Diagnosis/Treatment

- **ESR** is almost always elevated.
- Obtain immediate MRI to confirm diagnosis.
- If MRI unavailable, a CT myelogram should be obtained.
- Antibiotics: Vancomycin and third generation cephalosporin
- Immediate surgical intervention

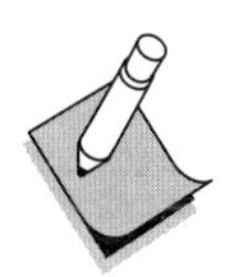

An elevated ESR/CRP in the patient with unexplained back pain should raise concern for spinal epidural abscess.

Diskitis

Diskitis is an inflammatory process of the intervertebral disc space, often due to viral or bacterial (*Staphylococcus aureus*) infection. It is usually seen in children under the age of 10. Risk factors include spinal surgical procedures, systemic infections (eg, UTI), and immunocompromise.

Symptoms/Exam

- Moderate to severe local pain and radicular symptoms
- Children often present with sudden onset of back pain and refusal to walk
- Fever (in most)
- Neurologic deficits are uncommon

Diagnosis/Treatment

- MRI
- Intravenous antibiotics

Spinal Neoplasm

Most commonly due to metastasis or direct spread from lung cancer, breast cancer and lymphoma

Symptoms/Exam

- Symptoms commonly localized to thoracic spine
- Characterized by pain that is worse at night

Diagnosis

- Plain X-rays are abnormal in most patients.
- MRI is confirmative.

Treatment

Includes high-dose steroids, radiation and surgery, depending on suspected pathology and degree of compression

Transverse Myelitis

Spinal cord dysfunction due to viral infection, autoimmune or idiopathic cause

Symptoms/Exam

- Characterized by a transverse level of sensory impairment, paraplegia and sphincter disturbance

DIFFERENTIAL

- Spinal cord tumors, Guillain-Barré syndrome

DIAGNOSIS/TREATMENT

- MRI to exclude compressive lesion
- Steroids (uncertain benefit)
- Only 50% have fair to good recovery.

Syringomyelia

Syringomyelia results from a CSF fluid collection (syrinx) within the spinal cord. Any location is possible, but it is most commonly seen in the cervical spine in association with Arnold-Chiari malformation.

SYMPTOMS/EXAM

- Depend on location of syrinx
- Pain
- **Disassociative anesthesia:** Loss of pain and temperature sensation with preservation of proprioception and light touch
- Weakness, spasticity

DIAGNOSIS/TREATMENT

- MRI
- Treated with surgery, if progressive symptoms

> A 55-year-old male presents with complaint of progressive weakness of arms and legs and dry mouth. ROS is positive for significant weight loss over the preceding months. Exam is significant for proximal muscle weakness that improves with repeated use. This is most consistent with which disease of the neuromuscular junction?
>
> Lambert-Eaton myasthenic syndrome, where antibodies form to the neuromuscular junction. This may be a solitary disease, but has also been seen in association with underlying malignancy.

NEUROMUSCULAR DISORDERS

The neuromuscular unit is made up of the anterior horn cells, the peripheral nerve, the neuromuscular junction, and the muscle. Neuromuscular disorders are a large group of disorders that result in degeneration and atrophy of muscles or nerve tissue. They can be grouped based on the location of pathology (Table 15.15).

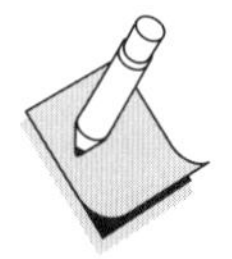

Campylobacter jejuni gastroenteritis is a common precursor to GBS.

Guillain-Barré Syndrome

GBS is primarily an **acute demyelinating disorder of the peripheral nerve**. Variants include early cranial nerve findings and ataxia, primary sensory involvement, and autonomic involvement.

TABLE 15.15. Grouping of Neuromuscular Disorders Based on Location of Pathology

LOCATION OF PATHOLOGY	COMMON DISEASES
Anterior horn cells	Spinal muscular atrophies
Peripheral nerve	Demyelinating polyneuropathies (eg, Guillain-Barré syndrome, diphtheria) Distal symmetric polyneuropathies (eg, diabetic, alcoholic) Radiculopathies and plexopathies (eg, brachial plexopathy) Mononeuropathies (eg, Saturday night palsy) Mononeuropathy multiplex Amyotrophic lateral sclerosis
Neuromuscular junction	Myasthenia gravis Lambert-Eaton myasthenic syndrome Botulism Tick paralysis
Skeletal muscle	Myopathies Muscular dystrophies Periodic paralysis

PATHOPHYSIOLOGY

- Antecedent illness (viral or ***Campylobacter jejuni*** gastroenteritis, URI) → autoimmune response → damage to myelin sheath → symptoms.

SYMPTOMS/EXAM

- Antecedent illness followed by latent period of days to weeks
- Classic presentation is **ascending symmetric paresthesias and motor weakness** with peak symptoms within 3 weeks of onset.
  - Relatively acute onset
  - **Decreased deep tendon reflexes**
  - Variable sensory loss
  - Normal rectal tone
  - May progress to ventilatory failure
- Less common findings (seen in half of patients):
  - Autonomic dysfunction (eg, urinary retention)
  - Cranial nerve involvement (including 7th nerve palsy)

DIFFERENTIAL

- Tick paralysis (examine thoroughly for ticks)
- Lyme disease

DIAGNOSIS

- Suspect based on clinical presentation.
- Electrodiagnostic testing
- Cerebrospinal fluid analysis
  - Classic picture = markedly elevated protein with up to 100 lymphocytes/ μL.
  - Often normal, when early

The classic CSF finding in GBS is a markedly elevated protein with up to 100 lymphocytes/uL.

TREATMENT

- Supportive therapy
- Close observation of respiratory function with forced expiratory volume (FEV_1) monitoring
- Prophylactic intubation or ventilatory support if
  - Decreased FEV_1 below 100% predicted
  - CO_2 retention

Diphtheria

A toxin-mediated multisystem illness caused by *Corynebacterium diphtheriae*

PATHOPHYSIOLOGY

- Respiratory or skin (tropical climates or poor hygiene) infection with *C. diphtheriae* → exotoxin release →
  - Local membrane formation.
  - Peripheral neuropathy → neurologic symptoms.

SYMPTOMS/EXAM

- Respiratory infection
  - Symptoms indistinguishable from pharyngitis, tonsillitis
  - Adherent, grayish-white to grayish-black membrane visible at site of infection
    - Sharply demarcated borders
- Skin infection
  - Clinically similar to chronic skin ulcers/wounds
    - Grayish membrane present

COMPLICATIONS

- Airway obstruction from membrane formation
- Neurologic
  - Weakness → paralysis (often starts with paralysis of the soft palate).
  - Dysphagia and dysarthria
- Myocarditis
- Nephritis

Diphtheria:

Exudative pharyngitis with progressive weakness. Treat with diptheria antitoxin.

DIAGNOSIS

- Suspect and treat based on clinical examination.
- Culture is confirmative.

TREATMENT

- Diptheria antitoxin.
- Antibiotics (penicillin or erythromycin).
- Supportive care.

Diabetic Distal Symmetric Polyneuropathy

The most common type of peripheral neuropathy. It is a gradually progressive disease process (years) due to microvascular injury to the nerve.

SYMPTOMS/EXAM

- **Distal, symmetric**, stocking glove distribution of sensory and motor dysfunction
  - Pain and paresthesias
  - Loss of deep tendon reflexes
- Typically involves lower extremities and moves proximally
  - Before reaching knees → fingertips involved
- May involve any peripheral nerve
  - Gastrointestinal → dysphagia, diarrhea
  - Genitourinary → incontinence, impotence

DIFFERENTIAL

- Other causes of distal symmetric polyneuropathy include:
  - Alcoholic neuropathy
  - HIV neuropathy
  - Toxic and metabolic neuropathy (eg, B_{12} deficiency, medications)

DIAGNOSIS

- Primarily based on clinical exam findings and exclusion of toxic-metabolic causes

TREATMENT

- Tricyclic antidepressants, carbamazepine and/or gabapentin to control pain
- Improve glycemic control

Isolated Mononeuropathies

Neuropathy involving a single peripheral nerve; most commonly due to compression of the nerve or trauma (Table 15.16)

Carpel tunnel syndrome is uniquely associated with multiple conditions:

- Diabetes mellitus (most common)
- Hypothyroidism
- Pregnancy
- Amyloid
- Arthritis
- Obesity

DIAGNOSIS

- Mostly a clinical diagnosis
- Carpel tunnel provocative testing
  - Tinel's sign: Tapping at volar wrist → symptoms.
  - Phalen's sign: Holding wrist in flexion for 30–60 seconds → symptoms.
- Electrodiagnostic studies if confirmation needed

TREATMENT

- Once compression is relieved, most mononeuropathies will resolve spontaneously over a period of weeks.
- **Radial mononeuropathy**
  - Splint wrist in **60° of dorsiflexion**.

TABLE 15.16. Common Peripheral Mononeuropathies Related to Trauma or Compression

MONONEUROPATHY	LOCATION OF INJURY	CLINICAL FINDINGS
Radial ("Saturday night palsy")	Mid-humerus.	Wrist and finger drop. Numbness over 1st dorsal interosseus muscles.
Ulnar	Elbow (cubital tunnel or ulnar condylar groove)—most common Wrist (Guyon's canal).	Paresthesias to 4th and 5th digits. Inability to tightly adduct fingers or grasp with thumb Claw hand is the result of paralysis of the ulnar nerve.
Median ("Carpal tunnel syndrome")	Wrist (carpal tunnel).	Pain and paresthesias in palmar aspect of thumb, index, 3rd and $^1/_2$ of 4th digits Thumb weakness. Thenar atrophy and ulnar deviation.
Sciatic	Buttock.	Inability to flex knee Inability to flex or extend ankle (→ footdrop)
Lateral femoral cutaneous ("Meralgia paresthetica")	Inguinal ligament.	Dysesthesia and numbness to upper thigh
Common peroneal nerve	Proximal fibula.	Numbness to web space between great and 2nd toe. Footdrop

NEUROLOGY

- Ulnar mononeuropathy
  - Corticosteroid injection may help.
  - May require surgical intervention if persistent
- **Median mononeuropathy**
  - Wrist splinting in **neutral position**
  - Corticosteroid injection into carpel tunnel
  - Oral corticosteroid burst
  - Surgery for persistent severe symptoms
- Sciatic and common peroneal mononeuropathy
  - Splint ankle at 90° with posterior splint.

Mononeuropathy Multiplex

Mononeuropathy multiplex is characterized by the presence of multiple mononeuropathies. Unlike isolated mononeuropathies, it is not due to compression/trauma.

ETIOLOGIES

- Most common = diabetes mellitus
- Most serious = vasculitis (must be considered in all cases)
- Others include inflammatory/autoimmune disorders, Lyme disease (late), HIV, toxic, neoplastic.

DIFFERENTIAL

- **Plexopathies:** On detailed examination these can be mapped to the brachial or lumbosacral plexus.
  - Symptoms will involve distal and proximal extremity.
  - May be due to trauma, radiation, malignancy, viral infection (lumbosacral)

SYMPTOMS/EXAM

- Pain and weakness in multiple peripheral nerves (eg,. sciatic, common peroneal, radial, femoral)
  - Asymmetric

DIAGNOSIS

- Electrodiagnostic studies
- Sural nerve biopsy if diagnosis in question

TREATMENT

- Treat underlying disorder (eg, steroids for vasculitis).
- Treat associated neuropathic pain (eg, amitriptyline, carbamazepine, gabapentin).

Amyotrophic Lateral Sclerosis

ALS is a disorder characterized by upper motor neuron disease in addition to lower motor neuron pathology.

PATHOPHYSIOLOGY

- Anterior horn cell neuronopathy → peripheral nerve findings.
- Loss of Betz cells in the CNS motor cortex → upper motor neuron findings.

SYMPTOMS/EXAM

- Lower motor neuron involvement
  - Muscle fasciculations and atrophy
  - Muscle cramps
  - Asymmetric distal weakness
- Upper motor neuron involvement
  - Hyperreflexia and clonus
  - Spasticity
  - Positive Babinksi
- Serious complications and or death result from progressive respiratory muscle weakness (→ respiratory failure) or dysphagia (→ aspiration).

The hallmark of ALS is the presence of both upper motor neuron and lower motor neuron signs and symptoms.

DIAGNOSIS

- Electrodiagnostic testing

TREATMENT

- Supportive therapy
- Disease-modifying agent (rizulon)

Myasthenia Gravis

Myasthenia gravis is an autoimmune **disorder of the neuromuscular junction**.

PATHOPHYSIOLOGY

- Antibodies against acetylcholine receptors at the neuromuscular junction → destruction of receptors → decrease in available receptors.

SYMPTOMS/EXAM

- Fatigable muscle weakness
  - **Repeated muscle use increases weakness.**
  - Weakness is improved after rest.
- Ocular muscle weakness is common → ptosis, diplopia, blurred vision.
- Dysarthria and dysphagia may be present.
- Exacerbated by heat, improved by cold
- **Acute myasthenic crisis** = respiratory failure requiring mechanical ventilation.
  - Triggers include infection, medications.

DIFFERENTIAL

- Lambert-Eaton myasthenic syndrome
- Botulism

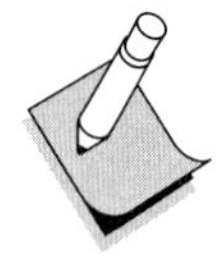

Myasthenia gravis: *Muscle weakness, worse with repeated use and commonly involving ocular muscles; treat with cholinesterase inhibitors and immunosuppressive agents*

DIAGNOSIS

- Suspect based on clinical examination.
- Edrophonium (Tensilon) test:
  - Edrophonium is a short-acting acetylcholinesterase blocking agent → increased acetylcholine available at neuromuscular junction → improvement in measured ptosis (and other symptoms).
  - Test dose must be administered first.
  - Have atropine ready in case of excessive cholinergic symptoms.
- Serologic testing for acetylcholine receptor antibodies
- Electromyographic testing.

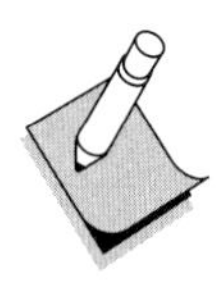

Acute myasthenic crisis: *Acute ventilatory failure, requiring mechanical ventilation; treat with plasma exchange and/or IVIG*

TREATMENT

- Cholinesterase inhibitors → increased circulating acetylcholine → symptom control.
  - Pyridostigmine, neostigmine
  - Should NOT be used during myasthenic crisis!
  - Excessive administration → cholinergic crisis with *weakness*, tachycardia, excessive secretions, etc.
- Immunosuppressive agents for chronic control
- Thymectomy
  - May induce early or late (2–5 years) remission of disease
- Plasmapheresis (plasma exchange) and intravenous immune globulin (IVIG) for acute exacerbations

Lambert-Eaton Myasthenic Syndrome

Lambert-Eaton myasthenic syndrome is an autoimmune disorder of the neuromuscular junction. About half the time it is associated with cancer (small cell carcinoma of the lung, lymphoma).

PATHOPHYSIOLOGY

- Antibodies → inadequate release of acetylcholine at neuromuscular junctions → symptoms.

SYMPTOMS/EXAM

- Proximal (primarily leg) **muscle weakness that improves with repeated stimulation**
- Autonomic symptoms (dry mouth, impotence)

DIAGNOSIS

- Clinical presentation
- Electrodiagnostic testing

TREATMENT

- Treat underlying malignancy, when present.
- Immunosuppressive agents
- Plasmapheresis and IVIG, if severe

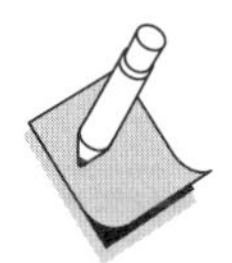

Lambert-Eaton myasthenic syndrome:
Proximal muscle weakness that improves with repeated stimulation; treat with immunosuppressive agents or plasmapheresis/IVIG, if severe

Botulism

Botulism is a toxin-mediated disorder of the neuromuscular junction.

PATHOPHYSIOLOGY

- Toxin produced by *Clostridium botulinum* → presynaptic inhibition of acetylcholine release at the neuromuscular junction.
  - Infants may ingest spores (**honey is a common agent**) → bacteria germinate in GI tract and produces toxin.

SYMPTOMS/EXAM

- Onset 6–48 hours after ingestion of toxin or *Clostridium botulinum* spores
- Classic presentation = descending flaccid paralysis.
  - **Diplopia, dysarthria, and dysphagia** occur early.
  - Progresses to generalized weakness; ventilatory failure may occur
  - May last for months
  - In children, may present as constipation, feeding difficulty, and hypotonia.
- Other anticholinergic symptoms may be present (dry skin, dilated pupils, increased temperature).
- Infantile botulism → lethargy, weakness/floppiness, poor feeding.

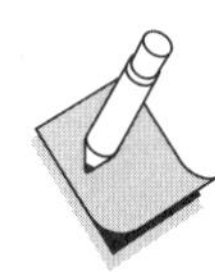

Botulism:
Descending flaccid paralysis with diplopia, dysarthria, and dysphagia occurring early; treat with horse serum antitoxin

DIAGNOSIS

- Clinical suspicion
- Electrodiagnostic testing
- Botulinum toxin testing of serum and stool

TREATMENT

- Supportive care
- Horse serum antitoxin

Tick Paralysis

Tick paralysis is a toxin-mediated disorder of the neuromuscular junction.

PATHOPHYSIOLOGY

- Tick toxin → decreased release of acetylcholine at neuromuscular junction → symptoms.

SYMPTOMS/EXAM

- Symmetric ascending paralysis

DIFFERENTIAL

- Other disorders at neuromuscular junction (botulism, myasthenia)

DIAGNOSIS

- Based on finding an attached feeding tick

TREATMENT

- Supportive
- Remove tick: Resolution of symptoms ranges from hours to days.

Polymyositis/Dermatomyositis

Polymyositis and dermatomyositis are both **inflammatory myopathies** of autoimmune etiology that produce muscle weakness. Dermatomyositis can occur in children.

SYMPTOMS/EXAM

- Chronic symmetric proximal muscle weakness
- Muscle pain and tenderness
- Dermatomyositis has additional skin findings including photosensitivity and extensor rashes.

DIAGNOSIS

- Electromyography and muscle biopsy confirm diagnosis.
- CK may (or may not) be elevated.
  - Significant rhabdomyolysis is unlikely.

TREATMENT

- Oral prednisone or cytotoxic drugs

Periodic Paralysis

Periodic paralysis is a disorder characterized by generalized muscle weakness due to muscle ion channel abnormalities.

- Hyperkalemic and hypokalemic periodic paralysis:
  - Most common
  - Familial
- Hyperthyroid periodic paralysis:
  - Secondary to related hypokalemia

SYMPTOMS/EXAM

- Episodic muscle weakness of rapid onset
- Flaccid paralysis of extremities

- Limited bulbar and ocular involvement
- Ventilatory failure is uncommon.

DIAGNOSIS

- Clinical diagnosis is based on personal and/or family history of similar episodes.
- ECG may show findings consistent with hyper- or hypokalemia.
- Serum K^+ levels

TREATMENT

- Supportive care
- Treat underlying electrolyte abnormalities.
- Treat hyperthyroidism, if present.

> A 30-year-old female presents to the ED complaining of pain with eye movement and visual changes in her right eye. She denies trauma or other complaints. Upon further history, the patient reports transient episodes of hand or leg weakness over the past few years. She has never seen a physician for this. On examination, the pupillary response to light is decreased in the affected eye and fundoscopic examination shows a blurred optic disc. What is the treatment for this patient's presenting illness?
>
> This patient likely has MS and is presenting with optic neuritis. Intravenous (not oral) steroids is the recommended treatment.

MULTIPLE SCLEROSIS

PATHOPHYSIOLOGY

Genetic and environmental factors → inflammatory reaction → regions of CNS demyelination with sparing of axons.

SYMPTOMS/EXAM

- Characterized by episodic neurologic dysfunction that onsets rapidly, then slowly resolves
- May involve any aspect of the CNS (cranial nerve findings, motor weakness, cerebellar dysfunction, cognitive changes, bowel/bladder dysfunction)
- **Optic neuritis** is often the presenting finding and is the most common cranial nerve finding; it is characterized by eye pain that is worse with eye movement followed by scotoma of central vision.
- **Internuclear ophthalmoplegia:** Abnormal horizontal eye movements due to lesion of the medial longitudinal fasciculus; may also be seen (less commonly) in brainstem vascular lesions, hypertensive crisis, trauma, cocaine use, and SLE
- **Uhthoff phenomenon:** Small increases in body temperature (eg, exercise, fever) → worsened symptoms.
- **Lhermitte phenomenon:** Electric shock sensation down spine with flexion of neck

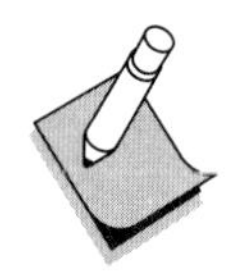

Multiple sclerosis:
Neurologic symptoms separated by "space and time"

DIAGNOSIS

- Suspect in patients with two episodes of differing neurologic symptoms occurring at different times.
- MRI may show multiple white matter lesions (better than CT).
- Lumbar puncture: CSF cell counts, protein and glucose are typically normal; CSF may show oligoclonal bands of IgG and/or myelin-based proteins.

TREATMENT

- High-dose methylprednisolone burst with taper for acute exacerbations

PARKINSON DISEASE

Parkinson disease is a chronic neurodegenerative disease of the elderly resulting from damage to dopaminergic neurons in the substantia nigra. Environmental and genetic factors play a role.

> Parkinson disease findings—
> **TRAP**
> **T**remor
> **R**igidity
> **A**kinesia
> **P**ostural instability

SYMPTOMS/EXAM

- Four characteristic findings:
  - Resting tremor ("pill-rolling")
  - Cogwheel rigidity
  - Bradykinesia or akinesia
  - Postural instability
- Other common findings include depression, muscle fatigue.

DIAGNOSIS

- Based on clinical findings
- CT/MRI is not definitive.

TREATMENT

- Agents to increase CNS dopamine and anticholinergics to decrease central muscarinic activity; see Antiparkinsonism Drugs, Chapter 6.

COMPLICATIONS

- Include dementia, falls, DVT/PE, aspiration

CHAPTER 16

Psychobehavioral Disorders

Maryam B. Shapland, MD

THE DSM-IV CLASSIFICATION

The DSM-IV classification aids in making a comprehensive assessment of disease and in organizing complex clinical disorders.

Axis I: Clinical syndromes of mental disorders (eg, schizophrenia, depression)

Axis II: Personality disorders and developmental disorders

Axis III: General medical conditions (eg, diabetes, hypertension)

Axis IV: Psychosocial and environmental stressors or problems

Axis IV: Global assessment of functioning

THE EMERGENCY CARE OF PSYCHIATRIC PATIENTS

The Emergency Petition (EP)

An emergency petition is indicated for patients who require immediate treatment to save their lives or to prevent imminent serious harm to themselves or to others. It is also indicated when an unanticipated situation arises where the patient's behavior presents an immediate and serious threat to the safety of the patient, other patients, and staff.

The **two essential elements** of an EP are: (1) a serious and imminent situation exists because of (2) the patient's psychiatric condition.

Indications for Seclusion and Restraint

- To prevent **clear and imminent** harm to patient or others
- To prevent significant disruption to treatment program and physical surroundings
- To assist in treatment as part of ongoing behavioral therapy
- To **decrease sensory overstimulation**
- To comply with patient's voluntary reasonable request

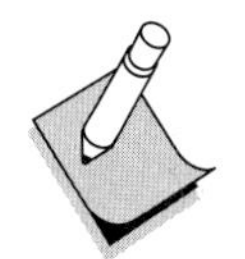

The presence of dangerousness without severe mental illness is not sufficient to involuntarily hospitalize a patient. Such persons are the responsibility of the police, NOT the psychiatrist!

Indications for Involuntary Hospitalization/Civil Commitment

- **Mentally ill**
- **Danger** to self or others
- Unable to provide basic needs of food, clothing, and shelter, ie, **gravely disabled**

A patient likely to sign out against medical advice (AMA) should be involuntarily hospitalized if the clinician believes the criteria have been met for involuntary commitment.

SUBSTANCE ABUSE DISORDERS/ADDICTION

Substance Abuse

Definitions

- **Intoxication:** Reversible substance-specific syndrome, with maladaptive behavioral or psychological changes that are due to the effect of the substance on the central nervous system (CNS)
- **Tolerance:** Repeated exposure **requires a larger dose** to produce intoxication, and the initial dose produces less intoxication.

- **Withdrawal:** Signs and symptoms opposite of intoxication when drug is discontinued.
- **Abuse:** Social or medical problems that result from substance use (relationship problems, liver disease from alcohol use) but without presence of dependence.
- **Dependence**
  - Physical dependence: Presence of **tolerance** or emergence of **withdrawal** symptoms.
  - Psychological dependence: The **craving** experienced or drug-seeking behavior.

*Alcoholism has a genetic component: Close relatives of alcoholics have **four times the risk** of alcoholism.*

> A 55-year-old man is brought in by EMS after being "found down" on the street. There are no signs of trauma and there is a strong odor of alcohol on his breath. What laboratory abnormalities are associated with heavy alcohol use?
>
> Increased GGT, increased MCV, AST > ALT, coagulopathy.

Alcohol

Alcohol use is very prevalent in society. **Lifetime risk for the general population is 15%.**

CAGE:

Have you ever felt that you should **Cut down** on your drinking?
Have people ever **Annoyed** you by criticizing your drinking?
Have you ever felt bad or **Guilty** about your drinking?
Have you ever had a drink first thing in the morning to steady your nerves or get rid of a hangover? (**Eye opener**)

Risk Factors

Male sex, ages 25–34, **psychiatric disorder** (antisocial personality disorder, mania, and schizophrenia), **homelessness**

The Medical Cost of Alcoholism

- Alcoholics have a 10- to 15-year shorter life span.
- Cardiac: Decreased occurrence of CAD, but increased risks of hypertension, dilated cardiomyopathy, arrhythmias
- Endocrine: Pancreatic insufficiency (glucose intolerance), increased ACTH, glucocorticoid, or catecholamine release, decreased testosterone synthesis (male hypogonadism)
- Metabolic: Hyperlipidemia, hypoglycemia, gout, immune compromise, electrolyte imbalance, vitamin deficiencies, coagulopathy
- GI: **Most common cause of liver failure** in the United States and worldwide from alcoholic hepatitis and cirrhosis; can also get gastritis, stomach or duodenal ulcers, esophageal varices causing GI bleeds
- Cancer: Increased risk of esophageal, stomach, pancreatic, and breast cancer
- Neuro: Peripheral neuropathy, cognitive deficits, memory impairment, Wernicke-Korsakoff syndrome
- Women: More prone to cirrhosis, and pregnant women have an increased risk of IUGR and fetal alcohol syndrome (FAS)

Standardized tests such as CAGE have been found to have higher sensitivity than BAC, breath smell, patient self-report, or patient complaint.

Symptoms/Exam

Screening for Alcoholism

CAGE screening tool is an internationally recognized tool for identifying alcoholics.

Score < or = 1 → further assessment, or = > 2 → highly specific for alcohol dependence

The blood alcohol concentration (BAC)

After the consumption of a standard drink (12 oz of beer, 5 oz of wine or 1.25 oz of 80 proof liquor), the BAC will peak within 30 minutes. The resulting BAC is determined by gender and weight. Two standard drinks will typically raise the BAC to 0.05% in a 70-kg male (higher in females). In most states, 0.08% is considered legally intoxicated.

A nontolerant patient's BAC typically correlates with a particular presentation (see Table 16.1). However, an alcohol-dependent person will exhibit tolerance to increased levels of blood alcohol.

Alcohol is metabolized at a constant rate, ie, zero order kinetics. A typical rate of metabolism is 0.01–0.02% per hour. However, there is great variability in an individual's ability to metabolize alcohol. Experienced drinkers may metabolize alcohol as fast as 0.04% per hour, but patients with advanced liver disease will metabolize slower.

ALCOHOL INTOXICATION

SYMPTOMS/EXAM/DIAGNOSIS

- Recent ingestion of alcohol
- Maladaptive behavior such as sexual or aggressive behavior, impaired judgment, labile mood, impaired social/occupational functioning
- Physical signs such as slow or slurred speech, incoordination, unsteady gait, nystagmus, impairment of attention or memory, stupor or coma
- Rule out other medical conditions.

DIFFERENTIAL

Opioid intoxication, sedative/hypnotic use, toxic overdose (clonidine, organophosphates, phenothiazines), carbon monoxide poisoning, hypoglycemia, hypoxia, CNS infections, postictal states, pontine hemorrhage

TREATMENT

- ABCs (intubate if airway not protected)
- Supportive care: IV fluids or banana bag (magnesium, thiamine, folate, multivitamin), dextrose, and electrolyte repletion if indicated
- Imaging if trauma is suspected
- Antipsychotic agent for behavioral control if indicated

TABLE 16.1. BAC Correlated With Typical Presentation in Nontolerant Alcohol-Intoxicated Patient

BAC (mg/dL)	CLINICAL PRESENTATION
30	Attention difficulties, mild euphoria
50	Coordination problems
100	Typical drunk-driving parameter, ataxia
200	Confusion, decreased consciousness
>400	Seizure, coma, could result in death

(Reproduced, with permission, from Hillard R, et al. *Emergency Psychiatry*. New York: McGraw-Hill, 2004:140.)

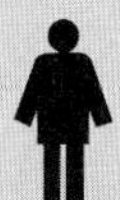

A 64-year-old man comes to the ED complaining of "feeling shaky." He is normotensive, HR is 104, and exhibits tremulousness. His last drink was 12 hours ago. How would you treat his symptoms?

IV/O_2/monitor, banana bag, benzodiazepines, observe closely for seizures.

An alcohol-abusing patient with a first seizure should be treated and evaluated as any patient with a first-time seizure.

ALCOHOL WITHDRAWAL

SYMPTOMS/EXAM/DIAGNOSIS

- Recent (few hours to few days) decrease or cessation of alcohol.
- Two or more of the following:
  - Autonomic hyperactivity (increased BP, HR >100, sweating)
  - Tremulousness
  - Nausea/vomiting
  - Psychomotor agitation
  - Insomnia
  - Anxiety
  - Grand mal seizures (**usually at least 24 hours after last drink**)
- Rule out other medical condition.
- See Table 16.2 for major symptoms of alcohol withdrawal.

DIFFERENTIAL

For alcohol-related seizures: Acute intoxication, metabolic abnormalities (hypoglycemia, hypo/hypernatremia, hypocalcemia), infections, trauma, cerebrovascular accident (CVA), benzodiazepine/barbiturate withdrawal, noncompliance with anticonvulsants

TABLE 16.2. Major Symptoms of Alcohol Withdrawal

	ONSET AFTER LAST DRINK	SYMPTOMS/SIGNS	TREATMENT
Mild withdrawal	6–8 hours	Coarse tremors, nausea, anxiety, tachycardia, hypertension, insomnia, irritability.	Supportive care, benzodiazepines.
Seizures	6–48 hours	Brief **generalized tonic-clonic seizures**, no aura, can have 1–3 in a short postictal period; status epilepticus can occur in about 3%	Supportive care, benzodiazepines Most resolve spontaneously. Can progress to delirium tremens (DTs).
Hallucinations	24–48 hours	Visual or tactile, **sensorium can be clear in early stages** but accompanied by disorientation/anxiety in late stages	Supportive care, benzodiazepines for hyperadrenergic signs and symptoms; not necessarily followed by DTs but are parts of the DT symptomatology
Delirium tremens	3–5 days	Severe autonomic hyperactivity, profound confusion, hallucinations, paranoid ideation, fever, diaphoresis, incontinence, mydriasis.	Benzodiazepines (may need to start a drip) admit to ICU

TREATMENT

- ABCs, IV/O_2/monitor, banana bag (thiamine, folate, multivitamins)
- Benzodiazepines are the mainstay of treatment.
- β-Blockers or clonidine may be used to control autonomic hyperactivity.
- Haldol or other antipsychotics may be used as an adjunct to benzodiazepines for delirium, delusions, or hallucinations (but be careful because it can lower the seizure threshold).
- Anticonvulsant use is typically not indicated unless the patient has a known seizure disorder.
- Admit if pt has >2 seizures in the ED.

DELIRIUM TREMENS

DTs usually occur in patients with a history of heavy, long-term alcohol use. About 5% of patients who withdraw from alcohol will proceed to DTs, **which usually begin 3–5 days after cessation.**

RISK FACTORS

- **History of DTs**
- BAC >300 upon presentation
- **Alcohol withdrawal seizures** upon presentation
- **Comorbid medical illness** (cardiovascular, pulmonary, renal disease, infection, electrolyte abnormalities)

DIFFERENTIAL

Sepsis, meningitis, hypoxia, **hypoglycemia**, hepatic failure, intracranial bleed

DIAGNOSIS

Symptoms are similar to severe alcohol withdrawal except these patients exhibit autonomic instability, disorientation, visual or tactile hallucinations, paranoid ideation, and delirium. Coma and death may result.

TREATMENT

Treatment includes supportive care, aggressive use of **benzodiazepines** (may need to start a continuous infusion). All patients with DTs will **need to be admitted to the ICU.**

Diagnosis of Wernicke encephalopathy–

Wernicke
Nystagmus and opthalmoplegia
Incoordination, ataxia
Confusion

WERNICKE ENCEPHALOPATHY

Occurs in heavy drinkers and severely malnourished patients, secondary to **thiamine (vitamin B_1) deficiency**. Consideration for Wernicke encephalopathy should be given to patients with any evidence of **long-term alcohol abuse or malnutrition or who present with altered mental status.**

In addition, hypotension or hypothermia (due to autonomic and temperature dysregulation) may occur.

TREATMENT

Thiamine! (The question about whether this should be given before glucose is controversial).

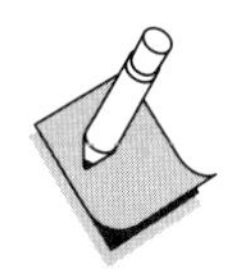

*Remember to give magnesium! **A hypomagnesemic state may be resistant to thiamine administration.***

KORSAKOFF'S SYNDROME/PSYCHOSIS

This is also due to **thiamine deficiency**. This is a progression of Wernicke encephalopathy and results in **confabulation** due to anterograde and retrograde memory impairment.

TREATMENT

Thiamine! **When in doubt, treat.** There is little risk and significant benefit by giving thiamine.

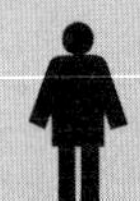

A 28-year-old pregnant woman, EGA 30 weeks, presents with cocaine toxicity. How are pregnant patients treated and what obstetrical complications are associated with cocaine use?

Treatment includes supportive care, benzodiazepines, and monitoring of fetal heart tones. Complications include altered uteroplacental blood flow secondary to vasoconstriction, resulting in increased incidence of spontaneous abortion, abruption placentae, fetal prematurity, and intrauterine growth retardation.

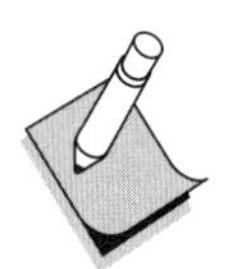

*Cocaine is primarily **metabolized by plasma cholinesterase**. Cocaine use can be fatal in patients with a relative deficiency of this enzyme!*

Cocaine

PATHOPHYSIOLOGY

Cocaine has both local anesthetic and CNS stimulant effects.

- Blocks the fast sodium channels in the cell membrane → inhibits conduction of nerve impulses → local anesthesia
- Also enhances the effects of excitatory amino acids and blocks the presynaptic reuptake of norepinephrine (NE), dopamine, and serotonin → sympathetic activation

SYMPTOMS

Cocaine intoxication: Euphoria, **hypervigilance**, anxiety, tension or anger, impaired judgment, impaired social or occupational functioning

Effects of cocaine intoxication are shown in Table 16.3.

DIFFERENTIAL

Amphetamine use, ephedrine use, alcohol withdrawal, sedative/anxiolytic withdrawal, opioid withdrawal.

DIAGNOSIS

- Diagnosed clinically
- Labs may show elevated cardiac markers, metabolic acidosis, renal failure, and rhabdomyolysis.
- Urine toxicology will be positive for cocaine metabolites if cocaine was used in the past 24–72 hours if after single dose; 7–12 days after repeated high doses; depends on acute/chronic cocaine use.
- ECG/CXR/head CT if indicated

TREATMENT

- IV/O_2/monitor
- Treat symphatomimetic si/sx with benzodiazepines.

TABLE 16.3. Effects of Cocaine Intoxication

ORGAN SYSTEM	EFFECTS
Cardiovascular	Has **quinidine-like effects** causing QRS widening and QT prolongation Large doses cause a direct toxic effect on the myocardium causing bradycardia, wide-complex dysrhythmias, myocarditis, and hypotension. α-Adrenergic–mediated coronary **vasoconstriction** occurs causing myocardial infarction and cardiomyopathy. Hypertension and **tachycardia** Aortic rupture, aortic and coronary artery **dissection**
Neurological	Hyperadrenergic state causes **pupillary dilatation**, hyperthermia, and **psychomotor agitation**. Severe hypertension and cerebral vasoconstriction cause intracerebral hemorrhages (ICH), seizures, CVAs, coma, confusion. Muscle weakness, dystonias, and dyskinesias can occur from inhibition of nerve impulses.
Pulmonary	Seen with crack cocaine use: pulmonary hemorrhage, pulmonary edema, pneumonitis, asthma, barotrauma (pneumothorax, pneumomediastinum)
Gastrointestinal	Toxicity seen with "**body packers**" (patient swallows multiple bags of well-concealed cocaine for smuggling purposes) and "**body stuffers**" (patient swallows one hastily wrapped bag to avoid police arrest); can also see mesenteric vasoconstriction resulting in ischemia
Renal	Increased creatinine phosphokinase (CPK) can cause rhabdomyolysis and acute renal failure. Renal infarction can also occur.

- **Avoid haldol, droperidol, chlorpromazine → can lower seizure threshold** and cause dysrhythmias and hyperthermia.
- Treat hyperthermia with rapid evaporative cooling.
- Aggressive IV fluids to prevent/treat rhabdomyolysis
- **Avoid β-blockers** in cocaine chest pain → can cause an unopposed α adrenergic state, thus worsening vasoconstriction.
- Treat wide complex tachydysrhythmias and QRS prolongation with sodium bicarbonate.
- Treat hypertension with **phentolamine** or sodium nitroprusside.

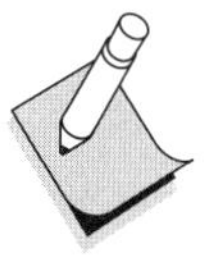

Body packers or stuffers should receive activated charcoal and polyethylene glycol (Go-LYTELY) for decontamination. If the patient shows signs of intoxication, immediate surgical consultation should be made!

Amphetamines

- **Derivatives of phenylethylamine**
- Enhances the release and blocks the reuptake of **catecholamines** and may directly stimulate catecholamine receptors
- **Induces release of serotonin centrally,** which accounts for the hallucinogenic properties of MDMA (3,4-methylenedioxy-N-methylamphetamine) ie, "ecstasy"
  - MDMA can cause hypertension, hyperthermia, and dehydration, which can lead to excessive water drinking and profound hyponatremia.
  - MDMA can also cause seizures.
  - Treat MDMA toxicity with IV fluids, active cooling, and benzodiazepines.
- **Methylphenidate [Ritalin]**, a widely prescribed drug for Attention Deficit Disorder (ADD), is an amphetamine derivative and is now becoming a drug of abuse.

EPHEDRINE

- Has both **α- and β-adrenergic activity** caused by release of dopamine and NE from neuronal stores
- Widely available in health food stores
- Can cause severe cardiovascular and neurologic toxicity, psychosis, hypertension if abused

PHENYLPROPANOLAMINE

- A **peripheral α-adrenergic agonist** that causes significant vasoconstriction with hypertension and reflex bradycardia
- Has been **withdrawn from the market** secondary to associated intracranial hemorrhage

Opioids

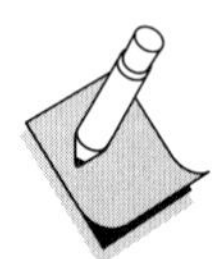

Pupillary constriction is not always present as patients can get mydriasis from coingestants or anoxia. Furthermore, meperidine, propoxyphene, and pentazocine may dilate the pupils.

Opiates properly refer to products derived from opium alkaloids (eg, morphine, codeine) and nonalkaloids (eg, heroin). **Opioids** are any drug that has morphine-like effects by binding to the opioid receptors in the CNS (eg, propoxyphene, methadone).

SYMPTOMS/EXAM

Symptoms vary with dose and frequency of use. Patients typically present with psychomotor agitation or retardation, impaired judgment and attention, drowsiness or coma, slurred speech, respiratory depression.

DIFFERENTIAL

Alcohol intoxication, sedative/hypnotic use, toxic overdose (clonidine, organophosphates, phenothiazines), carbon monoxide poisoning, hypoglycemia, hypoxia, CNS infections, postictal states, pontine hemorrhage

DIAGNOSIS

Diagnosis is clinical. **Classic triad is coma, miosis, and respiratory depression.**

TREATMENT

Remember to check an acetaminophen level on patients with possible ingestion of an opioid-acetaminophen combination.

- ABCs, IV/O_2/monitor, dextrose stick
- Narcan is a pure antagonist that can be administered via IV, IM, SC, SL, or via the endotracheal tube. It is effective in life-threatening overdoses or if the diagnosis is uncertain.
  - Onset of action is 1–2 minutes.
  - Duration is about 20–60 minutes. Repeated boluses or an infusion may be necessary, especially for long-acting opioids such as methadone.
  - Begin with small doses 0.2–0.4 mg to avoid acute withdrawal.
- Observe for 4–6 hours in the ED, and admit those with long-lasting ingestion, those requiring an infusion or repeated boluses.

ACUTE LUNG TOXICITY

- A rare complication of opioid toxicity
- Suspect in any patient with **tachypnea, rales, decreased O_2 saturations with normal cardiac silhouette on CXR**

- Treatment is positive pressure oxygenation, intubation if indicated, and use of PEEP.

OPIOID WITHDRAWAL

- Symptoms/exam: Include anxiety, nausea/vomiting, lacrimation, rhinorrhea, papillary dilatation, piloerection, diaphoresis, diarrhea, yawning, and insomnia
- Treatment: Can give clonidine, antiemetics, antidiarrheal agents, and refer to treatment center; buprenophrine best used in conjunction with a drug recovery center

Phencyclidine (PCP) and Hallucinogens

PCP is a dissociative anesthetic that is **structurally related to ketamine**. It is a **glutamate agonist** at the NMDA (N-methyl-D-aspartate) receptor. **Dextromethorphan** has similar effects to PCP.

SYMPTOMS/EXAM

- Peak effects occur approximately 15–30 minutes after inhaling PCP and can be up to 2 hours after oral doses.
- Symptoms/Exam: Variable. Patient can present with behavioral problems (anger, aggression, irritability), impaired judgment, **vertical or horizontal nystagmus**, hypertension, tachycardia, CNS depression or stimulation, physical violence, catatonia, coma, or seizures. **Pupil size is also variable**.

DIFFERENTIAL

Alcohol withdrawal or intoxication, trauma, meningitis, hypoglycemia, hypoxia, sedative/hypnotic withdrawal, acute psychosis, other intoxication (cocaine, amphetamine)

DIAGNOSIS

Diagnosis is clinical. Toxicology studies are not useful (chronic PCP users can test positive long after last use).

TREATMENT

Treatment is supportive. Give benzodiazepines for seizures, IV fluids for rhabdomyolysis, cooling for hyperthermia and activated charcoal for oral PCP use. Other medical causes need to be ruled out.

OTHER HALLUCINOGENS

See Table 16.4.

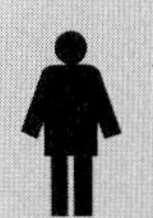

A 30-year-old woman on chronic benzodiazepines presents with autonomic hyperactivity, tremulousness, nausea/vomiting, transient visual, tactile, and auditory hallucinations, and proceeds to have a grand mal seizure. What is the most important consideration in the treatment of this patient?

This is benzodiazepine withdrawal, and benzodiazepine administration is indicated. This patient can be very tolerant and may require large doses for treatment of her symptoms.

TABLE 16.4. **Characteristics of Hallucinogens**

Drug	Duration of Action (hours)	Clinical Features	Complications	Treatment
MDMA (3,4-methylenedioxy-*N*-methylamphetamine	8-24	Mydriasis, sympathomimetic symptoms, euphoria, nausea, dry mouth, ataxia, musclespasm	Hypertension, hyperthermia, rhabdomyolysis, dehydration Excessive water drinking and hyponatremia Seizures	IV fluids, cooling, supportive care, benzodiazepines
LSD (derived from fungus *Claviceps purpurea*)	8–12	Mydriasis, sympathomimetic symptoms, muscle spasm	Persistent psychosis, "flashbacks" or hallucinogen persisting perception disorder	Supportive care, benzodiazepines
Psilocybin (derived from mushrooms of *Psilocybe* genus)	4–6	Mydriasis, sympathomimetic symptoms, nausea	Seizures (rare), hyperthermia (rare)	Supportive care, benzodiazepines
Mescaline (a phenylethylamine found in Mexican peyote cactus)	6–12	Mydriasis, sympathomimetic symptoms, abdominal pain, vomiting, dizziness	Rare	Supportive care, benzodiazepines
Marijuana	2–4	Tachycardia, conjunctival injection, impaired motor coordination	Rare	Supportive care, benzodiazepines

(Adapted, with permission, from Tintinalli JE, Kelen, GD, Stapczynski SJ. *Emergency Medicine: A Comprehensive Study Guide,* 6th ed. New York: McGraw-Hill, 2004:1080.)

Sedative/Hypnotics/Anxiolytics

Includes benzodiazepines, benzodiazepine-like drugs, barbiturates, and barbiturate-like drugs, carbamates

Symptoms/Exam

Inappropriate behavior, mood lability, slow, slurred speech, unsteady gait, incoordination, nystagmus, impairment in attention/memory, stupor, coma; can also see bradycardia, bradypnea, hypotension

Differential

Alcohol intoxication, CVA, head trauma, opioid intoxication, hypoglycemia, hypoxia

Diagnosis

Clinical diagnosis; urine and blood toxicology can be positive for up to a week with long-acting substances and chronic use

Treatment

- Supportive care
- ABCs; consider need for airway protection.

- Benzodiazepines and barbiturates are most often coingested with other agents. Consider giving dextrose, narcan, thiamine, and performing gastric lavage and/or activated charcoal.
- Flumazenil is a selective benzodiazepine antagonist that can **cause generalized seizures in patients with chronic benzodiazepine dependence. It can also increase intracranial pressure (ICP).**

Flumazenil is contraindicated in the unknown overdose patient and in patients with increased ICP.

MOOD AND THOUGHT DISORDERS

Acute Psychosis

SYMPTOMS/EXAM

Delusions, prominent hallucinations, disorganized speech, disorganized or catatonic behavior. A **brief psychotic disorder** is defined as psychotic symptoms lasting >1 day but <1 month. **Schizophreniform disorder** is defined as psychotic symptoms lasting 1–6 months (see Figure 16.1).

DIFFERENTIAL

Delirium, substance use/intoxication, schizophrenia, psychotic disorder secondary to a medical condition (hypoxia, hypoglycemia, hepatic or renal disease, metabolic abnormalities, endocrine disorder, neurologic condition such as CVA, multiple sclerosis, infection), mood disorder with psychotic features

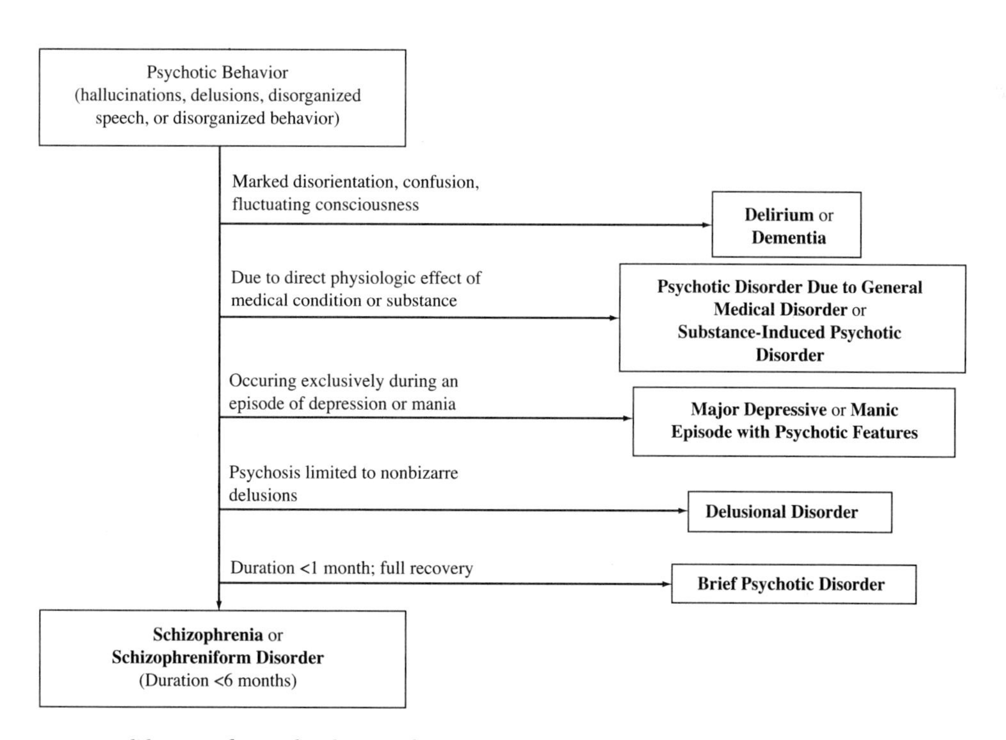

FIGURE 16.1. Decision tree for evaluating psychosis.

(Reproduced, with permission, from Tintinalli JE, Kelen, GD, Stapczynski SJ. *Emergency Medicine: A Comprehensive Study Guide*, 6th ed. New York: McGraw-Hill, 2004:1809.)

Diagnosis

Clinical diagnosis; check labs, head CT, and cerebrospinal fluid if indicated

Treatment

A patient who presents with brief psychotic disorder has a **high risk of suicide.** Any patient with new-onset psychosis needs to be evaluated by a psychiatrist and/or admitted after organic causes are ruled out.

A 24-year-old man is brought to the ED by his mother for hearing voices "telling me that the day of doom is coming." He is also becoming increasingly paranoid and believes that others are "out to get me because I speak the truth." He is diagnosed with new-onset schizophrenia. What are the risk factors for schizophrenia?

Multiple factors are associated with this disease. Those with family history (**first-degree relatives of patients with schizophrenia have 10 times the risk of developing schizophrenia**), brain abnormalities, low socioeconomic class, and those born in winter months living in northern climates have an increased risk of disease.

Schizophrenia

Symptoms/Exam

See Table 16.5.

Differential

- Same as for acute psychosis if new onset schizophrenia
- **Schizoaffective disorder:** Psychosis occurs exclusively during an episode of mania or depression.

TABLE 16.5. Signs and Symptoms of Schizophrenia

Phase	Signs/Symptoms	Treatment
Prodromal Phase	Social isolation, new interest in religion/philosophy, restlessness, difficulty concentrating	Experimental studies designed to train patients on appropriate social behavior
Positive symptoms	Delusions, hallucinations, strange behaviors, incoherent thought process, grossly disorganized or catatonic behavior	Antipsychotics, outpatient therapy, inpatient treatment if new onset, suicidal, or severe psychosis
Negative symptoms	Flat affect, decreased fluency, and productivity of thought and speech, social withdrawal, decrease in goal-directed behavior	Atypical antipsychotics, group therapy, inpatient if new onset, suicidal, or severe symptoms
Residual phase	Occurs between episodes of psychosis, patient retains flat affect and continues to hear voices	Outpatient and group therapy

- **Schizophreniform disorder**: Symptoms present for <6 months.
- **Schizoid personality disorder**: Voluntary social withdrawal with no signs of psychosis
- **Schizotypal personality disorder**: Odd, magical thinking with no signs of psychosis

Diagnosis/Treatment

See above.

Complications

- **Ten percent risk of suicide** (there is an increased risk for those with recent hospital discharge or in the postpsychotic period)
- Forty percent risk of concurrent substance abuse
- Long-term use of antipsychotics can cause extrapyramidal symptoms, dystonia. Decrease doses and administer diphenhdyramine, benztropine.
- Tardive dyskinesia (TD) may also be seen with use of antipsychotics. Consider switching to atypical antipsychotics (which have lower incidences of TD when compared to typical antipsychotics).
- Watch out for neuroleptic malignant syndrome (NMS). (See "Neuroleptic Malignant Syndrome.")

A 45-year-old Caucasian man with a history of diabetes and coronary artery disease presents to the ED with suicidal ideation. He is married with two children, has no personal history of mental illness but has a sister with a depression and previous suicide attempts. He reports that he lost his job recently and is feeling hopeless that he'll be able to provide for his family. What is his risk for suicidality?

High! (He has 7 of 11 risk factors.)

Major Depression and Suicide

Affects about **10–25% of women** and 5–12% of men. **Lifetime risk of suicide is 15%.**

Risk Factors for Suicide

- Age (adolescent and elderly)
- Male gender
- Poor physical health
- History of mental illness
- Caucasian
- Feeling of hopelessness, helplessness
- Isolation
- Unemployment or stressful work situation
- Poor financial situation
- Previous suicide attempt
- Family history of completed or attempted suicide

Symptoms of major depression—

SIGECAPS

Sleep (hypersomnia or insomnia)
Interest (lost of interest or pleasure in activities)
Guilt (feelings of worthlessness or inappropriate guilt)
Energy (decreased)
Concentration
Appetite
Psychomotor agitation or retardation
Suicidal ideation

Symptoms/Exam

One or more depressive episodes (at least 2 weeks of depressed mood or loss of interest, accompanied by four or more additional symptoms of depression).

Differential

Mood disorder secondary to neurological (Alzheimer disease, multiple sclerosis (MS), Huntington disease), endocrine (hypothyroidism), metabolic conditions, substance abuse, dementia, bereavement, adjustment disorder, postoperative/cardiac patients

Diagnosis

Diagnosis is clinical and by history. Also eliminate potential other medical etiologies, eg, check TSH, CBC, etc.

Treatment

Admit all suicidal patients and patients at high risk for suicide. Otherwise, treat with antidepressants (starting them in the ED is controversial) with close follow-up/therapy.

Grief Reaction

- Bereavement after loss of a loved one is normal.
- Illusions (seeing loved one briefly), guilt, and weight loss can occur.
- **Severe symptoms typically resolve after 2 months and moderate symptoms after 1 year.**
- Prolonged symptoms (>1 year) that include marked functional impairment, morbid preoccupation with worthlessness, suicidal ideation, psychotic symptoms, and psychomotor retardation are abnormal and should prompt immediate psychiatric evaluation.

Dysthymic Disorder

At least 2 years of depressed mood (1 year for children and adolescents) for more days than not, and without any 2-month asymptomatic period. Needs outpatient psychiatric evaluation unless patient is suicidal. Treatment often involves combination drug therapy along with individual and/or group psychotherapy.

Bipolar Disorder

Symptoms/Exam

- **Bipolar I**: One or more manic episodes or mixed episodes
- **Bipolar II**: One or more major depressive episodes accompanied by at least one hypomanic episode
- **Manic syndrome**: **Elation or irritability**, feels "top of the world" with **decreased need for sleep**, increased activity, **rapid pressured speech**, racing thoughts, **grandiose ideas**; patient may quickly become hostile, irritable, and argumentative

Differential

Mood disorder secondary to neurological (temporal lobe epilepsy), endocrine (hyperthyroidism), metabolic conditions, substance abuse, dementia, psychotic disorders

DIAGNOSIS

Diagnosis is clinical and by history. Also eliminate potential other medical etiologies (see above).

TREATMENT

Admit patients with suicidality and acute psychosis; mood stabilizers (lithium, select anticonvulsants), antipsychotics if indicated. Outpatient therapy.

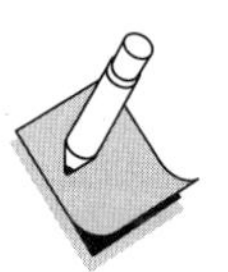

Onset after age 45 or presence of atypical symptoms during an episode of anxiety (loss of consciousness, loss of bowel or bladder control, headache, altered speech, focal neurologic symptoms, amnesia) suggest an organic cause!

Anxiety Disorders

See Table 16.6.

TABLE 16.6. Anxiety Disorders

DISORDER	SYMPTOMS/EXAM	DIFFERENTIAL	DIAGNOSIS	TREATMENT
Generalized anxiety disorder (GAD)	Six months of persistent/excessive anxiety and worry about a broad range of topics	Rule out: 1. Organic causes such as hyperthyroidism, hyperparathyroidism, pheochromocytoma, vestibular dysfunction, seizure disorder, acute coronary syndrome 2. CNS stimulants such as caffeine, cocaine, amphetamines 3. Other psychiatric condition (depression, psychosis, schizophrenia, bipolar disorder, or other anxiety disorder)	Diagnosis is clinical. Rule out other causes! Rule out all likely medical etiologies (eg, check ECG, lytes, CXR).	Cognitive behavioral therapy (CBT), group therapy, **long-acting benzodiazepines**, anxiolytic agents (eg, Flonazepam) selective serotonin reuptake inhibitor (SSRI)
Panic disorder	Recurrent, unexpected panic attacks followed by at least 1 mo of persistent concern about having another panic attack	**Endocrine:** Hypoglycemia, hypo/hyperthyroidism, hyperparathyroidism, pheochromocytoma **Neurologic:** Seizure disorders, vestibular disorders, vestibular dysfunction, neoplasms **Pharmacologic:** Acute intoxication, medication-induced symptoms **Cardiovascular:** Arrhythmias, MI **Psychiatric:** GAD, obsessive-compulsive disorder (OCD), posttraumatic stress disorder (PTSD)	Same as for GAD	SSRI, short-acting benzodiazepines, anxiolytic agents, β-blockers, desensitization, "flooding" therapy (CBT)

TABLE 16.6. Anxiety Disorders (*Continued*)

DISORDER	SYMPTOMS/EXAM	DIFFERENTIAL	DIAGNOSIS	TREATMENT
		Age of onset usually late adolescence to mid-30s.		
Phobic disorder	Clinically significant anxiety provoked by exposure to a specific feared object or situation leading to avoidance behavior	Panic disorder, PTSD, GAD	Same as for GAD	CBT (exposure-response prevention therapy), desensitization, SSRI, short-acting benzodiazepines, β-blockers (eg, propanolol), anxiolytic agents (eg, alprazolam)
Obsessive compulsive disorder (OCD)	Repetitive thoughts (obsessions) that cause marked anxiety or distress and/or mannerisms (compulsions) that serve to neutralize and relieve anxiety (but only temporarily)	Delusional disorder, schizophrenia, GAD.	Same as for GAD	CBT (exposure-response prevention therapy), SSRI, clomipramine; higher doses than those for depression usually required
Posttraumatic stress disorder	Reexperiencing an extremely traumatic event accompanied by symptoms of increased arousal, hypervigilance, and by avoidance of stimuli associated with the trauma; **patients typically have no history of panic attacks.**	Depression, GAD, adjustment disorder (patients have stress, anxiety, behavioral changes that are related to a specific trigger **but do not have reexperiencing, avoidance, and increased arousal**).	Same as for GAD	CBT, individual/group therapy (especially helpful), SSRI, sleep agents, long-acting benzodiazepines.

*"**La belle indifference**" (patient unconcerned about condition) no longer diagnostic of conversion disorder but can be seen.*

A 15-year-old girl presents to the ED after seeing a friend hit by a car and reports sudden paralysis of the left leg immediately after the incident. She was not involved in the accident. Her neurologic exam is significant for no voluntary movement of the left leg although sensation is intact. Upon motor exam, she has a positive thigh adductor test (when the examiner places her hands on the patient's bilateral inner thighs and asks her to adduct against resistance, both of legs adduct). What is her diagnosis?

Conversion disorder.

Somatoform Disorders

See Table 16.7.

TABLE 16.7. Somatoform Disorders

Disorder	Symptoms/Exam	Differential	Diagnosis	Treatment
Conversion Disorder (rare, F > M, adolescence)	**Usually involves neurologic/orthopedic manifestations** (paralysis, seizures, blindness), sudden onset of single symptom related to severe stress	Rule out organic pathology first (MS, SLE, Lyme disease, polymyositis, toxins). Check labs or imaging if indicated.	Clinical diagnosis; no physical findings related to symptom found, and exam is inconsistent with known anatomic or pathophysiologic states	Reassurance; supportive care; refer for outpatient medical and psychiatric follow-up
Somatization Disorder (F > M, adolescent–30s)	Wide variety of complaints and long complicated history of medical problems with no apparent medical cause; a pan-positive review of systems, repeated visits	Rule out organic causes if indicated.	Clinical diagnosis.	Reassurance, close outpatient medical and psychiatric follow-up; minimize number of providers and ensure a single one is taking the lead on treatment plan
Hypochondriasis	Patient is preoccupied with fears of serious illness that persist despite appropriate medical evaluation and reassurance.	Rule out organic causes.	Clinical diagnosis.	Reassurance, close outpatient medical and psychiatric follow-up; minimize number of providers and ensure a single one is taking the lead on treatment plan

Fictitious Disorders

See Table 16.8.

TABLE 16.8. Factitious Disorders

Disorder	Symptoms/Exam/Diagnosis	Differential	Treatment
Drug-seeking behavior	Most common complaints are back pain, headache, extremity pain, and dental pain. Common techniques include lost prescription, impending surgery, factitious hematuria, self-mutilation, multiple drug allergies. **Secondary gain is to obtain pain medication.**	Rule out real medical illness. Strike a balance between sufficient workup and exhaustive unnecessary tests/procedures.	Refuse drug, consider need for alternative medication/treatment, refer for drug counseling.
Malingering	**This is strongly linked with antisocial personality disorder.** There is marked discrepancy between patient's complaints and objective findings, with poor cooperation during exam or a history of poor compliance.	Somatization disorder; same as for drug-seeking behavior	Close outpatient follow-up.

TABLE 16.8. Factitious Disorders (*Continued*)

Disorder	Symptoms/Exam/Diagnosis	Differential	Treatment
	Secondary gain may be obvious (eg, patient is homeless or incarcerated). Patient may complain of mental illness because this is more difficult to disprove.		
Munchausen syndrome (M > F, ages 20–40 yr.)	Patients view themselves as important people, usually have extensive knowledge of medical terminology. There is significant **"pseudologica fantastica"** (pathologic lying) about medical illnesses, which are difficult to diagnose or disprove (eg, taking warfarin to induce bleeding). **Secondary gain is to subject him or herself to unnecessary tests to secure the "sick role."**	Same as for drug-seeking behavior	Early confrontation, close outpatient follow-up
Munchausen syndrome by proxy (MSBP) (Rare, perpetrator is usually the biological mother)	Child has significant history of failure-to-thrive, with persistent presentation for medical treatment. Illness is concocted by perpetrator (eg, injection of feces into IV line), and symptoms/signs cease when child is separated from perpetrator. **Secondary gain is prolonged contact with health care providers at the expense of her child.**	Same as for drug-seeking behavior	This is child abuse. Child Protective Services (CPS) needs to be notified immediately. There is a **high risk of maternal suicide associated with confrontation**; arrange psychiatric care for mother.

EATING DISORDERS

Eating disorders affect **5–10% of adolescent girls** and young women in the United States, and up to 1% of males.

Anorexia Nervosa

Symptoms/Exam/Diagnosis

- Refusal to maintain body weight over a minimum normal weight for age and height (**BMI <17.5**)
- Intense fear of becoming obese even when underweight
- **Misperception of body weight, shape, or size**
- Absence of at least **three consecutive** menstrual cycles (primary or secondary amenorrhea)
- Chronic findings are emaciated appearance, brittle hair and nails, lanugo, bradycardia, hypothermia.

Treatment

- Volume repletion and gradual correction of electrolyte imbalances
- **Avoid refeeding syndrome** secondary to aggressive refeeding: Rapid electrolyte shifts, hypophosphatemia, hypokalemia, hypomagnesemia cause severe cardiopulmonary and neurologic sequelae.
- Admit patients with extreme weight loss, severe metabolic disturbance, psychiatric disorders, poor familial/social support, complex medical problems and those who have failed outpatient therapy.

- Outpatient therapy includes psychotherapy (both individual and group) and antidepressants.

Bulimia

SSRIs are the antidepressants of choice for eating disorders, particularly bulimia.

Symptoms/Exam/Diagnosis

- Minimum of **two episodes of binge eating per week for at least 3 months**
- Feeling of lack of control over behavior during eating binges
- Regular self-induced vomiting, use of laxatives, strict dieting, fasting, vigorous exercising
- Persistent overconcern with body shape and weight
- Physical exam significant for parotid and **submandibular gland enlargement**, dental enamel erosion, **Russell sign** (calluses over the dorsal aspect of the fingers), posterior pharyngeal abrasions, facial petechiae, scleral hemorrhage, stress fractures

Treatment

Same as for anorexia

Eating Disorder, Not Otherwise Specified (NOS)

Diagnosis

- All criteria for anorexia except the patient is still menstruating and has normal weight
- All criteria for bulimia but decreased in frequency or duration
- Binge eating disorder, chewing/spitting out of food, eating large amounts of food

Treatment

Same as for anorexia/bulimia

VIOLENCE/ABUSE/NEGLECT

Child Abuse

Risk Factors

Domestic violence, poverty, child's medical condition, mental illness, history of abuse and substance abuse in parent

Symptoms/Exam

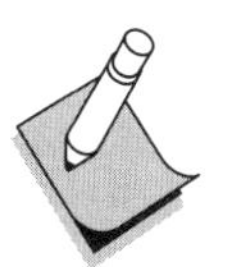

A sexually transmitted disease (STD) in a prepubescent child is highly suspicious for sexual abuse!

- Look for cutaneous manifestations such as bruises that are not over bony prominences; area of erythema in specific shapes, cigarette burns, bites, immersion burns on buttocks and legs. (See Figures 16.2 and 16.3.)
- **Shaken baby syndrome**: Usually children <2 years presenting with lethargy, vomiting; exam shows retinal hemorrhages, skeletal fractures
- Sexual abuse: Look for perianal tears or fissures, acute tears of hymen, vaginal petechiae, or hematomas.

Differential

Mongolian spots, coagulopathy, coining/cupping, impetigo, toxic epidermal necrolysis, herpes simplex virus, osteogenesis imperfecta, accidental trauma, urethral prolapse, priapism

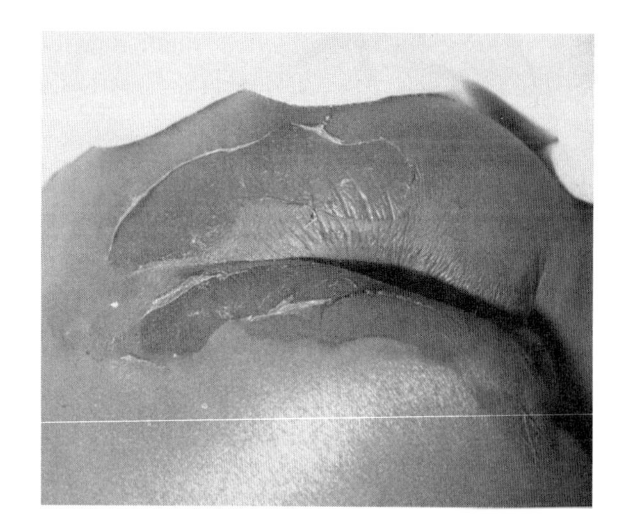

FIGURE 16.2. Burns on buttocks.

(Reproduced, with permission, from Weinberg S, et al. *Color Atlas of Pediatric Dermatology*, 3rd ed. New York: McGraw-Hill, 1998:240.)

DIAGNOSIS

- History and physical exam
- Skeletal survey, ophthalmologic exam, head CT if indicated
- Fractures that raise suspicion of abuse:
  - Any fracture in a child <2 years old
  - Fracture of rib, scapula, vertebral body, spinous process, sternum (see Figure 16.4)
  - Metaphyseal injuries, including a **chip fracture or bucket-handle fracture**
  - Skull fracture
  - Spiral or transverse diaphyseal fracture (any long bone fracture on a perambulatory child)
  - Fractures of different ages

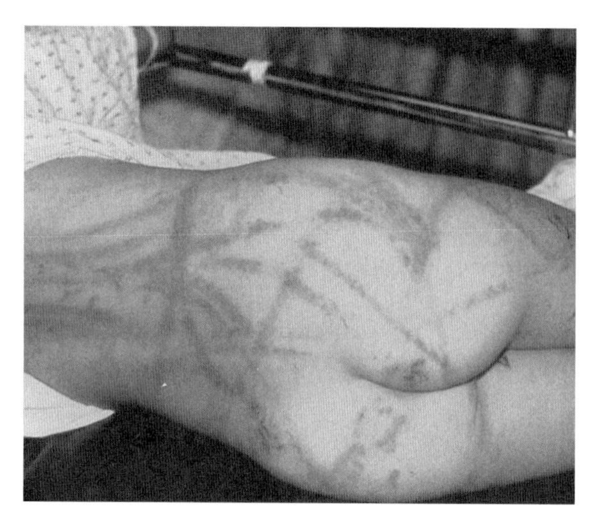

FIGURE 16.3. Loop marks from hanger.

(Reproduced, with permission, from Weinberg S, et al. *Color Atlas of Pediatric Dermatology*, 3rd ed. New York: McGraw-Hill, 1998:240.)

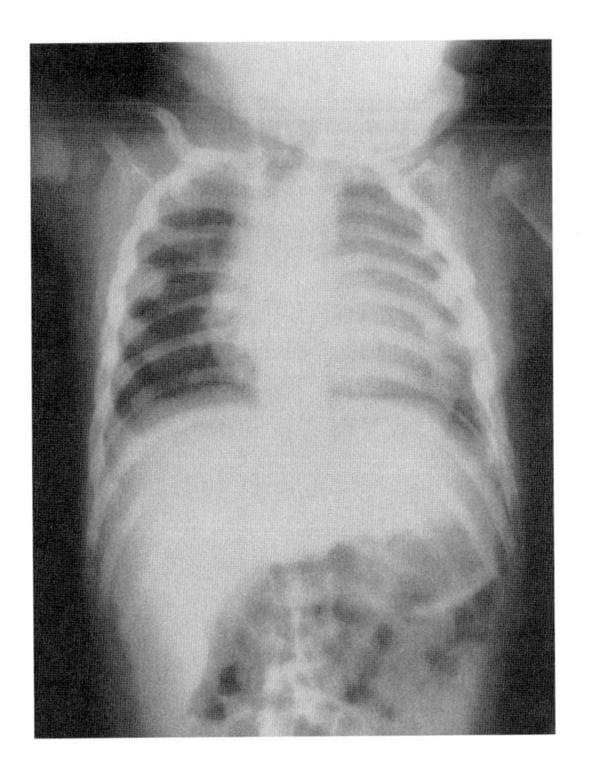

FIGURE 16.4. Rib fractures.

(Reproduced, with permission, from Skinner HB, et al. *Current Diagnosis and Treatment in Orthopedics*, 4th ed. New York: McGraw-Hill, 2006: 644.)

TREATMENT

Treat injuries. Child Protective Services should be immediately contacted.

Intimate Partner Violence and Abuse (IPVA)

IPVA crosses all demographic and socioeconomic boundaries. Victims are usually women but are increasingly male.

RISK FACTORS

Partner with alcohol or substance abuse problems, recent unemployment or intermittent employment, history of police arrest, low educational attainment, or having experienced abuse as a child

SYMPTOMS/EXAM

- Patient presents with physical injuries, most commonly of **head, neck, face, chest, breasts, and abdomen.**
- Patient also can present with a wide variety of medical conditions, with pain as a common presenting symptom (eg, headache, pelvic pain, vaginal infections, depression, anxiety).

DIAGNOSIS

Suspect IPVA if stated mechanism of injury does not correlate with physical exam. **Ask patient directly!**

TREATMENT

- Assess immediate risk (victims are at highest risk when they attempt to leave the relationship).
- Document patient's description of the event and current and past injuries.
- Refer to social work while in the ED.

Elder Abuse and Neglect

Elder abuse is increasing but continues to be underreported and under recognized.

Elder abuse is associated more with personality problems of caregivers (substance or alcohol dependence, mental illness) than with situational stress.

RISK FACTORS

Caregiver overwhelmed, frustrated, or resentful; elder is disabled or has worsening cognitive impairment

SYMPTOMS/EXAM

- **Sudden onset of behavior symptoms** (depression, confusion, anxiety)
- Caregiver refuses to leave patient alone with physician.
- **Unexplained delay in seeking treatment or previous unexplained injuries** (bruises, burns, fractures)
- Lack of physical care (poor personal hygiene, malnutrition, soiled beddings or clothing, decubiti)
- **Patient appears fearful of caregiver**, and caregiver has an attitude of indifference or anger toward him/her.
- Caregiver is overly concerned with cost of treatment.

DIAGNOSIS

- Look for injuries, bruises.
- Check for STDs.
- Directly question patient regarding abuse (alone).

TREATMENT

Treat illness and injuries. Notify adult protective services immediately!

Sexual Assault

Male sexual assault is now 10% of all sexual assault.

SYMPTOMS/EXAM/DIAGNOSIS

- Obtain data about assault tactfully (victims should not have to relive every detail).
- Do a thorough and compassionate physical exam, with a rape kit if available.
- **Toluidine blue** detects small vulvar tears, and **Wood's lamp** detects semen stains.
- Chances of finding forensic evidence >72 hours are slim to none.

TREATMENT

- Treat all injuries.
- Pregnancy prophylaxis
- STD/HIV prophylaxis
- Counseling in the ED, arrange for close follow-up

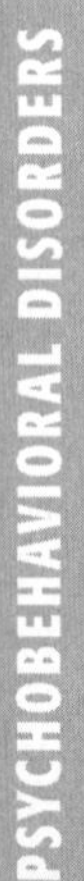

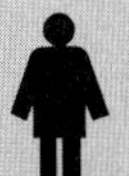

A 55-year-old woman with a history of depression treated with phenelzine presents to the ED after drinking Chianti wine at dinner. What is the hallmark symptom of the tyramine reaction?
Severe occipital or temporal headache.

Complications of MAOI toxicity, although rare, include intracranial hemorrhage and myocardial infarction. Do a head CT for persistent, severe headache or focal neurological findings, and an ECG on all patients with chest pain!

Monoamine Oxidase Inhibitor (MAOI) Toxicity

Monoamine oxidase (MAO) is a major enzyme in the metabolism of norepinephrine, dopamine, and serotonin. MAO also decreases the availability of absorbed dietary biogenic amines (tyramine) in the body via hepatic and intestinal metabolism (see Table 16.9).

TABLE 16.9. MAOI Toxicity

Toxicity	Onset	Symptoms/Exam	Differential	Treatment
MAOI overdose	Can be delayed up to 24 hr	Agitation, mydriasis, rigidity, hyperthermia, coma, hyperreflexia, nystagmus, seizures, tachycardia, hypertension; can cause hypotension and bradycardia if severe	Symphatomimetic or PCP intoxication, alcohol or sedative withdrawal, CVA, ICH, meningitis, encephalitis, serotonin syndrome, neuroleptic malignant syndrome, heat stroke, acute coronary syndrome (ACS), pheochromocytoma, thyroid storm, malignant hyperthermia.	▪ Activated charcoal/ gastric lavage for overdose ▪ Supportive care ▪ Phentolamine and nitroprusside for severe hypertension. ▪ Nifedipine or prazosin for moderate hypertension. ▪ Lidocaine for ventricular arrhythmias ▪ Avoid β-blockers and Ca channel blockers (unopposed α receptor stimulation, can also worsen hypotension and bradycardia). ▪ IV fluids for rhabdomyolysis ▪ Dantrolene for life-threatening hyperthermia. ▪ Benzodiazepines for agitation ▪ Observe for 4–6 hr, admit for those with persistent symptoms.
Tyramine reaction	15–90 min after ingestion	Rapid onset of severe occipital/ temporal headache, hypertension, diaphoresis, mydriasis, neck stiffness, neuromuscular excitation, palpitations, chest pain.	Same as for MAOI overdose	Same as for MAOI overdose
MAOI drug interaction	Minutes to hours	MAOI have interactions with multiple drugs, namely, Meperidine, dextromethorphan, tramadol, and SSRI can precipitate **serotonin syndrome**	Same as for MAOI overdose	Same as for MAOI overdose

TABLE 16.9. **MAOI Toxicity (*Continued*)**

Toxicity	Onset	Symptoms/Exam	Differential	Treatment
		(need at least a 2-wk "washout" period after stopping MAOIs). Indirect acting symphatomimetics (ephedrine, guanethedine, pseudoephedrine) can also cause a tyramine-like reaction.		

Since the development of newer antidepressants, MAOIs are reserved for atypical or refractory depression. There are five MAOIs approved in the United States: selegiline (antiparkinsonian), phenelzine and trancyclopromine (antidepressants), fluazolidane (antibiotic), and procarbazine (antineoplastic).

Serotonin Syndrome

Can be caused by any drug (or combination of drugs) that increase central serotonin transmission by stimulation of the 5-HT_{1A} and 5-HT_2 postsynaptic receptors; most cases occur at therapeutic levels of drugs (see Table 16.10)

Symptoms/Exam

Typically **rapid onset of muscle rigidity (lower extremities > upper extremities)**, **hyperthermia**, diaphoresis, **confusion/disorientation**, agitation, myoclonus, **tremor**, ataxia, hypertension, tachycardia, tachypnea, anxiety, coma

Differential

Same as for MAOI toxicity

Diagnosis

Diagnosis is clinical. **Serotonin syndrome is easily missed or misdiagnosed.** Rule out other causes.

Treatment

- Stop offending drug.
- Supportive care/ABCs
- Activated charcoal/gastric lavage if overdose
- Up to 25% will need intubation and ventilatory support.
- Benzodiazepines for muscle rigidity
- IV fluids for rhabdomyolysis
- Cyproheptadine (an antiserotonergic agent) for severe cases

Neuroleptic Malignant Syndrome (NMS)

Onset occurs about 2 weeks after initiation of typical and atypical antipsychotic drugs, although this reaction has also been seen in patients on a stable drug regimen.

Risk factors

Rapid drug loading, high dosage, increase in dosage, use of **high potency antipsychotic (droperidol, haloperidol, loxapine)**, parenteral form, dehydration, previous episodes of NMS

TABLE 16.10. Serotonergic Potential of Various Drugs

Extreme Potency	Moderate Potency	Low Potency	None
Amitriptyline	Amphetamine	Amantadine	Acetaminophen
Citalopram	Buspirone	Bromocriptine	Granisetron
Clomipramine	Cocaine	Bupropion	Metoclopramide
Dexfenfluramine	Desipramine	Carbamazepine	Morphine
Dextromethorphan	Doxepin	Cisapride	NSAIDs
Fenfluramine	Levodopa	Codeine	Ondansetron
Fluoxetine	LSD	Pentazocine	Salicylates
Fluvoxamine	Mescaline	Pergolide	
Imipramine	Mirtazapine	Reserpine	
Isocarboxazid	Nefazodone		
L-Tryptophan	Nortriptyline		
5-Hydroxytryptophan (5-HTP)‡	St. John's wort‡		
Lithium	Sumatriptan		
MDMA	Trazodone		
Meperidine			
Moclobemide*			
Pargyline†			
Paroxetine			
Phenelzine			
Selegiline			
Sertraline			
Tramadol			
Tranylcypromine			
Venlafaxine			

(Reproduced, with permission, from Tintinalli JE, Kelen, GD, Stapczynski SJ. *Emergency Medicine: A Comprehensive Study Guide,* 6th ed. New York: McGraw-Hill, 2004:1038.)

*Not available in the United States.

†No longer manufactured in the United States.

‡Over-the-counter herbal product.

Note: The serotonergic potential of the drugs listed was determined by both objective and subjective criteria and can be influenced by different doses and formulations.

Abbreviations: LSD = lysergic acid diethylamide; MDMA = 3,4-methylenedioxymethamphetamine; NSAIDs = nonsteroidal anti-inflammatory drugs.

Symptoms/Exam/Diagnosis

Severe muscle rigidity and hyperthermia plus two or more of the following: diaphoresis, dysphagia, tremor, incontinence, altered mental status, mutism, tachycardia, increased or labile blood pressure, leukocytosis, increased creatinine phosphokinase

Differential

Same as for MAOI toxicity

Treatment

- Stop offending drug.
- Supportive care/ABCs
- Activated charcoal/gastric lavage for overdose
- Benzodiazepines for agitation and muscle rigidity
- Refractory cases may need paralysis (**use a nondepolarizing paralytic like vecuronium or rocuronium**!) and intubation.
- Active cooling
- The use of dantrolene and dopaminergic agents such as bromocriptine and amantadine are controversial.

Complications

Dysrhythmias, renal failure, seizures, pneumonia, DIC, death

Acute Dystonic Reaction

Symptoms/Exam/Diagnosis

- Involuntary muscle movements and spasms of the face, neck back, and extremities, occurring with the first few days of treatment of an antipsychotic drug
- **Oculogyric crisis:** Continuous rotatory eye movements
- **Laryngeal dystonia**: Rare throat-tightening sensation resulting in difficulty breathing and swallowing; can be life threatening

Treatment

Stop or decrease dose of drug. Administer diphenhydramine for control of acute reaction. Use benztropine to prevent recurrence. Consider changing to atypical antipsychotic agent.

Disulfram Reaction

Symptoms/Exam/Diagnosis

- Patients treated with disulfram (Antabuse) who then drink alcohol experience skin flushing, nausea/vomiting, headache, chest and abdominal discomfort, diaphoresis, vertigo, palpitations, and confusion about 15–30 minutes after alcohol use.
- Severe reactions may cause hypotension, seizures, and dysrhythmias.
- This is secondary to increased acetaldehyde from inhibition of aldehyde dehydrogenase.

Treatment

Supportive care, IV fluids, and dopamine for hypotension; observe or admit for severe symptoms

CHAPTER 17

Dermatology

Mitzi A. Dillon, MD

EXFOLIATIVE DERMATITIS (ERYTHRODERMA)

SYMPTOMS/EXAM

- Presence of erythema and scaling involving >90% of skin surface (see Table 17.1)
- Systemic complaints of pruritis, chills, and LAD on exam

ETIOLOGY

- Caused by drugs, chemical agents, underlying systemic or cutaneous disease; can have abrupt onset when associated with drugs, contact allergen, or malignancy

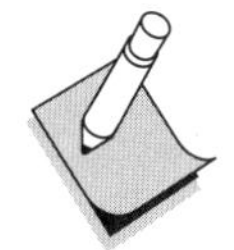

Exfoliative dermatitis is distinguished from other desquamating diseases by a feeling of skin tightness, scaly skin, and large areas of involvement.

DIFFERENTIAL

- Primary dermatologic disease (psoriasis, atopic dermatitis, seborrheic dermatitis)
- Infection (SSSS, dermatophyte, scabies)
- Drug reaction (most commonly allopurinol, amoxicillin, carbamazepine, phenobarbital, phenytoin, sulfonamides, or vancomycin)
- Malignancy (lymphoma)

TREATMENT

- Emergent dermatology consultation, hospital admission, correct hypothermia and hypovolemia, systemic corticosteroids

TABLE 17.1. Primary Lesions

Lesion	Description
Macule	Flat, nonpalpable, circumscribed lesion <5 mm in diameter
Patch	Flat, nonpalpable, circumscribed lesion >5 mm in diameter
Papule	Palpable, circumscribed lesion <5 mm in diameter, raised above skin surface
Plaque	Palpable lesion >5 mm in diameter, raised above skin surface
Nodule	Firm lesion arising in subcutaneous tissue <2 cm in diameter
Tumor	Firm lesion arising in subcutaneous tissue >2 cm in diameter
Vesicle	Raised, fluid-filled, superficial lesion <5 mm in diameter
Bulla	Raised, fluid-filled, superficial lesion >5 mm in diameter
Pustule	Pus-filled superficial lesion <5 mm in diameter
Abscess	Pus-filled lesion arising in subcutaneous tissue >5 mm in diameter
Wheal	Evanescent, raised, round, or flat-topped lesion caused by edema

COMPLICATIONS

- Disruption of dermis can lead to water loss, excessive heat loss, and high-output CHF due to widespread vasodilatation.
- Mortality is approximately 30%.

URTICARIA (HIVES)

SYMPTOMS/EXAM

- Hives are pruritic, erythematous wheals of varying size that are **transient**, lasting <24 hours. Urticaria becomes chronic when recurrent eruptions occur for >6 weeks.

The standard epinephrine dose for anaphylaxis is 0.3 mg IM (usually given as 0.3 mL of 1:1000). Remember 1 mg is a cardiac arrest dose—don't give this much to patients with a pulse.

ETIOLOGY

- Most frequent causes are infection (especially viral), drugs (PCN, sulfonamides, NSAIDs, ACE inhibitors), food (shellfish, fish, eggs, nuts), and idiopathic. Emotional stress, exercise, and excess heat or cold exposure are also causes.

TREATMENT

- Avoid cause, supportive treatment includes cold compresses, first- or second-generation H_1-receptor blockers. H_2-receptor blockers and prednisone can be added when chronic or unresponsive to first-line treatment. Epinephrine when associated with anaphylaxis (ie, hypotension, wheezing, or difficulty breathing).

ERYTHEMA MULTIFORME (EM)

SYMPTOMS/EXAM

- This erythematous, papular rash appears over 72 hours, most commonly on hands and forearms (palmar and dorsal surfaces) but also occurs on feet, face, and lower extremities, usually <10% BSA. There is great variation, but typically >100 lesions are present.
- Papules may evolve to **target lesions** with a characteristic central dusky or purple zone surrounded by a pale ring and then third erythematous halo.
- Discrete **oral lesions** are present in ~50% of patients.

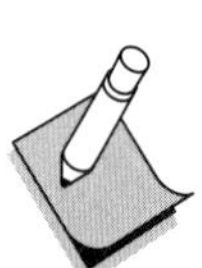

Rashes that commonly appear on the palms: Erythema multiforme, drug eruption, secondary syphilis, RMSF, hand, foot and mouth disease, scabies.

DIFFERENTIAL FOR RASHES ON THE PALMS

- EM: Target lesions evolve over 72 hours.
- Rocky Mountain spotted fever: Erythematous/hemorrhagic macules and papules
- Drug eruption: Lesions occur minutes to several hours after drug administration. They recur in the same area when the offending drug is given. They may be circular, violaceous, or edematous plaques that resolve with macular hyperpigmentation.
- Secondary syphilis: Scaling papular eruptions
- Scabies: Papules and burrows, mainly in web spaces, intensely pruritic
- Hand, foot, and mouth disease: Small, discrete vesicles; patients usually <10 years old

CAUSES

- Drugs: Antibiotics, anticonvulsants, sulfonylureas, allopurinol, NSAIDs, barbiturates
- Infections: HSV, mycoplasma, hepatitis, strep, TB
- Collagen vascular disorders: RA, SLE
- Malignancies: Leukemia, lymphoma, carcinoma

DIFFERENTIAL

- SJS: Skin and oral lesions are more severe involving 10–30% BSA, two or more mucosal sites involved in SJS
- Urticaria: Lesions migrate (EM lesions are fixed, persists >24 hours)

TREATMENT

- Treat cause (treat infection, acyclovir decreases recurrences in patients with HSV).
- Oral antihistamines to reduce stinging and burning of skin
- Hospitalize patients with impaired intake due to oral involvement.
- Local wound care with wet compresses (Burrows solution)
- Epinephrine not effective
- Steroids controversial

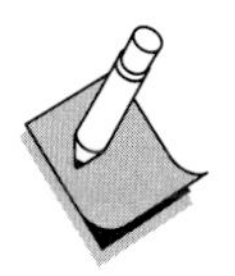

Four erythemas:

1. *Erythema marginatum–migratory annular and polycyclic erythematous eruption, cutaneous manifestation of acute rheumatic fever*
2. *Erythema migrans–expanding red lesion with central clearing at site of tick bite, Lyme disease*
3. *Erythema multiforme–target lesions, ± mucosal involvement, many causes*
4. *Erythema nodosum–tender, raised red nodules on legs, many causes*

STEVENS-JOHNSON SYNDROME

A severe expression of erythema multiforme, though not as severe as toxic epidermal necrolysis (see Figure 17.1)

SYMPTOMS/EXAM

- More common in children, peak incidence in second decade of life
- Starts with a prodrome of upper respiratory symptoms, malaise, fever, vomiting, and diarrhea; patient appears ill

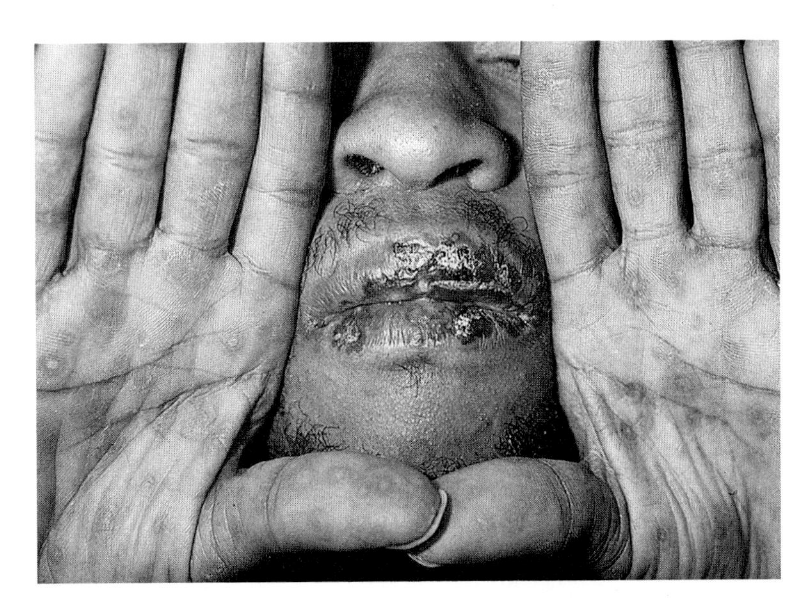

FIGURE 17.1. Stevens-Johnson syndrome. Note the target lesions on the hands of this patient. (See also color insert.)

(Reproduced, with permission, from Knoop KJ, Stack LB, Storrow AB. *Atlas of Emergency Medicine*, 2nd ed. New York: McGraw-Hill, 2002:379.)

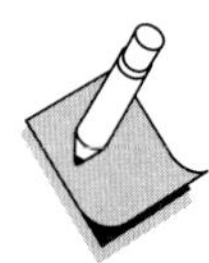

"Target lesion" classically refers to the bright red borders and central petechiae of erythema multiforme and Stevens-Johnson syndrome, but is also used to describe erythema migrans, the primary lesion in Lyme disease.

- After 1–14 days, abrupt onset of symmetric red macules, which progress to extensive areas of skin necrosis, usually <10% BSA; may have **targetlike cutaneous lesions**
- Oral mucosa extensively denuded with hemorrhagic crust on lips; may have compromised airway due to sloughing of respiratory epithelium
- Involvement of **two or more mucosal sites** (eyes, mouth, vagina, urethra, anus)
- Multisystem involvement may include arthritis, arthralgias, hepatitis, myocarditis, and nephritis.

CAUSES

- Majority due to drug reactions (NSAIDs, sulfonamides, anticonvulsants, antibiotics)
- Bacterial and fungal infections (rare)

TREATMENT

- Admit to ICU or burn unit.
- Identify underlying cause; withdraw offending drug.
- Skin care, fluid/electrolyte correction
- Ophthalmology mandatory for patients with eye involvement
- IVIG and steroids controversial

COMPLICATIONS

- Mortality up to 10% related to sepsis, GI hemorrhage, fluid/electrolyte imbalances
- Long-term morbidity due to scarring, blindness, renal tubular necrosis/RF

TOXIC EPIDERMAL NECROLYSIS

Five dangerous rashes:
Hives associated with ***anaphylaxis***
Petechiae due to ***meningococcemia***
Erythema due to ***TEN*** *or* ***SSSS***
Macules starting on wrists/ankles due to ***RMSF***
Woody induration and pain due to ***necrotizing fasciitis***

Rare, potentially fatal, adverse cutaneous drug reaction considered by most to be related to erythema multiforme and Stevens-Johnson syndrome but more severe; defined by **>30% BSA** involved; affects all age groups and both sexes, but most common in the elderl; HIV-positive individuals are at a 1000-fold higher risk for TEN

SYMPTOMS/EXAM

- 1–3 day prodrome with fever, cough, sore throat, and malaise
- Abrupt onset of a generalized, dusky, tender, erythematous macules, and patches that coalesce and slough in large sheets causing widespread, progressive exfoliation; progression is variable, can be rapid (<24 hours) or take days
- Purulent conjunctivitis and painful erosions in the oral and genital skin
- Positive **Nikolsky sign:** Tangential pressure results in spontaneous epidermal detachment
- Involvement of the mucous membranes including the GI and respiratory tract common

CAUSES

- Drug reactions (penicillin, sulfonamides, fluoroquinolones, anticonvulsants, allopurinol, oxicam NSAIDs)
- Infections
- Idiopathic

TREATMENT

- Same as SJS with **burn care center admission**, airway observation for possible oral mucosal sloughing, aggressive fluid rehydration, antibiotics only when infection is present
- Steroids are not recommended.
- Mortality rate is 30–40% due to infection, fluid loss, and electrolyte disturbances.

IMPETIGO

Divided into two clinical types:

1. Impetigo contagiosa
   - Caused by *Staphylococcus aureus* and group A streptococci
   - Superficial vesicles and pustules covered with **honey colored crusts** (see Figure 17.3)
2. Bullous impetigo
   - Caused by epidermolytic, toxin-producing S. *aureus*
   - Flaccid vesicles and bullae up to 3 cm in diameter

SYMPTOMS/EXAM

- Superficial bacterial infection of the epidermis commonly around the nose and mouth of children <6 years old
- Predisposing factors include poor hygiene, warm weather, overcrowding, and breaks in skin barrier from abrasions or insect bites.

TREATMENT

- Systemic and topical antibiotics are equally successful, with systemic preferred for more extensive infections. Neither treatment prevents the rare development of acute glomerulonephritis.
- Topical mupirocin 2% ointment
- Systemic treatment: Previously treated with cephalexin, oxacillin. Due to prevalence of CA-MRSA, current recommendations are for TMP-SMZ or clindamycin.
- Meticulous hygiene can prevent the spread.

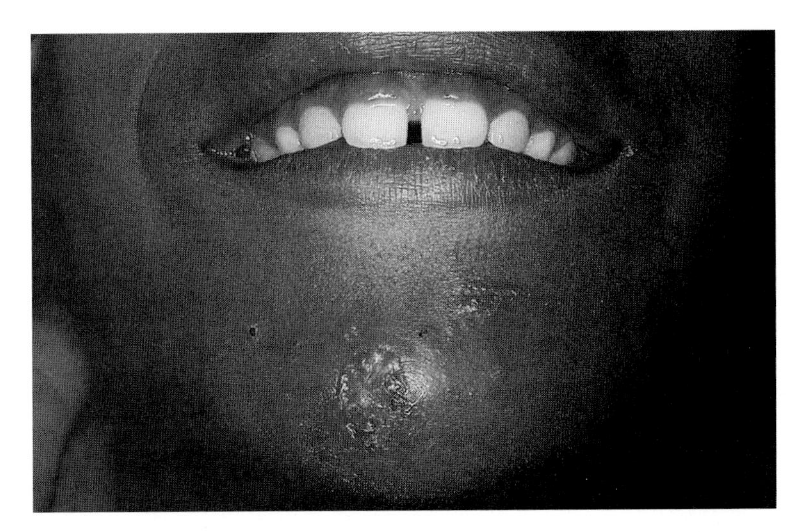

FIGURE 17.2. Impetigo.

(Courtesy of Michael J. Nowicki, MD as reproduced, with permission, from Knoop KJ, Stack LB, Storrow AB. *Atlas of Emergency Medicine*, 2nd ed. New York: McGraw-Hill, 2002:444.)

COMPLICATIONS

- **Very contagious**, easily spreading to surrounding skin and other young children
- Lymphadenitis, acute poststreptococcal glomerulonephritis (seen in 1% during epidemics)

STAPHYLOCOCCAL SCALDED SKIN SYNDROME (STAPHYLOCOCCAL EPIDERMAL NECROLYSIS)

SYMPTOMS/EXAM

- Usually in children <6 years old with S. *aureus* infections of the conjunctiva, nasopharynx, or umbilicus
- Caused by an **exotoxin** produced by S. *aureus* that is released into the bloodstream causing superficial separation of the skin and widespread **painful erythema and blistering**.

DISEASE COURSE

- Phase One: Sudden appearance of tender erythema with sandpaperlike texture prominent in perioral, periorbital, and groin regions and in skin creases of the neck, axilla, popliteal, and anticubital regions; mucous membranes are not affected
- Phase Two: Exfoliative phase begins on second day of illness. Minor trauma causes skin to wrinkle and peel off. There is positive Nikolsky sign. Large flaccid, fluid-filled bullae and vesicles appear, which easily rupture and are shed in large sheets. Underlying skin resembles scaled skin.
- Phase Three: After 3–5 days the skin desquamates, leaving normal skin in 10–14 days.

DIFFERENTIAL

- TEN: Associated with use of medication, occurs in adults, involves mucous membranes
- TSS
- Exfoliative drug eruptions
- Localized bullous impetigo

TREATMENT

- Generalized disease requires hospitalization and parenteral abx
- Fluid resuscitation, correct electrolyte abnormalities, identify and treat source of staph infection with penicillinase-resistant penicillins such as oxacillin or vancomycin (depending on prevalence of CA-MRSA); steroids are not recommended
- Skin care with bland emollients

COMPLICATIONS

- 3% mortality in children
- Disease is very rare in adults, is associated with renal failure and immunosupression, and a higher mortality rate >50%.

TOXIC SHOCK SYNDROME

SYMPTOMS/EXAM

- Toxic shock syndrome presents as acute febrile illness with high fever (>102°F), myalgias, vomiting, diarrhea, headache, and pharyngitis. Rapid progression to hypotensive shock can occur.

- Disease is accompanied by diffuse, nonpruritic, scarlitiniform exanthem that starts on trunk and spreads centrifugally. Subsequent desquamation may occur.
- Other manifestations include conjunctival hyperemia, strawberry tongue, erythema and edema on palms and soles, hair shedding, and nail loss. Desquamation of hands and feet commonly occurs 1–2 weeks after onset of illness.

A strawberry tongue is seen with toxic shock syndrome, Kawasaki disease, and scarlet fever.

ETIOLOGY

- Linked with exotoxin-producing S. *aureus* and severe group A B-hemolytic streptococcal infections; associated with **tampon use**, nonsurgical wounds (lacerations, burns, ulcers), surgical wounds, and **nasal packs**

DIAGNOSIS

- Rapid onset of high fever and hypotension
- Skin rash: Diffuse, blanching, macular erythema, with nonexudative mucous membrane inflammation; pharyngitis, "Strawberry tongue," conjunctivitis, or vaginitis can be seen
- Involvement of at least three organ systems (GI, muscular, CNS, renal, hepatic, or hematological)

DIFFERENTIAL

- Scarlet fever, streptococcal toxic shock syndrome (STSS), staphylococcal scalded skin syndrome, Kawasaki disease, exfoliative drug eruptions

TREATMENT

- IV fluids, ventilatory support, pressors, penicillinase-resistant penicillins, or vancomycin (if CA-MRSA suspected), drainage/debridement of infected sites

STREPTOCOCCAL TOXIC SHOCK SYNDROME

SYMPTOMS/EXAM

- Affects mostly healthy people between 20 and 50 years old
- This uncommon syndrome involves multiple organ systems with fever, hypotension, and skin findings of edema, erythema, or bullae. Desquamation occurs less commonly than in Staph TSS.

ETIOLOGY

- Invasive soft-tissue *Streptococcus pyogenes* (group A streptococcus) infections, such as cellulitis or myositis (look for elevated CK as evidence of myonecrosis)

TREATMENT

- Inspect skin for source of infection and palpate muscles for tenderness suggestive of myositis or fasciitis.
- Aggressive management of source of infection with I&D and debridement if necessary
- Parenteral nafícillin, oxacillin, or vancomycin or a first-generation cephalosporin
- Clindamycin is thought to inhibit production of bacterial toxins and is considered to be first-line treatment by some.

CONTACT DERMATITIS

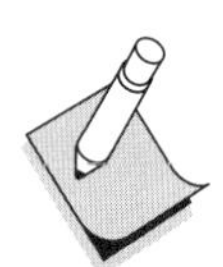

Rashes with discrete distributions (wrist, ears, neck, belly button, fingers) suggest contact dermatitis.

Contact dermatitis is an inflammatory reaction of the skin to a chemical, physical, or biological agent. Clothing, jewelry, soaps, plants (including poison ivy/oak), and topical medications (such as neomycin) are all causes. See papules, vesicles, or bullae on an erythematous base, often in a linear configuration. Treat by avoiding cause and with topical or oral steroids.

Plant Contact Dermatitis

SYMPTOMS/EXAM

- Itching, burning, redness, and vesiculobullous formations occur 7–12 days after first exposure. Often distribution is linear due to branch or leaf rubbing along skin. Reactions may occur in <12 hours in individuals with prior exposure.

ETIOLOGY

- Poison ivy (*Toxicodendron radicans*), poison oak, and poison sumac are the most common causes. Other species in the Anacardiaceae family (including mango tree, cashew nut tree) may also cause dermatitis.
- The oil urushiol, common to all these plants, induces an allergic response in approximately 70% of the population.

TREATMENT

- Wash all contaminated skin and clothing with soap and water.
- Antipruritic and topical therapies (oatmeal baths, ultrapotent topical steroids, sedating antihistamines at night) are indicated. Oral steroids may be necessary in patients with severe reactions. Taper over 1–2 weeks.

DIAPER RASH

SYMPTOMS/EXAM

- Candidal diaper dermatitis is characterized by moist red patches with well-demarcated borders and **satellite papules or pustules**. Usually involves inguinal folds. Occurs in moist occluded areas exacerbated by heat, moisture, friction, and the presence of urine or feces.
- Diaper rash may also be due to irritant- or allergic-contact dermatitis. These prefer the convexities (buttocks, thigh, abdomen, and perianal area) and spare the inguinal creases. However, discriminating between these causes may be difficult.

TREATMENT

- Regular cleaning of skin and air exposure will treat most cases.
- Consider Burrows solution for exudative lesions, topical anticandidal agents such as nystatin with overlying zinc oxide paste for candidal infections, and topical corticosteroids for irritant/contact dermatitis.

PRESSURE ULCERS (DECUBITUS ULCERS)

Pressure ulcers cause significant morbidity in the elderly and the bed bound, eg, obese, neurological impairment, postoperative patients particularly in nursing homes and in the ICU.

SYMPTOMS/EXAM

- **Stage 1:** Intact skin, local tissue erythema
- **Stage 2:** Penetrate the epidermis or dermis but not the subcutaneous tissue
- **Stage 3:** Extend through the dermis into the subcutaneous tissue
- **Stage 4:** Extend beyond the subcutaneous tissue through to the deep fascia and may involve muscle and bone

DIFFERENTIAL

Cellulitis

DIAGNOSIS

- Clinical diagnosis is based mainly on physical exam.
- Stage 4 ulcers are often underestimated due to fistula formation, eg, a seemingly superficial skin defect may mask extensive deep tissue necrosis. Eschar may also make it difficult to determine depth of wound.

TREATMENT

- **Prevention:** Ideal positioning of bed-bound patients, position changes at least every 2 hours, pressure reducing devices
- **Treatment:** Fundamentals include proper nutrition, pain management, reducing tissue pressure, maintaining a moist environment, wound debridement, and fighting infection.
  - **Stage 1:** More intensive prevention measures
  - **Stage 2:** Occlusive or semipermeable dressing to maintain moist wound environment; avoid wet to dry dressings
  - **Stage 3:** Remove necrotic tissue, manage infections, and maintain moist wound environment.
  - **Stage 4:** Undermining and tunneling in consultation with wound specialist, eg, plastic surgeon

COMPLICATIONS

- Common in stage 3 and 4 ulcers
- Chronic pain, depression, social isolation
- Cellulitis and osteomyelitis especially with MRSA, VRE, and multiple-resistant Gram-negative bacilli leading to bacteremia, sepsis, and death
- Rare: Fistulas, heterotrophic calcification, systemic amyloidosis, squamous cell carcinoma

DRUG ERUPTIONS

ETIOLOGY

- Appear within 1 to 2 weeks after an offending drug is taken, except or PCN, which can take longer
- Most drug eruptions are type IV delayed, cell-mediated reactions, but drug eruptions resulting from type I, II, and III reactions also occur.

SYMPTOMS/EXAM

- Exanthematous: Resemble erythematous, morbilliform, skin eruptions from viral or bacterial infections, widespread symmetric maculopapular eruptions

- Eczematous: Resemble contact dermatitis but are more extensive, erythematous, or papular eruptions that can become vesicular eg, topical medication with prior sensitization
- Vasculitic: Urticarial papules or palpable purpura that can ulcerate due to immune-complex mediated vasculitis; purpuric lesions may rarely be from bone marrow suppression or platelet destruction
- Photosensitive:
  - Phototoxic: Sulfonamides, sulfonylureas, thiazide diuretics, tetracyclines taken in adequate amounts cause sunburn appearance on sun-exposed areas of skin; nonimmunologic
  - Photoallergic: Antigen formation from drug causing delayed response of 2 weeks or longer after exposure to drug and sunlight; eczematous and intensely puritic (eg, chlorpromazine, promethazine, chlordiazepoxide)
- Fixed drug reactions: Appear and reappear in the same sites after repeat exposure to the same drug; sharply marginated oval or round lesions (eg, tetracyclines, sulfonamides, NSAIDs)

TINEA

Etiology

- Dermatophytoses, superficial fungal infections of the outer keratin layer of skin, hair, nails, are caused by fungal species from one of three genera (*Trichophyton*, *Microsporum*, and *Epidermophyton*); more common in warm, moist environments; not markedly contagious except for tinea capitus

Diagnosis

- Usually can be diagnosed clinically
- Confirmation may be achieved with microscopic identification of branching hyphae after KOH prep or Wood's lamp evaluation showing yellow-green fluorescence; most useful for tinea capitis.

Treatment

- Topical antifungal agents are usually effective. Systemic therapy (griseofulvin, itraconazole, or terbinafine) required for infections of the hair and nails and for recalcitrant disease.
  - Tinea barbae: Beard and neck
  - Tinea capitis: Scalp
  - Tinea corporis: Ringwormlike configuration on the body with sharply marginated, annular lesions with raised or vesicular margins and central clearing
  - Tinea cruris: Groin and pubic region
  - Tinea pedis: Athlete's foot
  - Kerion: Dermatophytic infection of the scalp that appears as an indurated, boggy plaque with overlying pustules; treated the same as tinea capitis (oral antifungals) with the addition of prednisone 1 mg/kg/day for 1–2 weeks (see Figure 17.3)
  - Tinea unguium (onychomycosis): Nails
  - Tinea versicolor: Superficial infection caused by *Pityrosporum ovale*; causes scaling patches of various colors, pink, tan white usually on the chest and trunk; treated with selenium sulfide shampoo, imidazole creams, or oral ketaconazole

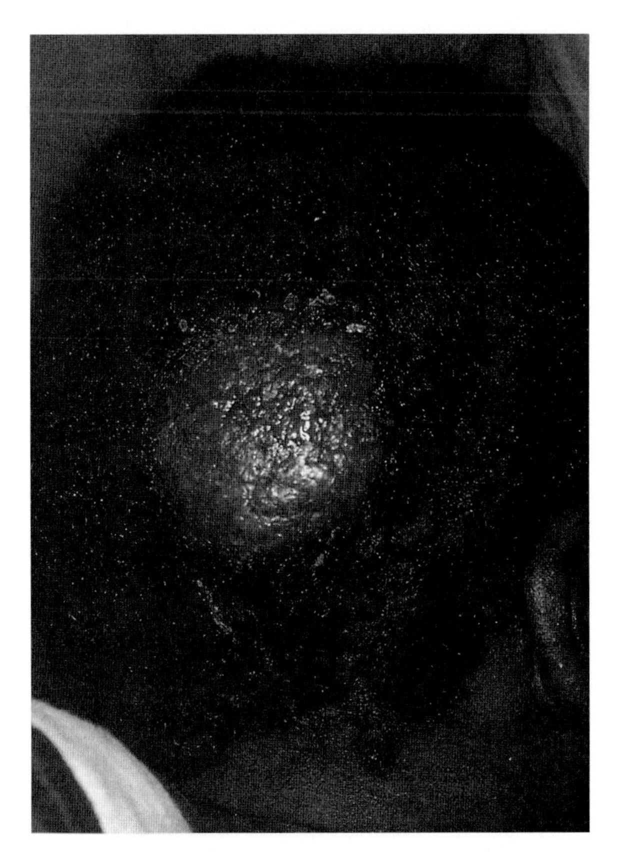

FIGURE 17.3. Kerion with occipital boggy swelling and hair loss.

(Courtesy of Anne W. Lucky, MD as reproduced, with permission, from Knoop KJ, Stack LB, Storrow AB. *Atlas of Emergency Medicine*, 2nd ed. New York: McGraw-Hill, 2002:445.)

ORAL THRUSH

SYMPTOMS/EXAM

- Oral thrush is a *Candida* infection consisting of patches of white material covering an erythematous base on the buccal mucosa, tongue, palate, or tonsils. Typically, these lesions are easy to remove, revealing an underlying erythematous base.
- This infection is most common in newborns during the first week of life. In adults **immunosuppression** should be considered in the absence of dentures or antibiotic use.

TREATMENT

- **Nystatin** suspension applied to the oral mucosa 4–5 times/day. Clotrimazole troches dissolved in the mouth can be used in adults. In severe cases, systemic antifungals may be necessary.

A Mexican immigrant complains of tender, swollen, red nodules on the lower legs. What rash is suggested by this description? What's the next step?

Erythema nodosum. Patient needs further evaluation (start with a review of systems) for causes of erythema nodosum, including tuberculosis and coccidiomycosis.

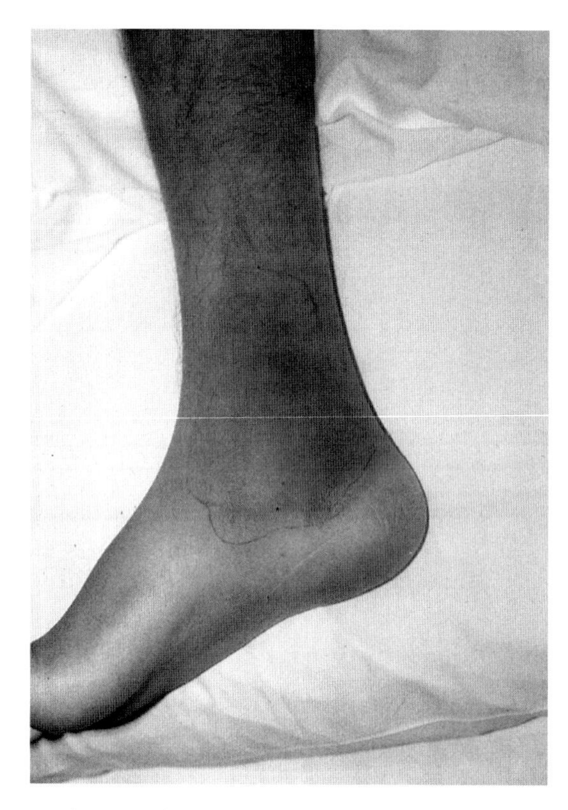

FIGURE 17.4. Erythema nodosum.

(Reproduced, with permission, from Tintinalli JE, Kelen GD, Stapczynski JS. *Emergency Medicine: A Comprehensive Study Guide*, 6th ed. New York: McGraw-Hill, 2004:1531.)

ERYTHEMA NODOSUM

SYMPTOMS/EXAM

- Inflammatory reaction of the subcutaneous fat causing numerous, tender, erythematous nodules most commonly on the pretibial area of the **lower extremities**; lesions may turn yellow-purple and resemble bruises (see Figure 17.4)
- Most common in young women, with female-to-male ratio of 4:1
- Ulceration is not a typical feature and may suggest an alternative diagnosis.

> ***Causes of Erythema NODOSUM:***
>
> **NO** known cause: Even after a thorough evaluation, the cause of EN remains unknown in 40–60% of cases.
> **D**rugs (OCP, sulfonamides, PCN, vaccines)
> **O**ther (Coccidiodomycosis, TB, Herpes, EBV, pregnancy)
> **S**trep (most common)/**S**arcoidosis
> **U**lcerative colitis/inflammatory bowel disease
> **M**alignancy (leukemia, lymphoma)

TREATMENT

- Symptomatic treatment includes bed rest, leg elevation, and NSAIDs.
- Additional treatment depends on underlying cause.

PITYRIASIS ROSEA

SYMPTOMS/EXAM

- Pruritic, but otherwise a benign self-limited illness
- Multiple 1- to 2-cm-diameter, salmon-colored oval plaques following the ribs in a "Christmas tree" pattern on the trunk
- In half of cases, a larger solitary lesion called a "herald patch" precedes the other lesions by 7 days.

ETIOLOGY

- Unknown

DIFFERENTIAL

- Secondary syphilis
- Pityriasis rosea–like drug reaction (captopril, barbituates)

TREATMENT

- Supportive, topical steroids

PEMPHIGUS VULGARIS

SYMPTOMS/EXAM

- Symptoms include bullous lesions in the mouth and lips that erode and leave painful ulcers (see Figure 17.5).
- Subsequently, small, flaccid bullae form anywhere on the body. They erode easily, forming widespread, **confluent erosions** that are often secondarily infected.
- Nikolsky sign is positive. New blisters may be formed by tangential pressure on intact dermis.

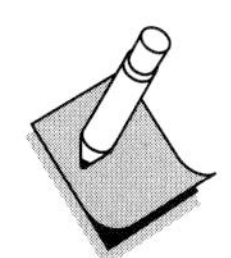

Nikolsky sign is positive in blistering disease with a very superficial blister, in particular toxic epidermal necrolysis, staphylococcal scalded skin syndrome, and pemphigus vulgaris.

ETIOLOGY

- The disease affects both sexes equally, and is most common in 40- to 60-year-olds. The cause is unknown, but use of penicillamine and captopril have been associated with its development.

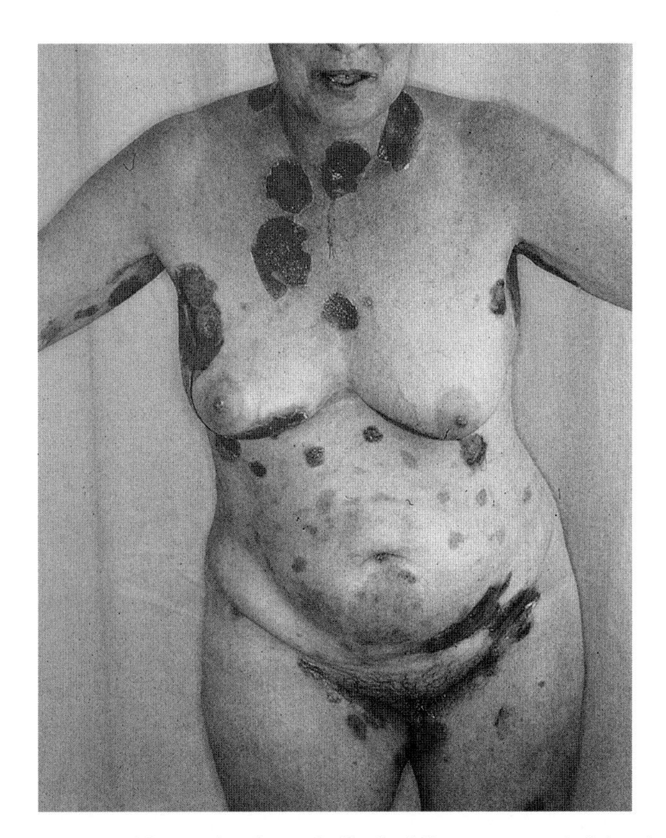

FIGURE 17.5. Pemphigus vulgaris. Typically the blisters are eroded, leaving painful erythematous lesions.

(Courtesy of James J. Nordlund, MD as printed in Knoop KJ, Stack LB, Storrow AB. *Atlas of Emergency Medicine*, 2nd ed. New York: McGraw-Hill, 2002:424.)

DIAGNOSIS

- Positive Tzanck test showing acantholytic cells, confirmed by serum immunofluorescence

TREATMENT

- Pain control, local wound care, antibiotics for secondary infection, and oral steroids
- Prior to steroid introduction the mortality rate was 95% due to spread of disease, secondary infection, dehydration, and thromboembolism. The mortality rate is now 10–15%.

BULLOUS PEMPHIGOID

Bullous pemphigoid is a chronic autoimmune blistering disease. Patients are typically older than pemphigus patients (>60 years old) and blister formation occurs deeper (within the epidermal basement membrane). Prognosis is better than for pemphigus vulgaris.

SYMPTOMS/EXAM

- Large, tense blisters (1–4 cm) arise from normal or pink, urticarial appearing skin. Affected skin may be intensely pruritic. Ulceration and tissue loss can follow.
- Axilla and groin are commonly affected sites.
- Oral lesions are rare.
- Due to the depth at which blisters form, Nikolsky sign is **negative** in bullous pemphigoid.

TREATMENT

- Limited disease: Nicotinamide, doxycycline, and ultrapotent topical steroids
- Extensive disease: Oral steroids, methotrexate

SYPHILIS

ETIOLOGY

- *T. pallidum* infection from direct contact with an infected individual

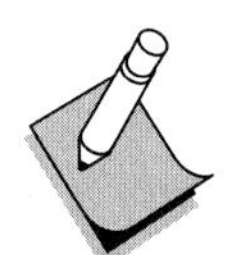

Treponema pallidum *is a spirochete, a flagellated Gram-negative bacteria. Other spirochetes include* Leptospira *sp. (Leptospirosis) and* Borrelia burgdorferi *(Lyme disease).*

SYMPTOMS/EXAM

- Primary stage: **Painless**, usually single chancre (1 cm ulcer with clean base and raised borders) on genitalia or in mouth (see Figure 17.6)
- Secondary: 3–6 weeks later sore throat, fever, malaise, LAD, and rash; dull pink-red papular rash starts on trunk and flexor surfaces of the extremities and spreads to the **palms and soles**
  - Condyloma lata: Secondary syphilis infection in the genital area with a moist, flat, verrucous appearance
- Tertiary: 3–20 years after initial infection; nervous system, cardiovascular involvement, and widespread granulomatous lesions (gummas)

DIAGNOSIS/TREATMENT

- Penicillin or doxycycline; for details, see “Infectious Disease,” in Chapter 8

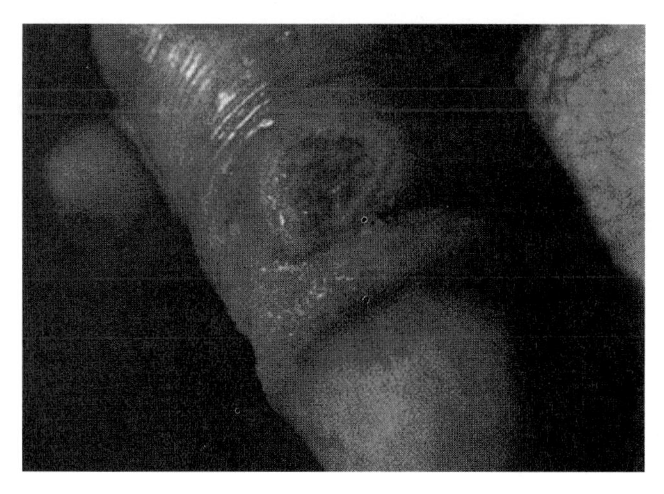

FIGURE 17.6. Primary syphilis penile chancre. (See also color insert, Figure 18.2.)

(Reproduced, with permission, from Wolff K, Johnson RA, Suurmond D. *Fitzpatrick's Color Atlas & Synopsis of Clinical Dermatology*, 5th ed. New York: McGraw-Hill, 2005:915.)

CONDYLOMA ACUMINATUM

- Genital warts, caused by sexually transmitted papillomavirus; soft, fleshy growths on the skin of the genital, perianal, or anal canal regions
- Malignant transformation to squamous cell carcinoma may occur.
- If recurrent, atypical, large, or occurs in HIV-positive patient, may require biopsy to rule out malignancy

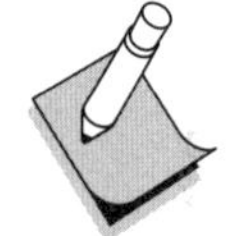

Condyloma lata = secondary syphilis. Condyloma acuminatum = HPV.

DISSEMINATED GONOCOCCAL INFECTION

SYMPTOMS/EXAM

- Fever, migratory arthritis, and rash are the common presentation of disseminated gonococcal disease (see Figure 17.7).

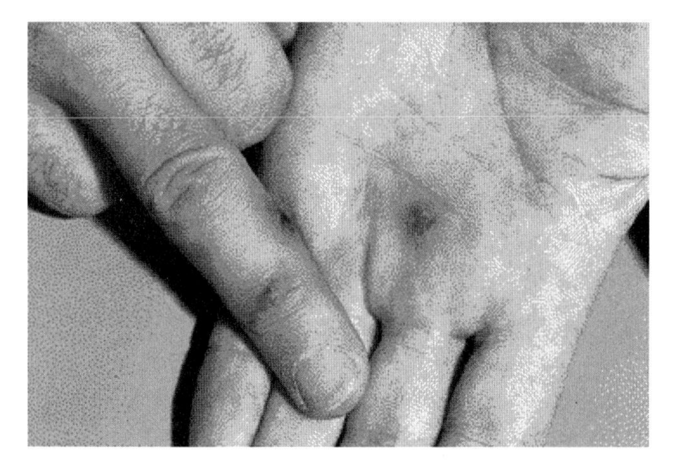

FIGURE 17.7. Disseminated gonococcal infection. Hemorrhagic, painful pustules near small joints of hands and feet.

(Reproduced, with permission, from Wolff K, Johnson RA, Suurmond D. *Fitzpatrick's Color Atlas & Synopsis of Clinical Dermatology*, 5th ed. New York: McGraw-Hill, 2005:910.)

- Multiple lesions around the **periarticular areas of the extremities**, beginning as tender erythematous or hemorrhagic papules that change into **pustules** and vesicles with an erythematous halo, which then scab over in 4–5 days.
- Gonococcal tenosynovitis primarily affects larger joints (knees, elbows, wrists, ankles, and hands).

DIAGNOSIS/TREATMENT

- Often treated in ED based on clinical findings
- Ceftriaxone 125 mg IM for uncomplicated disease, 250 mg IM for PID, and 1 g IV q day × 10 days for disseminated infection; see Chapters 8 and 12 for details

MENINGOCOCCEMIA

ETIOLOGY

- *Neisseria meningitides*
- Affects primarily young children and young adults

*Waterhouse-Friderichsen syndrome is **acute adrenal insufficiency** caused by hemorrhage in patients with meningococcemia.*

SYMPTOMS/EXAM

- Fever, severe HA, AMS, N/V, arthalgias, stiff neck and rash
- The classic rash is petechiae found on the trunk, extremities, palms, soles, and mucous membranes (see Figure 17.8).
- It evolves into angulated purpuric papules, patches and plaques with gray necrotic centers, a pathognomonic finding for meningococcal infection.
- Fulminant meningococcal disease presents with sudden prostration, petechiae with large areas of ecchymosis and shock, and can be complicated by **purpura fulminans**, a severe form of DIC.

TREATMENT

- Vancomycin and ceftriaxone
- All household contacts, day-care contacts, and exposed hospital personnel should receive prophylactic antibiotic treatment with **rifampin**.

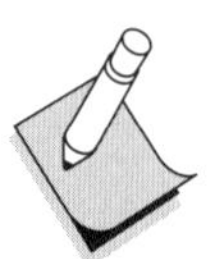

Ill-appearing + petechiae = ceftriaxone and vancomycin. Other diseases may cause this, but meningococcemia is at the top of the list.

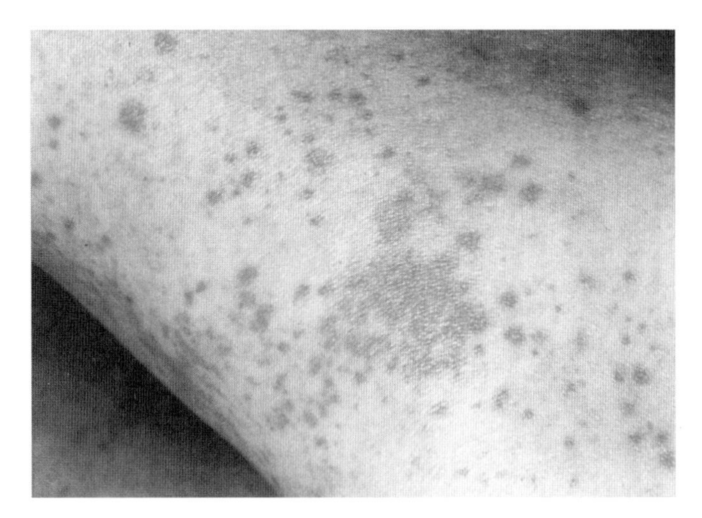

FIGURE 17.8. Meningococcemia. Early findings include petechiae evolving into a purpuric lesion.

(Reproduced, with permission, from Tintinalli JE, Kelen GD, Stapczynski JS. *Emergency Medicine: A Comprehensive Study Guide*, 6th ed. New York: McGraw-Hill, 2004:1519.)

HERPES

Etiology

- Herpes simplex virus is transmitted through direct contact or infected secretions (saliva or genital).
- Patients with eczema are at elevated risk for widely disseminated eruptions of HSV.
- Neonatal herpes is acquired during delivery.

Symptoms/Exam

- Small, thin-walled, **grouped vesicles** on an erythematous base
- HSV-1 primarily causes oral lesions throughout the mouth (unlike herpangina, which are posteriorly located); after primary infection a recurrence of lesions usually occur on the lower lip triggered by local trauma, sunburn, or stress. Prodrome of local LAD, pain, and tingling may occur with lesions appearing within 2 days.
- HSV-2 mainly causes genital lesions.
- A **Tzanck** smear may be used to confirm the diagnosis. Tzanck smears are also positive with varicella/herpes zoster.

Treatment

- Oral acyclovir can shorten duration of symptoms. Topical penciclovir is not effective.
- For sexually transmitted HSV, abstinence is the only method for absolute prevention, condoms are only effective if they cover all lesions; asymptomatic viral shedding still occurs with suppressive drug therapy.
- Herpes simplex virus keratitis (usually due to HSV 1) is a leading cause of corneal blindness. It most commonly presents with a **dendritic** corneal ulcer. Topical or oral antivirals with or without topical steroids are used, depending on location of infection within the cornea.

HERPETIC WHITLOW

- Herpetic whitlow is a primary or recurrent HSV-1 or HSV-2 infection of the finger causing painful vesicles on a digit that coalesce and may appear to contain pus, but instead contain necrotic epithelial cells.
- It must not be misdiagnosed as a paronychia and incised, which can delay healing and allow secondary infection.
- Treat with local wound care and pain control.

CHICKENPOX (VARICELLA-ZOSTER VIRUS, HUMAN HERPES VIRUS 3)

Symptoms/Exam

- Prodrome of 1–2 days of low-grade fever and malaise is followed by appearance of clear vesicles on an erythematous base, described as "**dew drops on a rose petal.**"
- The vesicles, which can be anywhere on the body including the mucous membranes, then scab over in various stages. The rash moves from the trunk out to the extremities. **Multiple stages of lesions** on the same body part is characteristic of chickenpox.
- Chickenpox may cause congenital defects if infects pregnant woman in first trimester.

TREATMENT

- Oral acyclovir
- Chickenpox is highly contagious from 5 days before the appearance of the rash to five days after the appearance of the vesicles.
- Susceptible pregnant women should be given varicella-zoster immune globulin within 96 hours of exposure to prevent first and second trimester effects to the fetus, which include limb atrophy, scarring, and CNS, and ocular manifestations.

SHINGLES

ETIOLOGY

- Reactivation of the latent VZV
- Key risk factor is advanced age (>75 years old).

SYMPTOMS/EXAM

- Identical to chickenpox in appearance but lesions have a **unilateral dermatomal** distribution, with thoracic and lumbar areas being most common
- Lesions appear simultaneously and remain in **congruent stages of healing**.
- Infection begins as prodrome of headaches, photophobia, malaise, itching/tingling/pain in the affected area for 1–3 days followed by maculopapular rash → vesicular rash → pustules → ulcers → crusting. The course of the disease is approximately 2 weeks.
- Cranial nerve involvement may cause herpes zoster ophthalmicus if involving the ophthalmic branch of CN V and is a vision-threatening condition that requires ophthalmology consult.
- Occasionally lesions on the tip of the nose (**Hutchinson sign**) may be seen before ocular involvement.
- **Ramsay Hunt syndrome** or herpes zoster oticus classically presents with ear pain, facial paralysis (due to CN VII inflammation), and herpetic lesions of the ear canal or auricle. The presentation may mimic Bell palsy, the pathophysiology for Bell palsy may involve VZV, and both Bell palsy and Ramsay Hunt syndrome are treated with oral acyclovir and steroids.

Hutchinson sign = VZV reactivation of ophthalmic branch of CN V, lesion on tip of nose.

Ramsay Hunt syndrome = VZV reactivation of CN VII, lesion in ear canal

TREATMENT

- Systemic analgesia, antivirals, and steroids

EXANTHEMS

Exanthems are skin eruptions that occurs as a symptom of a general disease. Of those mentioned here, RMSF and scarlet fever are treated with antibiotics; the rest are viral and are treated supportively (see Table 17.2).

Rocky Mountain Spotted Fever

- Caused by *Rickettsia rickettsii*, which is harbored in tick saliva and transmitted during a tick bite

TABLE 17.2. Exanthems

EXANTHEM	KEY ASPECTS	CUTANEOUS FEATURES
Rocky Mountain spotted fever	Palm and sole involvement	Petechial lesions begin on wrists and ankles.
Scarlet fever	Strawberry tongue	**Sandpaper rash**, pastia lines (red lines in skin folds)
Measles/rubeola	Cough, coryza, and conjunctivitis	Lesions begin on head esp. behind the ears, then generalize.
Roseola	High fever precedes rash	Fine papular rash appears when fever defervesces
Rubella	LAD Arthralgias	Lesions begin on face, generalize, then disappear within 3 days.
Erythema infectiosum	Arthralgias	**Slapped cheek** appearance
Hand, foot, and mouth disease	Oral lesions that ulcerate	Palm and sole vesicles

- Found throughout North, Central, and South America, particularly the southeastern parts of the United States; **not particular to the Rocky Mountain area**
- Begins with HA, N/V, fever (>39°C), and malaise. On the second to the fourth day, erythematous macules with central petechiae appear on the wrists and ankles and then spread onto the trunk.
- Lesions on the palms and soles are characteristic.
- Systemic symptoms in severe cases, most frequently neurologic (seizures, palsies) or pulmonary (cough, dyspnea, pleural effusions)
- Antibiotic of choice is doxycycline. Chloramphenicol is also effective but has more severe side effects.

Scarlet Fever

- Caused by group A streptococcus
- Abrupt onset of fever, exudative pharyngitis (most common site of bacterial invasion), palatal petechiae, strawberry tongue, and lymphadenopathy (see Figure 17.9)
- A characteristic trait of this disease is a fine maculopapular rash with an erythematous background ("**sandpaper rash**") and pastia lines (petechiae in skin folds).
- Treatment PCN
- Complications include acute rheumatic fever and poststreptococcal glomerulonephritis.

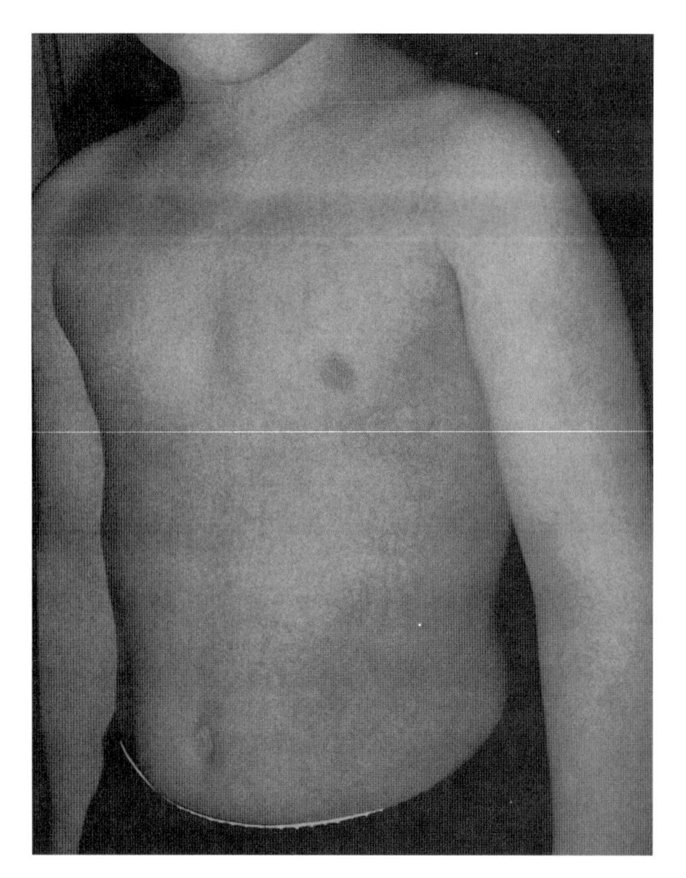

FIGURE 17.9. Scarlet fever.

(Reproduced, with permission, from Knoop KJ, Stack LB, Storrow AB. *Atlas of Emergency Medicine*, 2nd ed. New York: McGraw-Hill, 2002:455.)

Measles (Rubeola)

- Highly contagious viral illness spread by infectious droplets. Starts with fever up to 40.5°C, then cough, coryza, and conjunctivitis.
- **Koplik spots** (pathognomonic of the disease) appear on the buccal mucosa opposite the lower molars as small, irregular, bright red spots with bluish-white centers.
- Cutaneous eruption begins on third day of illness with maculopapular erythematous lesions beginning on head especially behind the ears and around the hairline and progressing to feet.

ROSEOLA INFANTUM (EXANTHEMA SUBITUM OR SIXTH DISEASE)

- Caused by human herpes virus; majority of cases occur between 6 months and 3 years.
- Illness starts with abrupt onset of high fever (104–105°F) although infant seems well. **Defervescence of fever** is associated with onset of rose pink macules and papules 2–3 mm in diameter, which blanch on pressure and rarely coalesce, appear on the trunk, and then spread to the extremities, and may be accompanied by lymphadenopathy.
- The rash disappears over 1–2 days.
- Febrile seizures may rarely occur.

Rubella (German Measles)

- Viral illness characterized by fever, exanthem (cephalocaudad), and lymphadenopathy (cervical, postcervical, suboccipital, postauricular)
- The rash is red to pink maculopapules that appear first on the face and then spread rapidly down. The lesions on the trunk may coalesce, but the ones on the extremities do not. The rash usually disappears after 3 days and may rarely have associated fine desquamation.
- Can cause congenital deafness or cardiac defects when occurs in pregnant women in first trimester

> ***Congenital infections—***
>
> **TORCHES**
> **T**oxoplasmosis
> **R**ubella
> **C**ytomegalovirus
> **H**erpes
> **S**yphilis

Erythema Infectiosum (Fifth Disease)

- Caused by parvovirus B19 infection
- Most common in children 4–10 years old, the disease may begin with mild prodrome of systemic symptoms and occasional fever then characteristic red macular exanthem on cheeks (**"slapped-cheek"** appearance) with circumoral pallor. Four days later, an erythematous reticular (lacelike) rash starts on the arms and moves to the trunk, buttocks, and thighs. Arthritis and arthralgias occur in 10% of patients.
- Papular purpuric glove and stocking syndrome is a separate manifestation that affects young adults. Hallmark findings are edema and erythema of palms and soles, with petechiae and purpura. Oral erosions and petechiae may occur as well.
- The disease is spread by respiratory tract infection, no longer infectious by time exanthem appears.

Hand, Foot, and Mouth Disease

- Hand, foot, and mouth disease is caused by coxsackie virus, enterovirus. Highly contagious, it occurs both as isolated events and as **epidemics**.
- Initial infection includes fever, anorexia, malaise, and sore mouth. Oral lesions appear 1–2 days later and cutaneous lesions shortly thereafter. **Oral lesions** are vesicles on an erythematous base which ulcerate. They occur on the buccal mucosa, tongue, **soft palate**, and gingiva but spare the lips.
- Cutaneous lesions start as red papules that change to gray vesicles about 3–7 mm in size. They are found on the palms and soles but may also be found on the dorsum of hand and feet and on the buttocks.
- Complications include aseptic meningitis, myocarditis, pulmonary edema, and orchitis.

INFESTATIONS

Pediculosis

- Infestation is by parasitic blood sucking insect (louse) on various body regions.
- Adult lice are the size of sesame seed and live up to 30 days on infested individual feeding on blood and living up to 2 days on inanimate objects.
- Transmission is through direct contact with infected individuals or their objects such as bedding, clothing, combs, or brushes.
- Pruritis is a common feature as an irritant response to lice saliva or excreta.
- Diagnosis is made by identifying louse nits (eggs) or live lice securely attached to hair shafts (head lice) or in seams of clothing (body lice).

TREATMENT

- **Permethrin** 1% rinse or 5% cream is first-line therapy. All close contacts should be treated. Clothing, linens, hairbrushes, carpets, sofas, and similar items should be heated to temperatures of 65°C for 15–30 minutes. Exposure to infested items should be avoided for 2 weeks before reuse.
- Lindane 1% lotion is second-line therapy. There is concern about neurotoxicity causing seizures in children.

Scabies

ETIOLOGY

- Scabies is a highly contagious, pruritic skin disorder caused by mite, *Sarcoptes scabiei.*
- The disease is transmitted through direct contact with an infected individual but less commonly occurs from contact with contaminated objects, which scabies can live on for 2–3 days.

SYMPTOMS/EXAM

- Mites live within the epidermis of the skin and make tunnels within the skin for laying eggs. **Burrows** are wavy, threadlike, grayish white and 1–10 mm in length is a pathognomonic sign.
- Intense pruritus and small erythematous papules with associated excoriations are also common.
- Typical sites of involvement include the **interdigital web spaces** of hands and feet. Penile and scrotal lesions are common in men. Areolae, nipple, and genital areas are commonly affected in women.
- If mite burden becomes high (millions) a form called crusted scabies develops and an immunocompromised state should be suspected.

TREATMENT

- Topical scabicides should be applied from head to toe, excluding scalp. Fingernail areas, web spaces, and the umbilicus should be thoroughly treated. **Permethrin,** 5% cream or lindane, 1% lotion are equally effective if left on overnight. Lindane is neurotoxic in infants, children, and pregnant mothers. All close contacts should be treated and linens washed and dried in a drier on high heat. A second treatment should be done 7 days after the first to kill any nymphs that have hatched from eggs.
- 5–10% precipitated sulfur in petrolatum base has been used in pregnant women because of its presumed low toxicity.
- Pruritus and lesions can persist for 2–4 weeks after successful treatment due to irritant reactions against residuum of dead mites.

CHAPTER 18

Renal and Genitourinary Emergencies

Liza J. Cadnapaphornchai, MD

A 5-year-old male presents to the ED with 3 days of "brown urine" and facial swelling. One week earlier he had experienced a URI with fevers and sore throat. On examination, he is mildly hypertensive and has periorbital edema but is otherwise normal. His BUN and creatinine are elevated. What UA findings would confirm your suspicion of poststreptococcal glomerulonephritis?

Proteinuria, dysmorphic RBCs, and RBC casts.

PROTEINURIA

Proteinuria can be divided into four basic groups: Glomerular (increased glomerular permeability), tubular (decreased tubular reabsorption), overflow (excess production exceeding normal kidney capabilities), and functional (benign causes).

SYMPTOMS/EXAM

- Varies with underlying cause
- As most cases are functional, exam is often normal.
- Patients with glomerular proteinuria classically present with edema, ranging from dependent peripheral edema to anasarca.
- Ask about history of recent viral or systemic illness, change in medications, hypertension, diabetes, cardiac, or renal disease.

DIAGNOSIS

- Evaluate urinalysis to look for markers of disease:
  - RBC casts and hematuria → glomerulonephritis (GN).
  - Fatty casts or oval fat bodies → nephrotic syndrome.
  - WBCs, WBC casts without bacteria → interstitial nephritis.
  - Hyaline casts → benign causes.
- Obtain BUN/Cr in patient with evidence of underlying renal disease.

TREATMENT

- Depends on underlying etiology
- Patients at minimum need primary care follow-up to evaluate for persistent proteinuria.

Nephrotic Syndrome

A form of glomerular proteinuria characterized by nephrotic-range proteinuria (3.5 g/24 hours), hypoproteinemia, hyperlipidemia, and peripheral edema, it may be caused by a primary glomerular disease process or secondary to diabetes, lupus, etc.

SYMPTOMS/EXAM

- Gradual onset of edema
- Foamy urine, due to high levels of protein

DIAGNOSIS

- Based on characteristic clinical and laboratory findings

- Peripheral edema
- Proteinuria—3+ or 4+ on dipstick
- Fatty casts or oval fat bodies on UA: Related to associated hyperlipidemia
- Hypoproteinemia

- BUN and creatinine are often normal.

TREATMENT

- May include fluid restriction, IV diuretics

COMPLICATIONS

- Increased risk of thrombosis
  - The most notable is **renal vein thrombosis**, characterized by hematuria, flank pain, and worsening renal function.

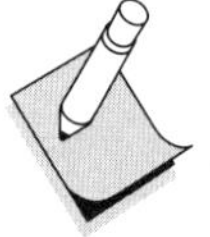

Renal vein thrombosis should be considered in all patients with nephrotic syndrome presenting with hematuria, flank pain, and worsening renal function.

HEMATURIA

Hematuria can be microscopic or gross in nature. Microscopic hematuria is defined as >3 RBC/hpf on spun urine sediment, while gross hematuria correlates to 1 mL of blood in 1 L of urine. Gross hematuria has a higher incidence of serious underlying pathology.

Hematuria can be thought of as belonging to four main groups:

- Traumatic
- Hematologic: eg, coagulopathy, sickle cell disease
- Renal: eg, glomerulonephritis, AVM
- Postrenal: eg, stones, bladder carcinoma, BPH, UTI

Table 18.1 lists the most common etiologies of hematuria by age group.

SYMPTOMS/EXAM

- Vary with underlying etiology

TABLE 18.1. Common Causes of Hematuria by Age

Common Causes of Hematuria by Age	
<20 yr	Glomerulonephritis
	UTI
20–40 yr	GU trauma
	Malignancy
	Stone
	UTI
40–60 yr	Carcinoma (bladder, kidney)
	Stone
	UTI
	BPH (males)

TABLE 18.2. Clinical Clues That Suggest a Particular Diagnosis in Patients With Hematuria

CLINICAL FINDINGS	DISEASE
Dysuria, frequency	UTI
Hearing loss	Alport syndrome
Hemoptysis	Goodpasture syndrome
Recent URI	Glomerulonphritis or IgA nephropathy
Proteinuria, RBC casts	Glomerulonephritis
Petechiae/purpura, schistocytes on smear	Hemolytic uremic syndrome (children) or thrombotic thrombocytopenic purpura [TTP] (adults)
Nephrotic syndrome, flank pain	Renal vein thrombosis
Third World country	*Shistosomiasis*

- The character of hematuria may help localize the source.
  - Blood clots indicate a nonglomerular source.
  - Brown-colored urine indicates a renal source.
  - Occurring with initiation of voiding or between voids suggests urethral source.
  - Occurring at the end of voiding suggests a source in the bladder neck or prostatic urethra.
  - Occurring throughout the urinary stream suggests a source proximal to the urethra.
- Table 18.2 lists clues from the clinical presentation that suggest a particular diagnosis in patients with hematuria.

DIAGNOSIS

- Obtain UA, BUN/Cr, CBC in all.
  - Gross hematuria will be dipstick positive for protein.
- Other studies as indicated based on clinical suspicion and severity of bleeding, including coagulation studies, urine culture, renal imaging (CT, USN), cystoscopy.

DIFFERENTIAL

- **Pseudohematuria**: Can be due to ingestion of beets, berries, medications (rifampin, pyridium), porphyrias
- Rhabdomyolysis: Presence of myoglobin in urine → urine dipstick positive for heme, but negative for RBCs.

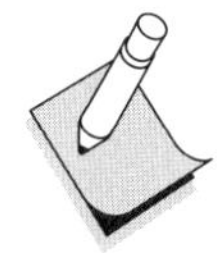

If a urine dipstick is positive for heme but no RBCs are seen on microscopic urinalysis, consider rhabdomyolysis.

TREATMENT

- Depends on underlying cause.
- Patients with bladder outlet obstruction from clot formation require three-way foley catheter placement and bladder irrigation.

ACUTE RENAL FAILURE

Acute renal failure (ARF) describes a sudden decline in kidney function marked by the accumulation of nitrogenous waste products, disturbances of fluid balance, and a wide range of other metabolic disturbances. It is classified according to underlying pathophysiology into three groups: **Prerenal**, **intrinsic,** and **postrenal** (see Table 18.3 and Table 18.4).

TABLE 18.3. Classification and Causes of Acute Renal Failure

PRERENAL	INTRINSIC RENAL	POSTRENAL
Hypovolemia Volume redistribution Decreased effective cardiac output Medications	Glomerulonephritis Acute interstitial nephritis (AIN) Acute tubular necrosis (ATN) Vascular causes	Urinary tract obstruction (at any level)

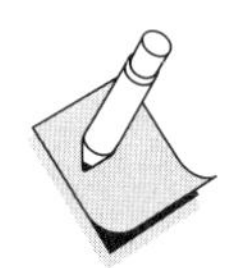

The primary cause of community-acquired acute renal failure is hypovolemia.

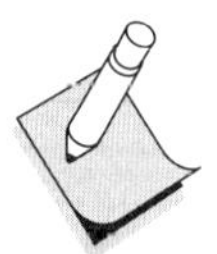

Suspect bilateral renal artery stenosis in patients with acute renal failure after initiating ACE inhibitor therapy.

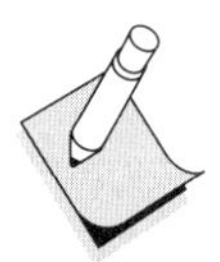

Prerenal acute renal failure is associated with a low U_{Na} (<20 mEq/dL) and a low FE_{Na} (<1%).

Prerenal

Prerenal acute renal failure occurs as a result of decreased renal perfusion. It is the most common reason for acute renal failure in the nonhospitalized patient.

CAUSES

Causes of prerenal ARF include:

- **Hypovolemia:** Hemorrhage, vomiting and diarrhea, diuretic therapy
- **Volume redistribution:** Third-space sequestration, sepsis, hypoalbuminemic states
- **Decreased effective cardiac output:** Myocardial infarction, valvular disease, cardiomyopathy
- **Medications that limit glomerular perfusion:** ACE inhibitor or prostaglandin (NSAID) use

SYMPTOMS/EXAM

Will vary depending on underlying etiology

TABLE 18.4. Urinary Indices in Acute Renal Failure

			INTRINSIC RENAL		
	PRERENAL	ACUTE TUBULAR NECROSIS	ACUTE GLOMERULONEPHRITIS	ACUTE INTERSTITIAL NEPHRITIS	POSTRENAL
Serum BUN/Cr ratio	>20:1	<20:1	>20:1	<20:1	>20:1
U_{Na} (mEq/L)	<20	>20	<20	Variable	Variable
FE_{Na} (%)	<1	>2	<1	Variable	Variable
Urine osmolality	Increased	<350	Increased	Variable	< 350
Urinalysis	Normal or hyaline casts	Granular (muddy brown) casts, renal tubular casts	Dysmorphic RBCs, RBC casts, proteinuria	WBC, WBC casts, eosinophils	Normal

DIAGNOSIS

- BUN/Cr ratio > 10:1.
- Evidence of **increased renal Na^+ conservation**:
  - Urinary Na^+ (U_{Na}) concentration < 20 mEq/dL.
  - Fractional excretion of sodium (FE_{Na}) < 1%.

$$FE_{Na} = \frac{\text{Urine Na} \times \text{Plasma Cr}}{\text{Plasma Na} \times \text{Urine Cr}} \times 100$$

  - May be impaired in patients with chronic renal failure (CRF) or diuretic use
- Increased urine osmolality
- Urinalysis: Normal with occasional hyaline casts
- No evidence for obstruction on renal ultrasound

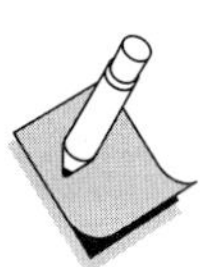

A low U_{Na} indicates intact urinary concentrating ability and the presence of a stimulus to conserve Na^+.

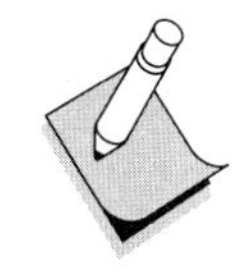

Evaluating urinary sodium indices is not helpful in patients with underlying chronic renal failure or diuretic use.

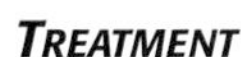

TREATMENT

- Treat underlying cause (eg, correct hypovolemia, augment cardiac output).
- Discontinue offending drugs: NSAIDs, ACE inhibitors.
- Correct electrolyte imbalances.
- Dialyze as needed.

Intrinsic

Intrinsic acute renal failure results from pathology of the glomerulus, interstitium, or renal tubule.

CAUSES

Causes of intrinsic ARF include:

- **Glomerulonephritis**
- **Acute interstitial nephritis**
- **Acute tubular necrosis**
- **Vascular disease**

GLOMERULONEPHRITIS

Glomerulonephritis is a renal disease characterized by inflammation of the glomeruli. It may be a primary process, as in poststreptococcal glomulonephritis, or secondary to underlying systemic disease, such as lupus, Goodpasture syndrome, and systemic vasculitis. Most cases are seen in the pediatric population.

SYMPTOMS/EXAM

- Patients may be asymptomatic at time of diagnosis.
- Symptoms include dark urine, hematuria, edema, hypertension.

DIAGNOSIS

- The characteristic findings on urinalysis include hematuria, dysmorphic RBCs, proteinuria, and, most importantly, **RBC casts.**
- Proteinuria may be nephrotic range.
- Renal biopsy is definitive.

TREATMENT

- Antibiotics if poststreptococcal etiology
- Supportive care, control BP
- Steroids and other immunosuppressives are used to treat underlying systemic disease (when present), but are not indicated in poststreptococcal GN.

ACUTE INTERSTITIAL NEPHRITIS

Acute interstitial nephritis results from interstitial inflammation, most commonly in response to medication, but is also associated with infections and autoimmune disease. The most commonly implicated medications include:

- Penicillins
- Diuretics
- Anticoagulants
- NSAIDs

SYMPTOMS/EXAM

- Fever and rash may be present.

DIAGNOSIS

- Elevated BUN/Cr
- Presence of eosinophils, WBCs, and WBC casts on UA
- Renal biopsy is definitive.

TREATMENT

- Discontinue offending agent.
- Steroids if significant renal impairment
- Renal function generally returns to baseline over weeks.

ACUTE TUBULAR NECROSIS

The most common cause of hospital-acquired ARF, this is (generally) reversible injury to the renal tubule due to:

- **Renal ischemia:** Surgery, trauma, sepsis
- **Nephrotoxic agents:** Aminoglycosides and radiocontrast agents are most common offenders.
  - Risk factors for contrast-induced ATN include renal insufficiency, diabetes, intravascular volume depletion, and higher dose of contrast material.
- **Pigments:** Myoglobin, hemoglobin

DIAGNOSIS

- Characterized by the loss of urinary concentrating ability
  - $U_{Na} > 20$
  - $FE_{Na} > 2\%$
  - Urine osmolality = serum osmolality.
- Urinalysis is positive for granular (muddy brown) casts and renal tubular casts.

- Suspect rhabdomyolysis if urine is dip positive for heme, but negative for RBCs.

TREATMENT

- Treat underlying precipitating cause or discontinue offending agent.
- **N-Acetylcysteine** may help prevent ATN in high-risk patients receiving radiocontrast agents.
- Administer crystalloid, mannitol, and alkalinize urine if pigment induced.
- Renal function typically recovers over days to weeks.

VASCULAR DISEASE

Vascular disease of the kidney may be macrovascular (eg, renal artery occlusion, AAA) or microvascular (eg, embolus, malignant hypertension, hemolytic uremic syndrome, TTP). Hemolytic uremic syndrome (HUS) will be discussed further.

HEMOLYTIC UREMIC SYNDROME

Hemolytic uremic syndrome is a disease characterized by microangiopathic hemolytic anemia, thrombocytopenia, and acute renal failure. It is one of the most common causes of acute renal failure in children under the age of five. Thrombotic thrombocytopenic purpura is similar in pathophysiology, but occurs primarily in adults and characteristically has prominent neurologic involvement (vs renal involvement in HUS).

ETIOLOGY

HUS most commonly occurs following infection with *Escherichia coli serotype O157:H7*. Other infectious agents and toxins have also been implicated including *Shigella*, *Salmonella*, *Campylobacter*, and *Yersinia*.

HUS = microangiopathic hemolytic anemia, thrombocytopenia, and acute renal failure.

SYMPTOMS/EXAM

- Prodrome of fever, vomiting, abdominal pain, and diarrhea (often bloody)
- Onset of pallor with petechial or purpural rash
- Decreased urinary output
- CNS symptoms (minority of patients): Stroke, seizures, coma

DIAGNOSIS

- Anemia (Hgb <8 g/dL) and thrombocytopenia
- PT and PTT normal
- Renal failure
- Peripheral smear: **Schistocytes**

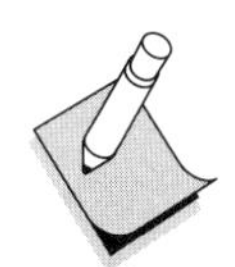

HUS most commonly follows infection with E. coli *serotype O157:H7. A history of abdominal pain and diarrhea is common.*

TREATMENT

- Treat complications of acute renal failure (dialysis as needed).
- Careful rehydration
- PRBC transfusion if Hgb < 6 g/dL)
- Platelet transfusion only if significant bleeding or need for invasive procedure
- **Plasma exchange if CNS symptoms**

Postrenal Acute Renal Failure

CAUSES

Results from obstruction at any level of the urinary tract:

- **Urethral obstruction:** Phimosis or stricture
- **Bladder obstruction:** BPH, stones, clot, tumor, neurogenic bladder, posterior urethral valve
- **Intrarenal/ureteral obstruction:** Kidney stone, crystalline precipitation, tumor, iatrogenic, papillary necrosis

SYMPTOMS/EXAM

- Vary with underlying cause

DIAGNOSIS

- Renal ultrasound to confirm presence of upper or lower tract obstruction
- Urine indices and BUN/Cr ratios are typically unhelpful.
- Urinalysis is often normal.
- Obtain retrograde urography if bilateral ureteral obstruction is suspected.

TREATMENT

- Relieve obstruction (eg, Foley for bladder outlet obstruction).
- Correct electrolyte imbalances.
- Dialyze as needed.

CHRONIC RENAL FAILURE

Chronic renal failure is a wide spectrum of disease defined as permanent loss of renal function of >3 months' duration. It is staged based on the estimated glomerulofiltration rate (GFR). End-stage renal disease (ESRD, now termed *kidney failure*) is the final endpoint where GFR is <10% and clinical symptoms of uremia will ensue without dialysis or transplant.

SYMPTOMS/EXAM

- Symptoms of uremia are often nonspecific, including anorexia, nausea, and vomiting, declining mental function.
- **Uremic frost**
  - Deposition of urea from evaporated sweat
  - Fine white powder on skin
- **Volume overload/pulmonary edema**
- **Hypertension**
- **Renal osteodystrophy**
  - Due to loss of Vitamin D_3 production and secondary hyperparathyroidism
  - Bone pain, muscle weakness, fractures
- **Pericarditis**
  - Suspect tamponade in **any** ill-appearing patient with ESRD.
  - Early tamponade may manifest as hypotension during dialysis.
- **Systemic calcification**
  - Occurs when calcium-phosphate product ($Ca^{2+} \times PO_4$) is >**70–80**
  - Deposition of calcium in joints (pseudogout) or small vessels (ischemia and necrosis)
- **Anemia**
  - Normocytic, normochromic
  - Due to decreased erythropoietin production and RBC survival time

- **Bleeding**
  - Multifactorial: Decreased platelet function, altered von Willebrand factor
  - May include *subdural hematomas*, GI bleeding
- **Encephalopathy**
  - May include mental status changes, hiccups, asterixis (hand flapping with dorsiflexion), and myoclonic twitching
- **Hyperkalemia (see Chapter 14)**
- **Metabolic acidosis**
- **Immunosuppression**
- **Peripheral neuropathy**
  - Sensorimotor

TREATMENT

- If patient is not ESRD, look for and treat reversible causes of renal failure ("acute on chronic renal failure").
- Usual management of HTN, pulmonary edema, hyperkalemia
- Dialysis
- Renal transplantation
- Acute bleeding:
  - **DDAVP:** First-line, stimulates release of vWF from endothelial cells
  - **Cryoprecipitate:** Contains factors I (fibrinogen), II (fibronectin), VIII, XIII, and vWF
  - **Conjugated estrogens:** Increases platelet reactivity and decreases nitric oxide generation
  - **Transfusion of PRBCs:** To hematocrit of 30%

A 45-year-old female with ESRD presents to the ED complaining of shortness of breath. Her last dialysis was 1 day prior via a recently place right arm AV fistula. She does receive erythropoietin replacement therapy. As part of your physical examination, you temporarily occlude her dialysis access site and observe a drop in her heart rate. What diagnosis does this finding support?

The drop in heart rate with occlusion of the dialysis access site is termed Branham sign, which indicates a high-output heart failure from excess flow through the AV fistula. The diagnosis can be confirmed with Doppler ultrasound.

DIALYSIS-RELATED EMERGENCIES

Dialysis can be in the form of hemodialysis (HD) where an artificial membrane filters solute and fluids, or peritoneal dialysis (PD) where the peritoneal membrane serves as the dialysis membrane. HD allows for faster exchange of solute and fluids.

Indications for Emergent Dialysis

Indications for emergent dialysis are listed in Table 18.5.

Indications for emergent dialysis—

AEIOU
Acidosis
Electrolyte (K >6.5, BUN >100, Creatinine >10)
Ingestions
Overload (fluid)
Uremia

TABLE 18.5. Indications for Emergent Dialysis

Severe acid-base disturbance (metabolic acidosis)
Severe electrolyte disturbance (hyperkalemia, hypercalcemia)
Certain toxic ingestions
Volume overload (pulmonary edema, severe HTN)
Uremia (pericarditis, twitching, N/V, encephalopathy)

Complications of Hemodialysis

Hypotension

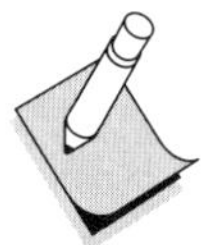

Always consider serious causes (eg, tamponade, MI, hyperkalemia) when evaluating the patient presenting with "hypotension during dialysis."

Commonly due to fluid shifts and often resolves spontaneously or with a small fluid bolus. Be sure to consider serious causes: Tamponade, infection, MI, bleeding, hyperkalemia, air embolism, anaphylaxis.

Bleeding

Dialysis-related bleeding may be due to underlying platelet dysfunction of ESRD or HD associated transient thrombocytopenia and anticoagulation.

Treatment

- DDAVP, cryoprecipitate, conjugated estrogens and transfusion as with chronic renal failure (above)
- **Protamine:** To reverse heparin, if overanticoagulation is a concern

Dialysis Disequilibrium Syndrome

Due to rapid changes in body fluid composition and osmolality, typically when first starting HD; occurs during or immediately after the dialysis session

Symptoms/Exam

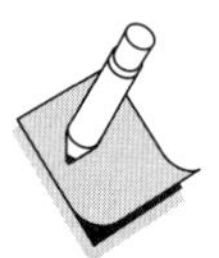

Dialysis disequilibrium is due to transient decrease in blood osmolality and resultant fluid shifts.

- Often includes headache, nausea/vomiting, muscle cramping
- If severe: Altered mental status, seizures, and coma from cerebral edema

Treatment

- Symptoms generally resolve over several hours, but may be treated with mannitol, if severe.

Fistula-Specific Problems

Fistula-specific problems include:

- **Puncture site bleeding:** The most common complication
- **True aneurysms:** Rare and rarely rupture

- **Pseudoaneurysms:** Typically present with swelling, bleeding, or infection.
- **Thrombosis**
- **High-output heart failure**
  - Branham sign: A drop in HR with temporary compression of HD access site

Treatment

- Treat puncture site bleeding with direct pressure, application of gel foam soaked in thrombin, other medications/transfusion as listed above.
- Obtain vascular surgery consult for suspected pseudoaneurysm, thrombosis, uncontrolled bleeding, or high-output heart failure.
- Direct thrombolytic injection or angiographic clot removal (within 24 hours) can be used to treat thrombosis.

Vascular Access Infection

Can occur in HD catheters or fistulas (grafts > native vein); typically result from Gram-positive organisms such as *Staphylococcus*, but Gram-negative infections are also seen

Symptoms/Exam

- Fever or history of documented bacteremia
- Absence of local signs does **not** rule out vascular access infection.

Treatment

- Obtain blood cultures.
- Parenteral antibiotics: Intravenous vancomycin to cover staphylococcal infection and gentamycin or third generation cephalosporin to cover Gram-negatives (if suspected).

> A 50-year-old female on peritoneal dialysis, presents to the ED with complaint of fever, abdominal pain, and cloudy PD fluid. On examination, she is well appearing and afebrile, but has a diffusely tender abdomen. The dialysis catheter site is normal. What peritoneal fluid cell counts would confirm your suspicion of peritonitis?
>
> Greater than 100 WBC/mm^3 with >50% neutrophils. A positive Gram stain can also confirm the diagnosis.

Peritonitis

Peritoneal dialysis-related peritonitis is commonly due to Gram-positive organisms (*Staphylococcus* and *Streptococcus*), followed by Gram-negative bacteria and (rarely) anaerobes and fungi. If the culture shows multiple organisms, suspect bowel perforation.

Symptoms

- Fever, abdominal pain, cloudy PD fluid

Diagnosis

- PD fluid with: >100 WBC/mm^3 with >50% neutrophils *or* a positive Gram stain.

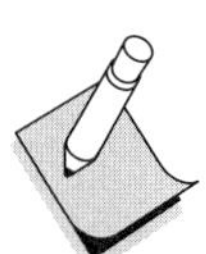

The most common organisms in PD-related peritonitis = Staphylococcus *and* Streptococcus.

Treatment

- Intraperitoneal (not IV) antibiotics: Vancomycin or third-generation cephalosporin

RENAL TRANSPLANT COMPLICATIONS

Renal transplants have survival rates of 96% at 1 year and 91% at 3 years.

Infections

Infections are most common during the first 6 months following transplant surgery (when immunosuppressant doses are highest) and are the most common cause of morbidity and mortality in the first posttransplant year.

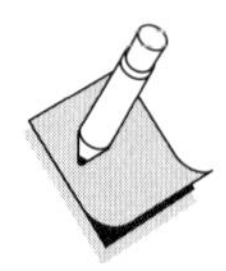

CMV is the most common life-threatening infection in solid organ transplant patients.

ETIOLOGY

- Overall bacterial infections are most common.
- Immediately following surgery: Typical bacterial postoperative organisms (*Staphylococcus, Streptococcus, E. coli*).
- Months 1–6: Highest incidence of viremia and opportunistic infections, most notably *CMV* infection, but also EBV, HSV, herpes zoster, *Pneumocystis carinii*, *Listeria* meningitis, and fungal sepsis.

SYMPTOMS/EXAM

- Varies with underlying etiology.
- CMV: Fever spikes, malaise, arthralgias, lymphadenopathy, pneumonitis, retinitis, hepatitis
- Primary EBV: Mononucleosis-like syndrome

DIAGNOSIS

- CXR, UA, CBC, chemistries, blood cultures, urine cultures, viral PCR

CMV infections are treated with gancyclovir or foscarnet.

TREATMENT

- Depends on suspected underlying cause
- CMV: Gancyclovir or foscarnet
- Primary EBV: Reduce immonosuppression, acyclovir
- HSV or herpes zoster: Acyclovir
- Fungal sepsis: Amphotericin

Graft Rejection

Types of rejection:

- *Hyperacute:* Occurs within minutes to hours after transplant surgery and results in graft destruction
- *Acute:* Occurs within 1–12 weeks following surgery, mediated through attack by T lymphocytes against antigen donor tissues
- *Chronic:* Results from nephrosclerosis and subsequent ischemia to the graft

SYMPTOMS/EXAM

- Low-grade fevers, malaise
- Worsening hypertension, increased creatinine
- Weight gain, peripheral edema
- Tenderness to palpation over the graft

Differential

- Includes renal artery stenosis, cyclosporine or tacrolimus toxicity, obstruction, UTI

Diagnosis

- Suggested in setting of elevated BUN/Cr
- Allograft biopsy is definitive.
- Rule out other causes with UA, immunosuppressant levels, renal ultrasound.

Treatment

- High-dose steroids
- Antibody preparations directed at attacking T lymphocytes causing allograft rejection (eg, OKT3)

The differential of acute renal transplant rejection?

Renal artery stenosis

Cyclosporin or tacrolimus toxicity

Obstruction

UTI

NEPHROLITHIASIS

Types of stones (see Table 18.6):

- **Calcium oxalate (most common)**
- **Struvite**
- **Uric acid**
- **Cystine**

Acute Renal Colic

Renal stones most commonly become symptomatic when they obstruct the ureter, causing renal colic. Complete obstruction may cause irreversible damage after 1–2 weeks.

There are five sites along the ureter where calculi are likely to cause obstruction: Calyx of kidney, ureteropelvic junction, pelvic brim, **ureterovesicular junction (most common)**, and vesicle orifice.

TABLE 18.6. Renal Stones

Stone Type	Pathophysiology
Calcium oxalate (most common)	↑ Ca^{2+} production (hyperparathyroidism, neoplasm, sarcoid, RTA). ↑ Oxalate absorption (inflammatory bowel disease).
Struvite	Infection with urea-splitting bacteria (*Pseudomonas, Klebsiella, Staphylococcus, Proteus*) May cause staghorn calculi and alkaline urine
Uric acid	↑ Uric acid excretion in the urine (gout, leukemia, or high protein diet). Low urine pH supports stone formation.
Cystine (rare)	Inborn errors of metabolism

RENAL AND GENITOURINARY EMERGENCIES

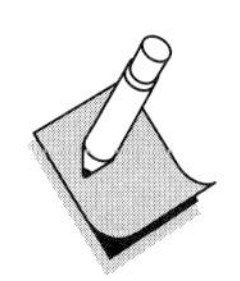

Five sites of ureteral obstruction:

Calyx of kidney

Ureteropelvic junction

Pelvic brim

Ureterovesicular junction (most common)

Vesicle orifice

SYMPTOMS/EXAM

- Abrupt onset of extreme colicky flank pain radiating to the groin.
- Patients frequently are unable to lay still.
- Nausea/vomiting, urinary urgency, and frequency may occur.
- Fevers and chills if concomitant infection.

DIFFERENTIAL

- The most critical diagnosis in differential is AAA.
- **Acute papillary necrosis**
  - Ischemic necrosis of the renal papillae → sloughed papillae, which may lead to obstruction and infection.
  - Seen most commonly in patients with diabetes mellitus, sickle cell disease, and chronic NSAID use.
- Other considerations include pyelonephritis, testicular torsion.

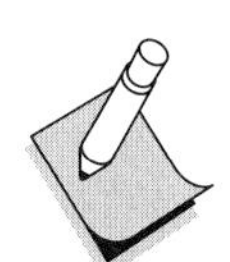

Uric acid stones are radiolucent.

DIAGNOSIS

- Hematuria is common (gross or microscopic), but absence of RBCs does **not** exclude stones.
- Urinary pH:
  - pH > 7.6 → suspect urea-splitting organisms.
  - pH < 5 → suspect uric acid crystalluria.
- Bacteriuria suggests infection.
- BUN/Cr—if solitary kidney, transplant, chronic renal failure.
- Imaging:
  - **Plain radiographs**—low specificity; calcium, struvite and cystine stones are radiopaque.
  - **Helical CT**—standard imaging modality; can identify other pathology, no contrast, rapid.
  - **IVP**—provides functional information; findings consistent with obstruction: *delayed nephrogram*, *columnization* (entire ureter visible), *hydronephrosis*; requires IV contrast.
  - **Ultrasound**—less reliable for small stones; can be used in pregnant or pediatric patients.

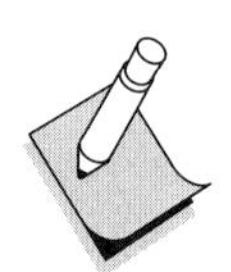

On the boards, suspect AAA in any patient over 50 presenting with flank pain!

TREATMENT

- Supportive care with IV fluids and analgesia
  - NSAIDs are first line: Shown to decrease both renal capsular pressure (through decreased GFR) and ureterospasm
- Stones <5 mm: Likely to pass spontaneously within 4 weeks
- Stones >8 mm: Unlikely to pass, often require lithotripsy or surgical intervention
- Medical expulsive therapy may be helpful:
  - Ureteral antispasmodic: Tamsulosin (Flomax)
  - Anti-inflammatory agent: Prednisone
- Urology follow-up
- Admission criteria:
  - Obstruction with concomitant infection
  - Intractable pain or vomiting
  - Urinary extravasation
  - Solitary kidney
  - Acute renal insufficiency
  - Severe underlying disease

A healthy 70-year-old female presents with 4 days of dysuria and urgency. On clinical examination there is no evidence for pyelonephritis. UA shows many WBCs and bacteria, + leukocyte esterase, + nitrite, and few RBCs and epithelial cells. Is this patient a candidate for a 3-day course of antibiotic therapy?

No. She needs a 7-day regimen. A 7-day regimen is recommended for pregnant women or those with >7 days of symptoms, comorbid conditions such as diabetes, previous or recurrent UTI, or >65 years old.

URINARY TRACT INFECTION/PYELONEPHRITIS (ADULTS)

Urinary tract infection (UTI) is an infection of the urinary tract. With the exception of the neonatal period, UTIs are more common in females than males.

DEFINITIONS

Cystitis: Inflammation of the bladder; may be bacterial or nonbacterial

Complicated UTI: UTI associated with underlying disease that may put the patient at risk for a broader spectrum of pathogens or an increased rate of failure of short course antibiotic therapy (see Table 18.7)

Pyelonephritis: Infection of the renal parenchyma and collecting system

ETIOLOGY

- Organisms causing UTIs usually ascend the urethra from the perineum.
- *E. coli* is the dominant pathogen, followed by *Staphylococcus saprophyticus*. Less common organisms include *Proteus*, *Klebseilla*, and *Enterobacter*.
- Patients at risk for unusual organisms include institutionalized or hospitalized patients and complicated UTIs.

TABLE 18.7. Complicated UTIs

Complicated UTIs
Men
Elderly
Pregnant women
Serious medical disease
Immunosuppression
Recent hospitalization
Treatment failure
Structural urinary tract abnormalities
Pyelonephritis
Indwelling catheter
Recent instrumentation

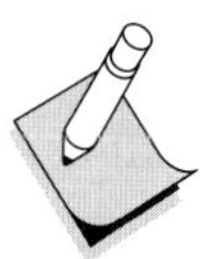

*The presence of **any** bacteria in an unspun urine sample is significant.*

SYMPTOMS/EXAM

- Urgency, dysuria, hematuria
- Flank pain, back pain, suprapubic pain
- Fever

DIAGNOSIS

- **Pyuria:** Significant at >2–5 WBC/hpf in women and >1–2 WBC/hpf in men
- **Bacteriuria:** Significant for *any bacteria* in an unspun urine sample or >15/hpf on spun samples
- **Urine dipstick leukocyte esterase:** Indicates presence of WBCs; negative result does not rule out infection.
- **Urine dipstick nitrite:** Indicates presence of Gram-negative bacteria; negative result does not rule out infection.
- **Urine culture:** Definitive test; indicated for all complicated UTIs; positive if >100 CFU/mL of known uropathogen

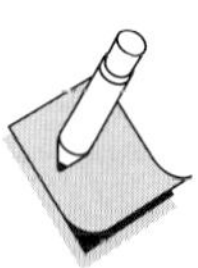

The presence of nitrite on urine dipstick indicates the presence of Gram-negative organisms.

DIFFERENTIAL

- Nonbacterial cystitis: Due to inflammation (radiation, interstitial cystitis, medications)
- Urethritis: *Clamydia* is commonly implicated pathogen.
- Prostatitis
- Vaginitis

TREATMENT

Urethritis or prostatitis is most likely cause of dysuria or pyuria in sexually active young male, not UTI.

- Antibiotic therapy (see Table 18.8)
- Criteria for admission:
  - Extremes of age
  - Systemic toxicity
  - Renal failure
  - Obstruction
  - Intractable vomiting or pain
  - Complicated UTI: Have lower threshold if questionable
- **Pregnancy**: Treat asymptomatic bacteriuria as UTI.
- **Diabetes and sickle cell disease**: Patients are at an increased risk of papillary necrosis, abscess formation, and microvascular complications.
- **Indwelling catheters**: Replacement of the catheter can eliminate bacteria in many patients.

Asymptomatic bacteriuria in pregnancy should be treated as a UTI.

COMPLICATIONS

- Complications include perinephric abscess or obstruction; CT is preferred method of evaluation.

URETHRITIS

Inflammation of the urethra, it is most commonly due to ***Chlamydia trachomatis*** or ***Neisseria gonorrhoeae* (GC)**, but other organisms include *Ureaplasma urealyticum*, *Trichomonas vaginalis*, herpesvirus, or candida.

TABLE 18.8. Antibiotic Therapy in UTI

CONDITION	ANTIBIOTIC (INITIAL THERAPY)	THERAPY DURATION (TOTAL)
Acute uncomplicated cystitis	Trimethoprim/sulfamethoxazole *or* Fluoroquinolone	3 days
Acute uncomplicated cystitis with comorbid conditions	Trimethoprim/sulfamethoxazole *or* Fluoroquinolone	7 days
Acute uncomplicated pyelonephritis	Mild to moderately ill:	
	■ Oral fluoroquinolone *or*	7 days
	■ Trimethoprim/sulfamethoxazole	14 days
	Hospitalized:	
	■ IV fluoroquinolone *or* ampicillin/ gentamycin	14 days
Complicated UTI	Mild to moderately ill:	
	■ Oral fluoroquinolone *or* trimethoprim/ sulfamethoxazole	14
	Hospitalized:	
	■ IV ampicillin/gentamycin *or* imipenemcilastin *or* fluoroquinolone	14 days
Pregnancy	Amoxicillin or trimethoprim/ sulfamethoxazole (not in late third trimester) *or* nitrofurantoin	7 days
Pregnant with pyeolonephritis	Hospitalized: IV gentamycin *or* ceftriaxone	14 days

SYMPTOMS/EXAM

- Though most patients have dysuria and urethral discharge, occasional patients are asymptomatic.

DIAGNOSIS

- Nucleic acid amplification test of first-voided urine or urethral swab, *or*
- Culture of urethral secretions

TREATMENT

- Regimen must be effective at treating both GC and chlamydia: Ceftriaxone (IM) *or* cefixime for GC and doxycycline *or* azithromycin for chlamydia.
- Fluoroquinolones are no longer recommended due to a high prevalence of N. *gonorrheae* resistance.
- Metronidazole can be considered in patients with persistent symptoms despite treatment for GC and chlamydia, or if otherwise indicated.

RENAL AND GENITOURINARY EMERGENCIES

ACUTE BACTERIAL PROSTATITIS

ETIOLOGY

- **Patients <35 years**: Sexually transmitted pathogens *C. trachomatis and*/or *N. gonorrhoeae* (GC) predominate.
- **Patients ≥35 years:** Most often caused by Gram-negative organisms, predominantly *E. coli*. Mixed bacterial infections are uncommon. Suspect an **acute exacerbation of chronic prostatitis** if there is a history of recurrent UTIs.
- Tuberculosis should be considered in the presence of renal TB.

SYMPTOMS/EXAM

- Fever/chills.
- Perineal or low back pain.
- Urgency, dysuria, frequency, urinary retention.
- Tender swollen prostate that is firm and warm to the touch (avoid prostatic massage as it may precipitate bacteremia).

DIAGNOSIS

- Clinical examination is key to diagnosis.
- Urine culture may help isolate organism.

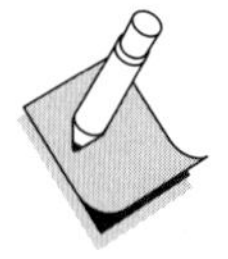

Prostatitis

<35 years: Think STD.

≥35 years: Think E. coli; *needs prolonged antibiotic therapy.*

TREATMENT

- Supportive care with analgesia, antipyretics, hydration.
- Antibiotics:
  - Age <35 years: Ceftriaxone (IM × 1) or ofloxacin (× 10 days) and doxycycline (× 10 days)
  - Age ≥35 years: Fluoroquinolone or trimethoprim/sulfamethoxazole for 2–4 weeks
  - Chronic bacterial: Fluoroquinolone × 4 weeks or trimethoprim/sulfamethoxazole for 1–3 months
- **Avoid** urethral catheterization, use suprapubic catheter if urinary retention occurs.
- Parenteral antibiotics and admission if patient appears toxic

PENILE ULCERS

Sexually transmitted diseases are the likely cause of isolated penile ulcers. Table 18.9 outlines the organisms, diagnosis, and treatment. See Figures 18.1–4.

DIFFERENTIAL

- In the setting of genital ulceration **and** oral ulcerations consider Behçet disease, Stevens-Johnson syndrome, Reiter syndrome, pemphigus vulgaris.
- Others causes of isolated genital unceration include lymphoma, carcinoma, vasculitis, fixed drug eruption, trauma.

DIAGNOSIS

- Diagnosis is often clinical.
- Syphilis is diagnosed by dark-field examination, direct fluorescent antibody testing, and serology.

TABLE 18.9. Sexually Transmitted Penile Ulcers

DISEASE	ORGANISM	CLINICAL	PAINFUL?
Chancroid	*Haemophilus ducreyi*	Sharply demarcated ulcer with undermined edges; often multiple; "Kissing lesions;" suppurative inguinal nodes	Yes
Herpes	Herpes simplex virus	Grouped vesicles on red base form shallow ulcers.	Yes
Syphilis	*Treponema pallidum*	Painless, indurated ulcer; heals spontaneously	No
Lymphogranuloma venereum	*Chlamydia trachomatis*	Transient, painless ulcer; followed by unilateral (mostly) inquinal adenopathy which may suppurate	No
Granuloma inguinale (donovanosis)	*Calymmatobacterium granulomatis*	Subcutaneous nodule(s), becomes beefy red, highly vascular ulcer(s).	No

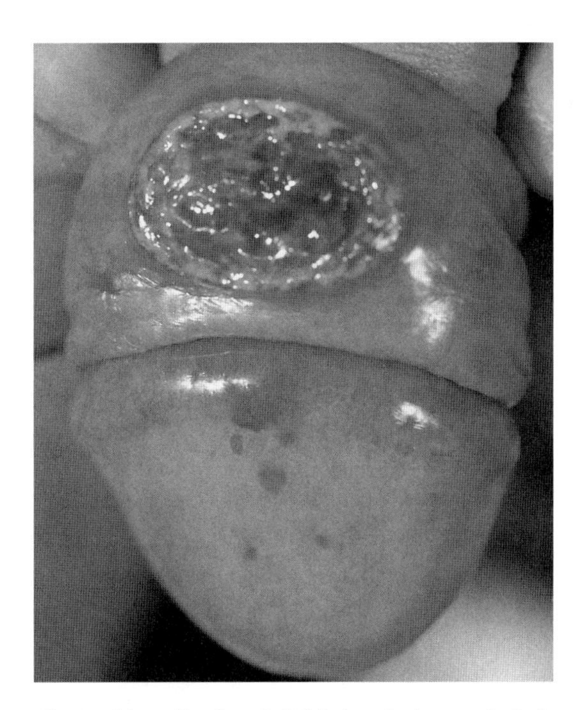

FIGURE 18.1. Chancroid penile ulcer. Painful sharply demarcated ulcer with undermined edges. (See also color insert.)

(Courtesy of Professor Alfred Eichman, MD as reproduced, with permission, from Wolff K, Johnson RA, Suurmond D. *Fitzpatrick's Color Atlas and Synopsis of Clinical Dermatology*, 5th ed. New York: McGraw-Hill, 2005:926.)

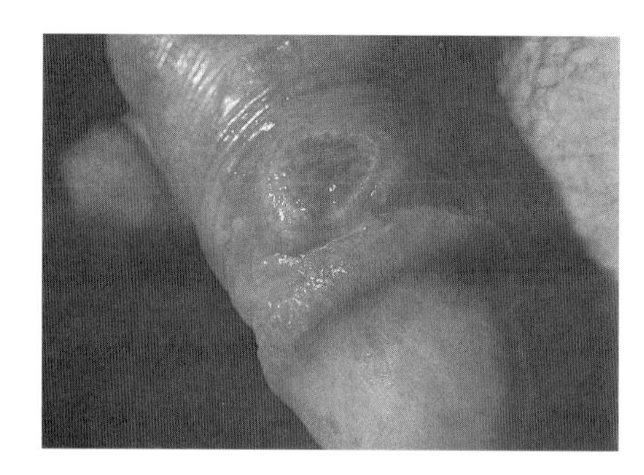

FIGURE 18.2. Syphilis. Painless, indurated chancre. (See also color insert.)

(Reproduced, with permission, from Wolff K, Johnson RA, Suurmond D. *Fitzpatrick's Color Atlas & Synopsis of Clinical Dermatology*, 5th ed. New York: McGraw-Hill, 2005:915.)

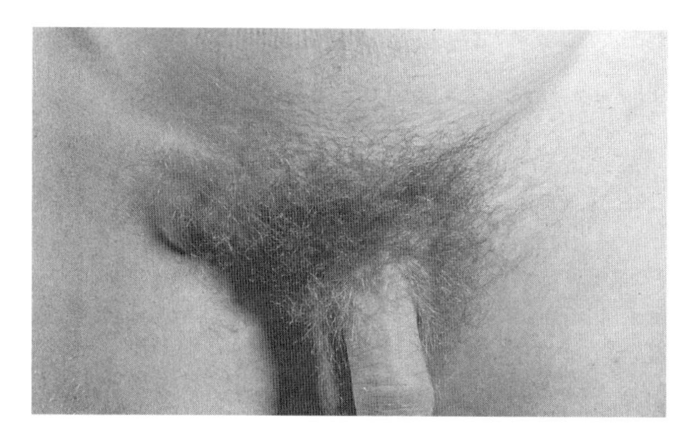

FIGURE 18.3. Lymphogranuloma venerum. Unilateral tender lymphadenopathy. (See also color insert.)

(Reproduced, with permission, from Wolff K, Johnson RA, Suurmond D. *Fitzpatrick's Color Atlas & Synopsis of Clinical Dermatology*, 5th ed. New York: McGraw-Hill, 2005:935.)

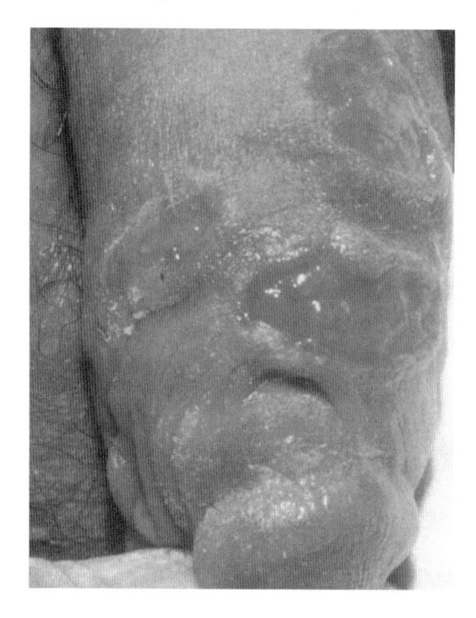

FIGURE 18.4. Granuloma inguinale. Beefy red, highly vascular, painless ulcers. (See also color insert.)

(Reproduced, with permission, from Kasper DL, Braunwald E, Fauci AS, Hauser SL, Longo DL, Jameson JL. *Harrison's Principles of Internal Medicine*, 16th ed. New York: McGraw-Hill, 2005:933.)

TABLE 18.10. **Treatment of Sexually Transmitted Genital Ulcers**

Chancroid	Azithromycin *or* ceftriaxone or ciprofloxin
Herpes	Acyclovir
Syphilis	Benzathine penicillin G IM
Lymphogranuloma venereum	Doxycline
Granuloma inguinale	Doxycline *or* Trimethoprim/sulfamethoxazole

- Lesions can be swabbed and cultured for bacterial and viral identification.
- Chlamydia can also be diagnosed via nucleic acid amplification testing of swab, lymph node aspirate, and urethral or urine samples.
- Special Chlamydia typing is required to verify strain.

TREATMENT

- Antibiotics: For STD-associated genital ulcers (see Table 18.10)

EPIDIDYMITIS

Inflammation or infection of the epididymis, epididymitis is due to retrograde (**not** hematogenous) spread of bacteria and may spread to involve the testicle (**epididymo-orchitis**). Common etiologic organisms vary with age. Less commonly, syphilis and TB may be associated with epididymitis.

- **Prepubertal boys:** Infection with Gram-negative bacteria due to congenital structural urinary tract pathology
- **Men <35 years:** *Chlamydia* and N. *gonorrhea*
- **Men ≥35 years:** Gram-negative organisms, predominantly *E. coli*

SYMPTOMS

- Gradual onset of pain that may begin in the flank or suprapubic area and progress to scrotal pain.
- Fevers/chills
- Dysuria, urgency, frequency

EXAM

- Swollen, tender epididymis
- **Prehn sign**: Relief with elevation of the scrotum
- Whole testicle may be swollen if associated orchitis
- Cremasteric reflex is present.

DIAGNOSIS

- Mostly clinical
- Urine culture if prepubertal or over 35 years
- Urethral swab if under 35 years
- Ultrasound to rule out torsion, as indicated

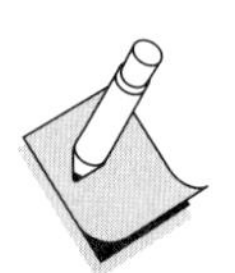

Epididymitis exam findings:
Swollen tender epididymis
Relief with elevation of scrotum (Prehn sign)
Normal cremasteric reflex

TREATMENT

- Supportive care with analgesia, bed rest, elevation of scrotum
- Antibiotics
  - **Prepubertal boys**: Augmentin or trimethoprim/sulfamethoxazole
  - **Men <35 years**: Ceftriaxone and doxycycline
  - **Men ≥35 years**: Fluoroquinolone
- Referral to urologist
- Criteria for admission:
  - Immunocompromised
  - Intractable pain
  - Complicating abscess
  - Failure of therapy
  - Bacteremia
  - Bilateral involvement

ORCHITIS

Orchitis is an acute infection involving the testis. It most commonly is due to secondary spread of bacterial epididymitis (see above) but may be viral in nature, most commonly due to mumps. Orchitis is typically unilateral (even viral).

SYMPTOMS/EXAM

- Testicular pain, swelling, and tenderness
- Pain may be out of proportion to exam findings
- Fevers/chills
- If mump related, may be associated with parotitis and other nonspecific viral symptoms

DIAGNOSIS

- As with epididymitis, above

TREATMENT

- If viral, supportive therapy only
- If bacterial, treat as above for epididymitis.

A 19-year-old male is crossing his campus to class and experiences sudden onset of L flank and testicular pain. He has a history of kidney stones and reports that this pain is as severe as with previous kidney stones. On presentation to the ED, he has minimal costovertebral angle tenderness, minimal left lower quadrant tenderness, and a diffusely tender L testicle with loss of cremasteric reflex. What is the first test that should be ordered?

Testicular ultrasound with Doppler. Obtain immediate urologic consultation. Although testicular torsion usually occurs following strenuous activity, it may occur after minimal exertion or even during sleep. Pain is usually severe and felt in the left lower quadrant, inguinal canal, or testes. On examination, the involved testis is usually firm and tender and rides higher than the unaffected testicle.

TESTICULAR TORSION

The tunica vaginalis normally surrounds the testicle and attaches to the scrotal wall and epididymis posteriorly, anchoring the testicle in place. In patients at risk for testicular torsion, the tunica vaginalis attaches higher up on the spermatic cord, leaving a redundant spermatic cord and a mobile testicle (*bell-clapper deformity*). Torsion occurs with twisting of the testicle on the spermatic cord resulting in venous, or rarely, arterial occlusion. This results in rapid swelling and edema of the testis.

SYMPTOMS

- May occur at any age, but peaks in the first year of life and at puberty
- About half may report similar pain that resolved spontaneously.
- Severe onset of unilateral testicular pain that occurs with trauma, strenuous activity, or sleep
- Nausea/vomiting, abdominal pain
- Urgency, frequency, and dysuria

EXAM

- Elevated (or **"high-riding"**) testicle with a **transverse lie**
- **Loss of the cremasteric reflex**
- Tender, firm, swollen testicle
- Prehn sign (relief of pain with elevation of testicle) is *not* reliable in differentiating torsion from epidymitis.
- Bell-clapper deformity (horizontal lie) of contralateral testicle

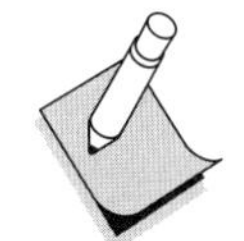

The loss of the cremasteric reflex is the most accurate sign of testicular torsion.

DIAGNOSIS

- Torsion is a clinical diagnosis, but if this diagnosis is equivocal, Doppler ultrasound or radionuclide scanning can be used to evaluate blood flow to the testicle.

TREATMENT

- Immediate urology consult
- Supportive care with analgesia
- Attempt manual detorsion (medial to lateral twisting or "open-book") method.
- Definitive surgical intervention with exploration and possible orchiopexy

A 60-year-old diabetic male presents to the ER complaining of 2 days of scrotal pain. On examination, the patient has tenderness to palpation of the underside of the scrotum and the perineum, with slight erythema. The patient's pain seems out of proportion to his physical exam findings, and the nurse is concerned that he may be drug-seeking. What diagnosis should be strongly considered in this patient?

Fournier gangrene should be considered, especially in a diabetic male. The patient may complain of scrotal, rectal, or genitalia pain out of proportion to examination findings of warmth, erythema, and edema. Mortality in these patients is about 20%.

FOURNIER GANGRENE

Fournier gangrene is a rapidly progressing, necrotizing infection of the scrotum, penis, or perineum, sparing the testicles. It usually occurs secondary to direct spread from infections in the perirectal area, urogenital tract, or skin of the genitalia. Predominant organisms are *Bacteroides fragilis* and *E. coli*, but may also include streptococci, staphylococci, and Clostridia (rarely fungal or anaerobic). These infections occur most commonly in patients with diabetes, immunosuppression, obesity, malignancy, chronic steroid use, or chronic alcoholism.

Symptoms

- Scrotal pain or itching are early symptoms.
- Fever, malaise, and intense perineal swelling develop.

Exam

- Patients are often toxic appearing, with marked tachycardia.
- Hypotension is common.
- Involved skin is tender to palpation and may have crepitus, erythema, edema, or frank necrosis (see Figure 18.5).

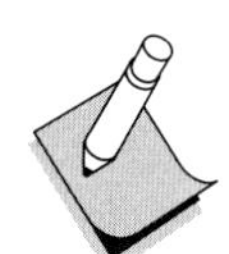

Definitive therapy for Fournier gangrene is wide surgical debridement.

Diagnosis

- With strong clinical suspicion, imaging only delays treatment.
- If the diagnosis is equivocal, CT or MRI scanning can be used to demonstrate fluid collections in deep fascial planes or gas within the tissue.

Treatment

- Aggressive supportive care
- Broad spectrum antibiotics: Imipenem-cilastin + vancomycin
- Emergent surgical debridement

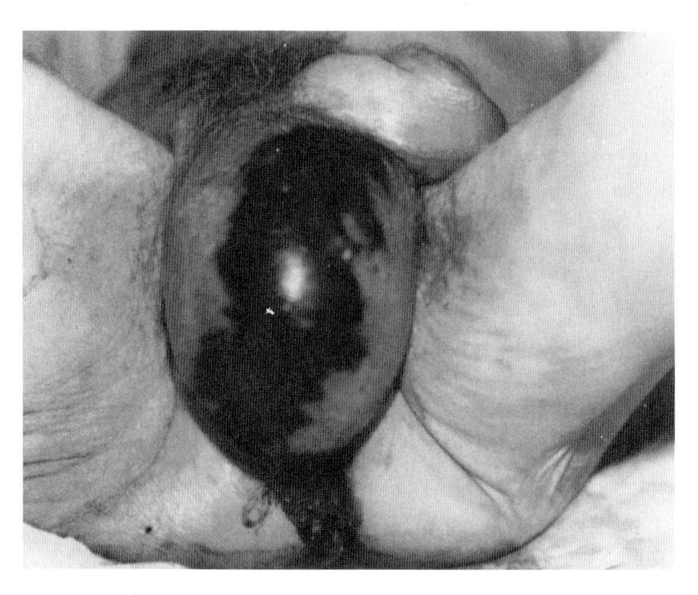

FIGURE 18.5. Fournier gangrene.

(Reproduced, with permission, from Tintinalli JE, Kelen GD, Stapczynski JS. *Emergency Medicine: A Comprehensive Study Guide*, 6th ed. New York: McGraw-Hill, 2004:615.)

BALANITIS/BALANOPOSTHITIS

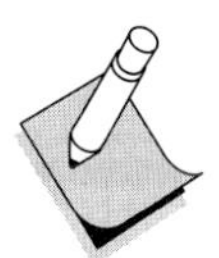

Balanitis = inflammation of the glans penis.

*Balanoposthitis = inflammation of the glans penis **and** foreskin.*

Most common cause = Candidal infection.

Results from inflammation of the glans penis (**balanitis**) or the glans and foreskin (**balanoposthitis**). The primary cause is infection, most commonly *Candida*. Contributing factors include diabetes, local trauma or irritation, contact dermatitis, poor hygiene.

SYMPTOMS/EXAM

- Pain, discharge, and itching are common symptoms.
- The glans may appear erythematous and tender to palpation.
- The foreskin may be adherent or may reveal foul or purulent discharge when retracted.

DIAGNOSIS

- The diagnosis is primarily clinical.
- KOH prep to identify *Candida* sp.
- D-stick to evaluate for diabetes

TREATMENT

- Improve hygiene.
- Apply topical antifungal ointment.
- Antibiotics (Keflex) if presence of cellulitis
- Treatment of diabetes or underlying immunosuppressive condition

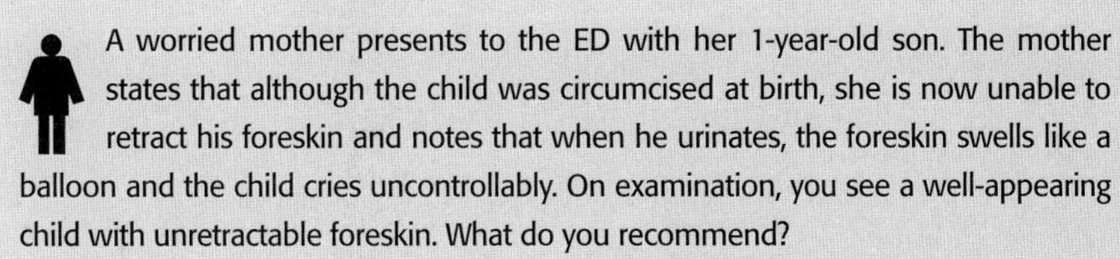

A worried mother presents to the ED with her 1-year-old son. The mother states that although the child was circumcised at birth, she is now unable to retract his foreskin and notes that when he urinates, the foreskin swells like a balloon and the child cries uncontrollably. On examination, you see a well-appearing child with unretractable foreskin. What do you recommend?

The child likely has a secondary phimosis. Daily cleaning of the foreskin and topical steroids are standard therapy in cases of phimosis. However, with ballooning of the foreskin upon voiding, revision of the circumcision is recommended.

PHIMOSIS

Phimosis is a constriction of the foreskin resulting in an inability to retract the prepuce over the glans. This is usually physiologic (resolves by age 4) but may occur as a result of trauma, infections, poor hygiene, or chemical irritation.

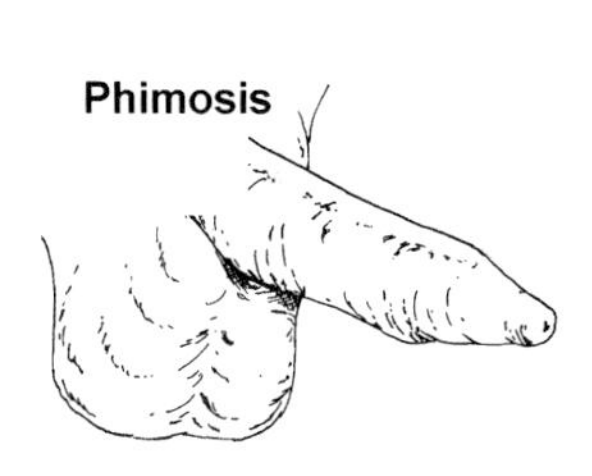

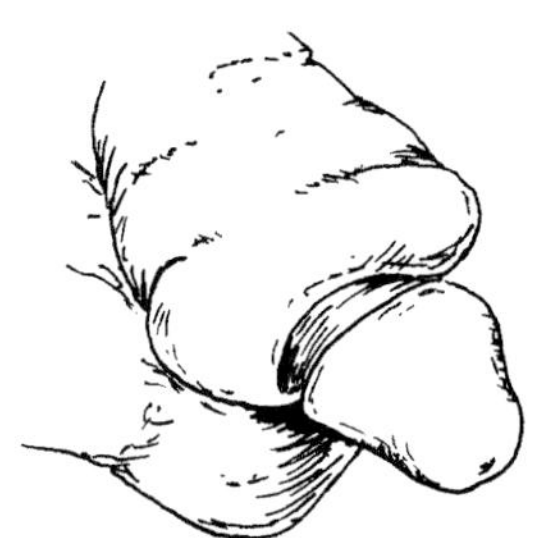

FIGURE 18.6. Phimosis and paraphimosis.

(Reproduced, with permission, from Tintinalli JE, Kelen GD, Stapczynski JS, *Emergency Medicine: A Comprehensive Study Guide*, 6th ed. New York: McGraw-Hill, 2004:615.)

SYMPTOMS/EXAM

- Pain at the penis, hematuria, abnormal urinary stream, bulging of the foreskin with urination
- Examination classically shows unretractable foreskin with occasional obstruction of the preputial meatus (see Figure 18.6).

DIAGNOSIS

- Diagnosis is based on clinical examination.

TREATMENT

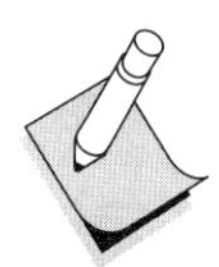

Phimosis Treatment

Daily cleaning of foreskin

Topical steroids

Immediate intervention if outlet obstruction or vascular compromise develops

- Gentle, but not forceful, retraction of the foreskin
- Improved hygiene
- Topical steroids for 4 to 6 weeks (very effective)
- Dilation of the meatus with forceps if signs of urinary outlet obstruction
- Dorsal split procedure or circumcision in cases of vascular compromise
- Admission for patients with urinary obstruction, evidence of systemic infection, or vascular compromise

PARAPHIMOSIS

Paraphimosis occurs when the proximal foreskin cannot be reduced distally over the glans penis, resulting in distal vascular congestion. This is a true urologic emergency.

SYMPTOMS/EXAM

- Patient often reports inability to replace foreskin back over glans (see Figure 18.6).
- Exam reveals a flaccid proximal penis with erythema and engorgement distal to the obstruction.

DIAGNOSIS

Diagnosis is largely based on clinical examination.

TREATMENT

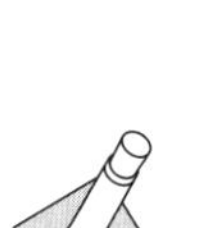

Paraphimosis is a true urologic emergency! Manual reduction with firm pressure for 5–10 minutes is the initial treatment.

- Supportive care with analgesia
- Dorsal penile nerve block as needed
- Manual reduction with firm pressure to the glans for 5–10 minutes to reduce edema and slide foreskin distally
- Dorsal slit procedure if manual reduction is unsuccessful
- Circumcision
- Admission for patients unable to void spontaneously

A 25-year-old male with history of schizophrenia presents to the ED with priapism. He was recently started on risperdal and has a history of cocaine use. On examination, the corpora cavernosa are rigid and tender with palpation. What is the most appropriate initial therapy?

This patient is presenting with low-flow (ischemic) priapism, likely related to risperdal and cocaine use. This is a true urologic emergency. Immediate intervention includes terbutaline (SQ or PO) and pseudoephedrine (PO) and immediate urologic consultation for corpus cavernosum aspiration and diluted phenylephrine injection.

PRIAPISM

The penis is composed of two corpora cavernosa and the corpus spongiosa surrounding the urethra. With normal erection the corpora cavernosa fill with well-oxygenated blood (which on blood gas analysis has the appearance of arterial blood).

Priapism is defined as persistent painful erection unrelated to stimulation or desire. Priapism is divided into two types: **Low-flow (ischemic) priapism** (most common) and **high-flow (nonischemic) priapism.**

Low-Flow (Ischemic) Priapism

Low-flow (ischemic) priapism occurs secondary to venous stasis and blood pooling in the corpora cavernosa with resulting ischemia. This type is **most common** and is a **true emergency.**

Predisposing Factors for Low-flow Priapism:

- **Sickle cell disease**
- **Malaria**
- **Cancer**
  - Leukemia, multiple myeloma
- **Illicit drug use**
  - Cocaine, ecstasy, marijuana
- **Medications**
  - Antihypertensives, anticoagulants, psychiatric medications
- **Penile injection for erectile dysfunction**
  - Phentolamine, prostaglandin

SYMPTOMS/EXAM

- The corpora cavernosa are *rigid and tender* with palpation.

DIAGNOSIS

- Primarily based on presence of predisposing factor and clinical exam
  - CBC may be used to screen for hematologic malignancy.
- Tests that may confirm diagnosis, if in question:
  - Corpus cavernosum blood gas showing hypercarbia, hypoxia, and acidosis
  - Ultrasound showing diminished cavernous blood flow

TREATMENT

- Emergent urology consult
- Supportive care with analgesia and ice packs to perineum; IV hydration
- Aspiration of the corpus cavernosum
- Injection of 1 mL of diluted phenylephrine (100–500 μg/mL) into the corpus cavernosum with repeated attempts q 3–5 minutes
- Terbutaline (SQ or PO) and pseudoephedrine (PO) have been used with some success and may be tried while preparing for aspiration/injection.
- Systemic treatment of underlying disorders

COMPLICATIONS

- Permanent erectile dysfunction

High-Flow (Nonischemic) Priapism

High-flow (nonischemic) priapism occurs secondary to unregulated corpora cavernosum arterial inflow.

RENAL AND GENITOURINARY EMERGENCIES

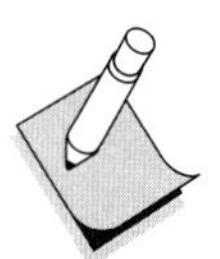

With high-flow (nonischemic) priapism the penis is semierect and painless. Observation alone is often effective.

SYMPTOMS/EXAM

- Predisposing factor: Recent history of straddle or groin injury, spinal cord lesions
- The penis is *semierect and painless.*
- Perineal compression with the thumb (blocking arterial inflow) may cause detumescence (**Piesis sign**).

DIAGNOSIS

- Rule out low-flow state, as above.

TREATMENT

- Urology consult
- Observation alone may be effective as there are few long-term consequences.
- Selective angiography to control arterial inflow
- Surgical ligation of fistula

PENILE FRACTURE

Rupture of the tunica albuginea surrounding the corpus cavernosum as a result of blunt trauma to the erect penis (see Figure 18.7)

SYMPTOMS/EXAM

- Patient reports a "snapping sound" followed by rapid detumescence.
- The penis appears swollen, deformed, tender, and discolored.

DIAGNOSIS

- Primarily clinical
- Retrograde urethrogram can be used to evaluate for associated urethral injury.

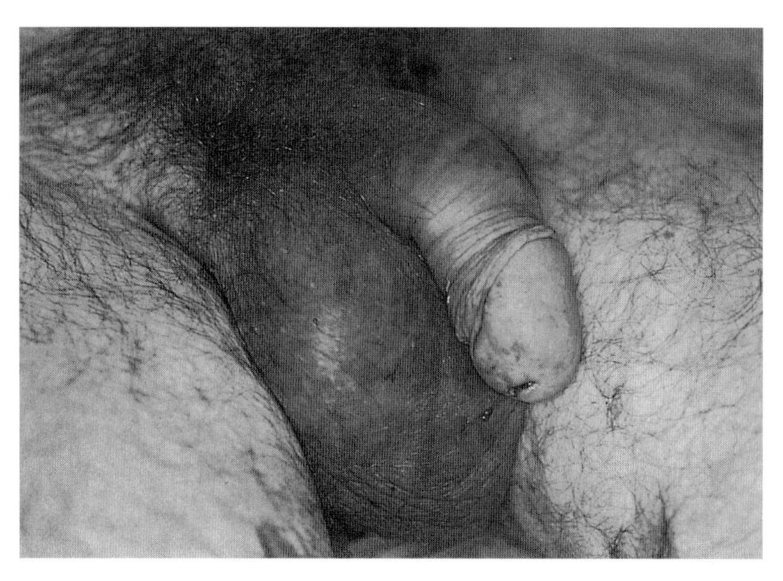

FIGURE 18.7. Penile fracture. Swollen, deformed, and discolored penis. (See also color insert.)

(Reproduced, with permission, from Knoop KJ, Stack LB, Storrow AB. *Atlas of Emergency Medicine*, 2nd ed. New York: McGraw-Hill, 2002:228.)

TREATMENT

- Supportive care with analgesia
- Suprapubic catheter if urinary drainage needed
- Immediate urologic consult for surgical repair

TESTICULAR MASSES

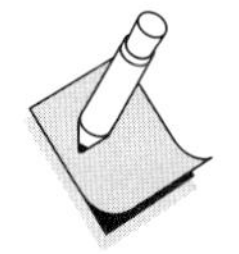

Hydroceles transilluminate with a homogenous glow.

Hydrocele

A collection of fluid in the tunica vaginalis. Communicating hydroceles occur when the processus vaginalis fails to obliterate and leaves a potential space between the peritoneum and scrotum. Noncommunicating hydroceles result from an imbalance between the production and absorption of fluid by the tunica vaginalis.

SYMPTOMS/EXAM

- Scrotal fullness, which may be accompanied by pain with palpation
- Transillumination may illustrate a homogenous glow without presence of shadows.

DIAGNOSIS

- Doppler ultrasound can be used to identify and determine the cause of hydrocele.

TREATMENT

- Supportive care
- Urology referral for possible surgical intervention

Varicocele

Varicocele is a collection of venous varicosities of the spermatic veins due to incomplete drainage of the pampiniform plexus. It is most common in adolescent males. Suspect IVC compression or thrombosis if R sided and obstruction of the L renal vein from renal cell carcinoma if L sided.

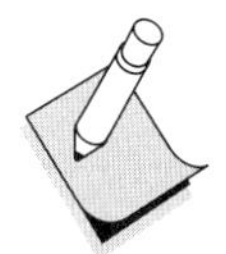

On examination varicoceles feel like a "bag of worms."

SYMPTOMS/EXAM

- Scrotal mass or swelling
- "Bag of worms" with examination and palpation superior and posterior to the testis

DIAGNOSIS

- Clinical examination with abdominal CT if suspected vascular compression

Tumors

Most commonly seminomas, but also may be embryonal cell cancer or teratoma

SYMPTOMS/EXAM

- Hallmark is *asymptomatic* testicular mass, firmness, or induration.
- Exam may show scrotal swelling or a palpable mass.

DIAGNOSIS

- Ultrasound can confirm the presence of a mass.

Painless testicular mass = cancer until proven otherwise.

TREATMENT

- Urgent urologic referral

Appendageal Torsion

The testicle has four appendages. Torsion of the **appendix testis** (90%) and the **appendix epididymis** (8%) account for virtually all cases of appendageal torsion. The appendix testis attaches to the upper pole of the testes and the appendix epididymis to the head of the epididymis. Appendageal torsion is most frequently seen in preadolescent boys.

SYMPTOMS

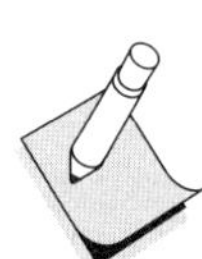

- Acute onset of scrotal pain with a discrete painful testicular or epididymal mass
- Less commonly, associated with nausea/vomiting, dysuria, urgency, or frequency

"Blue-dot sign" with transillumination of scrotal skin = appendageal torsion.

EXAM

- Tender and discrete scrotal "nodule"
- Blue-black dot when present with transillumination of the testicle (blue-dot sign) is pathognomonic (see Figure 18.8).

DIAGNOSIS

- Primarily clinical
- Doppler ultrasound and radionuclide scanning that illustrates decreased blood flow to the appendage

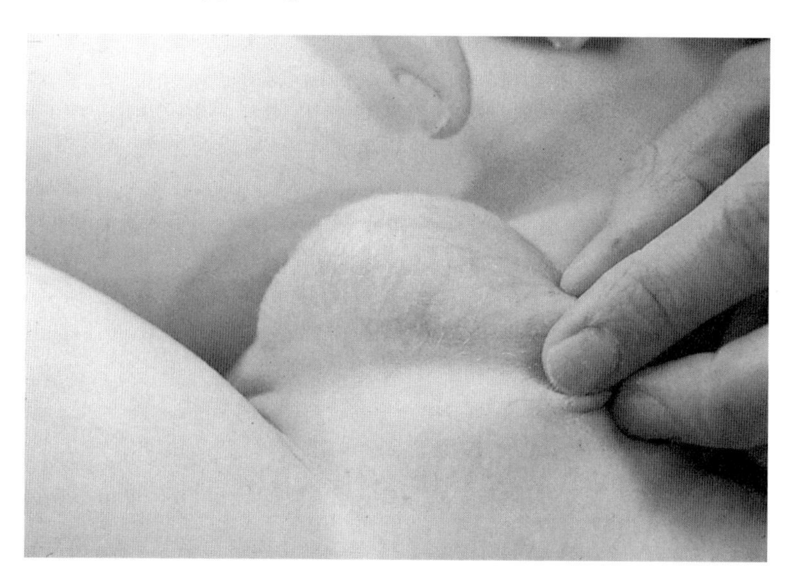

FIGURE 18.8. Blue-dot sign indicating appendageal torsion. (See also color insert.)

(Courtesy of Javier A. Gonzalez del Rey, MD as published in Knoop KJ, Stack LB, Storrow AB. *Atlas of Emergency Medicine*, 2nd ed. New York: McGraw-Hill, 2002:220.)

TREATMENT

- Supportive care only with analgesia, bed rest, scrotal elevation
- Surgical exploration in severe cases

Inguinal Hernia

Inguinal hernias peak in a bimodal distribution, before 1 year of age and then after age 40. They can be direct or indirect. A hernia is clinically significant when it becomes incarcerated (nonreducible) or strangulated.

Direct inguinal hernias protrude DIRECTLY through the transversalis fascia and external ring.

INDIRECT INGUINAL HERNIA

- Protrudes through the internal ring, *lateral* to the inferior epigastric vessels due to a congenitally patent processus vaginalis

DIRECT INGUINAL HERNIA

- Protrudes directly through the transversalis fascia and the external inguinal ring *medial* to the inferior epigastric vessels
- Are acquired hernias

SYMPTOMS/EXAM

- Often asymptomatic
- Pain and tenderness if incarceration occurs
- Nausea and vomiting if resultant bowel obstruction
- More toxic appearance with peritonitis or shock if strangulation develops

DIFFERENTIAL

- Includes femoral hernia, testicular torsion, testicular tumor, hydrocele

DIAGNOSIS

- Typically a clinical diagnosis
- Abdominal radiographs if obstruction or perforation is suspected

TREATMENT

- Incarcerated hernia should be reduced via Trendelenberg position, sedation, and gentle pressure.
- A nonreducible hernia or suspicion of strangulation warrants immediate surgical consultation.
- Inguinal hernias in infants and children have a higher risk of incarceration and should be repaired shortly after diagnosis is made.

ACUTE URINARY RETENTION

Acute urinary retention is defined as the sudden inability to pass urine. May be caused by obstruction, neurogenic causes, or medications (see Table 18.11).

SYMPTOMS

- Abdominal discomfort and distention (unless neurogenic)
- Hesitancy, decreased force of stream, straining with voiding, sensation of incomplete emptying in patients with obstructive etiology
- Dysuria, urgency, frequency, or discharge with infection

TABLE 18.11. Causes of Acute Urinary Retention

Penile obstruction	Meatal stenosis Paraphimosis Phimosis
Urethral obstruction	Foreign body Hematoma Severe urethritis Stricture Tumor
Prostate obstruction	BPH Cancer Severe prostatitis
Neurogenic causes	Diabetes Multiple sclerosis Cauda equina syndrome
Medications	α-Adrenergic agents Antihistamines Anticholinergics Antispasmodics TCAs

EXAM

- Findings vary with cause of obstruction (eg, enlarged prostate c/w BPH).
- Abdominal tenderness
- Palpable bladder (if containing > 150 mL)

DIAGNOSIS

- UA to evaluate infection, tumor, calculi
- BUN and creatinine to evaluate renal function

TREATMENT

- Supportive care with analgesia
- Placement of a 16- or 18-inch French urethral catheter or Coudé catheter
  - Do **not** clamp catheter.
- Bladder aspiration if Foley catheter cannot be placed and urology consultant is unavailable
- Observation of patients with chronic retention for the development of postobstructive diuresis (4–6 hours)
- Discharge with catheter in place and follow up with urology.
- Antibiotics for infection, as needed
- Avoidance of offending drug or surgical treatment of obstruction as indicated

CHAPTER 19

Procedures and Skills

Ana Paola Uranga, MD, MBA

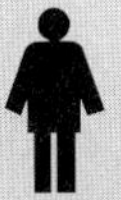

A patient with breast cancer presents with a BP of 60/30, muffled heart sounds, and distended neck veins. Cardiac monitor shows electrical alternans. Which diagnostic test is indicated? Which therapeutic intervention follows?

Cardiac ultrasonography to confirm pericardial effusion followed by pericardiocentesis.

Pericardiocentesis

INDICATIONS

- Hemopericardium
- Pericardial effusion with tamponade
- Pneumopericardium

CONTRAINDICATIONS

- Relative: Immediately available definitive treatment modalities, ie, pericardial window

TECHNIQUE

- Use ultrasound guidance when available to identify greatest fluid collection.
- Cardiac monitoring with defibrillator on hand during procedure
- 7.5- to 12.5-cm 18-Ga needle or Intracath needle should be used.
- Parasternal approach: Needle is inserted perpendicular to the skin in the left fifth intercostal space. Insertion either just lateral to the sternum or 3–4 cm from the sternum should be used to avoid injury to the internal mammilary artery.
- **Subxyphoid approach:** Needle is inserted between the xyphoid process and the left costal margin at a 30–45° angle to the skin aiming toward the left shoulder (see Figure 19.1).
- Parasternal approach has less chance of injury to right atrium but more chance of lung injury compared to subxyphoid approach. During "blind" pericardiocentesis, the subxyphoid approach is recommended.
- An ECG lead attached to the needle will show a current of injury (typically ST elevation) when the needle touches the ventricular wall. When this occurs, withdraw the needle until the injury pattern is no longer present.
- Needle will penetrate the pericardium about 6–8 cm beneath the skin in adults and <5 cm in children.
- Obtain CXR to evaluate for pneumothorax.

COMPLICATIONS

- Failure to yield fluid ("dry tap")
- Myocardial injury possibly leading to hemopericardium
- **Coronary vessel laceration leading to myocardial infarction and/or hemopericardium**
- Dysrhythmia
- Pneumothorax
- Pneumoperitoneum

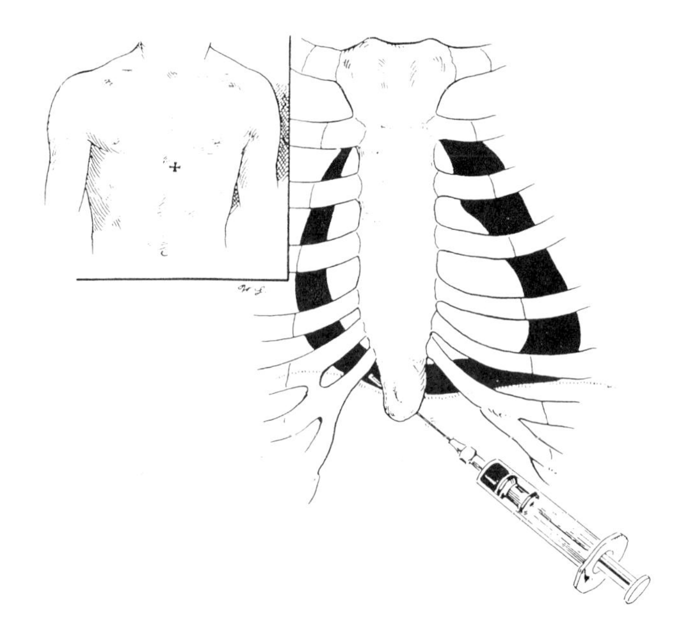

FIGURE 19.1. Subxyphoid approach for pericardiocentesis.

(Reproduced, with permission, from Wilson RF. Injury to the heart and great vessels. In: Henning RS, ed. *Critical Care Cardiology*. New York: Churchill Livingstone, 1989.)

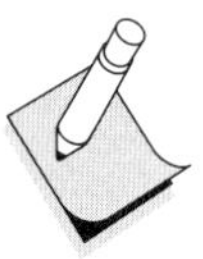

Cardiac tamponade is one of the five Hs and five Ts that represent the most common and potentially ***treatable causes of PEA****.*

INTERPRETATION OF RESULTS

- Removal of even 30–50 mL may result in marked clinical improvement.
- Except in trauma or ventricular wall rupture, pericardial fluid should have a lower hematocrit than venous blood, otherwise suspect that the needle has entered a cardiac chamber (most likely the right ventricle).
- Injection of a small amount of contrast under fluoroscopy can disclose intracardiac placement.

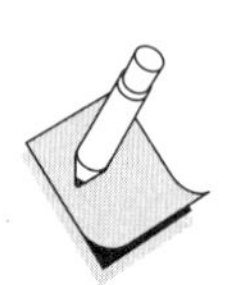

The intercostal neurovascular bundle underlies each rib. During thoracentesis or thoracostomy, ***enter the chest just above the rib*** *to avoid the neurovascular bundle.*

Thoracentesis

INDICATIONS

- Evacuation of air: Anterior approach
  - Temporary treatment of tension pneumothorax
  - Treatment of stable pneumothorax
- Evacuation of fluid: Posterior approach
  - Analysis of pleural effusion
  - Treatment of symptomatic pleural effusion or tension hydrothorax

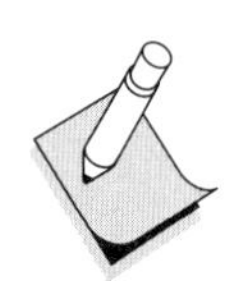

A tension pneumothorax is treated with either immediate thoracostomy or with thoracentesis ("needle decompression") followed by thoracostomy.

CONTRAINDICATIONS

- Absolute: Needle insertion through an infected area
- Relative: Readily available tube thoracostomy if needed
- Bleeding diatheses or on anticoagulants when treating stable PTX

TECHNIQUE

- Evacuation of air: Anterior approach
  - Patient supine, head elevated 30°
  - 14- to 18-Ga needle with or without catheter

  - Needle is inserted in second intercostal space, midclavicular line over third rib to avoid nerve/vessel damage.
  - Rush of air will confirm placement, catheter, if used, can be advanced over needle.
  - Attach to one-way drainage system to prevent pneumothorax reaccumulation.
    - Sterile glove finger can be used as a one-way valve tied to needle at one end with small hole on other end.
- Evacuation of fluid: Posterior approach
  - Patient sitting upright:
    - 18- to 22-Ga needle is inserted at midscapular line or posterior axillary line below the top of the fluid determined by percussion, but not below eight intercostal space. Catheter (if used) is then advanced.
  - Patient supine with head elevated:
    - 18- to 22-Ga needle is inserted at midaxillary or posterior axillary line in the fourth or fifth intercostal space.

COMPLICATIONS

- Pneumothorax
- Diaphragmatic, liver, intercostal nerve/vessel, or spleen injury

INTERPRETATION OF RESULTS

- For diagnostic thoracentesis, send for LDH, glucose, protein, cell count, and differential.
- If needed, send for amylase, triglyceride level, cholesterol, complement, RF, CEA, G-stain, cultures, AFB, fungal cultures, cytology, pH.
- Exudate: Inflammation causing increased capillary permeability (pneumonia, TB, CA, other)
  - Fluid/plasma protein >0.5
  - Fluid/plasma LDH >0.6
  - Fluid LDH >200 IU/mL
  - Fluid protein >3 g/dL
  - Specific gravity >1.016
- Transudate: Ultrafiltrates of plasma through intact capillaries (CHF, cirrhosis, hypoproteinemia, other)
  - Fluid/plasma protein <0.5
  - Fluid/plasma LDH <0.6
  - Fluid LDH <200 IU/mL
  - Fluid protein <3 g/dL
  - Specific gravity <1.016

Thoracostomy Tube

INDICATIONS

- Pneumothorax
- Hemothorax
- Hemopneumothorax

CONTRAINDICATIONS

- Relative:
  - Adhesions/blebs
  - Recurrent pneumothorax
  - Need for open thoracotomy
  - Bleeding diathesis

Technique

- Head of bed is elevated 30–60°.
- Arm should be secured over patient's head.
- Local anesthesia and procedural sedation should be used.
- 2- to 4-cm incision is made at fourth or fifth intercostal space, midaxillary line (see Figure 19.2A).
- Blunt dissection is performed with long closed Kelly clamp above rib to avoid nerve/vessel damage (see Figure 19.2B).
- Place finger through hole and feel for lung to confirm you've entered the pleural space. This key step increases the likelihood that the tube will enter the pleural space. (See Figure 19.2C.)
- Use finger to guide tip of Kelly-clamped chest tube into pleural space.
- Insert chest tube posteriorly and toward lung apex (see Figure 19.2D).
- Connect to regulated suction (typically beginning at 20 cm H_2O).
- Secure with sutures (0 or 1-0 silk), gauze, and tape.
- Confirm placement with CXR.

Complications

- Diaphragm, spleen, lung, cardiac, vascular, or liver injury
- Subcutaneous placement of chest tube

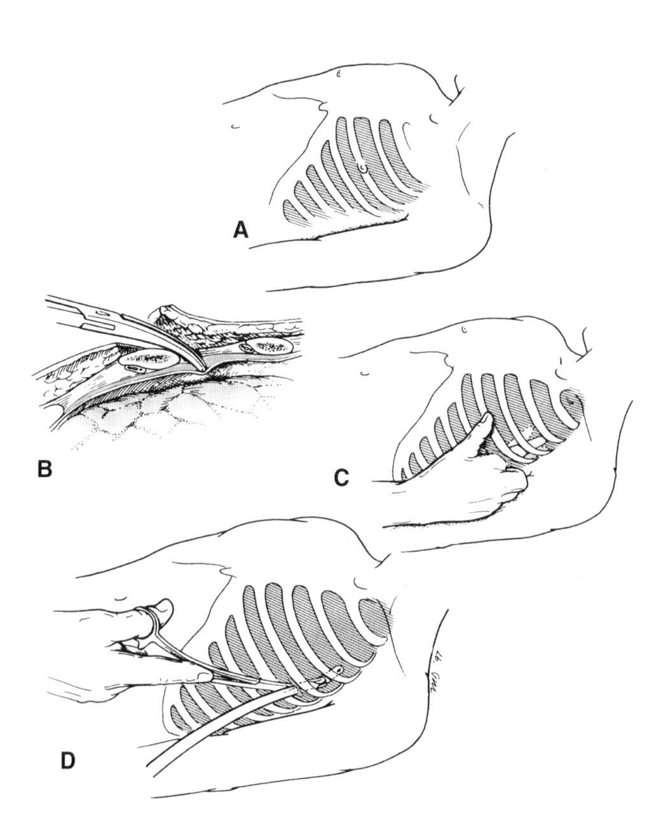

FIGURE 19.2. (A) Site of thoracostomy tube insertion. (B) Blunt dissection with Kelly clamp. (C) Finger confirmation of hole into pleura. (C) Insertion of thoracostomy tube.

(Reproduced, with permission, from Brunicardi FC, Andersen DK, Billiar TR, Dunn DL, Hunter JG, Matthews JB, Pollock RE, Schwartz SI. *Schwartz's Principles of Surgery*, 8th ed. McGraw-Hill, 2005:131.)

INTERPRETATION OF RESULTS

- Air return (rush) confirms pneumothorax.
- Blood return confirms hemothorax, as long as the blood is coming from the pleural space.
- An air leak is either due to significant air movement from the lung into the pleural space or a leak in the tubing. Temporarily clamp the tube near to the chest—if the leak persists, it is in the tubing not the patient.

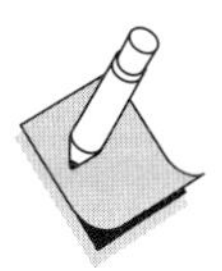

Don't advance a chest tube after it's been placed—it's better to place another tube than risk introducing bacteria into the chest.

Emergency Department Thoracotomy

INDICATIONS

- Patients with **penetrating chest or abdominal trauma** who are pulseless but have electrical cardiac activity may benefit.
- Blunt trauma patients with vital signs in the field and organized electrical activity in the ED may benefit from ED thoracotomy.
- Goals are to relieve cardiac tamponade, cross-clamp descending aorta for control of abdominal hemorrhage, control hemorrhage from heart or great vessels, and provide effective cardiac compressions.

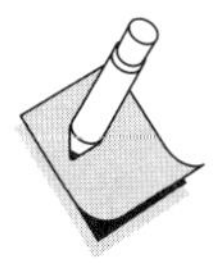

Don't clamp a chest tube except to look for an air leak—clamping a chest tube exposes the patient to the risk of tension pneumothorax.

CONTRAINDICATIONS

- Blunt trauma patients who require over 15 minutes of prehospital CPR and any trauma patient who is apneic, pulseless, and in asystole are unlikely to benefit from this intervention.

TECHNIQUE

- Patient should be intubated and, if possible, analgesia and deep sedation should be provided.
- NGT should be placed to help differentiate esophagus from aorta.
- Incision using No. 20 blade is made into the left chest between fourth and fifth ribs: Just inferior to the nipple in men or along the inframammary fold in women (see Figure 19.3A).
- Incision extends from sternum to posterior axillary line cutting down through pectoralis and serratus muscles.
- Once the pleural space is entered, ventilations are temporarily stopped to allow the lung to collapse away from chest wall.
- Place chest wall retractor (rib spreader) to spread ribs. The crank should be placed laterally, so that the incision can be extended across the sternum into the right chest if necessary.
- If exam suggests any possibility of tamponade, perform pericardiotomy: Lift pericardial sac near diaphragm with forceps, make a small incision with scissors, and extend the incision cephalad along anterior pericardium **parallel to the phrenic nerve** (see Figure 19.3B).
- Aortic cross-clamping used when SBP <70 mm Hg: Identify aorta which lies anterior to vertebral column. Place a vascular clamp around the aorta or occlude aorta with digital pressure (see Figure 19.3B).
- Retract pericardium to examine heart for injury and repair with staples or sutures (see Figure 19.3C).

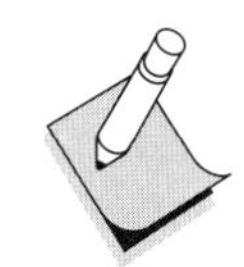

Typically, operative treatment of bleeding is required in patients with initial chest tube blood loss of >1500 mL or >200–300 mL/hour thereafter.

COMPLICATIONS

- Injury to intrathoracic structures (internal mammilary artery, phrenic nerve, coronary arteries, aorta, esophagus)
- Ischemia of spinal cord, liver, bowel, and kidneys with cross clamping aorta or of cerebral hemorrhage or LVF if pressure elevation is excessive

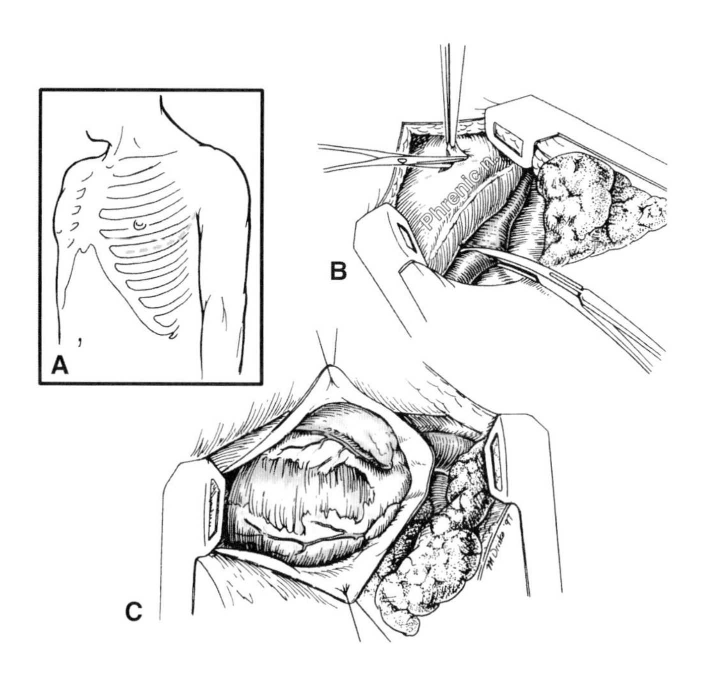

FIGURE 19.3. (A) Site of incision for thoracotomy. (B) Clamping of descending thoracic aorta and site of pericardial window. (C) Visualization of the heart for repairs.

(Reproduced, with permission, from Brunicardi FC, Andersen DK, Billiar TR, et al. *Schwartz's Principles of Surgery*, 8th ed. New York: McGraw-Hill, 2005:134.)

The ideal candidate for ED thoracotomy is a victim of a stab wound to the anterior chest or abdomen who arrests after arriving in the ED due to cardiac tamponade. Get into the chest and relieve the tamponade. If the patient regains a pulse, sedate the patient—this hurts!

- Infection
- Injury or disease transmission to healthcare workers.

INTERPRETATION OF RESULTS

- SBP after the first 30 minutes of resuscitation predicts outcome. Patients with SBP >110 mm Hg within 30 minutes have good survival rates and neurologic outcomes. Those with SBP >85 mm Hg will likely have brain damage, and those with SBP <70 mm Hg will likely not survive.

A woman with a family history of sudden cardiac death presents following a syncopal episode. ECG shows intermittent polymorphic ventricular tachycardia and a QT interval of 600 milliseconds. What is the rhythm disturbance? Which treatments are indicated?

Torsades de pointes. Treat with intravenous magnesium. Consider overdrive pacing at 140 bpm.

Transcutaneous Cardiac Pacing

INDICATIONS

- Treatment of hemodynamically unstable bradydysrhythmias that have not responded to atropine
- Initial stabilization of the patient in the ED while arranging for transvenous pacemaker

- May be used to treat refractory tachydysrhythmias by overdrive pacing
- May be preferable to transvenous pacing in patients who have received thrombolytic agents

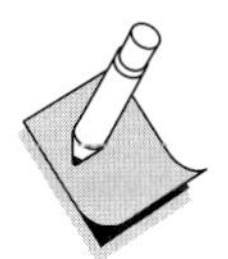

With transcutaneous pacing, increase to 40 to 60 mA to get capture. With transvenous pacing, get capture at 5 mA, then decrease the amps. Once you lose capture, increase by 2.5 times to ensure consistent capture.

CONTRAINDICATIONS

- In conscious patients with hemodynamically stable bradycardias, transcutaneous pacing is unnecessary.

TECHNIQUE

- The anterior electrode is placed at the point of maximal impulse on the left chest wall. The second electrode is placed directly posterior to the anterior electrode.
- Set the rate to 60–70 bpm. Then slowly increase the output current from the minimal setting until capture is achieved on ECG monitor, usually 42–60 mA.

COMPLICATIONS

- Dysrhythmia induction
- Soft tissue discomfort with the potential for injury

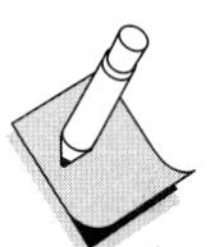

When pacing, always confirm electrical capture seen on the monitor by palpating a pulse. Electrical capture without a pulse equals PEA.

INTERPRETATION OF RESULTS

- Feel for a pulse and check BP to confirm that the electrical capture seen on the monitor results in improved perfusion.

Transvenous Cardiac Pacing

INDICATIONS

- Bradycardias: Sick sinus syndrome, second- and third-degree heart block, atrial fibrillation with symptomatic slow ventricular response, pacemaker malfunction
- Tachycardias: Supraventricular dysrhythmias, ventricular dysrhythmias

CONTRAINDICATIONS

- Bradycardic, hypothermic patients should be rewarmed first, then paced if condition does not improve.

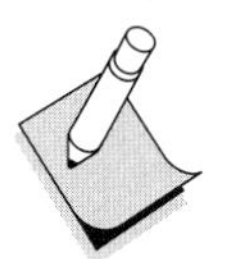

When a magnet is placed over a permanent pacemaker, the pacemaker will temporarily revert to an asynchronous, fixed-rated pacing usually at a rate of 60 bpm.

TECHNIQUE

- Pacemakers can be placed through brachial, subclavian, femoral, or internal jugular veins.
- Patient should be connected to an ECG machine and pacemaker to record chest V lead. The distal terminal of pacing catheter (negative or "–" lead) must be connected to the V lead of the ECG machine to be used as an intracardiac exploring electrode
- Introducer sheath is passed over the guidewire, then pacing wire is inserted about 10–12 cm into selected vein. If a balloon-tipped catheter is used, the balloon is inflated after the catheter enters the SVC.
- Lidocaine may be needed to desensitize the myocardium from catheter induced ectopy.
- The ECG recorded from the electrode tip localizes the position of the tip of the pacing electrode. The ECG complex varies depending on which chamber is entered, with negative forces seen when the catheter tip is above the atrium and diminished amplitude seen if the catheter tip enters the IVC or the pulmonary artery.

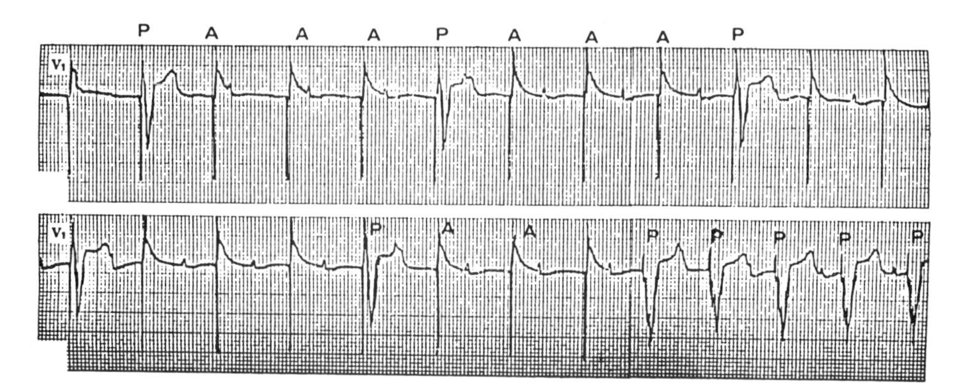

FIGURE 19.4. Pacing with intermittent capture. "P" indicates paced beats; "A" indicates pacer artifact without capture.

(Reproduced, with permission, from Tintinalli JE, Kelen GD, Stapczynski JS. *Tintinalli's Emergency Medicine: A Comprehensive Study Guide*, 6th ed. New York: McGraw-Hill, 2004:136.)

- Once ventricular endocardial contact is made, the catheter is disconnected from the ECG machine and connected to the pacing generator. Set to a rate of 80 bpm, or 10 bpm faster than underlying ventricular rhythm. If capture does not occur, the pacer must be repositioned.
- Testing threshold (the minimum current necessary to obtain capture) is ideally < 1.0 mA and usually between 0.3 and 0.7 mA. Set to 5 mA and reduce until capture is lost; this threshold amperage is increased by 2.5 times to ensure consistent capture (usually between 2 and 3 mA).
- Introducer sheath is then removed and catheter secured to the skin. CXR and ECG are obtained for evaluation of placement/capture.

COMPLICATIONS

- Inconsistent pacing, infection, pneumothorax, arterial puncture, arrhythmias, perforations, pulmonary embolism, bleeding, DVT
- In general, transvenous pacemakers fire automatically at a controllable rate. They do not have an atrial lead and do not have a sensing component, so they do not suffer from the problems of oversensing or undersensing.

INTERPRETATION OF RESULTS

- Appropriate pacing and CXR indicate proper placement. If the catheter is within the right ventricle, a left bundle-branch pattern with left axis deviation should be evident in paced beats (see Figure 19.4).

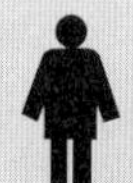

While you're placing a subclavian line your patient becomes agitated, hypoxic, tachycardic, and hypotensive. CXR shows Westermark sign (focal oligemia). What's the diagnosis? Treatment?

Air embolism. Clamp the central line. Reposition the tip of the line 2 cm below SVC-RA junction and aspirate. Place the patient in left lateral decubitus position and Trendelenburg. Consider hyperbaric therapy.

Central Venous Catheterization

Indications

- Need for CVP monitoring
- Need for rapid volume resuscitation
- Need for emergent venous access
- Need for nonemergent venous access in patients with poor or no peripheral access
- Need to infuse hyperalimentation or other concentrated solutions
- Need for emergent hemodyalisis

Contraindications

- Relative:
  - Distorted local anatomy or landmarks or previous radiation therapy
  - Cellulitis, burns, abrasions over insertion site
  - Suspected proximal vascular injury
  - Bleeding disorders or patient on anticoagulants

Technique

- Use strict sterile technique to reduce infectious complications.
- Seldinger (guidewire) technique: Thin-walled needle is used to introduce a guidewire into the vessel lumen. A catheter is placed over the guidewire and once it is in place, the guidewire is removed.
- Ultrasound guidance is strongly recommended for the IJ approach and may be useful for femoral approach. It is also useful for obese patients and patients with a history of multiple access at that site. The use of ultrasound has been shown to increase the rate of successful first puncture, increase patient satisfaction, decrease the number of attempts, decrease the time to perform the procedure, and lower the complication rate.
- Subclavian: Patient is placed in **Trendelenberg position**. Vein lies posterior to the medial third of the clavicle. Aim needle toward suprasternal notch. Vein is entered at a depth of 3–4 cm (see Figure 19.5).
- Internal jugular: Patient is placed in Trendelenberg position and head is turned slightly away from puncture site. The vein usually lies anterior and lateral of the carotid artery just deep to the SCM muscle at the level of the thyroid cartilage. Vein can be accessed medial to the SCM aiming toward ipsilateral nipple (anterior approach), lateral to the SCM aiming towards sternoclavicular notch (posterior approach), and between the sternal and clavicular heads of the SCM (central approach) (see Figure 19.5).
- Femoral: Patient is supine. Vein lies medial to femoral artery below the inguinal ligament. Palpate femoral pulse and place needle just medial to it below inguinal ligament.

During IJ central line insertion, ultrasound helps you find the internal jugular vein and avoid the common carotid artery.

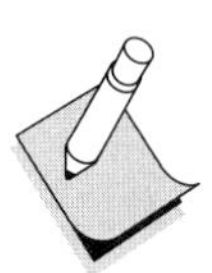

For IJ and subclavian lines, use Trendelenburg to increase intrathoracic pressure and decrease the risk of an air embolism.

Complications

- Pneumothorax, hydrothorax (higher with SC access)
- Vein or artery laceration, bleeding/hematomas that can compress airway (IJ)
- Arterial puncture (higher with IJ access)
- Air embolism
- Infections (higher with femoral vein access)
- Dysrhythmias

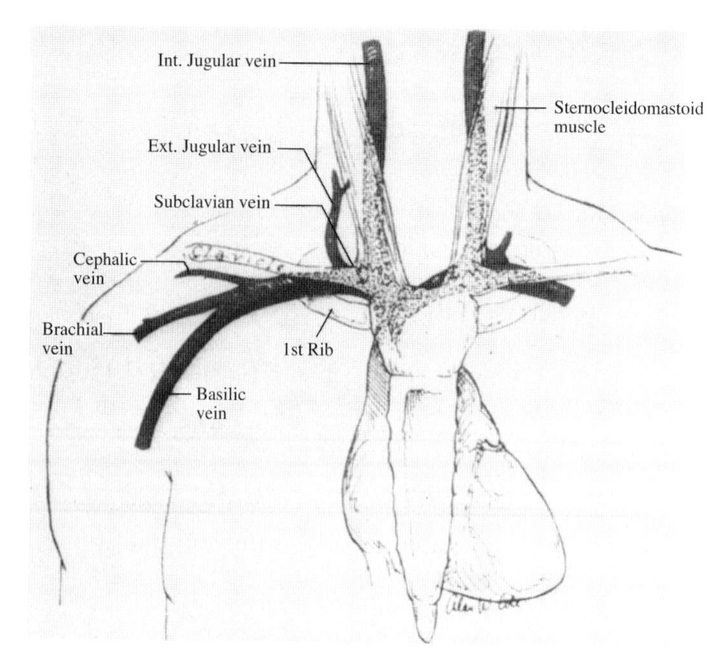

FIGURE 19.5. Anatomy of thoracic veins.

(Reproduced, with permission, from Tintinalli JE, Kelen GD, Stapczynski JS. *Tintinalli's Emergency Medicine: A Comprehensive Study Guide*, 6th ed. New York: McGraw-Hill, 2004:126.)

Interpretation of Results

- The return of pulsatile flow signifies arterial puncture.
- Dysrhythmias signal irritation of atria or ventricles. Guidewires and catheters should be pulled back until dysrhythmias stop.
- Vein has been entered successfully when a flashback of dark venous blood that flows freely into the syringe is obtained.
- CXR will show appropriate placement of subclavian and internal jugular catheterization.

Venous Cutdown

Indications

- Inability to access peripheral veins, including scalp veins in infants
- Emergent access as well as long-term venous access

Contraindications

- Less invasive alternatives are available.
- Infection over site or injury proximal to cutdown site

Technique

- Greater saphenous vein can be accessed:
  - At the ankle, 1 cm anterior to the medial maleolus
  - At the knee, 1–4 cm below the knee and immediately posterior to the tibia
  - Below the femoral triangle, 3–4 cm distal to the inguinal ligament, the saphenous vein is easily isolated from the surrounding fat.
- Basilic vein is generally cannulated at the antecubital fossa 2 cm above and 1–3 cm lateral to the medial epicondyle on the anterior surface of the upper arm.

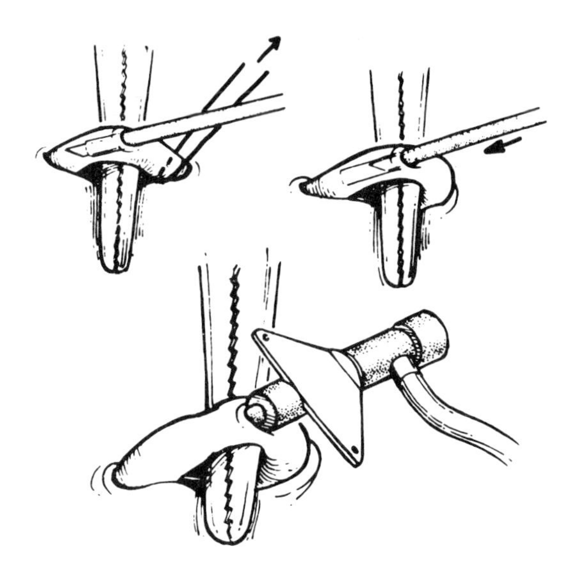

FIGURE 19.6. Venous cutdown technique.

(Reproduced, with permission, from Tintinalli JE, Kelen GD, Stapczynski JS. *Tintinalli's Emergency Medicine: A Comprehensive Study Guide*, 6th ed. New York: McGraw-Hill, 2004:130.)

- Cephalic vein can be accessed in the antecubital fossa at the distal flexor crease.
- External jugular vein is superficially located on the SCM muscle. This is not recommended as a first-line venesection site because potential airway management problems, risk of injury to the greater auricular nerve, cervical spine immobilization frequently prohibits access to the area, and it is potentially a hazardous procedure in the uncooperative patient.
- Tourniquet placed proximal to cutdown site. A skin incision is made perpendicular to vein's course and vein is exposed with blunt dissection. A tie is placed distally. Vein is then incised until lumen is entered. Over-the-needle catheter is placed through incision. Ties are removed, incision is closed and catheter is sutured in place and dressed (see Figure 19.6).

Complications

- Local hematoma, infection, embolization, wound dehiscence, and injury to adjacent structures

Interpretation of Results

- Vein has been successfully entered when a flashback of dark, free flowing venous blood is seen.

Intraosseous Infusion

Indications

- Need for emergent, rapid vascular access when venous access is not available, especially in children, infants, or newborns

A bone with an interruption in the cortex (ie, fracture, recent prior intraosseous site, or placement of intraosseous needle through the entire bone) should not be used for intraosseous infusion.

CONTRAINDICATIONS

- Osteoporosis and osteogenesis imperfecta increase fracture risk.
- Fractured bone leads to extravasation of infused fluid (an absolute contraindication).
- Recent prior use of the same bone for IO infusion also leads to extravasation.
- Needle insertion through cellulitis, infection, or burns

TECHNIQUE

- Can be placed in proximal tibia, distal tibia, distal femur, and in adults, the sternum.
- Use sterile technique.
- On the proximal tibia, the anteromedial surface is used, approximately 1 to 3 cm (two finger widths) below the tuberosity on the medial, flat surface of the tibia. This location is far enough from the growth plate to prevent damage. A needle is directed away from the joint space and rotary motion is applied with pressure. The distance from the skin through the cortex of the bone is rarely >1 cm in an infant or child (see Figure 19.7).
- The distal tibia, a preferred site in adults, may also be used in children. The site of needle insertion is the medial surface at the junction of the medial malleolus and the shaft of the tibia, posterior to the greater saphenous vein.
- The distal portion of the femur is occasionally used as an alternate site, but it is more difficult to palpate bony landmarks. The needle should be inserted 2 to 3 cm above the external femoral condyles in the anterior midline.

COMPLICATIONS

- Osteomyelitis, mediastinitis (especially in children)

INTERPRETATION OF RESULTS

- Aspiration of blood and marrow contents confirms position. Many times, particularly during cardiac arrest, blood aspiration is not possible.
- The needle's ability to stand **upright without support** and infuse fluids that flow easily without evidence of swelling or extravasation also confirms position

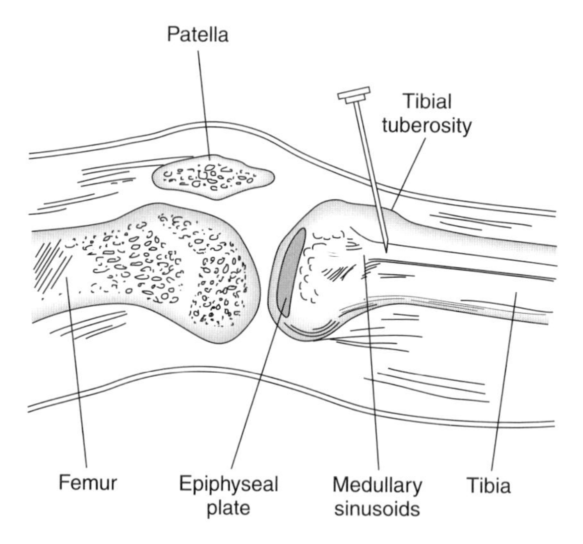

FIGURE 19.7. Insertion of intraosseous needle in the proximal tibia.

(Reproduced, with permission, from Morgan GE, Mikhail MS, Murray MJ. *Clinical Anesthesiology*, 4th ed. New York: McGraw-Hill, 2006:989.)

Umbilical Vein Catheterization

INDICATIONS

- Vein: Need for emergent vascular access in newborns. The umbilical vein remains patent for about a week after birth.
- Artery: Need for frequent monitoring of arterial blood gases and BP.

CONTRAINDICATIONS

- Peripheral access obtainable in newborn

TECHNIQUE

- Use standard sterile technique to place a purse-string suture at base of umbilicus. Cord is cut with a scalpel 1 cm from the base.
- The vein is at 12 o'clock and is thin walled with a large lumen. The urachus may persist but can be differentiated from the vein by presence of urine. The catheter is advanced 1–2 cm beyond the point at which good blood return is obtained. (See Figure 19.8.)
- The **two arteries have thick walls and smaller lumens**. Artery must be dilated with repeated passes and forceps. Use a 3.5–5 Fr catheter and advance toward the feet. The tip should be placed anywhere from T6 to the lower border of the L3 vertebra on X-ray.

COMPLICATIONS

- Bleeding, infection, vessel perforation
- Air embolization, especially during catheter removal
- Thromboembolism, aortic thrombosis, aortic aneurysm, peritoneal perforation

INTERPRETATION OF RESULTS

- Easy aspiration of blood confirms placement in vein lumen.
- X-ray of an umbilical vein catheter demonstrates placement in IVC (the line should go toward the head). An X-ray of an umbilical artery catheter should show the line going away from the head.

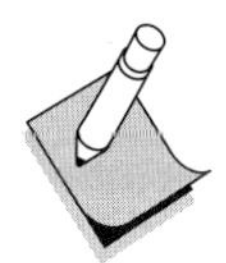

Intraosseous access is a bridge to venous access in critically ill patients. Once definitive intravenous access is obtained, the intraosseous line should be removed.

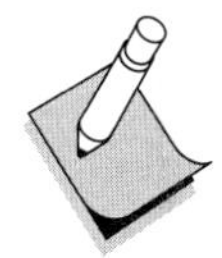

There is only one umbilical vein, and that is what you want to access to provide treatment to an ill newborn.

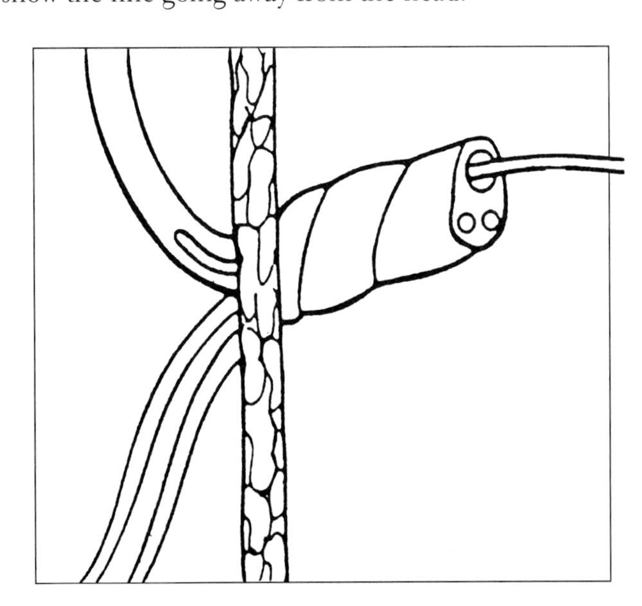

FIGURE 19.8. Cross section of umbilical cord showing location of vein and arteries.

(Reproduced, with permission, from Tintinalli JE, Kelen GD, Stapczynski JS. *Tintinalli's Emergency Medicine: A Comprehensive Study Guide*, 6th ed. New York: McGraw-Hill, 2004:73.)

Arterial Catheterization

Indications

- Need for frequent monitoring of arterial blood gases
- Need for continuous BP monitoring or inability to use indirect blood monitoring.
- Need for use of vasoactive agents/inotropes

Contraindications

- Strict: Inadequate circulation to the extremity, Raynaud syndrome, Buerger disease, full-thickness burns
- Relative: Patient on anticoagulants, coagulopathy, overlying cellulitis, partial thickness burns, inadequate collateral flow

Technique

- Standard sterile technique should be used and when possible, local anesthesia.
- The radial, brachial, femoral, axillary, and ulnar arteries are usual sites for arterial puncture. Pediatric sites include the dorsalis pedis, temporal arteries, and umbilical artery in newborns.
- Allen's test is performed prior to radial artery cannulation to ensure collateral flow from ulnar artery.
- Cannulation is usually placed with an over-the-needle catheter with or without a guidewire. Larger vessels, such as femoral, always use needle puncture of the artery followed by the catheter placed over a guidewire (Seldinger technique).
- The arterial pulsation is palpated with the index and middle fingers and the vessel course identified. The skin is punctured distal to the palpated pulse under the index finger. The needle is advanced slowly at a 30° angle with the skin. For larger arteries, the Seldinger/guidewire technique is used to cannulate the vessel.
- Ultrasound or handheld Doppler can be used to assist in cannulation.

Complications

- Bleeding, thrombosis leading to ischemia, infection

Interpretation of Results

- Once in the artery, the syringe plunger for blood gas collection should rise on its own due to arterial pressure.
- The arterial wave form has a distinctive dicrotic notch on the down slope, caused by the closure of the aortic valve.

ABDOMINAL AND GASTROINTESTINAL PROCEDURES

Paracentesis

Indications

- Decompressive therapy to relieve the cardiorespiratory and gastrointestinal manifestations of tense ascites
- Diagnostic test for patients with new onset ascites or to determine presence of infection in patients with chronic ascites

CONTRAINDICATIONS

- Relative: Coagulopathy (though even patients who have platelet levels <50000/mm^3 and prothrombin times >20 seconds have very few complications)
- Absolute: Infection or engorged veins over site

TECHNIQUE

- Patient is placed supine or in left lateral decubitus position. Sterile technique is used. Local anesthesia is applied at entry site. Ultrasound may be used to confirm presence of ascites and avoid bowel injury, though "blind taps" have a very low complication rate.
- Possible sites of entry are 2 cm below the umbilicus in the midline or 4–5 cm cephalad and medial to the anterior superior iliac spine. Avoid the inferior epigastric artery, which runs from the midpoint of the inguinal ligament to the umbilicus.
- An over-the-needle fenestrated catheter is inserted perpendicular to skin. The "Z tract" method can be used wherein the skin is pulled ~2 cm caudad, then the needle is inserted, and the skin is released when fluid flows from needle. After the needle is removed, the catheter is taped to the skin and connected to a vacuum bottle.
- Fluid is routinely sent for cell count, culture, and Gram stain but can also be sent for protein, glucose, LDH, amylase, albumin, TB culture, cytology, triglycerides, and bilirubin.
- When performing a therapeutic paracentesis, consider intravenous albumin if volume of ascites removed exceeds 5 L. Hemodynamic compromise may occur with removal of large amounts of fluid.
- Intravenous albumin is also part of the treatment of patients with SBP.

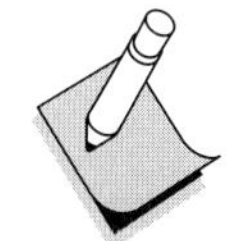

Review medications for patients receiving a therapeutic paracentesis. A low sodium diet and increased doses of furosemide and spironolactone are usually indicated.

COMPLICATIONS

- Persistent leakage of fluid from site (which can be remedied by a single suture), hematoma, perforation of vessels/viscera, peritonitis or abdominal wall abscess

INTERPRETATION OF RESULTS

- Peritoneal fluid containing **>250 PMN/μL** is used by many authorities as presumptive evidence of **SBP**. However, other cutoffs have been described including WBC count >250 WBC/μL with >50% polymorphonuclear leukocytes.
- WBC count <250 WBC/μL, with predominant mesothelial cells occurs with cirrhosis.
- WBC count >1000 WBC/μL with variable cell types occurs with neoplasms.

Rectal Foreign Body Removal

INDICATIONS

- All rectal foreign bodies (FB) should be removed when diagnosed.

CONTRAINDICATIONS

- Severe abdominal pain or signs of perforation
- Nonpalpable rectal FBs require surgical consultation.
- Insufficient experience or equipment

TECHNIQUE

- An X-ray may be useful to confirm the presence of a FB and to define its size and position.
- Patient assumes knee-chest or lateral decubitus position.
- IV sedation and/or perianal block may be required.
  - Perianal block: Local infiltration is administered circumferentially around the anus in the submucosal tissue.
- Perform direct rectal examination (DRE) to gauge position/orientation of FB.
- Application of suprapubic pressure while patient performs a valsalva maneuver may deliver FB.
- If unsuccessful, an anoscope, rigid sigmoidoscope, vaginal speculum, or retractor can be inserted into the anus to visualize FB clearly. An instrument can then be used to secure and remove the FB along with the anoscope as a single unit.
- If a vacuum is created between FB and mucosa, it must be released by distending the rectal wall around the FB with air. This can be done using a sigmoidoscope or a Foley catheter passed beyond the FB and balloon inflated.

COMPLICATIONS

- Failure to remove FB
- Mild mucosal edema and rectal bleeding are common.
- **Perforation or deep mucosal tear** require hospitalization.
- Cracking or shattering of glass FB may require surgical exploration and retrieval.

INTERPRETATION OF RESULTS

- Removal of intact FB under direct visualization without abdominal pain, fever, or severe bleeding indicates successful removal.

Diagnostic Peritoneal Lavage

INDICATIONS

- To determine or exclude the presence of intraperitoneal hemorrhage in the hemodynamically unstable blunt or penetrating trauma patient
- Useful when ultrasound is unavailable, is technically difficult, or results are indeterminate, especially when the patient is hemodynamically unstable
- May be useful in evaluating patient with CT demonstrating free fluid without evidence of solid organ damage

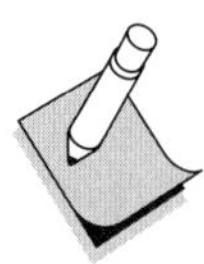

Consider DPL for blunt trauma victims with free fluid on ultrasound and obvious signs of liver disease and suspected ascites. A DPL with no blood may spare the patient a nontherapeutic exploratory laparotomy.

CONTRAINDICATIONS

- **Relative:**
  - Prior abdominal surgery or infections, obesity, coagulopathy, second or third trimester pregnancy

TECHNIQUE

- Stomach and bladder should be decompressed. Patient is supine. Sedation and analgesia provided if appropriate. Use sterile technique.
- In the open technique, a 4- to 6-cm incision is made infraumbilically in the midline to reach the linea alba. A 2- to 3-mm opening is made in the linea alba in the semiopen technique and extended in the fully open

technique for direct visualization of the peritoneum. Clips are placed to grasp each side of the rectus fascia to lift it and advance the catheter caudally into the peritoneum. The fully open technique is preferred when more direct view is needed such as with pelvic fractures, pregnancy, prior abdominal surgery, infections, and obesity.

- In the closed technique, a guide needle is inserted into the peritoneal cavity in the infraumbilical midline. The Seldinger (guidewire) method is then used to allow over-the-wire placement of a catheter.
- In the event of second- or third-trimester pregnancy, a suprauterine approach is used. With pelvic fractures, a supraumbilical approach should be used.
- Once cathether is in place, aspiration is attempted. If 10 mL of frank blood is aspirated, the DPL is positive and terminated. If there is little or no blood, the cavity is lavaged with 1 L of NS or LR in adults or 15 mL/kg in children. Fluid is then allowed to return to bag by gravity.

Complications

Infection, hematoma, wound dehiscence, bowel/bladder/vascular injury

Interpretation of Results

- **Immediate aspiration of 10 mL of blood** is considered positive.
- RBC counts >100,000/mm^3 is considered positive after lavage with 1 L of NS.
- When the diaphragm is at risk of injury as with penetrating chest trauma the RBC criterion should be lowered to 5000/mm^3 to maximize sensitivity for isolated injury to this structure.

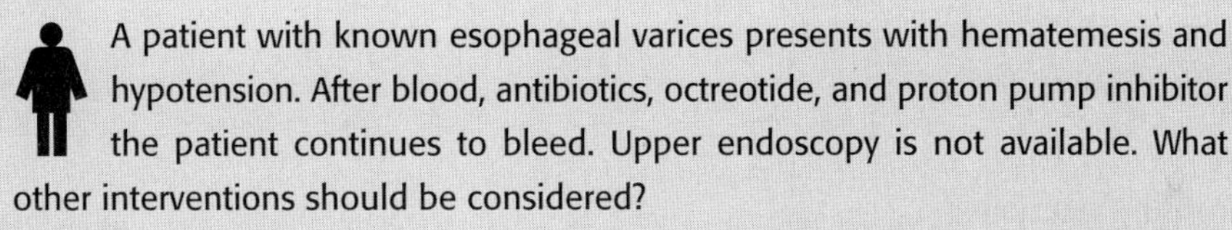

A patient with known esophageal varices presents with hematemesis and hypotension. After blood, antibiotics, octreotide, and proton pump inhibitor the patient continues to bleed. Upper endoscopy is not available. What other interventions should be considered?

Balloon tamponade of gastroesophageal varices may serve as a bridge to upper endoscopy in patients with massive upper GI bleeds. Surgical consultation should also be obtained for possible operative intervention.

Balloon Tamponade of Gastroesophageal Varices

Indications

- Patient with known portal hypertension or prior variceal hemorrhage with substantial ongoing upper GI bleeding despite optimal medical therapy and for whom endoscopy is unavailable

Contraindications

- Endoscopy readily available

Technique

- Sedation should be provided during procedure. Head of bed should be elevated to 45° if possible or placed in left lateral decubitus position.
- Stomach is evacuated with gastric lavage, NGT removed.
- Currently there are two types of gastroesophageal balloon tamponade (GEBT) tubes available: The three-lumen Sengstaken-Blakemore tube (gastric balloon, esophageal balloon, and gastric aspiration) and the four-lumen Minnesota tube (which adds an esophageal aspiration port).

- All balloons are collapsed and balloon ports clamped. Tube is then passed through mouth/nose into stomach. Suction is applied to gastric and esophageal aspiration lumens and position confirmed by X-ray. Increments of 100 mL of air are introduced through the gastric balloon inflation lumen until the recommended total volume (usually 500 mL) fills the gastric balloon. The intragastric balloon pressure is monitored. If high, balloon is likely in the esophagus and should be deflated and replaced into stomach. Once the gastric balloon is inflated, the tube is pulled back until the resistance of the diaphragm is firmly felt and the proximal end is secured using a traction device.
- If blood is still detected in the gastric aspiration port (or in the esophageal aspiration port on a four-lumen tube) after lavage, the esophageal balloon should be inflated to the pressure recommended in the accompanying instructions (generally 30 to 45 mm Hg).
- After bleeding has been controlled by the tamponade, the pressure in the esophageal balloon is generally reduced by 5 mm Hg every 3 hours until an intraesophageal balloon pressure of 25 mm Hg is achieved without ongoing bleeding.

Complications

- Ulceration of mucosal surfaces, mucosal ischemia inducing esophageal necrosis, aspiration pneumonia, asphyxiation, duodenal rupture

Interpretation of Results

- Pressure should be maintained at the lowest level that will stop bleeding from each of the aspiration suction ports.

NEUROLOGIC PROCEDURES

Lumbar Puncture

Indications

- Evaluate for: Infection, SAH, demyelinating CNS process, or carcinomatous/metastatic disease.
- Therapy for: Pseudotumor cerebri (idiopathic intracranial HTN), normal pressure hydrocephalus.

Contraindications

- Absolute: Infection near the puncture site
- Relative: Increased ICP due to space occupying lesion
- Relative: Lateralizing signs (hemiparesis), uncal herniation (unilateral third nerve palsy with AMS)
- Relative: Bleeding diathesis

Opening pressures are only useful when the LP is done on a recumbent patient. On seated patients, the pressure will usually be higher than normal and does not reflect the ICP.

Technique

- Patient positioning: Lateral decubitus or seated position
- Needle placement: L2–3 to L5–S1 interspaces in adults, L4–L5 or L5–S1 in infants (cord ends at L3 level at birth)

Complications

- Bleeding: Spinal epidural/subdural hematoma
- Herniation

- Infection/abscess
- Headache/backache
- Late onset of epidermoid tumors of the thecal sac

INTERPRETATION OF RESULTS

- Normal opening pressure (accurate in lateral decubitus position)
  - **60–200 mm H_2O (6–20 cm H_20) in adults**
  - 10–100 mm H_2O in children <8 years old
  - 30–60 mm H_2O in neonates
    - Low OP = CSF leak, dehydration.
    - High OP = overproduction, infection, bleeding, tumor, falsely elevated with sitting position/valsalva/crying.
- Normal color = clear.
  - Xanthochromia/yellow = seen in SAH, hyperbilirubinemia.
- Cells
  - Normal WBC = <5 cells/mm^3 in adults with <3 PMN/mm^3, <20 cells/mm^3 in neonates with < 1 PMN/mm^3.
    - Elevated WBC = bacterial/fungal infection, leukemia, vasculitis.
    - PMN predominance = bacterial infection.
  - Normal RBC = < 10 cells/mm^3.
    - Elevated RBC = SAH, traumatic tap.
- Normal glucose = 45–80 mg/dL.
  - Decreased in bacterial/TB meningitis or CNS tumors
- Normal protein = <45 mg/dL in adults, <20 mg/dL in children.
  - Increased in bacterial/TB meningitis, blood (SAH or traumatic taps), multiple sclerosis, and Guillain-Barré syndrome
- Miscellaneous
  - India ink = cryptococcus.
  - VDRL/RPR = neurosyphilis.
  - PCR for HSV or CMV infections

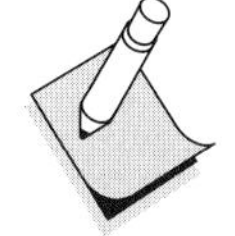

Both multiple sclerosis and Guillain-Barré syndrome can raise CSF protein levels.

> A patient with a history of hydrocephalus presents with headache. What imaging tests do you order? How do you evaluate shunt function?
>
> Radiologic shunt series and head CT. Compress shunt to confirm normal flow. Perform LP or tap shunt if any sign of infection.

Ventriculoperitoneal (VP) Shunt Evaluation

ETIOLOGY

- Obstruction is the most common cause of shunt malfunction. Presenting symptoms may be nonspecific (nausea, change in behavior). Proximal obstructions, often from choroid plexus within the catheter, are more common than distal obstructions. Distal obstruction of VP shunts may be due to thrombus.
- About 8% of VP shunts become infected. The infection most often results from ulceration of the skin overlying the valve. Skin organisms (*Staphylococcus epidermidis* and *S. aureus*) are the most common bacteria isolated.

INDICATIONS

- To evaluate cause of shunt malfunction
- To evaluate cause of increased ICP in a VP shunt patient

CONTRAINDICATIONS

- None

TECHNIQUE

- Obtain radiologic shunt series, which includes AP/lateral skull, AP chest, and AP abdominal X-rays to evaluate for kinking, disconnections or breaks in catheter.
- Palpate the shunt along temporal area of head. Compress the shunt reservoir. The reservoir should refill over 15–30 seconds.
- A head CT may show ventricular dilation, which suggests shunt obstruction. A comparison film is useful.

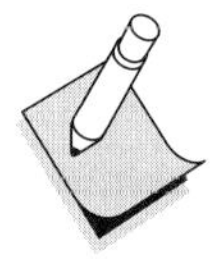

In pregnant women with cardiac arrest and unknown gestational age, if the fundus of the uterus is palpated above the umbilicus, assume that the fetus is viable.

COMPLICATIONS

None

INTERPRETATION OF RESULTS

- If the valve fills slowly (>30 seconds) and can be compressed easily, the obstruction is proximal to the valve. If the valve is not compressible, blockage is either at the valve or distal to it.
- Patients with VP shunt infections require directed antibiotic therapy. Often the shunts must be removed.

PERIMORTEM CESAREAN SECTION

INDICATIONS

- Cesarean delivery must be considered in any woman who suffers a cardiac arrest after 24 weeks' gestation and is unresponsive to brief resuscitation.
- Cesarean section performed within 5 minutes of death of the mother usually results in an excellent neonatal outcome; from 5 to 10 minutes, good; from 10 to 15 minutes, fair; and from 15 to 20 minutes, poor.

CONTRAINDICATIONS

- **Relative:**
  - Performance of the procedure before the point of fetal viability at approximately 24 weeks is not indicated.
  - Absence of obstetric backup immediately at hand

There is no evidence that perimortem C-section worsens maternal outcome, and there are both theoretical reasons and some evidence suggesting it may improve maternal outcome.

TECHNIQUE

- CPR should be begun at the time of maternal cardiac arrest and be continued until after delivery of the infant.
- A midline vertical incision is made through the abdominal wall extending from the symphysis pubis to the umbilicus and carried through all abdominal layers to the peritoneal cavity.
- A small (approximately 5 cm) vertical incision is made through the lower uterine segment until amniotic fluid is obtained or until the uterine cavity is clearly entered.
- The infant is then gently delivered, the mouth and nose suctioned, and the cord clamped and cut. The infant may require active resuscitation measures including bag-valve mask, intubation, CPR, and/or administration of medications including epinephrine, naloxone, dextrose 10%, IVF, or bicarbonate depending on the situation (see Figure 19.9).

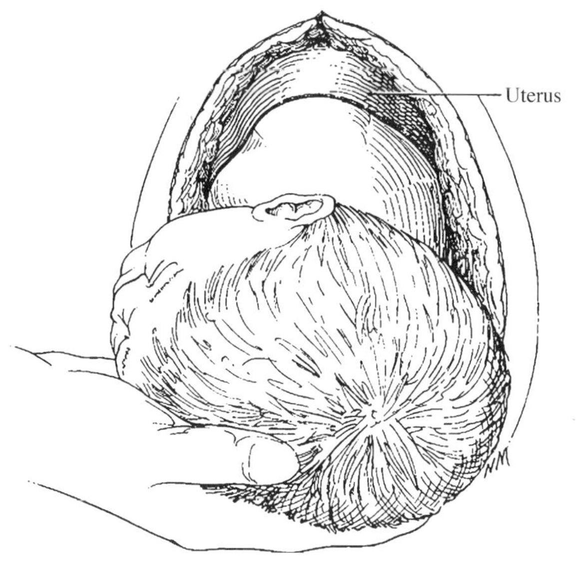

FIGURE 19.9. Delivery of neonate with perimortem cesarean section.

(Reproduced, with permission, from Cunningham FG, Leveno KL, Bloom SL, Hauth JC, Gilstrap LC, Wenstrom KD. *Williams Obstetrics*, 22nd ed. New York: McGraw-Hill, 2005:597.)

Complications

- Maternal death or poor neurologic outcome
- Neonatal death or poor neurologic outcome

Interpretation of Results

- Traditionally, Apgar scores are used in the standard newborn evaluation. A score of 7–10 is considered normal, while 4–7 might require some resuscitative measures, and a baby with Apgars of 3 and below requires immediate resuscitation.

> **APGAR** score—invented by Dr. Virginia Apgar
> **A**ppearance—blue/pink; body/pink
> **P**ulse—absent/< 100/> 100
> **G**rimace—no response/ grimace/pulls away
> **A**ctivity—none/ flexion/active movement
> **R**espirations—absent/ weak/strong

ANESTHESIA

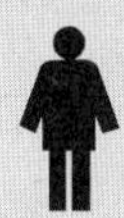

A young woman presents with a laceration of the upper right lip after being bitten by her dog. How would you anesthetize this wound prior to examination, irrigation, and possible closure?

Infraorbital nerve block.

Local Anesthesia

Indications

- Used for the majority of minor surgical procedures such as excision of skin lesions, incision of abscesses, and suturing of wounds

Contraindications

- Local infiltration distorts the tissues that will be incised or repaired, making it undesirable in areas requiring precise anatomic alignment (eg, some lip repairs).
- Epinephrine can theoretically cause ischemia and gangrene and should be avoided in digital blocks, penis, tip of nose, or earlobe.

TECHNIQUE

- Pain from local anesthesia can be diminished by using a small needle, ie, <25-gauge, slow infiltration, buffering the local anesthetic with bicarbonate (do not use with bupivacaine because the combination will crystallize), warming the local anesthetic to body temperature, and injecting into the wound margins (instead of intact epidermis).
- Anesthetic agents: 0.5–2% lidocaine, 0.5–1% procaine, 0.25% bupivacaine (Marcaine), 1% diphenhydramine (Benadryl). Higher concentrations do not provide additional benefit.
  - Lidocaine is most commonly used because of its excellent activity profile, low allergenicity and toxicity, user familiarity, and ready availability.
    - Onset: 2–5 minutes, duration: 1–2 hours
  - Procaine is useful for patients who are allergic to amide anesthetics.
  - Bupivacaine is used because of its prolonged duration and may be preferred for prolonged procedures, or for short procedures that may be interrupted in a busy ED.
    - Onset: 2–5 minutes, duration: 4–6 hours
- Epinephrine: Prolongs anesthesia duration. Epinephrine also provides excellent wound hemostasis and slows systemic absorption and therefore may be useful for areas with increased vascular supply (ie, scalp lacerations).
  - Phentolamine, which produces postsynaptic α-adrenergic blockade, can be used to reverse epinephrine-induced tissue ischemia in a dose of 0.5–5 mg diluted 1:1 with saline infiltration.
- Sodium bicarbonate: Works by increasing the ratio of nonionized to ionized molecules, which either renders the pain receptors less sensitive or causes a more rapid diffusion of solution into the nerve and a shorter time to anesthetic onset.

COMPLICATIONS

- True allergic reactions account for only 1–2% of all adverse reactions.
  - Ester solutions (procaine, tetracaine), which produce the metabolite *para*-aminobenzoic acid (PABA), account for the great majority of these reactions.
  - Amide solutions (lidocaine, bupivacaine) are rarely involved and it is usually the preservative methylparaben (MPB), which is structurally similar to PABA, that is responsible.
  - As with any allergic or anaphylactic reaction, symptoms include pruritis, urticaria, swelling, laryngospasm, bronchospasm, and even seizures, coma, and respiratory arrest.
- Epinephrine can cause headache, hypertension, palpitations, tremors, tachycardia, diaphoresis, and cardiac arrest.

INTERPRETATION OF RESULTS

- Local anesthesia is achieved when the patient no longer feels the tip of the needle in area requiring suturing/procedure. Typically, pressure sensation will remain intact.

Regional Nerve Blocks

INDICATIONS

- Regional nerve blocks are effective for closing facial lacerations, especially those of the lips, the forehead, and the midface, where the swelling caused by local infiltration is undesirable (see Table 19.1 and Figures 19.10A and B). They are also useful for providing anesthesia to the hands and feet.
- Regional blocks are also useful for the control of dental pain.

TABLE 19.1. Regional Nerve Blocks

Technique	Injection Location/Anatomy	Tissues and/or Teeth Affected	Comments
Supraperiosteal injection (local infiltration)	Anesthetic will diffuse across the bone to reach the nerve root of the involved tooth.	Any maxillary tooth	Straightforward, highly successful; ideal for relief of a toothache
Mental nerve block	Inside the mouth, adjacent to the foramen below the second premolar	Buccal soft tissues from second mandibular premolar to midline; skin of lower lip and chin	Technically simple, highly successful; ideal for repairing lower-lip lacerations
Infraorbital (anterior superior alveolar) nerve block	Inside the mouth, opposite the upper second bicuspid and directed toward the foramen, a depth of approximately 2.5 cm on inferior border of infraorbital ridge	Maxillary teeth and buccal soft tissues from midline through canine; upper lip, lateral aspect of nose, and lower eyelid; maxillary premolars	Highly safe and successful; ideal for repairing lacerations to upper lip
Posterior superior alveolar nerve block	Distal to the distal buccal root of the upper second molar toward maxillary tuberosity at depth of 2–2.5 cm	Entire second and third maxillary molars	Highly effective but carries significant risk of hematoma, so frequent aspiration during injection is crucial
Inferior alveolar nerve block	In the pterygomandibular triangle, at a point that is 1 cm above the occlusal surface of the molars	All mandibular teeth to midline; anterior 2/3 of tongue and floor of oral cavity; distribution of mental nerve	Failure rate 15–20% even in experienced hands; extremely useful and, when successful, extremely effective
Ophthalmic (V_1) nerve block	Near the supraorbital notch, above a midline pupil, along the superior orbital rim	The forehead and the scalp back to the lamboid suture	Suturing or debridement of the forehead, scalp, or delicate upper eyelid
Median nerve block	On the radial border of the palmaris longus tendon just proximal to the proximal wrist crease	The anterior palm, the anterior thumb, index finger, and middle finger	Suturing or debridement of the hand and/or palm
Ulnar nerve block	On the ulnar aspect of the wrist at the proximal palmar crease and is directed horizontally under the *flexor carpi ulnaris*	Fourth and fifth digits	Suturing or debridement of the fourth and fifth digits
Digital nerve blocks	Can be administered in the finger, in the web space between the fingers, or between the metacarpals on both sides of the bone	Any digit	Epinephrine should not be used since it vasoconstricts digital blood supply.

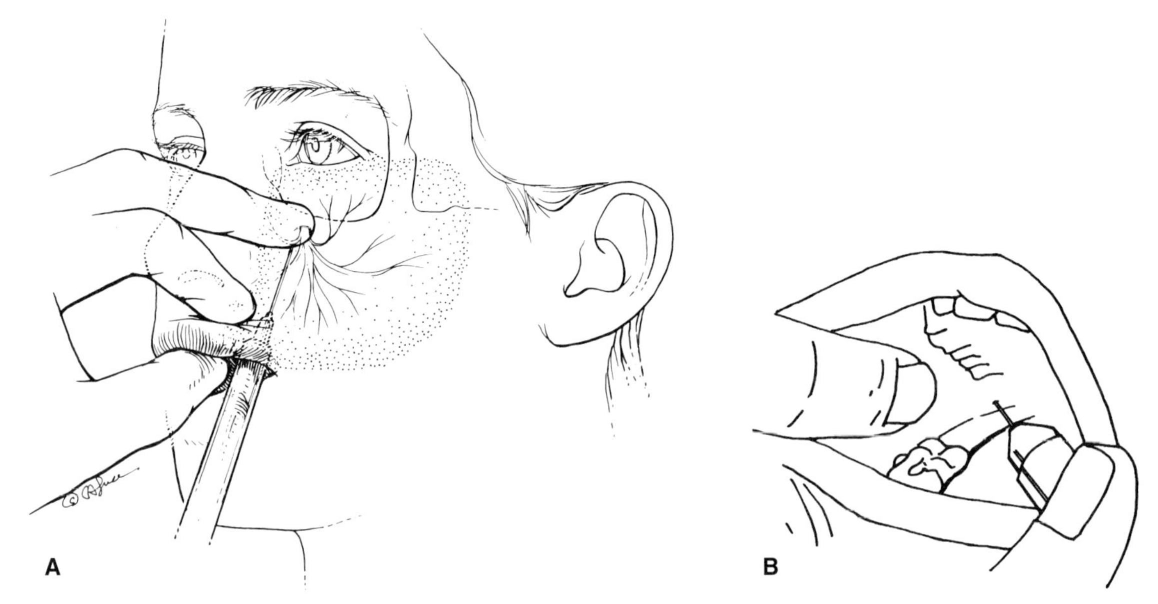

FIGURE 19.10. Insertion site for needle during (A) infraorbital nerve block and (B) inferior alveolar nerve block.

(Reproduced, with permission, from Tintinalli JE, Kelen GD, Stapczynski JS. *Tintinalli's Emergency Medicine: A Comprehensive Study Guide*, 6th ed. New York: McGraw-Hill, 2004:273.)

Contraindications

- Infection overlying site of injection

Technique

Complications

- Placement of the needle or injection of liquid into the nerve or a foramen can produce pain and neurovascular damage.
- For the posterior-superior alveolar nerve block, puncture of the pterygoid plexus and hematoma formation should the syringe not be aspirated before injection. Also, if the needle were advanced too far posteriorly, a Division II block of cranial nerve V will result.
- For the inferior alveolar block—injection of anesthetic posteriorly in the region of the parotid gland, which will anesthetize the facial nerves, will cause temporary facial paralysis (similar to a Bell palsy) that results in inability to close the eyelid. Should this occur, the eye must be protected until the local anesthetic has worn off (approximately 2–3 hours or up to 10–18 hours if marcaine is used).

Interpretation of Results

- Anesthesia of intended area signifies successful nerve block.

Procedural Sedation

Indications

- To relieve the pain and anxiety associated with diagnostic and therapeutic procedures performed in various settings
- To allow the provider to perform procedures in uncooperative patients
- To facilitate fracture and dislocation reductions by causing muscle relaxation

CONTRAINDICATIONS

- Lack of support staff or monitoring equipment
- Comorbidities (ie, cardiac, hemodynamic, or respiratory compromise)
- Recent (<2 hours) food intake

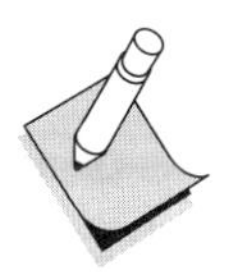

Ketamine should not be used in patients with: Closed head injury, globe rupture, recent URI.

TECHNIQUE

- Assess airway, cardiopulmonary status, gastrointestinal status (to prevent aspiration).
- Have necessary equipment in the room: O_2, nonrebreather mask, bag-valve mask, suction, oral airway, intubation materials including laryngoscope and ET tubes, and cardiac resuscitation equipment and medications.
- Monitoring is essential for procedural sedation: Oxygenation (via pulse oximetry), ventilation (via capnography), and hemodynamic status (including BP and cardiac rhythm) should all be monitored.
- Informed consent should be obtained and documented for elective procedural sedation in awake patients.
- Give appropriate medication in appropriate doses to achieve level of procedural sedation (see Table 19.2).
- Pharmacology (see Table 19.3)

COMPLICATIONS

- Delayed awakening: Usually due to prolonged drug action, but consider also hypoxemia or hypercarbia
- Agitation: Usually due to pain, or paradoxical or emergence reactions
- Nausea and vomiting: Sedative agents, premature administration of oral fluids after procedure
- Tachycardia: Pain, hypovolemia, impaired ventilation
- Bradycardia: Vagal stimulation, opioids, hypoxia
- Hypoxia: Laryngospasm, airway obstruction, oversedation

TABLE 19.2. Continuum of Sedation and Analgesia (Levels of Procedural Sedation)

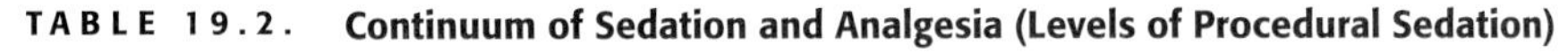

Level	Patient Response	Ventilatory Response	Cardiovascular Response
Minimal	Anxiolysis	Maintained	Maintained
Moderate (formerly "conscious sedation")	Depression of consciousness Responds purposefully to commands	Maintained	Maintained
Deep	Not easily aroused Responds purposefully to repeated stimuli	May be impaired	Maintained
General anesthesia	Cannot be aroused even by painful stimuli	Impaired	May be impaired

PROCEDURES AND SKILLS

TABLE 19.3. **Drug Characteristics Used in Procedural Sedation**

Drug	Onset Time	Duration	Adverse Effects	Notes
Versed **Children:** 0.1 mg/kg IV Adults: 0.03–0.1 mg/kg IV	3 min IV	30 min IV	Paradoxical hyperexcitability in children Apnea Hypotension	Hypotension Can reverse with flumazenil
Propofol 1 mg/kg IV	30–45 s IV	20–75 min IV	Apnea Hypotension Bronchospasm	
Etomidate 0.1–0.3 mg/kg IV	30–60 s IV	3–5 min IV	Myoclonus, adrenal suppression with multiple doses	Can cause myoclonus or laryngospasm
Methohexital 1–2 mg/kg IV	1 min IV	15 min IV	Apnea Hypotension	
Ketamine Children: 1–2 mg/kg IV; 2–4 mg/kg IM	1 min IV 5 min IM	10–20 min IV 15–45 min IM	Laryngospasm, emergence reaction, increased ICP, hypersalivation	Give atropine or glycopyrrolate to suppress hypersalivation, benzodiazepines to prevent emergence reaction or cardiovascular instability
Fentanyl 1–1.5 μg/kg IV	3 min IV	30 min IV	Apnea	Can reverse with naloxone, nalmefene
Atropine Children: 0.01 mg/kg IM or IV Min 0.1 mg Max 0.5 mg	30–60 s IV 5 min IM	2 hours	Tachycardia Anticholinergic symptoms	Use in children <5 year-old to counteract vagal effects of ketamine
Glycopyrrolate 0.004 mg/kg IV/IM	1 min IV 15–30 min IM	2–7 hours	Tachycardia Anticholinergic symptoms	Use in children <5 year-old to counteract vagal effects of ketamine
Flumazenil Children: 0.01 mg/kg IV Adults: 0.2 mg IV	<30 s IV	30–60 min IV	Unmasking of seizures	
Naloxone Children: 0.01 mg/kg IV Adults: 0.4–2 mg IV/IM	1–2 min IV 2–5 min IM	1–4 hours	May precipitate withdrawal reactions	May require repeat dosing due to short duration

- To be discharged, patients should be alert and oriented (or returned to age-appropriate baseline), vital signs should be stable and patient should be escorted by a reliable adult who will observe them after discharge. Absent lower extremity injuries, patients who walk in should walk out.

OPHTHALMOLOGIC PROCEDURES

Lateral Canthotomy

Indications

- Retrobulbar hemorrhage resulting in acute loss of visual acuity, increased IOP, and proptosis
- An IOP >40 mm Hg (normal IOP is 10–21 mm Hg)
- In patients with retrobulbar hemorrhage with afferent pupillary defect, ophthalmoplegia, cherry-red macula, optic nerve head pallor, or severe eye pain

Contraindications

- Suspected globe rupture: Hyphema, irregular pupil, exposed uveal tissue, and/or limited extraocular movements
- Tonometry and globe palpation are also contraindicated in patients with an open globe injury.

Technique

- Use local anesthesia and conscious sedation with or without paralysis so that patient doesn't move during procedure.
- Clear debris with NS
- Crimp skin at the lateral corner of patient's eye with hemostat, pick up skin of lateral orbit and use scissors to make a 1- to 2-cm incision from lateral corner of the eye and extending laterally.
- Visualize lateral canthus tendon by pulling down on inferior lid and with scissors pointing away from the globe, dissect the inferior lateral canthus tendon and cut it.
- If IOP remains elevated (>40 mm Hg), cut the superior portion of the lateral tendon.

Complications

- Iatrogenic globe injury, bleeding, and infection
- Irreversible vision loss can occur if retina ischemia time is >90–120 minutes.

Interpretation of Results

- The afferent pupillary defect, or Marcus Gunn pupil, is tested using the swinging flashlight test. The test is positive when the affected pupil dilates in response to light (the other normal pupil also dilates when light is shone in the affected eye). Both pupils constrict when the light is shone in the normal eye. The Marcus Gunn pupil results from injury to the afferent fibers of cranial nerve II of the defective eye, while the efferent signals from cranial nerve III to both eyes are uninjured.
- A successful procedure is marked by improved visual acuity, resolution of a previously detected afferent pupillary defect, and decrease in IOP to below 40 mm Hg.

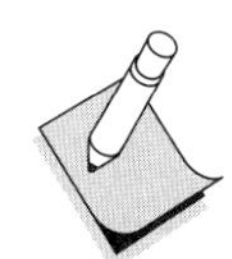

Causes of an afferent pupillary defect: Glaucoma, retrobulbar hematoma, retinal pathology, optic neuritis/MS

IOP Measurement

Indications

- To confirm the diagnosis of acute angle-closure glaucoma
- To determine the ocular pressure after blunt ocular injury, or in patients with iritis

Contraindications

- Relative:
  - Examination of infected eyes unless a sterilized cover can be used
  - The presence of corneal defects that may be further injured with tonometry.
- Absolute:
  - Suspected penetrating ocular injury

Technique

- Topical ocular anesthesia (proparacaine) must be instilled prior to procedure.
- Several methods of measuring intraocular pressure:
  - Applanation tonometry: Measures the pressure required to create a flat surface on the globe as determined by visual inspection of globe; method used by the Goldmann tonometer
  - Electronic indentation tonometry: Used by the Tono-Pen
  - Impression tonometry: Measures depth of deflection of cornea created by a known weight; used by the Schiotz tonometer
  - Pneumotonometry (air puff tonometry): Measures deflection of the cornea in response to a puff of air

Complications

- Corneal abrasions
- Transmission of infection
- Extrusion of ocular contents with penetrating injuries

Interpretation of Results

- Normal IOP is 10–20 mm Hg
- A reading of >20% reliability using the Tono-Pen reflects an unreliable measurement, which should be repeated.

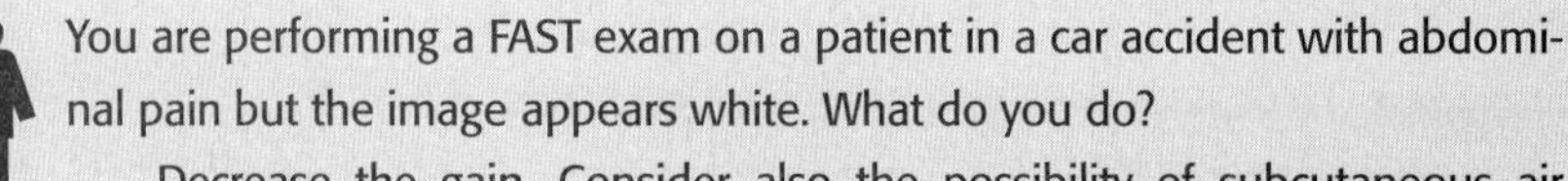

You are performing a FAST exam on a patient in a car accident with abdominal pain but the image appears white. What do you do?

Decrease the gain. Consider also the possibility of subcutaneous air from a pneumothorax.

ULTRASOUND

Indications

- Ultrasound is useful in the evaluation of
  - Cholecystitis
  - Abdominal aortic aneurysm
  - Ectopic pregnancy
  - Pericardial tamponade
  - Hemoperitoneum

- Cardiac electromechanical dissociation
- Hydronephrosis
- Tendons, bursae, cartilage, synovium, synovial fluid, and bone
- Fetus during routine and emergency prenatal care
- Foreign bodies in soft tissues or eyes

- To guide cannulation of vessels, aspirate fluid collections within cavities (eg, pericardium, pleurae, bladder, or joints), and locate soft tissue foreign bodies in the skin, soft tissues, or eyes
- To mark the site for skin puncture or provide continuous real-time visualization throughout a procedure

CONTRAINDICATIONS

- Lack of sonographic training and experience

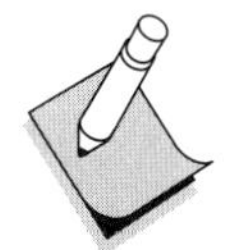

Medical diagnostic ultrasound uses sound between 3 and 20 MHz (10^6 times per second). This is above the upper limit for the human ear to hear sound of 20 KHz (10^3 times per second).

TECHNIQUE

- Lower-frequency probes (3–7 MHz) are used for viewing deeper structures but produce lower resolution images.
- Higher-frequency probes (7–20 MHz) are used for viewing superficial structures and provide higher resolution images.
- The "gain" controls the amplification of the returning signal. High gain will cause the image to appear white, low gain will produce dark images.
  - The depth gain control is a set of slide bars that allow you to set individual gains (brightness) at different levels.
- The "magnify" function causes the field to be magnified with the skin surface remaining in the image.
- The "zoom" function causes the boxed area of interest to be magnified. Other portions of the image are cut.

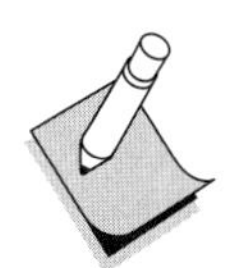

Use a low frequency probe to see deep structures. For example, a 3.5-MHz probe is appropriate for a FAST exam.

COMPLICATIONS

- Ultrasound is generally considered safe because it does not produce cancer-causing ionizing radiation. However, prolonged ultrasound causes increased inflammatory response and heats soft tissue.

INTERPRETATION OF RESULTS

- Catheters, wires, and needles appear as brightly reflective structures within fluid-filled anechoic spaces.
- Arteries and veins appear as anechoic circular structures when viewed in the transverse plane. Veins are easily compressed, arteries are less easily compressed, and veins filled with clot are noncompressible.

ORTHOPEDIC PROCEDURES

Extensor Tendon Repairs

INDICATIONS

- The optimal time for repair of tendons is within 24 hours of injury, but tendons can be repaired up to 2 weeks later.
- **Zone 4:** Area over the dorsal proximal phalanx between the metacarpophalangeal (MCP) and proximal interphalangeal (PIP) joints
- **Zone 5:** Tendon (area over the MCP joint) caused by a clean, sharp object rather than human bite. This area is also often referred to a hand surgeon.
- **Zone 6:** Tendon (dorsal hand) injuries

CONTRAINDICATIONS

- Relative:
  - Zones 1 and 2 consist of the area over the DIP joint and the middle phalanx, respectively. These usually require a hand surgeon consultation.
    - Mallet finger deformity: Unopposed action of the flexor digitorum profundus tendon due to disruption of the terminal extensor mechanism resulting in inability to extend at the distal interphalangeal (DIP) joint
  - Zone 3 tendon (the area over the PIP joint) with penetration into the joint; if tendon is not carefully repaired, it can result in long-term deformity
    - Boutonniere deformity: Rupture of the central slip leading to unopposed flexion of flexor digitorum superficialis tendon at the PIP joint and extension of the DIP joint
- Absolute:
  - Zones 7 and 8 (dorsal wrist and forearm) injuries are not repaired in the ED because risk of adhesions following repair and possible retraction of tendons past retinaculum that make repair difficult.

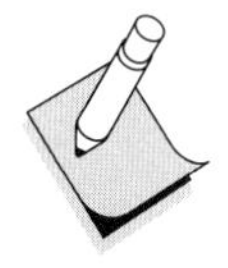

Use nonabsorbable suture to repair tendons.

TECHNIQUE

- Assess neurovascular status of injured hand and fingers.
- Obtain X-ray to evaluate for associated fractures/dislocations.
- Visualize location of tendon injury and locate both ends to be repaired.
- Larger tendons may allow sutures to pass through the core of the tendon but smaller tendons require a modified Kessler or Bunnell core suture technique with 4-0 nonabsorbable suture.
- After repair of a lacerated extensor digitorum commmunis (EDC) tendon in zone 6, a volar splint should be applied so that the wrist is in 45° of extension, the affected MCP joint is in neutral (0° of flexion), and the unaffected MCP joints are in 15° of flexion. The PIP and DIP joints should be allowed full range of motion.
- There are inadequate data to prove the value of prophylactic antibiotics for extensor tendon injuries, and no standard of care exists. If doubt exists concerning contamination and potential for infection, antibiotics should be given.

COMPLICATIONS

- Infection
- Tendon rupture
- Restriction of PIP and MCP joint flexion due to tendon shortening or adhesions

INTERPRETATION OF RESULTS

- Return of tendon function demonstrates adequate repair. However, all patients will need reevaluation and most require assistance with improving range of motion.

Arthrocentesis

INDICATIONS

- To obtain synovial fluid for analysis in order to differentiate joint disease caused by crystal-induced arthritis or septic arthritis
- To determine if an intra-articular fracture is present

- To determine if a laceration communicates with the joint space.
- To relieve pain from hemarthrosis by removing blood from joint space.

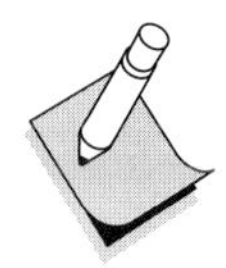

If you suspect septic arthritis, perform an arthrocentesis. No other test allows you to exclude the diagnosis with confidence.

CONTRAINDICATIONS

- Absolute: Infection in the tissues overlying the puncture site
- Relative: Known bacteremia that may lead to hematogenous spread of bacteria into the joint

TECHNIQUE

- Always use sterile technique to prevent infection.
- Local anesthesia can be used to reduce pain of procedure.
- Ultrasonography may be used to assess for the presence and location of synovial fluid.
- **Elbow:** The elbow is flexed to 90° with forearm pronated and palm flat on a table. A 22-Ga needle is inserted from the lateral aspect distal to the lateral epicondyle and directed medially.
- **Shoulder:** The patient should sit upright with the arm at the side and his or her hand in the lap. A 20-Ga needle is inserted at a point inferior and lateral to the coracoid process and is directed posteriorly toward the glenoid rim.
- **Knee:** The knee can either be fully extended or flexed to 15–20° by placing a towel under the knee to open up the joint space. The foot is kept perpendicular to the floor. An 18-Ga needle is inserted at the midpoint or superior portion of the patella approximately 1 cm medial to the anteromedial patellar edge. The needle is directed between the posterior surface of the patella and the intercondylar femoral notch.
- **Ankle:** The patient is positioned supine with the foot plantar flexed. A 20- to 22-Ga needle is inserted at a point just medial to the anterior tibial tendon and directed into the hollow at the anterior edge of the medial malleolus. The needle must be inserted 2 to 3 cm to penetrate the joint space.
- Studies usually obtained include cell count with differential, crystal analysis, Gram stain, bacterial culture and sensitivity analysis, and synovial fluid glucose measurement. Less frequently obtained studies include protein measurement, rheumatoid factor analysis, fungal and acid-fast stains, lyme titer, fungal and tuberculous culture, and complement analysis.

COMPLICATIONS

- Infection, bleeding, allergic reaction to local anesthesia

Pseudogout is caused by calcium **P**yrophosphate crystals that are **P**ositively birefringent.

INTERPRETATION OF RESULTS

- WBC >50,000/mm^3 is highly suggestive of a septic joint. WBC >50,000/mm^3 may be seen with gout. The presence of crystals, the absence of bacteria on Gram stain and culture, and the clinical presentation should help differentiate between septic and crystal-induced synovitis.
- A high percentage of neutrophils on the differential suggests a septic joint even if WBC <50,000/mm^3.
- Joint fluid-to-serum glucose ratio <50% suggests a septic joint.
- Crystal analysis: Gout is caused by monosodium urate crystals, which are negatively birefringent. Pseudogout is caused by calcium pyrophosphate crystals, which are positively birefringent.
- Presence of fat globules in joint fluid indicates presence of a fracture extending into the joint.

Splints and Casts

Indications

- To immobilize fractures/tendon injuries and maintain bony alignment in order to facilitate the healing process
- To decrease pain and protect extremity from further injury

Contraindications

- Casts should not be placed on swollen or recent injuries that may become swollen and cause compartment syndrome of that limb.

Technique

- Splints are placed over stocking and cushion and wrapped with elastic bandage (see Table 19.4).

Complications

- Dermal damage from splint/cast due to insufficient cushioning
- Compartment syndrome leading to ischemic limb due to constrictive cast/bandage
- Burns from plaster or fiberglass during hardening process
- Infection, dermatitis, joint stiffness

Interpretation of Results

- Always assess and document neurovascular status before and after splinting.
- Patients who return to the ER with pain at the site of a splint or cast need to have the splint or cast removed to allow examination of the extremity

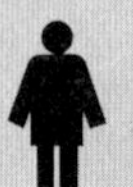

An 8-year-old boy falls backward off a swing. He is diagnosed with a supracondylar fracture, splinted, and sent home with next-day orthopedic follow-up. The child returns to the ED the same evening complaining of arm pain. What limb-threatening diagnosis must be considered?

Compartment syndrome.

PROCEDURES AND SKILLS

Compartment Pressure Measurement

Indications

- Evaluation of patients with suspected compartment syndrome based on: Tight muscle compartment in patients with extremity trauma or bleeding, pain out of proportion to exam, paresthesias, or otherwise unexplained limb ischemia
- Limb may be salvageable for up to 10–12 hours, but with very high pressures, the time period may be as little as 4 hours.

Contraindications

- Infection overlying site of needle insertion

Technique

- Use sterile technique and local anesthesia.
- The compartment to be measured should be at the same level as the heart.

TABLE 19.4. Splints for Various Extremity Injuries

SPLINT	INJURIES	CONSTRUCTION	NOTES
Long arm splint	Elbow and proximal forearm injuries	Splint posterior proximal arm down to hand at MCP joint.	Elbow is flexed. Provide sling.
Double sugar-tong splint	Elbow and forearm injuries	Two pieces: First splint from posterior MCP joint around elbow and back to anterior MCP joint. Then splint medial proximal humerus around elbow to lateral humerus.	Elbow is flexed. Prevents pronation and supination of the forearm which is preferable for distal forearm and elbow fractures Provide sling.
Volar splint	Hand and wrist injuries	Splint from palm at MCP joint along volar forearm to just proximal to elbow.	Wrist in slight extension
Sugar-tong splint	Distal radius and ulnar injuries	Splint from posterior MCP joint around elbow and back to anterior MCP joint.	Prevents pronation and supination of the forearm.
Thumb spica splint	Scaphoid, lunate, thumb, and first metacarpal injuries	Splint from distal to Interphalangeal thumb joint to mid forearm.	Position hand as if it was holding a glass.
Ulnar gutter	Little and ring fingers, and fourth and fifth metacarpals	Incorporate the little and ring fingers to mid forearm along medial forearm.	With boxer's fractures, MCP joint should be flexed to 90°.
Radial gutter splint		Splint radial aspect of forearm from distal IP joint of index finger to mid forearm.	
Swathe and sling shoulder immobilizer	Proximal humerus fractures, reduced shoulder dislocations	Sling supports weight of arm; swathe immobilizes arm.	
Knee immobilizer	Ligamentous injuries of the knee		
Posterior knee splint	Mild to moderate knee injuries	Splint form below buttocks crease to above the ankle of posterior leg.	Alternatively, two parallel splints placed along each side of the leg and foreleg can immobilize lateral and medial collateral ligaments.
Posterior ankle splint	Distal fibula and tibia, ligaments, and reduced ankle dislocations	Splint from plantar surface of metatarsal heads to posterior foreleg up to fibular head.	Ankle is flexed to 90°.
U-splint (sugar-tong ankle splint)	Ankle injuries	Splint from fibular head under plantar surface of foot to medial side of foreleg.	Immobilizes the medial and lateral ligaments

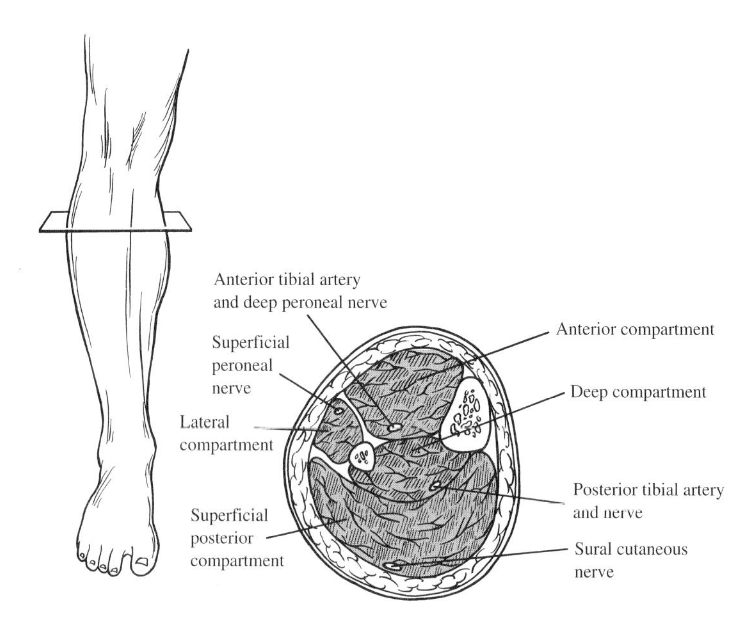

FIGURE 19.11. The four compartments of the lower leg.

(Reproduced, with permission, from Tintinalli JE, Kelen GD, Stapczynski JS. *Tintinalli's Emergency Medicine: A Comprehensive Study Guide*, 6th ed. New York: McGraw-Hill, 2004:1747.)

- Needle placement is perpendicular to the skin:
  - Lower Leg (see Figure 19.11)
    - Anterior compartment: Needle entry point is 1 cm *lateral* to the anterior border of the tibia.
    - Deep posterior compartment: Needle entry point is just posterior to the medial border of the tibia.
    - Lateral compartment: Needle entry point is just anterior to the posterior border of the fibula
    - Superficial posterior compartment: Needle entry point is 3–5 cm on either side of a vertical line drawn down the middle of the calf at the junction between the proximal and middle thirds of the lower leg.
  - Forearm (see Figure 19.12)
    - Volar compartment: Needle entry point is just medial to the *palmaris longus.*
    - Dorsal compartment: Needle entry point is 1–2 cm lateral to the posterior aspect of the ulna.
- Pressures can be measured either with an arterial line pressure measurement system or with a Stryker Intracompartmental pressure monitor system.

Complications

- Infection, pain, inaccurate readings, exacerbation of compartment syndrome by injection of fluid into compartment

Interpretation of Results

- Falsely elevated pressures may be a result of needles placed into tendons or fascia, plugged catheters, or faulty electronic systems. Falsely low readings may result from bubbles in the lines or transducer, plugged catheters, or faulty electronic systems.

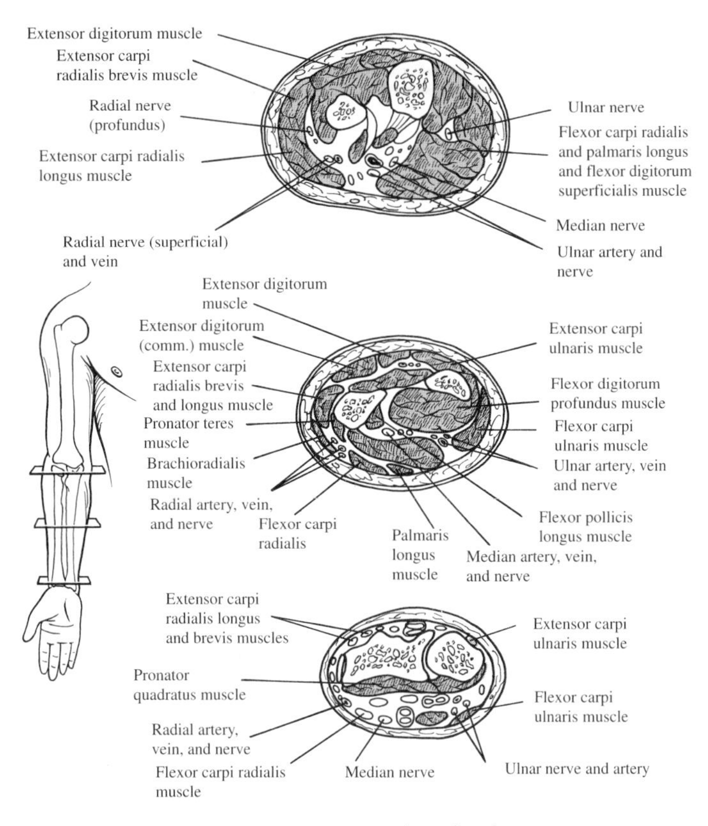

FIGURE 19.12. Forearm compartments at various levels.

(Reproduced, with permission, from Tintinalli JE, Kelen GD, Stapczynski JS. *Tintinalli's Emergency Medicine: A Comprehensive Study Guide*, 6th ed. New York: McGraw-Hill, 2004:1747.)

- Proper needle placement can be confirmed by seeing a rise in pressure during digital compression of the compartment just proximal or distal to the needle insertion site, or by contraction of muscle in compartment being measured.
- Compartment pressure of 30 mm Hg is considered by some to be diagnostic of compartment syndrome. However, this is an imperfect test with both false positives and false negatives. Interventions should be informed by history, exam, and compartment pressure measurements.
- Fasciotomy is the standard treatment for compartment syndrome. However, compartment syndrome may be treated with hyperbaric O_2 therapy. Additionally, compartment syndrome resulting from **snake bites should not be treated with fasciotomy**.

SUPRAPUBIC CATHETERIZATION

INDICATIONS

- Men with urethral stricture or complex prostatic disease
- Trauma patient with evidence of urethral injury including **blood at the meatus, a high-riding prostate**, or scrotal or perineal hematoma: Traditionally, in these patients no attempt at urethral catheterization should be made until a retrograde urethrogram is performed to evaluate the integrity of the urethra.

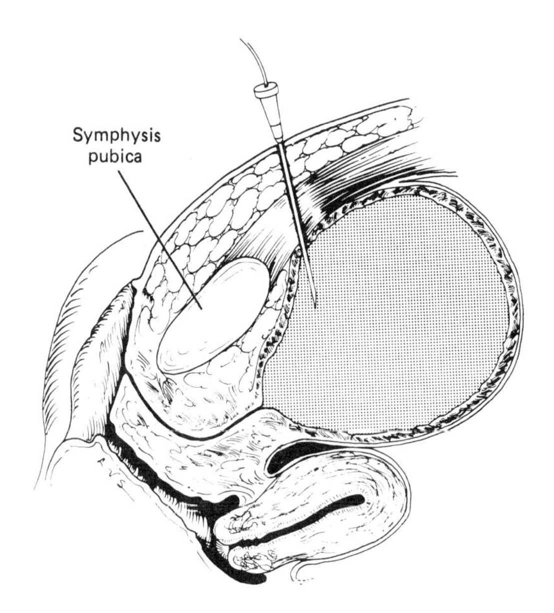

FIGURE 19.13. Insertion site of catheter during suprapubic catheterization.

(Reproduced, with permission, from Stone CK, Humphries RL. *Current Emergency Diagnosis & Treatment*. 5th ed. New York: McGraw-Hill, 2004:128.)

CONTRAINDICATIONS

- Avoid placing in patients whose bladder is not full enough to visualize or is not definable due to previous surgery or radiation. Ultrasound is useful in determining bladder position.

TECHNIQUE

- Use sterile technique and local anesthesia. If necessary, conscious sedation should be provided.
- The needle is placed approximately 2–3 cm above the pubic symphysis directed toward the pelvis and advanced slowly while aspirating until urine is easily aspirated (see Figure 19.13).
- Once the bladder is located, the Foley is placed over a guidewire and sheath.

COMPLICATIONS

- Bowel perforation, intraperitoneal/extraperitoneal extravasation, infection, obstruction of tubing, tubing comes out, ureteral catheterization

Patients with pelvic fractures and either a high-riding prostate or blood at the urethral meatus should have a retrograde urethrogram (RUG) for evaluation of urethral injury. If present, place a suprapubic catheter.

INTERPRETATION OF RESULTS

- Aspiration of urine from the catheter confirms placement.

ABSCESS INCISION AND DRAINAGE (I+D)

INDICATIONS

- Definitive treatment of a soft tissue abscess (antibiotics alone are ineffective)

CONTRAINDICATIONS

- Incision prior to localization of pus (may extend infection)

TECHNIQUE

- Ultrasound may be used to guide incision or needle aspiration.
- Regional blocks are preferred to local anesthesia as local anesthetic agents function poorly in the low pH of infected tissue and local injection is painful. Conscious sedation may be appropriate.
- Patients at risk for endocarditis should receive IV antibiotics prior to I+D.
- Abscess is incised along total length of the cavity for noncosmetic areas. For cosmetic areas a stab incision or simple aspiration may be attempted.
- The abscess should be probed to break open loculations with hemostat or hemostat wrapped in gauze.
- Irrigate and gently pack cavity with gauze.
- Prescribe packing change periodically and follow up in 1–3 days.
- The use of antibiotics following I+D is a clinical decision that depends on host factors (immunocompromised status, diabetes) and wound characteristics (associated cellulitis).

COMPLICATIONS

- Bleeding
- Extension of infection
- Recurrence

INTERPRETATION OF RESULTS

- Drainage of pus indicates correct localization of pus but follow-up must be provided to ensure progression of adequate drainage.

CHAPTER 20

EMS and Disaster Medicine

Jacqueline Ward-Gaines, MD, FACEP

ORIGINS OF EMERGENCY MEDICAL SERVICE

A need for an extension of emergency care in the community grew into what we know today as the EMS system. EMS was established in the 1960s.

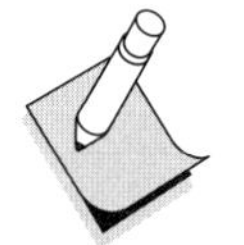

The Highway Safety Act of 1966 established the initial government funding for prehospital services.

Important steps in the development of EMS (see Table 20.1):

- **Highway Safety Act** (1966)
  - Authorized the U.S. Department of Transportation (DOT) to develop prehospital services
  - Established the National Highway Traffic Safety Administration (NHTSA)
- **Emergency Medicine Services Act** (1973)
  - Provided government funding and training for states to develop regional, county, and local EMS systems
  - Identified 15 essential components of an EMS system (see Table 20.2)
- **Development of communication and ambulance standards** (1973–1974)
  - 911 system
  - Dedicated radio frequencies for EMS
  - Federal specifications for ambulances
- **Emergency Medical Treatment and Active Labor Act (EMTALA)** 1985
  - Part of the Consolidated Omnibus Budget Reconciliation Act (COBRA)
  - Penalized emergency departments that refused care
- **Trauma Care Systems Planning and Development Act** (1990)
  - Authorized government funds to states for development of trauma systems

EMS DESIGNS

Multiple EMS designs exist and depend on the type of community served. In general, there should be one ambulance per every 7000–10,000 people.

- **Volunteer model:** Used primarily in rural areas where there are no funds to pay personnel

TABLE 20.1. Origins of Emergency Medical Service

YEAR	LEGISLATION	EFFECT	KEYWORD
1966	Highway Safety Act	Funding of prehospital services (via U.S. Department of Transportation) National Highway Traffic Safety Administration	DOT NHTSA
1973	Emergency Medical Services Act	Government funds and training for states to develop EMS systems	Funding Components
1973–1974	Establishment of communication and ambulance standards	911 system Established dedicated EMS radio frequencies and ambulance specifications	911
1985	Emergency Medical Treatment and Active Labor Act	Penalized emergency departments that refused patients	EMTALA COBRA
1990	Trauma Care Systems Planning and Development Act	Government funds to states for trauma systems	Trauma

- **Public utility model:** Allows a local government to contract all their calls to a *private* company that provides basic life support (BLS) and/or advanced life support (ALS); the government oversees and regulates performance
- **Third service model:** A separate municipal department owns, operates, and staffs ambulances
- **Fire station–based model:** Public fire department provides all EMS services
- **Combined public/private model:** eg, fire department provides first response with transportation to hospital provided by private ambulance service

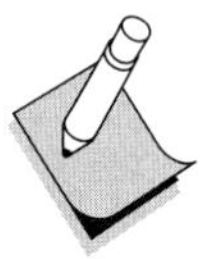

In a multitiered EMS system the level of response (BLS or ALS) depends on the nature of the call.

All models provide first responders, but the response after that varies:

- **Single-tier system:** Provides *only* BLS **or** ALS (including EMT-I and EMT-P) response
- **Multitiered system:** Provides a mixed BLS/ALS response
  - Is becoming less common

In a single-tier EMS system only one level of response (eg, BLS) is provided for every call.

COMPONENTS OF AN EMS SYSTEM

The Emergency Medical Service Act of 1973 identified 15 essential components of an EMS system. (See Table 20.2. Shaded entries are discussed in this chapter.)

Training

Multiple levels of EMS training and credentialing exist (see Table 20.3).

- **First responders (FR)**
  - Firefighters, police officers, community EMS responders: First to arrive on scene
  - Are trained in CPR, BLS, and basic trauma care
- **Emergency medical technician basic (EMT-B)**
  - The lowest EMT level
  - Can perform BLS, automated external defibrillation (AED), basic assessments, and assist in medication administration
- **Emergency medical technician intermediate (EMT-I)**
  - Addition of IV access, endotracheal intubation, and manual defibrillation
- **Emergency medical technician paramedic (EMT-P)**
  - The most advanced EMT level
  - Can perform advanced airway procedures, needle decompression of chest, ECG interpretation, external pacing, and advanced drug therapy

EMT-B providers can assist in medication administration and provide BLS, AED, and basic care.

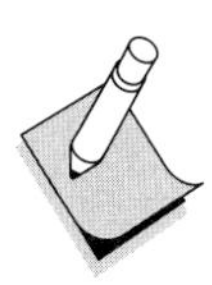

EMT-P providers can perform advanced drug therapy, ECG interpretation, external pacing, surgical airway, and needle decompression of chest.

Communication

After activating the system via 911, goal is to get BLS to scene in 4 minutes and ALS in 8 minutes. An **enhanced 911** system displays the caller's telephone number and address.

The emergency medical dispatcher must

- Take and triage call
- Alert appropriate unit
- Address location
- Assist victim until arrival

Communication must also be available between hospital and field or dispatch center via designated radio frequencies.

TABLE 20.2. **Fifteen Essential Components of an EMS System**

Acronym	Component
The	Training
M	Manpower
D	Disaster plan
Calls	Communication
For	Facilities
A	Access to care
Medical	Mutual aid
Technician	Transportation
2	
C	Critical care units Customer participation
People	Public safety
Perform	Patient transfer
C	Coordinated patient record
P	Public education
R	Review and evaluation

(Shaded entries are discussed in this chapter.)

Facilities

There are three categories of hospital facilities:

- Vertical
  - Describes a level of care provided at the hospital
  - Is not standardized
    - Level 1 trauma center: Most sophisticated, with all specialty services immediately available 24 hours a day
    - Level 3 nursery: Most sophisticated NICU services
- Horizontal
  - Describes the specialty care provided at the hospital (eg, neurosurgery, burn, cardiac care, trauma)
- Circular
  - Transfer agreements among hospitals of different vertical and horizontal levels so they can get to most appropriate care (eg, regionalization of trauma centers)

TABLE 20.3. EMS Training Levels

Provider	Hours of Training	Skills
First responders	40	CPR and BLS Basic trauma care
Emergency medical technician basic	110	FR training, plus: Basic assessment skills Automated external defibrillation May assist in medication administration
Emergency medical technician intermediate	300–400	Addition of IV access Endotracheal intubation Manual defibrillation
Emergency medical technician paramedic	1000–12,000	EMT-I, plus: Surgical airway Needle decompression of chest Advanced drug therapy including ACLS ECG interpretation External cardiac pacing

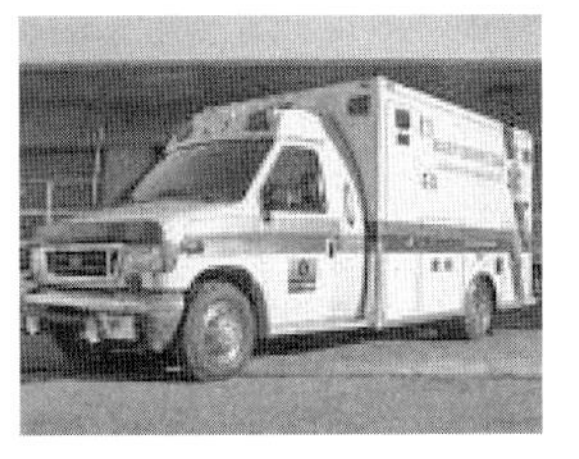

FIGURE 20.1. Type I ambulance.

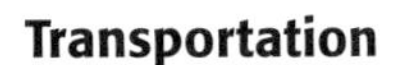

Transportation

GROUND TRANSPORTATION

- Ground transportation is used for the majority of acutely ill or injured patients.
- Manned by two persons of varying training levels

There are three types of ambulances:

- Type I (see Figure 20.1): Pick-up chassis with a separate modular compartment to carry equipment, personnel, and patient but **no passageway** between driver and patient
- Type II (see Figure 20.2): Van chassis with raised roof and other modifications
- Type III (see Figure 20.3): Pickup chassis with an integrated modular patient care compartment

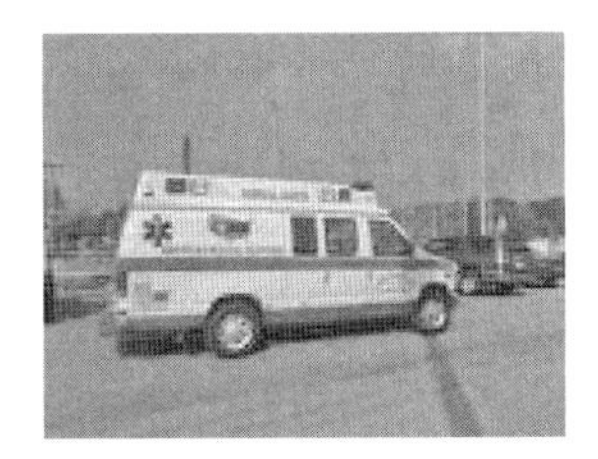

FIGURE 20.2. Type II ambulance.

ROTARY-WING AIR TRANSPORTATION

- Range of 50–150 miles
- Use when travel time >30 minutes to hospital and rapid transport is essential.
- Limited by poor weather

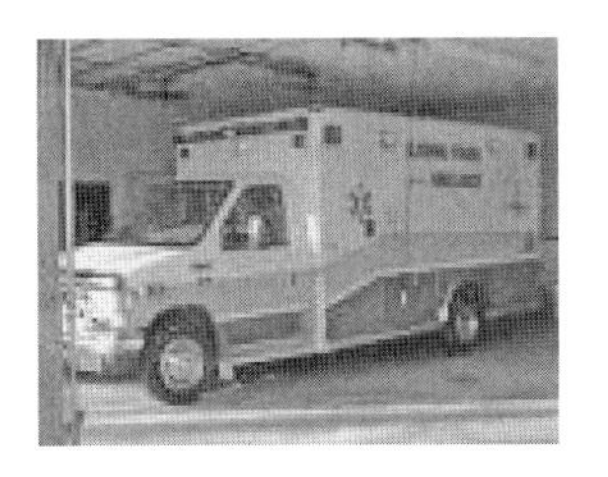

FIGURE 20.3. Type III ambulance.

FIXED-WING AIR TRANSPORTATION

- For distances >100 miles, when rapid transport is essential
- Limited by weather, lack of runways, refueling
- Possible altitude problems for the patient, eg, pneumothorax, ET cuff, balloon catheters
  - There are **no** absolute contraindications to air transport.

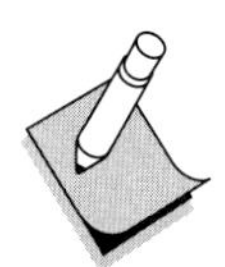

An impaired patient cannot refuse prehospital care.

Patient Transport

- Refusal of care: The main litigation against EMS, lawsuits number approximately 1 per 24,000 calls.
  - Impaired patient cannot refuse.
  - Competent patient may sign waiver form with online medical physician consultation.
- On-scene physician: Can assist with EMS protocols after identity check
  - If on-scene physician assumes full medicolegal responsibility then he may take control, but must follow patient to hospital.

Public Education

Includes public safety initiatives such as household poisoning prevention and child car seats

Review and Evaluation

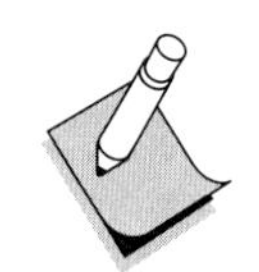

Direct medical control = providing direction to EMTs during actual patient care.

The EMS medical director is a physician who provides administrative and medical oversight for an EMS system.

Means of medical control and evaluation:

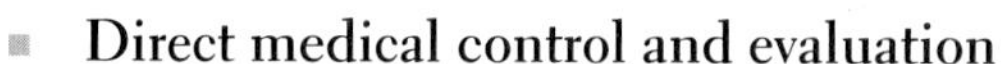

- **Direct medical control and evaluation**
  - In-field observation
  - Online medical orders
- **Indirect medical control and evaluation**
  - **Prospective** via development of standing orders, medical care protocols, and training
  - **Retrospective** via review of ambulance runs, quality assurance through EMS training

> Denver EMS gets a call that there was an explosion at Mile High Stadium, with an unknown number of injured victims. Source of the explosion is unclear. Backup is en route. What would define this event as a medical disaster?
>
> This event would be defined as a disaster if the local health care system is unable to meet the needs of the event. It is not determined by the absolute number of victims or type of event (eg, man-made explosive).

DISASTER

A medical disaster is defined as an event that overwhelms the response capabilities of the community.

- It **is not** defined by the absolute number of victims or type of event (natural or man-made).
- It **is** defined by the health care system's ability to meet the needs of the event.

With most disasters, patients generally arrive to the ED over a short period of time with the majority having only minor injuries, not requiring advanced trauma services.

TABLE 20.4. Disaster Classification

LEVEL	PROJECTED NEED	RESPONSE TIME
I	Local resources only	Hours
II	Regional resources, which may take up to 1 day	Up to 1 day
III	Statewide or federal assistance required	Up to 3 days

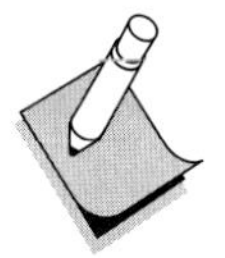

Classic disaster terminology: Three levels, based on projected need for resources

Classic terminology:

- May be further divided into **internal** (within the hospital) and **external** (outside the hospital grounds)
- Are often classified by level (see Table 20.4)

PICE classification: Four stages, 0–III, based on potential for further victims, state of local resources, and extent of geographic involvement

Newer nomenclature: **Potential injury-creating event (PICE;** see Table 20.5)

- A new term created to eliminate the confusion over the word "disaster"
- Describes an event based on the following three modifiers:
  - Potential for **additional victims**
  - Whether the **local resources** are overwhelmed and need augmentation or reconstitution
  - Extent of **geographic involvement** (local to international)
- The PICE stage predicts the need for outside aid.

Disaster Preparedness

The Joint Commission on Accreditation of Health Care Organizations (JCACO) requires all hospitals to have a written plan for both internal and external disasters and to perform practice drills twice yearly.

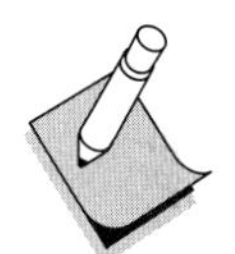

JCAHO phases of disaster preparedness: Mitigation, preparedness, response, implementation

A disaster plan must have:

- Flexibility
- Structure, such as normal daily operating procedures
- Coordination with adjacent community areas
- Input from EMS, police, medical community, and local government
- Media liaison
- Four phases: Mitigation, preparedness, response (activation, implementation), recovery (see Table 20.6)
  - Must address both internal and external event response

TABLE 20.5. Potential Injury-Creating Event Classification

	A	B	C
PICE STAGE	POTENTIAL FOR FURTHER VICTIMS?	STATE OF LOCAL RESOURCES?	EXTENT OF GEOGRAPHIC INVOLVEMENT
0	No = static	Controlled (= **ok**)	Local
I	Yes = dynamic	Disrupted	Regional
II		Paralyzed	National
III			International

TABLE 20.6. Phases of Disaster Preparedness

Phase	
Mitigation	Activities to lessen impact of a *potential* event
Preparedness	Identifying resources, training, drills
Response	
Activation	Notification for response Organization of incident command post Assessment of event
Implementation	Scene: Search and rescue, triage and transport, definitive management ED: Coordinating treatment
Recovery	Scene withdrawal Debriefing Return to normal operations

Disaster Triage

A means of assigning priority of treatment for the injured; must be an ongoing process

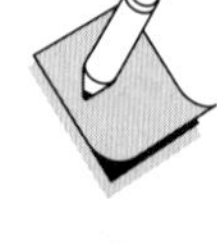

In disaster triage, a patient who is unsalvageable is triage category "black."

Simple Triage and Rapid Treatment (START)

(See Table 20.7.)

- For routine multicasualty triage
- Green category = those able to walk away from the scene.
- Each remaining victim undergoes a quick assessment of **respirations, perfusion, and mental status.**
- Red = need for immediate care (eg, severe mental status changes, HR > 120 or capillary refill >2 seconds or RR > 30).
- Yellow = not Red or Green, delayed care appropriate.
- Black = unsalvageable or dead.

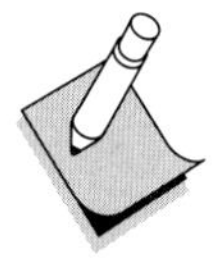

A disaster triage category "red" patient requires immediate care.

Secondary Assessment of Victim Endpoint (SAVE)

- For catastrophic numbers of casualties, to identify patients who may benefit from field intervention

TABLE 20.7. Multicasualty Triage Categories

Black ("Dead")	Unsalvageable or dead
Red ("Immediate")	First priority
Yellow ("Delayed")	Second priority
Green ("Minor")	Walking wounded

- Three categories:
  - Those who are unsalvageable.
  - Those who will survive regardless of care
  - Those who will benefit from field intervention

Disaster Response

Prehospital phase, important components include:

- Incident Command System = the standard emergency management system for a single scene disaster. It has five components:
  - Incident command: The **incident commander** has overall management responsibility for the incident.
  - Operations (tactical activities, managing resources)
  - Planning
  - Logistics (providing resources)
  - Financing
- Communications: Number 1 problem during disasters
- Health considerations: Storing dead, mechanisms for water/food supplies

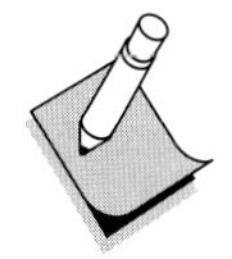

The standard prehospital management system for a single scene disaster = Incident Command System.

Hospital phase, important components include:

- **Control center:** Near, but not in ED, to monitor all activities
- **Plan activation:** Must have rapid plan to get necessary personnel
- **Treatment areas:** Correspond to triage categories and where continued triage is ongoing
- **Documentation:** Critical information only
- Security: Control perimeter, establish ingress and egress routes
- **Waiting areas:** Separate for patients, police, and media

Disaster Response Organizations

Table 20.8 summarizes the federal response resources that are available.

TABLE 20.8. Disaster Response Organizations

ORGANIZATION	RESOURCE PROVIDED
Department of Homeland Security	Federal Emergency Management Agency (FEMA) State and local assistance
National Disaster Medical System (NDMS)	Federally coordinated system of government and private institutions Disaster medical assistance teams (DMATs)
Centers for Disease Control	Public health emergency preparedness and response
Department of Veterans Affairs	Highly trained disaster medical personnel
Urban search and rescue	Highly trained medical, fire, and rescue personnel
Metropolitan Medical Response Systems	Personnel and equipment to enhance local planning and disaster response
The military	Response personnel

A rabbit hunter shows up in a rural Arkansas ED complaining of a sore on his right finger that will not heal even though his wife has been tending to it. The patient also complains of swollen lymph nodes in the same arm pit. What is the likely diagnosis?

Ulceroglandular tularemia. Tularemia is commonly called "rabbit fever" due to its association with lagamorphs and rodents. Diagnosis can be made on clinical findings, but confirmed with antibody titers or PCR. Streptomycin is the antibiotic of choice.

BIOLOGICAL WEAPONS OF MASS DESTRUCTION

Typically divided into three groups: Bacteria, viruses, and toxins. All share the ability for aerosol dispersal.

The agents considered to have the most severe potential (Class A agents) include:

- *Bacillus anthracis* (anthrax)
- *Yersinia pestis* (plague)
- *Variola major* (smallpox)
- *Francisella tularensis* (tularemia)
- *Clostridium botulinum* (botulism): See "Botulism" in Chapter 8.
- Filoviruses and arenaviruses (viral hemorrhagic fevers)

Anthrax

Organism: *B. anthracis*, a Gram-positive spore-forming bacterium

- Appears as long chains, resembling bamboo or boxcars (see Figure 20.4)

Anthrax is found worldwide in grass-eating mammals that ingest or inhale the spores while feeding. In normal circumstances, humans may become infected by eating infected animals or through contact (skin or inhalation) with spores on the fur or hide of animals (eg, woolsorter's disease).

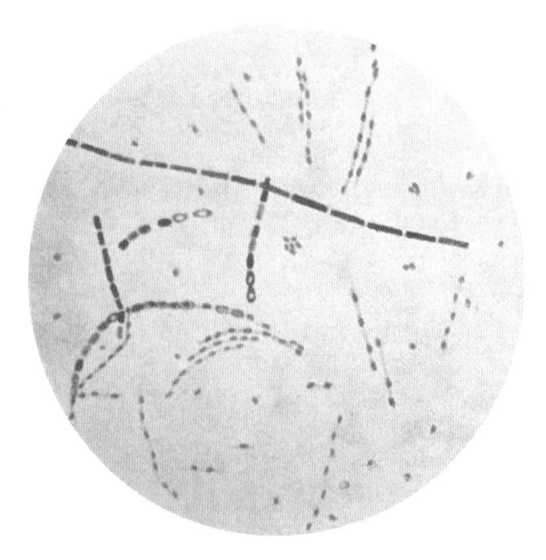

FIGURE 20.4. *Bacillus anthracis.*

(Reproduced, with permission, from Grey MR, Spaeth KR, *The Bioterrorism Sourcebook.* New York: McGraw-Hill, 2006:194.)

Forms of disease:

- **Cutaneous anthrax**
  - Most common
- **Pharyngeal or gastrointestinal anthrax**
- **Inhalational anthrax**
  - Most deadly

PATHOPHYSIOLOGY

- Exposure to spore via skin or (worse) inhalation → spores germinate into bacilli → transported to **regional lymph nodes** → **release toxins** → symptoms.

Prevention

- Vaccine available to military at risk only
- Ciprofloxacin or doxycycline prophylaxis for 30 days (with vaccination) or 60 days (no vaccination)

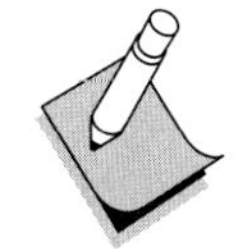

Cutaneous anthrax is the most common form of anthrax. Inhalational anthrax is the most deadly form of anthrax.

SYMPTOMS/EXAM

Cutaneous Anthrax

- Painless papules that become vesicular with significant edema
- Progresses to ulcerated black eschar after 1 week (see Figure 20.5)
- Constitutional symptoms and lymphadenopathy

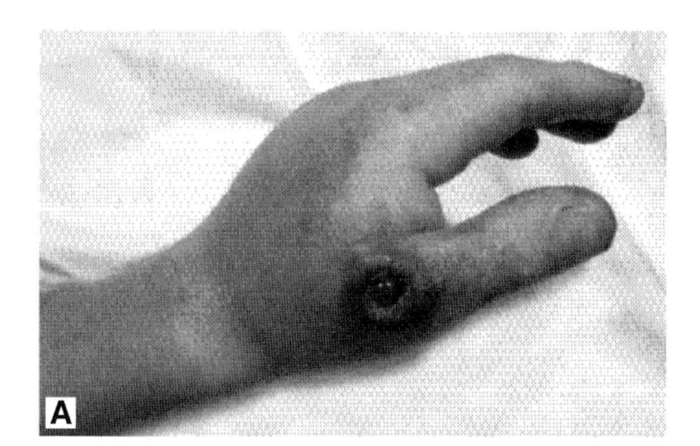

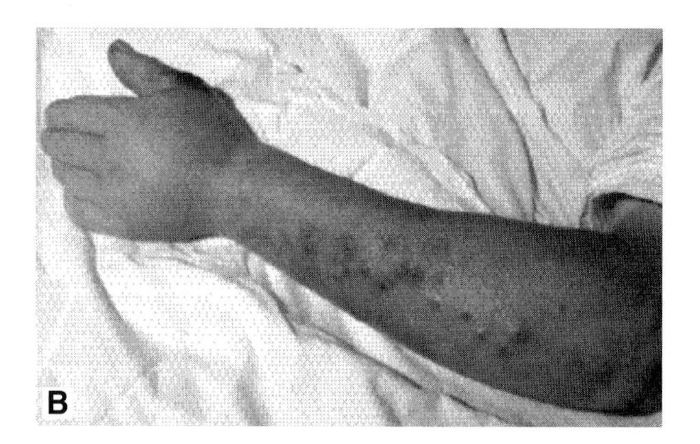

FIGURE 20.5. Cutaneous anthrax. (A) A black eschar with a central hemorrhagic ulceration on the thumb associated with massive edema of the hand. (B) A nodular lymphangitis extending proximally from the primary lesion on the thumb.

(Reproduced, with permission, from Wolff K, Johnson RA, Suurmond D. *Fitzpatrick's Color Atlas & Synopsis of Clinical Dermatology*, 5th ed. New York: McGraw-Hill, 2005:631.)

Pharyngeal or Gastrointestinal Anthrax

- Ulcers and edema of pharynx followed in 5 days by abdominal pain, upper and lower GI bleeding

Inhalational Anthrax

- Mild flu-like symptoms that rapidly progress to respiratory distress and septic shock

DIAGNOSIS

- Primarily a clinical diagnosis
- CXR (inhalational disease, see Figure 20.6)
  - Mediastinal lymphadenopathy (CT is more sensitive than CXR)
  - Possible pleural effusions
  - May be clear of infiltrates
- Gram stain and culture of skin lesions
- Tissue or pleural fluid evaluation

Anthrax treatment requires prolonged (60 days) antibiotic therapy.

TREATMENT

- Supportive and symptomatic care
- Simple cutaneous anthrax (nontoxic): Ciprofloxacin, doxycycline, or amoxicillin
- Toxic patients or inhalational disease; require triple antibiotic therapy
  - Ciprofloxacin or doxycycline *plus*
  - Two other antibiotics (eg, rifampin, clindamycin)
- Antibiotic therapy must continue for 60 days.

Plague

Organism: Y. *pestis*, a Gram-negative bacillus.

Plague is normally a disease of rodents transmitted to humans by inhalation of flea feces or bite of infected flea.

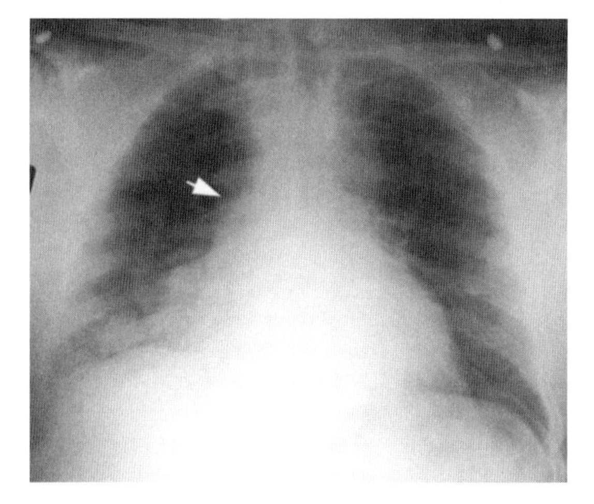

FIGURE 20.6. Inhalational anthrax. Arrow indicates mediastinal lymphadenopathy.

(Reproduced, with permission, from Mayer TA, et al. "Clinical Presentation of Inhalational Anthrax Following Bioterrorism Exposure: Report of 2 Surviving Patients." *JAMA*. 2001;286:2549–2553.)

Forms of disease:

- **Bubonic** (skin)
  - Bacilli migrate to regional lymph nodes → bubo.
- **Pneumonic** (inhalational)
  - Most common
  - May be transmitted person to person
- **Septicemia** (from secondary dissemination)

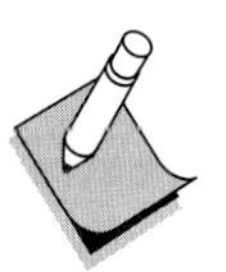

Pneumonic plague is due to inhalation of Y. pestis *(Gram-negative bacillus), normally found in flea feces.*

SYMPTOMS/EXAM

Bubonic Plague

- Two to three days incubation followed by:
  - Regional **painful** lymph node inflammation and necrosis (bubo, see Figure 20.7)
  - Fevers, chills, malaise
  - Will disseminate over next week in 50% (if untreated) → septicemia

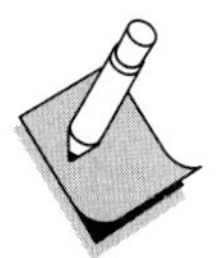

Half of untreated patients with bubonic plague will develop septicemia from bacterial dissemination.

Pneumonic Plague

- Two to three days incubation followed by:
  - Abrupt onset of fevers, chills, and flulike illness
  - Severe pneumonia in 24 hours
  - Patients may develop meningitis, liver injury, coagulation disturbances, and gangrene in extremities (black death).

Septicemic Plague

- Characterized by endotoxemia, shock, DIC, and coma

DIAGNOSIS

- Suspect in any healthy individual who develops overwhelming Gram-negative sepsis.
- Gram stain and culture all body fluids.

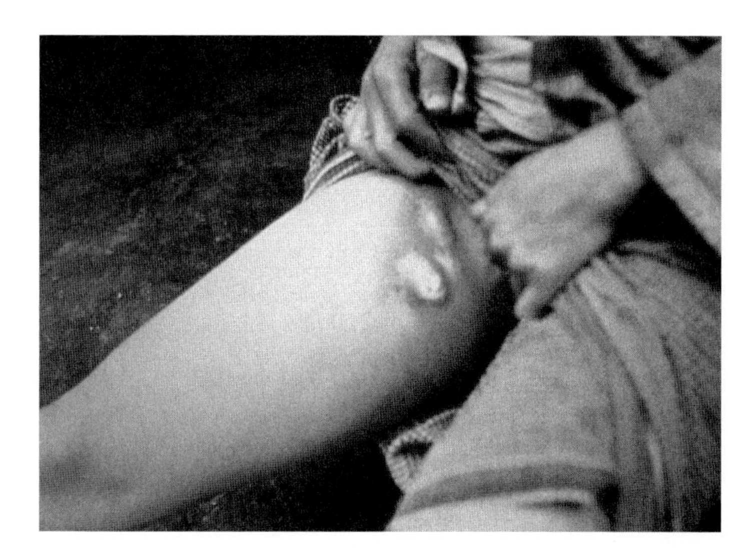

FIGURE 20.7. Plague: An inguinal bubo.

(Courtesy of the CDC.)

Treatment

- Isolate patients.
- Do **not** incise and drain fluctuant lymph nodes (aspiration **ok**).
- Antibiotics: Multiple choices available
- Mild bubonic may be treated at home.
- Prophylaxis: Same drugs for 7-day course

Smallpox

Organism: *V. major*, a large DNA virus

Was successfully eradicated in 1980 with small pox vaccine, but United States and Russia have viral repositories for research purposes

There are several clinical forms of disease:

- **Variola major and minor**—90% of cases
  - The classic form of disease
- **Hemorrhagic smallpox**
- **Malignant smallpox**

Symptoms/Exam

Variola Major and Minor

- Incubation period of 2 weeks, followed by:
- Constitutional symptoms
- Maculopapular rash (see Figure 20.8)

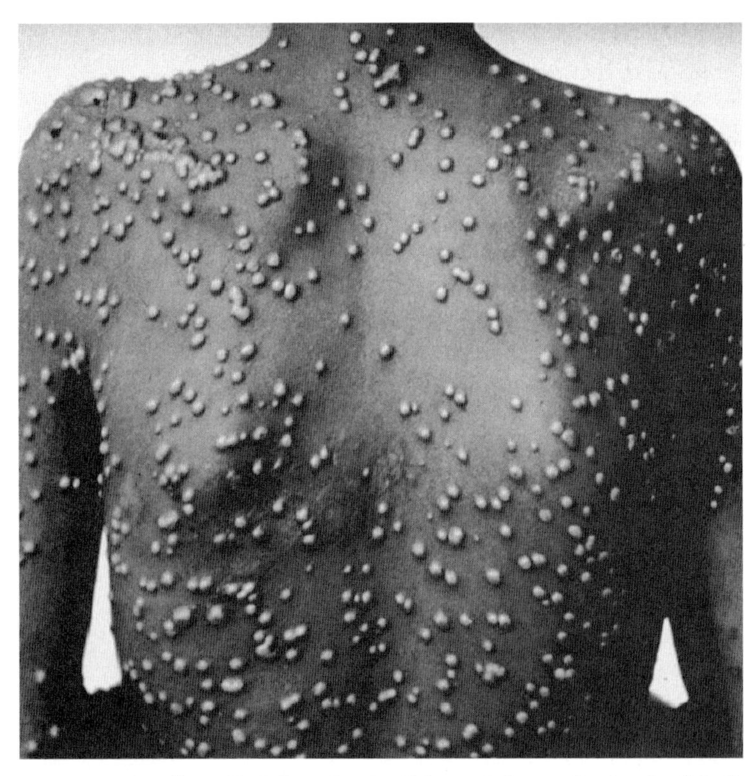

FIGURE 20.8. Smallpox: Variola major. Mutiple pustules on the trunk, all in the same stage of development.

(Reproduced, with permission, from Wolff K, Johnson RA, Surrmond D. *Fitzpatrick's Color Atlas & Synopsis of Clinical Dermatology*, 5th ed. New York: McGraw-Hill, 2005:771.)

- Begins in mouth
- Predilection for face, then spreads distally
- Involves palms and soles
- Changes from vesicular to pustular with **all lesions in same stage**

Hemorrhagic Smallpox

- Quicker and more toxic course
- Petechiae and hemorrhage (not pox)
- Ninety percent mortality

Malignant Smallpox

- Also quicker and more toxic course
- Lesions are flatter and never progress to pustules.

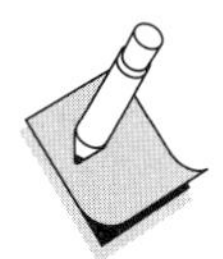

Classic smallpox lesions change from maculopapules → vesicles → pustules with all lesions in the same stage of development.

DIAGNOSIS

- CDC clinical diagnosis algorithm (see Table 20.9):
  - Major criteria:
    - Febrile prodrome
    - Classic smallpox lesions
    - Lesions in same stage of development
  - Minor criteria:
    - Centrifugal distribution of pustules
    - Toxic appearance
    - First lesions in mouth, face, or forearms
    - Slow evolution of lesions
    - Pustules on the palms and soles
  - Three major → presumed disease.
  - Two major or one major and four minor → probable disease.
  - Fewer than four minor → disease not likely.
- Laboratory PCR identification of variola DNA in a clinical specimen

TABLE 20.9. CDC Clinical Criteria for Diagnosing Smallpox

Major criteria
Febrile prodrome
Classic smallpox lesions
Lesions in the same stage of development
Minor criteria
Centrifugal distribution of pustules
Toxic appearance
First lesions in mouth, face, or forearms
Slow evolution of lesions
Pustules on the palms and soles
Three major → presumed disease
Two major or one major and four minor → probable disease
Fewer than four minor → disease not likely

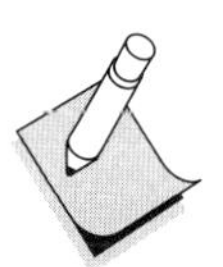

Vaccinia immunoglobulin is given to limit the complications of smallpox vaccination (not disease).

TREATMENT

- Isolate patient.
  - Very contagious until all scabs fall off
- Exposed persons → vaccinate within 3 days to prevent or attenuate disease.
  - Vaccinia immunoglobulin is given simultaneously with vaccine and redosed as needed to limit complications of vaccination.
- Antivirals are being investigated as treatment.

Tularemia

Organism: *F. tularensis*, a Gram-negative intracellular bacterium

Tularemia (commonly called "rabbit fever") is transmitted primarily from ticks, lagomorphs, and rodents via direct contact or ingestion of infected water, soil, or fomites.

Several forms exist depending on route of contact:

- **Localized disease** with regional lymph node involvement:
  - Ulceroglandular: Most common
  - Glandular: Second most common
  - Oculoglandular
  - Oropharyngeal
- **Invasive and generalized disease**:
  - Typhoidal
  - Pulmonary

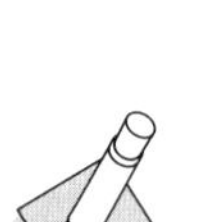

The most common form of Tularemia = ulcerogladular.

SYMPTOMS/EXAM

- Multiple presentations are possible depending upon which form is present (see Table 20.10).

TABLE 20.10. Clinical Findings in Tularemia

Localized Disease	
Ulceroglandular disease	Ulcerated skin lesion Regional (sometimes generalized) lympadenopathy Fever
Glandular tularemia	Regional lymphadenopathy without skin lesion
Oculoglandular tularemia	Conjunctivitis with preauricular adenopathy
Oropharyngeal tularemia	Severe pharyngitis with cervical lymphadenitis
Invasive and Generalized Disease	
Typhoidal tularemia	Fevers, chills GI symptoms No skin lesions
Pulmonary tularemia	Fevers, chills Nonproductive cough, shortness of breath

- In localized disease:
  - Ulcerated skin (see Figure 20.9), conjunctivitis, or pharyngitis with associated regional lymphadenopathy, **or**
  - Regional lymphadenopathy alone
- Typhoidal tularemia:
  - Fevers, chills, GI symptoms without skin lesions
- Pulmonary tularemia:
  - Fevers, chills, nonproductive cough, shortness of breath

DIAGNOSIS

- Based on clinical findings
- Antibody titers, rapid PCR

TREATMENT

- Isolation is **not** required.
- Antibiotic: Streptomycin is drug of choice.
- Prophylaxis = doxycycline.

Viral Hemorrhagic Fever

Organisms: Filoviruses and arenaviruses

Normally transmitted via mosquitoes, rodents, or their parasites

SYMPTOMS/EXAM

- Incubation period from 4 to 21 days, followed by:
  - Fevers, myalgias, prostration
  - Petechial hemorrhage, DIC
  - Multisystem organ dysfunction, cardiovascular collapse

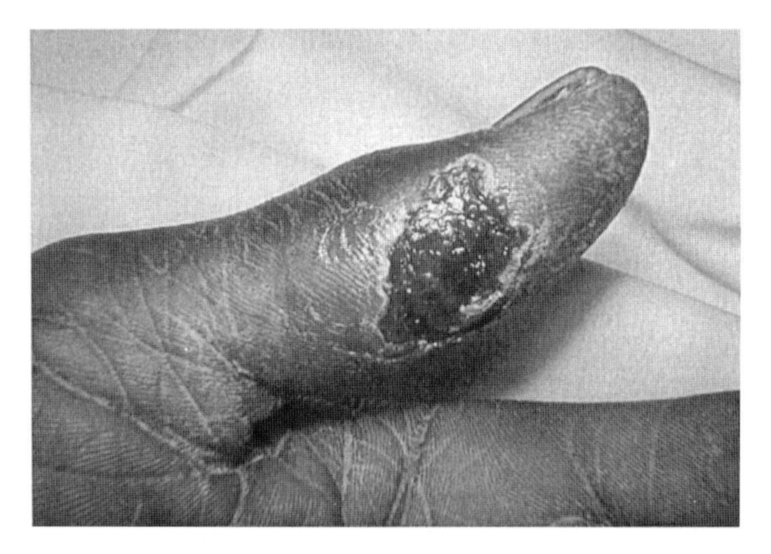

FIGURE 20.9. Tularemia: Ulcerated skin lesion.

(Courtesy of the CDC.)

DIAGNOSIS

- ELISA or PCR

TREATMENT

- Supportive care
- Antiviral: Ribavirin
- Prophylaxis: Ribavirin

CHEMICAL WEAPONS OF MASS DESTRUCTION

Agents include nerve agents, vesicants, and blood agents (cyanide: see Chapter 6.)

Nerve Agents

Nerve agents are organophosphates and include sarin, soman, VX.

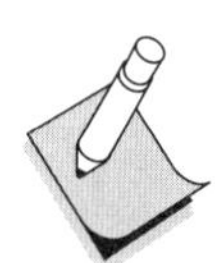

Nerve agents (sarin, soman, VX) inhibit acetylcholinesterase producing a cholinergic toxidrome.

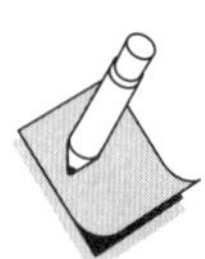

Antidotes to nerve agent poisoning = atropine and pralidoxime.

PATHOPHYSIOLOGY

- Inhibit acetylcholinesterase → accumulation of acetylcholine at muscarinic and nicotinic receptors → cholinergic toxidrome.

SYMPTOMS/EXAM

- Cholinergic toxidrome (SLUDGE): Salivation/sweating, lacrimation, urination, defecation, GI distress, emesis
- Miotic pupils
- Fasciculations, muscle weakness, apnea
- Altered mentation or seizures

DIAGNOSIS

- Based on history of exposure and clinical presentation

TREATMENT

- Supportive care
- **Atropine** dosed to secretion control (may require 2–4 mg at frequent intervals)
- **Pralidoxime** chloride (2-PAM) to reverse paralysis
- **Benzodiazepines** for seizures

Vesicants

Agents that induce blistering via cellular damage, including mustard

SYMPTOMS/EXAM

- Local skin effects: Severe pain, vesicle formation, and inflammation to site of contact
  - Skin injury resembles second-degree burn.
- Inhalation effects: Pharyngeal edema and pulmonary necrosis → varying degrees of respiratory distress
- Systemic effects: Bone marrow suppression

TREATMENT

- Skin and mucous membrane decontamination with irrigation
- Supportive care

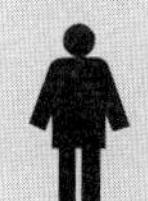

A nuclear physicist presents to the ED after total-body radiation exposure of uncertain dose. On arrival he appears acutely ill with nausea, vomiting, and disorientation. What can you predict regarding his likely clinical course?

The rapid onset of prodromal and CNS symptoms indicates an extremely high-exposure dose. This patient will likely develop refractory hypotension, circulatory collapse, and death in 24–72 hours despite aggressive intensive care.

RADIATION INJURIES

Most radiation exposures occur accidentally in an industrial setting, with the most common overall site of injury = hands.

Types of exposure:

- **Contamination:** Either external via skin or internal via inhalation or ingestion
  - These patients are "radioactive."
  - For example, the recent intentional poisoning of a former Russian agent with Polonium-210
- **Irradiation**
  - Patients pose no risk to other people.

PATHOPHYSIOLOGY

- **Ionizing radiation** (alpha particles, beta particles, neutrons, gamma rays) has short wavelength, high frequency, and high energy
- High-level exposure → direct cell death.
- Low-level exposure → formation of free radicals → breakage of DNA and RNA strands → cell injury and/or death.
- Rapidly dividing cells (bone marrow, GI, and reproductive) are most sensitive.

Lethal dose 50 (LD_{50}) is the dose that will kill 50% of the exposed population within 60 days = approximately 450 radiation-absorbed dose (rad) or 4.5 gray (Gy).

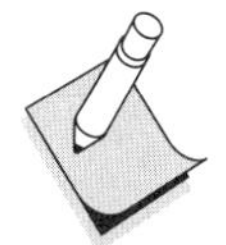

Higher radiation exposure is associated with earlier prodrome phase and shorter latent phase.

Local Skin Exposure

Results in cutaneous changes ranging from erythema to overt skin necrosis and ulceration, depending on dose

Acute Radiation Syndrome (ARS)

Occurs after whole body ionizing radiation exposure to a dose of >2 Gy. It is divided into three phases: Prodromal, latent, and manifest illness (see Table 20.11).

PRODROMAL PHASE

- Autonomic nervous system response to radiation
- Primarily gastrointestinal symptoms: N/V, diarrhea
- Higher exposure = earlier, longer, and more severe symptoms, including bloody diarrhea.

TABLE 20.11. Acute radiation syndrome

Approximate Dose	Onset of Prodrome	Duration of Latent Phase	Manifest Illness
>2 gy (200 rad)	Within 2 days	1–3 weeks	Hematopoietic syndrome with pancytopenia, infection, and hemorrhage; survival possible
>6 gy (600 rad)	Within hours	<1 week	GI syndrome with dehydration, electrolyte abnormalities, GI bleeding, and fulminant enterocolitis; uniformly fatal
>30 gy (3000 rad)	Within minutes	None	Cardiovascular/CNS syndrome with refractory hypotension and circulatory collapse; fatal within 24–72 h

(Reproduced, with permission, from Tintinalli JE, Kelen GD, Stapczynski JS, *Emergency Medicine: A Comprehensive Study Guide*, 6th ed. New York: McGraw-Hill, 2004:56.)

Latent Phase

- Symptom-free interval, prior to onset of bone marrow suppression
- Generally lasts 2–4 weeks
- Again, higher exposure = shorter latent period.

Manifest-Illness Phase

- Consists of the following "syndromes" that occur with increasing radiation dose:
  - **Hematopoietic syndrome**
    - Bone marrow suppression with resultant complications
    - Survival likely with appropriate care
  - **Gastrointestinal syndrome**
    - Reappearance of GI symptoms
    - Survival possible with aggressive care
  - **Cardiovascular/CNS syndrome ("neurovascular")**
    - Altered mentation and hypotension typically occurring immediately following exposure
    - Universally lethal with death in 24–72 hours

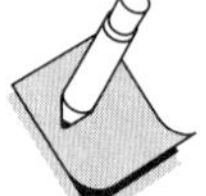

Estimating exposure dose after whole body radiation: Timing of onset of prodromal symptoms (earlier = higher dose) and/or Timing of onset of lymphocyte depletion (earlier/rapid = higher dose)

Diagnosis

- Exposure history
- A Geiger-Mueller counter can detect all contaminating ionizing radiation (depending on model).
- The actual exposure dose is often not known, but can be estimated by clinical or laboratory findings ("biologic dosimetry"):
  - The timing of onset of prodromal symptoms.
    - No vomiting by 4 hours → nonlethal dose.
    - Vomiting in <2 hours → serious/lethal dose.
  - Timing of onset of lymphocyte depletion
    - Rapid decline (over hours) = serious/lethal dose.

TABLE 20.12. Predicting Survival After Radiation Injury

PROGNOSIS	ABSOLUTE LYMPHOCYTES (AT 48 HOURS)
Good	>1200/mm^3
Fair	300–1200/mm^3
Poor	<300/mm^3

TREATMENT

- Immediate decontamination, as needed:
  - Remove clothing (will remove the majority of contamination), wash skin.
  - Enhance elimination of ingested particles (cathartics, lavage etc).
  - Blocking agents: eg, potassium iodine for radioactive iodine exposure
  - Chelating agents: eg, calcium disodium edetate and penicillamine for radioactive lead exposure
- Supportive care
- The absolute lymphocyte count at 48 hours is the best predictor of survival (see Table 20.12).

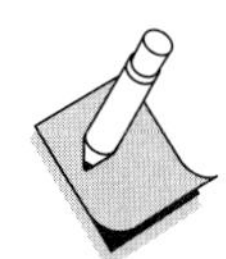

The absolute lymphocyte count at 48 hours can be used to predict survival.

COMPLICATIONS

- Delayed malignancy
- Mutagenesis in offspring

BLAST INJURIES

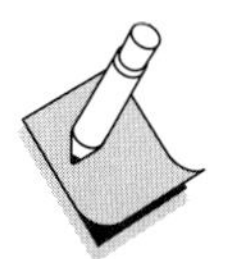

Primary last injury = blast pressure wave. Secondary blast injury = projectiles from the explosion. Tertiary blast injury = blunt trauma from explosion.

Primary Blast Injury

- Barotrauma resulting from the blast pressure wave
- Air-containing structure is most commonly affected (ears, lung, intestines).

Secondary Blast Injury

- Results from solid projectiles from the explosive itself or the surrounding structures

Tertiary Blast Injury

- Seen when victim is thrown against a solid structure or caught in a structural collapse
- Most lethal injury

Most common blast injury = tympanic membrane (TM) rupture at the pars tensa. This predicts other significant injury.

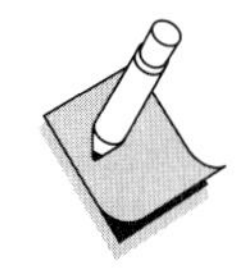

TM rupture predicts other significant injury.

SYMPTOMS/EXAM

- Depends on organs involved and presence of secondary or tertiary injuries

Primary Blast Injury

- Ear involvement: Hearing loss, vertigo, nystagmus, and TM rupture
- Pulmonary

- Barotrauma (pneumothorax, air embolism, pneumomediastinum)
  - Pulmonary hemorrhage: Increasing respiratory distress and poor air exchange
- Intestinal
  - Less common than ear or lung injury
  - Intestinal wall hemorrhage and edema → abdominal pain, N/V.

Secondary and Tertiary Blast Injury

- Findings of penetrating injuries, boney fractures/dislocations, closed head injuries
- If suicide bomber, possible human foreign material embedded

DIAGNOSIS

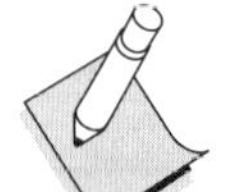

Following blast injury, obtain abdominal CT if any GI symptoms are present.

- Standard trauma evaluation
- Careful evaluation to rule out primary blast injury:
  - CXR in all cases
  - Chest CT if significant pulmonary symptoms
  - Abdominal CT if any GI symptoms

TREATMENT

- Supportive care
- Treat associated injuries.
- Risk of pneumothorax and air embolism is particularly high in blast lung injury.
  - Minimize peak airway pressures and allow permissive hypercapnea in ventilated patient.
  - Immediate hyperbarics if suspected air embolism
- Consider Hepatitis B vaccine and IgG if suicide bomber.

CHAPTER 21

Legal Issues

Hugh F. Hill III, MD, JD, FACEP, FCLM

Licensure

To Become a Licensed Physician, You Must

- Successfully complete a required course of education in a school that is licensed and accredited
- Pass a standardized examination.
- Fulfill the requirements of your government.
- Obtain at least one state's permission to practice.

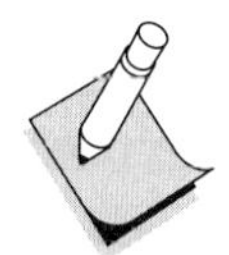

*Medical licenses are granted and regulated by **states**.*

To Become a Board-Certified Emergency Physician, You Must Also

- Complete a required course of training in an accredited postgraduate emergency medicine residency program approved by the Accreditation Council for Graduate Medical Education (ACGME).
- Pass a qualifying examination and an oral certification exam as specified by the American Board of Emergency Medicine (ABEM).

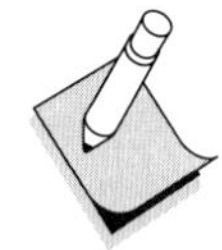

Licensure is general, but hospital privileges are specific.

State medical practice statutes vest authority in state medical boards, which control access to licensure and regulate in the public's interest, subject to judicial review. Courts usually cannot be persuaded to intervene unless the physician has exhausted administrative remedies. Unlike in the podiatric, chiropractic, dental, or other professions, medical licenses are **unrestricted.** Any licensed physician can perform neurosurgery or even practice emergency medicine—if he can convince a hospital to allow it. There is no right to a medical license, but courts have overturned state requirements that unconstitutionally discriminate, such as U.S. citizenship and minimum length of residency requirements. Applicants must establish credentials, competence, and character to the state board's satisfaction, and pay a fee.

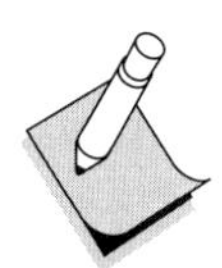

Adverse action against a license or privilege holder can become the basis of similar or even more severe action by other institutions—Win one, win one; lose one, lose all.

Grounds for Denial of License, as Well as Basis for Revocation, Sanction, and Discipline of Established License Holders Include

- Fraudulent or false application statements
- Conviction of a felony
- Suspension or reduction of hospital privileges
- Unprofessional conduct, eg, disruptive behavior
- Immoral conduct, eg, sexual activity with patients

State boards of medicine discipline small numbers of physicians, only 2–3%. Critics of our profession's commitment and ability to police itself suggest that up to 10% of physicians may be impaired.

> A newly hired emergency physician is scheduled to work tonight, but the state has not yet issued his license. Can he work his shift?
>
> No. In addition to likely violating the group's contract with the hospital and medical staff rules regarding privileges, it would violate state law that prohibits practicing medicine without a license.

Credentialing

Hospital credentialing is specific to each institution. A committee of physician colleagues and administrators grants an approved list of activities, especially procedures based on education, training, and experience. Hospitals may accept ABEM certification as a sufficient indicator of competence, but they do not have to. When new techniques and technologies are introduced, physicians must often demonstrate knowledge and skills. State boards, insurors, regulatory agencies, and others organizations may use credentialing, or denial and revocation of credentials by one another, as a basis for adverse action on payment, participation, and even licensing.

COMPLIANCE AND CONFIDENTIALITY

Although the word compliance in common usage has much wider meaning, in health law it refers to conformity with rules, especially federal medical billing rules and patient confidentiality laws.

Billing

Billing for services requires both the CPT® (Current Procedural Terminology) and International Classification of Diseases (ICD) codes. One overly simple way to look at the two is that the CPT is what you did and the ICD is why you did it.

CURRENT PROCEDURAL TERMINOLOGY

- Basis of Evaluation and Management (E&M) codes
- Owned and published by the American Medical Association
- Enforced by Medicare
- Five levels of E&M codes plus the critical care code
- Insurers insist on the codes in all billing submissions.

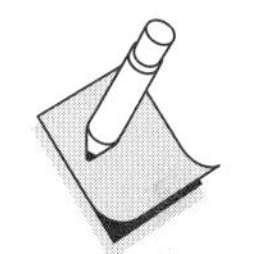

A medical bill submitted in your name can subject you to penalties and fines for lack of compliance.

Billing for services not performed is fraud, if intentional. Fraud is a form of theft and subjects the physician to fines and other penalties. The more common problem for physicians is error. It often results from use of billing agencies or the hospital's system. Even honest error can subject the physician, not the billing company, to investigation by insurers, principally Medicare or Medicaid. Investigators come to the hospital and review a number of charts. If inaccurate or unsupported coding is found, the percentage of that finding can be applied to all bills in a given period. Errors are discovered through automated review, focused medical review, and random audits.

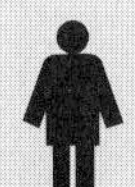

An ED patient in police custody is being discharged and the officer wants a copy of the medical record. Can you give it to him?

Only if the patient/arrestee consents.

Confidentiality and HIPAA

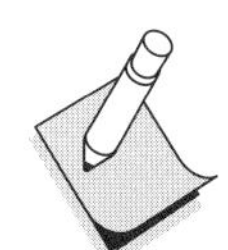

Disclosures of confidential health information must comply with the privacy rule of HIPAA.

The Health Insurance Portability and Accountability Act of 1996 (HIPAA) was intended to:

- Standardize health information transfers
- Require identification numbers for providers, health plans, and employers
- Protect confidential protected health information

The direction to address protected health information (PHI) was included because of fears that electronic transfers and ID numbers could be misused. So the law penalized disclosures of confidential health information that are not authorized in writing by the patient and violate the privacy rule. PHI includes (but is not limited to) name, postal address, telephone numbers, e-mail addresses, social security numbers, medical record numbers, health plan beneficiary numbers, vehicle identifiers, driver's licenses, and biometric identifiers such as facial photographs and fingerprints.

The concept of confidentiality and the risk of civil liability that guided physicians and hospitals in the past is now subsumed in HIPAA compliance rules. The Secretary of Health and Human Services imposes civil monetary penalties for violation of any HIPAA requirement, up to $25,000 per disclosure.

Important Points About HIPAA and Confidentiality

- Any release of PHI to another health provider eg, getting information from another hospital, must be accompanied by a signed release from the patient.
- Mandatory reporting requirements to an agency (eg, a local health authority) must include a written note of such disclosure in the patient's medical record.
- Police do **not** have automatic access to a patient's medical record.
- Disclosures for the purposes of treatment or "health care operations" are permitted, except for **psychotherapy notes,** which have a special status. Disclosures for billing are allowed, but may be limited by "minimum necessary" rules.

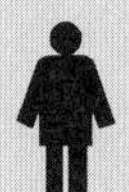

Tom is more drunk than usual, or is he? His head CT shows an epidural hematoma. Does the neurosurgeon need consent before she drills?

No, unless his family is readily available.

CONSENT AND REFUSAL OF CARE

Precedents in the law regarding informed consent appear in the category of suits for "battery," defined as a harmful or offensive unpermitted touch. In the medical context, touch is expected, but without consent, the emergency physician can be liable for battery. All injuries resulting from the touch are injuries for which the victim could sue even if there is no malpractice.

Consent can be

- Expressed
  - Verbally
  - Written form
- Implied

Informed Consent

Obtaining informed consent should be considered:

- When the procedure is extraordinary, ie, not routine for most patients
- When the procedure carries significant risks
- When it is the community standard, ie, situations where others do it
- Where hospital rules require it

In general, the patient or a substituted decision maker should know:

- The **nature of the procedure** being proposed
- The **expected outcome**
- The **risks** of the proposed procedure
- The **natural history**, eg, what may happen if the procedure is not attempted
- What **alternatives** exist

The law contains two tests that address how much detail to present with these items:

1. The reasonable physician standard.
The first test courts used was to ask was: What would a reasonable physician tell a patient? This professional standard is like a "standard of care" analysis for negligence, requiring expert testimony.

2. The reasonable patient standard.
Many states now ask juries: "What would a reasonable patient want to know before undergoing the procedure?" Predictably, this shift has meant more litigation and initially left providers guessing or overreacting.

When a patient cannot consent, do not think that consent is no longer necessary. Instead, think that consent is not possible. Then, in situations of emergency or waiver, for example, you will know that you have to document the reasons obtaining consent was not possible.

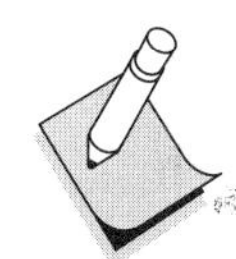

A signed form can be a manifestation of, but not a substitute for, actual consent.

The signed form or the chart note is not informed consent. It is a representation of what information was communicated. The documentation should include the essential characteristics of an informed consent.

Caution dictates that documentation include complete lists of risks and alternatives discussed, but this is impractical. In obtaining informed consent always include risks of death, permanent limb and organ impairment, all serious and severe possibilities, and temporary minor adverse results that occur >5% of the time. Precise means of injury and causation do not need to be disclosed in detail.

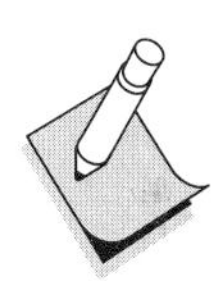

*The Emergency Exception is **not** a blanket covering all ED patients. Do not presume this exception applies unless the patient cannot communicate and the treatment must take place **immediately**.*

Most forms require the **signature of a witness**. If you want the witness to be able to testify as to what was said in the informed consent session, that person has to be present throughout the conversation. More commonly, the witness is only confirming that the patient signed the document, and has to be present only for the signing.

THE EMERGENCY EXCEPTION DOCTRINE

In extreme situations, emergency physicians may treat the patient without consent **only if all of the three** following conditions are met:

- The patient is unable to express his or her wishes.
- The patient has a condition that demands **immediate** attention.
- No family or other substitute decision maker is immediately available to consent.

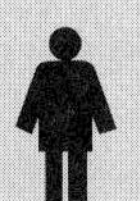

The nurse objects to getting Dick's consent for the procedure. "He'll freak out and try to leave." Can you skip informing Fred for his own good?

No.

THERAPEUTIC PRIVILEGE

Another exception to the requirement for informed consent that appears in both statutes and case law is therapeutic privilege. If the information and discussion would be dangerous for the patient, they can be limited. This may be helpful to other specialists who have established relationships with their patients, but is not useful to emergency physicians.

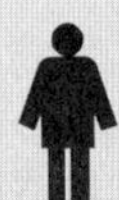

Harry says, "I don't wanna know. Just do it." If you use this exception, document witnessed offers to inform **and** the patient's mental ability to make this choice.

WAIVER

Patients sometimes respond, "Whatever you say, doctor. I trust you." Both case law and statute recognize that a patient's rejection of attempts to give information is a defense to a suit. Witnessed notes in the chart and signed statements from the patient can help prove the patient insisted on not knowing.

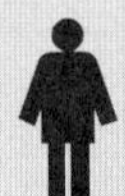

Tonight, Fred is obviously intoxicated, but he has a fever and seems more impaired than his blood alcohol level indicates. Can he consent to a lumbar puncture?

No, he lacks the mental capacity.

Capacity to Consent

The capacity to consent requires

- **Physical ability** to perceive and respond to information, and
- **Mental ability** to process, prioritize, and exercise judgment

Capacity is always contextual. So sometimes emergency physicians have to assess—and document—a patient's capacity. A patient need not be fully functioning constantly, in every respect, to meet this standard. **Lucid moments may allow valid consent**.

The law sometimes presumes that the individual's status invalidates the capacity to consent. The most common situations of this type involve minors and the mentally incompetent.

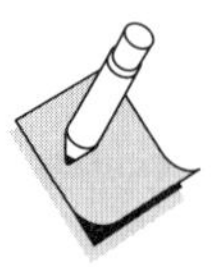

The capacity to make a decision requires that the patient have the ability to understand what is proposed and the consequences of accepting or rejecting the intervention.

States Can Make Exceptions Including:

- Emancipated minors: Minors with dependent children, who are self-supporting, or have court-approved independence from parents
- Minors seeking medical attention for:
  - Reproductive issues
  - Communicable diseases
  - Drug abuse

Substituted Consent

Since the law often restricts who may consent for incapacitated patients, the family member or other person who is most available may not be the right source.

If a court has declared the patient to be under guardianship including making medical decisions, or if a patient prior to their infirmity has signed advance directives and authorized a substitute decision maker, the person to ask for consent is obvious.

Without a court order or advance directives, physicians sometimes look to the "next-of-kin." Many states have statutes prescribing which relative and in what order. These statues may track the order of inheritance of those who die without a will. They do not identify individuals within a class; for example, two siblings may have equal authority. Lack of consensus among family and others who claim to be empowered to consent or refuse is dangerous for the provider.

Refusal to Consent

Apart from emergency situations and other contexts where patients do not have the capacity to decide, patients have the right to refuse treatment. The patient's values may be strange to the physician, but must be respected. Unusual philosophical or religious beliefs do not necessarily mean that the patient lacks capacity. However, a choice clearly inconsistent with a patient's lifelong value system does raise questions about capacity.

Refusal has to be informed, comparable to consent. In the context of an informed consent counseling session, this will not be difficult. The provider is already discussing the risks and alternatives, including refusing to do anything, and the risks of those alternatives. Sensitivity to the legal issues and extra effort are required when routine procedures are rejected informally.

Treat refusal of recommended care like informed consent. Make it an "informed refusal."

Make the discussion an informed refusal session, to the extent the patient will allow. Patients who don't want to listen or who leave before any discussion are still a potential problem, and their rejection of information should be documented. Patients who are willing to listen should be warned of the risks they are taking by refusing care or choosing a nonrecommended option.

In an emergency, patients still have the right to self-determination, but if they lack the capacity to decide, you may proceed if there is no time to find a surrogate or obtain a court order. Remember to include the risks to the patient of force, if they are physically resisting, in your considerations. As soon as you can, write a note explaining why you proceeded without consent. Court orders and surrogate identification will usually be sought after admission, often with the help of the hospital's legal counsel. **Regardless of how you reach your conclusion, if the court is not involved, documentation must support it.**

Some people do not have the capacity to consent or refuse because of their status:

- **Minors** are the most obvious category, and usually a parent is available to consent. Beware the pediatric patient who appears with some other relative or friend—you cannot assume that someone other than a parent has the authority to approve care for the child.
- **Victims of infectious disease**, for example, can have treatment forced on them for public health reasons.
- **Incarcerated patients**. Police may bring in a suspected drunken driver and demand that blood be drawn for testing. In these situations, avoid establishing a physician-patient relationship. If the person asks about other health issues, make it clear that you are not taking care of him, and those questions should be addressed to his own physician. If the person refuses the treatment

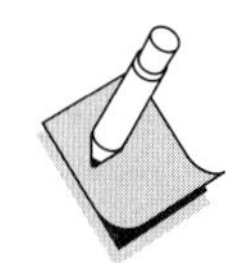

People in another's custody, be it police, family, or nursing home, are not automatically unable to refuse treatment.

apparently required by law, you must decide how comfortable you are proceeding without a specific court order. Arrestees and incarcerated prisoners have not automatically lost the right to refuse medical care.

Patients Who Refuse Treatment or Leave Against Medical Advice Should Have the Following Documented in the Medical Record

- Mental capacity to refuse treatment
- Understanding of the risks of refusing treatment and explanation of alternative treatment, if any
- Discharge instructions if appropriate
- Follow-up care options if appropriate

EMERGENCY MEDICAL TREATMENT AND ACTIVE LABOR ACT (EMTALA)

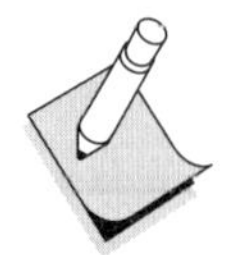

EMTALA focuses on medical screening and stability, not simply financial motivations for transfers.

At its most basic, EMTALA mandates that unstable patients cannot be discharged or transferred except for medical necessity.

The Emergency Medical Treatment and Active Labor Act:

- First appeared in the 1986 Consolidated Omnibus Budget Reconciliation Act (COBRA)
- Discourages poor and high-risk patients from being transferred from one ED to another for financial advantage
- Encourages "**equal**" treatment for patients, not necessarily appropriate treatment
- Is **not malpractice law**
- Mandates that hospitals keep **on-call lists** of specialty physicians

EMTALA Basics

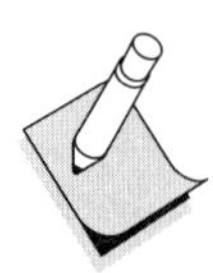

Patients must have screening and stabilization before discharge from the ED.

- Any patient presenting to an emergency department has the right to a **medical screening exam (MSE)** to determine if an emergency medical condition (EMC) exists without regard to the patient's ability or willingness to pay for any services rendered.
- If an EMC exists, the hospital must, given its resources including staff and facilities, **stabilize the condition.** The term "stabilize" means to assure that no material deterioration of the condition is likely to result from or occur during the transfer, or to deliver the baby and placenta.
- If the hospital cannot stabilize the condition, the staff are further obligated to **transfer the patient** to a facility that can.

An EMC Is One Where:

- Any delay in treatment would cause loss of body functions or impairment to organs or limbs. The regulation offered examples of such symptoms: severe pain, psychic disturbances, and/or symptoms of substance abuse.
- A pregnant woman is contracting and there isn't time to transfer her before she delivers, or the transfer may pose a threat to mother or child. In reality, if a woman is in active labor in the emergency department, she should deliver in that hospital.

An MSE:

- **Is not triage!** MSE requires the usual workup including ancillary tests and consultations as necessary to determine if an EMC exists.

- Can be performed by anyone the hospital designates as its standard of practice; in practice, this is usually the physician, but it can be a delegate, ie, nurse, physician assistant, etc.

Transfers, When the EMC Is Not Yet Stabilized, Cannot Take Place Unless:

- The patient or representative requests it, knowing the risks and the hospital's EMTALA obligations, or
- The transferring physician certifies the benefits outweigh the risks, and
- The transfer is medically appropriate

An Appropriate Transfer Includes the Following Elements:

- The transferring hospital must do all it can to **minimize the risks of transfer**.
- The receiving hospital has **available space and personnel** and has agreed to take the case.
- The transferring hospital sends **copies of records**, including the name and address of any on-call physician who has refused or failed to appear within a reasonable time to help stabilize the patient.
- The transfer must use qualified personnel and equipment.
- Medical records must be maintained by the hospital for a period of 5 years from the date of transfer.

If a receiving hospital, such as burn or shock-trauma units, has capacity, it cannot refuse "appropriate transfers." This leaves open the possibility of rejecting inappropriate transfers, but many authorities point to the difficulty of proof and suggest a "Just Say Yes" policy.

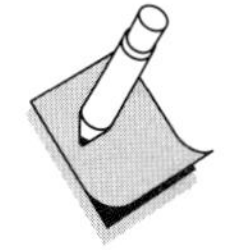

Referral center hospitals, eg, burn centers, with capacity cannot refuse transfers.

The New Regulations of 2003 Made the Following Modifications:

- A **dedicated emergency department** is any hospital-owned or controlled facility that is:
  - Licensed by the state as an emergency department
  - Held out to the public or advertised as seeing emergency medical conditions without appointment, **or**
  - One-third or more of its outpatient visits in the previous year were for EMCs without appointment.
  - Previous amendments to the regulation considered **all hospital-owned and operated ambulances** and any property within **250 yards of the campus** as "coming to the hospital"
- **On-call requirements** for hospitals were relaxed; allow for one specialist to take call for several hospitals simultaneously as long as there is a backup plan in case the specialist is unavailable.
- A hospital's EMTALA obligation ends with hospital admission.
- **Nonemergent conditions** do not invoke an EMTALA obligation. For example, patients coming for suture removal are exempt from EMTALA.
- Normal registration processes may be followed as long as screening and stabilizing treatment are NOT delayed.
- **Hospital ambulances** are **not** subject to community-wide EMS protocols on hospital diversion.
- **Bioterrorism emergencies** are **exempt** from EMTALA regulations.

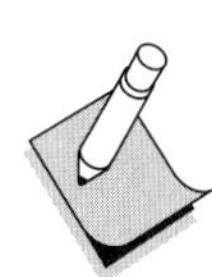

Civil monetary penalties are not covered by malpractice insurance.

EMTALA Violations

Enforcement of EMTALA is complaint driven. To that end, the law requires hospitals receiving transfers to report violations within 72 hours. EMTALA is enforced by the Office of the Inspector General. Civil penalties include:

- A hospital that negligently violates an EMTALA requirement may have to pay up to $50,000 per violation.
- The responsible emergency physician and the on-call physician who negligently violate may also have to pay up to $50,000 per violation. **Civil money penalties such as EMTALA are not covered by malpractice insurance.**
- Violation may result in loss of Medicare/Medicaid billing privileges for the hospital.

LIABILITY AND MALPRACTICE

Statute of Limitations is time limits in which to file a claim for malpractice. They vary from state to state but are usually within 2 or 3 years from the date of the injury or when they discover the negligence. These statutes carry exceptions for disability, legal minority or mental illness, but even these extensions are not open-ended.

Most potential cases are rejected by at least one lawyer. Of those filed, some are settled, some dismissed by judges, and some—estimates suggest only ~10%—go to trial. Of malpractice trials, physician defendants win more than half. The numbers also suggest that most emergency physicians will be sued at least once in their professional lifetimes.

The Legal Process

REQUIRED ELEMENTS OF A MALPRACTICE LAWSUIT

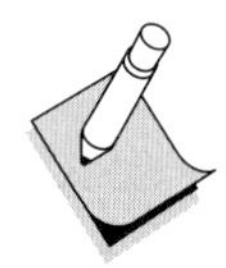

Negligence forms the basis of most malpractice cases.

To Get to a Jury, Plaintiff Must Offer Proof That:

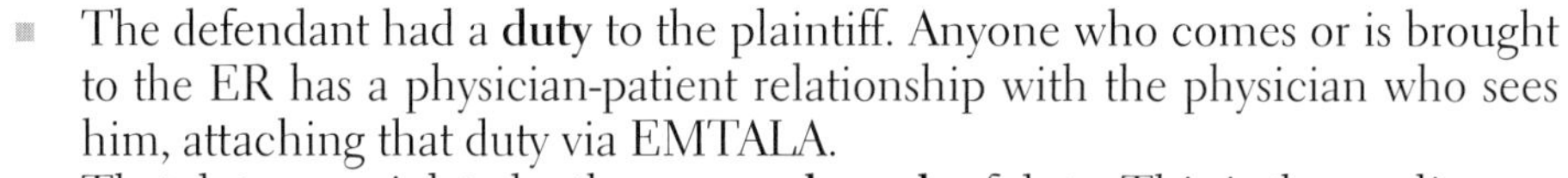

- The defendant had a **duty** to the plaintiff. Anyone who comes or is brought to the ER has a physician-patient relationship with the physician who sees him, attaching that duty via EMTALA.
- That duty was violated—there was a **breach** of duty. This is the negligence in a medical negligence case.
- The plaintiff was injured—there were **damages**. What would the plaintiff's condition have been if the duty had been fulfilled? If the outcome would have been the same, there are no damages.
- There was a causal link between the breach and the damages—there was **causation**. It's not enough to say that the injury would not have occurred without the negligence. This link has to be something more than "but for," but less than locked-in inevitability.

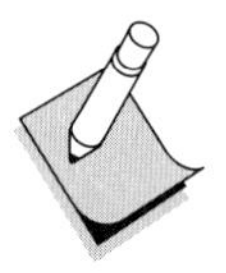

The four main elements of a lawsuit:
Duty
Breach of duty
Damages
Causation

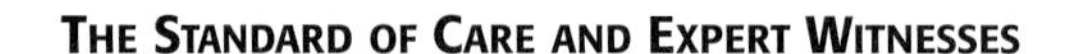

THE STANDARD OF CARE AND EXPERT WITNESSES

In a malpractice suit, the standard against which physicians are judged is:

"How would a reasonable emergency physician have performed in the same or similar circumstances?"

This national standard does not demand the highest skill, although physicians have set themselves up against that threshold by advertising the highest or best practices. And the standard depends on what is actually done, not a theoretical ideal. **Internal guidelines and policies** for quality assurance and peer review are often protected by statute, but any information accessible to plaintiffs may potentially be used in litigation. Admission of **expert testimony** remains at the discretion of the judge. At least one state requires emergency physician experts in malpractice cases against EPs. Medical malpractice involves a professional standard. The expert answers the question above about standard of care. The expert is also usually asked about the causation element—did the claimed negligence cause the harm?

Standard of Proof

Judges instruct juries that, to find for the plaintiff, they must conclude that there was duty, breach of duty, damages, and causation "more likely than not," ie, preponderance of the evidence. This is a significantly **lower** threshold than the criminal standard of "beyond a reasonable doubt."

The burden of proof for a malpractice case is the preponderance of evidence.

Compensation

Juries award the plaintiff damages, which are the amount of the verdict. The amount of damages is intended to make the victim of malpractice whole. Lost income and medical bills are "actual" damages; pain and suffering compensation, and punitive damages are "noneconomic" damages. Lawyers estimate potential verdict amounts based on all involved factors, but sometimes use a rule of thumb that applies a multiplier to the more easily demonstrated real damages.

$$\text{Potential damages} \sim= 5 \times \text{actual damages}$$

In addition to actual damages, a plaintiff may be entitled to **punitive damages,** which may be awarded if the jury feels that the conduct of the defendant was particularly loathsome and unprofessional. In usual cases, however, the verdict should be sufficient for the plaintiff to break even. The plaintiff should never come out ahead of where she would have been had the malpractice not occurred. Tort reform efforts often seek caps on the possible amount of noneconomic damages.

Insurance

There are two types of insurance policies:

- **Occurrence**: Coverage for errors or omissions in a case occurring during the life of the policy, no matter when the suit is eventually filed
- **Claims made**: Coverage only if there is a claim made (or, sometimes, a report of an incident) during the coverage period of that policy or renewal of that policy

The latter of these is cheaper and has become much more common. If an emergency physician leaves a group, he should make sure that renewals will include him, or that the group will buy a "**tail**" covering later filed suits. Effectively the tail converts a claims made into an occurrence policy.

Right to Approve Settlement. An anxious defendant can always demand that the insurer offer policy limits to any plaintiff, but most policies today do **not** provide for any control by the physician or group policyholders. Insurers want to be able to make economic choices about settlement, free of the visceral and professional concerns driving physician defendants.

Security of Coverage. Large commercial insurers have moved out of the malpractice market. Many malpractice companies have failed. The cheapest insurance is not always the best. Insurance companies buy insurance themselves, and their coverage may become imperiled. Companies invest the premiums they collect and often make more money on investments than from the premium versus expense ratio. When the investment cycle is negative, another malpractice insurance "crisis" follows.

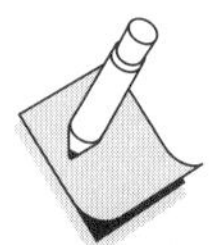

Claims-made malpractice insurance should be renewed or have tail coverage purchased.

Domestic insurers are inspected and regulated by state insurance commissioners. Offshore companies can be less secure. Some hospitals insist that staff and contract physicians and physician groups carry U.S. insurance, and usually at required minimum face amounts.

REPORTING: RESPONSIBILITIES TO THE WHOLE OF SOCIETY

There are no areas of medical practice where a patient's interests and societal interest collide more obviously. Both physicians and the public good are served by encouraging the sick and injured to seek help. But the patient has the right to confidentiality and privacy. Limited revelations are permitted by patients and allowed by law. Other disclosures are required by law, which varies greatly by state.

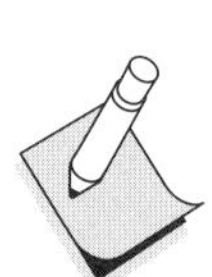

The lists of conditions that must be reported varies from state to state.

States structure reporting laws two ways. The state government enacts laws requiring physicians to report, sometimes specifying conditions or injuries, and states delegate to regulatory agencies responsibility for identifying what is to be reported and how. They infrequently carry criminal penalties for failure to report, but they are a legal requirement.

Penalties and civil liability can follow failure to report.

Communicable and Infectious Disease

This is the germinal type of reportable disease. To report the condition to public health authorities and attempt to reduce the spread of the disease, physicians required legal cover to avoid lawsuits regarding breech of confidentiality. The law takes away any decision-making once the diagnosis is made; even if the patient demands otherwise, the doctor has to report. Many hospitals identify lab personnel as reporting officers and admitted patients' reports are often handled by inpatient caregivers. But emergency physicians still retain shared responsibility for compliance with the laws.

Typical State Reporting Lists Include:

- Sexually transmitted infections, including HIV
- Community outbreaks, eg, food poisoning
- Illnesses related to foreign travel, eg, malaria
- Suspected biological terrorist threats, eg, anthrax
- Animal bites

Results of Criminal Activities

Assault

Not all injuries that are or could be the result of assault must, or even can, be reported. At present, five states do not have reporting requirements for assault-related injuries. Forty-two states connect the report to injuries from weapons, usually guns only, but knives and even martial arts weapons have been included.

Domestic Violence

This form of assault often causes a dilemma for emergency physicians. Many of the victims do not want reports made. There are reporting rules that include injuries resulting from domestic violence in only 7 states. In many states, if the patient does not want a report made, you cannot call the police. However, some states require reporting of injuries that appear to be intentionally inflicted.

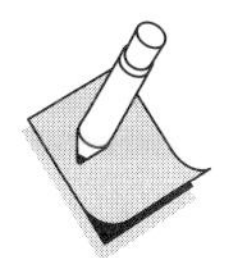

Except in a small handful of states, emergency physicians may not report rapes or domestic violence not involving a lethal weapon, over the victim's objection.

Child Abuse

This is another form of assault, but it deserves its own category because the reporting rules are clearer and more consistent. Children cannot decide that they do not want an assault reported. They still have privacy interests, but the society's interests in protecting children are universally understood and accepted. **All states have laws protecting children and require mandatory reporting of child abuse.** Some even include express immunity from suit for reporting health professionals. In all jurisdictions, the good faith communication is privileged.

There Are Still Some Variations for Emergency Physicians to Learn When They Go to a New State to Practice

- Definition of "child" may vary with statutory language or by reference to other concepts, such as emancipated minors.
- What constitutes abuse is inconsistent. Generally it is any nonaccidental serious physical injury inflicted by any adult responsible for the child. Some states include neglect as a form of abuse.
- Mechanisms of reporting vary. Sometimes, the staff member tells the authority in charge of the hospital. Many states require a verbal report followed by a written one.

Child abuse is one of only two situations where patients may be held in the ED against their and their parents' wishes, the other being the patient who lacks capacity and puts himself at immediate great risk by leaving. Sometimes the only way ED staff can assure protection for the child is to arrange admission. Hospitals have been successfully sued for failing to report abuse in children who are subsequently reinjured. Criminal penalties for failing to report appear in many state laws.

Elder Abuse

Neglect can also present as apparent self-care deficit. Many states now have adult protection laws, some for all adults, some only above a stated age. These reporting rules usually call for initial contact with a social service agency, like adult protective services.

Monitoring

Births and deaths involve forms and certification best left to hospital officials or personal physicians. **Adverse drug** and **device event** reporting is voluntary, unless hospital rules require it. Some reports are made by notations kept in logs distinct from the medical record and those logs submitted periodically or simply kept for access by reviewing authorities. Examples include the EMTALA mandated log of those who "come to the emergency department" and **trauma** registries. Other situations involve purported physician or hospital misdeeds.

RISK MANAGEMENT

Physicians and hospitals attempt to "manage" risks, acknowledging the impossibility or relative undesirability of perfect prevention. In health care, the frequency of suit is low but the potential for loss is mind-numbingly huge. **Research has shown that only one factor correlates with outcome: Severity of injury.**

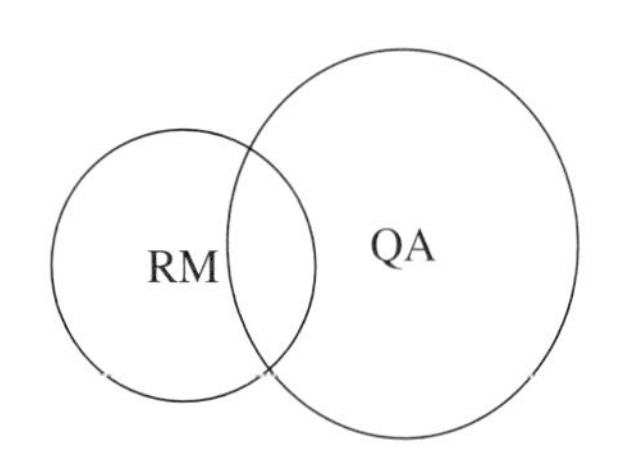

FIGURE 21.1. Risk management and quality assurance: overlapping effect.

We all want optimum quality care for all our patients. When we try to reduce medical error or make other care-focused efforts, we follow the expected path of the healer (and other fiduciary, learned-intermediary roles), placing the best interest of those for whom we are responsible above our own. In so doing, we also, we hope, reduce our chances of being sued.

The overlap between the quality assurance (QA) and risk management (RM) is extensive. Some argue the two are coincidental. But the perspective and intention are undeniably different. Quality assurance protects the patient. Risk management protects the provider. Some examples of both:

RM and QA

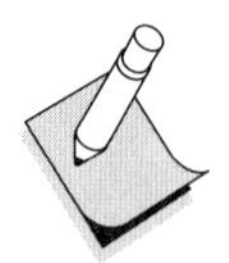

Quality assurance protects the patient. Risk management protects the provider.

- Maintaining and enhancing knowledge and skills
- Efforts to deliver best possible care
- Maintaining safe setting
- Records that communicate well
- Patient and family relations

Given the Unscientific Basis for the Exercise and the Pitfalls Surrounding the Attempt, Physicians May be Justifiably Discouraged, But We Still Have to Try. The Foci of RM in EM Are

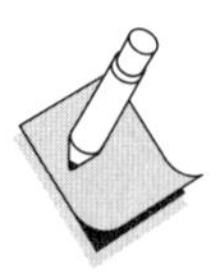

Managing risk involves more than medical malpractice.

- Care of boarded patients
- Compliance, fraud, and abuse
- Consent and refusal, capacity and holding patients
- Contracts
- Dealing with complaints and concerns
- ED colleagues and staff performance, qualifications, and safety
- EMS communications and relations
- EMTALA
- Follow-up after discharge
- High-risk clinical situations
- How patients and families perceive the EP and the ED
- Insurance
- Malpractice
- Patient and family expectations
- Preparedness
- Records adequacy, accessibility, and confidentiality
- Reporting, mandated and disallowed
- The physical facility, supplies, and equipment
- Transitions, at shift change and on admission, admitting orders
- Triage, flow, delays

From various sources, the following clinical conditions appear most often associated with malpractice claims:

- Failure to diagnose/treat AMI
- Missed fractures
- Wound care, including missed vital structure injury and infections

- Misdiagnose of abdominal pain or failure to diagnose
- Failure to diagnose, treat meningitis
- Missed appendicitis
- Delay in diagnosis of spinal cord injury
- Delayed identification or missed CVAs
- OB disasters
- Testicular torsion
- Eye conditions/injuries resulting in loss of vision
- Airway obstruction

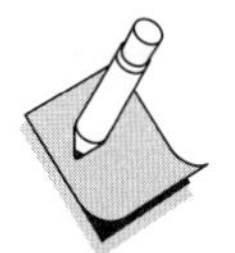

The most expensive clinical error alleged in emergency medicine malpractice cases is the missed MI.

The most expensive clinical error alleged in EM malpractice cases is missed MI. It may not be the most frequent, but incidence combined with severity yields top cost status for this claim.

Index

D

E

F

G

H

I

J

K

L

N

O

P

S

T

U

V

W

Y

Z